Operative Neurosurgical Techniques
Indications, Methods, and Results

Operative Neurosurgical Techniques
Indications, Methods, and Results
Volume 2

Edited by

Henry H. Schmidek, M.D., F.A.C.S.
Professor of Surgery
University of Vermont College of Medicine, and
Chief of the Neurosurgical Service
Medical Center Hospital of Vermont
Burlington, Vermont

and

William H. Sweet, M.D., D.Sc., F.A.C.S.
Professor of Surgery
Harvard Medical School, and
Emeritus Chief of the Neurosurgical Service
Massachusetts General Hospital
Boston, Massachusetts

GRUNE & STRATTON
A Subsidiary of Harcourt Brace Jovanovich, Publishers
New York   London
Paris   San Diego   San Francisco   Sao Paulo
Sydney   Tokyo   Toronto

Library of Congress Cataloging in Publication Data

Main entry under title:
Operative neurosurgical techniques indications,
    methods, and results.

    Includes bibliograhical references and index.
    1. Nervous system—Surgery. I. Schmidek, Henry H.
II. Sweet, William Herbert, 1910—   . [DNLM: 1. Neuro-
surgery—Methods. WL 368 061]
RD593.063   1983   617'.48   82-15431
ISBN 0-8089-1440-5 (set)

Grune & Stratton, Inc.
111 Fifth Avenue
New York, New York 10003

Distributed in the United Kingdom by
Academic Press Inc. (London) Ltd.
24/28 Oval Road, London NW 1

Library of Congress Catalog Number 82-15431
International Standard Book Number 0-8089-1440-5

Printed in the United States of America

This book
is affectionately dedicated to
Elizabeth Sweet, Mary Schmidek,
Ian, Alexandra, Jared, and Robin.

CONTENTS

Volume 1

Volume 2

PREFACE

The gratifying response accorded *Current Techniques in Operative Neurosurgery* by the neurosurgical community suggested to the editors that a more comprehensive text modeled on the first book would be appropriate. The previous publication arose from the proceedings of a seminar, and the content was limited to constraints inherent in that forum.

This new two-volume text addresses the indications, operations, intraoperative considerations, and results of the various forms of surgical intervention within the central and peripheral nervous system. It incorporates revised and updated chapters from the previous book, as well as new sections on anesthetic management, pediatric neurosurgery, surgery of the scalp and skull, head injuries, benign and malignant brain tumors, vascular disorders, functional neurosurgery, surgery of the cranial and peripheral nerves, and surgery of the spinal column and spinal cord.

There are also several sections of the book in which alternative surgical approaches to the same problem are presented. These deal with areas in which the decision to use a particular approach may be a difficult one and where it was felt that the presentation of these different points of view could be helpful to the neurosurgeon. Some of these sections are on the surgical management of intraventricular tumors, neoplasms of the pineal region, and acoustic neurinomas. Also included in this volume are discussions of some techniques that are still experimental, such as the stereotactic clipping of aneurysms, or procedures that are of potential importance but have not been widely used within the neurosurgical community, such as neurosurgical endoscopy or the use of intraspinal opioids in the control of pain.

In the five years since the publication of the previous text there has been an evolution in our thinking about the different procedures. The majority of those that were selected for inclusion before remain unchanged, at least in regard to their indications and anticipated outcome. Some of the operations, however, have been abandoned by even their most enthusiastic proponents. Posterior lumbosacral coagulation has not stood the test of time, and should be included in that category, whereas the balloon obliteration of certain intracranial vascular abnormalities has developed into a major technical advance.

In the same five-year interval a highly undesirable change in neurosurgical practice has been taking place in the United States—namely, a frightening escalation in the number of malpractice lawsuits and in the amount of awards given by juries or in out-of-court settlements reached before or during trial. The testimony and statements on behalf of plaintiffs by neurosurgeons is playing no small role in the increasing magnitude of the problem. We ourselves have given formal opinions that have incriminated our professional colleagues and have seen such opinions followed by massive out-of-court settlements for plaintiffs, yet we think the maintenance of professional integrity permits no other course when it is dictated by one's best professional judgment. One must differentiate, however, between negligence on the one hand and acceptable error or an acceptable course of action that would not have been that of the opinion-giver on the other hand. Having considered various approaches to a problem and having decided on the best one to teach, those of us who are teachers may elect to carry that teaching into the courtroom. There such didacticism is decidedly out of place. The expert witness should decide only whether the patient's management was so seriously deviant as to constitute negligence. Some of our best surgeons are giving testimony for plaintiffs, which is nothing short of outrageous.

Unfortunately we address this problem incompletely in our decision to include alternative surgical modes of management. This might well have been pursued more extensively, but we could not include every acceptable modus operandi in these volumes and still have a text of wieldy size.

We also have not emphasized the number and types of complications that may occur in the hands of the average neurosurgeon in any given situation. This is because we don't know those numbers, and nearly all of us reporting series of patients select our better not worst cases, so that the surgical literature necessarily presents an overly optimistic picture. The only reports that approach depiction of the entire scene are those arising from cooperative studies from many services. The tactic of having a compilation of reports from different centers, each designated only by a code number, would doubtless give us a truer notion of our problems and discourage expert witnesses from insisting on too rosy a level of performance as the standard we should invariably attain. We hold the view that no profession can be practiced without error by anyone.

We would like to thank each of the contributors for the very substantial effort involved in preparing their contributions, and, in addition, we would like to thank the editorial staff of Grune & Stratton for doing a superb job with the production of this book.

Henry H. Schmidek, M.D.
William H. Sweet, M.D.
September 3, 1982

CONTRIBUTORS

Mounir N. Abou-Madi, M.B., Ch.B., F.R.C.P.(C) *Department of Anesthesiology, Montreal Neurological Hospital and Institute; and McGill University, Montreal, Quebec, Canada*

John E. Adams, M.D. *Department of Neurological Surgery, University of California, San Francisco, California*

Phil A. Aitken, M.D. *Division of Ophthalmology, University of Vermont College of Medicine, Burlington, Vermont*

Melvin G. Alper, M.D., F.A.C.S. *Departments of Ophthalmology and Neurological Surgery, The George Washington University School of Medicine and The Washington Hospital Center, Washington, D.C.*

A. L. Amacher, M.D. *Division of Neurological Surgery, University of Western Ontario, London, Ontario, Canada*

Ronald I. Apfelbaum, M.D. *Leo M. Davidoff Department of Neurological Surgery, Albert Einstein College of Medicine; and Montefiore Hospital and Medical Center, Bronx, New York*

Michael L. J. Apuzzo, M.D. *Department of Neurological Surgery, University of Southern California School of Medicine, Los Angeles, California*

Donald P. Becker, M.D. *Division of Neurological Surgery, Medical College of Virginia, Virginia Commonwealth University, Richmond, Virginia*

Perry Black, M.D. *Department of Neurosurgery, Hahnemann Medical College and Hospital, Philadelphia, Pennsylvania*

Ronald Brisman, M.D., F.A.C.S. *New York Neurological Institute, Columbia-Presbyterian Medical Center, College of Physicians and Surgeons, Columbia University, New York, New York*

William A. Buchheit, M.D. *Department of Neurosurgery, Temple University Health Sciences Center, Philadelphia, Pennsylvania*

Robert C. Cantu, M.D. *Neurological Service, Department of Surgery, Emerson Hospital, Concord, Massachusetts*

Paul H. Chapman, M.D., F.A.C.S. *Neurosurgical Service, Massachusetts General Hospital, Boston, Massachusetts*

Shelley N. Chou, M.D., Ph.D. *Department of Neurosurgery, University of Minnesota Hospitals, Minneapolis, Minnesota*

Kemp Clark, M.D. *Division of Neurological Surgery, University of Texas Health Science Center at Dallas, Dallas, Texas*

Edwin W. Cocke, Jr., M.D. *Department of Otolaryngology, University of Tennessee Center for Health Sciences; and The Baptist Memorial Hospital, Memphis, Tennessee*

Laurence H. Coffin, M.D. *Division of Cardiothoracic Surgery, University of Vermont College of Medicine, Burlington, Vermont*

William F. Collins, M.D. *Section of Neurosurgery, Yale University School of Medicine, New Haven, Connecticut*

Louis W. Conway, M.D. *Department of Neurosurgery, Arnett Clinic and Hospital, Lafayette, Indiana*

Dennis W. Coombs, M.D. *Department of Anesthesiology, Dartmouth-Hitchcock Medical Center, Hanover, New Hampshire*

Robert M. Crowell, M.D. *Department of Neurosurgery, University of Illinois, Chicago, Illinois*

Charles W. Cummings, M.D. *Department of Otolaryngology, University of Washington, Seattle, Washington*

Gerard Debrun, *Department of Radiology, Massachusetts General Hospital, Boston, Massachusetts*

Tomas E. Delgado, M.D. *Department of Neurosurgery, Temple University Health Sciences Center, Philadelphia, Pennsylvania*

Patrick J. Derome, M.D. *Hôpital Foch, La Celle-St. Cloud, France*

R. M. Peardon Donaghy, M.D., D.Sc., F.A.C.S. *Division of Neurosurgery, University of Vermont College of Medicine, Burlington, Vermont*

Edward F. Downing, M.D.   *Neurological Institute of Savannah, Savannah, Georgia*

Charles G. Drake, M.D., F.R.C.S.(C).   *Department of Surgery, The University of Western Ontario, University Hospital, London, Ontario, Canada*

Mel H. Epstein, M.D., F.A.C.S.   *Department of Neurological Surgery, The Johns Hopkins Hospital, Baltimore, Maryland*

Bernard E. Finneson, M.D., F.A.C.S.   *Low Back Pain Clinic, Crozer-Chester Medical Center, Chester, Pennsylvania; and Department of Neurological Surgery, Hahnemann Medical College, Philadelphia, Pennsylvania*

Edwin G. Fischer, M.D.   *Department of Neurosurgery, Children's Hospital Medical Center, and the Harvard Medical School, Boston, Massachusetts*

Gale Gardner, M.D.   *Department of Otolaryngology, University of Tennessee Center for Health Sciences; and the Baptist Memorial Hospital, Memphis, Tennessee*

Barry E. Gerald, M.D.   *Department of Otolaryngology, University of Tennessee Center for Health Sciences; and the Baptist Memorial Hospital, Memphis, Tennessee*

Philip L. Gildenberg, M.D., Ph.D.   *Division of Neurosurgery, University of Texas Medical School at Houston, Houston, Texas*

J. Leonard Goldner, M.D.   *Division of Orthopaedic Surgery, Duke University School of Medicine, Durham, North Carolina*

Francisco B. Gomes, M.D.   *Division of Neurological Surgery, University of Vermont College of Medicine, Burlington, Vermont*

Robert L. Grubb, Jr., M.D.   *Department of Neurology and Neurological Surgery, Division of Radiation Sciences, The Edward Mallinckrodt Institute of Radiology; and McDonnell Center for Studies of Higher Brain Function, Washington University School of Medicine, St. Louis, Missouri*

John E. Hall, M.D.   *Department of Orthopedic Surgery, Children's Hospital Medical Center and Harvard Medical School, Boston, Massachusetts*

Robert R. Hansebout, M.D., F.R.C.S.(C)., F.A.C.S.   *Neurological Service, McMaster University and St. Joseph's Hospital, Hamilton, Ontario, Canada*

Robert Harbaugh, M.D.   *Section of Neurosurgery, Dartmouth-Hitchcock Medical Center, Hanover, New Hampshire*

Russell W. Hardy, Jr., M.D.   *Department of Neurological Surgery, Cleveland Clinic, Cleveland, Ohio*

Yoshio Hosobuchi, M.D.   *Department of Neurological Surgery, University of California School of Medicine, San Francisco, California*

Edgar M. Housepian, M.D.   *Department of Neurological Surgery, College of Physicians and*

Surgeons, Columbia University; and the New York Neurological Institute, Columbia-Presbyterian Medical Center, New York, New York

Leslie P. Ivan, M.D.   *Division of Neurosurgery, Children's Hospital of Eastern Ontario, Ottawa, Ontario, Canada*

Dean B. Jacques, M.D.   *Huntington Institute of Applied Medical Research; and California Institute of Technology, Pasadena, California*

Jonas Johnson, M.D.   *Department of Otolaryngology, University of Pittsburgh, Pittsburgh, Pennsylvania*

Edward I. Kandel, M.D., D.Sc.   *Neurosurgical Clinic, Institute of Neurology, Moscow, U.S.S.R.*

John P. Kapp, M.D., Ph.D.   *Department of Neurological Surgery, University of Mississippi School of Medicine, Jackson, Mississippi*

T. T. King, M.D., F.R.C.S.   *Department of Neurosurgery, The London Hospital, Whitechapel, London E.1., England*

Edward R. Laws, Jr., M.D.   *Department of Neurosurgery, Mayo Medical School, Mayo Clinic, Rochester, Minnesota*

Robert D. Leffert, M.D.   *Department of Orthopaedic Surgery and Department of Rehabilitation Medicine, Massachusetts General Hospital; and Harvard Medical School, Boston, Massachusetts*

Paul M. Lin, M.D.   *Department of Neurological Surgery, Temple University Health Science Center, Philadelphia, Pennsylvania*

Peter C. Linton, M.D., F.A.C.S.   *Division of Plastic Surgery, University of Vermont, College of Medicine, Burlington, Vermont*

Robert Lippert, M.D.   *Department of Neurological Surgery, University of California Medical Center, San Francisco, California*

L. Dade Lunsford, M.D.   *Department of Neurological Surgery, University of Pittsburgh School of Medicine, University Health Center of Pittsburgh, Pittsburgh, Pennsylvania*

Harold Lutes, O.D., B.S.   *Huntington Institute of Applied Medical Research; and California Institute of Technology, Pasadena, California*

Ghaus M. Malik, M.B., B.S., F.A.C.S.   *Department of Neurological Surgery, Henry Ford Hospital, Detroit, Michigan*

Joseph C. Maroon, M.D., F.A.C.S.   *Department of Neurological Surgery, University of Pittsburgh School of Medicine, University Health Center of Pittsburgh, Pittsburgh, Pennsylvania*

Robert E. Maxwell, M.D., Ph.D.   *Department of Neurosurgery, University of Minnesota Hospitals, Minneapolis, Minnesota*

Joseph W. McSherry, M.D., Ph.D. *Department of Neurology, University of Vermont College of Medicine, Burlington, Vermont*

Arnold H. Menezes, M.D., F.A.C.S. *Division of Neurosurgery, University of Iowa Hospitals, Iowa City, Iowa*

Lester A. Mount, M.D., F.A.C.S. *New York Neurological Institute and Columbia-Presbyterian Medical Center and College of Physicians and Surgeons, Columbia University, New York, New York*

John F. Mullan, M.D. *Department of Neurosurgery, Pritzker School of Medicine, University of Chicago, Chicago, Illinois*

Robert G. Ojemann, M.D. *The Neurosurgical Service, Massachusetts General Hospital and the Harvard Medical School, Boston, Massachusetts*

Michael S. Olin, M.D. *Neurosurgical Service, Division of Neurosurgery, University of Vermont College of Medicine, Burlington, Vermont*

Robert E. Palmer, M.D. *University of Tennessee Center for Health Sciences; and The Baptist Memorial Hospital, Memphis, Tennessee*

Dwight Parkinson, M.D. *Department of Neurological Surgery, Faculty of Medicine, University of Manitoba, Winnipeg, Manitoba, Canada*

Russel H. Patterson, Jr. *Division of Neurological Surgery, Cornell University Medical College, New York, New York*

Sydney J. Peerless, M.D., F.R.C.S.(C). *Division of Neurosurgery, The University of Western Ontario, University Hospital, London, Ontario, Canada*

David G. Peipgras, M.D. *Department of Neurologic Surgery, Mayo Clinic, Mayo Medical School, Rochester, Minnesota*

Vyacheslav V. Peresedov, M.D. *Neurosurgical Clinic, Institute of Neurology, Moscow, U.S.S.R.*

Robert N. Pilon, M.D. *Department of Anesthesiology, Athens General Hospital, Athens, Georgia*

Charles E. Poletti, M.D. *Neurosurgical Service, Massachusetts General Hospital and Harvard Medical School, Boston, Massachusetts*

Kalmon D. Post, M.D. *New York Neurological Institute and the College of Physicians & Surgeons, Columbia University, New York, New York*

Eugene A. Quindlen, M.D. *Division of Neurosurgery, University of South Carolina School of Medicine, Columbia, South Carolina*

Ralph Rashbaum, M.D. *Division of Neurosurgery, University of Pennsylvania School of Medicine and Pennsylvania Hospital, Philadelphia, Pennsylvania*

Robert A. Ratcheson, M.D. *Division of Neurological Surgery, School of Medicine, Case Western Reserve University, Cleveland, Ohio*

Michael J. Redmond, M.B., B.S., F.R.A.C.S. *Department of Neurologic Surgery, Mayo Graduate School of Medicine, Rochester, Minnesota*

Albert L. Rhoton, Jr., M.D. *Department of Neurological Surgery, University of Florida College of Medicine, Gainesville, Florida*

Howard A. Richter, M.D. *Division of Neurosurgery, Lankenau Hospital and the Thomas Jefferson Medical College, Philadelphia, Pennsylvania*

James T. Robertson, M.D. *Department of Neurosurgery, University of Tennessee Center for Health Sciences; and The Baptist Memorial Hospital, Memphis, Tennessee*

Robert A. Robinson, M.D. *Professor Emeritus of Orthopedic Surgery, Johns Hopkins University School of Medicine, Baltimore, Maryland*

Maurice I. Saba, M.D. *Division of Neurosurgery, American University of Beirut, Beirut, Lebanon*

Richard L. Saunders, M.D. *Division of Neurosurgery, Dartmouth-Hitchcock Medical Center, Hanover, New Hampshire*

Henry H. Schmidek, M.D. *Division of Neurosurgery, University of Vermont College of Medicine and the Medical Center Hospital of Vermont, Burlington, Vermont*

R. Michael Scott, M.D. *Department of Neurosurgery, Tufts University School of Medicine; and New England Medical Center, Boston, Massachusetts*

David Seligson, M.D. *Department of Orthopedic Surgery, University of Vermont College of Medicine, Burlington, Vermont*

Bertram Selverstone, M.D. *Division of Neurosurgery, Brown University; and Miriam and Roger Williams Hospitals, Providence, Rhode Island*

C. Hunter Shelden, M.D. *Huntington Institute of Applied Medical Research; and California Institute of Technology, Pasadena, California*

Frederick A. Simeone, M.D. *Division of Neurosurgery, University of Pennsylvania School of Medicine; and Chief, Department of Neurosurgery, The Elliot Neurological Center of the Pennsylvania Hospital, Philadelphia, Pennsylvania*

Dennis D. Spencer, M.D. *Section of Neurosurgery, Yale University School of Medicine, New Haven, Connecticut*

Bennett M. Stein, M.D. *Department of Neurological Surgery, College of Physicians and Surgeons, Columbia University; and Director of Service, Department of Neurosurgery, Columbia-Presbyterian Medical Center, New York, New York*

William H. Sweet, M.D., D.Sc., D.H.C.   *Neurosurgical Service, Massachusetts General Hospital and the Harvard Medical School, Boston, Massachusetts*

Lindsay Symon, M.D.   *Neurological Surgery, Institute of Neurology, National Hospital, London, England*

Edward Tarlov, M.D.   *Department of Neurosurgery, Lahey Clinic Medical Center, Burlington, Massachusetts*

Ronald R. Tasker, M.D.   *Division of Neurosurgery and Department of Surgery, Toronto General Hospital and University of Toronto, Toronto, Ontario, Canada*

John McLellan Tew, Jr., M.D.   *Mayfield Neurological Institute, Cincinnati, Ohio*

William D. Tobler, M.D.   *Mayfield Neurological Institute, Cincinnati, Ohio*

Davy Trop, M.D., F.R.C.P.(C).   *Department of Anesthesiology, Montreal Neurological Hospital and Institute; and McGill University, Montreal, Quebec, Canada*

Merlin L. Trumbull, M.D.   *Department of Otolaryngology, University of Tennessee Center for Health Sciences and The Baptist Memorial Hospital, Memphis, Tennessee*

Sumio Uematsu, M.D.   *Department of Neurosurgery, The Johns Hopkins University School of Medicine, Baltimore, Maryland*

James Q. Urbaniak, M.D.   *Division of Orthopaedic Surgery, Duke University School of Medicine, Durham, North Carolina*

John C. VanGilder, M.D., F.A.C.S.   *Professor and Chairman, Division of Neurosurgery, University of Iowa Hospitals, Iowa City, Iowa*

Harry van Loveren, M.D.   *Mayfield Neurological Institute, Cincinnati, Ohio*

Steven L. Wald, M.D.   *Division of Neurosurgery, University of Vermont and Medical Center Hospital of Vermont, Burlington, Vermont*

Lester J. Wallman, M.D.   *Division of Neurosurgery, University of Vermont and Medical Center Hospital of Vermont, Burlington, Vermont*

Carrie L. Walters, M.D.   *Division of Neurosurgery, Medical Center Hospital of Vermont; and The University of Vermont College of Medicine, Burlington, Vermont*

John Ward, M.D.   *Division of Neurological Surgery, Medical College of Virginia, Virginia Commonwealth University, Richmond, Virginia*

Donald H. Wilson, M.D.   *Section of Neurosurgery, Dartmouth-Hitchcock Medical Center, Hanover, New Hampshire*

Kenneth E. Wood, M.D.   *Division of Orthopaedic Surgery, Duke University School of Medicine, Durham, North Carolina*

R. Lewis Wright, M.D.   *Neurological Surgery, Stuart Circle Hospital; and St. Mary's Hospital, Richmond, Virginia*

David Yashon, M.D., F.A.C.S., F.R.C.S.(C).   *Division of Neurological Surgery, Ohio State University, Columbus, Ohio*

Henry A. Young, M.D.   *Division of Neurosurgery, Medical Center Hospital of Vermont, Burlington, Vermont*

Nicholas T. Zervas, M.D.   *Neurosurgical Service, Massachusetts General Hospital and Harvard Medical School, Boston, Massachusetts*

Operative Neurosurgical Techniques
Indications, Methods, and Results

CHAPTER 45
Surgical Management of Diseases of The Extracranial Carotid Artery

Robert A. Ratcheson   Robert L. Grubb, Jr.

THE VARIED AND COMPLEX DANGERS presented by atherosclerotic lesions of the carotid artery bifurcation are widely appreciated. Many of these lesions obstruct blood flow to the cerebral hemispheres, while others are hemodynamically insignificant but have the potential to produce ischemic cerebral damage because of distal embolization from diseased intima. Although both embolic and hemodynamic mechanisms play important roles in cerebral ischemia and infarction, embolization appears to be the dominant factor in the carotid system. These emboli may originate from focal accumulations of lipid-laden, intimal smooth-muscle cells surrounded by an intracellular matrix of lipid, collagen, elastic fibers, and proteoglycans, which become altered as a result of hemorrhage, calcification, cell necrosis, and thrombosis.[1] In the cervical carotid artery these lesions usually occur at or near the bifurcation of the common carotid artery. The etiology of the underlying disease—atherosclerosis—and the factors that render these lesions active, remain poorly understood. At the present time surgical therapy of these lesions offers the most direct and efficient mechanism for removing the source of cerebral emboli and for restoring cerebral blood flow when the lesion produces a critical stenosis. Treatment cannot be directed only toward removal of an anatomic abnormality, however, but must include consideration of the multiple problems introduced by the patient's physiologic state and collateral cerebral circulation. In certain situations a patient will be better served by treatment with anticoagulants or agents that suppress platelet aggregation. A number of conditions of non-atherosclerotic etiology also affect the cervical carotid artery and may interfere with cerebral blood flow or serve as a nidus for thrombus formation and cerebral embolization. For many of these conditions, the role of surgical therapy is not well defined.

Diagnosis and Patient Selection

All lesions of the carotid artery that are angiographically identified do not represent a significant risk to an individual patient. The decision to perform carotid endarterectomy must therefore rely upon an accurate correlation of clinical symptomatology and angiographic findings arrived at through an understanding of the influence of anatomic variations upon the cere-

Division of Neurological Surgery, Case Western Reserve University, School of Medicine, Cleveland, Ohio, and Department of Neurology and Neurological Surgery, Washington University School of Medicine, St. Louis, Missouri

bral circulation and a knowledge of the pathophysiology of occlusive extracranial and intracranial vascular disease. Medical and surgical factors that increase the risk of surgery must also enter into the decision whether to perform carotid endarterectomy or to treat the patient medically.

Indications

The primary indication for carotid endarterectomy is the angiographic demonstration of a stenotic or ulcerated lesion in the extracranial carotid artery that is compatible with the patient's cerebrovascular symptomatology. Presenting symptoms may include any and all of the spectrum of cerebral and ocular ischemia. Patients with amaurosis fugax, central retinal artery occlusion, carotid distribution transient ischemic attacks (TIAs), prolonged reversible ischemic neurologic deficits (PRINDs), and mild to moderate fixed neurologic deficits are at risk for further hemispheric ischemic damage. All patients having cerebrovascular symptoms should be evaluated to determine their specific risk of stroke. Those patients at the greatest risk, including patients with frequent TIAs, stuttering-stroke symptomatology, or an acute onset of mild to moderate neurologic deficit, should be evaluated on an urgent basis. Patients having infrequent cerebral episodes are at unknown risk but should be evaluated without undue delay. The evaluation of each patient should include an assessment of surgical risk factors for carotid endarterectomy. At the present time there is no noninvasive test that can reliably depict all the conditions of the cervical carotid artery that may be responsible for the cerebral symptomatology. A number of diagnostic techniques currently under development may dramatically alter the approach to the patient threatened with cerebral infarction in the future, but for now cerebral angiography is the only reliable study that will accurately demonstrate extracranial and intracranial vascular lesions. Therefore, definitive angiographic studies should not be delayed by noninvasive medical evaluation, unless there is evidence to implicate an etiology other than extracranial or intracranial vascular disease.

In most instances the administration of intravenous heparin will prevent further ischemic episodes until angiography can be performed under optimal conditions. Anticoagulation, however, does not guarantee that a patient will not suffer additional symptoms and permanent sequelae. We prefer to perform angiography immediately after appropriate medical evaluation and computerized tomographic (CT) scanning of the head has been completed. If stenosis with a residual lumen less than 1 mm is found, or if intraluminal thrombus is found, surgery usually is performed on an urgent basis. If ulceration or plaque formation is demonstrated in the appropriate carotid artery, a patient without neurologic deficit will undergo surgery at the next elective opportunity. When the cervical carotid artery contains a nonstenotic lesion with only shallow ulceration, it is our preference to treat these patients with warfarin anticoagulant therapy. On occasion, despite adequate anticoagulation, such patients will have persistent symptoms and will require carotid endarterectomy (Fig. 45-1).

The indications for surgical therapy in a large group of patients, which includes those with asymptomatic cervical bruits, asymptomatic angiographic lesions, and vertebrobasilar symptoms associated with carotid artery stenosis, are controversial. The natural history of patients with asymptomatic cervical bruits is not clearly defined,[2-4] and further investigation of these patients is not recommended; rather, their course and the bruit should be followed closely. If a change in the character of the bruit is noted, further study is advised. Frequently the neurosurgeon must decide whether to treat an asymptomatic lesion that has been demonstrated angiographically during investigation of a contralateral symptomatic lesion. With the exception of unusual circumstances, dictated by the pattern of collateral circulation or accessibility of the lesion, treatment should be directed toward the symptomatic side. As the natural history of asymptomatic lesions also is not well defined,[5-7] carotid endarterectomy should be restricted to those lesions having a residual lumen of 2 mm or less or lesions with evidence of multiple intraluminal irregularities that could produce eddies that interrupt normal laminar blood flow and predispose the lesion to further ulceration and thrombus formation. On occasion, patients with

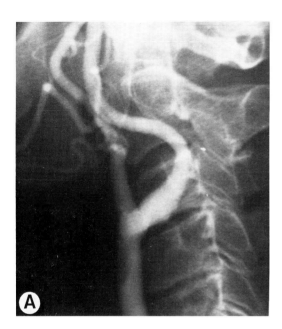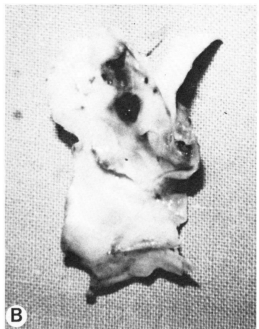

Fig. 45-1   A. A left-carotid angiogram of a patient who experienced sudden-onset transient dysphasia and weakness of the right arm. Fairly smooth, shallow irregularities are visible near the carotid bifurcation. The patient was treated with warfarin, but suffered a further episode of dysphasia and clumsiness of the right arm, which partially improved. **B.** The atheroma that was removed surgically from the left carotid artery of the patient. Intraluminal thrombus, not apparent on standard angiographic views, was found attached to an ulcer crater.

symptoms of vertebrobasilar insufficiency will benefit from carotid endarterectomy if it is demonstrated that an insufficient posterior circulation blood flow may be augmented by removing a critical carotid stenosis. These patients must be carefully evaluated to determine the competence of the circle of Willis and collateral blood flow.

Cerebral Angiography

Good-quality angiography is an absolute necessity in evaluating patients for carotid endarterectomy. It is important that the origin of the cerebral vessels in the thorax and the cervical and intracranial distribution of the carotid arteries all are well visualized. Neurologic consequences are not proportional to the size of a carotid lesion, and the angiographic appearance is often an unreliable predictor of the presence of active ulceration with shallow erosion of endothelium and the accumulation of thrombus and debris. The chances of a nonstenotic angiographic lesion containing active elements are higher if its presence can be correlated with appropriate clinical symptomatology. In our surgical experience, greater than 90 percent of the atherosclerotic plaques occurring in a carotid artery ipsilateral to a hemisphere affected by a TIA or monocular visual loss will be ulcerated and contain platelet aggregates and thrombus. When surgery is performed for asymptomatic cervical carotid lesions, irregularities identified angiographically often are found to be smooth and endothelialized.

Preoperative Preparation

Before operation the cardiopulmonary status of the patient must be carefully evaluated. Detailed attention must be given to maintenance of adequate intravascular volume. During preoperative evaluation, patients may become hypovolemic as a consequence of fluid redistribution caused by bedrest, the diuresis induced by hyperosmolar contrast agents administered for angiography and CT scanning, and the prohibition of fluid intake in preparation for these tests. In some instances it is necessary to supplement the patient's intravascular volume with intravenous fluid or albumin on the night before surgery. When possible, patients with severe chronic obstructive pulmonary disease, angina at rest, or recent myocardial infarction are treated with anticoagulant or platelet-suppressing agents rather than surgery.

Surgical Management

Satisfactory results following carotid endarterectomy have been reported with a variety of surgical techniques. The operation requires careful attention to technical details, and certain specific principles are essential to achieve a consistently favorable outcome. It is important to adequately expose the distal internal carotid artery to permit direct visualization of the entire extent of an atheromatous plaque. The following technique has been used and continuously modified by the authors and by the neurosurgical residents who have assisted them and who, in turn, have been assisted in performing this operation.

The surgery is performed under "balanced" anesthesia achieved by the intravenous administration of supplementary narcotics and the inhalation of a mixture of 50% nitrous oxide and 50% oxygen. Pancuronium is administered for muscle relaxation. An arterial line is placed in the radial artery after an Allen test has been performed. Nasotracheal intubation, which allows greater mobility of submandibular structures, is carried out when it is anticipated that high dissection will be required for distal exposure. Blood pressure is maintained at a normal or slightly elevated level throughout the procedure. Undesirable elevations of blood pressure are controlled by the administration of small amounts of halothane or enflurane. Phenylephrine is used to raise blood pressure when indicated. $PaCO_2$ is maintained in the normal range to avoid both the reduction of cerebral blood flow associated with hypocarbia and the theoretical possibility of luxury perfusion occurring around an ischemic area as a result of hypercapnia.

The patient is positioned with the head slightly extended and turned 45° away from the side to be operated upon. The incision is made along the anterior border of the sternocleidomastoid muscle to a point 1 cm posterior to the angle of the jaw; from here the incision is gently curved toward the mastoid process (Fig. 45-2). Careful attention is given to hemostasis during the dissection as systemic anticoagulation will be employed later. The platysma is divided and sharp dissection is continued along the medial border of the sternocleidomastoid muscle until the carotid sheath is encountered. The sheath is entered with care to avoid manipulation of the bifurcation. The internal jugular vein is identified, and dissection is continued medial to the vein (Fig. 45-3). The common facial vein and other large bridging veins may require double ligation and division. Dissection of the common carotid artery is performed with minimal disturbance of adjacent tissues in order to avoid injury to the recurrent laryngeal nerve. The artery is isolated with a right-angle gallbladder clamp and secured with a Silastic tape passed through a rubber catheter. When use of an internal shunt is anticipated, an umbilical tape is placed about the artery proximal to the Silastic tape.

The carotid bifurcation is identified and 0.1 cc of 1% lidocaine is injected into the region of the carotid sinus nerve to prevent reflex bradycardia and hypotension resulting from sinus manipulation. The bifurcation is left undisturbed in its adventitial bed, and the external carotid artery is dissected free, isolated distally, and secured with a Silastic tourniquet. The origin of the superior thyroid artery is exposed for a few millimeters with care taken to avoid the underlying superior laryngeal nerve (Fig. 45-3). The superior thyroid artery is temporarily occluded by wrapping it twice with a 2-0 silk suture under tension. Other branches of the external carotid artery having a proximal origin can be handled in a similar fashion. In many instances it is necessary to divide the ansa hypoglossi during distal exposure of the internal carotid artery in order to mobilize the hypoglossal nerve without traction. Division of the ansa hypoglossi is without clini-

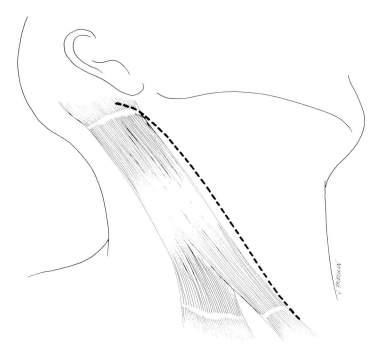

Fig. 45-2. The position of the neck and the location of the skin incision for carotid endarterectomy.

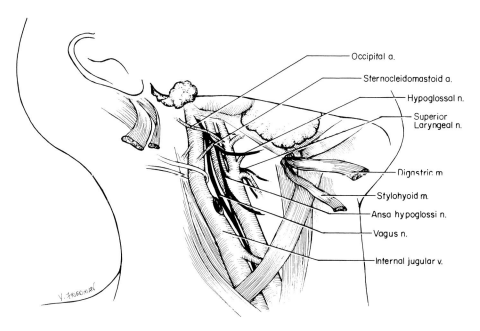

Occipital a.

Sternocleidomastoid a.

Hypoglossal n.

Superior Laryngeal n.

Digastric m

Stylohyoid m.

Ansa hypoglossi n.

Vagus n.

Internal jugular v.

Fig. 45-3. The relationship of the carotid artery to adjacent vascular and neural structures.

cal effect. In most cases the internal carotid artery is mobile immediately distal to the carotid bulb and is easily freed from surrounding tissue. Just distal to the bifurcation, however, the adventitia often adheres more strongly to the arterial wall, and it is helpful to initially enter the correct plane distal to the bulb. When the diseased segment of the vessel extends beyond the bulb into the distal internal carotid artery, this segment may be more difficult to dissect free. As seen in Figure 45-3, the vagus nerve lies posterior and lateral to the carotid artery. In rare instances, however, its position may be anterior to the carotid, where it is vulnerable to injury unless its presence is anticipated. It is often necessary to expose the lower pole of the parotid gland, which can be undermined and retracted superiorly to allow additional exposure. Care should be taken to avoid entering the glandular stroma, as this can lead to postoperative sialorrhea. The marginal mandibular branch of the facial nerve, which supplies the lower lip, passes through the substance of the inferior pole of the parotid gland. Retraction of the inferior pole may produce paralysis of the homolateral lip, which is nearly always transient and usually clears in 6 to 10 weeks. Additional exposure of the artery is facilitated by dividing the posterior belly of the digastric and, rarely, the stylohyoid muscle in addition to the sternocleidomastoid artery and vein, the so-called "sling vessels," as they cross the hypoglossal nerve. These structures and branches of the occipital artery and vein may limit mobilization of the hypoglossal nerve superiorly and away from the vessel. It may be necessary to mobilize the occipital artery and occasionally to divide it in order to gain additional length. These maneuvers allow the internal carotid artery to be exposed to within 1 cm of the base of the skull. The digastric muscle is easily repaired if tagged at the time of division. The common, internal, and external carotid arteries are isolated away from the diseased segment of the vessel in order to avoid embolization of friable plaque and thrombus (Fig. 45-4A). At times it is necessary to dissect free the posterior aspect of the bifurcation. When ulceration has penetrated the media and involves the posterior adventitia, the bifurcation must be mobilized in order to repair the artery. In some circumstances adequate exposure only can be obtained by dividing the nerve to the carotid sinus with mobilization of the entire bifurcation. Dissection should be performed immediately adjacent to the carotid artery in order to avoid injury to the superior laryngeal nerve, which lies beneath the bifurcation (Fig. 45-3). Injury to this nerve may result in mild hoarseness and cough with subjective complaints of an inability to clear the throat. When the internal carotid artery lies directly posterior to the external carotid artery, access to the internal carotid artery and the surgical assistant's view can be improved by tilting the operating table to the contralateral side.

After the artery and its major branches are isolated, the patient is given 5000 U of heparin intravenously. The external carotid artery is occluded with a large aneurysm clip and the common carotid artery is occluded with an appropriately angled DeBakey vascular clamp.

An intraoperative shunt is not used routinely. We rely upon the angiographic evaluation of the circle of Willis and the intraoperative measurement of carotid artery stump pressure to aid in the selection of patients in whom a shunt should be employed. We believe that in certain cases an intraoperative shunt provides an added margin of safety. The stump pressure is measured through a 23-gauge needle inserted into the common carotid artery just below the level of the angiographically identified disease. When the mean pressure is below 50 mm Hg, a shunt is used during arterial occlusion if it does not interfere with dissection of the plaque. The distal internal carotid artery is occluded with a large aneurysm clip and an incision is made in the common carotid artery with a small scalpel blade, beginning at the point in the common carotid artery where the stump pressure was measured. The arteriotomy is extended with an angled Potts scissors (Fig. 45-4B) into the internal carotid artery and carried through the involved area into the region of relatively normal intima (Fig. 45-5A). If a shunt is to be used, one of appropriate size is chosen and inserted into the distal internal carotid artery. If bleeding about the shunt persists, the Silastic loop is gently tightened about the shunt. The shunt is back-bled, placed in the common carotid artery and loosely secured by the Silastic loop that is placed around the common carotid artery. This will prevent vigorous bleeding and allow optimal positioning of the shunt, which can then be secured by tightening the umbilical tape (Fig. 45-5B). On some occasions the

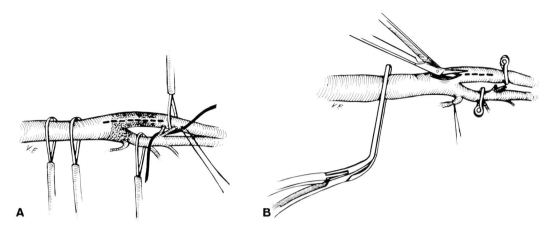

Fig. 45-4. Steps in the exposure and isolation of the carotid artery and placement of the arteriotomy.

ascending pharyngeal artery will originate from the posterior aspect of the distal common carotid artery which causes back-bleeding that may obscure the surgical field. This can be controlled by compressing the tissue lying between the internal and external carotid arteries without
disturbing the bifurcation. With advanced atherosclerotic plaque formation, a well-defined
plane demarcating atheromatous intimal changes from the relatively uninvolved media can be
visualized at the edge of the arteriotomy. The plane of dissection usually is carried distally into
the internal carotid artery with a small blunt dissector (Fig. 45-5C). Often the plaque will end at
the distal carotid bulb and feather off from normal intima, which is adherent to the vessel wall.
If the bifurcation is high or atheroma extends beyond the bulb, as in Figure 45-6, it may be necessary when a shunt is used to remove the shunt when the distal plaque is dissected from the arterial wall. During this period of time blood pressure should be elevated. Dissection of the intact
plaque proceeds into the common and external carotid arteries. While in most cases separation
of plaque from uninvolved media is facilitated by initial removal from the internal carotid artery, in some instances, often determined by the exact location of atheroma, it will be easier to
start the dissection in the common carotid artery. Circumferential dissection around the plaque
extending into the external carotid orifice defines a plane between the diseased and normal arterial wall. The end of the external carotid plaque often can be blindly reached with a dissector. In
some instances, however, it will be necessary to temporarily remove the aneurysm clip occluding
the external carotid artery in order to deliver the entire plaque. The plaque is separated from the
common carotid media and sharply amputated (Fig. 45-5D). The remaining cuff of intima,
which may be thickened, will be pressed against the vessel wall by the force of the arterial flow. It
is unnecessary to place tack sutures in the cuff if the distal intima is adherent and not thickened.
When the intima is not securely attached, simple longitudinal 7-0 silk sutures extending over the
intimal cuff are placed, with care being taken to avoid buckling the arterial wall (Fig. 45-5E).
When the atherosclerotic disease process produces shallow intimal ulceration with fibrin and
thrombus accumulation, it may be considerably more difficult to determine the appropriate
plane for dissection. In these cases the use of magnification is very helpful. The distal extent of
the plaque will not be prominent and it may be necessary to sharply divide the intima with microscissors. After the plaque is removed, the artery is irrigated with heparinized saline and carefully inspected for any loose fronds of tissue.

On occasion, ulcerations extend through the media to involve the adventitial layer. When
the artery is of sufficiently large size it may be possible to repair the vessel by plication without
compromising the lumen. If this is not feasible, a patch graft should be used.

Closure is done with a continuous 5-0 or 6-0 suture. Because of its handling characteristics,
Prolene* is preferred, but this suture material has the disadvantage of requiring a number of

*Prolene Blue Monofilament Polypropylene Suture, Ethicon, Inc. Somerville, NJ.

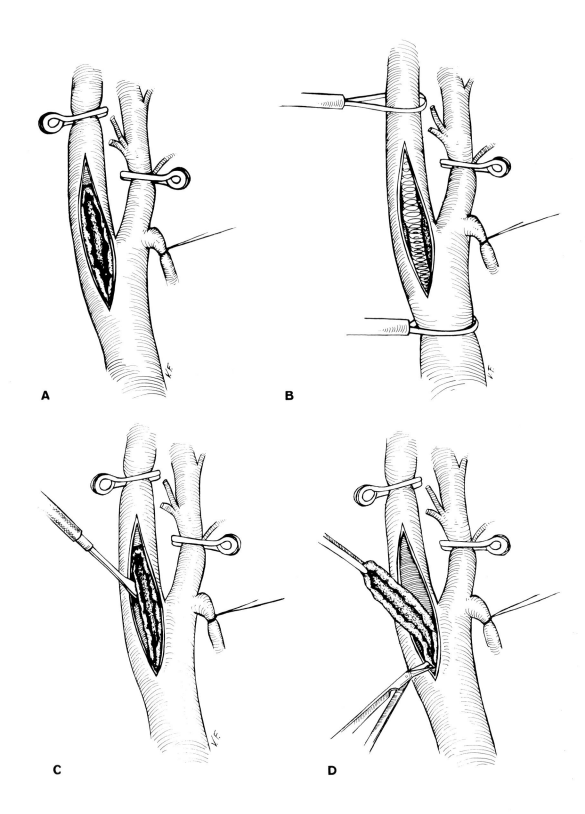

A

B

C

D

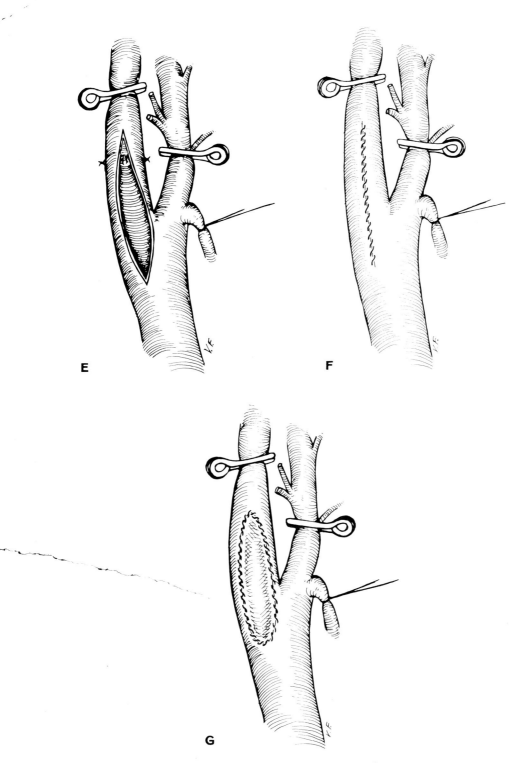

Fig. 45-5. The surgical steps in carotid endarterectomy.

knots to be placed in order to secure the ends. In the distal internal carotid artery, the space between running sutures may be smaller than the bulk of the knot, thus interfering with a tight suture line. To ensure competency of the suture line, the following technique is used: A suture is placed at the distal extreme of the arteriotomy and secured with two overhand knots. Another suture is placed immediately proximal to the first and also secured with two knots. Both ends of the distal suture then are tied to the trailing end of the proximal suture. This same procedure is repeated at the proximal end of the arteriotomy. The arteriotomy is closed with the proximal suture, beginning at the distal internal carotid artery. Individual sutures are placed close to each other, accurately approximating the layers of the arterial wall. The individual loops of suture have a tendency to roll over and it is essential that each loop be tightened perpendicular to the vessel wall in order to prevent leakage. The internal and common carotid arteries are back-bled, the vessels again are occluded, and closure is completed by tying a final backhand suture, using the suture placed at the proximal end of the arteriotomy, to the running suture (Fig. 45-5F). A shunt, when used, is removed before closing the final centimeter of the arteriotomy. We do not routinely use a vein or synthetic patch for closure unless the internal carotid artery is particularly small and simple closure may compromise the lumen (Fig. 45-5G). Placement of a graft is also effective in preventing the kinks that may occur as a result of the artery being removed from its bed. Occluding clamps are removed first from the external carotid artery, followed by removal of the clamps on the common carotid artery, which allows any air and debris to be flushed up the external carotid system. The aneurysm clip then is removed from the distal internal carotid artery. Hemostasis is encouraged by holding warm abdominal lap pads over the suture line, followed by cold irrigation. In those instances where brisk bleeding from the suture line is encountered, it may be necessary to seal the vessel with a 6-0 Prolene suture passed through a Teflon pledget. This last maneuver has the potential of causing a narrowing of the internal carotid artery and is best avoided by careful attention to the original closure. Hemostasis of the suture line will present little problem if sutures are placed close together and spaced evenly. A soft Silastic drain is inserted through an inferior stab wound, the platysma is approximated, and skin closure is completed. The heparin that was administered previously is not reversed.

Bilateral carotid endarterectomies should be staged at least 3 weeks apart. Before the second operation the vocal cords and tongue should be checked for mobility as bilateral vocal cord or hypoglossal nerve pareses are serious and disabling complications. Blood pressure lability, which may accompany bilateral endarterectomy, may be avoided by increasing the time between the two procedures and by sparing at least one of the nerves to the carotid sinus.

Restenosis of the carotid bifurcation following endarterectomy is caused by myointimal proliferation, which is thought to be secondary to technically inadequate vessel closure or the postoperative build-up of platelet aggregates at the suture line. Surgery for this condition is tedious and at times difficult because of perivascular scarring, which can interfere with distal control of the internal carotid artery. Control may be achieved by inserting a small balloon catheter beyond the stenotic area and inflating it to provide intraluminal occlusion. Often the demarcation between obstructing lesion and uninvolved media cannot be seen; at times, however, a plane can be initiated with sharp dissection, and the tissue can be removed. A patch of Dacron or microporous polytetrafluoroethylene (Gore-tex) is placed to enlarge the arterial lumen and encourage continued vessel patency.

Postoperative Care

The patient must be monitored carefully following surgery, particularly during the first 24 hours. Vital signs and neurologic status are checked frequently during the initial 6 hours and then every hour for the first 24 hours. Pain is rarely a problem and is easily controlled with codeine. More potent analgesics should be avoided as they may depress respiratory function. Arterial blood gases are routinely checked in the early postoperative period. Respiratory function

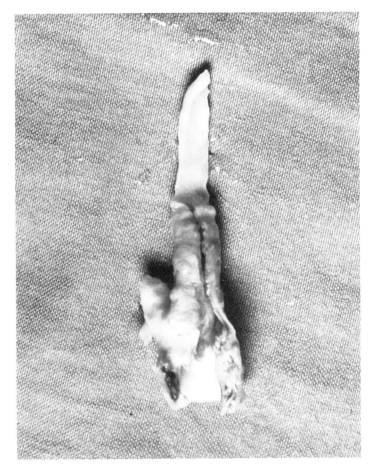

Fig. 45-6. Atherosclerotic plaque that was removed surgically, which extended beyond the carotid bulb.

must be carefully monitored, especially in those patients who have previously undergone a contralateral carotid endarterectomy. Bilateral procedures may result in the loss of carotid body function, leaving the patient without compensatory respiratory and circulatory response to hypoxia.[8] Pareses of the tenth and twelfth nerves also may contribute to postoperative respiratory problems. The operative area must be watched for the development of hematoma and airway obstruction. A hematoma that causes tracheal compromise and respiratory insufficiency requires immediate evacuation. The incidence of this complication can be decreased by connecting the wound drain to low-pressure suction for 12–18 hours.

Arterial blood pressure changes and cardiac arrhythmias must be recognized and treated promptly because of the high incidence of coexistent coronary artery disease. Arterial blood pressure is maintained at normal or mildly elevated levels. Blood pressure is often labile following carotid endarterectomy because of carotid baroreceptor dysfunction,[9,10] and a significant number of patients will develop early postoperative hypotension that often will respond to fluid replacement. More severe decreases must be corrected promptly to avoid carotid thrombosis. Intravenous fluids including colloid solutions and blood are used to expand systemic blood volume. If these measures fail, vasopressors are administered. Patients remain at bedrest for 18–24 hours before being allowed to sit up, because of the potential instability of blood pressure. Even then, assuming the upright position may cause a significant fall in pressure. When the patient tolerates the sitting position, ambulation is begun. Some patients will develop hypertension in the

Table 45-1. Causes and Rates of Morbidity and Mortality for Carotid Endarterectomy Based on 165 Procedures in 150 Patients

Cause	Percent
Operative mortality	
Myocardial infarction	2
Operative morbidity	
Permanent neurologic deficit	2
Transient neurologic deficit	4
Permanent vocal cord paralysis	1
Transient palsy of the 7th, 10th, 12th and cervical sympathetic nerves	6
Neck hematoma (requiring re-exploration)	1
Wound infection	1
Pulmonary embolus	1
Pulmonary hemorrhage	1
Asymptomatic intimal flap	1
Combined rates of mortality and permanent neurologic deficit	4

postoperative period. Mild elevations are safely tolerated, but severe degrees must be vigorously treated to prevent the development of an intracerebral hemorrhage or cerebral edema, especially in patients who have suffered a recent cerebral infarction.

Therapy of cerebrovascular atherosclerotic disease does not end with carotid endarterectomy. Long-term treatment with antiplatelet drugs, while not proven to be of benefit, is recommended. Risk factors, including cardiac disease, hypertension, diabetes mellitus, obesity, hyperlipidemia, and cigarette smoking must be reduced.

Complications

The complications of carotid endarterectomy are listed in Table 45-1. The incidence of complications is low when attention is given to the details of patient selection, intraoperative management, and postoperative care.[11,12]

The occurrence of a new neurologic deficit as a result of carotid endarterectomy is a serious complication. The majority of intraoperative deficits are thought to be caused by embolization from ulcerated atherosclerotic lesions during dissection and manipulation of the carotid artery. Intraoperative ischemia, either secondary to hypotension or to inadequate collateral circulation during carotid occlusion, also may result in neurologic deficit. By avoiding decreases in blood pressure during anesthesia and by using techniques to enhance cerebral perfusion, including induced hypertension and temporary intraluminal bypass, the incidence of cerebral ischemia is reduced. In the early postoperative period, neurologic deficit can be caused by cerebral emboli originating from platelet aggregates at the suture line and denuded media. Severe postoperative hypotension may predispose the artery to this thrombus formation. If the patient develops a postoperative neurologic deficit, angiography should be performed immediately, and the patient should be returned to the operating room to correct abnormalities such as occlusion of the carotid vessels, thrombus formation at the endarterectomy site, and dissection of a distal intimal flap that obstructs flow in the internal carotid artery. If angiography cannot be performed immediately, the patient should be returned directly to the operating room.

Figure 45-3 demonstrates the major cranial nerves and their branches that are often encountered during exposure of the carotid artery. Others lie near the area of dissection. These include the hypoglossal nerve, the vagus nerve with its superior and recurrent laryngeal branches, the marginal branch of the facial nerve, and the cervical sympathetic trunk. Fortunately, postoperative pareses of these nerves are rarely permanent and their incidence can be greatly reduced by meticulous dissection techniques and by avoiding vigorous retraction.

Disruption and aneurysm formation occasionally occur after carotid endarterectomy. The incidence of these complications is higher when synthetic patch grafts are used to close the arteriotomy, especially if a deep wound infection occurs. Infection following carotid endarterectomy is rare.

Because of the high incidence of associated coronary artery disease, myocardial ischemia and cardiac arrythmias are not infrequently encountered during and after carotid endarterectomy. Myocardial infarction is the leading cause of operative mortality (Table 45-1).

Following surgery many patients experience headaches ipsilateral to the endarterectomy site.[13] These headaches are usually self-limited, rarely lasting more than a few days. An infrequent complication is postoperative seizures,[14] which are frequently focal in nature and associated with paroxysmal lateralizing epileptiform discharges on EEG. These seizures are resistant to anticonvulsant therapy and have been attributed to restoration of flow in a previously ischemic zone, representing a manifestation of reactive hyperemia.[15] Another likely explanation is cerebral embolization.[16] If seizures occur, cerebral angiography should be performed.

The complications we have encountered in a series of 165 procedures performed on 150 consecutive patients on our service are listed in Table 45-1. The 3 postoperative deaths were due to myocardial infarction. Four patients had a new or increased permanent neurologic deficit following surgery. In 2 patients the deficits were mild.

Sundt and his co-workers[16] have published an analysis of 712 carotid endarterectomies in which they related the rate of mortality and serious morbidity to preoperative risk factors. Neurologically stable patients without major medical or angiographically determined risks incurred no mortality and had a 1.2 percent incidence of myocardial infarction and a 0.6 percent incidence of minor stroke. Neurologically unstable patients with or without associated major medical or angiographic risks suffered the highest rate of neurologic complications following operation, having a 4.2 percent incidence of major stroke and a 2.1 percent incidence of minor stroke.

Outcome of Carotid Endarterectomy

The long-term outcome of carotid endarterectomy is difficult to evaluate. The wide variation in severity of preoperative neurologic deficits and the natural history of improvement of strokes without treatment make it difficult to assess the role of endarterectomy in neurologic recovery. In selected patients with mild, stable strokes, carotid endarterectomy appears to lower the incidence of recurrent strokes and possibly has been responsible for improvement in neurologic function beyond that expected from the natural course of the disease.[17] The role of carotid endarterectomy in patients with TIAs is better defined. Carotid endarterectomy is effective in relieving the symptoms of TIAs and in lowering the incidence of stroke in selected patients. Only 1 of our patients had further TIAs in the distribution of the treated carotid artery following surgery. The majority of late deaths in patients undergoing carotid endarterectomy are of cardiac origin. While at the present time no increase in survival rate of surgical patients compared with control patients can be demonstrated,[18] it is believed that the avoidance of stroke significantly improves the quality of life.

Miscellaneous Conditions Affecting the Extracranial Carotid Arteries

Traumatic Injuries

Injuries to the carotid artery may result from penetrating injuries or, less frequently, from blunt trauma.[19,20] Penetrating neck injuries, usually from stab or missile wounds, most frequently involve the common carotid artery.[20] Findings of a local, at times pulsatile hematoma may accompany the injury. Arteriovenous fistulas are not uncommon. A significant number of patients will demonstrate a related neurologic deficit.

Patients suffering from hypotension as a result of blood loss from a suspected carotid artery injury require rapid resuscitation and immediate exploration of the neck to control hemorrhage.[21] Tracheal intubation is essential, as airway compromise by external compression from hematoma or massive internal bleeding may occur. When bleeding is controlled and the airway is not compromised, angiography should be performed to define the presence and extent of vascular injuries.[22] Information obtained from good-quality angiograms may be crucial in planning the surgical approach to a correctable vascular injury. While it has been suggested that early arterial repair in the presence of a neurologic deficit may lead to worsening of neurologic status,[23] most authorities believe that early exploration is essential for appropriate management.[24] Preoperative neurologic deficits often are permanent.[20,24] While penetrating injuries are frequently tangential, perforation and complete transection of the carotid artery also are seen. The method of operative repair is dictated by the nature of the injury to the vessel. Necrotic portions must be resected and intimal flaps excised. With some tangential wounds, arteriorrhapy or a vein patch graft may be sufficient for repair, especially when the common carotid artery is involved. End-to-end anastomosis of the artery with either a vein or a synthetic graft is required to repair more extensive arterial injuries. A temporary shunt is seldom needed and may interfere with repair. Clots should be evacuated from the distal stump of the artery by back-bleeding or by careful extraction with a Fogarty catheter. Heparin should be administered systemically during repair. When the injured artery cannot be adequately exposed for repair, ligation may be necessary to control hemorrhage. The presence of shock or coma before surgery is a grave prognostic sign.[24]

Blunt injuries of the carotid artery are uncommon, but when they are unrecognized they are associated with a high incidence of severe neurologic complications.[19,20] Often there is no evidence of direct trauma to the neck and the frequent association with closed head injury may obscure recognition of the carotid injury.[25] Direct blunt trauma to the neck that causes arterial damage frequently involves the carotid bifurcation, particularly in older patients with atheromatous disease. Extension and rotation of the neck because of head trauma may stretch the internal carotid artery over a transverse process of an upper cervical vertebra. Basilar skull fractures can disrupt the petrosal portion of the internal carotid artery, while intraoral trauma may be associated with injury to the internal carotid artery adjacent to the tonsillar fossa.

Suspicion of a blunt carotid artery injury may not arise until the patient develops focal neurologic symptoms—perhaps hours to weeks after the injury. Often neck swelling or a Horner's syndrome will be present and will serve as an early clue. The diagnosis should be corroborated by angiography. Surgical management is indicated if an appropriate accessible lesion is found.

Kinking

The clinical importance of elongation of the cervical carotid artery with looping and kinking is obscure. Although a number of surgical techniques have been developed to deal with this phenomenon, most surgeons question the need for surgery in the majority of cases.[26] Kinking or buckling of the carotid artery is due to atherosclerosis and is distinguished from coiling, which is thought to be a developmental abnormality.[27] Coiling in an exaggerated S-shaped curvature or circular configuration is a result of elongation and redundancy of the internal carotid artery and is often an incidental angiographic finding. Kinking, which consists of angulation of one or more segments of the artery, usually is associated with atherosclerotic disease at the carotid bifurcation. True kinking may, in rare instances, cause obstructive symptoms. In this situation, factors such as changes in neck position, blood pressure variation, and the presence of extracranial atherosclerotic occlusive disease may play a major role. In patients with recurrent cerebrovascular symptoms, resection of the kink should be considered only if it significantly reduces the arterial lumen and no other causative angiographic abnormality is found.[27,28] The head should be rotated during angiography to observe the effects on the kink. Symptomatic kinking is surgically managed by resection of the involved segment of the internal carotid artery with end-to-end anastomosis. At times it is necessary to reimplant the distal internal carotid artery into the common carotid artery.[29]

Aneurysms

Nondissecting aneurysms of the extracranial carotid artery are rare, but represent a serious entity that has the potential of causing death or stroke from rupture, thrombosis, or embolism.[29,30] In the past, syphilis and pharyngeal infections were the predominant cause of these aneurysms, but today they are most often associated with trauma or atherosclerosis. They may occur following carotid endarterectomy, most frequently when a patch graft has been employed in closure.[31] Patients usually present with a pulsatile cervical mass and bruit. These lesions should be resected. The involved arterial segment is excised and replaced with a synthetic or vein graft. Rarely, a saccular aneurysm can be transected through its stalk and the carotid artery repaired directly.

Dissecting extracranial carotid artery aneurysms constitute a small group of lesions that usually occur above the carotid bifurcation.[32-34] Some cases are clearly related to a predisposing factor such as trauma, angiography, and fibromuscular dysplasia, but many have a spontaneous onset with an obscure etiology. The dissection may occur bilaterally, often forming pseudoaneurysms. Symptoms and signs are ascribed to three basic mechanisms: disruption of sympathetic fibers within the wall of the carotid artery, accumulation of thrombi on areas of intimal disruption that lead to cerebral emboli, and reduction in cerebral blood flow due to stenosis or occlusion of the carotid artery.[32] Initial symptoms may include unilateral head and face pain associated with an ipsilateral Horner's syndrome,[35] TIAs, and stroke. The diagnosis is made by angiography.

A number of therapeutic approaches have been used in small groups of patients. Operative management includes segmental resection and grafting, thrombectomy and endarterectomy, dilatation, carotid ligation, and extracranial–intracranial bypass.[32,36] The distal extent of dissection in the majority of cases, however, can make direct surgery hazardous and can lead to undesirable clinical results. Patients surviving an extracranial carotid artery dissection often have a stable or improving course, although if aneurysmal changes are present, some evidence of the lesion may persist.[33] The recommended initial treatment is anticoagulation to prevent thromboembolic events. Serial angiography has shown that many of these lesions will resolve when treated in this manner.

Fibromuscular Dysplasia

Fibromuscular dysplasia of the internal carotid arteries often is an incidental angiographic finding.[17] This condition is most commonly seen in women in their third and fourth decades. The lesions are frequently bilateral, and nearly always located in the distal part of the cervical internal carotid artery extending to or beyond the base of the skull. The proximal 2.5 cm of the internal carotid usually is spared.[37] There is a recognized association with fibromuscular hyperplasia of the renal arteries, hypertension, and multiple intracranial aneurysms. In older patients, associated atherosclerotic lesions near the carotid bifurcation are more likely to be the source of cerebrovascular symptoms. Surgical treatment should be directed toward the atherosclerotic plaque. In patients without associated lesions, symptoms of cerebrovascular insufficiency have been attributed to fibromuscular dysplasia. In these patients surgical treatment will vary with the location of the lesion. In most cases it is impossible to expose the normal distal internal carotid artery with a cervical approach, and techniques of graded arterial dilation using instruments such as rigid biliary dilators,[38,39] coronary artery dilators,[17] and small Fogarty catheters[29] have been employed. A short arteriotomy is made in the common carotid artery just proximal to the bifurcation. Progressively larger dilators are passed through the arteriotomy to the end of the diseased segment of the internal carotid artery at the base of the skull. Satisfactory results have been reported with these techniques in selected patients.[17]

Summary and Conclusions

In selected patients, carotid endarterectomy is a relatively safe and effective means of preventing cerebral infarction caused by atherosclerotic occlusive and embolic disease of the extracranial carotid artery. Patients who have a cerebral ischemic event and who have a significant amount of hemispheric neurologic function at risk should undergo cerebral angiography following appropriate medial evaluation and determination of surgical candidacy. Among the factors influencing a decision to treat a patient surgically are the correlation of clinical and angiographic features, collateral cerebral circulation, and medical and surgical risk factors. Satisfactory surgical results require precise attention to technical details. Measures must be taken to avoid intraoperative embolization and ischemia and to ensure continued vessel patency by direct visualization of the distal extent of atheromatous involvement of the internal carotid artery. Rapid correction of postoperative abnormalities of cardiovascular and respiratory status will diminish the rate of serious complications during this period. The patient with atherosclerotic cerebrovascular disease must have continued treatment of identifiable risk factors following carotid endarterectomy.

REFERENCES

1. Ross R, Glomset JA: The pathogenesis of arterosclerosis, Part 1. *N Eng J Med 295*:369–376, 1976
2. Hammond JH, Eisinger RP: Carotid bruits in 1,000 normal subjects. *Arch Intern Med 109*:109–111, 162
3. Fields WS: The asymptomatic carotid bruit: operate or not? Current concepts of cerebrovascular disease—stroke. *Stroke 9*:269–271, 1978
4. Heyman A, Wilkins WE, Heyden S, et al: Risk of stroke in asymptomatic persons with cervical arterial bruits: a population study in Evans County, Georgia. *N Engl J Med 302*:838–841, 1980
5. Moore WS, Boren G, Malone JA, et al: Asymptomatic carotid stenosis: Immediate and long-term results after prophylactic endarterectomy. *Am J Surg 138*:228–233, 1979
6. Levin SM, Sondheimer FK, Levin JM: The contralateral diseased but asymptomatic carotid artery: to operate or not?: an update. *Am J Surg 140*:203–205, 1980
7. Johnson N, Burnham SJ, Flanigan DP, et al: Carotid endarterectomy: A follow-up study of the contralateral non-operated carotid artery. *Ann Surg 188*:748–752, 1978
8. Wade JG, Larson CP Jr, Hickey RF, et al: Effect of carotid endarterectomy on carotid chemoreceptor and baroreceptor function in man. *N Engl J Med 282*:823–829, 1970
9. Bove EL, Fry WJ, Gross WS, et al: Hypotension and hypertension as consequences of baroreceptor dysfunction following carotid endarterectomy. *Surgery 85*:633–637, 1979
10. Tarlov E, Schmidek H, Scott RM, et al: Reflex hypotension following carotid endarterectomy: mechanism and management. *J Neurosurg 29*:323–327, 1973
11. Thompson JE: Complications of carotid endarterectomy and their prevention. *World J Surg 3*:155–165, 1979
12. Dunsker SB: Complications of carotid endarterectomy. *Clin Neurosurg 23*:336–341, 1976
13. Messert B, Black JA: Cluster headache, hemicrania, and other head pains: Morbidity of carotid endarterectomy. *Stroke 9*:559–562, 1978
14. Wilkinson JT, Adams HP Jr, Wright CB: Convulsions after carotid endarterectomy. *JAMA 244*:1827–1828, 1980
15. Sundt TM, Houser OW, Sharbrough F, et al: Carotid endarterectomy: Results, complications, and monitoring techniques, in Thompson RA, Green JA (eds): *Advances in Neurology, Vol. 16.* New York, Raven Press, 1977, pp 97–119
16. Sundt TM: Extracranial occlusive cerebral vascular disease, in Wilson CB, Hoff JT (eds): *Current Management of Neurologic Disease.* New York, Churchill-Livingston, 1980, pp 191–201
17. Thompson JE, Talkington CM: Carotid endarterectomy. *Ann Surg 184*:1–15, 1976
18. Toole JF, Janeway R, Choi K, et al: Transient ischemic attacks due to atherosclerosis: A prospective study of 160 patients. *Arch Neurol 32*:5–12, 1975
19. Krajewski LP, Hertzer NR: Blunt carotid artery trauma. *Ann Surg 191*:341–346, 1980
20. Rubio PA, Reul GJ Jr, Beall AC, Jr. et al: Acute carotid artery injury: 25 years experience. *J Trauma 14*:967–973, 1974
21. Ledgerwood AM, Mullins RJ, Lucas CE: Primary repair vs. ligation for carotid artery injuries. *Arch Surg 115*:488–493, 1980

22. O'Donnell VA, Atik M, Pick RA: Evaluation and management of penetrating wounds of the neck: The role of emergency angiography. *Am J Surg 138*:309–313, 1979
23. Bradley EL III: Management of penetrating carotid injuries: An alternative approach. *J Trauma 13*:248–265, 1973
24. Unger SW, Tucker WS Jr, Mrdeza MA, et al: Carotid arterial trauma. *Surgery 87*:477–487, 1980
25. Heilbrun MP, Ratcheson RA: Multiple extracranial vessel injuries following closed head and neck trauma: case report. *J Neurosurg 37*:219–223, 1972
26. Perdue GD, Barreca JP, Smith RB, et al: The significance of elongation and angulation of the carotid artery: a negative view. *Surgery 77*:45–52, 1975
27. Desai B, Toole JF: Kinks, coils, and carotids: A review. *Stroke 6*:649–653, 1975
28. Connolly JE: Discussion: Kinking of internal carotid artery. *Am J Surg 134*:88, 1977
29. Cooley DA, Wukasch DC: *Techniques in Vascular Surgery.* Philadelphia, W. B. Saunders Co., 1979, pp 20–44
30. Coleman PG, Kittle GF: Aneurysms of the common carotid artery. *Surg Clin N Amer 53*:231–240, 1973
31. Smith RB III, Perdue GP, Collier RH, et al: Post-operative false aneurysms of the carotid artery. *Am Surgeon 36*:335–341, 1970
32. Friedman WA, Day AL, Quisling RG, et al: Cervical carotid dissecting aneurysms. *Neurosurgery 7*:207–214, 1980
33. Luken MG III, Ascherl GF Jr, Correll JW, et al: Spontaneous dissecting aneurysm of the extracranial internal carotid artery. *Clin Neurosurg 26*:353–375, 1978
34. Fisher CM, Ojemann RG, Roberson GH: Spontaneous dissection of cervico-cerebral arteries. *Can J Neurol Sci 5*:9–19, 1978
35. Mokri B, Sundt TM Jr, Houser OW: Spontaneous internal carotid dissection, hemicrania, and Horner's syndrome. *Arch Neurol 36*:677–680, 1979
36. Ehrenfeld WK, Wylie EJ: Spontaneous dissection of the internal carotid artery. *Arch Surg 111*:1294–1301, 1976
37. Sandok BA, Houser OW, Baker HL, et al: Fibromuscular dysplasia: Neurologic disorders associated with disease involving the great vessels in the neck. *Arch Neurol 24*:462–466, 1971
38. Morris GC, Lechter A, DeBakey ME: Surgical treatment of fibromuscular disease of the carotid arteries. *Arch Surg 96*:636–643, 1968
39. Ehrenfeld WK, Wylie EJ: Fibromuscular dysplasia of the internal carotid artery. *Arch Surg 109*:676–681, 1974

CHAPTER 46
Surgical Management of Extracranial Lesions of the Vertebral Artery

Edward F. Downing

THE PROBLEM OF VERTEBROBASILAR INSUFFICIENCY long has been overshadowed by the problem of carotid insufficiency. The unqualified acceptance[1] of this attitude is no longer acceptable, however. The dogmatic attitudes of the neurologic world have contributed to this state of affairs, which, in our experience, is not justified.

Sorenus in 98 AD described what is known today as vertebrobasilar insufficiency in his syndrome of dizziness, tinnitus, and ataxia. It was not until 1955, however, that Millikan and Siekert[2] further elucidated the modern-day syndrome of vertebrobasilar insufficiency in their classical paper. The first successful vertebral artery endarterectomy was done in 1959 by DeBakey et al.[3] and by Cate and Scott.[4] Since then, references to this procedure in the literature have been scanty.[5-7] Natali et al.[8] reported 13 cases, and Cormier and Laurian[9] reported the treatment of 119 vertebral elongations. In 1968, Morris et al.[10] reported on 365 vertebral reconstructions out of 2900 extracranial reconstructive operations. In our material vertebral operations form approximately 10 percent of the total carotid operations.

There are certain distinguishing characteristics of the symptoms produced by extracranial vertebral artery disease compared with those produced by occlusive disease of the intracranial vertebral and basilar arteries. The symptoms produced by extracranial disease are almost uniformly reproducible by mechanical maneuvers of the cervical spine and are almost exclusively mechanical in nature. In the management of extracranial vertebral disease, there are two key indications for surgical treatment:

1. The isolated posterior circulation, meaning no contribution to the vertebrobasilar system is made from the posterior communicating arteries on either side. It has been well demonstrated by Drake* that both vertebral arteries can be ligated in the cervical region if there is adequate collateral circulation from the posterior communicating arteries from the carotid circulation.
2. Symptoms that can be reproduced by mechanical maneuvers. Our experience is limited to patients who fulfill these two criteria and has resulted in the routine alleviation of the patient's symptoms.

Muller et al., Greitz,[11] 1966, and the American Joint Study[12] all have shown that stenosis and occlusion of the vertebral artery is approximately two-thirds as common as occlusion of the

Neurological Institute of Savannah, Savannah, Georgia
*Personal communication.

internal carotid artery. This also has been confirmed by the work of Hutchinson and Yates. Stenosis at the origin of the vertebral artery has a much greater significance in the development of symptoms than lateral osteophytes, which the author has never seen produce vertebrobasilar symptoms. The tortuosities in stenosis of the vertebral artery are still not sufficiently appreciated, even though Rieben has shown by flow studies in the vertebral artery that a mechanical effect on the speed of flow is produced by movements of the head and cervical spine.[1] This obstruction or even interruption of blood flow can be more severe when there is stenosis and tortuosity of the vertebral artery, thus this finding is of importance in the illness. It is the author's opinion that operable causes of vertebrobasilar insufficiency at the proximal segment of the vertebral artery bear much more attention.

Clinical Considerations

In our experience of over 50 cases of vertebrobasilar insufficiency, dizziness has been present in 80 percent of the patients; ataxia in 45 percent; bilateral visual disturbance in 40 percent; and motor sensory changes in 25 percent. Headaches, drop attacks, and mental changes rarely have been present.

Before invasive investigation of patients with symptoms of vertebrobasilar insufficiency is performed, a cardiac etiology of the symptoms is ruled out. All patients in our series have been investigated with arch aortography and four-vessel, selective retrograde cervical and intracranial arteriography. It is mandatory that views of the origin of both vertebral arteries be obtained, preferably with 104 Cine radiography, as it is that views of the intracranial vertebral and basilar circulation along with bilateral internal carotid series be obtained in order to determine the patency of the posterior communicating arteries. We have elected not to operate on any patient in whom the posterior communicating arteries were patent unless the symptoms, in our opinion, were embolic in origin, which has been rare.

The pathology in this series consists of the following types of lesions.

1. Severe atherosclerotic stenosis of the origin of the vertebral artery.
2. Extraluminal compression of the vertebral origin, producing severe stenosis from fibromuscular bands.
3. Bilateral, second-portion vertebral stenosis from extraluminal compression of the arteries caused by hypertrophied scalene muscles (some have questioned whether this may be an early form of fibromuscular hyperplasia of the vertebral artery).
4. Combined, severe, ulcerative occlusive disease of the proximal subclavian and vertebral origin.
5. Subclavian steal syndrome.

We have tended not to operate on unilateral stenotic lesions of the vertebral origin when the contralateral vertebral artery has been widely patent unless the stenotic lesion was subtotal in character. If the unilateral vertebral lesion has been subtotal in character and the contralateral vertebral artery has been widely patent, we have recommended endarterectomy on the basis of preventing impending occlusion of the vertebral artery, which in our experience has been the most common cause of the Wallenberg syndrome.

Figure 46-1 illustrates the most common cause of symptomatic extracranial vertebral stenosis, that being an hourglass-shaped, severe, occlusive lesion at the origin of the vertebral artery. This represented over 80 percent of the patients in our series. We have treated this lesion with transsubclavian vertebral artery endarterectomy.

Figure 46-2 represents stenosis of the origin of the vertebral artery from extraluminal fibromuscular bands. You will note that this differs from the atherosclerotic narrowing of the origin of the vertebral artery in that the narrowing of the artery is from one side only, always the me-

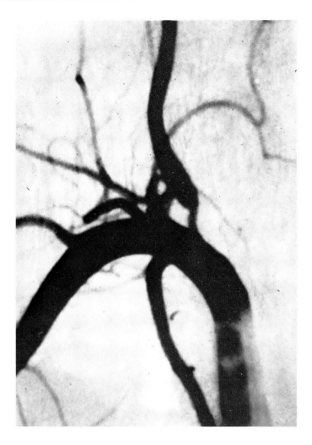

Fig. 46-1.   A severe occlusive lesion at the origin of the vertebral artery. Note the hourglass shape.

dial side, as opposed to the hourglass-type constriction, which is secondary to intraluminal atherosclerotic plaquing. Careful evaluation of this angiographic configuration has led us to this conclusion. The surgical treatment for this lesion is simply a scalenotomy, with care being taken to be sure that all of the fibromuscular bands of the posterior aspect of the posterior scalene muscle has been lysed. After this has been done, care must be taken to palpate with vascular forceps to be sure that there is not an intraluminal atherosclerotic plaque, which in our experience has not been present. This thesis has been verified with postoperative angiography and with intraluminal inspection of the vertebral arteries.

Figure 46-3 represents bilateral stenosis of the second portion of the vertebral artery, just proximal to the entrance into the transverse foramen. We have seen 3 such cases and all have been present in extremely short, stocky, and muscular individuals. The symptoms have been uniformly reproducible by simply extending the neck. It is interesting to note that all 3 of these patients were timber cutters. This type of lesion has been treated with bilateral extraluminal decompression of the vertebral artery from its origin to its entrance into the transverse foramen.

Figure 46-4 represents the postoperative angiography of Figure 46-3, after extraluminal decompression of both vertebral arteries. Some people have suggested this could be treated simply by intraluminal dilatation; however, we have had no experience with that procedure.

Figures 46-5 and 46-6 represent stenosis of the vertebral origin combined with severe ulcerative stenotic disease of the proximal subclavian. Because an endarterectomy at the origin of the vertebral artery in this situation would only form a funnel to channel emboli to the basilar circulation from the proximal subclavian, we have treated this lesion with amputation to the vertebral

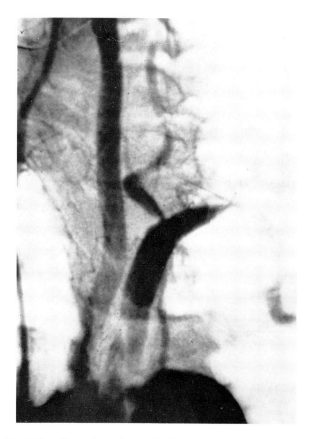

Fig. 46-2. Stenosis at the origin of the vertebral artery from extraluminal fibromuscular bands.

artery at its origin and end-to-side anastomosis to the ipsilateral common carotid artery. The postoperative angiogram of the end-to-side vertebral-to-common carotid anastomosis of the patient shown in Figures 46-5 and 46-6 is shown in Figure 46-7.

Figure 46-8 represents a patient who had severe stenosis of the origin of the left vertebral artery that arose from the aortic arch. The right vertebral artery was totally occluded and there were no posterior communicating arteries present. This patient also was treated with vertebral amputation and end-to-side anastomosis of the left vertebral artery into the left common carotid artery with alleviation of symptoms.

Figure 46-9 is a subtraction arch study of a subclavian steal. Figure 46-10 shows the postoperative angiogram of this patient, after he was treated by an extrathoracic common carotid-to-subclavian bypass graft.

Operative Considerations

Vertebral Endarterectomy

In my opinion, one of the main reasons that vertebral endarterectomy has not become as popular as carotid endarterectomy has been the uniformly poor results produced in the 1960s. The reasons for these results are two-fold. (1) The early surgical attempts at vertebral artery reconstruction were focused directly on the vertebral artery at its origin. The vertebral artery is a very thin artery once the atherosclerotic plaque is removed and does not lend itself well to direct surgery at all. (2) The suture material used in the early operations was large in size.

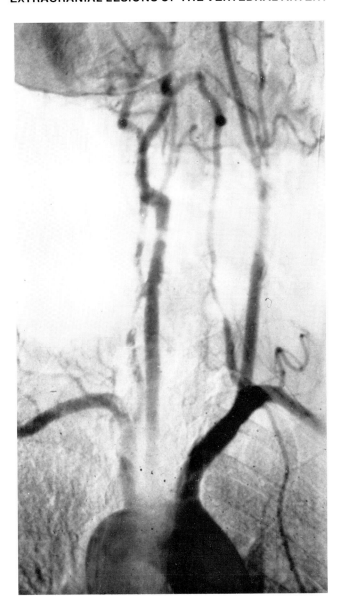

Fig. 46-3. Bilateral stenosis of the second portion of the vertebral artery.

The surgical approach that I have chosen to use in this series avoids both of these problems. The approach has been an indirect approach through the subclavian artery across from the vertebral orifice, and 7-0 suture material is used. Figure 46-11 shows the skin incision, which consists of a 10-cm incision parallel to and just above the clavicle from the sternal notch laterally. The entire sternocleidomastoid muscle must be taken down just adjacent to its insertion on the clavicle. This is done by doubly clamping the sternocleidomastoid once it has been completely dissected free by blunt dissection with four large, curved Kelly clamps. The muscle then is sectioned with the cutting current and the ends are coagulated with the coagulating current. The medial and lateral halves of the muscle are individually mattress sutured with 0 silk suture, both distally and proximally. These sutures then are left long, and the muscles are allowed to retract. Figure 46-12 shows the exposure after the sternocleidomastoids have been transected with the internal jugular vein coming into view, which on some occasions may have to be ligated because of

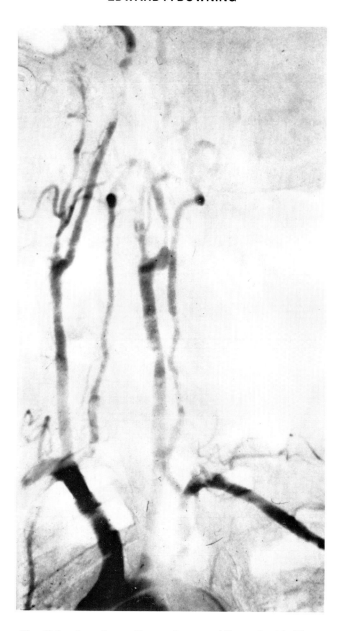

Fig. 46-4. A postoperative angiogram of the patient in Figure 46-3 after extraluminal decompression of the vertebral arteries.

its position in the wound. It usually can be retracted out of the way, along with the phrenic nerve, which runs anterior to the anterior scalene muscle. The scalene fat pad has been removed at this point to allow visualization of the scalene muscle, the phrenic nerve, and the brachial plexus. The phrenic nerve generally is retracted either medially or laterally with a 0.25-inch Penrose drain, with care being taken to retract as little as possible. The scalene muscles then are completely transected. Figure 46-13 shows the scalene muscles after transection with the dome of the subclavian artery coming into view. The dome of the subclavian artery then is exposed along with the thyrocervical trunk (Fig. 46-14), the internal mammary artery, and the origin of the vertebral artery. It is necessary to reflect the subclavian approximately 2.5 cm proximal to the origin of the vertebral artery and approximately 2.5 cm distal to the thyrocervical trunk or

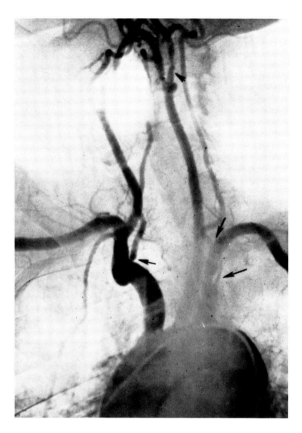

Fig. 46-5.   Stenosis of the origin of the vertebral artery combined with severe ulcerative stenotic disease of the
proximal subclavian artery.

internal mammary, whichever is the most distal. Once this exposure is obtained, the patient is
fully heparinized. The vertebral artery then is dissected free for approximately 3 cm, which will
always be distal to the plaque. The plaque is always situated at the origin and is always very short
in nature, as opposed to the rather long plaque of the internal carotid origin. The internal mammary artery, the thyrocervical trunk, and the distal vertebral artery then are temporarily occluded with Scoville aneurysm clips, following which the proximal subclavian and distal subclavian arteries are temporarily occluded with large, angled, vascular occlusion clamps (Fig. 46-15),
following which a 2-cm incision is made in the subclavian artery just opposite the origin of the
vertebral artery. After this has been done, tenting sutures are placed in each leaf of the subclavian artery (Fig. 46-16) and a No. 11 blade is used to make a circumferential incision in the
plaque around the origin of the vertebral artery. Then, with careful teasing with a small dissector, the plaque is removed in toto by the intussusception, pull-down technique. The fact that lesions of the vertebral origin are always short and are situated at the origin of the vertebral artery
makes this technique feasible. After the funnel-shaped plaque has been removed from the origin
of the vertebral artery, care is taken to be sure there are no loose intimal tags distally in the vertebral artery and also distally in the subclavian artery. Occasionally it will be necessary to use tacking sutures in the rather thick atheromatous plaque in the subclavian artery to prevent distal
dissection. If tacking sutures are needed, double-armed, No. 6 arterial silk sutures are used. After the plaque has been removed along with all intimal tags and the intimal edges have been taken
care of, the arteriotomy is closed with a running, 7-0 Prolene suture. Figure 46-17 shows the operative field after the vertebral plaque has been removed and the subclavian closed with a 7-0

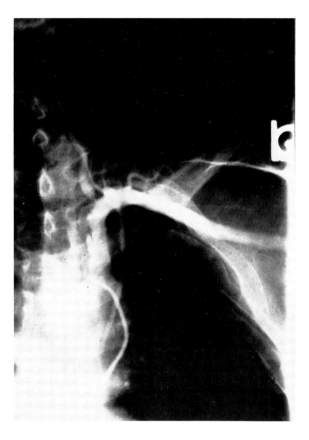

Fig. 46-6. Stenosis of the origin of the vertebral artery combined with severe ulcerative stenotic disease of the proximal subclavian artery.

Prolene suture before removal of the clamps. After the arteriotomy has been closed, the vertebral artery is opened first to allow back-bleeding into the operative site. This also is done after the plaque is removed before the arteriotomy is closed.

After the vertebral has flooded the operative site and hemostasis of the suture line has been ascertained, the temporary Scoville aneurysm clip is placed back on the vertebral artery. The clamps then are removed from the subclavian artery proximally, then distally, followed by removal of the aneurysm clips from the internal mammary, the thyrocervical trunk, and, lastly, the vertebral artery. A 0.25-inch Penrose drain is brought out through a stab wound and the sternocleidomastoid muscles are reconstructed with the 0 silk sutures that previously had been placed in a mattress fashion at the beginning of the operation. After these sutures have been tied, approximately six additional 0 silk sutures are used to reconstruct the sternocleidomastoid. The platysma and the subcuticular layers then are closed with 4-0 Tycron and the skin is closed with Steri-strips. The drain is removed 12 hours postoperatively. The usual clamp time of the vertebral artery has been approximately 15 to 20 minutes; however, on one occasion, a clamp time of 35 minutes was necessary in the absence of the contralateral vertebral artery without producing any ischemia.

Postoperatively, the patients are treated with aspirin and Persantine on a long-term basis and the operative anticoagulation is not reversed. This operative procedure has not produced any new ischemic attacks and has relieved preoperative symptoms that were mechanically reproducible in every occasion. It has been my experience that temporary diaphragmatic paralysis has been present almost uniformly, but has never persisted for more than 6 weeks and has never

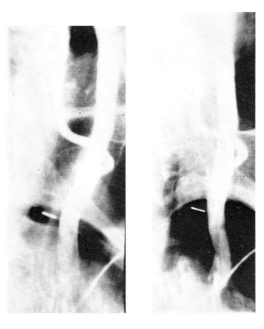

Fig. 46-7. Postoperative angiograms of the patient in Figures 46-5 and 46-6 after end-to-side anastomosis of the vertebral artery to the common carotid.

been symptom producing. The only complication that we have encountered has been a thoracic duct fistula, which required reoperation and ligation. When operating on the left side, the thoracic duct must be adequately ligated to prevent this complication.

Subclavian Steal

The recommended surgical procedure of choice for the treatment of subclavian steal syndrome[13,14] is the extrathoracic common carotid–subclavian bypass. Figure 46-18 illustrates the operative technique for this procedure. Story* and Fein[15] have advocated treatment of the subclavian steal by end-to-side, vertebral-to-common carotid anastomosis. Long-term follow-up results are not available at this time for this variation of treatment, and until they are available, the extrathoracic bypass is the procedure of choice. There are certain technical points that must be vividly adhered to, however, in order to avoid complications with this procedure. When the bypass graft is anastomosed to the common carotid artery, either an exclusion clamp should be used or a temporary internal bypass should be placed in the common carotid artery in order to avoid occluding this artery more than a minute or two while the anastomosis is being made. This is an extremely important technical consideration because the deleterious results of early repairs of subclavian steal syndrome were almost uniformly related to ischemia in the carotid distribution from prolonged clamping of the carotid artery.

Combined Subclavian–Carotid Stenosis

The surgical approach to this combined lesion is exactly the same as in a vertebral endarterectomy down to the exposure of the vertebral origin. After the vertebral origin has been exposed, the common carotid artery, which is immediately adjacent, is exposed. The vertebral artery is amputated at its origin with a 2-0 silk ligature. Distally, the vertebral artery is temporarily occluded with a Scoville aneurysm clip, and a small, vascular, exclusion clamp is used to par-

*Personal communication.

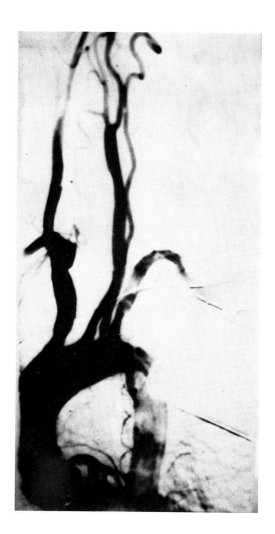

Fig. 46-8. Severe stenosis of a left vertebral artery that arises from the aortic arch.

tially occlude the common carotid artery, following which a vertical arteriotomy is made and an
end-to-side anastomosis in a running fashion with 7-0 Prolene sutures after two corner-
anchoring sutures have been placed. After the end-to-side anastomosis has been completed, the
temporary clip on the distal vertebral artery is removed to allow flooding of the operative site to
test the anastomosis. After this has been done and the anastomosis has been ascertained to be
adequate, the partial exclusion clamp is removed from the common carotid artery. By using the
partial exclusion clamp, flow in the common carotid has not been interrupted at all. The closure
from this point on is exactly the same as in the previously described vertebral endarterectomy
procedure.

Figure 46-19 illustrates preoperative and postoperative angiograms of a tightly stenotic lesion of the vertebral origin. The left side of the figure demonstrates a subtotal occlusion of the

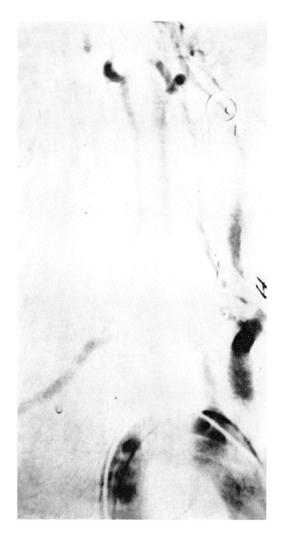

Fig. 46-9. A subtraction arch study of a subclavian steal.

origin of the left vertebral artery, and the right side of the figure represents a postoperative angiogram showing the widely patent vertebral orifice.

Many patients have asymptomatic vertebral stenotic disease, which is incidentally found on
angiography performed for other reasons. Figure 46-20 represents a patient who was studied because of asymptomatic bruits before a coronary artery bypass and was demonstrated to have bilateral occlusion of the internal carotid arteries and bilateral vertebral artery occlusion with
reconstitution of the left vertebral artery via the muscular branches of the left thyrocervical
trunk. This patient illustrates why extracranial vertebral artery reconstruction surgery should
not be recommended for any patient who is asymptomatic or whose symptoms cannot be reproduced by mechanical maneuvers. If these operative indications are adhered to, the postoperative
results strongly suggest that a more active, aggressive attitude should be adopted toward reconstructive surgery of the vertebral artery.

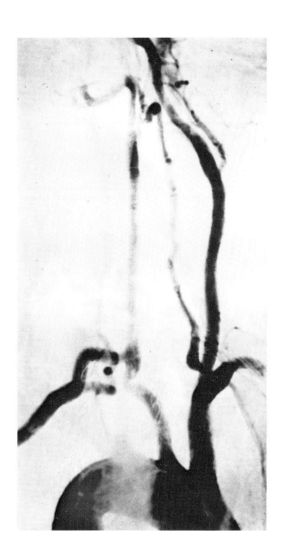

Fig. 46-10. A postoperative angiogram of the patient in Figure 46-9 after treatment by
an extrathoracic common carotid-to-
subclavian artery bypass graft.

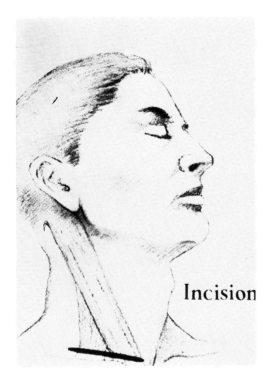

Fig. 46-11. The line of incision for vertebral endarterectomy.

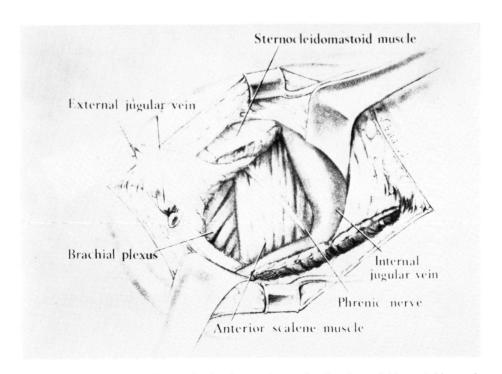

Fig. 46-12. The exposure for vertebral endarterectomy after the sternocleidomastoid muscle has been transected and the internal jugular vein is visible.

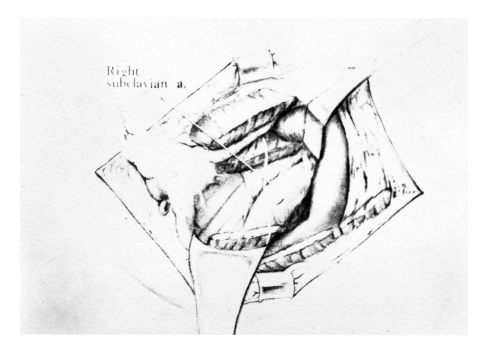

Fig. 46-13. The exposure after transection of the scalene muscle. The dome of the subclavian artery is visible.

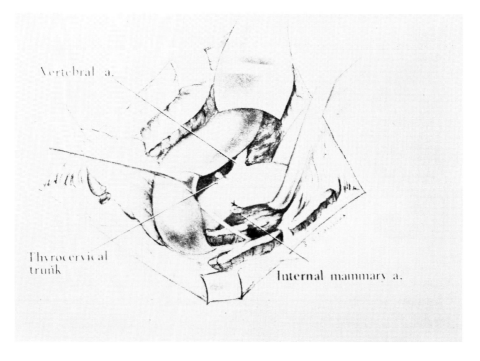

Fig. 46-14. The dissection continues along the dome of the subclavian, the thyrocervical trunk, the internal mammary artery, and the vertebral artery.

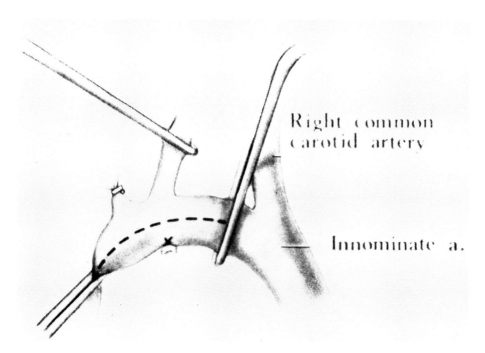

Fig. 46-15.   The line of incision in the subclavian artery opposite the origin of the vertebral artery.

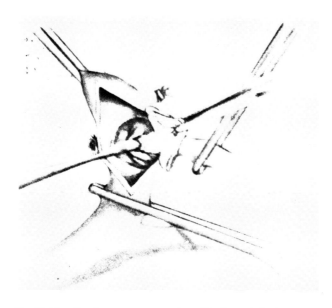

Fig. 46-16.   Tenting sutures are placed in the subclavian artery and a No. 11 blade is used to excise the plaque in the origin of the vertebral artery.

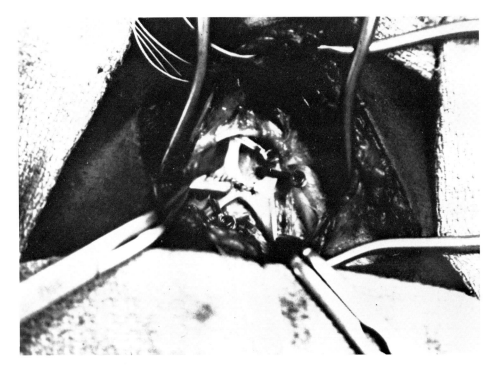

Fig. 46-17.   The operative field after the plaque has been removed and the subclavian artery
closed with 7-0 Prolene sutures.

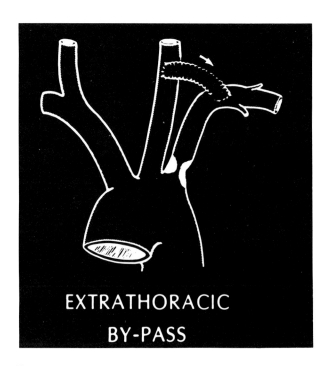

Fig. 46-18.   A diagram of the technique of extrathoracic common carotid–subclavian artery bypass for the
treatment of subclavian steal.

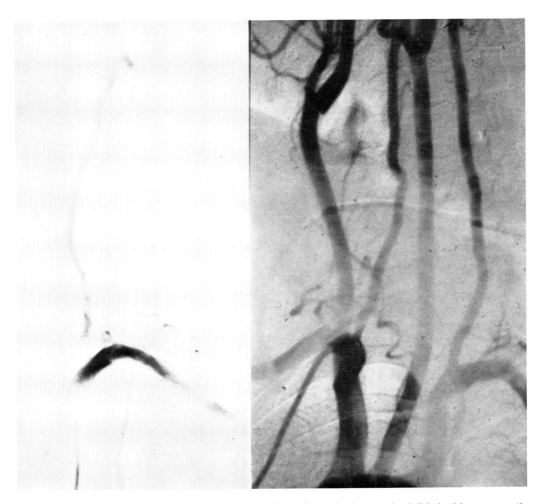

Fig. 46-19. (Left) Subtotal occlusion of the origin of the left vertebral artery is visible in this preoperative angiogram. (Right) A postoperative angiogram demonstrates a widely patent vertebral orifice.

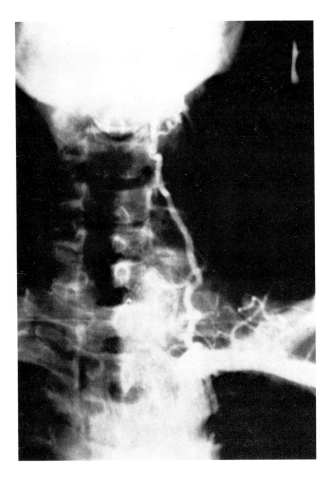

Fig. 46-20. Bilateral occlusion of the internal carotid arteries
and the vertebral arteries was noted in this patient
who was undergoing studies because of asymptomatic bruits noticed before coronary bypass surgery. Note that the left vertebral artery has been
reconstituted via muscular branches of the left
thyrocervical trunk.

REFERENCES

1. Rieben FW: *Zur Orthologie und Pathologie der Arteria Vertebralis.* Sitzungsberichte der Heidelberger Akad. Wiss., math-nat. Kl. Berlin, Springer-Verlag, 1973, pp 95–132
2. Millikan CH, Siekert G: Studies in cerebrovascular disease: I. The syndrome of intermittent insufficiency of the basilar arterial system. *Proc Staff Meet Mayo Clin 30*:61, 1955
3. DeBakey ME, Crawford ES, Cooley DA, et al: Surgical considerations of occlusive disease of innominate, carotid, subclavian, and vertebral arteries. *Ann Surg 149*:690–710, 1959
4. Cate W, Scott RH Jr: Cerebral ischemia of central origin: relief by subclavian-vertebral artery thromboendarterectomy. *Surgery 45*:19–30, 1959
5. Berguer R, Audaya LV, Bauer RB: Vertebral artery bypass. *Arch Surg 3*:976–979, 1976
6. Castaigne P, Lhermitte F, Gautier JC, et al: Arterial occlusions in the vertebrobasilar system: a study of 44 patients with postmortem data. *Brain 96*:133–154, 1973
7. Fisher CM, Gore I, Okalie N, et al: Atherosclerosis of the carotid and vertebral arteries—extracranial and intracranial. *J Neuropathol Exp Neurol 24*:455–476, 1965
8. Natali J, Maraval M, Kiefer E: Surgical treatment of stenosis and occlusion of the internal carotid and vertebral arteries. *J Cardiovasc Surg 13*:4–15, 1972
9. Cormier JM, Laurian C: Surgical management of vertebral-basilar insufficiency. *J Cardiovasc Surg 17*:205–223, 1976
10. Morris GC Jr, Crawford ES, DeBakey ME: The vertebral artery in cerebral anoxia, in de la Camp B, Linder HF, Trede M, et al (eds): *Joint Meeting, Munich, 1968,* Berlin, Springer-Verlag, 1969, pp 42–49
11. Hutchinson EC, Acheson J: *Strokes, Natural History, Pathology, and Surgical Treatment.* London, W.B. Saunders, 1975
12. Marshall J: *The Management of Cerebrovascular Disease.* (3rd ed) Oxford, Blackwell, 1976
13. Editorial: A new vascular syndrome—"The Subclavian Steal." *N Engl J Med 265*:912, 1961
14. North RR, Fields WS, DeBakey ME, et al: Brachial-basilar insufficiency syndrome. *Neurology 12*:810, 1962
15. Fein JM: Vertebral artery transposition for vertebrobasilar insufficiency. Presented at the 50th Meeting of the American Association of Neurological Surgeons, Boston, April, 1981

CHAPTER 47
Direct Brain Revascularization

Robert M. Crowell

ISCHEMIC CEREBRAL INFARCTION is the result of decreased cerebral blood flow caused by arterial occlusion. Surgical revascularization of the brain therefore is a logical approach to the prevention of ischemic stroke.

Indirect revascularization of the brain by carotid endarterectomy can often benefit patients with extracranial occlusive disease.[1] Atherosclerotic occlusive disease, however, frequently affects intracranial arteries, which are inaccessible to carotid endarterectomy.[2] Rational surgery for such cases is direct cerebral revascularization, including cerebral embolectomy and various bypass procedures. These delicate and refined operations have become feasible since the development of microneurosurgery.[3-5] Although the indications for such procedures have not yet been firmly established, the early results are encouraging, especially for superficial temporal artery–middle cerebral artery (STA–MCA) bypass. This chapter reviews the procedures for direct cerebral revascularization; STA–MCA bypass is described in some detail.

Procedures

Middle Cerebral Artery Embolectomy

Embolectomy represents the most direct surgical treatment for embolic occlusion of the middle cerebral artery (MCA) (Fig. 47-1).[6-8] The surgeon may remove the embolus and restore patency of the MCA using microsurgical techniques. Reversible cerebral ischemia, however, often ripens to irreversible infarction faster than the surgeon can open the occlusion, and thus medical measures are needed to extend the period of reversibility. MCA embolectomy, at present, cannot be recommended as standard therapy.

Long Grafts

Bypass grafting is a reasonable surgical approach for occlusive disease of the internal carotid artery (ICA) that is inaccessible (Fig. 47-2). A number of authors have recommended interposition of free grafts between large arteries in the neck and the intracranial arteries (ICA or MCA) to provide immediate high-flow revascularization. The initial results with saphenous vein grafts between the common carotid artery and the intracranial internal carotid artery were disappointing, with high morbidity and low patency.[9-10] More recent experience with the interposi-

Department of Neurological Surgery, University of Illinois College of Medicine, Chicago, Illinois. The author wishes to acknowledge the help of Mrs. Edith Tagrin, who did the line drawings, Georgia Frederic, who helped prepare the manuscript, and Dr. R. G. Ojemann, who provided constructive criticism.

This work was supported in part by Teacher-Investigator Award NS11001, and Grants NS10828 and NS13165 from the National Institute for Neurological and Communicative Disorders and Stroke.

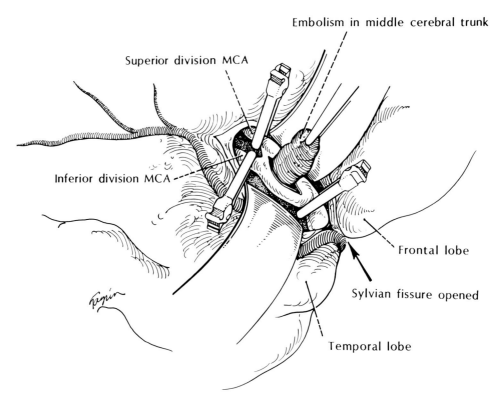

Fig. 47-1. Middle cerebral embolectomy. The right sylvian fissure has been split to expose the MCA. The embolus is removed through a microsurgical arteriotomy, which then is closed with a microsuture technique.

tion of grafts between the common carotid artery or the subclavian artery and a cortical branch of the MCA have been more promising.[11] Use of the cortical branch of the MCA will likely diminish complications of long grafting. Further experience will be required before this technique is established.

Occipital Artery–Posterior Inferior Cerebellar Artery (Occipital–PICA) Bypass

Recently occipital–PICA bypass (Fig. 47-3) has been developed for revascularization of the posterior circulation.[12-14] The technical feasibility and relative safety of occipital–PICA bypass have been established, but its clinical indications are as yet unknown.

Other Techniques

Several alternative conduits have been suggested for direct revascularization of the MCA. These include the middle meningeal artery[15] and the occipital artery.[16]

Indirect revascularization may be achieved by the application of vascularized omentum to the brain[17-18] or the insertion of the ligated superficial temporal artery into the subarachnoid space. Late angiograms have shown fine collateral channels emanating from neck grafts, but the functional significance and impact on subsequent stroke are unknown.

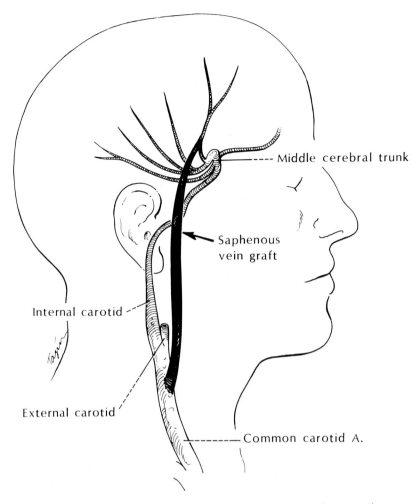

Fig. 47-2. Long graft. A free graft of saphenous vein is interposed between the common carotid artery and a branch of the MCA. Long grafts give high-flow revascularization of the anterior circulation, but indications remain uncertain.

Superficial Temporal Artery–Middle Cerebral Artery (STA–MCA) Bypass

STA–MCA bypass is the most promising and widely used form of cerebral revascularization. By applying microsurgical techniques, Donaghy and Yasargil first performed STA–MCA bypass on humans in 1967.[3-5] Refinements in the technique have included the use of interrupted sutures for greater precision,[19] use of the angular branch of the MCA for maximal flow,[2,16] and a linear incision over the STA to avoid necrosis of the flap edge.[20]

The therapeutic role of STA–MCA bypass has not been fully defined. The procedure carries a low risk in selected cases, and appears to diminish the incidence of transient ischemic attacks (TIAs) and infarction.[2-5,16,19-21] Studies of regional cerebral blood flow (rCBF) and metabolism have been reported to assist in defining the indications for the operation.[22-23] A cooperative randomized controlled study, the Extracranial–Intracranial (EC–IC) Bypass Study, is under way to clarify indications for STA–MCA bypass.[24-25] The tentative indications are listed in Table 47-1 in descending order of establishment.

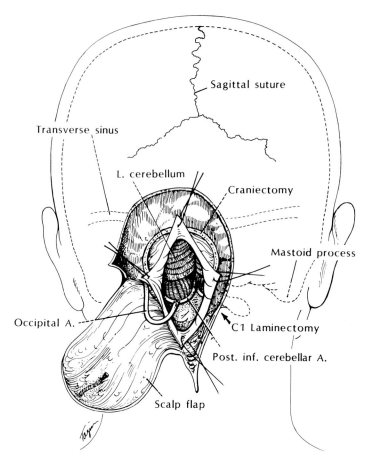

Fig. 47-3. Occipital–PICA graft. A suboccipital craniectomy and a C1 laminectomy provide exposure of the caudal loop of the PICA. Anastomosis of the occipital artery to the PICA provides new
collateral to the posterior circulation.

Preoperative Evaluation

Patient history is often crucial in establishing the need for a bypass. Transient ischemic attacks (TIAs) may signal insufficiency of the MCA, particularly in the setting of demonstrated occlusion of the internal carotid artery antedating the attacks. Attacks of amaurosis fugax have
been taken as an indiciation for bypass. Low flow in the border zone of the MCA is suggested by
TIAs that come on as the patient stands up or that include shaking of the limbs, especially the
lower limbs. Particularly ominous as harbingers of stroke are spells present on arising and those
lasting longer than 1 hour.

Physical examination should include careful quantitative neurologic examination, as documented in the EC–IC bypass study, to permit an estimate of the surgical impact to be made
through follow-up examinations. The vascular examination should include careful palpation of
the branches of the STA; if no pulse can be felt, the vessel is probably not suitable for anastomosis. Dynamic palpation of the facial pulses may give an indication of virtual or complete occlusion of the ICA or the ophthalmic artery.

Preoperative studies include EKG, serum cholesterol, and serum triglycerides. We routinely
obtain medical consultation regarding management of cardiac status, blood pressure, and risk
factors for atherosclerosis. Computed tomographic (CT) scanning identifies cerebral infarctions
and unanticipated pathology, i.e., hemorrhage or tumor which may preclude bypass surgery.
Studies of rCBF and metabolism may help to establish the indications for revascularization.[22-23]

Table 47-1. Tentative Indications for Direct Brain Revascularization in Descending Order of Establishment

Presentation	Angiography	Comment
(1) TIAs	ICA occlusion	Esp. promising if TIAs continue after angiogram.*
	Siphon stenosis	Natural history unknown.*
	Stenosis of the MCA	Medical treatment may be better.*
(2) Giant aneurysm	(Planned) occlusion of the ICA	Certainly helpful in some cases, but some may not require bypass. CBF studies may guide selection.
(3) Dementia, generalized hypoperfusion	Multiple occlusions, poor collateral supply	Anecdotal data. Some patients may improve.
(4) Moyamoya disease	Multiple occlusions, cloudlike collateral supply	Anecdotal data. Future strokes may be diminished in some patients.
(5) "Slow stroke"	Occlusion of the ICA	Only anecdotal data; some patients may improve with bypass.
(6) Amaurosis fugax	Stenosis or occlusion of the ICA	Conflicting reports regarding future strokes. Medical treatment may be better.
(7) Fixed stroke	Occlusion of the ICA	Anecdotal data suggests some patients may improve.
(8) Acute stroke	Occlusion of the ICA (or MCA)	Anecdotal data. No striking improvement.

*The EC-IC study should help to clarify these.

The keystone of evaluation is three-vessel angiography, which is used to delineate cerebrovascular occlusions, collateral circulation, and potential bypass vessels. In some cases, delayed films may show reconstitution of the carotid siphon with reflux to the upper cervical ICA, a sign that suggests the carotid occlusion may be opened surgically.[1] Multiple filling defects in branches of the MCA suggest embolic occlusions that probably cannot be helped by STA–MCA anastomosis. Poor collateral circulation to a symptomatic hemisphere suggests a hemodynamic mechanism. Failure of the MCA branches to opacify via collateral routes need not imply the lack of a suitable recipient branch at surgery. Careful study of the angiogram usually permits identification of the best vessels for anastomosis. The larger branch of the STA—usually the frontal—is selected, and when this is less than 1 mm in diameter, the occipital artery may be chosen instead. In the setting of a tiny STA and a proximally branching occipital artery, a short vein graft may be interposed between the STA (or the occipital artery) and the recipient branch of the MCA.[21]

Operative Technique

Anesthesia

Anticoagulant drugs are omitted preoperatively. Heparin is discontinued 12 hours before surgery, and aspirin or dypyridamole are discontinued, preferably 1 week before surgery. Some surgeons prefer to maintain antiplatelet therapy through the perioperative period, but we have experienced marked intraoperative oozing with this practice that required platelet transfusion (10 units) in order to achieve hemostasis. Using modern anesthetic technique, antihypertensive medication, including propranolol or reserpine, may be maintained throughout the operation. Diphenylhydantoin is begun the day before surgery (300 mg daily) to ensure prophylactic blood levels of anticonvulsant in the immediate postoperative period.

Atropine and droperidol are given as premedication, and the patient's legs are wrapped with Ace bandages before induction. General endotracheal anesthesia is used, usually halothane or a balanced technique (nitrous oxide, Innovar, and muscle relaxant). Controlled ventilation is preferable for maintenance of arterial P_{CO_2} in the range of 35–40 torr. Precordial electrodes provide continuous EKG monitoring. Arterial blood pressure is monitored continuously, with a radial arterial catheter on a Tektronix portable oscilloscope. Infusions of colloid, phenylephrine, or nitroprusside are used to maintain blood pressure in the normal range for the individual patient during induction and surgery. Arterial blood gases are sampled, and P_{O_2} is maintained over 80 torr by adjustment of the concentration of inspired O_2. A Foley catheter is used only in particularly lengthy procedures, i.e., a double anastomosis or exploration of the occluded cervical ICA before STA–MCA bypass. Oxacillin is administered just before incision and for 24 hours postoperatively in divided doses of 2 gm intravenously every 6 hours.

Positioning

The operative side of the head is shaved before the induction of anesthesia, and the course of the STA is marked with a marking pen, since the pulse may be harder to delineate after induction. The patient is positioned supine with the head turned away from the operative side. The table is flexed slightly to bring the head above the level of the heart. A small roll serves to elevate the shoulder on the operative side. The head of the anesthetized patient is fixed in a 3-point (Mayfield) headrest. Frequently the operating table may need to be tilted with the "side" adjustment to bring the temporal squama parallel to the floor.

Instruments

Several microsurgical instruments are essential in addition to the usual craniotomy kit. The Zeiss operating microscope (OPMI-1) is preferred, with a 250-mm objective, 160-mm angled binocular tubes, and 12.5-X high-eyepoint eyepieces. The stereoscopic binocular observer tube is attached to the scope via the small beam splitter. The assistant is positioned on the left (for a right-handed surgeon), to allow the surgeon's hand free access to the scrub nurse. A No. 5 Dumont jeweler's forceps, adapted for bipolar coagulation, is needed for precise hemostasis near the bypass vessels. A No. 5 Dumont jeweler's forceps and a 5-inch iris scissors serve well to prepare the small arteries for anastomosis. Kleinert-Kees miniature clips are ideal for temporarily occluding the cortical arteries with minimal trauma. A 10-mm straight Heifetz clip is satisfactory for temporary occlusion of the origin of the STA. Miniature Gelpi retractors are helpful in maintaining satisfactory exposure. A curved, sharp Rhoton microscissors is used to fashion the cortical arteriotomy. Fine Silastic tubing (0.025-inch O.D.) serves as a stent for the MCA during surgery. The anastomosis is performed with a curved 8-inch Rhoton needle holder and 10-0 monofilament nylon suture on a BV-6 needle (Ethicon).

Incision

Before shaving and preparing the scalp, the course of the STA is scratched into the skin over the previous pen marking. The position of the recipient branch of the MCA likewise is marked. In general we prefer linear incisions to a scalp flap. Linear incisions permit rapid preparation of the STA and avoid the possibility of scalp necrosis, which may occur with a flap. One or two linear incisions may be needed, depending upon the branch of the STA that is selected

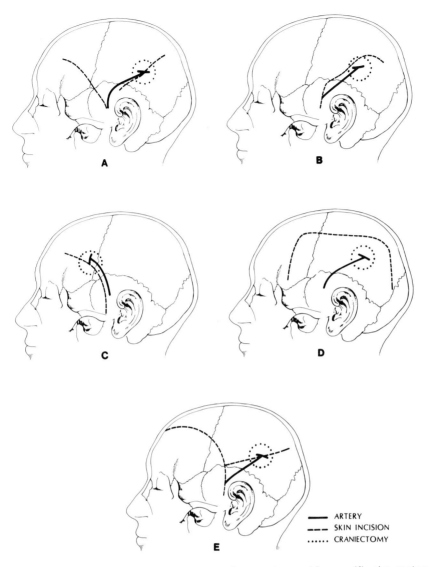

Fig. 47-4. STA–MCA bypass. A variety of approaches may be used for specific circumstances. **A.** Most commonly, two linear incisions permit anastomosis of the largest branches, namely the frontal branch of the STA and the angular branch of the MCA. **B.** Sometimes a parietal branch of the STA is larger and is therefore used. **C.** Occasionally the frontal STA is joined to a frontal branch of the MCA. **D.** A scalp flap gives the widest perusal and selection of the STA branches; also, a double bypass can be performed with this exposure. **E.** When a craniotomy for an aneurysm is to be used, a T-incision may be used for the bypass.

and occasionally on the branch of the MCA that is chosen (Fig. 47-4). Most frequently the frontal branch of the STA and the angular branch of the MCA are the largest and thus the best arteries available for anastomosis (Fig. 47-4A). The angular branch may be used with safety even on the dominant hemisphere. Occasionally, the posterior branch of the STA (Fig. 47-4B) or a frontal branch of the MCA will be selected for bypass (Fig. 47-4C). When a pterional (or other) approach to an intracranial aneurysm is needed, a modified flap, as shown in Figure 47-4E, may provide an exposure for all of the contemplated surgical maneuvers. Although one might anticipate ischemia at the tips of scalp flaps, as shown in Figure 47-4E, we have not experienced this problem.

The initial incision is made over the STA with the magnification microscope set at 10x.

Portable Mayo stands support the surgeon's arms on either side, and the seated surgeon and assistant link arms to provide comfortable access to the operative site for all four hands. A subcutaneous injection of local anesthetic is omitted. The initial incision with a No. 15 blade is made over the distal STA down to the subcutaneous fat to avoid injury to the trunk of the STA. Then the surgeon and assistant elevate the scalp tissue with Adson forceps, and the plane just superficial to the STA is developed with Metzenbaum scissors. When the proper plane is chosen, the STA is readily exposed over a length of 8–10 cm.

STA Preparation

Small scalp flaps, about 1 cm wide, are elevated on each side of the STA (Fig. 47-5). The adventitia is incised with a No. 15 blade about 2 mm to each side of the STA and down to the temporalis fascia. Small bleeders are electrocoagulated away from the STA with bipolar cautery. Branches larger than 0.5 mm are divided between 6-0 silk ligatures. To facilitate these maneuvers, the surgeon uses a knife and forceps, and the assistant uses a sucker and bipolar cautery. A few spreading movements with the Metzenbaum scissors develop the plane between the STA and the temporalis fascia, thus completing isolation of the vessel. After isolation of the recipient branch of the MCA (described below), the tip of the STA is prepared. Satisfactory graft length of the STA is confirmed; this is usually at least 8 cm and includes an extra amount to facilitate suturing of the back wall. Heifetz clips are applied at both ends, the distal end is crosscut, and heparinized saline is flushed into the STA via a No. 20 Medicut catheter. This irrigation flushes out blood and helps to identify bleeders for coagulation. When a large proximal side branch is available, the irrigation catheter may be tied into the branch to permit intermittent irrigation of the STA during anastomosis and to permit bypass pressure measurements to be made after completion of the graft. The tip of the STA then is freed of adventitia for a length of 1 cm. The tip is beveled with two straight snips in a fish-mouth fashion that is designed to maximize the anastomotic ostium. If atheromatous intima should separate from the muscularis, a second effort at beveling often permits the two layers of the artery to remain adhered. After the tip of the STA is prepared, flow is measured into a beaker and the artery again is flushed with heparinized saline.

When a flap technique is used (Fig. 47-4D or E), the STA is isolated from the adventitia by sharp dissection down to the fat and the hair follicles, where a plane is established superficial to the vessel. In some cases, the STA segment must be led from one incision to another. A tunnel is prepared by blunt dissection between the galea and the temporalis fascia. The tip of the STA is pulled through the tunnel with a terminal silk tie. Twists and kinks in the STA segment are carefully avoided.

MCA Preparation

Generally the angular branch of the MCA is used, which lies about 6 cm rostral to the external auditory canal. When the frontal branch of the STA is used, however, the angular branch is exposed through a separate incision (Fig. 47-4A). Temporalis muscle is opened with cutting cautery, which also can be used to elevate the periosteum. When a frontal branch of the MCA is to be used, an incision and exposure in this area are employed, as shown in Figure 47-4C. When an aneurysm approach via a bone flap is anticipated, as in Figure 47-4E, the scalp flaps are raised as shown, but the incision through the temporalis muscle is best made from the proximal STA to the assumed location of the angular artery in order to facilitate routing of the graft before closure.

A small craniotomy flap, about 7 cm in diameter, is fashioned over the recipient artery with a power drill and a craniotome. We have found this method faster and safer than either craniectomy or trephine. The bone edges are waxed, and the dura is opened in a cruciate fashion. Additional bone may be rongeured away if no suitable recipient branch is identified. When a suitable vessel is exposed, three drill holes are made in the bone edge for eventual bone flap replacement, and dural-to-pericranial sutures are placed.

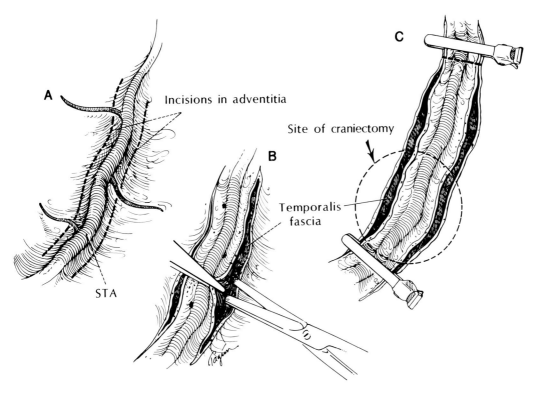

Fig. 47-5. STA–MCA bypass technique: Preparation of the STA. **A.** Exposure. **B.** Undermining. **C.** Mobilization.

The arachnoid next to the MCA is cut with microscissors under 16-x magnification (Fig. 6A). With the bipolar cautery set low (0–15), up to three tiny side branches may be coagulated and cut as needed to prepare a 1-cm length of artery. Generally, one or two larger side branches can be preserved by using temporary clips. A strip of rubber dam is placed under the MCA to protect the cortex.

Final preparation of the MCA is achieved at 25-x magnification, with the prepared tip of the STA in full view. Kleinert-Kees clips are placed on the branch of the MCA at least 8 mm apart (Fig. 47-6B). A slender oval arteriotomy is made in the MCA, with a single snip of the microscissors, the length corresponding to the width of the end of the STA (Fig. 47-7A). The vessel is irrigated with heparinized saline. A stent of fine Silastic tubing is inserted into the vessel.

Anastomosis

The end of the STA is positioned against the opening in the MCA with the end aiming back toward the origin of the MCA to promote flow throughout the territory of the MCA. The Rhoton needle holder and jeweler's forceps are used to place interrupted 10-0 nylon sutures in each corner (Fig. 47-7B). Forceps are used primarily as a counter pressor during suturing, and the vessel wall is handled as little and as gently as possible. Squeezing the intima is particularly avoided. An additional 6 to 8 interrupted sutures are placed in the front wall (Fig. 47-8A), and these are tied down after all have been placed to give maximum accuracy. The bites are a bit larger on the STA side to promote slight eversion and intima-to-intima apposition. Sutures must accurately include the intima of the STA, which may be thickened and separated from the muscularis. Inside-to-outside passage of the needle through the STA is recommended when an intimal flap threatens. Sutures are placed slightly closer together near the corners where leaks are more common. Keeping the area dry facilitates handling the sutures, and keeping the needle in view on the rubber dam minimizes time lost in searching for it.

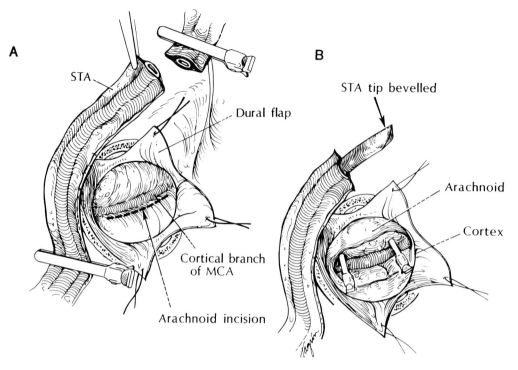

Fig. 47-6. STA–MCA bypass technique: Preparation of vessels. **A.** A craniotomy and opening of the dura expose the cortical branch of the MCA. The STA is cut to the proper length. **B.** The arachnoid is opened and clips are applied. The tip of the STA is freed of adventitia and tailored.

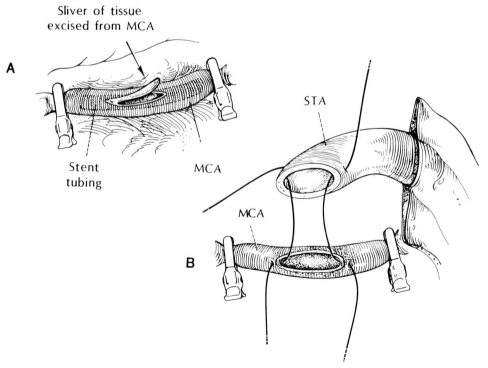

Fig. 47-7. STA–MCA bypass technique: arteriotomy. **A.** A sliver of the MCA is excised with scissors and a stent is inserted. **B.** Interrupted corner sutures appose the STA to the MCA.

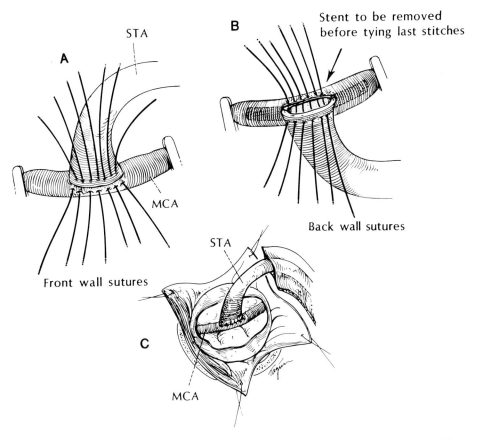

Fig. 47-8. STA–MCA bypass technique: Anastomosis. **A.** Interrupted sutures are placed in the front wall; the sutures are tied after all have been placed. **B.** The back wall sutures are placed. The front wall suture line is inspected and the stent is removed before the last sutures are tied. **C.** The completed anastomosis.

The STA is reflected aside to reveal the back wall of the anastomosis. The front-wall suture line is inspected from inside to confirm accurate suture placement. Then 6 to 8 interrupted sutures are used to complete the back wall (Fig. 47-8B). Before the last two sutures are tied, the tube stent is gently removed, and the three vascular limbs are opened briefly to check flow and expel air. The final sutures then are tied down.

The distal clip on the MCA is removed first, then the proximal. Under 25-x magnification, the suture line is inspected for leaks. A major leak requires a stitch; suture line ooze will stop without additional stitches. The rubber dam is folded over the suture line, and a cottonoid is used to provide pressure for 1 to 2 minutes. In some cases a collar of Gelfoam may secure hemostasis of the suture line. Finally, the clip on the STA is removed to begin augmented cerebral flow. Graft pressures may be measured where a suitable side branch of the STA has been cannulated: with a clip distal to the cannulated branch, pressure in the STA is determined; with a clip proximal to the branch, pressure in the MCA is measured. Graft flow may be estimated with an electromagnetic flow probe and meter, but great care must be exercised to avoid injuring the STA with the flow probe.

Closure

The dura is loosely approximated with 4-0 silk sutures. A Gelfoam pledget is used to cover the exposed dura and surround the distal STA segment. After the graft is routed smoothly and without kinking, the bone flap is trimmed with rongeurs (sometimes extensively) to avoid contact with the STA, and then is wired in place. The temporalis muscle and fascia are approximated as separate layers with interrupted 3-0 coated Vicryl; great care must be taken to avoid compression of the graft. The wound is irrigated with Bacitracin solution and closed with interrupted sutures of 3-0 coated Vicryl in the galea and continuous 5-0 nylon sutures in the skin. When the viability of the scalp edge is in question, closure using interrupted 5-0 nylon without tension offers the best chance for avoiding necrosis. A small dressing is applied together with a sign warning against pressure and a mark to indicate a palpable pulse.

Postoperative Management

Postoperatively (24–48 hours), blood pressure is carefully maintained in the normal range for the individual patient with the aid of a radial arterial cannula and infusions of colloid, pressors, or nitroprusside. In the event of deterioration, which is rare in these patients, CT scanning can be used to identify hemorrhage or infarction, and angiography can be used to assess patency of the graft and the collateral circulation. A postoperative EKG is obtained to check for myocardial ischemia. Patients are gradually mobilized after 48 hours, and blood pressure is controlled with oral agents as needed. Diphenylhydantoin (300 mg/day) is given as an anticonvulsant. Aspirin (300 mg) and dipyridamole (25 mg) are given twice daily for 6 months to foster graft patency. Angiography is performed at 1 week to assess patency of the anastomosis. Careful management of risk factors continues indefinitely.

Illustrative Cases

Case 1.   MCA stenosis; STA–MCA bypass to eliminate TIA. This 58-year-old right-handed executive experienced 3 episodes of marked dysphasia lasting up to 30 minutes. There were no other neurologic symptoms. On admission his blood pressure was 130/80 and the neurologic examination was entirely normal. Complete cerebral angiography disclosed a stenosis of the left middle cerebral artery with a residual lumen of about 1 mm.

As part of the EC/IC Bypass Study, the patient was randomized to surgery. A left STA–MCA bypass was performed. Two linear incisions were used, one over the frontal branch of the superficial temporal artery, the other over the angular gyrus area. Intraangular arterial pressure was found to be 90/40 torr at a time when the STA pressure was 150/70 torr. An electromagnetic flow meter confirmed flow of about 35 cc/min through the graft. A postoperative angiogram disclosed filling of four middle cerebral branches via the graft (Fig. 47-9). The patient was discharged on aspirin (300 mg) and Persantine (25 mg) b.i.d. There were no further spells of cerebral dysfunction over a 12-month follow-up period.

Comment: The alarming TIAs referable to stenosis of the MCA in this patient ceased after STA–MCA bypass. The smooth postoperative course is typical for patients with this lesion. A similar course could result with medical therapy, however. The EC–IC Bypass Study should help clarify the role of bypass surgery for symptomatic stenosis of the MCA.

Intraoperative cortical artery pressure was moderately decreased (90/40 torr) compared with STA pressure (150/70 torr). This significant gradient may be correlated with excellent postoperative filling of the MCA via the graft. Such correlation often has been noted, but in some cases metabolic parameters, rather than hemodynamics, have correlated with postoperative angiographic filling via the graft.[23]

Case 2.   Multiple occlusions and right frontal infarct; cessation of TIAs and mental improvement after bypass. This 68-year-old right-handed male junior high school principal became confused and disoriented, but returned to normal within 24 hours. Over the ensuing several days there was intermittent confusion. On one occasion he could not find his way from his bedroom to the bathroom. Later, toilet paper was unwound in the bathroom in a confused fashion. The patient became apathetic and used his left hand little. Neurologic examination in a local hospital showed a mild hemiparesis on the left with mild confusion and disorientation. An isotope brain scan showed right frontal uptake. A CT scan showed a right frontal cerebral infarction in the territory of the middle cerebral artery.

Examination on admission showed a blood pressure of 160/90 torr. The neurologic examination showed marked apathy, lethargy, and disorientation to time, but gait and motor power were normal. He was unable to give answers to simple questions regarding the President of the United States, American history, or his chosen field of endeavor. Cere-

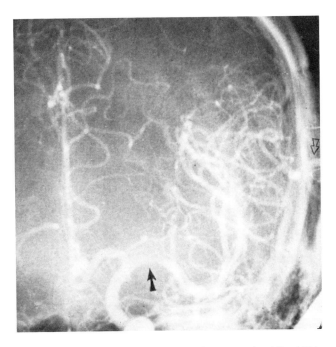

Fig. 47-9. Case 1: STA–MCA bypass for stenosis of the MCA. A postoperative left carotid angiogram shows stenosis (filled arrow) of the left MCA and a patent STA–MCA bypass (open arrow). Severe episodes of dysphasia ceased after surgery (see text).

bral angiography showed an occlusion of the right internal carotid artery. The left internal carotid artery was likewise occluded at its origin. The right vertebral artery was markedly stenotic at its origin, and the left vertebral artery was occluded near its origin with reconstitution via cervical muscular collateral. The middle cerebral arteries and anterior cerebral arteries were both filled in retrograde fashion from the posterior cerebral arteries bilaterally. A Xenon blood flow study and positron emission tomography showed generally decreased blood flow, particularly in the right cerebral hemisphere. Cortical function examination showed a decline from a previously superior intellectual capacity with some preservation of crystallized learning; this was best in verbal reasoning. An EEG showed delta slowing in the right hemisphere.

A right superficial-temporal to angular-bypass graft was performed. Pressure in the angular artery was 50/20 torr, and pressure in the superficial temporal artery was 140/80 torr. Flow through the graft was at least 90 cc/min. The postoperative course was smooth. Postoperative angiography (Fig. 47-10) showed filling of at least six branches of the right middle cerebral artery and of the right anterior cerebral artery, with flash filling into the left middle cerebral territory. The patient was discharged on aspirin (300 mg) and Persantine (25 mg) b.i.d. Six months after surgery, at follow-up examination, the patient was bright and alert without neurologic deficit. Both he and his wife insisted that his mental capacity was much improved since surgery and he considered returning to work as a junior high school principal. Repeat cortical function examination showed modest improvement vis-à-vis preoperative testing.

Comment: The TIAs ceased and mentation improved in this patient after STA–MCA bypass. Revascularization for symptomatic generalized hypoperfusion has been reported, but the role of surgery in such cases is not yet clear. In this case, the existence of TIAs helped us decide for surgery. Neuropsychologic testing in bypass cases may be helpful in refining indications for surgery. A marked pressure gradient across the anastomosis correlated with excellent angiographic filling postoperatively.

Case 3. Stenosis of the ICA progressing to occlusion after bypass. This 57-year-old right-handed male barber experienced 6 attacks, lasting up to 10 minutes, of numbness of the left corner of the mouth and drooping of the left corner of the mouth with weakness in the left hand. The neurologic examination was normal. Cerebral angiography showed a tight stenosis of the internal carotid artery at the level of C2; the residual lumen was judged to be about 1.5 mm. The patient was placed on sulfinpyrazone (200 mg t.i.d.), but the attacks persisted, occurring approximately every other day. Neurologic examination remained normal. A right STA–MCA anastomosis was performed. Cerebral angiography

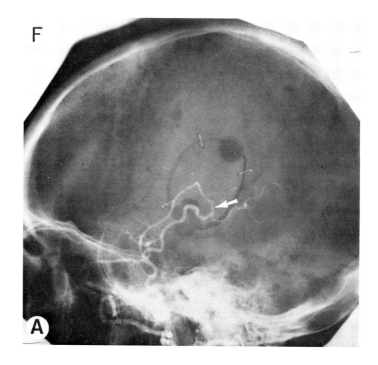

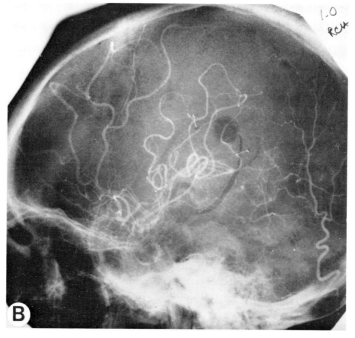

Fig. 47-10.   Case 2: Bypass for multiple occlusions and dementia. A postoperative left carotid angiogram shows **A** a patent bypass (arrow), **B** widespread filling of branches of the left MCA, and **C**
some contralateral filling of the ACA and MCA (arrow) from the
graft. This patient's spells ceased after surgery, and mentation
improved (see text).

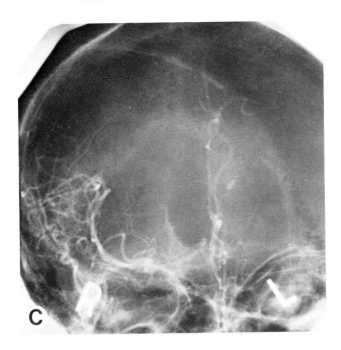

showed filling of two branches of the MCA via the graft. The patient was discharged on aspirin (300 mg) and Persantine (25 mg) 4 times per day.

Over the ensuing 6 months, the patient experienced 5 attacks of numbness at the left corner of the mouth, lasting up to 5 minutes. Six months after surgery the patient suddenly developed weakness in the left arm, face, and leg. Examination showed a moderate left hemiparesis with the left arm 7/10, the face 5/10, and the leg 9/10. Cortical sensory discrimination was intact. Angiography showed complete occlusion of the internal carotid artery and excellent filling from the bypass graft into seven branches of the MCA. Injection of the left internal carotid artery gave only flash filling of the right middle cerebral artery. A CT scan showed low density in the right parietal area. Over the course of several days the patient improved steadily. Six months after discharge, he had minimal slowing of finger tapping on the left and otherwise normal neurologic examination. He has returned to work full time as a barber, managing his own shop.

Comment: This patient had persistent TIAs heralding occlusion of the ICA and cerebral infarction. No other patient in this series had persistent TIAs after bypass. When TIAs recur despite patent bypass, Coumadin therapy is probably warranted to ward off infarction.

The relation of the bypass to the stroke is unclear: the bypass may have diminished the pressure gradient across the stenosis of the ICA, provoking subsequent occlusion. On the other hand, the vigorously functioning graft may have protected against a more extensive infarction.

Complications

There have been no operative deaths in this series of cases. Two operative strokes are reported below (see Results). This brings the overall major complication rate of stroke and death to 2 cases in 45, or 4 percent serious morbidity or mortality. Other major reported complications, not encountered in this series, include subdural[26] and intracerebral[27] hemorrhage.

Minor complications occurred in 9 of our cases (20 percent). Wound infection occurred in 1 individual in whom a Teflon plate had been implanted as a cranioplasty. Antibiotics and removal of the Teflon plate allowed the wound to heal nicely; the patient remained intact, and the postoperative angiogram showed patency. We have since omitted the Teflon cranioplasty and instituted perioperative antibiotic coverage, and we have encountered no further infections. Necrosis of the scalp edge occurred in 2 early cases in which excessive tension on the suture line was present. Since that time, we have used only the incisions diagrammed in Figure 47-4, and the wounds have been closed without tension using the plastic suture technique, and there have been no other necroses of scalp edges. Seizures occurred in 2 cases and were readily controlled with anticonvulsant therapy postoperatively. Since that time we have placed all patients on prophylactic anticonvulsants after surgery for a period of 6 months. Transient neurologic worsening has occurred in the early postoperative period in 3 individuals. All 3 were treated with steroid and antiaggregate therapy with resolution of deficits. Myocardial ischemia was demonstrated on a postoperative EKG in 1 patient with known coronary artery disease, although the patient developed no symptoms. Overall, these nine minor complications (20 percent) led to no lasting deficits in any patient.

Results

Patency

Patency in this series was documented angiographically in 45 of 49 grafts studied (92 percent). Technical errors led to thrombosis in 2 cases. In 1 case, the very first in the series, insufficient attention was paid to the routing of the graft through muscle and bone. Compression of the graft by these structures led to asymptomatic thrombosis. In another patient, the STA segment was cut too short, leading to tension on the suture line. Although an initial angiogram showed only minor irregularity at the site of the anastomosis, occlusion occurred 3 months later, with obstruction of the cortical vessel and a mild stroke. Two intraoperative thromboses were noted, both in patients who were found to have marked hypercoagulability (spontaneous aggregation of platelets). Technical errors were not identified in these two instances. Multiple efforts to open these occlusions were unsuccessful, as in thrombosed experimental grafts. Fortunately, no neurologic sequela was noted in either case.

On the basis of these experiences, we believe that avoiding technical errors (particularly graft tension or compression) can avoid occlusions and complications. Additionally, preoperative anticoagulation with antiplatelet agents might avoid thrombosis in hypercoagulable individuals, although intraoperative bleeding in these patients might be a problem.

Late Strokes

Delayed stroke occurred despite a functioning bypass graft in 3 cases (6.7 percent). In 2 of these 3 cases, occlusion of an intracranial internal carotid artery that was previously markedly stenotic had occurred since surgery. Mild strokes resulted in both of these cases, despite improved filling of the MCA via the graft, as compared with immediate postoperative studies. We have observed this type of occlusion once without symptoms. In another case, a mild stroke occurred in the face of a functioning graft and poor cerebral collateral circulation. In these cases, STA–MCA bypass may have promoted occlusion of the ICA, protected against infarction, or both (see Case 3 above).

In 2 cases (4 percent), late strokes seemed unrelated to the bypass surgery. In 1 case, a lacunar infarction, probably in the internal capsule, occurred on the opposite side 2 years after surgery, leading to a mild stroke. In another patient with an occluded bypass, late thrombosis of the ICA led to a severe stroke and death. These cases underline the importance of care for the total patient, which may include antihypertensive medication and normalization of other risk factors.

Functional Outcome

Overall, these patients did well functionally. Twenty-three patients (51 percent) remained normal over the follow-up period. Fourteen cases (31 percent) were judged to have good results, with minimal neurologic deficit and the ability to maintain their preoperative functional level. This gives a combined rate of 82 percent for excellent and good results.

Table 47-2. Complications From STA-MCA Bypass

Complication	No. of Patients
Minor	
Infection	1
Scalp edge necrosis	2
Seizures	2
TIA	3
Myocardial ischemia	1
Total	9 (20%)
Major	
Stroke	2 (4.4%)
Death	0 (0%)
Total	2 (4.4%)

Poor results were recorded in 6 patients (13 percent). Four of these cases were regarded as poor functionally before surgery. A single patient went from good status to poor status in relation to surgery; this individual suffered a mild stroke related to occlusion of the bypass. The other patient who went from good to poor postoperatively did so in relation to contralateral lacunar infarction. This series of 50 bypass grafts included no deaths directly attributable to surgery. Two patients succumbed from unrelated causes late after the bypass operation: one from occlusion of the ICA and cerebral infarction (see above) and the other from pneumonia.

Discussion

Personal experience with 50 grafts in 45 patients has been encouraging and parallels the results of others[3-5,16,19,21,28-29] (Tables 47-1, 47-2, and 47-3). Patency has been high (92 percent), and serious complications infrequent (4 percent). Technical improvements should increase patency and decrease complications (see above). Overall, the risk of STA–MCA bypass surgery appears to be small and the patency rates excellent.

The impact of bypass surgery on subsequent cerebral ischemia and infarction is more difficult to determine. Our own experience shows that delayed stroke occurred in 3 cases (6.7 percent) despite a satisfactorily functioning bypass graft. In an additional 2 cases (4 percent), late strokes occurred that seemed unrelated to bypass surgery. The overall rate of late strokes was

Table 47-3. Results of STA-MCA Bypass in 49 Patients

Result	No. of Patients
Patency	45 (91.8%)
Late strokes	
Despite bypass	3 (6.7%)
Unrelated to bypass	2 (4.0%)
Total	5 (10.7%)
Functional outcome	
Excellent	23 (51.0%)
Good	14 (31.0%)
Poor	6 (31.0%)*
Died	2 (4.0%)**

* 4 were poor preoperatively
** Both unrelated to bypass

10.7 percent over an average follow-up of 4 years, or about 2.7 percent per year. According to Whisnant, the rate of stroke in patients with TIAs is about 5 percent per year. There is thus a suggestion that bypass surgery may diminish the frequency of strokes in patients with TIAs. From the standpoint of statistical validation, the most satisfactory procedure is a comparison of control and treated patients in a randomized clinical study. Such an endeavor is presently under way in the form of the International Extracranial–Intracranial Bypass Study.[24-25] It is hoped that the results of this study, to be made available in the next several years, will indicate the impact of bypass grafting on cerebral ischemia and infarction. Only this sort of factual information can give us a statistical validation of the indications for STA–MCA bypass surgery.

Bypass seems helpful in preventing ischemia where occlusion of the ICA is carried out in the treatment of giant ICA aneurysms in the presence of poor native collateral supply.[30-31] The precise role of bypass surgery in this setting has not yet been defined. Evidence has been presented suggesting that ischemic damage may occur long after carotid occlusion for aneurysm. Cerebral blood flow determinations may be useful in determining which patients require bypass to supplement native collateral supply.

Regarding emergency STA–MCA bypass grafting, our small experience and reports from the literature indicate mixed results.[32-33] In most reported cases, however, conditions have not been ideal; a long delay between the onset of symptoms and surgery, or the presence of occlusive material in lenticulostriate branches, likely determined a bad result. Emergency direct cerebral revascularization is a rational concept that awaits several technical developments: (1) A rapid test for tissue viability is needed to identify reversible cases; positron tomography scanning may permit such case selection. (2) A method must be found to extend the period of reversibility until blood flow is restored; a number of methods under study hold promise (barbiturates,[34] hypertension, and hemodilution). (3) Techniques for revascularization must be improved by decreasing the time of surgery and increasing the volume of flow; synthetic long grafts and tissue adhesives may someday provide rapid high-flow revascularization.

The role of bypass surgery remains uncertain for several other conditions, including amaurosis fugax with occlusion of the ICA,[35] moyamoya disease,[36-37] chronic (moderate) cerebral infarction,[38-39] and dementia secondary to multiple cerebrovascular occlusions.[40] Further data is needed to clarify these potential indications.

REFERENCES

1. Ojemann RG, Crowell RM, Fisher CM, et al: Surgical treatment of extracranial carotid occlusive disease. *Clin Neurosurg* 22:214–263, 1975
2. Chater N, Mani J, Tonnemacher K: Superficial temporal artery bypass for cerebrovascular occlusive disease. *Cal Med* 119:9–13, 1973
3. Donaghy RMP, Yasargil MG: *Micro-Vascular Surgery.* Stuttgart, Georg Thieme Verlag, 1967
4. Yasargil MG: *Microsurgery Applied to Neurosurgery.* Stuttgart, Georg Thieme Verlag, 1968
5. Yasargil MG, Krayenbuhl HA, Jacobson JH: Microneurosurgical arterial reconstruction. *Surgery* 67:221–233, 1970
6. Welch K: Excision of occlusive lesions of the middle cerebral artery. *J Neurosurg* 13:73–80, 1956
7. Chou SH: Embolectomy of middle cerebral artery. *J Neurosurg* 20:161–163, 1963
8. Garrido E, Stein BM: Middle cerebral artery embolectomy. Case Report. *J Neurosurg* 44:517–521, 1976
9. Woringer E, Kunlin J: Anastomose entre la carotide primitive et la carotide intra-cranienne on la Sylvienne par greffon selon la technique de la suture suspendue. *Neurochirurgie* 9:181–188, 1963
10. Lougheed W, Marshall BM, Hunter M, et al: Common carotid to intracranial internal carotid bypass venous graft. *J Neurosurg* 34:114–118, 1971
11. Story JL, Brown WE Jr, Eidelberg E, et al: Cerebral revascularization: common carotid to distal middle cerebral artery bypass. *Neurosurg* 2:131–135, 1978
12. Khodadad G: Occipital artery-posterior inferior cerebellar artery anastomosis. *Surg Neurol* 5:225–227, 1976
13. Sundt TM Jr: Intracranial bypass grafts for vertebral-basilar ischemia. *Mayo Clin Proc* 53:12–18, 1978
14. Sundt TM Jr, Piepgras DG: Occipital to posterior inferior cerebellar artery bypass surgery. *J Neurosurg* 48:916–928, 1978
15. Miller CF II, Spetzler RF, Kopaniky DJ: Middle meningeal to middle cerebral arterial bypass for cerebral revascularization. Case report. *J Neurosurg* 50:802–804, 1979

16. Chater N, Popp J: Microsurgical vascular bypass for occlusive cerebrovascular disease: review of 100 cases. *Surg Neurol 6*:115–118, 1976

17. Yonekawa Y, Yasargil MG: Brain vascularization by transplanted omentum: a possible treatment for cerebral ischemia. *Neurosurgery 1*:256–259, 1977

18. Goldsmith HS, Duckett S, Chen W-F: Prevention of cerebral infarction in the monkey by omental transposition to the brain. *Stroke 9*:224–229, 1978

19. Reichman OH, Davis DO, Roberts TS, et al: Anastomosis between STA and cortical branch of MCA for the treatment of occlusive cerebrovascular disease, in Marei FT (ed): *Reconstructive Surgery of Brain Arteries*. Budapest, Akademiai Kiado, 1974, pp 201–218

20. Robertson J: Personal communication, 1975

21. Tew JM: Reconstructive intracranial vascular surgery for prevention of stroke. *Clin Neurosurg 22*:264–280, 1974

22. Schmiedek P, Gratzl O, Spetzler R, et al: Selection of patients for extra-intracranial arterial bypass surgery based on rCBF measurements. *J Neurosurg 44*:303–312, 1976

23. Grubb RL, Ratcheson RA, Raichle ME, et al: Regional cerebral blood flow and oxygen utilization in superficial temporal-middle cerebral artery anastomosis patients. *J Neurosurg 50*:733–741, 1979

24. McDowell FH: The Extracranial/Intracranial Bypass Study. *Stroke 8*:545, 1977

25. Barnett HJM, Peerless SJ, McCormick CW: In answer to question: "As compared to what?" A progress report on the EC/IC bypass study. *Stroke 11*:137–140, 1980

26. Reichman OH: Complications of cerebral revascularization. *Clin Neurosurg 23*:318–335, 1976

27. Heros RC, Nelson PB: Intracerebral hemorrhage after microsurgical cerebral revascularization. *Neurosurg 6*:371–375, 1980

28. Sundt TM Jr: Bypass surgery for vascular disease of the carotid system. *Mayo Clin Proc 51*:677–692, 1976

29. Samson DS, Boone S: Extracranial-intracranial (EC-IC) arterial bypass: past performance and current concepts. *Neurosurgery 3*:79–86, 1978

30. Ammerman BJ, Smith DR: Giant fusiform middle cerebral aneurysm: successful treatment utilizing microvascular bypass. *Surg Neurol 7*:255–257, 1977

31. Iwabuchi T, Kudo T, Hatanaka M, et al: Vein graft bypass in treatment of giant aneurysm. *Surg Neurol 12*:463–466, 1979

32. Crowell RM, Olsson Y: Effect of extracranial-intracranial vascular bypass graft on experimental acute stroke in dogs. *J Neurosurg 38*:26–31, 1973

33. Crowell RM: Emergency STA–MCA bypass for acute focal cerebral ischemia, in Schmiedek P et al (eds): *Microneurosurgical Anastomoses for Cerebral Ischemia*. Berlin, Springer-Verlag, 1977

34. Smith AL, Hoff JT, Nielsen SL, et al: Barbiturate protection in acute focal cerebral ischemia. *Stroke 5*:1–7 1974

35. Kearns TP, Siekert RG, Sundt TM Jr: The ocular aspects of bypass surgery of the carotid artery. *Mayo Clin Proc 54*:3–11, 1979

36. Amine ARC, Moody RA, Meeks W: Bilateral temporal-middle cerebral artery anastomosis for moyamoya syndrome. *Surg Neurol 8*:3–6, 1977

37. Karosawa J, Kikuchi H, Furuse S, et al: Treatment of moyamoya disease with STA–MCA anastomosis. *J Neurosurg 49*:679–88, 1978

38. Holbach K-H, Wassmann H, Hoheluchter KL: Reversibility of the chronic post-stroke state. *Stroke 7*:296–300, 1976

39. Holbach K-H, Wassmann H, Hoheluchter KL, et al: Differentation between reversible and irreversible post-stroke changes in brain tissue: Its relevance for cerebrovascular surgery. *Surg Neurol 7*:325–331, 1977

40. Ferguson GG, Peerless SJ: Extracranial-intracranial arterial bypass in the treatment of dementia and multiple extracranial arterial occlusion. Presented at the 26th Annual Meeting of the Congress of Neurological Surgeons, New Orleans, October 28, 1976

CHAPTER 48
Surgical Management of Lesions of the Dural Venous Sinuses

R. M. Peardon Donaghy

TRAUMA OF THE DURAL SINUSES of a severity sufficient to warrant surgical consideration is more common among the military than in civilian life, but the occurrence, nonetheless, is common enough to merit familiarity with the forms of therapy.[1] On occasion, therapy could prove lifesaving.

Although there are five single and six sets of paired venous sinuses within the cranium,[2,3] only one of the former—the superior longitudinal or superior sagittal sinus—and two of the latter—the cavernous and the lateral or transverse sinuses—have a frequency of trauma and a specificity of therapy sufficient to suggest individual consideration.

The aims of surgical interference include:

1. The control of hemorrhage.
2. The elimination of compressive obstruction.
3. The reinstitution of normal blood flow.
4. The elimination of abnormal vascular communications.

In general, a venous channel may be sacrificed during surgery and not repaired or reconstituted if there is adequate venous drainage of the area by an alternate route. Ordinarily the superior longitudinal sinus may be ligated with impunity along the anterior one-third of its course, for example, but ligation in the posterior two-thirds, especially posterior to the rolandic fissure, is likely to lead to increasing intracranial pressure, often with alarming rapidity (Fig. 48-1).[3-5] If the patient's condition permits, presurgical evaluation of venous drainage and its pattern in the area may be accomplished by angiography. If the patient's condition does not permit such presurgical examination, such information may be gained by intraoperative sinography. In performing sinography, care must be taken to confine the contrast medium to the interior of the sinus, since the medium may be an intense irritant to the cerebral cortex.

A corollary to the above general principle is that the loss of a large venous drainage channel that serves an area that does not have other drainage facilities may portend a grave emergency. A lateral or transverse sinus should not be occluded unless there is adequate drainage from the opposite side. Likewise, should a cervical wound cause injury to an internal jugular vein, the vein should not be permanently ligated until patency of the opposite internal jugular vein has been confirmed or provision made for whatever bypass procedure will allow for adequate drainage.[6,7]

Division of Neurosurgery, University of Vermont College of Medicine, Burlington, Vermont

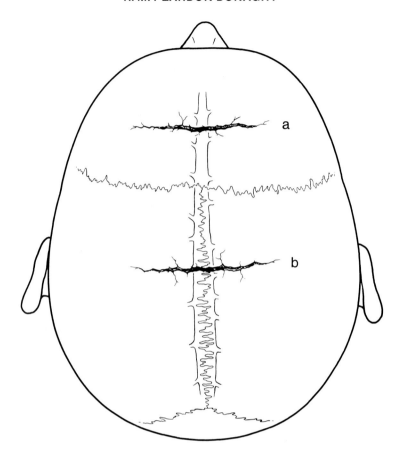

Fig. 48-1. The sinus beneath fracture A probably can be ligated safely if it is damaged beyond easy repair. The sinus beneath fracture B probably cannot be ligated without serious consequence. The surgeon should be prepared to handle a disrupted sinus before embarking upon exploration.

Control of Hemorrhage

Puncture wounds or small openings into a major sinus usually do not pose a severe problem since the wound is small, bleeding is at venous pressure, and, if the bleeding occurs on the external surface of the sinus, it is often tamponaded against the skull. Moreover, since bleeding usually occurs at a fracture line, the site is apparent.

Simple puncture or short linear tears may be sutured directly (Figs. 48-2 and 48-3). Larger or irregular tears may require patching. The adjacent dura is an excellent source of patch material (Figs. 48-4, 48-5, and 48-6).

Elimination of Compressive Obstruction

A rare situation but one of great danger to the patient may occur when a small amount of bleeding occurs between the fracture line and the external surface of the sinus. If the clot exerts enough pressure upon the sinus to obstruct it, and the dura does not strip away from the skull sufficiently to relieve it, intracranial pressure may develop very rapidly if the sinus has no adequate collateral drainage. There may not be enough time for angiography, and the lesion may

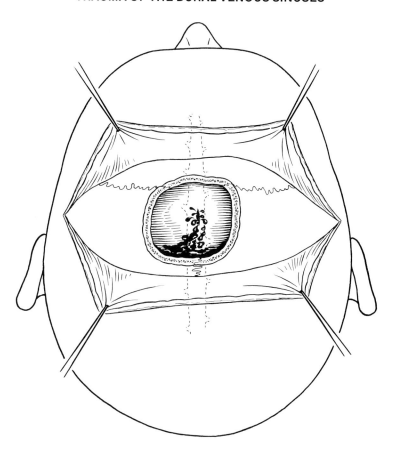

Fig. 48-2.   Bleeding from a small rent in a sinus.

not be demonstrable in other studies. The essential thing is to keep this danger in mind. Immediate decompression at the fracture site may be lifesaving. Once decompressed, flow in the sinus should be confirmed before closing the wound, lest thrombus within the sinus remain unrecognized. Flow in the sinus can be confirmed by aspirating at the site, or by angiography or sinography.

On occasion one may find the sinus totally disrupted or even a portion of the sinus avulsed. A clot may be dislodged in exploring the wound, allowing for brisk hemorrhage from the open sinus ends. A maneuver that has been of great value is to quickly control the hemorrhage by inserting a finger beneath the sinus and exerting pressure outward against the intact skull while an assistant performs the same maneuver at the opposite end of the wound (Figs. 48-7, 48-8, and 48-9). Care should be exercised not to tear bridging veins. The maneuver should not be done blindly except in the most urgent of circumstances. Usually, adequate washing and suction provide adequate visibility.

Once the hemorrhage is controlled, we have found it expedient to introduce a siliconized vascular T-tube, with each end secured in the sinus by a single encircling suture (Figs. 48-10, 48-11).

Flow is now re-established in the sinus. Flow can be monitored in either direction, and the T-tube can be used to introduce heparin or for sinography. Most important, the acuteness of the emergency has been met and one can now plan the reconstruction or replacement if this is necessary.[8,9]

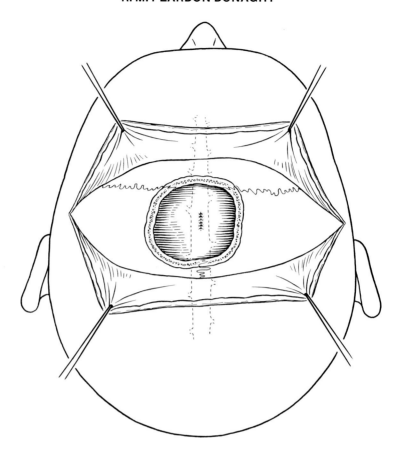

Fig. 48-3.   Repair of a linear rent by direct suture.

Reinstitution of Normal Flow

Several techniques are available for reinstituting normal flow.

Dural Tunnel

If the missing segment is short (1.00–1.25 cm), a dural tunnel can be fashioned to bridge the defect (Fig. 48-12). The advantages of the dural tunnel are (1) the dura is an autogenous tissue, and (2) it is locally available. The disadvantages are (1) the procedure is time-consuming and flow in the sinus is interrrupted during the suturing of the graft; (2) the graft does not have an intimal lining; and (3) dura from some surface must be sacrificed.

Venous Replacement Graft

A graft of the required length may be obtained from a vein of an extremity. The advantages of this graft are (1) long defects may be bridged; (2) the tissues are autogenous; and (3) it is a vascular structure and has an intimal lining. The disadvantages are (1) it is time-consuming and flow is interrupted while the graft is being placed; (2) it is not locally available and an additional and separate incision must be made in the arm or leg; (3) the vein contains valves that must be removed, or at least the segment must be oriented so that it allows flow in the proper direction; and (4) the vein does not have stiff walls as the sinus does, and hence may collapse if negative pres-

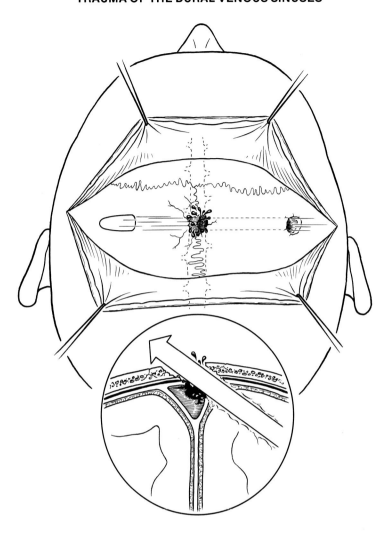

Fig. 48-4.   Loss of a portion of a sinus wall from a gunshot wound.

sure develops within the sinus.[10] The adventitia, however, may be sutured to surrounding dura or periosteum to lessen the likelihood of this problem (Fig. 48-13).

Replacement by an Intimal-Lined Stent

A section of siliconized vascular T-tube is cut of sufficient diameter to just fit inside the orifice of the open sinus and that is slightly longer than the defect.[9] Holes are cut at intervals through the walls of the stent. A piece of vein from an extremity, slightly longer than the stent, is passed through the stent and the ends are folded back over the end of the stent and held by a ligature at each end.

The disadvantages of the method are (1) the stent wall itself is a foreign body and one is reluctant to introduce a foreign body into a wound. The foreign material is not in contact with the bloodstream, however. (2) The valves must be removed from the vein segment that lines the stent, or at least the stent must be so oriented to allow flow in the proper direction past the valves. The advantages of the method are (1) the lining of the stent is vascular and autogenous; (2) placing the stent into the sinus to replace the T-tube already in place can be done in a very few minutes and hence, flow is interrupted for a very short time; and (3) the segment will not collapse

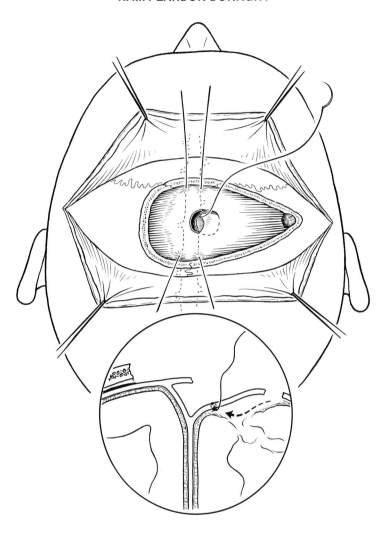

Fig. 48-5. Patch of a sinus wall, using adjacent dura.

since the lining of the vein is held by traction sutures over the wall of the stent and through the holes in the stent wall to the adventitia of the graft segment (Figs. 48-14, 48-15, and 48-16).

Based upon observations of Sawyer and Pate,[11-13] Mullan,[14] and Schwartz,* a technique was developed to help prevent thrombosis in the relatively slow-flowing sagittal sinus after grafting or the introduction of a prosthesis.

After completion of the graft or positioning of the prosthesis, three platinum wires (.003 inch) are sutured into the sinus at either end of the graft or prosthesis so that a portion of the wire is in contact with the bloodstream within the sinus. The ends of the wire are left long. A third wire is similarly placed in the center of the graft or prosthesis. Fine polyethylene tubing is placed over the wire to provide insulation from the tissue, and the three wires are twisted together at their free ends and attached to the negative pole of a 9-V battery.

A similarly insulated wire is attached to the positive pole of the battery and soldered at its other end to a chest electrode (a U.S. 25-cent piece) that is attached to the chest wall by adhesives with an EKG conducting gel between the 25-cent piece and the skin. The position of the chest electrode is changed daily to prevent skin irritation beneath it.

Personal communication.

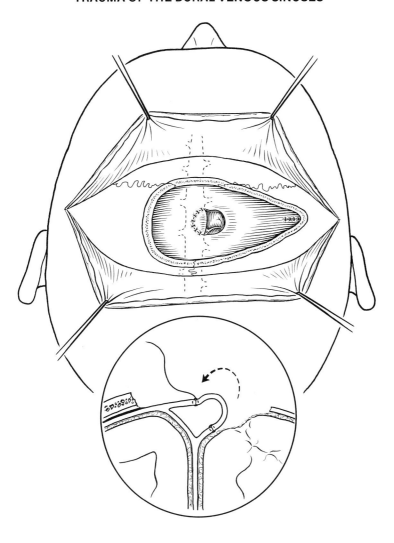

Fig. 48-6. Completed patch of the sinus in Figure 48-5.

By this means a negative current is provided at the intima of the sinus for 5 to 7 days. After that time the wires are removed from the sinus under direct vision by reopening the skin incision.

Elimination of Abnormal Vascular Communications

The most common example of an abnormal vascular communication is the artery–vein communication seen in trauma to the wall of the internal carotid artery during its course through the cavernous sinus. This is not an infrequent complication of injuries to the frontal area. This complication may not occur at the time of the initial trauma but becomes apparent when a pulsating exophthalmos develops on the injured site, resulting in audible bruit over the area and swelling and chemosis of the conjunctiva. The mechanism is simply that the carotid artery has begun to leak but, since it is encased at its point of rupture within the various venous channels of the cavernous sinus, it bleeds within the dural confines of the sinus. Hence, patients do not bleed to death since they are bleeding into their own bloodstream, albeit from an arterial to a venous structure. The fact that the venous structure of the sinus now contains blood at close to arterial

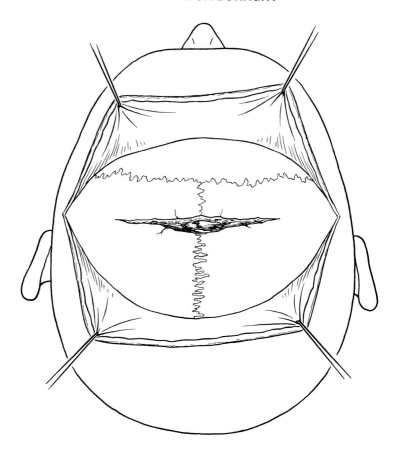

Fig. 48-7. Wide fracture line warning the surgeon that the underlying sinus may be extensively torn.

pressures accounts for most of the symptomatology. The distention of the venous components of the sinus and back pressure upon the orbital veins give rise to the proptosis of the eye with swelling and chemosis of the conjunctiva. The jet of arterial blood in the carotid artery into the venous structure of the cavernous sinus accounts for the bruit.

Therapeutic Choices

Nonsurgical choices.   There is no satisfactory nonsurgical answer to the problem of an abnormal vascular communication. This opinion is based upon history of the disorder. Although in a small number of such cases the communication sealed spontaneously, in the greater proportion there was gradually increasing proptosis and conjunctival edema, paralysis of the extraocular muscles, and diminished vision. Useful function of the ipsilateral eye is frequently lost (20 percent).

Surgical choices.   Ligating the cervical carotid artery reduces the arterial pressure in the carotid artery at the site of the arterial tear, hence favoring thrombosis and sealing of the communication. The advantages of this procedure are (1) it is simply and easily performed; (2) it does not require craniotomy; and (3) it can be performed under local anesthesia. The disadvantages are (1) it has a high failure rate. Because of retrograde flow in the distal internal carotid artery, the syndrome may persist. It may be somewhat less severe or may slowly worsen. (2) It is

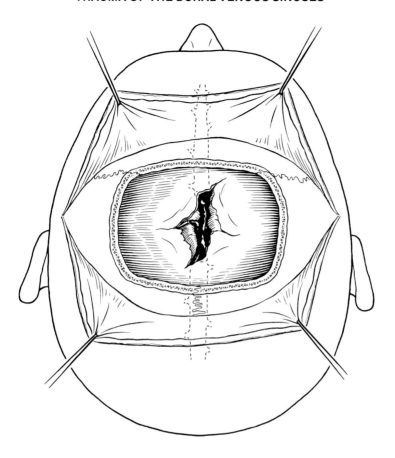

Fig. 48-8. Exposed sinus revealing a clot at the torn sinus ends and at the mouth of a torn bridging vein.

often accompanied by significant complications such as embolism or ischemia, resulting in neurologic deficit such as hemiplegia.

Trapping has perhaps been the most widely used method of surgical therapy, at least until very recent years. It consists of ligating either the internal carotid artery or the common carotid artery in the neck and the intracranial internal carotid artery, thus trapping the leaking area between the occlusions and reducing flow and pressure at the site of communication, thereby promoting thrombosis at this site.

The relative popularity of this method is not because it is without risk but rather because there has been a fair measure of success with it and because it is the least complicated of a number of procedures that have complication rates. This procedure, along with the newer procedures, also has a significant failure rate, however. In the case of trapping, failure may be caused by collateral flow via the ophthalmic arteries, hypophysial vessels, small communicators from the opposite side, or persistent trigeminal arteries.

To perform trapping, the internal or common carotid artery is exposed in the neck. An umbilical tape is placed about it so that a tourniquet or an arterial clamp, such as a Selverstone or Crutchfield, can be applied.

If the patient is being operated upon under general anesthesia, the vessel is allowed to remain fully open until the patient has recovered from the anesthesia. Then the vessel is occluded, either slowly or rapidly depending upon the preference and experience of the surgeon. The patient is continuously monitored and if untoward symptoms develop, the device can be immedi-

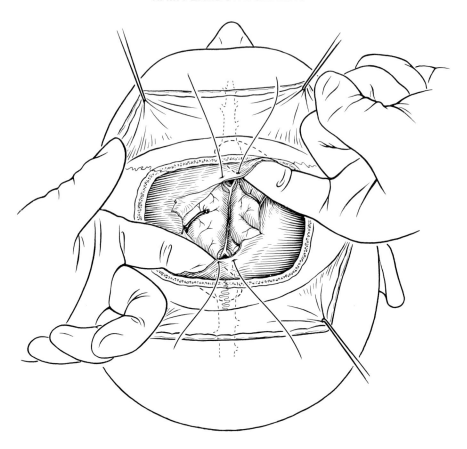

Fig. 48-9.   Maneuver for control of hemorrhage following expulsion of a clot.

ately released. (Not all neurologic deficits recover on release, but many do.) When the vessel is completely closed, the patient is monitored for 24 to 48 hours. If no untoward symptoms develop, the external portion of the clamp may be disconnected and the vessel permanently ligated. Some prefer to ligate doubly and to section the vessel; others leave it in continuity. The common carotid artery is preferred as the ligation site by many neurosurgeons. The approach is easier and is alleged to have a lower complication rate than the internal carotid approach, although it also is alleged to have a higher failure rate.

The intracranial clipping of the internal carotid artery then can be performed as a second operation if the communication persists. Such clipping should be proximal to the posterior communicating artery to allow the circulation of that vessel to remain in continuity with the distal internal carotid, the anterior choroidal artery, and the anterior and middle cerebral arteries of that side.

Some surgeons prefer to do both the cervical operation and the craniotomy at the same time because they feel there is a lower incidence of embolization that way. This depends largely on the surgeon's experience. It is difficult to argue with a high success rate in the hands of an individual and improper to advocate persistence in the face of misfortune.

The following procedures have been performed but no series was of great size, and extensive experience is not available. The interested reader is encouraged to consult the reference literature or to seek the advice of the innovator.

With the advent of the cervical carotid to intracranial internal carotid shunt, a method was presented for trapping the carotid and cavernous fistula[15] while at the same time preserving blood flow to the distal internal carotid. Such procedures have so far been unsuccessful for tech-

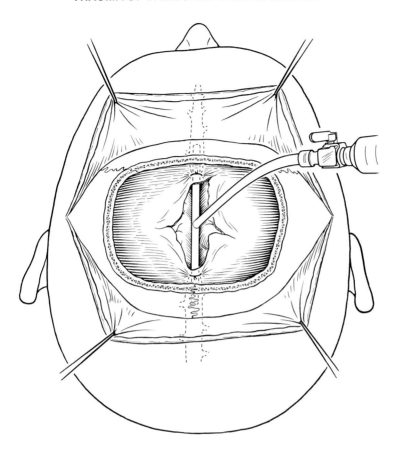

Fig. 48-10.   Siliconized vascular T-tube in a sinus.

nical reasons, but simulated surgery in the laboratory has an established success rate.[16-18] Theoretically, the success rate should be higher than in surgery for atherosclerotic disease since the distal internal carotid is not involved because of disease and since most artery–vein communications occur in young people who have good vessels in general except for the lesion that was induced by trauma.

Embolization

In 1940, Mixter[19] considered closing a carotid cavernous fistula by introducing a piece of muscle marked by a small silver clip, and attached to a long suture, into the cervical carotid artery and allowing it to enter the carotid siphon, with the thought that it would be sucked into the orifice of the communication and thus block it. Should it have passed beyond the site, it could have been recovered by traction upon the suture. There had been no laboratory preparation for this procedure and Mixter never did use it, but he did a good deal of thinking about it. In more recent years, however, embolization has been tried with muscle, Gelfoam, etc.[20-22]

Balloon Embolization

Serbinenko has devised and successfully used a catheter with a detachable balloon that he introduces into the cervical carotid. Then, under roentgen control, he guides the balloon to the carotid rent and releases it from the catheter, allowing it to plug the communication.[23,24]

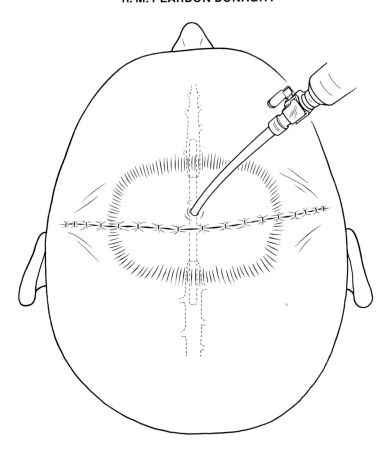

Fig. 48-11.   Wound is closed following introduction of T-tube.

Use of a Balloon in the Venous Channel

Mullan has reported using a balloon that he introduces into the venous channels leading to the sinus,[25] and Wright and Donaghy,[26] after unsuccessfully attempting to catheterize a series of cadavers via the superior petrosal sinus, did introduce such a balloon into the cavernous sinus via the ophthalmic veins. Although the balloon deflated, thrombosis occurred in the venous channels secondary to foreign body effect. Proptosis and extraocular movement improved, although the patient did not recover his sight.

Thrombosis via Positive Current

Mullan, using the experience of Sawyer,[11,13] has devised a method of introducing positive electric current into the venous structures leading from the sinus, thus promoting thrombosis.[25]

Parkinson has reported an elegant procedure based upon his anatomic research on the structure of the cavernous sinus.[27,29] In his procedure, the sinus is opened under cardiac arrest and the internal carotid artery rent is identified and repaired under direct vision. This procedure goes to the very heart of the problem. There is no question that the surgery is one of great magnitude, but the fact that it was conceived and then applied with some success testifies to the magnitude of the problem it was designed to correct.

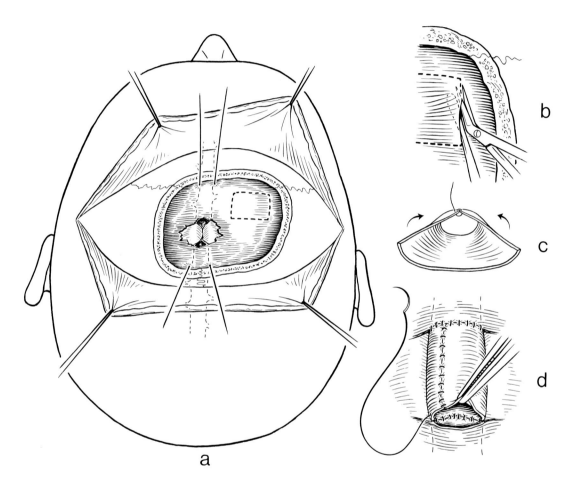

Fig. 48-12.   Formation of a dural tunnel. **A.** Sinus disruption. Outline of dural flap on right. **B.** Raising dural flap. **C.** Forming the dural tunnel. **D.** Completing the dural tunnel

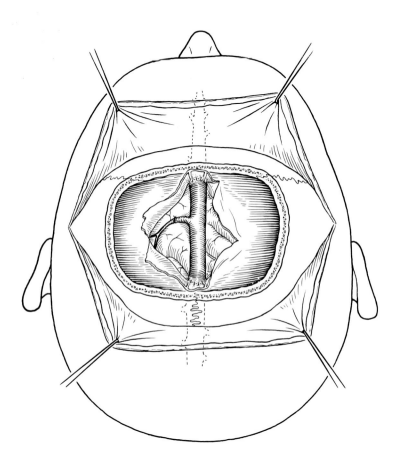

Fig. 48-13.   Vein graft in place, bridging a long sinus defect.

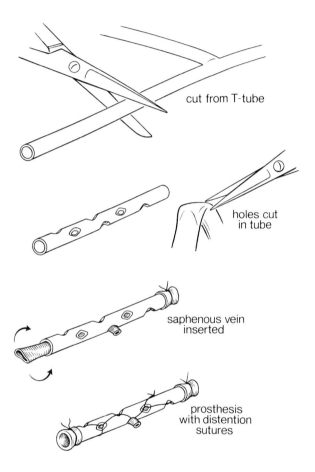

cut from T-tube

holes cut
in tube

saphenous vein
inserted

prosthesis
with distention
sutures

Fig. 48-14. Formation of an intimal lined stent.

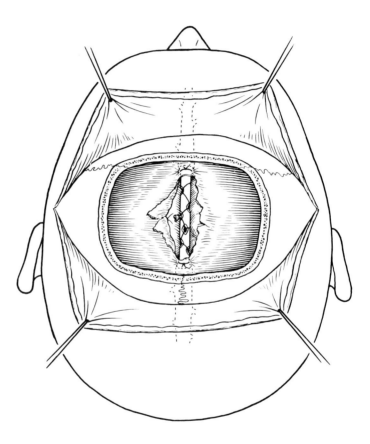

Fig. 48-15.   Stent in place following removal of a temporary T-tube.

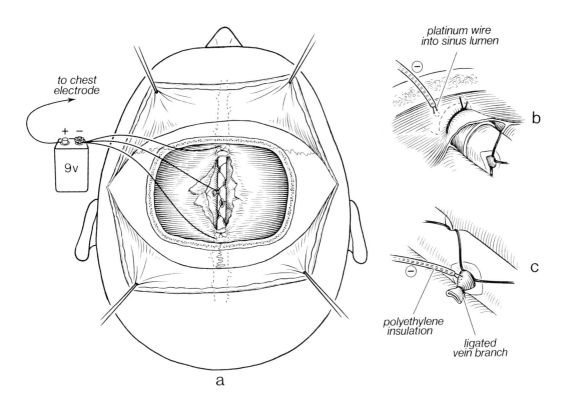

Fig. 48-16. Apparatus to provide 5 to 7 days of continuous negative current to the sinus intima.

REFERENCES

1. Kapp JP, Gielchinsky I: Management of combat wounds of the dural sinus. *Surgery 71*:913–917, 1972
2. Piersal GA (ed): *Human Anatomy, 8th ed.* Philadelphia, J. B. Lippincott, 1923, pp. 867–874
3. Browder J, Browder A, Kaplan H: The venous sinuses of the cerebral dura mater. *Arch Neurol 26*:175–180, 1972
4. Kaplan HA, Browder J: Atresia of the rostral superior sagittal venous channels. *Neurosurg 38*:602–607, 1973
5. Browder J, Kaplan HA: Venous drainage following ablation or occlusive isolation of the rostral superior sagittal sinus. *Surg Neurol 1*:245–251, 1973
6. Troup H, Tarkkanen J: Continuous recording of the sigmoid sinus pressure after radical neck dissection. *J Laryngol Otol 82*: 1013–1016, 1968
7. Fitz-Hugh GS, Robins RB, Craddock WD: Increased intracranial pressure complicating unilateral neck dissection. *Laryngoscope 76*:893–906, 1966
8. Kapp JP, Gielchinsky I, Petty C, et al: Internal shunt for use in reconstruction of dural sinuses: technical note. *J Neurosurg 35*:351–354, 1971
9. Donaghy RMP, Wallman LJ, Flanagan ME, et al: Sagittal sinus repair. *J Neurosurg 38*:244–248, 1973
10. Bonnal J, Brotchi J: Surgery of the superior sagittal sinus in parasagittal meningiomas. *J Neurosurg 48*:935–948, 1978
11. Sawyer PN, Pate JW: Bio-electric phenomena as an etiologic factor in intravascular thrombosis. *Am J Physiol 175*:103–107, 1953
12. Sawyer PN, Pate JW, Weldon CS: Relations of abnormal and injury electric potential differences to intravascular thrombosis. *Am J Physiol 175*:108–112, 1953
13. Sawyer PN, Pate JW: Electrical potential differences across the normal aorta and aortic grafts of dogs. *Am J Physiol 175*:113–117, 1953
14. Mullan S: Experience with surgical thrombosis of intracranial berry aneurysm and carotid cavernous fistula. *J Neurosurg 41*:657–670, 1974
15. Woringer E, Kunlin J: Anastomose entre la carotide primitive et la carotide intra-cranienne ou la sylvienne par greffon selon la technique de la suture suspendue. *Neurochirurgie 9*:181–188, 1963
16. Maroon J, Donaghy RMP: Experimental cerebral revascularization with autogenous grafts. *J Neurosurg 38*:172–179, 1973
17. Shields CB: Autogenous artery and vein grafts in common carotid suproclinoid carotid anastomoses. *J Microsurg 1*:114–119, 1979
18. Lougheed WM, Marshall BM, Hunter M, et al.: Common carotid to intracranial internal carotid bypass venous graft: technical note. *J Neurosurg 34*:114–118, 1971
19. Mixter, WJ: Personal communication, 1940
20. Treatment of carotid-cavernous fistula consisting of one stage operation by muscle embolization of the fistula's carotid segment, in Donaghy RMP, Yasargil MG (eds): *Microvascular Surgery.* Stuttgart, Georg Thieme Verlag, 1967, pp 151–167
21. Brooks B: The treatment of traumatic arteriovenous fistula. *South Med J 23*:100–106, 1930
22. Ohta T, Nishimura S, Kikuchi H, et al: Closure of carotid-cavernous fistula with polyurethane foam embolus: technical note. *J Neurosurg 38*:107–112, 1973
23. Serbinenko FA: Balloon catheterization and occlusion of major cerebral vessels. *J Neurosurg 41*:125–145, 1974
24. Picard L, Lepoire J, Montaut J, et al: Endoarterial occlusion of carotid-cavernous sinus fistulas using a balloon-tipped catheter. *Neuroradiol 8*:5–10, 1974
25. Mullan S, Brown FD, Patronas NJ: Treatment of carotid-cavernous fistulas by cavernous sinus occlusion. *J Neurosurg 50*:131–144, 1979
26. Wright S, Donaghy RMP: Unreported case.
27. Parkinson D: A surgical approach to the cavernous sinus portion of the carotid artery. Anatomical studies and case report. *J Neurosurg 23*:474–483, 1965
28. Parkinson D: Transcavernous repair of carotid-cavernous fistula. Case report. *J Neurosurg 26*:420–424, 1967
29. Parkinson D: Carotid cavernous fistula. Direct repair with preservation of the carotid artery. Technical note. *J Neurosurg 38*:99–106, 1973

CHAPTER 49
Surgical Management of Intracerebral Hemorrhage

David G. Piepgras　　　　Michael J. Redmond

STROKE IS THE THIRD MOST COMMON CAUSE OF DEATH in the United States after coronary heart disease and cancer, accounting for 11 percent of all deaths.[1,2] The annual incidence of spontaneous intracerebral hemorrhage is approximately 15 per 100,000.[3] The relative gravity of the problem of intracerebral hemorrhage is evident from its high morbidity and mortality: a 1-month survival rate of only 17 percent compared to 35 percent for subarachnoid hemorrhage and 73 percent for stroke resulting from cerebral thrombosis.[4]

Classification

Intracerebral hemorrhages may be classified as "symptomatic"—those caused by the rupture of an aneurysm or arteriovenous malformation (AVM), related to a known hematologic disorder or cerebral mass lesion—and "primary" intracerebral hemorrhages—those hemorrhages for which such underlying causes cannot be determined. Excluded from both of these categories are the relatively common traumatic and preterm neonatal intracerebral hemorrhages.

Primary Intracerebral Hemorrhage

The large majority of spontaneous intracerebral hemorrhages fall into the "primary" category, with hypertension most often implicated as the contributing factor. Ransohoff[5] has stated that hypertension is the cause in over 90 percent of single, sizable intracerebral hemorrhages; however, McCormick and Rosenfield,[6] in a prospective autopsy study, concluded that hypertension could be incriminated in only 25 percent of their patients with massive spontaneous intracerebral hemorrhages. Furlan et al.,[3] reviewing cases in an essentially white population over the past 20 years, found an 81 percent frequency of hypertension in their patients with primary intracerebral hemorrhage.

Although the exact pathologic lesion of hypertensive intracerebral hemorrhage remains a subject of discussion among neuropathologists, there is evidence to incriminate a degenerative process specific to small cerebral arteries, now described as lipohyalinosis[7] or fibrinoid necrosis.[8] The distribution of these changes match those sites at which the greatest incidence of intracerebral hemorrhage and lacunar infarcts occur. Consistent with this, sites of predilection for hypertensive intracerebral hemorrhage have been identified, with approximately half occurring in the striate body, 15 percent in the thalamus, 10 to 15 percent in the pons, 10 percent in the cerebel-

Department of Neurologic Surgery, Mayo Clinic, Mayo Medical School, and Department of Neurologic Surgery, Mayo Graduate School of Medicine, Rochester, Minnesota

747

lum, and 10 to 20 percent in the cerebral white matter.[5,9,10] The hemorrhage may be massive and fatal, or small with good recovery. It is characteristic of an intracerebral hemorrhage to dissect along tissue planes and tracts, separating and compressing the nervous tissue rather than destroying it. Extension into the ventricular system has been stated to be common, and according to Fisher,[10] occurs in 90 percent of the cases. This estimate was made in the era before computerized tomography (CT), however, and was undoubtedly based on findings of bloody cerebrospinal fluid or at autopsy. Interestingly, a series of CT studies in patients with ganglio-thalamic and lobar hematomas showed intraventricular or cisternal blood in only 9 percent and 20 percent of cases respectively.[11]

Clinical Presentation

The onset of symptoms in a patient with a primary intracerebral hemorrhage typically occurs abruptly while the patient is awake and active; prodromal symptoms are not typical.[10] Neurologic deficit develops progressively as the hemorrhage increases, usually becoming maximal in hours to days. Headache occurs in one-half to two-thirds of the patients and is commonly lateralized to the side of the hemorrhage. A declining level of consciousness occurs as the hemorrhage extends directly into the brainstem or because of increased intracranial pressure and secondary involvement of the brainstem.

For a more detailed review of the syndromes related to intracerebral hemorrhages at the various sites of predilection, the reader is referred to the excellent monographs of Fisher.[10,12] Emphasis should be placed, however, on the clinical profile of cerebellar hemorrhage inasmuch as correct diagnosis may be difficult early in its course and delayed treatment may prove fatal.[13] An acute complex of symptoms, including headache, nausea and vomiting, and inability to walk or stand, with signs of gait or appendicular ataxia, ocular disturbances, and peripheral facial palsy, should suggest the diagnosis, which can be readily confirmed by CT scan. These hemorrhages characteristically originate in or near one of the dentate nuclei where branches of the cerebellar arteries anastomose.[14] Extension of the hemorrhage into the vermis or opposite hemisphere may occur, and rupture into the fourth ventricle is not uncommon (Fig. 49-1).

The causes of primary brain hemorrhage other than hypertension and anticoagulants rarely are defined. Cerebral amyloid angiopathy has been recognized as a rare but important cause in aged patients.[8,15,16] The occurrence of single or multiple intracerebral hemorrhages in elderly, perhaps demented, nonhypertensive patients suggests amyloid angiopathy. In contrast to hypertensive hemorrhages, hematomas secondary to amyloid angiopathy tend to be near the cortical surface in the parietal and occipital lobes.[16] Amyloid angiopathy has also been implicated as the cause of cerebral hemorrhage after shunting procedures for what was clinically considered a normal pressure hydrocephalus.[17]

Symptomatic Intracerebral Hemorrhage

Symptomatic intracerebral hemorrhages most commonly are caused by aneurysms, arteriovenous malformations, or blood dyscrasias, but the bleeding also may be caused by a brain tumor or sepsis, or may be secondary to liver disease or other systemic illnesses. Intracerebral hemorrhages occurring in the anterior sylvian fissure and adjacent regions of the frontal and temporal lobes commonly are caused by middle cerebral or, less likely, internal carotid artery aneurysms (Fig. 49-2). Hematomas in the interhemispheric fissure and the medial aspect of the frontal lobe suggest an aneurysm of the anterior communicating artery as the source of bleeding. Intraventricular extension of the hemorrhage may occur from any aneurysmal site, but probably is more common in aneurysms of the anterior communicating and internal carotid arteries.[18] Lobar intracerebral hemorrhages may be primary (hypertensive), but their occurrence should al-

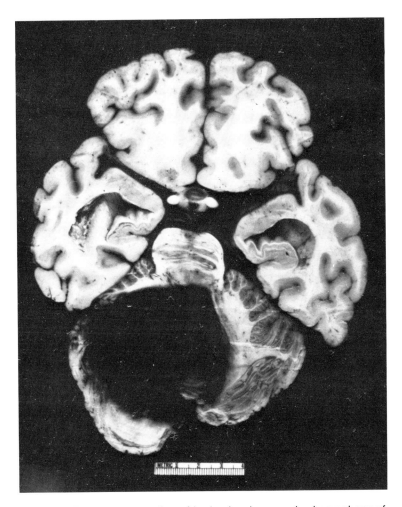

Fig. 49-1. A transverse section of brain showing massive hemorrhage of the cerebellar hemisphere with midline extension and rupture into the fourth ventricle.

ways raise the question of the underlying vascular abnormality, particularly an AVM (Fig. 49-3). Most underlying vascular lesions will be apparent on a contrasted CT scan or angiogram, but even if they are not visible on these studies, an occult vascular malformation may be the source and may be diagnosed only in a later angiogram[19] or at surgery or autopsy.

Spontaneous intracerebral hemorrhage may be the first symptom of a previously unsuspected cerebral neoplasm, but more commonly this develops acutely on a background of known malignancy or a course indicative of a progressive focal cerebral lesion. Although neoplasms account for only 2 to 3 percent of intracranial hemorrhage in series reported by Locksley[21] and Russell,[22] Scott[23] found primary or metastatic tumors as the cause in 10 percent of 80 patients operated on for spontaneous intracerebral hemorrhage. A wide spectrum of neoplasms producing intracerebral hemorrhage have been reported, the more common primary tumors being gliomas, angiomas, and meningiomas, and metastases including melanomas, bronchogenic carcinomas, and chorioepitheliomas.[5,23]

Massive intracerebral hemorrhage may occur in acute leukemias, particularly in association with extreme leukemic leukocytosis or "blast crisis." Hemorrhage probably results from a combination of cerebral vascular insults including perivascular infiltration by blast cells, an elevated blood viscosity, and microcirculation thrombosis and vasodilatation. In an attempt to prevent this complication, Dearth et al.[24] have advised emergency cranial radiation as well as other thera-

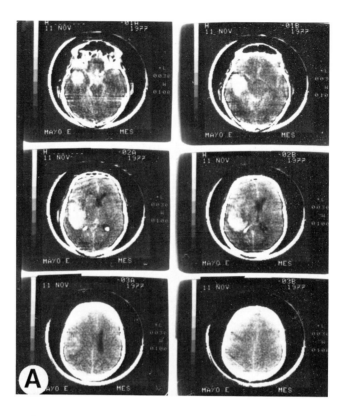

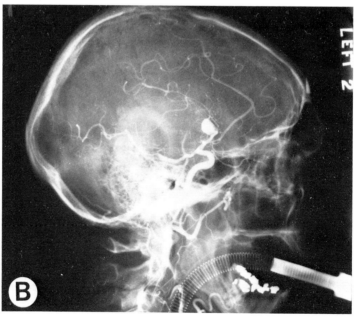

Fig. 49-2.   **A.** CT scan showing a left temporal intracerebral hemorrhage. **B.** Lateral view of an angiogram of the left carotid of the same patient, showing a large aneurysm of the left middle cerebral artery with elevation of the sylvian vessels caused by the temporal hematoma mass.

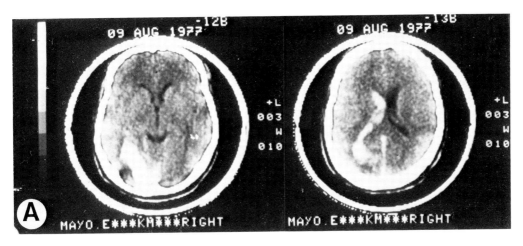

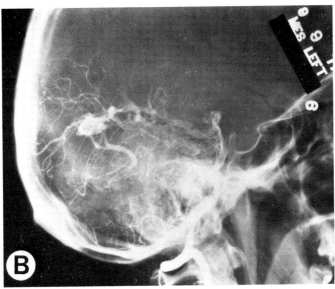

Fig. 49-3. A. CT scan demonstrating a hemorrhage of the left occipital lobe with intraventricular extension. **B.** Lateral view of an angiogram of the left vertebrobasilar system in the same patient. There is a moderate-sized occipital AVM filling from the left posterior cerebral artery and draining into the transverse sinus.

peutic measures for any patient with acute leukemia who has leukocyte count exceeding 100,000/cubic mm.

Intracranial hemorrhage is the leading cause of death in hemophiliac patients and poses a special challenge to the neurosurgeon. Approximately half of these hemorrhages are subdural or epidural. Intracerebral hemorrhage and its operative treatment have carried a high mortality in these patients and led Silverstein to state in 1960 that "the only worthwhile indication for surgical intervention in the treatment of intracranial hemorrhage in hemophiliacs is bleeding limited to the sub- or epidural spaces."[25] Since that time dramatic improvement in replacement therapy and methods for neutralization of factor VIII inhibitors have allowed the hematologist to render even the severe hemophiliac hemostatically competent so that the hemorrhage can be managed in accordance with basic neurosurgical principles. More recent series, therefore, show a marked improvement in the results of management of intracranial hemorrhage including intracerebral hematoma.[26,27] The reader is referred to specific authoritative references for guidelines on replacement therapy and operative management of the hemophiliac patient.[27-29]

An entirely separate category of intracerebral hemorrhage is the subependymal and intraventricular hemorrhages (SEH-IVH), which occur in preterm and, less frequently, full-term infants. With improved clinical recognition of the syndrome and, particularly, absolute diagnosis with CT scanning, SEH or IVH or both are now known to occur in 40 percent to 50 percent of newborn infants of less than 35 weeks gestation who require intensive care for more than 24 hours.[30] The majority of infants with SEH-IVH survive; Ahmann et al.[31] found a mortality rate of 28 percent in premature infants conforming to the above criteria, with hemorrhage the primary cause of death in 75 percent.

The onset of the hemorrhage typically occurs in the first several days of life, with a mean age of 38 hours.[32] Cases occurring in older infants have been recognized, although the etiology of the hemorrhage in these cases probably is different.[33] The hemorrhages are thought to arise from the periventricular germinal matrix area secondary to congestion, thrombosis, and disruption of the weakly supported capillaries and veins in this region.[30] In addition to prematurity, factors associated with high risk for SEH-IVH include hyaline membrane hypoxia, mechanical ventilation, and rupture of alveoli. It has been postulated that increased central venous pressure and decreased cerebral venous return caused by mechanical ventilation or rupture of alveoli leads to disruption of the germinal matrix microvasculature, which is already damaged by hypoxia and ischemia.[30] Clinical symptoms may be an abrupt deterioration with progression to death, or a stuttering course of deterioration followed by stabilization and improvement. A bulging fontanelle, seizures, decreased muscle tone, and abnormal eye signs may also be present. Of the infants surviving IVH, progressive hydrocephalus develops in about 20 percent, particularly in those infants who had more severe hemorrhages. This may resolve spontaneously or with medical management including serial lumbar punctures. In the study of Ahmann et al.[31] shunting was eventually required in only 2 of 12 patients.

Diagnosis and Prognosis

Prior to CT the diagnosis of intracerebral hemorrhage was made on the basis of clinical features aided by x-ray or echoencephalographic evidence of midline structure shift, a cautious lumbar puncture, and cerebral angiography. In spite of these measures, a "diagnostic impasse" sometimes existed "in as many as 30 percent of the patients presenting with acute cerebrovascular episodes"[34] for whom the critical difference between hemorrhage and infarction could not be readily distinguished, and expeditious treatment was therefore compromised. Now CT scanning allows rapid diagnosis of intracerebral hemorrhage, and, in addition to being the most definitive diagnostic test, also gives information regarding the exact site, extent, and possibly the cause of the hemorrhage, considerations that substantially affect the prognosis and management. CT scanning after contrast infusion may be very helpful in demonstrating the source of the intracerebral hemorrhage, particularly in cases of vascular malformation, tumors, and occasionally aneurysms. Although most cases of ganglio-thalamic hemorrhage are primary, Weisberg has advised contrasted CT for patients less than 40 years of age, those without a history of hypertension, those in whom maximal neurologic deficit developed after 4 hours or longer, those with prodromal symptoms, those with a history of neoplasm, endocarditis, or blood dyscrasia, and last, those whose noncontrasted CT had an atypical appearance.[11] Contrast examination is likewise indicated in all cases of lobar hemorrhage, cerebellar hemorrhage in young or nonhypertensive patients,[11,19] and the rare cases of multiple spontaneous intracerebral hematomas.[35]

CT is very useful in following cases of intracerebral hemorrhage, particularly those managed nonsurgically or in an expectant fashion (Fig. 49-4). Liquefaction and resorption of intracerebral hematomas may occur over several weeks,[34] while blood usually is cleared from the ventricles within 2 weeks.[18] Also, delayed development of communicating hydrocephalus is best diagnosed by CT.

Although some have advocated angiography in all cases of intracerebral hemorrhage to be

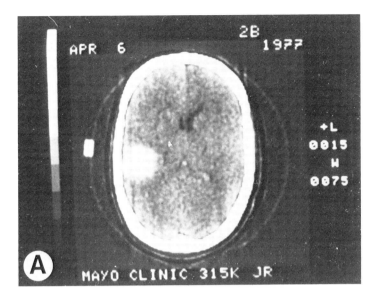

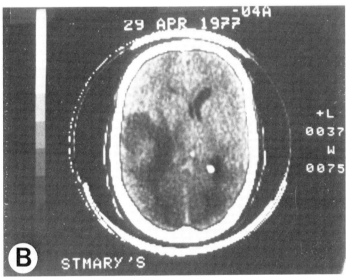

Fig. 49-4. **A.** CT scan demonstrating a moderate-sized, acute, primary, left posterotemporal intracerebral hemorrhage in a young man. His only neurologic deficit was moderate aphasia, and conservative therapy was elected. **B.** CT of the same patient 3 weeks later. The hematoma has liquefied, but there is now extensive surrounding edema with midline shift. The patient showed increased aphasia and papilledema, which resolved after craniotomy and evacuation of the liquefied clot.

treated surgically,[13] the authors would not consider this necessary in cases where there is a typical clinical and CT picture for primary intracerebral or cerebellar hemorrhage or in patients whose condition is deteriorating so rapidly that a delay in surgery seems contraindicated.

In an analysis of the CT scans of 300 patients with nontraumatic intracranial hemorrhage, Weisberg found 283 with intracerebral hemorrhage, 12 with subarachnoid bleeding, and only 5 with exclusively intraventricular hemorrhage.[11] The overall mortality in this series was 26 percent, similar to that of another series of intracerebral hemorrhage diagnosed with CT,[36] and markedly better than the 83 percent 1-month mortality for cases of cerebral hemorrhage reported by Whisnant[4] before the advent of CT diagnosis. This difference in mortality may be accounted for in part by the present-day CT diagnosis of milder cases of intracerebral hemorrhage previously misdiagnosed as ischemic stroke or subarachnoid hemorrhage. Thalamic-ganglionic hemorrhage was present in 232 of Weisberg's cases,[11] 81 percent of these being hypertensive patients. The mortality for patients with thalamic-ganglionic hemorrhage without ventricular extension was 25 percent but rose to 70 percent for those with ventricular extension. The mortality in patients with lobar hematomas was 20 percent with or without extension of the hemorrhage into the ventricular system. Ropper et al. found a 12 percent mortality in 26 cases of lobar hemorrhage.[19]

Extensive intraventricular hemorrhage caused by extension from a thalamic-ganglionic hypertensive hemorrhage or aneurysm rupture usually carries a grave prognosis. Little et al.[18] found an overall mortality of 83 percent in adult patients with intraventricular hemorrhage and a 100 percent mortality in those with "massive" extension into the ventricles. The latter group typically presented with sudden profound coma and neurologic deficits of pontomedullary dysfunction, and died within 48 hours. A second group of patients in the series of Little et al. developed sudden focal cerebral or cerebellar disturbance and secondary brainstem dysfunction; in these the mortality was 88 percent. A smaller group of patients with intraventricular hemorrhage had relatively mild symptoms and signs and followed a benign course with no mortality directly related to the hemorrhage.

In another recent series of patients with intraventricular hemorrhage diagnosed by CT, de Weerd[37] found an overall mortality of 53 percent, which rose to 63 percent if the hemorrhage extended into all ventricles and dropped to 38 percent if there was limited ventricular extension. Of the latter subgroup in de Weerd's series i.e., limited ventricular extension of the hemorrhage, 38 percent also survived with no disability.[37]

As in other series,[18,38,39] de Weerd found a close correlation between the clinical condition of the patient on admission and prognosis.[37] This fact has already been alluded to earlier in this chapter in reference to cerebellar hemorrhage. In the review of Ott et al.,[40] two-thirds of the patients suffering from cerebellar hemorrhage were responsive on admission, but one-half were comatose within 24 hours and 75 percent within one week of onset. With surgical intervention the mortality rate for cerebellar hemorrhage was only 17 percent if the patients were operated on while they were still in a responsive condition, but this rose to 75 percent for unresponsive patients. The prognosis for cerebellar hemorrhage in children has been found to be better than for adults despite the severity of the initial condition.[41,42]

Management

General Measures

With the widespread availability of CT, the diagnosis of intracerebral hemorrhage can now be readily established and early specific treatment initiated. The airway should be secured with intubation, if necessary, to avoid hypoxia and hypercarbia. Close observation of vital signs, neurologic status, and ventilation, pulmonary toilet, and fluid balance usually dictate the need for intensive care nursing of the acutely ill patient. If a coagulopathy is present, particularly that brought on by anticoagulant therapy, it should be expeditiously corrected with appropriate blood component transfusions and reversal medications. Hypertension should be treated aggressively[43] with intravenous infusions of nitroprusside for rapid reduction and optimal control of blood pressure in cases of extreme elevation, or intramuscular hydralazine hydrochloride when the need for a reduction in blood pressure is less acute. If there is evidence of increased intracranial pressure (ICP), treatment with urea, mannitol, or furosemide may be indicated and placement of an intracranial pressure (ICP) monitor should be considered to guide this therapy. Such monitoring and treatment may permit adequate control of intracranial hypertension in certain cases so that surgery may be avoided. If the elevation of intracranial pressure becomes refractory to medical treatment, surgery may be indicated.[44,45]

Surgical Therapy

The indications for and timing of surgical intervention for intracranial hemorrhage has been contentious. In 1961, McKissock et al.[46] published the results of a controlled clinical trial that compared the benefits of surgical therapy with those of aggressive conservative management. The overall mortality was 65 percent for the surgically treated group and 51 percent for the nonsurgically treated patients. The authors concluded: "We have been unable to demonstrate any benefit from surgery in regard to either mortality or morbidity."[46]

A uniform surgical management for primary intracerebral hemorrhage, including angiography and surgery within 24 hours on all patients with a demonstrable intracerebral hematoma mass, major focal neurologic deficit, and a depressed level of consciousness or signs of brainstem involvement, was reported by Luessenhop et al. in 1967.[38] Their overall mortality was 37 percent, and 32 percent for the surgically treated patients, considerably better than that reported by McKissock. In 7 of the 12 surgically treated patients who died and in several survivors, reaccumulation of a hematoma occurred and was considered the most important surgical complication. The operative mortality was 89 percent in capsular hemorrhage cases compared to 4 percent in those with lobar hematomas. Patients not moribund on admission had an operative mortality of only 8 percent.

Kaneo et al.[39] recently reported remarkable success with early evacuation of laterally situated hypertensive basal ganglia hemorrhages, stressing the importance of surgery within 7 hours of ictus, and microsurgical technique. Other authors have advocated a less urgent, or even delayed, elective evacuation of the intracerebral hematoma, citing higher mortality rates in patients on whom surgery was performed earlier.[47-50] This approach can be supported to some degree with the observations of Papo[44] and Janny et al.,[45] who monitored intracranial pressure in a series of patients with intracerebral hemorrhage and found that the intracranial pressure in these patients was generally only moderately elevated (less than 33 mm mercury) shortly after the ictus and gradually became normal over several weeks. After the surgical evacuation of the hematomas, there was a rapid but only temporary reduction in pressure, followed by an increase to its preoperative level.[45] Except in the most mildly and most severely affected patients, no definite correlation was found between ICP and clinical condition or outcome.[44] Such findings indicate that the damaging effects of intracerebral hemorrhage are caused more by the disruption of the brain by the hemorrhage than the secondary intracranial hypertension, and that the beneficial effect of evacuating a hematoma may be due more to the reduction in local tissue pressures and improved microcirculation than the reduction in the increased intracranial pressure. More recent experimental studies suggest that intracerebral hemorrhage rapidly induces secondary brain tissue edema, hemorrhage, and necrosis, which can be minimized or halted by hematoma evacuation within six hours.[56] Clinical experiences in certain patients such as exemplified in Figure 49-4 attest to the edemogenic properties of intracerebral blood.

In the final decision-making process regarding operative versus conservative management of a patient with intracerebral hemorrhage, the surgeon must consider multiple factors including the clinical condition of the patient, particularly the severity and progression of neurologic deficits, and the site and extent of the hemorrhage as indicated on CT scan. Patients of advanced age and poor nutritional status or those who have co-existent major life-threatening medical problems are not usually candidates for surgical intervention. The patient with an extensive basal ganglia hemorrhage who is deeply comatose with severely depressed or absent brainstem reflexes and faltering vital signs should also not be subjected to operation. Conversely, those patients who have a small hemorrhage causing stable neurologic deficit and little alteration in their level of consciousness can be expected to do well without surgery.

Ten to 50 percent[5,38] of the patients who present with intracerebral hemorrhage will be between these two extremes, however, and should be considered for surgery. If their level of consciousness is deteriorating or the lateralized deficit increasing, emergency surgery may be indicated. If there is a pronounced focal neurologic deficit or stable depression of level of consciousness and a significant mass exists caused by an intracerebral hematoma, especially one that is lobar or subcortical in location, evacuation of the clot should be carried out at the earliest convenient time. When predominently intraventricular hemorrhage is present and there is significant obtundation or evidence of increased intracranial pressure, ventricular drainage should be performed. An open evacuation of a solid clot also may need to be considered.[20]

Special mention should be made regarding the management of cerebellar hemorrhage, since its course is unpredictable and it can produce rapid deterioration and death. With this in mind, Ott et al.[40] advised immediate surgery for all patients with intracerebellar hemorrhage presenting in the first 48 hours after ictus and for most patients within a week of onset. In an analysis of patients with cerebellar hemorrhage confirmed by CT scan, Little et al.[51] concluded that immediate evacuation of the hematoma was indicated if there was evidence of brainstem compression, hydrocephalus, or if the hematoma was larger than 3 cm. Ojemann[52] had advised immediate evacuation of all large hematomas even when the neurologic status is stable and there is hydrocephalus and neurologic compromise. Although rare, evacuation of brainstem hematomas may be indicated in selected cases.[53,54]

Operative Technique

Evacuation of an intracerebral hemorrhage should be carried out through a full craniotomy that is adequate enough to expose the limits of the hematoma and that also makes it possible to identify and deal with unsuspected pathology such as a tumor, vascular malformation, or aneurysm that might be present. The cavity of the hematoma should be entered through a cortical incision that provides the most direct access yet the least injury to vital cortical areas, tracts, or blood vessels. The hematoma is evacuated with gentle suction and irrigation and forceps. Leaving some clot attached to the walls may be preferable to an overly aggressive removal with resultant injury to the adjacent brain or small vessels. Attention should be given during the removal to identifying a likely source for the hemorrhage such as an occult vascular malformation or a tumor, and suspicious-looking tissue fragments should be saved for thorough histologic examination. Magnification and illumination with the operating microscope are particularly helpful during evacuation and exploration of cavities of deep hematomas approached through a limited cortical incision. In rare instances a single artery may be identified as the source of hemorrhage and bleeding controlled with a clip or coagulation. Bleeding from the cavity walls can be controlled by temporarily applying cottonoid patties and hemostatic gelatin sponge, gauze, or fibrillar collagen.

Irrigating the cavity of the hematoma with a gentle saline lavage will reveal persistent bleeding sites. Meticulous hemostasis must be achieved and Ojemann[55] has advised temporarily elevating the blood pressure to hypertensive levels to help visualize any possible recurrent bleeding site.[55]

Postoperative Care

Postoperative care should follow routine neurosurgical principles. Blood pressure control should be continued to avoid severe hypertension. Extensive cerebral edema may be associated with acute intracerebral hemorrhage[56] and steroids may be of benefit in its treatment.

Neurologic deterioration in the early postoperative period suggests hematoma reaccumulation, whereas delayed deterioration, particularly in cases of intraventricular hemorrhage, may be due to hydrocephalus. Fortunately, computerized tomography has greatly facilitated the diagnosis of these conditions as well as more routine follow-up of intracerebral hemorrhages.

REFERENCES

1. Wolf PA, Dawber TR, Thomas HE, et al: Epidemiology of stroke. *Adv Neurol 16*:5–19, 1977
2. Kurtzke JF: Epidemiology of cerebrovascular diseases, in Siekert RG (ed): *Cerebrovascular Survey Report for Joint Council Subcommittee on Cerebrovascular Disease,* National Institute of Neurological and Communicative Disorders and Stroke and National Heart and Lung Institute. Rochester, MN, Whiting, 1976, pp 213–242
3. Furlan AJ, Whisnant JP, Elveback LR: The decreasing incidence of primary intracerebral hemorrhage: a population study. *Ann Neurol 5*:367–373, 1979
4. Whisnant JP, Fitzgibbons JP, Kurland LT, et al: Natural history of stroke in Rochester, Minnesota, 1945 through 1954. *Stroke 2*:11–22, 1971
5. Ransohoff J, Derby B, Kricheff I: Spontaneous intracerebral hemorrhage. *Clin Neurosurg 18*:247–266, 1971
6. McCormick WF, Rosenfield DB: Massive brain hemorrhage: A review of 144 cases and an examination of their causes. *Stroke 4*:946–954, 1973
7. Fisher CM: Cerebral miliary aneurysms in hypertension. *Am J Pathol 66*:2. 313–325, 1972
8. Okazaki H, Reagan JT, Campbell RJ: Clinicopathologic studies of primary cerebral amyloid angiopathy. *Mayo Clin Proc 54*:22–31, 1979
9. Freytag E: Fatal hypertensive intracerebral hematomas: A survey of the pathological anatomy of 393 cases. *J Neurol Neurosurg Psychiatry 31*:616–620, 1968
10. Fisher CM: Clinical syndromes in cerebral thrombosis, hypertensive hemorrhage, and ruptured saccular aneurysm. *Clin Neurosurg 22*:117–147, 1974
11. Weisberg L: Computerized tomography in intracranial hemorrhage. *Arch Neurol 36*:422–426, 1979
12. Fisher CM: Clinical syndromes in cerebral hemorrhage, in Fields WS (ed): *Pathogenesis and Treatment of Cerebrovascular Disease,* Springfield, IL, Charles C Thomas, 1961, pp 318–342
13. Rossi GF, Maira G: Comments on chapters 28 and 29. *Adv Neurol 25*:305–307, Raven Press, New York, 1979
14. Freeman RE, Onofrio BM, Okazaki H, et al: Spontaneous intracerebellar hemorrhage. Diagnosis and surgical treatment. *Neurology* (Minneapolis), *23*:84–90, 1973
15. Jellinger K: Cerebrovascular amyloidosis with cerebral hemorrhage. *J Neurol 214*:195–206, 1977
16. Rengachary SS, Racela LS, Watanabe I, et al: Neurosurgical and immunological implications of primary cerebral amyloid (congophilic) angiopathy. *Neurosurgery 7*:1–9, 1980
17. Torack RM: Congophilic angiopathy complicated by surgery and massive hemorrhage: A light and electron microscopic study. *Am J Pathol 81*:349–366, 1975
18. Little JR, Blomquist GA, Ethier R: Intraventricular hemorrhage in adults. *Surg Neurol 8*:143–149, 1977
19. Ropper AH, Davis KR: Lobar cerebral hemorrhages: Acute clinical syndromes in 26 cases. *Ann Neurol 8*:141–147, 1980
20. Pia HW: The surgical treatment of intracerebral and intraventricular haematomas. *Acta Neurochir 27*, 149–164, 1972
21. Locksley HB, Sahs AL, Sandler R: Report on the cooperative study of intracranial aneurysms and subarachnoid hemorrhage. Section 3 Subarachnoid hemorrhage unrelated to intracranial aneurysm and A-V malformation: A study of associated diseases and prognosis. *J Neurosurg 24*:1034–1056, 1966
22. Russell DS: The pathology of spontaneous intracerebral hemorrhage. *Proc R Soc Med 47*:689–693, 1954
23. Scott M: Spontaneous intracerebral hematoma caused by cerebral neoplasms. Report of 8 verified cases. *J Neurosurg 42*:338–342, 1975
24. Dearth JC, Fountain KS, Smithson WA, et al: Extreme leukemic leucocytosis (blast crisis) in childhood. *Mayo Clin Proc 53*:207 211, 1978
25. Silverstein A: Intracranial bleeding in hemophilia. *Arch Neurol 3*:141–157, 1960
26. Van Trotsenburg L: Neurological complications of haemophilia, in Brinkhaus KM, Hemker HC (eds): *Handbook of Hemophilia,* part 1. New York, American Elsevier, 1975, p 389
27. Gilchrist GS, Piepgras DG: Neurologic complications in hemophilia, in Hilgartner MW (ed): *Hemophilia in Children,* Littleton, MA, Publishing Sciences Group, 1976, p 79
28. Hilgartner MW: Current therapy, in *Hemophilia in Children,* Littleton, MA, Publishing Sciences Group, 1976, p 151
29. Olsen ER: Intracranial surgery in hemophiliacs. *Arch Neurol 21*:401–412, 1969
30. Dykes FD, Lazzara A, Ahmann P, et al: Intraventricular hemorrhage: A prospective evaluation of etiopathogenesis. *Pediatrics 66*:42–49, 1980
31. Ahmann PA, Lazzara A, Dykes FD, et al: Intraventricular hemorrhage in the high risk pre term infant: Incidence and outcome. *Ann Neurol 7*:118–124, 1980
32. Tsiantos A, Victorin L, Relier JP, et al: Intracranial hemorrhage in the prematurely born infant. *J Pediatr 85*:854, 1974
33. Mitchell W, O'Tuama L: Cerebral intraventricular hemorrhages in infants: A widening age spectrum. *Pediatrics 65*:35–39, 1980

34. Feindel W: Management of intracerebral hemorrhage. *Adv Neurol 25*:293–300, 1979
35. Weisberg L: Multiple spontaneous intracerebral hemorrhages. Clinical and computerized tomographic correlations. *Neurology (NY) 311*:897–900, 1981
36. Kinkel WR, Jacobs L: Computerized tomography in cerebrovascular disease. *Neurology (NY) 26*:924–930, 1976
37. de Weerd AW: The prognosis of intraventricular hemorrhage. *J Neurol 222*:45–51, 1979
38. Luessenhop AJ, Shevlin WA, Ferrero AA, et al: Surgical management of primary intracerebral hemorrhage. *J Neurosurg 27*:419–427, 1967
39. Kaneo M, Tokomi K, Yokoyama T: Early surgical treatment for hypertensive intracerebral hemorrhage. *J Neurosurg 46*:579–583, 1977
40. Ott KH, Kase CS, Ojemann RG, et al: Cerebellar hemorrhage: Diagnosis and treatment. A review of 56 cases. *Arch Neurol 31*:160–167, 1974
41. Erenberg G, Rubin R, Shulman K: Cerebellar haematoma caused by angiomas in children. *J Neurol Neurosurg Psychiatry 35*:304–310, 1972
42. Kazmiroff PB, Weichsel ME, Grinnell V, et al: Acute cerebellar hemorrhage in childhood: Etiology, diagnosis and treatment. *Neurosurgery 6*:524–528, 1980
43. Meyer J, Bauer R: Medical treatment of spontaneous intracranial hemorrhage by use of hypotensive drugs. *Neurology (NY) 12*:36–47, 1962
44. Papo I, Janny P, Caruselli G, et al: Intracranial pressure time course in primary intracerebral hemorrhage. *Neurosurgery 6*:504–510, 1979
45. Janny P, Colnet G, Georget A, et al: Intracranial pressure with intracerebral hemorrhages. *Surg Neurol 10*:371–375, 1978
46. McKissock W, Richardson A, Taylor J: Primary intracerebral hemorrhage: A controlled trial of surgical and conservative treatment in 180 unselected cases. *Lancet 2*:221–226, 1961
47. Paillas, JE, Alliez B: Surgical treatment of spontaneous intracerebral hemorrhage: Immediate and long-term results in 250 cases. *J Neurosurg 39*:145–151, 1973
48. Tedeschi G, Bernini FP, Cerillo A: Indications for surgical treatment of intracerebral hemorrhage. *J Neurosurg 43*:590–595, 1975
49. Cuatico W, Adib S, Gaston P: Spontaneous intracerebral hematomas. *J Neurosurg 22*:569–575, 1965
50. Benes V, Koukolik F, Obrovska D: Two types of spontaneous intracerebral hemorrhage due to hypertension. *J Neurosurg 37*:509–513, 1972
51. Little JR, Tubman DE, Ethier R: Cerebellar hemorrhage in adults: Diagnosis by computerized tomography. *J Neurosurg 48*:575–579, 1978
52. Ojemann RG: Comments in: Kazimiroff PB, Weichsel ME, Grinnell V, Young RF: Acute cerebellar hemorrhage in childhood: Etiology, diagnosis and treatment. *Neurosurgery 6*:524–528, 1980
53. Cioffi FA, Tomasello F, D'Avanzo R: Pontine hematomas. *Surg Neurol 16*:13–16, 1981
54. Murphy M: Successful evacuation of acute pontine hematoma. *J Neurosurg 37*:224–255, 1972
55. Ojemann RG, Mohr JP: Hypertensive brain hemorrhage. *Clin Neurosurg 23*:220–244, 1975
56. Suzuki J, Ebina T: Sequential changes in tissue surrounding ICH, in Pia HW, Langmaid C, Zierski J (eds): *Spontaneous Intracerebral Haematomas, Advances in Diagnosis and Therapy.* New York, Springer-Verlag, 1980, pp 121–128

CHAPTER 50
Surgical Management of Cranial Arteriovenous Malformations

Russel H. Patterson, Jr.

INTRACRANIAL VASCULAR MALFORMATIONS have been classified by McCormick[1,2] as telangiectases, varices, cavernous malformations, venous malformations, and arteriovenous malformations (AVMs). Some of the clinical and pathologic distinctions are summarized in Table 50-1.

Approximately 20 percent of strokes are associated with hemorrhage. Of these, the ratio of parenchymal brain hemorrhage to subarachnoid hemorrhage is approximately 3:1. Rupture of an AVM accounts for only 10 percent of the cases of subarachnoid hemorrhage.

Hemorrhage is the first sign of an AVM in approximately 50 percent of the of cases. Small AVMs tend to bleed and rebleed more than large ones, and the hematoma associated with a small AVM is likely to be larger than one associated with a large AVM. Seizures are a sign of an AVM in approximately one-third of the cases, and perhaps 10 percent of the patients with an AVM present with a hemorrhage associated with a seizure.[2-5]

AVMs are not a cause of classical migraine headache; however, they may produce a headache associated with an unusual aura that lasts into the phase of the headache or even comes on after the onset of the headache. AVMs also have been blamed for progressive neurologic deficit, but this is relatively rare, except possibly in those cases that involve the brainstem or those that produce progressive hemodynamic steals.

Approximately 80 percent of AVMs are detectable on an unenhanced computed tomogram, and almost all of them will be revealed on an enhanced scan.[6,7] AVMs may be situated anywhere in the brain, and their frequency in a given region approximates the ratio of the mass of the region with respect to the whole brain.

Preoperative Evaluation

Complete multi-vessel arteriography is the single most important aid in both diagnosing and planning surgery for the patient with an AVM. Since adequate treatment of the patient requires that all the vessels feeding *to* the malformation be completely obliterated, a *complete* arteriogram is necessary to document each and every feeder vessel. The angiogram also may reveal associated abnormalities such as tumor or aneurysm. Since 15 percent of AVMs are supplied by branches of the external carotid artery, preoperative studies should include information regarding the arteries that normally supply the extracranial compartment in addition to those supplying the intracranial compartment. Complete arteriography also includes such techniques as

Division of Neurological Surgery, Cornell University Medical College, New York, New York

Table 50-1. Classification of Vascular Malformations According to McCormick[1]

Telangiectasis: A small conglomeration of thin-walled capillaries separated by normal parenchyma. It is common in the pons or at the gray–white matter junctions and is only occasionally associated with hemorrhage.

Varix: A dilated anomalous or normal vein that is usually a singular structure with normal surrounding parenchyma. It occasionally is responsible for massive hemorrhage.

Cavernous malformation: A mass of sinusoidal vascular spaces; commonly a small mass in the cerebrum, with associated calcium with no parenchyma between vessels. It is an infrequent lesion in the brain that occasionally ruptures. Angiography may reveal only mass effect and no pathologic circulation.

Venous malformation: A mass of abnormal vessels, generally small, with no direct arterial feeders, but with a central draining vein. The abnormal vessels are separated by relatively normal parenchyma. This is one of the most common of the vascular malformations in the nervous system; only rarely is it a source of hemorrhage.

Arterio-venous malformation: A mass of abnormal vessels with enlarged arterial feeders and large draining veins. The anomalous vessels may have the histologic characteristics of arteries or veins. The mass tends to be wedge-shaped with a broad base on the cortical surface and the apex pointing to the ventricle. The parenchyma surrounding the abnormal vessels is commonly gliotic. This lesion is the most likely of the five forms of vascular malformation to hemorrhage; it may present in any anatomic location within the nervous system.

magnification, subtraction, rapid-sequence exposure, and multi-view radiography in order to obtain maximum arteriographic information. Information gained from computerized tomography (CT) and studies of regional cerebral blood flow sometimes provides additional helpful data concerning the neighboring brain as well as the dimensions of the AVM and its relation to nearby important anatomic structures.[6-8]

In addition to providing information about the morphology of an AVM, the neuroradiologist has assumed an important role in their treatment.[9] Many AVMs may be embolized preoperatively and significantly devascularized with Gelfoam, silicone beads, or injectable glues.[10-14] For AVMs with one or two major feeders, the feeders occasionally may be occluded just before surgery with the aid of an intravascular detachable balloon, as described by Debrun (see Chapter 53).[15] Inherent in all of these techniques is the risk that the development of collaterals, given sufficient time, will erode the gains made by embolization. Because of this, surgery should follow an embolization procedure within a few weeks. The hope is that the preoperative embolization will help the surgeon by devascularizing the mass, making removal easier and therefore safer for the patient. Embolization alone occasionally obliterates an AVM, but most often a few feeders remain. Partial embolization does not reduce the chances of recurrent hemorrhage, so surgery is almost always required.

Surgical Techniques Employed in the Management of AVMs

The ideal treatment of all AVMs is complete excision. Lesser measures, such as partial embolization and interruption of major feeding arteries, reduce the AVM only temporarily and offer *very* little protection from hemorrhage. Consequently, excision remains the primary form of therapy. The principles of surgery, while common knowledge, are nevertheless worth reiterating.

The craniotomy always should be large enough to expose and allow access to all the major arterial feeders and draining veins. The usual strategy is to begin by interrupting each important arterial feeder as close as possible to the AVM itself so as to avoid important branches that might also supply eloquent brain. Some have proposed beginning the attack on an AVM by cannulating and embolizing major feeding arteries under direct vision.[16] After cannulating the artery, an angiogram is taken to confirm that the artery supplies the AVM exclusively and not brain. Then the embolic material, usually cyanocrylate glue and Pantopaque in a 50-50 mixture, is injected. This strategy reduces the vascularity of the AVM at the price of either turning part of it into a hard mass, which may be difficult to remove, or glueing or encasing a possibly important nutrient artery from normal brain to the AVM. Using the ligated arterial feeder as a handle, one works toward a common final pedicle involving a primary, major venous drainage channel and a few deep arterial feeders, such as the choroidal arteries in the ventricle. In removing the AVM one must be careful to encircle all 360° of the mass as well as to remain within the gliotic plane between tumor and brain. Where a hematoma exists, it usually has dissected the natural plane of separation between tumor and brain. Suspicious-looking brain that is discolored or that contains small vascular channels most likely is a residual knuckle of the arteriovenous malformation and should be excised.

If the ventricle has been entered, as it usually is, it should be packed off with cottonoids to prevent blood from spilling into the ventricular system, which could lead to the development of hydrocephalus. In the case of an AVM that is nestled up against cranial nerves, it usually will peel off the involved cranial nerve with careful microdissection. When in doubt about clipping and dividing a vessel, a trial of occlusion by holding the vessel closed with the tips of forceps may provide sufficient evidence to make a decision. Local bleeding generally will be controlled with local packing and direct pressure, with or without the use of head-tilt or induced systemic arterial hypotension. Vessels traced into a deep sulcus may be sorted out with the aid of loupe magnification or the operating microscope.

In general, a single vessel that is surrounded by relatively normal parenchyma and that leads to the AVM is likely to be either a feeder or an artery supplying normal structures. A vessel among a series of vessels, with minimal parenchyma surrounding it, likely represents a primary portion of the AVM.

Large feeders are best dealt with by ligating them with metal clips and then sharply dividing them, since coagulation is unreliable. Hemostasis sometimes may be improved by applying Gelfoam, topical thrombin, or peroxide-soaked cotton balls locally. Lesions occupying the tips of the frontal or occipital poles, for example, may be dealt with either by partial lobectomy as described by Kempe[17] or Patterson et al.[18] Before closing the dura, it is useful to elevate the blood pressure to the range of 150 mm Hg systolic, which usually will precipitate bleeding from any residual portion of the malformation.

In order to remove an AVM from an eloquent area of brain, Garretson recommends operating under local anesthesia and identifying speech and motor areas by electrically stimulating the cerebral cortex. His results, which showed that 38 of 39 patients were able to resume their former occupations following complete excision of an AVM, are impressive.[19]

AVMs in Specific Locations

Dural

Intracranial AVMs may have an associated extracranial component communicating via the dura or scalp. Preoperative embolization followed by careful interruption of the dura near the venous sinuses is important. The major sinuses and veins should be preserved to prevent cerebral venous infarction postoperatively. After the intracranial portion is removed, the dura that has been excised is replaced with a graft, and consideration is given to the need for scalp flaps as well.[20-23]

Intraventricular

Intraventricular lesions generally are supplied primarily by choroidal vessels. After standard craniotomy and corticotomy the lesion is exposed through a generous window into the ventricle. After the foramen of Monro has been adequately packed off with cottonoids, the standard principles of excision then may be employed to remove the intraventricular lesion. Yasargil et al. have described the microsurgical excision of AVMs involving both the corpus callosum and the ventricle.[24]

Cerebellar Lesions

Cerebellar AVMs generally are amenable to excision via a wide suboccipital craniectomy and application of the principles outlined for cerebral AVMs. Some posterior fossa AVMs involve the lateral or sigmoid sinuses. If division of one of the major sinuses is anticipated, the best test for the safety of the maneuver is to obstruct the sinus temporarily and observe the brain. If sectioning the tentorium, the tentorium and cerebrum should be retracted together to avoid tearing the draining veins.

Cerebellopontine Angle–Brainstem AVMs

These lesions generally peel off of the cerebellum, brainstem, and cranial nerves as long as care is exercised to remain within the plane separating the AVM from normal brain. Some of these lesions, like AVMs of the spinal cord, sit in the subarachnoid cisterns or on the pial surface of the brain. Other AVMs, however, infiltrate the brainstem, in which case they are not removable, except perhaps by using circulatory arrest under deep hypothermia. Even then there is risk to functional nerve tissue. Cerebellopontine angle AVMs sometimes have to be approached by a combination subtentorial– supratentorial exposure. This approach provides satisfactory access to posterior cerebral and superior cerebellar arterial feeders, and as well allows adequate handling of vessels that may be straddling the tentorium. Detailed descriptions of surgical technique can be found in the literature.[4,25-26]

Postoperative Evaluation

Just as the morphology of the AVM cannot be documented without complete arteriography, neither can surgical cure be documented without arteriography. Residual lesions may be treated with follow-up surgery, additional embolization, and perhaps in some cases with the aid of radiation therapy.[27] Similarly, for lesions in inaccessible locations i.e., in the basal ganglia or thalamus, embolization, stereotactic treatment by means of heat or cold, or even radiation therapy may be necessary.[27]

Special Considerations

AVMs occasionally are associated with a tumor or with aneurysms. In the case of the associated tumor, the AVM may be dealt with first and the tumor removed either at the same or a second operation. In the case of associated aneurysms, the aneurysms are best dealt with during the primary attack or just preceding the primary attack on the arteriovenous malformation. Such lesions are often but not always located in the circulation proximal to the AVM. When they are located proximal to the AVM, they may be dealt with at the same operation. When an aneurysm is located in another area of the cerebral circulation, however, it should be treated first, unless there is clear-cut information (such as a computed tomogram) documenting hemorrhage from the AVM. A recent review by Gamache et al. summarizes the experience in this regard.[28]

REFERENCES

1. McCormick WF: The pathology of vascular ("arteriovenous") malformations. *J Neurosurg* 24:807–816, 1966
2. McCormick WF, Hardman GM, Boulter TR: Vascular malformation "angiomas" of the brain with special reference to those occurring in the posterior fossa. *J Neurosurg* 28:241–251, 1968
3. Paterson JH, McKissock W: A clinical survey of intracranial angiomas with special reference to their mode of progression and surgical treatment. A report of 110 cases. *Brain* 79:233–266, 1956

4. Patterson RH Jr, Gamache FW Jr: Arteriovenous malformations of the posterior fossa: a review, in Fein J, Flamm E, (eds): *Cerebrovascular Diseases,* New York, Springer-Verlag, 1981, pp 120–160

5. Perret G, Nishioka H: Report on the cooperative study of intracranial aneurysms and subarachnoid hemorrhage VI. Arteriovenous malformations. *J Neurosurg 25*:467–490, 1966

6. Pressman BD, Kirkwood JR, Davis DO: Computerized transverse tomography of vascular lesions of the brain. Part I. *Am J Roentgenol 124*:208–214, 1975

7. Terbrugge K, Scotti G, Eitheir R, et al: Computed tomography in intracranial arteriovenous malformation. *Radiology 122*:703–705, 1977

8. Debrun G, Chartres A: Infra and supratentorial arteriovenous malformation. A general review. *Neuroradiology 3*:184–192, 1972

9. Cromwell LD, Harris AB: Treatment of cerebral arteriovenous malformation. A combined neurosurgical and neuroradiological approach. *J Neurosurg 52*:705–708, 1980

10. Dubois PG, Kerber CW, Heinz ER: Interventional techniques in neuroradiology. *Radiol Clin N Am 17*:515–542, 1979

11. Djindjian R, Cophignon J, Theron J, et al: Embolization by superselective arteriography from the femoral route. Review of 60 cases 1. Technique, Indications, Complications. *Neuroradiology 6*:20–26, 1973

12. Kerber CW: Catheter therapy: fluoroscopic monitoring of deliberate embolic occlusion. *Radiology 125*:538–540, 1977

13. Kricheff I, Madayag M, Braumstein P: Transfemoral catheter embolization of cerebral and posterior fossa arteriovenous malformations. *Radiology 103*:107–111, 1972

14. Wolpert SM, and Stein BM: Catheter embolization of intracranial arteriovenous malformations as an aid to surgical excision. *Neuroradiology 10*:73–85, 1975

15. Debrun G, Lacour P, Caron JP: Balloon arterial catheter techniques in the treatment of intracranial disease, in Krayenbuhl H (ed): *Advances and Technical Standards in Neurosurgery,* Vienna: vol 4. Springer-Verlag, pp 131–145

16. Vlahovitch B, Fuentes JM: Embolization of cerebral angiomas by cerebral catheterization of cortical arteries, *Neuroradiology 11*:243–248, 1976

17. Kempe LG: Arteriovenous malformation, in *Operative Neurosurgery,* vol 1. New York Springer-Verlag, 1968, pp 244–263

18. Patterson RH Jr, Voorhies RM: Surgical approaches to intracranial and intraspinal arteriovenous malformations. *Clin Neurosurg 25*:412–424, 1978

19. Garretson NH: Surgery of arteriovenous malformations. Presented at the Sixth Joint Meeting on Stroke and Cerebral Circulation, Los Angeles. Feb. 12–14, 1981

20. Fernandez-Urdanibia J, Silvela J, Soto M: Occipital dural arteriovenous malformations. *Neuroradiology 7*:57–64, 1972

21. Houser OW, Baker HC, Rhoton AL, et al: Intracranial dural arteriovenous malformations. *Radiology 105*:55–64, 1972

22. Kosnik EJ, Hunt WF, Miller CA: Dural arteriovenous malformations. *J Neurosurg 40*:322–329, 1974

23. Manaka S, Izawa M, Nawata H: Dural arteriovenous malformations treated by artificial embolization with liquid silicone. *Surg Neurol 7*:63–65, 1977

24. Yasargil MG, Jain KK, Antic J, et al: Arteriovenous malformations of the splenium of the corpus collosum: microsurgical treatment. *Surg Neurol 5*:5–14, 1976

25. Drake CG: Surgical removal of arteriovenous malformations from brain stem and cerebellopontine angle. *J Neurosurg 43*:661–670, 1975

26. Patterson RH Jr, Fraser RA: Vascular neoplasms of the brainstem: a place for profound hypothermia and circulatory arrest. *Adv Neurosurg 3*:425–428, 1975

27. Steiner L, Leksell L, Greitz T, et al: Stereotactic radiosurgery in intracranial arteriovenous malformations. *Acta Neurochir (Suppl) 21*:195–209, 1974

28. Gamache FW Jr, Drake CG, Peerless SJ, Girvin JP: Intracranial arteriovenous malformations associated with intracranial aneurysm: a review. *J Neurosurg* (in press)

CHAPTER 51
Treatment of Multiple and Asymptomatic Aneurysms

Lester A. Mount   Ronald Brisman

THE TREATMENT OF MULTIPLE ANEURYSMS is in essence the treatment of asymptomatic aneurysms. All neurosurgeons agree that surgical treatment of symptomatic aneurysms is indicated, whenever possible. There is no unanimity of opinion regarding the treatment of asymptomatic aneurysm. Representative of the diversity of opinion, covering the past 23 years, are the following: Poppen and Fager[1] in 1959, Pool and Potts[2] in 1965, Hamby[3] in 1959, Pouyanne and associates in 1970[4] and 1973[5]. Moyes[6] in 1971, and Mount and Brisman in 1971[7] and 1973[8] advocated treatment of all intracranial aneurysms. Bjorkesten and Troupp[9] in 1960, Mc Kissock and coworkers[10] in 1964, and Paterson and Bond[11] in 1973 did not think treatment of an unruptured aneurysm was indicated, Heiskanen and Marttila[12] suggested clipping the asymptomatic aneurysm if it could be reached through the same approach used to treat the symptomatic aneurysm, but they did not advise a second operation to clip it. Drake stated that he "has long held the view that, provided the operation on a ruptured aneurysm has gone well, a nearby unruptured sac, known to be of operable size and position, should also be dealt with. If the one or more other unruptured aneurysms are remote or of a special nature, then they can be left for another operation" (p.274).[12]

Incidence

In 1955, Bigelow[14] collected 2737 patients with intracranial aneurysms, of which 10 percent were multiple. McKissock and associates,[10] in 1964, reported an angiographic incidence of multiplicity in 14 percent of 1686 cases and 28 percent in autopsy cases. In the Cooperative Study[15] 19 percent of 3321 clinically diagnosed cases were multiple and in the autopsy series, 22 percent. Because of the high incidence of multiplicity, complete, four-vessel arteriography is required in any patient with an intracranial aneurysm.

Clinical Material

Between 1958 and 1980 there were 197 patients with multiple aneurysms, representing an incidence of 19 percent. Eighty-one percent were females. The average age for the group was the same as that for patients with single aneurysms; 58 percent occurred between the ages of 40 and

Department of Neurological Surgery, New York Neurological Institute, Columbia-Presbyterian Medical Center, College of Physicians and Surgeons, Columbia University, New York, New York

Table 51-1. Location of 475 Aneurysms in 197 Patients

Internal carotid	309
Middle cerebral	89
Anterior cerebral and anterior communicating	45
Posterior circulation	32

59. Blood pressure was elevated in 32 percent. Subarachnoid hemorrhage was the presenting symptom in 74 percent.

Location of Aneurysms

One hundred ninety-seven patients had 475 aneurysms, 309 of the internal carotid artery (30 of which were intracavernous), 89 of the middle cerebral, 45 of the anterior cerebral or anterior communicating arteries, and 32 of the posterior circulation (Table 51-1). There were 122 patients with two aneurysms, 29 with three, 11 with four, and 2 with five. There were 96 patients with bilateral symmetric aneurysms. One patient had bilateral symmetric aneurysms of both internal carotid arteries within the cavernous sinus and both middle cerebral arteries.

Results of Treatment

In the Cooperative Study the mortality rate for nonsurgically treated patients was 70 percent of the 252 patients who had multiple aneurysms and subarachnoid hemorrhage and were followed a maximum of 3 years. In our series 49 patients were treated nonsurgically and in 65 one aneurysm was treated surgically. Sixty-six patients had 2 aneurysms treated by surgery, 9 had all three, 3 had all four, and 2 had all five (Table 51-2).

One hundred and sixteen patients did not have all their aneurysms treated, including 49 who had no surgical procedure at all. In this group there were good results in 59 percent, poor in 27 percent, and death occurred in 19 percent. (These results cannot be compared to those in surgically treated patients.) Of 81 patients with 186 aneurysms, all of which were treated surgically by intracranial clipping, muslin wrapping, plastic spraying, or extracranial carotid ligation, 95.2 percent had good results, 2.4 percent poor, and 2.4 percent died (Table 51-3). In the group of 60 patients with 138 aneurysms, all of which were treated intracranially (100 operations), there were good results in 96.8 percent, poor in 1.6 percent, and death occurred in 1.6 percent (Table 51-4). In 1 patient who died, both aneurysms were clipped at one operation. Today this patient would not be considered a satisfactory risk at the time he was operated upon. Forty patients had elective craniotomies to treat 48 unruptured (multiple) aneurysms, with good results in 39 cases

Table 51-2. Treatment

Aneurysms treated	No. of Patients
Nonsurgical	49
Surgical	
One aneurysm only	65
Both aneurysms	66
All three	12
All four	3
All five	2

Table 51-3. Results of Surgical Treatment in 81 Patients Having 186 Aneurysms

Result	Percentage of Patients
Good	95.2
Poor	2.4
Died	2.4

and no operative mortality (Table 51-5). The 1 patient with a poor result had an asymptomatic aneurysm of the middle cerebral artery at the origin of a large lenticulostriate artery. It was coated with Selverstone plastic material. This patient did well for 1 month and then developed sudden hemiparesis. Arteriography did not show the aneurysm or the lenticulostriate artery.

A severe neurologic deficit existed in 5 percent of the surgical patients and 18 percent of the nonsurgical patients at the time the decision was made as to whether to operate. Most of the patients treated conservatively were not operated upon because of the multiplicity of their aneurysms. This was thought, by some physicians, in the earlier part of the study (late 1950s), to contraindicate surgery. During this same period, some of the asymptomatic aneurysms were not treated surgically, as this was considered unnecessary by some doctors. The two groups are not comparable however.

Discussion

The question is how to treat the asymptomatic aneurysm. In 1897 Gowers[16] wrote: "If there is an aneurysm, the prognosis is extremely grave for no one knows how near or how far may be the fatal rupture."

How near the fatal rupture may be is shown by a patient with a ruptured aneurysm of the left middle cerebral artery and a 3 mm unruptured one that arose from the right internal carotid artery. Her course was stormy, with persisting arteriospasm, but eventually the middle cerebral artery aneurysm was clipped. The patient slowly made an excellent recovery, but she was debilitated and apprehensive when she was sent home for further recuperation before her second operation. Two days later she was readmitted with fatal rupture of the 3-mm aneurysm of the right internal carotid artery, which was found at autopsy.

How far the fatal rupture may be is illustrated by a patient with two aneurysms, one at each internal carotid artery bifurcation, demonstrated by arteriography. The symptomatic one was clipped. Twenty-three years later the other aneurysm ruptured and the patient died.

The precarious nature of the unruptured aneurysm is demonstrated by autopsy examination, which in one case showed necrosis, phagocytosis, and hemorrhage in the wall of the aneurysm, indicating that it would soon have ruptured.

An existing aneurysm remains a permanent threat to the patient as long as he lives. The natural history of the asymptomatic companion of a ruptured aneurysm indicates that there is continuing morbidity and mortality with each passing year. In this series of 158 patients, 99 from the literature was 59 of our own, the rate of subarachnoid hemorrhage was 10 percent and mor-

Table 51-4. Intracranial Surgical Treatment of 60 Patients Having 138 Aneurysms

Result	Percentage of Patients
Good	96.8
Poor	1.6
Died	1.6

Table 51-5. Intracranial Surgical Treatment of 40 Patients Having 48 Unruptured Aneurysms

Result	No. of Patients	Percentage of Patients
Good	39	97.5
Poor	1	2.5
Death	0	

tality was 4 percent in an average period of only 5 years (Table 51-6). The surgical results of the direct intracranial treatment of asymptomatic aneurysms were better. In 40 patients, 15 of Moyes and 24 of our own, there was no mortality and morbidity was 5 percent.

The intracranial treatment of an unruptured aneurysm is like an anatomic dissection and, as shown above, is very safe when magnification is used (microscope, loops, or both) and the operating team is skilled in aneurysm surgery. After treatment, the patient can resume his normal life style, without fear of the aneurysm rupturing.

When should the asymptomatic aneurysm be treated? If it is in the same operative field, it should be treated at the same time as the symptomatic aneurysm. If a second operation is required, it should be done at the earliest feasible time. The timing, however, as well as the decision to operate must be based on the patient's neurologic, mental, and medical status as well as the surgical accessibility of the aneurysm. Even the smallest aneurysms rupture; hence, the patient is in danger, regardless of the size of the aneurysm. The patient's physiologic age is more important than his chronologic age. Therefore, only physiologic status is considered important.

It is recommended that all intracranial aneurysms be treated by surgery, preferably by direct intracranial methods, when there is a reasonable chance of success. An illustrative case is that of a patient who had five aneurysms, all of which were treated successfully. These were located on each internal carotid artery, one on the middle cerebral, one on the anterior communicating, and one at the apex of the basilar artery.

Summary

One hundred and ninety-seven patients had a combined total of 475 aneurysms. Of 81 patients in whom all 186 aneurysms were treated surgically 95.2 percent had good results, 2.4 percent had poor results, and 2.4 percent died. In 60 patients who had all 138 of their aneurysms treated intracranially in 100 operations, the results were good in 96.8 percent, poor in 1.6 percent, and 1.6 percent died. Elective craniotomies to treat unruptured (multiple) aneurysms 40 produced good results in 39 of 40 patients and there was no mortality.

It is recommended that all multiple intracranial aneurysms be treated surgically, preferably by direct intracranial methods, when there is a reasonable chance of success.

Table 51-6. Natural History of Unruptured Aneurysms

Source	No. of Patients at Risk	Time (yr)	No. Patients SAH	Death
Heiskanen/Marttila	76	0.3-11	8	3
Mount/Brisman	59	0.1-10	4	1
Moyes	23	1.0-10	4	2
Total	158		16 (10%)	6 (4%)

SAH = Subarachnoid hemorrhage

REFERENCES

1. Poppen JL, Fager CA: Multiple intracranial aneurysms. *J Neurosurg 16*:581–589, 1959
2. Pool JL, Potts DG: *Aneurysms and Arteriovenous Anomalies of the Brain. Diagnosis and Treatment.* New York, Harper and Row, 1965, p 287
3. Hamby WB: Multiple intracranial aneurysms. *J Neurosurg 16*:558–563, 1959
4. Pouyanne H, Riemens V, Guerin J, et al: Less aneurysmes saculaires multiples du systeme carotidien. Indications et resultats de l'abord direct. *Neurochirurgie 16*:25–31, 1970
5. Pouyanne H, Banayan A, Guerin J, et al: Less aneurysmes sacculaires multiples du systeme carotidien supra clinoidien. Etude anatomoclinique et therapeutique. *Neurochirurgie 19:Suppl 1,* 1973
6. Moyes PD: Surgical treatment of multiple aneurysms and of incidentally discovered unruptured aneurysms. *J Neurosurg 35*:291–295, 1971
7. Mount LA, Brisman R: Treatment of multiple intracranial aneurysms. *J Neurosurg 35*:728–730, 1971
8. Mount LA, Brisman R: Treatment of multiple aneurysms—symptomatic and asymptomatic, *Clinical Neurosurgery,* vol. 21. Baltimore, Williams & Wilkins, 1974, pp 166–170
9. Bjorkesten G, Troupp H: Multiple intracranial arterial aneurysms. *Acta Chir Scand 118*:387–391, 1960
10. McKissock W, Richardson A, Walsh L, et al: Multiple intracranial aneurysms. *Lancet 1*:623–626, 1964
11. Paterson A, Bond MR: Treatment of multiple intracranial arterial aneurysms. *Lancet 1*:1302–1304, 1973
12. Drake CG, Girvin, JP: The surgical treatment of subarachnoid hemorrhage with multiple aneurysms, in Morley TP (ed): *Current Controversies in Neurosurgery.* Philadelphia, Saunders, 1976, pp 274–278
13. Heiskanen O, Marttila I: Risk of rupture of a second aneurysm in patients with multiple aneurysms. *J Neurosurg 32*:295–299, 1970
14. Bigelow NH: Multiple intracranial arterial aneurysms: an analysis of their significance. *Arch Neurol Psychiatry 73*:76–99, 1955
15. Sahs AL, Perret GE, Locksley HB, et al: Intracranial aneurysms and subarachnoid hemorrhage. A cooperative study. Philadelphia, Lippincott, 1969, p 50
16. Gowers WR: *A Manual of Diseases of the Nervous System,* vol 2. 2nd ed. Philadelphia, Blakiston, 1897, p 538

CHAPTER 52

Stereotactic Clipping of Arterial Aneurysms and Arteriovenous Malformations of the Brain

Edward I. Kandel   Vyacheslav V. Peresedov

GREAT ADVANCES IN THE SURGERY of cerebral arterial aneurysms and arteriovenous malformations (AVMs) have been achieved during the past two decades as a result of the development of microsurgical technique and modern anesthesiologic methods. In spite of that remarkable progress, however, many problems remain unsolved. In the case of arterial aneurysms, a direct attack very often is technically difficult because of the possibility of serious complications and mortality from rupture or arterial spasm. The risk to the patient increases greatly in acute stages of subarachnoid hemorrhage (SAH), in the presence of arterial spasm, or in cases of cerebral infarction or hematoma, which may be aggravated by the surgery.

In the case of AVMs there is a problem of palliative treatment. If the AVM is deep-seated, involves functionally important areas of the brain, or is of giant size, a direct attack may be dangerous or impossible. Statistics from the largest series of AVMs reported in the literature indicate that only about 45 percent of hemispheric malformations can be totally extirpated. In the remaining 55 percent radical extirpation is impossible and only palliative procedures can be applied. Many patients are considered untreatable by any known method.

These difficulties and disadvantages of common surgery have stimulated an intensive search for newer and safer methods of treating aneurysms and AVMs of the brain, including artificial embolization of aneurysms, the use of intravascular balloon catheters, and injection of suspended iron particles and the application of an external magnetic field.

Another new approach to the problem consists of using stereotactic techniques. Stereotactic techniques have undergone outstanding development during the past three decades. The first attempts to apply stereotactic methods for visual clipping of the feeding vessels of deep-seated and poorly accessible AVMs were made about 20 years ago.[1,2] The operations were done by the classic open approach. After an ordinary flap craniotomy had been performed, a stereotactic device was installed and a thin probe was introduced and directed toward the AVM. After the probe touched the AVM, a cortical incision was made and a routine approach to the lesion was performed using the probe as a guide. The clipping of vessels and the removal of the AVM was made *ad occulus*. Riechert and Mundinger[2] reported 4 cases of deep-seated AVMs successfully removed in this way.

It should be noted that the stereotactic method was used only to locate the AVM in these cases; all other manipulations, including clipping, were carried out under visual control with ordinary instruments.

Neurosurgical Clinic, Institute of Neurology, Moscow, USSR

In the past few years the technique of metallic thrombosis of arterial aneurysms of the brain was developed. Alksne and Rand,[3] using stereotactic methods, introduced a magnetic cannula 6 mm in diameter to the dome of an arterial aneurysm. The wall of the aneurysm was punctured with a fine needle inserted through the cannula and a suspension of iron particles was injected into the aneurysm, resulting in intra-aneurysmal thrombosis. Alksne and Smith[4] recently reported the results of stereotactic occlusion of anterior communicating artery aneurysms by means of an iron-acrylic mixture introduced into the carotid. Seventeen of 22 patients treated in this manner have shown complete thrombosis of the aneurysms.

Mullan[5] reported his experience in producing stereotactic intra-aneurysmal thrombosis by means of several fine steel needles inserted into the aneurysmal sac, after which positive direct electric current was applied. The results were satisfactory in most cases, but there were 4 postoperative deaths directly attributed to the procedure, while 8 patients showed incomplete obliteration.

Four patients with anterior communicating-anterior cerebral arterial aneurysms were operated upon by Samotokin and Hilko,[6] who stereotactically introduced thin electrodes into the aneurysms. This was followed by anodal electrolysis for 1 to 3 hours. The operation was combined with intravenous infusion of coagulants. In all cases the volume of the aneurysm was reduced by 30 to 40 percent, but complete thrombosis was not achieved. One case of successful stereotactic thrombosis of an anterior communicating artery aneurysm and another case of stereotaxic electrocoagulation of a single vessel feeding a small AVM in the frontal lobe of an 8-year-old child also have been reported.[7,8]

Despite encouraging results, the stereotactic methods of managing arterial aneurysms and AVMs is used seldom and has not been put into common neurosurgical practice. This situation prompted us to propose a new approach to the problem and to develop a "pure" stereotactic operation for clipping vessels or aneurysmal necks in deep areas of the brain through an ordinary burr hole.[9,10] The primary purpose of this method was to achieve a higher degree of safety in the surgery of aneurysms and AVMs.

Before its clinical use, the new method was tried in technical and animal experiments. The reliability of clipping was tested in a special model consisting of thin-walled silicone tubes. After being placed on the tube, the clips tolerated an elevation of the pressure in the system up to more than 300 mm Hg. In animal experiments the carotid or femoral arteries of dogs under general anesthesia were clipped with the device. The vessels were securely clipped in all cases. Morphologic controls demonstrated lack of damage to the vascular walls.

In another series of experiments the clips were introduced into the brains of dogs for different time intervals from several hours to 6 months. Morphologic investigations disclosed that the perifocal reaction of brain tissue was minimal.

Technical Equipment

The equipment for the new operative technique consists of two main components: a stereotactic apparatus and a special device for clipping.

The stereotactic apparatus has been described previously (Fig. 52-1).[11] It is relatively simple in design and use, compact and light weight. The patient is placed in the supine position on a head rest that has three plastic supports 5 cm in diameter. A metallic frame is installed on the head rest that consists of two semiarcs joined by two horizontal bars. The portion of the stereotactic apparatus that is not connected to the head rest also consists of two parts. The first part is a thin, square, metallic platform, which is fixed in a burr hole made in the convexity of the skull with the aid of a wrench. The main part of the stereotactic apparatus is attached to the platform. This part has two small perpendicular arcs graduated in degrees and the holder structure. There is a roller mechanism for guiding the fixation and direction of cannulas (electrode) or clipping devices of different diameters. The guide mechanism of the apparatus makes it possible to

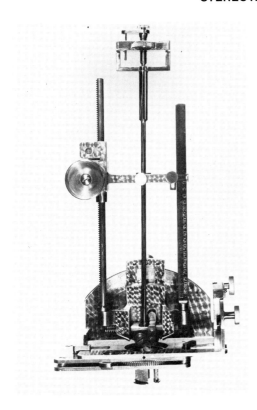

Fig. 52-1. The device for stereotactic clipping combined with the stereotactic apparatus.

insert the cannula or clipping instrument gradually into the brain and to fix it at any depth with an accuracy of ± 0.5 mm.

Our newly designed device for stereotactic clipping* consists of several parts (Fig. 52-2). The main part of the device is a stainless steel tube 17 cm long with the outer diameter of 3.2 mm. There is a conical narrowing inside the tip of the tube. It is this narrowing of the tube that opens and closes the clip. At the outer end of the tube there is a special structure, which consists of a shackle with two nuts. This controls opening and closing the clip and disconnecting the clip from the device after it has been applied to the vessel or aneurysm.

There are also two interchangeable metal pivots that are inserted into the tube. The first (guide) pivot has a thin terminal segment that protrudes from the end of the tube for several millimeters. The length of the segment that emerges from the tube tip is equal to the distance from the end of the tube to the ends of the clip blades when they are opened to their fullest extent. This pivot is installed in the tube, which is introduced stereotactically toward the target point in the brain. Once the target has been reached, the guide pivot is removed and a second (working) pivot with a special clip is inserted into the tube. The outer end of the second pivot has a scale graduated in millimeters that corresponds to the distance between the clip blade's as they open inside the brain.

Special removable stainless-steel clips of different size are available for use with the device. The length of the clips ranges from 10 to 17 mm, and the weight from 80 to 140 mg. The clips are of a crossing-spring or α design with parallel blades and can be used to clip vessels from 1 to 7 mm in diameter. It is important to note that the blades of a clip loaded into the 3-mm (I.D.) tube may be opened to a distance of about 8 mm.

The principle of action of the device is presented schematically in Figure 52-3. The surgeon chooses a suitable clip before the operation depending on the diameter of the artery or aneurysmal neck to be clipped as determined angiographically. The size of the clip is selected so that the

*USSR Patent No. 452336, US Patent No. 4241734

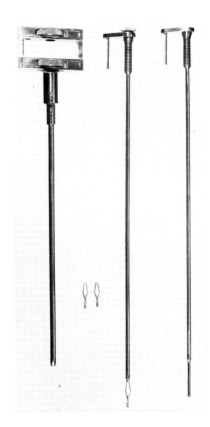

Fig. 52-2. The clipping device unassembled. Right: the tube with the special structure at the outer end for controlling clip movement; center: the second (working) pivot with a clip fixed in the grip on the pivot tip and two clips of different sizes; left: the first (guide) pivot with thin terminal segment.

width of the gap between its open blades exceeds the outer diameter of the vessel or the neck by 1.5 to 2 mm. The clip is easily attached to the tip of the working pivot before it is inserted into the tube. The fulcrum or loop of the clip is fixed in the grip of the working pivot. As the clip passes through the conical narrowing at the end of the tube, the shoulders of the loop are squeezed and the blades are opened as they emerge from the tube. When the clip loop moves past the narrow portion of the tube, the blades of the clip are closed by the spring action of the loop and the clip compresses the vessel or the aneurysmal neck. The schematic stages of clipping are shown in Figure 52-4.

Preoperative Calculations

After an exact diagnosis of the aneurysm or AVM has been made, preoperative calculations are made on angiograms in both projections. The aim of the calculations is to: (1) select the point of clipping (target point) of the feeding artery (or arteries) or the aneurysmal neck; (2) locate the point for the burr hole in the skull; and (3) determine the plane of approach for the open clip.

The target point must be chosen in accordance with several factors. In aneurysms, the target point is the neck, which has to be relatively long and narrow. The diameter of the neck at the target point is carefully measured so the degree of clip opening can be determined. Sometimes it is difficult to determine the target point because the neck is poorly visible in one or both projections. In such cases oblique angiograms are helpful.

In the case of AVMs the target may be at any point along the feeding artery (or arteries). As a rule, however, a point is selected beyond the last normal branch of the artery in the distal direction. A target point close to the AVM is desirable, but in many instances clipping a feeder close to the AVM may be dangerous because of the possibility of damaging angiomatous tissue or

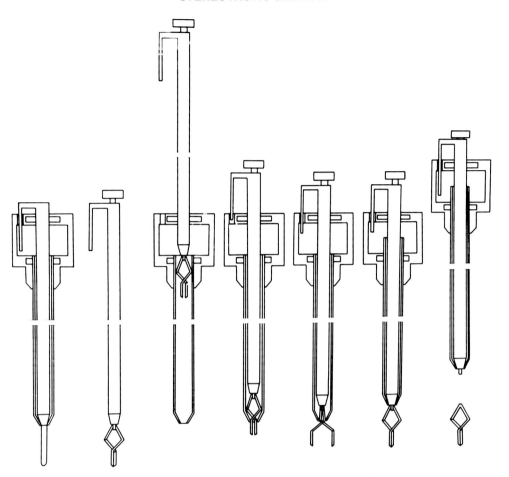

Fig. 52-3. A schematic representation of the principle of action of the clipping device (see text).

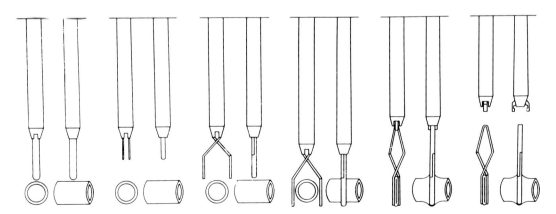

Fig. 52-4. The consecutive stages of clipping a vessel with the device (see text).

large draining veins coming from the vascular knot. Our experience has shown that clipping the hypertrophic feeding vessel quite proximal to the AVM leads to good results without any signs of neurologic deficit.

In making preoperative calculations, a knowledge of the following terms is useful: (1) target point (the center of the vessel or aneurysmal neck); (2) line of clipping (a line corresponding to the axis of the vessel or the neck); (3) line of approach (the axis of the clipping device); (4) angle of approach (the angle between 2 and 3 above); (5) plane of approach (the plane containing 2 and 3 crossing in 1); (6) plane of clipping (the plane contained by 3 perpendicular to 5); (7) axis of the burr hole (a line perpendicular to the center of the burr hole); and (8) angle of inclination (the angle between 7 and 3).

The selection of the target point and the line of clipping is made from angiograms in two projections. In choosing the center of the burr hole, which determines the location of the line of approach, one has to pay attention to the following factors: (1) the line of approach through which the tube will pass should not involve functionally important areas of the brain; (2) the best angle of approach is 90°, but it must not be less than 45° (if it is less than that critical value, the clip may slip); (3) the angle of inclination depends upon the construction of the stereotactic apparatus (in the case of our apparatus the angle must not be more than 20°). The details of the geometric calculations have been described previously.[10]

Before each operation the path of the tube of the device through different subcortical structures is analyzed with the aid of a Schaltenbrand and Bailey stereotactic atlas. The aim of the analysis is to avoid damage to functionally important structures.

Operative Technique

The operation is carried out with the patient under general anesthesia or neuroleptoanalgesia. Routine premedication is used. The patient's head is placed in the supine position on the stereotactic head-holder and fixed rigidly with two sharp pins. A sagittal line is drawn on the patient's skull and the preselected center for the burr hole is marked.

A catheter is inserted percutaneously into the carotid artery on the side of the aneurysm or AVM for intraoperative angiography.

A skin incision 4 to 5 cm long is made through the center marked for the burr hole. This incision can be placed at any point, but it is preferable to make it near the coronal suture. A burr hole 25 mm in diameter is made with a coronal trephine. The dura mater is incised. The stereotactic apparatus with the clipping device attached is fixed in the burr hole. The guide pivot is inserted into the device. After coagulation of the cortical point, the tube is introduced about 1 cm into the brain in the approximate direction of the target point.

The next stage of the operation is making the stereotactic calculations. Anterioposterior and lateral plain films are taken, and the preselected target point is transferred from the preoperative angiograms to the films taken on the operating table. Ordinary stereotactic calculations are made for the correct orientation of the clipping device. The calculations have to be made very carefully because the effectiveness of the clipping is obviously dependent upon the accuracy with which the target point can be reached. Two angles of correction in both projections are calculated and then are transferred to the protractors of the stereotactic apparatus.

Under the control of an image amplifier with a television monitor, the tube is introduced into the brain in the correct direction to the calculated depth until the tip of the guide pivot touches the target point. The guide pivot is now pulled out and is replaced by the working pivot, which carries a clip of the appropriate size. The clip is introduced to the tip of the tube.

Anteroposterior and lateral control angiograms are made. The target point on the preoperative angiograms then is transferred onto the newly obtained angiograms. If the angiograms confirm that the tip of the tube is in the correct position, the clipping device is oriented in the required plane for clip opening, as calculated before the operation. By turning a special ring on the shackle on the outer end of the device, the clip is pushed out of the tube and is opened in the immediate vicinity of the aneurysmal neck or the artery. The clip is opened by its compression in the tapered end of the tube. The distance between the clip blades in millimeters is checked on the scale on the end of the device. After the clip blades are opened to the required extent under the control of the TV monitor, angiograms again are made. If these show correct positioning of the clip, it is careful and slowly introduced a little deeper and applied to the vessel or aneurysmal neck.

At this stage of the operation the blood pressure is lowered to 50 to 70 mm Hg by intravenous injection of Arfonad. Further turning of the ring pushes the clip past the tapered end of the tube and closes it. The next angiogram should verify effective clipping.

Immediately after clipping, the patient is awakened so that normal function of the contralateral extremities can be confirmed. If this function is satisfactory, neuroleptoanalgesia is repeated and the blood pressure is increased gradually. The clip then is released from the pivot by pushing a button on the end of the working pivot. Under television control, the tube is withdrawn from the brain.

The stereotactic apparatus is released and removed. The bone "circus" is replaced and the wound is sutured. The duration of the clipping operation averages between 1.5 and 2 hours.

If it is necessary to clip two or more vessels, the entire procedure may be repeated as required.

The construction of the device provides for the opening and removal of a clip if the patient's condition is aggravated (for example, development of hemiparesis) or in case of failure such as partial or incorrect clipping. The clip may be opened and withdrawn into the tube by turning the ring of the end of the device in the opposite direction from applying the clip.

Clinical results

To date we have performed 42 stereotactic clipping operations on patients with cerebral aneurysms and AVMs in various locations. It should be emphasized that our patients as a rule endured the operation easily. The majority of patients were ambulatory 2 to 3 days after surgery. Postoperative angiography proved the success of the clipping of the vessel or aneurysm.

There were 3 complications in 42 operations. In one case there was moderate hemiparesis lasting several days, and in two cases in the early period of this study the clips slipped. In both of these cases a second successful clipping was performed. There was one mortality not directly related to the clipping operation; after successful clipping of a supraclinoid arterial aneurysm, the patient died from intracerebral hemorrhage because of the rupture of a second aneurysm in the same hemisphere.

Follow-up ranges from 4 months to 7 years. There was no rebleeding after surgery in all cases.

As our experience has shown cerebral blood flow (CBF) investigations before and after surgery appear to be the valid objective criterion for evaluating the effectiveness of stereotactic clipping operations in AVMs. It is well known that total and hemispheric CBF in the presence of an AVM is substantially increased. We study CBF by our modification of the Kety-Schmidt nitrous-oxide method. These investigations showed that highly increased CBF (from 130 percent to 340 percent of normal volume) decreased markedly after stereotactic clipping. In several cases of AVMs CBF became practically normal after surgery.

Below are several illustrative cases.

In our experience with stereotactic clipping of arterial aneurysms, the majority were aneurysms of the internal carotid artery at the site of its junction with the posterior communicating artery. These aneurysms are the most common of all intracranial aneurysms. The narrow necks of the majority of supraclinoid aneurysms make them particularly suitable to stereotactic clipping. The following case illustrates this point of view.

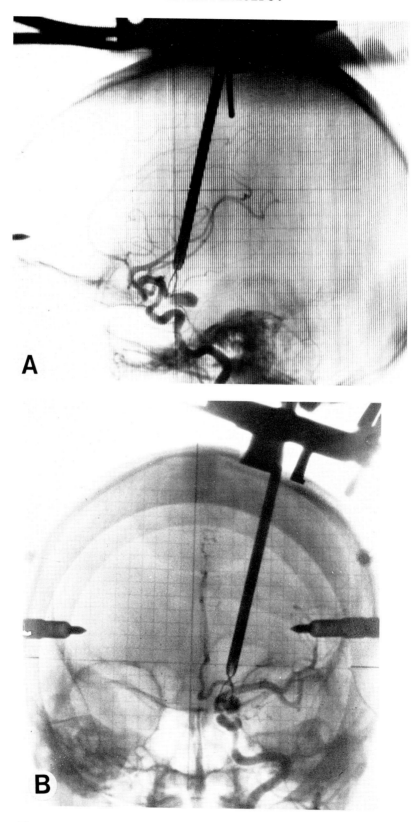

Fig. 52-5. Angiograms showing a supraclinoid internal carotid aneurysm during stereotactic clipping (A,B), and 2 weeks after surgery (C).

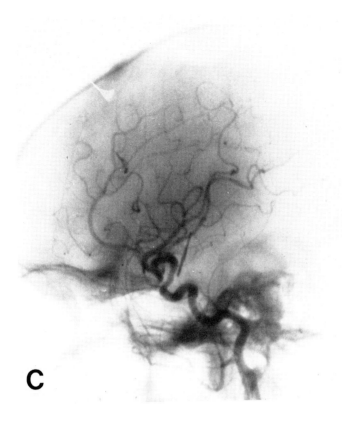

C

Case 1. A 49-year-old woman was admitted to our clinic after two severe subarachnoid hemorrhages (SAHs) 17 months and 1 month previously. Upon hospitalization her general condition was satisfactory. She had paralysis of the left third nerve, light hemiparesis of the right side, and signs of mild sensorimotor aphasia. Angiograms demonstrated a bilobed supraclinoid saccular aneurysm (14 × 7 mm in lateral projection) arising from the left internal carotid in the region of its junction with the posterior communicating artery (Figs. 52-5A and B). The neck of the aneurysm was narrow. These was mild spasm of the carotid.

Stereotactic clipping of the aneurysm neck was carried out under general anesthesia. A trephine opening was made 3 cm posterior from the coronal suture and 3 cm to the left of the midline. The stereotactic apparatus with the clipping device was installed in the opening, and a catheter was percutaneously introduced into the left common carotid. The target point (aneurysmal neck) was transferred from angiograms to the AP and lateral plain films and stereotactic calculations were made. The tip of the first pivot reached the target point at a depth of 76 mm. The guide pivot then was replaced by the working pivot with a compressed clip. The clip was placed on the aneurysmal neck, and its correct positioning was confirmed by control angiography. During the clipping the arterial pressure was lowered to 70 mm Hg.

The patient was awakened for several minutes in order to check movements in the contralateral limbs; no changes were noted. The clip was closed slowly by means of the ring on the external part of the clipping device. An additional control angiogram showed that the aneurysm neck had been clipped and that there was no filling of the aneurysm. The clip then was released and the device was withdrawn. The bone button was then put in place. The operation was performed under continuous television monitoring. The duration of the operation was 1 hour and 40 minutes. There were no postoperative complications and no neurologic changes. The patient was able to walk 3 days after surgery. Her aphasia and third nerve paralysis disappeared completely soon after the operation.

Control angiograms made 2 weeks after surgery demonstrated the elimination of the aneurysm (Fig. 52-5C). The lumen of the internal carotid artery at the level of the clip was not changed. Six years postoperatively the patient's condition is good.

Case 2. One week after a mild head injury, a 38-year-old woman was suddenly seized with severe headaches and vomiting but without loss of consciousness. Two weeks later the sharp headaches returned; these were centered mainly in the left fronto-orbital region. The same day full paralysis of the left third nerve developed.

Angiograms made immediately after admission to our clinic showed an aneurysm on the internal carotid at the point of its junction with the posterior communicating artery. Stereotactic clipping of the neck of the aneurysm, which was located at a depth of 77 mm from the cortex, was performed (Fig. 52-6A and B).

The postoperative course was uneventful. The patient was up and walking 4 days after the operation. A control an-

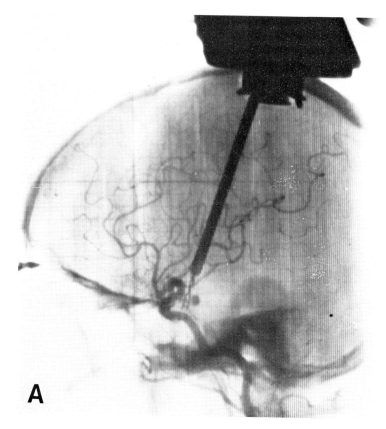

Fig. 52-6. Angiograms of a stereotactic operation on a supraclinoid aneurysm. (A) Before clipping, and (B) after stereotactic clipping.

giogram disclosed successful clipping of the aneurysm. A 2-year follow-up has shown complete recovery of third nerve function. There was no rebleeding during follow-up. The patient now works full time.

In spite of remarkable improvements in the results of direct attack of aneurysms of the anterior communicating artery the technical difficulties and rate of complications remain serious unsolved problems. Several neurosurgeons have proposed the open clipping of the dominant anterior cerebral artery in order to thrombose aneurysms of the anterior communicating artery. We believe that stereotactic clipping of the neck of such an aneurysm may be done in exceptionally rare cases but that stereotactic clipping of the dominant anterior cerebral artery is technically possible. The point of view is confirmed by the following case.

Case 3. A 44-year-old man began to suffer from sudden headaches and repeated vomiting, and on one occasion he lost consciousness for 3 hours. Initially he showed signs of meningeal irritation; he had slight pyramidal signs on the right side and bloody spinal fluid. After admission to our clinic 3 weeks later, he complained of a headache, but his general condition was good.

Right-sided axillary and carotid angiography disclosed a saccular, medium-sized aneurysm of the anterior communicating artery. Left carotid angiography showed no filling of the aneurysm, and the aneurysmal neck was not clearly visible. Since stereotactic clipping of the neck seemed technically impossible, clipping of the dominant right anterior cerebral artery was performed. A burr hole was made 1 cm anterior to the coronal suture and 3 cm to the right of the midline. The distance from the cortex to the target point was 62 mm. The clip was placed on the artery under television control.

A postoperative carotid angiogram showed that the clip had slipped and the aneurysm had refilled. A second stereotactic operation was done 2 weeks later through the same burr hole. The second clip was placed proximal to the first and 10 mm from the bifurcation of the internal carotid.

The postoperative course was free from complications. A subsequent left carotid angiogram showed that the right anterior cerebral artery was clipped and the aneurysm no longer filled. A control examination 5 years postoperatively, found the patient in excellent condition. He is working full time and has no complaints.

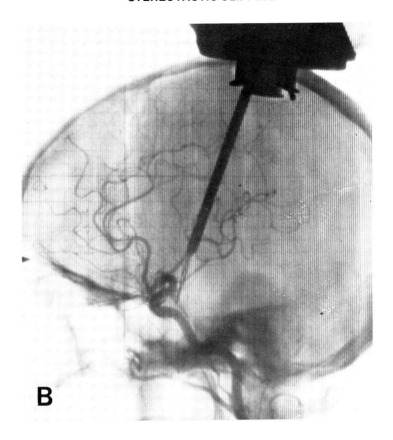

B

Aneurysms of the internal carotid bifurcation are an important surgical problem. The approach and direct attack on these aneurysms are associated with many technical difficulties. The following example illustrates the possibility of successful stereotactic clipping of such an aneurysm.

Case 4. A 48-year-old man suddenly developed severe headaches but without impairment of consciousness. A lumbar puncture was not done. About 1 month later the sharp headaches and pain in the right eye recurred. After 5 days a left-sided hemiplegia developed. The patient was admitted to our clinic; his general condition was serious. There was hemiplegia with decreased muscular tone and pathologic reflexes.

Angiography disclosed a sacular aneurysm of the internal carotid bifurcation. Marked spasm of the internal carotid and its main branches also was noted (Fig. 52-7A). The neck of the aneurysm was 2.5 mm in diameter.

After careful preoperative calculations, stereotactic clipping of the aneurysm was performed under general anesthesia (Fig. 52-7B). The depth of the target point was 77 mm.

There were no complications after the operation. Movement of left extremities gradually returned. The patient began to walk 3 weeks after the operation. A follow-up examination 6 months later showed light hemiparesis and the patient to be in good general condition.

The feeding vessels of AVMs may be successfully clipped by the stereotactic method. The cases described below confirm this point of view.

AVMs fed by the middle cerebral artery are very common. In cases in which the AVM is large and its location is in a functionally important cerebral area, radical extirpation may be dangerous and difficult. The following case illustrates successful stereotactic clipping of the main trunk of the middle cerebral artery proximal to the AVM.

Case 5. A 21-year-old woman suddenly developed sharp headaches and increased weakness in the right extremities. She then lost consiousness for 20 hours. Upon admission to our clinic there were paralysis of her right arm and deep paresis of the right leg, severe motor aphasia, marked papilledema, and bloody CSF.

Angiography demonstrated a large AVM located in the parietofrontal region and supplied by hypertrophic branches of the left middle cerebral artery (Fig. 52-8A). The AVM measured 4 × 3 × 2.5 cm.

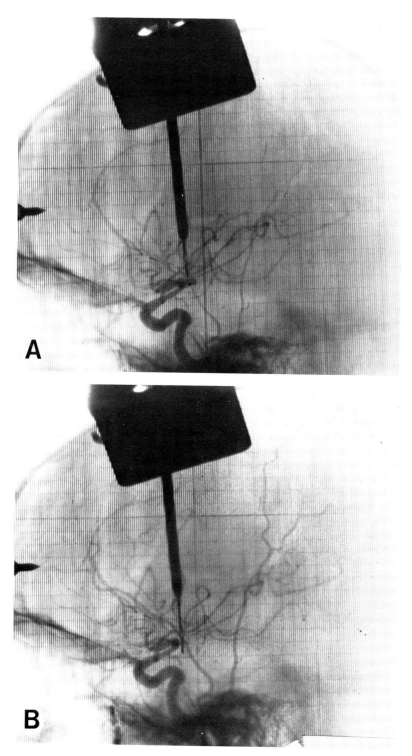

Fig. 52-7.   Angiograms of an aneurysm of the internal carotid bifurcation (A) before and (B) after stereotactic clipping

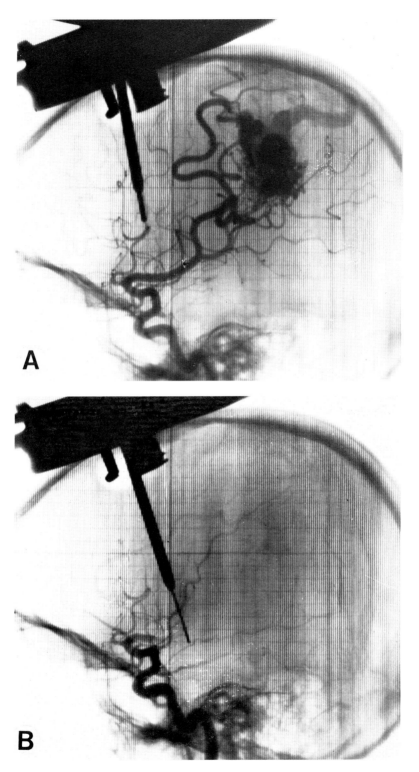

Fig. 52-8. Angiograms showing a large AVM supplied by a hypertrophic branch of the middle cerebral artery during the operation (A) and after clipping of the main trunk of the artery (B).

Stereotactic clipping was performed (Fig. 52-8B). The clip was put on M_1, the diameter of which at the target point was 3.5 mm; the distance from the surface was 58 mm. A control angiogram disclosed practically complete elimination of the AVM from the circulation. The postoperative course was free of complications. The severe neurologic deficit disappeared in 1 month. About 3 years after the operation the patient is in good condition without any compliants. There was no recurrent bleeding.

AVMs supplied mainly by the pericallosal artery are frequent in neurosurgical practice. These AVMs are located deep in the corpus callosum and often are marginally accessible to radical extirpation. The following case illustrates the possibility of clipping the pericallosal artery, which supplied an inoperable AVM of the corpus callosum and basal ganglia.

Case 6.   A 13-year-old boy suffered four severe intraventricular hemorrhages during the 4 years before admission. He was admitted to our clinic 3 weeks after the last hemorrhage. Angiography disclosed a medium-sized AVM involving the corpus callosum, the deep medial structures, and the posterior part of the third ventricle. The aneurysm was supplied mainly by the right pericallosal artery and, to a lesser extent, by branches of the right middle and both posterior cerebral arteries (Fig. 52-9A). The deep bilateral location of the aneurysm made it inoperable.

It was decided to clip the main feeder of the aneurysm—the pericallosal artery. Successful stereotactic clipping of the artery was performed. Control angiography showed that the AVM no longer filled through the artery (Fig. 52-9B). In comparison with the preoperative investigation, the CBF was markedly decreased. There were no postoperative complications. During the 7-year follow-up period there have been no hemorrhages and no epileptic seizures. The patient is in good condition. He was graduated from secondary school and is now working at a factory.

The next case is important for the evaluation of the clipping method. In this case the method was used to manage an AVM that undoubtedly could have been completely removed by classic open surgery. It is well known that AVMs supplied by one feeder are relatively rare. Their total extirpation usually may be achieved without great technical difficulties. Nevertheless, to study the possibilities of stereotactic clipping, we decided to employ it in a case in which the AVM was radically operable. It should be emphasized that stereotactic clipping totally eliminated the aneurysm from the circulation.

Case 7.   A 26-year-old man was admitted to our clinic several hours after a single subarachnoid-parenchymatous hemorrhage. The marked post-bleeding hemiparesis gradually disappeared. Angiography showed a small AVM (23 mm^3) in the right parietotemporal region. There was only one thin feeding branch arising from the middle cerebral artery (Fig. 52-10A). This branch was clipped by stereotactic technique (Fig. 52-10B). There were no complications in the postoperative period. Control angiography 3 weeks after the operation showed the complete exclusion of the malformation from the circulation. It is important to note that the second main branch of the middle cerebral artery, which was located very close to the first branch supplling the AVM, remained intact. Postoperative CBF studies demonstrated a return to normal figures.

About 7 years after surgery the patient is in good condition without neurologic deficit. He is working full time. Intracranial hemorrhage has not recurred.

Conclusion

Because the possibilities of the stereotactic method of clipping have not yet been fully investigated, the indications for using this new technique are not sharply defined. There are many situations in which a decision must be made depending on numerous factors—the type of aneurysm, its size and location, the size of the neck, anatomic structures around it, and many others.

Stereotactic clipping is advisable in carefully selected cases of arterial aneurysms and in cases of giant or deep-seated AVMs when direct attack may be dangerous or technically impossible. In selected cases of small AVMs fed by a single artery, stereotactic clipping may be a method of radical treatment.

The stereotactic technique has some important advantages. Stereotactic clipping operations are less dangerous and less traumatic than direct attack by open approach, and the method prevents serious complications due to possible rupture of the aneurysm, vascular spasm, or injured cerebral vessels.

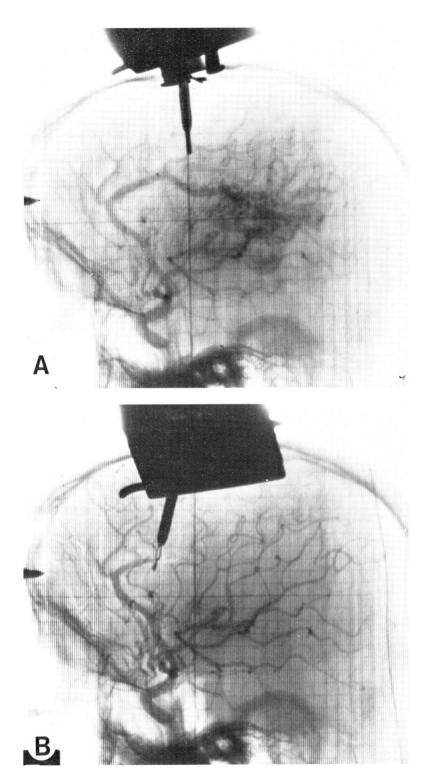

Fig. 52-9. Angiograms of an AVM supplied mainly by the pericallosal artery. (A) During the operation, and (B) after stereotactic clipping.

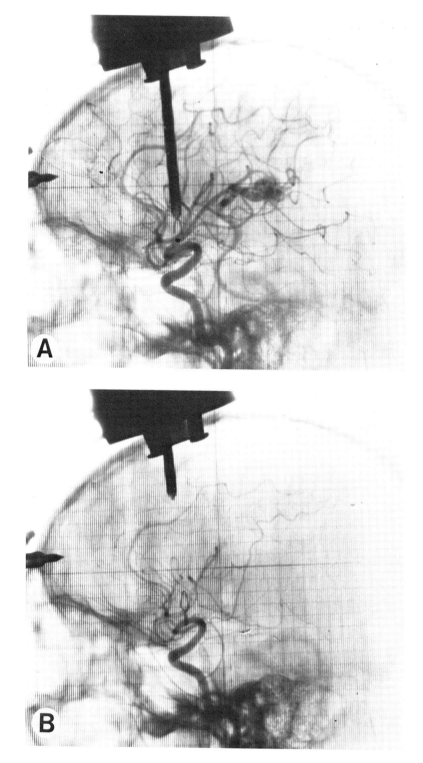

Fig. 52-10.   Angiograms of a small AVM supplied by only one branch of the middle cerebral artery. (A) Just before stereotactic clipping, and (B) after stereotactic clipping. The
aneurysm was totally excluded from the circulation.

REFERENCES

1. Guiot G, Rougerie J, Sachs M, et al: Repérage stéréotaxique de malformations vasculaires profondes intracérébrales. *Sem Hôp Paris 36*:1134–1143, 1960

2. Riechert T, Mundinger F: Combined stereotaxic operation for treatment of deep-seated angiomas and aneurysms. *J Neurosurg 21*:358–363, 1964

3. Alksne JE, Rand RW: Current status of metallic thrombosis of intracranial aneurysms. *Prog Neurol Surg 3*:212–229, 1969

4. Alksne JE: Stereotaxic occlusion of 22 consecutive anterior communicating artery aneurysms. *J Neurosurg 52*:790–793, 1980

5. Mullan S: Experiences with surgical thrombosis of intracranial berry aneurysms and carotid cavernous fistulas. *J Neurosurg 41*:657–671, 1974

6. Samotokin BA, Hilko VA: *Aneurysms and Arteriovenous Fistulas of the Brain.* (Rus) Leningrad, Meditsina, 1973

7. Cahan LD, Rand RW: Stereotaxic coagulation of a paraventricular arteriovenous malformation. Case report. *J Neurosurg 39*:770–774, 1973

8. Rand RW, Mosso JA: Treatment of cerebral aneurysms by stereotaxic ferromagnetic silicone thrombosis. *Bull Los Angeles Neurol Soc 38*:21–23, 1972

9. Kandel EI, Peresedov VV: Stereotactic clipping of an arterial aneurysm of the brain. (Rus) *Vopr Neirokhir 39*:13–15, 1975

10. Kandel EI, Peresedov VV: Stereotaxic clipping of arterial and arteriovenous aneurysms of the brain. *Acta Neurochir (Suppl) 30*:405–412, 1980

11. Kandel EI, New stereotactic apparatus and cryogenic device for stereotactic surgery. *Confin Neurol 37*:128–132, 1975

12. Kandel EI, Peresedov VV: Stereotaxic clipping of arterial aneurysms and arteriovenous malformations. *J Neurosurg 46*:12–23, 1977

CHAPTER 53
Treatment of Certain Intracerebral Vascular Lesions with Balloon Catheters

Gerard Debrun

THE BEST AVAILABLE TREATMENT for a cavernous carotid fistula is to release an inflated balloon into the cavernous sinus to occlude the fistula and preserve carotid blood flow, a procedure that was first carried out by Serbinenko.[1] Our own technique, in which an inflatable, detachable balloon is used, has been described,[2-6] but a more detailed presentation may be useful.

Technique

Making the Latex Sleeve

Stainless steel molds are available in different shapes and sizes (Ingenor, Paris, France); mold diameter vary from 0.2 to 1.0 mm. The mold is dipped in pure latex, then placed in an oven and treated with steam at 100°C for 30 minutes. The latex then is slipped off of the mold. The result is a small, latex, finger-shaped sleeve (Figs. 53-1 and 53-2A and B).

Making the Balloon

The latex sleeve is pulled over a catheter (catheter A, Fig. 53-2C), and tied onto it with a thin elastic thread cut from a latex glove. The thread is wound around the catheter 5 times. On the last loop around the catheter, three simple knots are made, and the two ends of the latex thread are cut close to the knot with scissors (Fig. 53-3). This may be easier to do under magnification. The part of the latex sleeve below the knot then is trimmed (Figs. 53-4 and 53-5).

Balloon Release System

The balloon is released by a second coaxial catheter, which is slipped over the first catheter and used to push the balloon off the end of the first catheter (Fig. 53-5). The aperture of the balloon is immediately closed by the rubber thread around its base.

The balloon may be filled with iodinated contrast medium and released without immediate leaking, but it progressively deflates (2 to 4 weeks) because the contrast medium passes through

Department of Radiology, Massachusetts General Hospital, Boston, Massachusetts

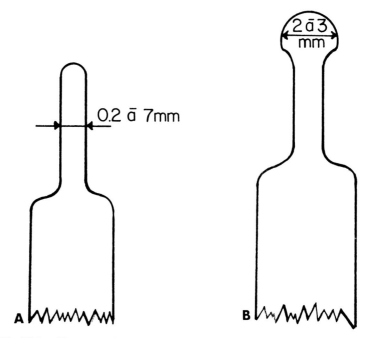

Fig. 53-1. Diagrams of the different shapes of stainless steel molds available for producing latex sleeves.

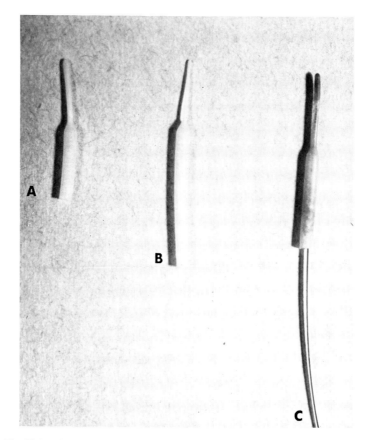

Fig. 53-2. **A.** and **B.** Two different shapes of latex sleeves. **C.** An inner catheter inserted into a latex sleeve.

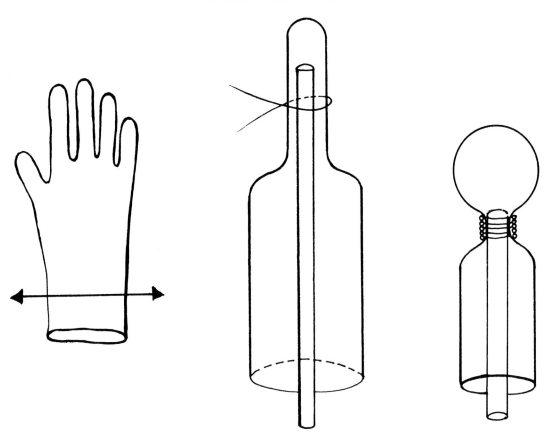

Fig. 53-3. Method of attaching the latex sleeve to the inner catheter. (Left) An elastic thread is cut from a latex glove. (middle, right) The elastic thread is wound around the sleeve on the catheter. After the thread has been wound around the sleeve 5 times, it is tied and the ends are trimmed close to the knots.

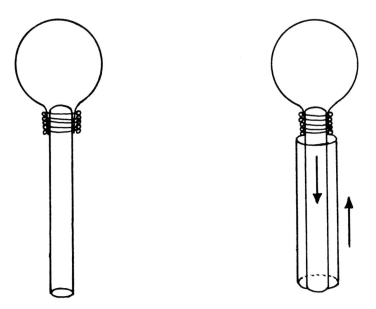

Fig. 53-4. **(Left)** The proximal part of the sleeve is trimmed close to the elastic thread. **(Right)** The coaxial outer catheter is slipped over the inner catheter.

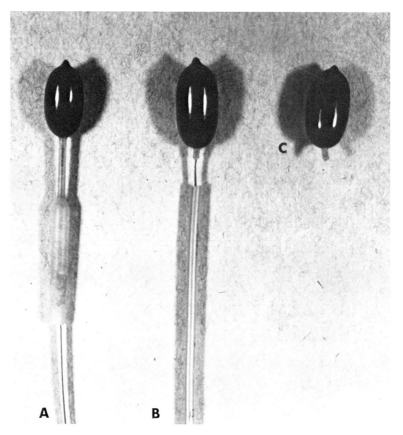

Fig. 53-5. **A.** The sleeve has been ligated over the inner catheter. **B.** The proximal part of the sleeve has been cut off. Both the ligature and coaxial outer catheter are visible. **C.** The balloon after it has been released.

the latex membrane of the balloon. For this reason, the iodinated contrast medium must be replaced with a polymerizing mixture so the balloon will retain its dimensions permanently.

Introducing the Coaxial Catheters into the Internal Carotid Artery

Both the inner catheter and the outer catheter are introduced into the internal carotid with an introducer, which is inserted by the Seldinger technique. The inside diameter (I.D.) of the introducer is 1.8 mm, which is wide enough to allow the catheters to be passed into the artery, as well as continuous infusions of isotonic glucose or iodinated contrast medium for preoperative angiographic control. For this purpose, a lambda-shaped (λ) pipe is attached to the rear end of the introducer (Fig. 53-6). The coaxial catheters are passed through the straight part of the λ-shaped tube. Blood loss around the outer coaxial catheter is prevented by a seal made of cotton soaked in heparinized jelly. A side arm also can be used.

The balloon can be made visible radiographically by injecting iodinated contrast medium into it when it is passed beyond the introducer. In order to visualize the balloon while it is in the introducer, a silver clip can be placed inside it before the inner catheter is placed in the sleeve. The clip is directed into the end of the sleeve. When the balloon has left the introducer and has been inflated with 0.05 ml of contrast medium, carotid blood flow and the thrust applied to the inner catheter are enough to drive the balloon into the carotid sinus.

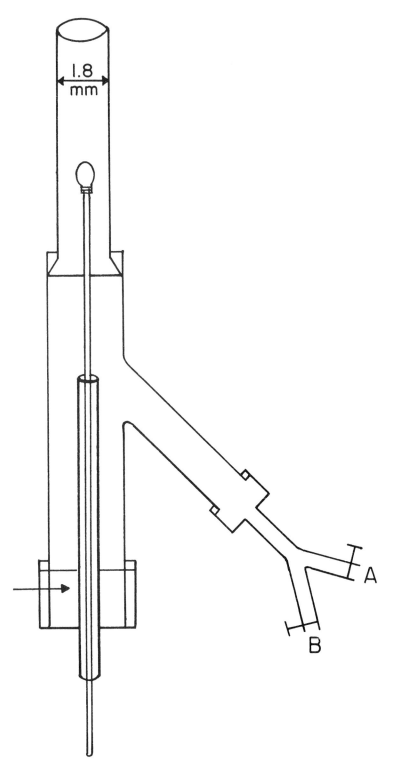

Fig. 53-6. A sketch of the introducer used to insert the catheter into the internal carotid. Note the lambda-shaped tube on the side of the introducer that allows the infusion of heparin **(A)** and contrast medium **(B).** Blood loss is prevented by a seal of cotton soaked in heparinized jelly (arrow).

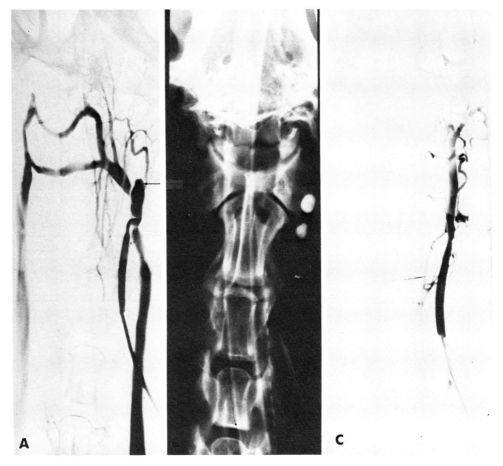

Fig. 53-7.   Occlusion of an experimental carotid jugular fistula in a dog. **A.** The jugular vein has been ligated above the fistula (arrow). The distal part of the carotid artery is not opacified because of
the shunt. **B.** The highest balloon has been released in the jugular vein; the lowest balloon is still
attached to the catheter. **C.** A control arteriogram after the second balloon has been released.
The fistula is occluded. The distal part of the carotid artery is now opacified.

Experimental Studies

In a series of experiments, carotid–jugular fistulas were created in dogs. One week later the
common carotid artery of each dog was punctured as far as possible below the fistula, and an introducer was placed in the artery. Carotid arteriography demonstrated the fistula (Fig. 53-7A).
The carotid artery was not opacified above the level of the fistula because of the shunt. The balloon catheter was introduced through the introducer, guided under fluoroscopy through the fistula into the jugular vein (Fig. 53-7B), and the balloon inflated until it occluded the fistula.
Carotid arteriography confirmed that the fistula remained occluded and that carotid blood flow
was preserved. The balloon was released, and additional arteriography was performed (Fig. 53-
7C) to ensure that the balloon remained inflated and in a good position, that the fistula was occluded, and that carotid blood flow was preserved. The carotid artery above the level of the
fistula was observed to be opacified.

Experimental carotid aneurysms also were created in dogs (Fig. 53-8), using a portion of
vein implanted on the cervical carotid artery. One week after implantation, the carotid artery
was studied arteriographically by means of a carotid introducer (Fig. 53-8A). If there was no evidence of spontaneous thrombosis of the aneurysm, the balloon catheter was introduced into the
aneurysm under fluoroscopy and the balloon inflated with iodinated contrast medium until its

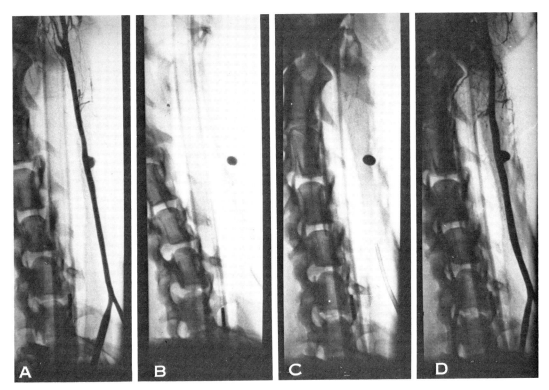

Fig. 53-8. Occlusion of an experimental carotid aneurysm in a dog. **A.** The aneurysm before treatment. **B.** The balloon inflated in the aneurysmal cavity; the catheter is still visible. **C.** The balloon has been released; carotid blood flow is preserved. **D.** Three weeks later the balloon is still opacified; the carotid artery is normal.

volume equaled that of the aneurysm (Fig. 53-8B). Maintenance of carotid blood flow was checked arteriographically before the balloon was released, because if the balloon was overinflated, it might have obstructed the carotid artery. The balloon then was released (Fig. 53-8C), and a final arteriogram was made to confirm that the carotid blood flow was preserved. At follow-up 3 weeks later, the balloons remained opacified and carotid blood flow was normal (Fig. 53-8D).

Clinical Indications

The ease with which the balloon is drawn into an arteriovenous shunt by the blood flow contrasts with the difficulty encountered when the balloon is inserted into an aneurysmal cavity. For this reason this technique is best reserved for use in treating posttraumatic carotid cavernous fistulas and the infrequent vertebrovertebral fistulas. A definitive clinical cure without impairing flow in the internal carotid artery can be achieved often enough and easily enough to make the use of a Fogarty catheter less satisfactory for these types of lesions. The goal of treatment is to place the balloon in the cavernous sinus on the venous side of the fistula and to inflate the balloon until the fistula is no longer visible on control angiograms while preserving blood flow in the carotid artery.

Spontaneous nontraumatic carotid cavernous fistulas are a different pathologic entity and the balloon technique is not indicated in their treatment. Generally, several small feeding vessels arise from the internal carotid artery in the cavernous sinus in addition to many feeding vessels arising from branches of the external carotid artery. The feeding vessels from the external carotid artery must be embolized. Weeks later the opthalmologic signs will have disappeared and in some cases arteriograms of the internal carotid may show that the feeding vessels from this branch also have disappeared.

For this reason the internal carotid artery of these patients must not be occluded surgically too soon. These fistulas are in fact dural AVM's and must be distinguished from the cavernous aneurysms spontaneously ruptured into the cavernous sinus which have to be treated with detachable balloons.

Surgery remains the best treatment for aneurysms because it is very difficult and hazardous to try to enter the neck of an aneurysm with the balloon catheter. Infraclinoid aneurysms of the carotid siphon, however, and certain basilar aneurysms cannot be operated upon, and in these cases the balloon technique should be considered. All of the complications we have encountered with the balloon technique have occurred during attempts to enter an aneurysmal cavity. No complications have been experienced in treating arteriovenous malformations (AVMs). It is useless and, indeed, dangerous to try to enter an aneurysm with the balloon if there is spasm. We have experienced one death from rupture of the aneurysmal sac under these conditions.

Brain angiomas that are not resectable without a major neurologic risk can be embolized with spheres or with bucrylate.* Bucrylate can probably induce more thrombosis and inflammatory reaction inside the nidus of the AVM than do Silastic spheres. The detachable balloon technique is not indicated in these situations because proximal occlusion of feeders has always proved to be useless in the treatment of AVMs.

We will successively describe the technique for treating and the results of the treatment of carotid cavernous fistulas, of vertebral fistulas, of giant unclippable aneurysms, and of AVMs of the brain.

Treatment of Posttraumatic Carotid Cavernous Fistulas

The first step in treating a posttraumatic carotid cavernous fistula with a detachable balloon inflated with a polymerizing substance is a thorough study of the location of the fistula by subtracted serial angiography (at least 3 films per second). Blood flow through the shunt generally is so rapid that the exact level of the fistula cannot be seen. Vertebral angiography with compression of the carotid artery in the neck feeding the fistula will, in most cases, opacify the carotid siphon by retrograde flow, and the level of the shunt will be visible (Fig. 53-9A and B). The contralateral carotid artery always is injected while the feeding carotid is compressed in order to determine if the blood supply to the cerebral hemisphere on the side of the fistula can be maintained by anastomosis via the circle of Willis should it become necessary to cut off flow in the carotid on the side of the fistula.

After the introducer has been placed in the internal carotid, the balloon catheter is moved. The balloon is inflated with 0.05 ml of iodinated contrast medium and its progress is followed under lateral fluoroscopy. It is difficult to follow the balloon through dense petrous bone, and television subtraction with video recording is helpful in these instances. As soon as the balloon has progressed beyond the petrous portion of the carotid canal, it once again can be seen quite easily. When it reaches the carotid siphon, it tends to be drawn upward by the flux through the fistula, and a slight flutter or a directional change indicates that it has entered the cavernous sinus. In the last case we treated, it was possible to push the balloon into the orbit through the superior ophthalmic vein.

If the balloon does not enter the cavernous sinus easily, it should be kept in the neighborhood of the suspected position of the fistula and small to-and-fro motions should be applied to the catheter as volume of the contrast medium in the balloon is varied. If these measures are not successful, the balloon must be replaced with a smaller one.

Once the balloon is inside the cavernous sinus, it must be inflated until the fistula is occluded, i.e., with about 0.20 ml of iodinated contrast medium. The tap on the inner catheter

*Bucrylate is available from Ethicon-Canada.

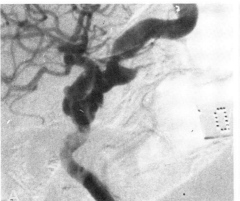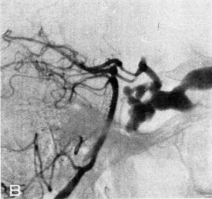

Fig. 53-9.   **A.** A right carotid cavernous fistula on a right carotid arteriogram. The exact level of the fistula cannot be seen. **B.** The same fistula with compression of the right carotid on a vertebral arteriogram. The fistula is clearly seen on the anterior curve of the carotid siphon.

then is closed. Preservation of carotid blood flow as well as closure of the fistula are confirmed by AP and lateral serial angiograms (the injection of contrast is carried out through the introducer [see Fig. 53-6B]). Any abnormality, such as leakage of contrast medium into the cavernous sinus or irregularity in carotid blood flow, implies that the amount of contrast medium in the balloon should be modified until perfect conditions are obtained. In a few cases all the procedures mentioned above may fail, probably because the aperture of the fistula is too small or is located in such a way that the balloon cannot enter it (Fig. 53-10). In this case the balloon should be released opposite the neck of the fistula to plug the carotid artery.

Final Release of the Balloon

Once the balloon is in final position, the balloon is deflated and the contrast medium it contained is carefully removed and measured. A small amount of the contrast medium in the inner

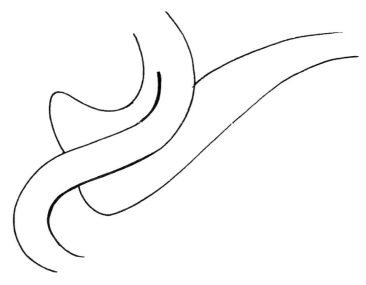

Fig. 53-10.   A diagram of a carotid cavernous fistula caused by dissection of the internal carotid artery; the fistulous aperture is located in such a way that introduction of a balloon is impossible.

catheter cannot be removed and will remain in the catheter when the polymerizing substance is injected.

The polymer substance we use, which is still in a trial stage, is a fluid silicone oil that is mixed with a catalyst just before it is injected. The viscosity of this substance increases after 1 minute, and it must be rapidly sucked into an insulin syringe (1.0 ml with 100 graduations), and the proper volume injected into the balloon immediately. We have tried to opacify the silicone oil with a small amount of tantalum powder, but the powder increases the viscosity of the silicone and can obstruct the inner catheter before the injection is completed. This approach has therefore not been pursued further.

Because the density of the contrast medium is higher than that of the silicone polymer, a layering effect will be seen in the inflated balloon.

Once the silicone has been injected, the tap of the inner catheter is closed. After a 10-minute interval, it is released. Then, the coaxial outer catheter is brought to the base of the balloon. A certain resistance can be felt that indicates that the catheter has reached the balloon. At this point traction is exerted on the inner catheter while the outer catheter is kept firmly in place; the release of the balloon can be felt distinctly. This step is controlled radiographically, and the balloon must not move at the time it is released.

Both catheters then are withdrawn from the introducer and new AP and lateral arteriograms are taken to check the final result.

The arteriograms must show that:

1. The balloon is in the cavernous sinus and outside the carotid artery.
2. The contrast medium used for the arteriogram is not leaking into the cavernous sinus.
3. Carotid blood flow is normal.

Sometimes it is impossible to use a polymerizing substance, and the balloon has to be inflated with contrast medium and detached. This happens whenever the dead space of the catheter is equal to or higher than the capacity of the balloon needed to occlude the fistula. It also should be noted that the dead space of the catheter is doubled when the treatment is done through the groin. This is the primary reason for performing the procedure through the neck. When the balloon must be inflated with contrast medium only, the fistula will be occluded immediately after injection, but the balloon will deflate in the weeks following the procedure. The fistula almost always remains occluded in these instances, but a false aneurysm can develop in place of the previously inflated balloon.

Results

Fifty-four traumatic carotid cavernous sinus fistulas have been treated with the detachable balloon technique in our clinic (Fig. 53-11).

The carotid blood flow was preserved in 67 percent of the cases. The remaining 33 percent, where the carotid artery did not remain patent, included patients in whom it was impossible to enter the cavernous sinus with the balloon (10 percent), patients who needed to have the carotid artery occluded as a second treatment because they either had intractable retro-orbital pain or oculomotor nerve palsy (15 percent), and patients who suffered severe stenosis of the carotid artery because the balloon bulged into the siphon (5 percent), and finally induced thrombosis of the carotid artery.

When the balloon was inflated with iodine material only, patients developed a false aneurysm in 50 percent of the cases. In most cases this pouch was asymptomatic (85 percent). In the remaining cases (15 percent) the patients either had intractable retro-orbital pain, which was immediately cured by occlusion of the carotid artery, or they had nonimproving oculomotor nerve palsy. Here, too, the oculomotor palsy was cured after permanent occlusion of the siphon. Oculomotor nerve palsies occurred in 6 cases and were always transient.

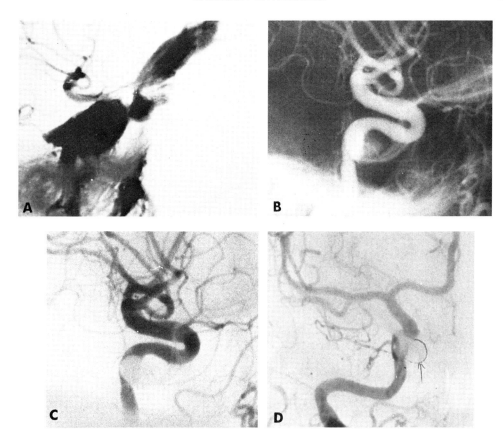

Fig. 53-11. **A.** A right posttraumatic carotid cavernous fistula. **B.** A control arteriogram. The fistula is occluded by a balloon inflated with silicone and released into the cavernous sinus. The level of iodinated contrast is visible. Carotid blood flow is preserved. **C.** A lateral view. **D.** The balloon is visible in the cavernous sinus on the left side of the carotid siphon.

There were no neurologic complications. The fistula was occluded in all cases but one, where there is still a minimal leak. The patient was asymptomatic and no further treatment has been required as yet.

Particular Cases

In two cases the patients previously had been treated by entrapment of the carotid artery and ligation of the internal carotid artery in the neck; these efforts had been unsuccessful. These two cases then were treated by direct exposure of the cavernous sinus. In one case bucrylate was injected into the carotid artery; in the other case the cavernous sinus was punctured and a balloon was released into the cavernous sinus. In both cases the results were satisfactory.

Whenever a fistula drains posteriorly through a wide inferior petrosal sinus, the treatment always should begin with a trial approach to the cavernous sinus in a retrograde manner through the jugular vein and inferior petrosal sinus, either with a Fogarty catheter (in which case the balloon is not detachable) or with the detachable balloon technique. Out of 4 patients in whom this treatment was attempted, 1 patient was cured and in 1 patient the cavernous sinus was occluded by the balloon but not the fistula because of partitions of the cavernous sinus. In the other 2 cases it was impossible to occlude the cavernous sinus.

Injection of bucrylate into the cavernous sinus, either with a calibrated-leak balloon introduced through the groin or by surgical exposure and puncture of the cavernous sinus, has been used by several authors. This seems to be a dangerous procedure, however, because of the risk of reflux of bucrylate into the carotid artery where the occlusion of the fistula begins. The amount of bucrylate that might pass through the fistula and return to the lungs also is unknown.

Treatment of Spontaneous Carotid Cavernous Fistulas

Spontaneous fistulas of the cavernous sinus are totally different from traumatic fistulas for many reasons. The patients often are elderly women; the fistula is often bilateral; the symptomatology generally is not prominent; and, the fistula often disappears spontaneously and may recur some years later.

The external carotid branches always are involved. In addition, there are abnormal communicating branches between the carotid siphon and the cavernous sinus.

The spontaneous rupture of a cavernous aneurysm is classical, but rare.

In young patients the fistula generally is a dural arteriovenous malformation of the cavernous sinus (Fig. 53-12).

Because the feeders from the internal carotid artery are numerous and small, there is no place for the detachable balloon. Branches of the external carotid artery must be embolized hyperselectively with particles of Gelfoam or Ivalon, or with bucrylate if it is a fast-flow AVM of the dura of the cavernous sinus. The permanent occlusion of the internal carotid artery must never be attempted first and is totally contraindicated. When the fistula is not completely occluded by embolization of the external carotid artery, a direct surgical approach to the cavernous sinus is the best way to save the carotid artery and to occlude the fistula, whatever the technique used (pieces of muscle, thrombogenic wire, or detachable balloon).

Seven patients with spontaneous carotid cavernous fistulas have been treated successfully on our service by embolization of the external carotid branches only. The carotid blood flow has been preserved in all cases and the fistula has been occluded. Figure 53-12 is an example of a dural AVM of the cavernous sinus that was totally obliterated by an injection of 0.5 ml of bucrylate into the internal maxillary artery.

One case of bilateral spontaneous carotid cavernous fistula has been totally cured on one side only, despite embolization of both external carotid arteries. The patient has a mild bruit on one side. Surgical treatment will be proposed in this case only if the patient's vision deteriorates or if double vision develops. Another patient, a 75-year-old woman who had progressive vision loss and did not wish to live with "that bruit in her head," was not embolized for technical reasons and had bilateral surgical plugging of the cavernous sinus with pieces of muscle. The clinical result was excellent.

There was one transient neurologic deficit in our series. In that case there was reflux of bucrylate into the internal carotid after embolization of the sphenopalatine artery.

Treatment of Vertebral Fistulas with the Detachable Balloon Technique

Congenital, traumatic, and iatrogenic vertebral fistulas are less frequent than carotid cavernous fistulas, but are an excellent prospect for use of the balloon technique. The balloon is detached in the vein and occludes the fistula, and the vertebral artery remains patent (Fig. 53-13). The size of the balloon needed is often larger than those used to treat a carotid cavernous fistula. A 9F introducer is introduced from the groin and positioned in the vertebral artery. It is not necessary to use a polymerizing substance because the false aneurysm that often develops in the cavernous sinus almost never develops during treatment of vertebral fistulas. Eleven cases have been totally cured, with preservation of the vertebral blood flow in 9 cases. No complications have occurred.

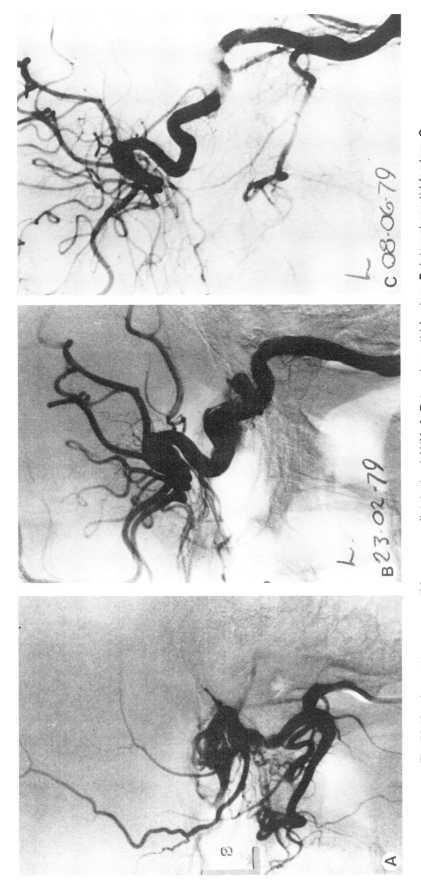

Fig. 53-12. A spontaneous carotid cavernous fistula-dural AVM. **A.** External carotid feeders. **B.** Internal carotid feeders. **C.** Four months after embolization of the internal maxillary artery with 0.5 ml of bucrylate. Complete disappearance of the dural AVM. Normal internal carotid artery.

801

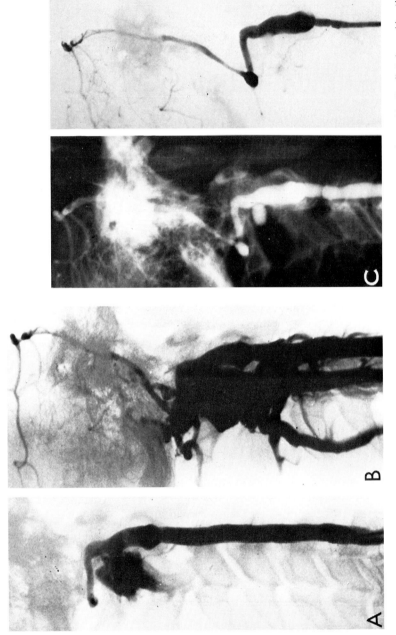

Fig. 53-13. **A.** and **B.** A congenital vertebrovertebral fistula at C1–C2. **C.** The balloon has been released in the fistula and is still opacified 8 days later. The fistula is occluded. The vertebral blood flow is preserved.

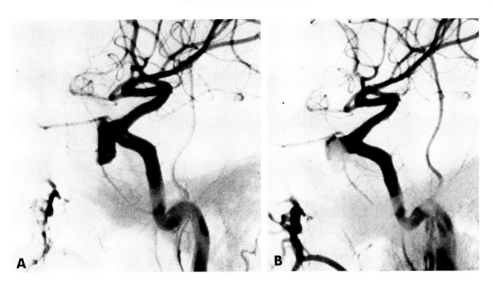

Fig. 53-14. **A.** An aneurysm of the carotid siphon in the cavernous sinus. **B.** One balloon has been released in the aneurysmal pouch, which is occluded.

Treatment of Aneurysms with the Detachable Balloon Technique

At the beginning of our experience with the balloon technique, we thought that it would be possible to occlude the sacs of many berry aneurysms. We found, however, that this was not the case. In one case of a giant aneurysm of the carotid bifurcation with spasm in a moribund patient, the sac burst during a trial entry of the neck. In another surgical case of an aneurysm of the bifurcation of the middle cerebral artery (MCA), the balloon stenosed the MCA and the patient suffered hemiplegia and died 3 days after surgical removal of the balloon. Based on this experience, we never treat an aneurysm with a detachable balloon if the aneurysm can be surgically clipped.

During attempts to occlude aneurysms of the cavernous portion of the internal carotid artery with preservation of the arterial flow, the procedures were long, difficult, and risky (Fig. 53-14).

There are many reasons for this: the patient risks death if the aneurysm bursts while the skull is closed. The balloon often bulges into the artery through the neck of the aneurysm and induces a stenosis of the artery that ends in a thrombosis. If the balloon is inflated with iodine material, the aneurysm fills again as soon as the balloon starts to deflate, even after 2 weeks. It is extremely difficult to get a balloon inflated with 100 percent polymerizing substance; because of the dead space of a single-lumen catheter, the balloon will always contain a certain amount of contrast medium (Fig. 53-15). A double-lumen catheter would allow a balloon to be inflated with silicone only (Fig. 53-16), but the double-lumen catheter is stiffer than a single-lumen catheter and makes it more difficult to enter the aneurysm. If the aneurysm is giant, the size of the uninflated balloon needed to occlude it is too large to pass easily through the introducer. Even if the balloon technique is successful, the aneurysm will be transformed into a solid mass that can induce compression of the surrounding neurologic and vascular structures. For all these reasons, the occlusion of unclippable aneurysms with balloons has been abandoned and replaced by simple permanent occlusion of the artery, which is done as close as possible to the neck of the aneurysm. A superficial temporal–middle cerebral artery bypass is done first whenever the patient cannot tolerate permanent occlusion of the artery. Because of the risk and the technical difficulties involved, we have never tried to occlude an unclippable basilar aneurysm.

Among 14 patients with aneurysms, 2 patients died, 2 patients had transient neurologic deficits, and 1 patient became blind in one eye. The best clinical results have been obtained in those

SINGLE LUMEN CATHETER

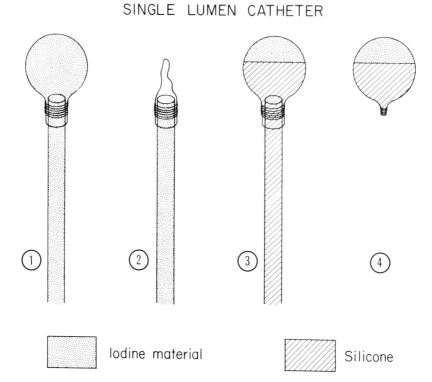

Iodine material   Silicone

Fig. 53-15.   Diagram of the single-lumen catheter. Because of the dead space of the catheter, the amount of iodine contrast equal to the dead space is reintroduced into the balloon when silicone is injected.

unclippable giant aneurysms of the carotid artery (cavernous, ophthalmic, bifurcation aneurysms) where the carotid artery was permanently occluded with a detachable balloon. Some of these patients underwent ligation of A1, or a bypass, or both.

Treatment of Brain AVMs with a Calibrated-Leak Balloon and Injection of Bucrylate

It is impossible to approach a cortical vessel distally with the Teflon catheter used for the detachable balloon technique. Teflon and even polyethylene is too stiff. Therefore it is necessary to use Silastic tubing that is so supple that it cannot be manipulated by pushing it; it has to be coiled in a holder and injected. There are two basic types of calibrated-leak balloons, Kerber balloons and Debrun balloons.

Calibrated Leak Balloons

The Kerber balloon[7,8] is a nondetachable Silastic balloon attached to the tip of radiopaque Silastic tubing. A calibrated leak located distally in the balloon allows a polymerizing substance to be injected into the balloon (Fig. 53-17). The tubing is coiled in a holder and a syringe containing 20 cc of saline is used to inject it through an introducer positioned in the internal carotid artery or the vertebral artery (Fig. 53-18). The catheter is totally flow directed and enters the vessel where the flow is the highest and the course is the straightest. This type of balloon is used to embolize arteriovenous malformations in the brain. Because the vessels feeding the AVM are dilated with a higher flow than the normal adjacent cortical branches, the balloon has a natural

DOUBLE LUMEN CATHETER

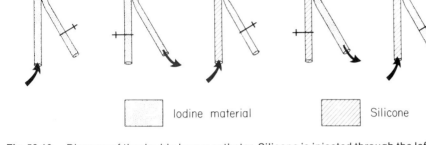

Iodine material		Silicone

Fig. 53-16. Diagram of the double-lumen catheter. Silicone is injected through the left lumen. The quantity of iodine contrast that is pushed into the balloon can be aspirated through the right lumen. The balloon can be inflated with 100% silicone.

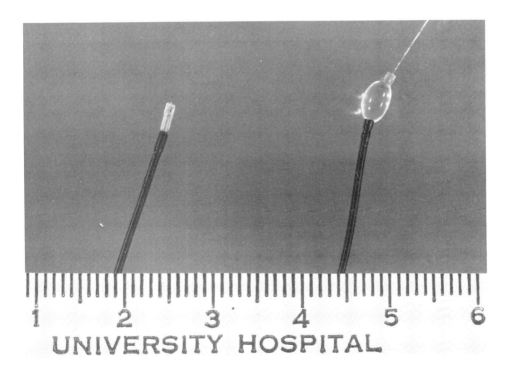

Fig. 53-17. Kerber's calibrated-leak balloon. Silastic balloon stuck to the tip of the Silastic tubing. The balloon cannot be detached.

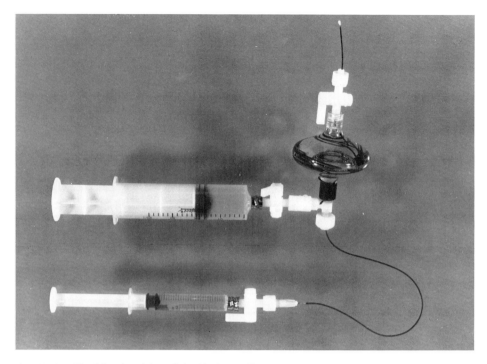

Fig. 53-18.   The Silastic tubing of the Kerber calibrated-leak balloon is coiled inside the transparent spin-top holder. The one-way stop cock is connected to the introducer positioned in either the internal carotid or the vertebral artery. The Silastic tubing is propelled by injecting 10 cc of saline with the 20-cc syringe.

tendency to follow the flow through those dilated feeders. When the Silastic tubing has been propelled by the syringe, the holder is removed and a small 25-gauge blunt needle is adapted to the proximal end of the Silastic tubing so that water-soluble iodinated contrast can be injected into it. The inflation and the positioning of the balloon can be followed by fluoroscopy.

In the best cases, the balloon will flow into one of the main cortical arteries feeding the AVM. After the catheter has been flushed thoroughly with pure dextrose, bucrylate can be injected into the balloon. The bucrylate solidifies when it contacts ionized solutions. The balloon must remain inflated during injection and until the bucrylate solidifies. The occlusion of the vessel during embolization is absolutely necessary in order to stop or decrease the flow through the AVM. If the balloon is not properly inflated during embolization or if it bursts immediately after the injection of the bucrylate has begun, there is a high risk of the draining veins of the AVM becoming occluded or of particles of bucrylate returning to the lungs. It is also critical that the injection of bucrylate is stopped at the appropriate point. This is generally when the progression of bucrylate through the network of the AVM decreases and when the bucrylate begins retrograde occlusion of the vessel through which the injection is done. The balloon must be deflated at that time and the catheter removed promptly but gently.

If the balloon cannot be deflated, it is safer to burst it intentionally before removing it. Removal of a bucrylate-filled balloon risks embolization of the normal cortical branches.

The solidification time of bucrylate depends upon the quantities of the components that are mixed together. Bucrylate is not spontaneously radiopaque. In order to properly control the injection of bucrylate through an AVM, the bucrylate must be mixed with tantalum powder and with an iodinated oil, such as Pantopaque. Two ampules of bucrylate (1 ml) mixed with 1 g of tantalum powder (1 μm particles) and 0.3 ml of Pantopaque will give a mixture of low viscosity that will solidify in 4 seconds.

In some instances, when all the Silastic tubing has been injected and the surgeon checks the position of the balloon under fluoroscopy, it is not visible intracranially. This is because a long length of the tubing has coiled in the internal carotid artery in the neck. In such a situation, the introducer must be pulled down until the tubing is uncoiled after the needle is connected to the tubing. Then a combination of gently inflating the balloon and pushing the introducer up will allow the balloon to progress.

There are several advantages to the calibrated-leak balloon technique. Embolization of a brain AVM or of a dural AVM can be accomplished by the intra-arterial route through the groin under local anesthesia. The patient is totally awake and cooperative. Progressive occlusion of an AVM can be achieved during two or three separate procedures, or three or four calibrated-leak balloons can be used during the same procedure. It depends on how easy it is to direct the balloons into the proper vessels. Three hours of working time is reasonable. After that period of time, generally both the patient and the neuroradiologist are exhausted, and it is safer to quit.

Another advantage is that any complications can be detected immediately. An angiogram is done at the end of each embolization.

The disadvantages of the technique include the fact that the routine use of bucrylate is not allowed by the United States Food and Drug Administration and its use is still experimental in the hands of a few experts. This glue can be extremely aggressive to normal tissues. White et al.[9] have demonstrated its toxicity in the celiac arteries of pigs. I have personally injected 50 kidneys of dogs and the anatomopathologist (Wallace) has found many necrotic areas of infarctions. This finding is totally different from the results obtained by injecting bucrylate into the abnormal network of vessels of an AVM. When injection of bucrylate is limited to the nidus of the AVM, neurologic symptoms do not occur in most cases.

The difficulty of having bucrylate solidify instantaneously in the AVM is that it carries the risk of having some of the bucrylate pass through the AVM and more or less occlude the veins (and possibly thrombose the longitudinal sinus, the torcular, or the straight sinus) or reach the lungs. Our policy after embolization of a brain AVM is to obtain a CT scan of the chest whenever we have seen bucrylate passing through the veins under fluoroscopy. In 1 case an amount of bucrylate was observed angiographically in the longitudinal sinus above the torcular but did not occlude it. The patient remained asymptomatic. In the same case a CT scan of the lungs showed a minimal number of dots of bucrylate in the lungs.

If bucrylate solidifies too quickly, there is a risk that the balloon will be stuck. Kerber has reported 3 cases where he could not remove the catheter at the end of the embolization. He removed one with a bent wire. A second patient was operated upon. A third lives with the Silastic tubing floating in his circulation. This complication occurred at the beginning of Kerber's clinical experience and has never happened since. This complication has happened twice in my experience. Both patients are alive and asymptomatic with the catheter left in place.

The biggest disadvantage with this type of balloon technique is the difference in the size of the balloons from one balloon to another, and in the same balloon, which becomes progressively larger after successive inflations and deflations. The risk of dissecting the vessel progressively increases as the balloon becomes larger and progresses distally in vessels that become smaller. If the balloon bursts when it is larger than the diameter of the vessel, the risk of dissection is extremely high. Several authors who have used this type of balloon have reported rupture of vessels. I have personally dissected the posterior cerebral artery five times, with subarachnoid and intracerebral bleeding in those 5 cases. Four patients have totally recovered; 1 died. I have unintentionally burst the balloon many times without complication, however, because the diameter of the vessel was large enough to accommodate the balloon (4 to 5 mm).

Until the quality of this Silastic balloon improves, the policy should be to use the technique only when the diameter of the feeding vessel of the AVM is 3 mm or more.

The Debrun calibrated-leak balloon technique uses the same latex covers that are used to make the detachable balloons. It is possible to make a hole at the tip of one of these balloon with a 25-gauge needle. This latex balloon then can be attached at the tip of a small Teflon or polyethylene catheter. The narrow portion of the sleeve also can grip the tip of a section of Silastic tubing similar to the Kerber catheter. (This tubing is used for brain AVMs.) (Fig. 53-19)

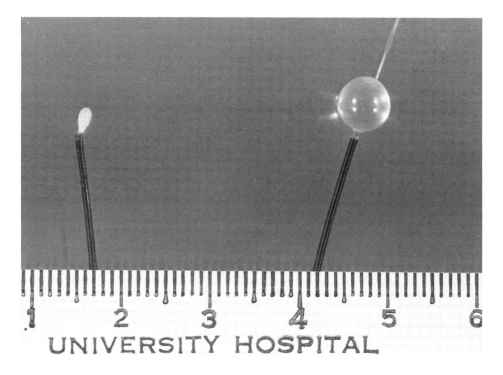

UNIVERSITY HOSPITAL

Fig. 53-19. Debrun's calibrated-leak balloon. The balloon is made of latex and grips the tip of a section of Silastic tubing. The balloon can be detached after injection of bucrylate through the leak.

The advantage in this method is the elasticity of the latex balloon compared with the stiffness of the Silastic balloon. By choosing a latex sleeve of small diameter (0.4 or 0.5 mm) it is possible to obtain inflated balloons that do not become wider than 3 mm and remain smaller in small vessels. The risk of rupturing the vessel is decreased. The balloon catheter permits maneuvering by pushing or pulling, and is more controllable than one of Silastic. It is used for embolization of branches of the external carotid artery. The disadvantage is that the leak cannot be calibrated as well in the latex balloon as in the Silastic balloon and also can become occluded by particles of tantalum powder faster than desired.

The Treatment of Brain AVMs

The treatment of brain AVMs would be easy if one could say which AVMs are the ones that must be embolized and how, which are the ones that must be resected, and which are the ones that must not be treated. There also is a place for proton beam therapy, cryotherapy, association of embolization, and surgery.

In fact, there is no rule in the treatment of brain AVMs. One neurosurgeon will consider a certain AVM resectable and another will say the reverse. There also is a natural tendency to treat all AVMs with the technique that the surgeon handles the best.

In general, however, AVMs that are considered unresectable are those AVMs invading the brainstem, the totality of the basal ganglion, or the rolandic and temporal areas of the dominant hemisphere. When these AVMs are accompanied by severe neurologic symptoms, embolization can be done either with Silastic particles or with bucrylate if feeders of reasonable size can be catheterized with the calibrated-leak balloon. Picard (unpublished report) has recently described the case of a patient who bled from a brainstem AVM. The patient was comatose and quadraplegic for many weeks and was considered locked in. Under family pressure, Picard attempted to

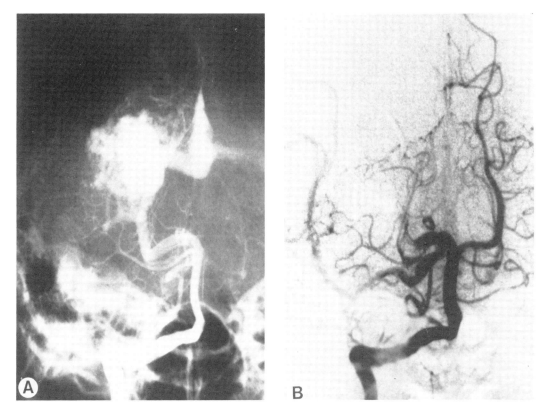

Fig. 53-20. **A.** An occipital brain AVM with one major feeder. The posterior cerebral artery could be embolized with minimal risk of neurologic deficit. **B.** After embolization with 0.5 ml of bucrylate, the AVM has completely disappeared. The patient had quadrantanopia after embolization.

embolize the AVM with particles of dura mater injected into one vertebral artery. Following treatment, the patient awoke and progressively improved. New embolizations were done. The steal through the AVM was tremendously decreased and the patient now can walk with the aid of canes.

It is impossible at this point to say whether surgery is safer and gives better long-term results than embolization with bucrylate in the case of a resectable AVM. It is almost certain that an AVM can be totally wiped out by bucrylate as in the case of an AVM with one main wide feeder (the best indication for balloon embolization) (Fig. 53-20).

We do not know the natural history of an asymptomatic AVM with precision. In many cases a long follow-up without any complications or with only a minor symptom occurs. In such cases the question of whether the risk of an embolization with its risk of stroke and the risk of rupturing the vessel should be taken remains unanswered.

Personally, I propose embolization for patients who have already bled, or who have permanent neurologic deficit, permanent migraines, or intractable seizures. If intra-arterial catheterization is impossible because the balloon does not go far enough and does not reach the nidus of the AVM, embolization can be done in the operating room and facilitate dissection of the AVM. The surgeon can expose one of the main feeders of the AVM, clip it, and inject bucrylate. The difficulty is in obtaining the necessary excellent x-ray facilities in the operating room, such as a C-arm, which is easy to maneuver, along with a good image intensifier connected to a video disc recorder. When the surgeon is working with the microscope, however, it takes time to clear the surgical field, and to protect it against septic mistakes. It is also difficult to avoid superposition of metallic objects on the skull. Embolization cannot be done blindly and must be followed under fluoroscopic control. It is essential that the catheter be inside an artery and not in a vein, and that the injection be done downstream.

The easiest AVM to embolize with the calibrated-leak balloon is one in which the number of main feeders does not exceed four or five, and where the caliber of the main feeders is 3 mm or more (thus decreasing the risk of rupturing the vessel).

When the three main trunks (posterior cerebral, middle cerebral, and anterior cerebral arteries) participate in the vascularization of the AVM, it is hopeless to expect complete occlusion of the entire nidus of the AVM, but embolization, even partial embolization, can decrease the steal and improve the patient. Embolization also can make surgical resection easier and safer.

Some AVMs are almost direct arteriovenous communications without the interposition of an abnormal network of vessels. This type of AVM must not be embolized with bucrylate because of the risk of venous thrombosis. The artery generally is enormous and any of the procedures that instantaneously interrupt the flow are dangerous, including the detachable balloon technique, which would seem to be one of the best ways to occlude the shunt.

We have selected 23 brain AVMs for embolization with bucrylate, 17 by endovascular technique with the calibrated-leak balloon and 6 by direct injection of bucrylate in one main feeder during surgical exposure.

In the group of 17 patients treated with the calibrated-leak balloon, the AVM always was huge, was fed by at least two main trunks (posterior cerebral and middle cerebral arteries), and was nonresectable without a major risk of huge neurologic deficit.

Complete obliteration was obtained in only 2 cases of occipital AVMs with one main feeder. Fifteen other cases have been obliterated only partially, but the steal has been reduced, the size of the remaining feeders has been decreased, and the surrounding normal cortical vessels have been better opacified. Two patients did not have bucrylate injection because of rupture of the vessel before injection of the glue.

The morbidity consists of 3 cases of permanent hemianopia and 4 cases of subarachnoid and intracerebral bleeding caused by rupture of the vessel. There was complete recovery in 3 cases. One of these cases was embolized 3 weeks later with an excellent result.

There is one death in this group; a patient with a hemispheric AVM. She died from rupture of the posterior cerebral artery by the calibrated-leak balloon before the bucrylate had been injected.

In the second group of 6 patients embolized during surgical exposure of the AVM, 5 of the AVMs were completely occluded, and 2 were resected after embolization. The AVM in these 2 cases was as hard as stone, but the dissection seemed to be easy with minimal bleeding. One AVM was partially occluded but not resected.

Two patients had transient neurologic deficits, 3 had permanent deficits (1 hemiparesis, 2 hemianopia).

There was no mortality in this group.

One patient had bucrylate in the longitudinal sinus close to the torcular, but has remained asymptomatic.

It seems that injection of bucrylate at surgery allows better occlusion of the AVM because it is possible to inject a higher quantity of bucrylate. The main risk is thrombosis of the sinuses. Some particles of bucrylate also can embolize the lungs, as a CT scan of the chest can demonstrate.

Conclusion

The detachable-balloon technique is indicated in two instances: traumatic carotid cavernous fistulas and vertebral fistulas. Spontaneous carotid cavernous fistulas cannot be treated with detachable balloons; they have to be treated by embolization of branches of the external carotid alone. Permanent occlusion of the internal carotid artery in these cases, which is done as the first therapeutic step, is contraindicated. Giant unclippable aneurysms have to be treated by occlusion of the vessel, and the patient may require a bypass if he cannot tolerate the permanent occlusion. Brain AVMs that cannot be resected without major neurologic risk and that are symptomatic can be embolized with bucrylate. Complete occlusion of AVMs can be expected by direct injection of bucrylate at surgery. Only partial occlusion is expected from embolization with the calibrated-leak balloon technique.

REFERENCES

1. Serbinenko FA: Balloon catheterization and occlusion of major cerebral vessels. *J Neurosurg* *41*:125–145, 1974
2. Debrun G, Lacour P, Caron JP, et al: Approche expérimentale du traitement des fistules carotido-caverneuses et des anévrysmes par la technique du ballonet gonflable et largable. Application chez l'homme. Communication faite à la Séance Commune des Sociétés Françaises de Neurochirurgie et de Neuroradiologie, Hôpital de la Salpêtrière, Paris, 4 Décembre, 1974
3. Debrun G, Lacour P, Caron JP, et al: Detachable balloon and calibrated leak balloon techniques in the treatment of cerebral vascular lesions. *J Neurosurg* *49*:635–649, 1978
4. Debrun G, Legre J, Kasbarian M, et al: Endovascular occlusion of vertebral fistula by detachable balloons with conservation of the vertebral blood flow. *Radiology* *130*:141–147, 1979
5. Debrun F, Lacour P, Vineula F, et al: Treatment of 54 traumatic carotid-cavernous fistulas. *J. Neurosurg* *55*:678–692, 1981
6. Debrun G, Fox A, Drake C, et al: Giant unclippable aneurysms: treatment with detachable balloons. *AJNR* *2*:167–173, 1981
7. Kerber CW: Intracranial cyanoacrylate. A new catheter therapy for arteriovenous malformations. *Invest Radiol* *10*:536–538, 1975
8. Kerber CW: Balloon catheter with a calibrated leak. *Radiology* *120*:547–550, 1976
9. White RI, Strandberg JV, Gross GS, et al: Therapeutic embolization with long term occluding agents and their effects on embolized tissues. *Radiology* *125*:677–687, 1977

CHAPTER 54
Techniques of Thrombosis of Carotid Cavernous Fistulae

John F. Mullan

THE SPONTANEOUS MORTALITY associated with carotid cavernous fistulae is low and results mainly from occasional nasal hemorrhage (3 percent). The incidence of neurologic deficit, in the form of hemiplegia or aphasia, is also low. Progressive ocular complications (70 percent), up to and including blindness, do occur.[1] Treatment therefore should be designed to prevent these ocular problems but should not invoke any measure traditionally prone to mortality, hemiplegia, or aphasia. Thus, traditional treatment, which involves some form of occlusion of the carotid artery, is conceptually undesirable and inadequate. Either the fistulous connection or the total venous sac must be shut off by a procedure that is virtually free from any risk of mortality, hemiplegia, or aphasia.

Detailed study of patients with fistulae has shown that each is different and that safe occlusion must be individually planned and may involve a variety of approaches and a variety of occlusive techniques.

The thrombogenic materials are:

1. Copper-clad steel needles
2. Phosphor bronze wire (0.005 mm in diameter)
3. Occlusive balloons
4. Conventional thrombogenic material (Gelfoam, oxidized cellulose, cotton).

It should be noted that an electric current is not advised in any instance.

Approaches to the carotid cavernous sinus are:

1. Anterior
2. Lateral
3. Posterior
4. Percutaneous transjugular

The types of fistulae that have been encountered are:

1. *Radiologically visible fistulous connections.* This is ideal and can be dealt with by stereotactic or direct insertion of copper-clad steel needles into the fistula, using the lateral approach.
2. *Fistulae that drain exclusively anteriorly into the ophthalmic vein.* This group directs its entire force into the orbit and produces severe orbital problems. It is the simplest to deal with. By the anterior approach, the point of junction between the ophthalmic vein and the sinus is entered, and the sinus is packed with conventional thrombogenic material. In some of these

Department of Neurosurgery, Pritzker School of Medicine, University of Chicago, Chicago, Illinois in which there is very little cavernous sinus component and the artery opens almost directly into the ophthalmic vein, copper-needle insertion might be adequate.

3. *Fistulae that drain exclusively posteriorly.* The posterior approach is a difficult one. Parkinson's triangle is devoid of nerves but the carotid artery lies in its depth, which is a problem for needle and wire insertion. We have used: (a) Direct insertion of wire or needles below and behind the third nerve, avoiding the artery by means of intraoperative angiography. (b) Direct insertion of thrombogenic material into the superior petrosal sinus and thence into the posterior cavernous sinus. The superior petrosal sinus is not always adequately developed. (c) Percutaneous retrograde insertion of an occlusive balloon via the jugular vein. The inferior petrosal sinus is not always adequately developed.

4. *Large fistulae of long standing.* These are relatively simple to manage. Their specific problem is that the carotid cannot be visualized initially by intraoperative angiography. They are approached by the lateral route. Wire is first inserted intradurally into the safe anterior inferior corner. Alternatively, the anterior inferior corner is packed by the anterior extradural approach. When this corner is occluded, the artery begins to show up on the arteriogram and further wire insertion can be carried out close to the artery, as indicated. These large fistulae may require 80 or more feet of wire.

5. *Smaller recent fistulae draining in all directions.* These usually require a combination of several approaches. They may be difficult.

6. *Bilateral fistulae.* These are approached as unilateral fistulae, one at a time.

7. *Fistulae with an intolerance to carotid compression.* It is believed that fistulae with this problem are not as dangerous as intact carotids with the same problem. Since carotid cavernous fistulae carry little spontaneous mortality or hemispheric morbidity, however, it seems unjustifiable to ever take any risk of hemispheric insufficiency. Therefore, in bilateral instances in which the contralateral side was treated by carotid occlusion, and in unilateral cases intolerant to compression, all risk of carotid spasm must be avoided. Copper needles, which might cause carotid spasm if inserted flush with the artery, should either be avoided or inserted at a few millimeters distance from the artery, even if a small pouch persists.

Problems

Two have been encountered:

1. Occlusion of the posterior exit from the sinus, before the anterior exit is sealed, exacerbates orbital symptoms and demands immediate attention.

2. Occlusion of both anterior and posterior exits without obliteration of the middle results in a central aneurysm, with resulting temporary nerve paralysis. This too requires further treatment once the condition is recognized.

Therefore, in planning the attack upon the fistula, the sequence and extent of each thrombogenic measure should be carefully determined. In general, it is desirable to complete unilateral occlusion in one stage, but staged occlusion is possible, either deliberately or if the initial procedure fails to achieve a complete result.

Technical Details

Superficial Temporal Artery Catheterization

Angiography is necessary for the lateral, posterior, and transjugular approaches but not for the anterior approach.

The essential components are: (a) use of intraluminal and perivascular papverine, (b) clear delineation of the lumen so that the catheter is not misplaced in the wall, (c) secure anchoring of

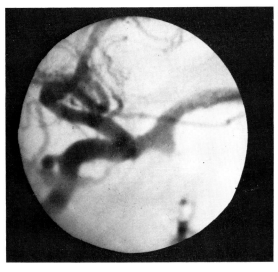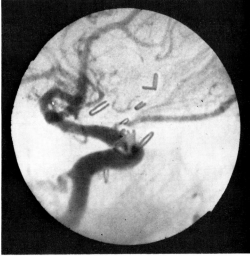

Fig. 54-1.   (left) Fistula drains almost entirely anteriorly.

Fig. 54-2.   (right) Fistula occluded by packing connection between ophthalmic vein and cavernous sinus.

the catheter by pleated brains attached to the artery wall and surrounding deep tissues so that the catheter cannot possibly become displaced, and (d) continuous heparinized irrigation.

Use of a carotid needle or catheter for angiography is not recommended during a prolonged operative procedure. The superior thyroid artery is a better alternative.

Anterior Approach

Through a simple low temporal craniotomy, the region of the foramen rotundum is located anteriorly in the extradural space. This guides the operator into the inferior orbital fissure. The bone between the superior and inferior orbital fissures is drilled out. The arterialized vein is seen running down from the roof of the orbit to the inferior fissure. Its presence at the point of entry into the sinus is confirmed by aspiration with a tuberculin syringe and fine needle. This point is entered with a fine scalpel, and the sinus is gently packed with Gelfoam, oxidized cellulose, or cotton. These materials have different degrees of rigidity and are used in combination to secure gentle packing of the anterior sinus. The bulk depends upon the size of the cavernous distention. Care should be taken that the packing does not slide anteriorly into the vein instead of into the sinus. (Figs. 54-1 and 54-2).

Lateral Approach

Through the low temporal craniotomy, the dura is opened and the temporal lobe is elevated after lumbar drainage and administration of mannitol. Radiologic markers are placed on the dura along the presumed path of the artery. Mental clips may be sewn to the dura. After angiography, phosphor bronze is inserted, by the method previously described,[2] through a point in the dura that is radiologically free from artery. If the artery is not defined on the initial angiogram, wire is inserted anteroinferiorly (or the anteroinferior corner is packed by the anterior extradural approach, as already described). Wire insertion is completed when resistance prevents further entrance. Thrombosis may be completed at this point or may require further minutes, hours, days, or, in one instance, even 3 months. Usually it is complete within an hour (Figs. 54-3 and 54-4).

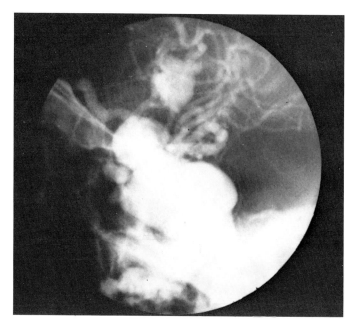

Fig. 54-3.   Fistula of 6 years' duration with greatly distended sinus and distended middle cerebral veins. Carotid obscured by sinus.

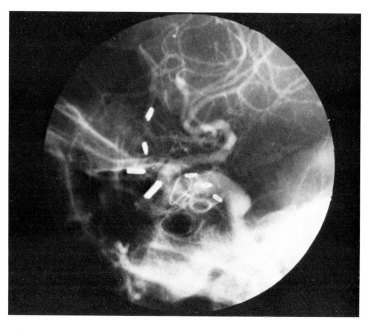

Fig. 54-4.   Cavernous sinus occluded by wire inserted first into the anterior inferior corner. Three posterior clips are dural markers.

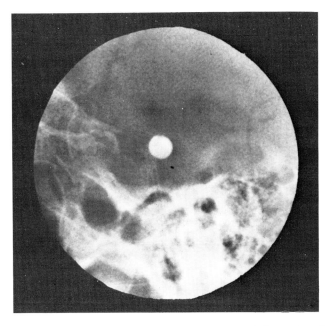

Fig. 54-5. Percutaneous transjugular, transinferior petrosal sinus insertion of balloon catheter. This is applicable to some fistulae from the region of the meningohypophyseal artery.

Posterior Approach

This also requires intraoperative angiography. It too is intradural. Wire or needles are inserted behind the radiographically outlined artery and below the visually identified third nerve. If conventional packing material is used, greater temporal retraction is necessary. The superior petrosal sinus is entered several millimeters behind its exit from the cavernous sinus, and the material is packed forward in a gentle manner. This has resulted in a temporary sixth-nerve palsy on one occasion.

Percutaneous Jugular Approach

A No. 5 Fogarty catheter has been used successfully. A No. 3 proved to be flexible. The catheter enters the lateral sinus preferentially. Appropriate manipulation usually guides it into the inferior petrosal sinus, but this attempt has not always been successful (Fig. 54-5).

Combined Approach

In most instances more than one approach is necessary for each individual fistula.

Results

In a previous study, 7 cases were reported and the techniques of stereotactic insertion of copper needles and craniotomy insertion of thrombogenic wire were described.[2] One temporary sixth-nerve palsy was encountered. We have since treated 17 additional patients. There was one temporary sixth-nerve palsy. In another recent patient the fistula was temporarily converted into an aneurysm. A partial ophthalmoplegia became complete and has again been resolved. There was no mortality and no sign of insufficiency of hemispheric blood flow in any patient.

REFERENCES

1. Hamby, WG: *Carotid Cavernous Fistula.* Springfield, IL, Charles C Thomas, 1966
2. Mullan S: Experiences with surgical thrombosis of intracranial berry aneurysms and carotid cavernous fistulas. *J Neurosurg 41*:657–670, 1974

CHAPTER 55

Surgical Management of Internal Carotid Artery Aneurysms within the Cavernous Sinus

Dwight Parkinson

SYMPTOMATIC SACCULAR ANEURYSMS of the internal carotid artery within the cavernous sinus may be either of developmental or traumatic origin. The developmental variety probably slightly outnumber the traumatic variety in occurrence, but together they total less than 5 percent of all intracranial aneurysms.[1-5] It is estimated that an equal number of asymptomatic aneurysms are found incidentally during angiography that is performed for other purposes, and still others may be overlooked at autopsy because they lie extradurally and are collapsed. The developmental variety occurs more frequently in females in a ratio of 14:3 and predominate in the groups over the age of 50 years.[2] They may be related to the normal branches of the parasellar carotid. Posteriorly, and above the sixth nerve, they should arise from the meningohypophyseal departure;[6] if below and posteriorly, they should arise from a persistent trigeminal remnant;[7,8] and if laterally placed, they might arise from the artery of the inferior cavernous sinus departure;[6] however, we have never been able to prove these relationships.

Diagnosis

Traumatic parasellar saccular aneurysms usually are associated with a basal skull fracture,[2,9] and may even be the residual of a spontaneous closure of a carotid fistula.[10,11] When present, Maurer's[12] triad of "unilateral blindness, orbital fracture, and delayed massive epistaxis following head injury" is diagnostic, but usually one or more of this triad is missing.[13-17]

The diagnosis of either type of aneurysm—traumatic or developmental—depends upon a suspicion that such a lesion may be present. Without epistaxis, there is no reliable bedside differentiation between an aneurysm and any other mass in this region.[18-35]

The signs and symptoms are anatomically logical.[14,19,20,29,36-40] Involvement of the first division of the fifth cranial nerve and of the third, fourth, and sixth cranial nerves is the earliest and most common sign.[41] Pain in the second division of the fifth nerve is less common, and involvement of the optic nerve and the third division of the fifth nerve is far less common.[42] Still less common again are exophthalmos, orbital venous engorgement, and intracranial mass effect.[43,44]

Jefferson's[16,45] classic description of the signs and symptoms remains relatively unchallenged. The occasional finding of a small pupil in association with a third-nerve palsy has been explained as being a result of the net of sympathetic nerves around the carotid being stretched or

Neurological Surgery, Faculty of Medicine, University of Manitoba, Winnipeg, Manitoba, Canada

otherwise disturbed by the aneurysm.[16,45-49] We believe this net around the carotid represents a sympathetic supply to, rather than from, the arterial wall.[50,51] Our work indicates that the largest residual of this sympathetic nerve, after supplying the carotid and other structures, then joins the sixth nerve, runs with it a few millimeters, and leaves to join the first division of the fifth nerve.[50-53] The small pupil probably results from interruption of this nerve of sympathetic continuation.[51,54] To date, there are no reports of altered patterns of sweating caused by involvement of the various divisions of the fifth cranial nerve.

The skull radiograms are abnormal in a very high percentage of symptomatic aneurysms. Erosion of the anterior clinoid, erosion of the lateral sphenoid sinus wall, and curvilinear calcification are the most frequent abnormalities.[30,55,56]

Although computed tomographic (CT) scans are used more frequently for all intracranial diagnosis, angiography remains the definitive procedure.[10,25,33,57-59] This study should demonstrate each of the arteries individually and be supplemented with cross-compression to better evaluate the presence or absence of an adequate anterior communicating artery. These studies also exclude the rare case of bilateral intracavernous aneurysms.[34,43,60]

Treatment

The first recorded surgical approach to an intracavernous aneurysm was that of Birley and Trotter,[61] who in 1928 ligated both the internal and external carotid arteries. Demoris and Lana-Peixoto[60] reported treating bilateral aneurysms by ligating one internal carotid artery and partially occluding the opposite one 3 years later with no ill effects.

Although most of the traumatic aneurysms and virtually all of the developmental sacs never bleed, the neurosurgeon's skill will be challenged to the utmost when confronted with an exsanguinating epistaxis. Initially, the hemorrhage must be brought under control.[12,39,62] During digital compression of the cervical carotid arteries, one must watch carefully for signs of cerebral ischemia and of ipsilateral retinal ischemia. If the hemorrhage persists with adequate digital compression, any retinal or hemispheric ischemia might be due to a steal,[63] and the carotid artery distal to the bleeding aneurysm must be brought under control. If the hemorrhage persists without evidence of retinal or hemispheric ischemia, the steal is neurologically innocuous, and probably results from the intracranial anastomosis of the meningohypophyseal arteries.[64] If the hemorrhage is brought under control and leaves no neurologic or visual deficit during digital compression (whether continuous or intermittent), one is relatively safe in ligating the internal carotid as a finite procedure. If, however, the hemorrhage stops during digital compression, and there is hemispheric or visual impairment, the surgeon faces a dilemma. In either case, we would favor exposing the common and internal and external carotid arteries under local anesthesia and determining whether the hemorrhage can be controlled and function preserved by clamping the common carotid artery or, preferably, the internal carotid artery by itself, leaving the external carotid collateral to supply circulation to the retina. Faced with a positive Matas test, but with the hemorrhage under control, a preliminary extracranial-intracranial bypass should be considered.

Although it has not yet been reported, it should be possible to get a guided balloon into the hemorrhaging opening[9] in order to control the aneurysmal hemorrhage and preserve the blood flow through the carotid artery.

Proximal ligation remains the treatment of choice for both traumatic and developmental saccular aneurysms within the cavernous sinus.[15,31,60,62,63,65-67] The clipping of the supraclinoid in addition to proximal ligation has been advocated in the hopes of further decreasing the turgor of the aneurysm, and thus diminishing or reversing the disturbance of the cranial nerve. Two authors have plicated the aneurysm after trapping the carotid artery in an effort to accomplish decompression of the cranial nerves.[3,65]

Until about 7 years ago our treatment was ligation and trapping, but as we developed more

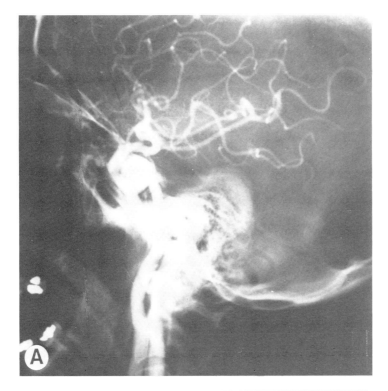

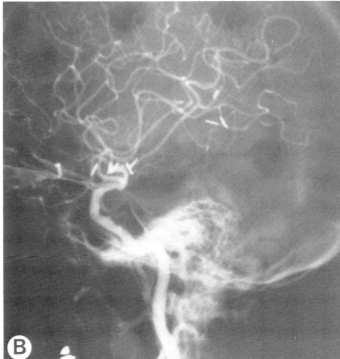

Fig. 55-1. **A.** and **B.** Pre- and postoperative angiograms demonstrating repair of a saccular aneurysm that had burst posteriorly and superiorly to become a fistula. (Reprinted from Parkinson D: Aneurysms of the cavernous sinus, in Pia HW, Langmaid C, Zierski J (eds): *Cerebral Aneurysms: Advances in Diagnosis and Therapy.* Berlin, Springer-Verlag, 1979, pp 80–81, with permission.

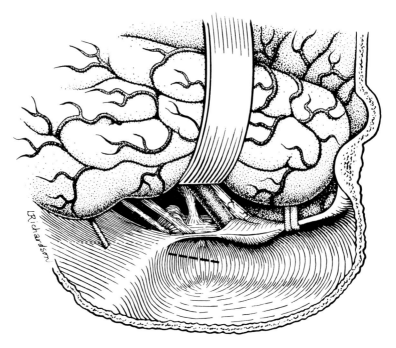

Fig. 55-2.   A drawing of the right middle fossa. The dashed line shows the
site and slope of the incision in the triangular space. Note that it
does not parallel the slope of the third and fourth nerves as the
brain is elevated, but rather the slope those nerves would follow
if the brain were not elevated.

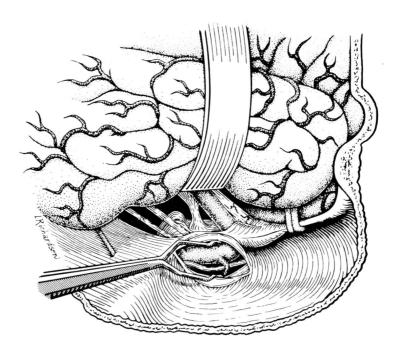

Fig. 55-3.   A drawing showing the exposure of normal structures through
the incision. The third and fourth nerves are elevated within the
upper dural margin, and the first division of the fifth nerve is visible in the down-turned lower margin. The sixth nerve is visible
within the space parallel to the first division of the fifth nerve.

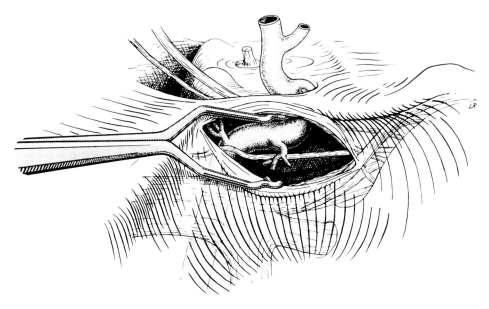

Fig. 55-4. A drawing giving an enlarged view of the exposure. The continuation of the first division of the fifth nerve and the third and fourth nerves along with the second and third divisions of fifth nerve below are ghosted-in.

confidence in our use of profound hypothermia with complete circulatory arrest while working on the direct repair of carotid cavernous fistulae,[6,68-71] it occurred to us that we should attempt the direct repair of one of these aneurysms. We have now repaired the aneurysm and successfully established a normal continuity of the carotid in 3 patients, one of whom subsequently died. Each patient had an intraoperative angiogram that confirmed satisfactory reconstruction of the carotid lumen with normal patency of that vessel (Fig. 55-1A and B).

Direct Surgical Repair

As with all surgical procedures, exposure is the first and most important consideration. Profound hypothermia provides a very excellent reduction in brain volume, but in addition, we place the patient in a lateral position to allow for spinal dainage as the exposure is developed. Mannitol is of questionable value in conjunction with cardiopulmonary bypass, although we have used this aid before starting the bypass. Once the dura is opened, it is of utmost importance to avoid bruising the temporal lobe.

Once the dural wall is exposed, the third nerve is identified as it appears over the free margin of the tentorium (Fig. 55-2). This nerve should be clearly in view during the placement of the incision in the lateral wall of the cavernous sinus and during the retraction and development of the next layer.[6] This exposure *should not be attempted* without first verifying the landmarks many time on cadavers (Figs. 55-3 and 55-4). It is better to incise the dura of the lateral wall of the cavernous sinus low rather than high since injury to a few fibers of the first division of the fifth nerve is of less importance than the risk of cutting the third or fourth nerves. As indicated in Figures 55-5 and 55-6, the triangular space is widened by any mass within it, which also obliterates the venous channels.[69,72-75] The sixth nerve is always pushed laterally and downward, parallel to the first division of the fifth nerve. Therefore, if no evidence of the first division of the fifth nerve is seen after incising the dura, the surgeon is probably well above both it and the sixth nerve since it is almost impossible to be inferior to the first division of the fifth nerve. If some fibers of the fifth nerve are noticed when the dural incision is made, they should be brushed inferiorly before the incision is enlarged.[70]

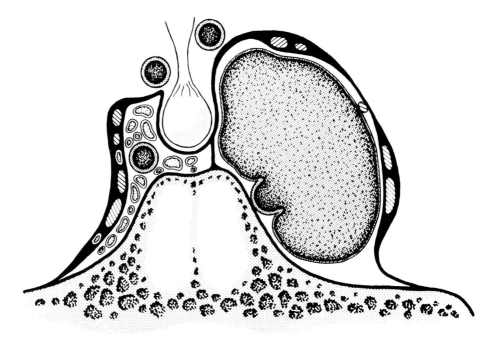

Fig. 55-5. A diagram of a coronal section indicating how the triangular space is widened by an aneurysm or any mass as on the right, and also how the venous channels are obliterated. The cross-hatched areas from above downward represent the third, fourth, and sixth nerves, and the first and second divison of the fifth nerve. On the left, the venous channels in the dural wall and within the parasellar space have a stippled center and plain walls.

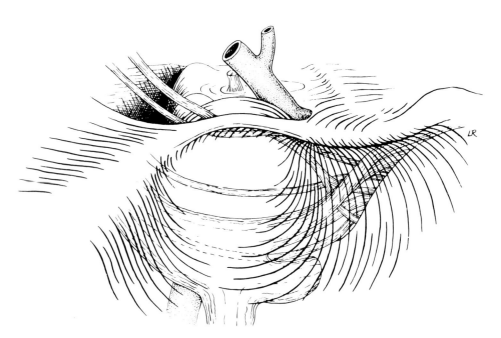

Fig. 55-6. A drawing demonstrating the lateral aspect and showing the widening of the triangular space with the third and fourth nerves again at the top, and the sixth nerve and first division of the fifth nerve bowed laterally and slightly downward.

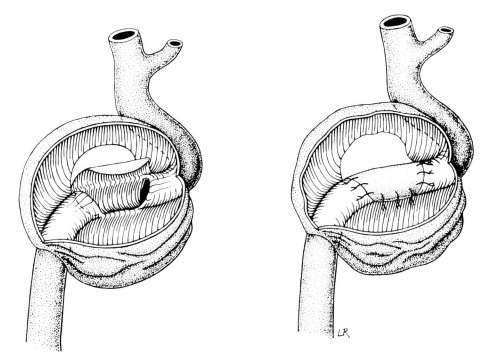

Fig. 55-7. A diagram of the repair procedure. A flap cut from the medial wall is rolled down and sutured. The remainder of the aneurysm wall is left in situ. The repair site then is packed lightly with Gelfoam and muscle, and the dural incision is closed.

The attenuation of the dura that is caused by the bulge of the intracavernous aneurysm often allows the first division of the fifth nerve to be seen through the dura. If not, it can often be felt by rubbing the blunt handle of the scalpel up and down in a vertical fashion;[70] the small ridge created by this nerve is palpable to the traverse of the knife handle. By centering at the point where the third nerve appears over the horizon, the incision can be safely extended forward for 1 cm parallel to the course of the third and fourth nerves. It must be remembered that with elevation of the temporal lobe, the third and fourth nerves assume a more vertical course, and it is the normal course that the incision must parallel, which is almost the slope of the free margin of the tentorium (see Fig. 55-2). If any fibers of the fifth nerve appear in the incision, they should be brushed inferiorly with the handle of the knife. Once the incision is 1 cm long, it can be extended forward by separating the fibers with a blunt hook; this minimizes the risk of cutting the third and fourth nerves above or the sixth nerve and first division of the fifth nerve as they converge to approach the superior orbital fissure. Posteriorly, there is no risk of cutting the cranial nerves, since they course farther apart in this area, but there is a risk of penetrating into the posterior fossa. It is always safe to expose posteriorly over a blunt hook, until the circumference of the aneurysm is sufficiently developed. Next, the dura should be separated up and down 2–3 mm to expose the surface of the aneurysm, thus further assuring against damage to the cranial nerves.

The aneurysm is opened after hypothermia and circulatory arrest have been induced. This is a safe procedure; however, the continued oozing of heparinized blood at the operative site when the circulation is restarted is a real problem that can be overcome only by waiting out the reversal of heparinization as the patient is warmed and the pump discontinued.

Technically, the aneurysmal site is best reinforced with a flap taken from the medial wall (Fig. 55-7) using 6-0 sutures in the arterial wall. This also avoids incising a cranial nerve, as they will be pushed up or down and laterally. The defect in the medial wall is patched with Gelfoam. We do not attempt to further remove the aneurysmal sac, as this would risk avulsing one of the cranial nerves. The area of repair on the carotid wall then is lightly packed with Gelfoam or muscle and the dural incision is closed with 4-0 Mersaline suture. The illumination and magnification of the operating microscope is of immense value throughout the procedure. We do not heparinize our patients postoperatively.

This procedure could be done by trapping the carotid artery without circulatory arrest, but we have been concerned about leaving an occluding clip or ligature on the carotid artery for any length of time for fear of causing an intimal lesion, which then might lead to thrombus formation. This may well be an unrealistic fear. If this operation was attempted by trapping alone without circulatory arrest, the minimal but obscurant retrograde bleeding from the meningohypophyseal and the ophthalmic arteries would have to be contended with. This should be easily controlled with a small pledget in the proximal and distal mouths of the aneurysmal opening.

We have never seen an aneurysm in this location with a neck to which a clip could be applied. All of the ones we have treated had enlarged the connection with the lumen in the manner diagrammed in Fig. 55-7. Some aneurysms possibly could be clipped—we just have not seen one. If the aneurysm could be clipped, this approach would not require any form of vascular occlusion, only the assurance that the cranial nerves had been brushed aside before the clip was applied.

REFERENCES

1. Alajouanine T, Thurel R, Nehlil J, et al: L'aneurysme due siphon-carotidien et son retentissement osseaux (reunion du trou optique et de la fente sphenoidale). *Rev Neurol (Paris) 92*:249–253, 1955
2. Brihaye J, Mage J, Verhiest G: Aneurysme traumatique de la carotide interne dans sa portion supraclinoidienne. *Acta Neurol Psychiatr Belg 54*:411–438,1954
3. Nakahara A, Asakura T, Kawabatake H, et al: A giant aneurysm of the internal carotid artery treated by intracranial direct surgery with a special reference to the anatomical relationship between the cavernous sinus and the internal artery. *Neurol Surg (Tokyo) 3*:783–789, 1975
4. Parkinson D, West M: Traumatic intracranial aneurysms. *J Neurosurg 52*:11–20, 1980
5. Verbruggen A: Subarachnoid hemorrhage. *Miss Valley Med J 77*:95–101, 1955
6. Parkinson D: A surgical approach to the cavernous portion of the carotid artery. Anatomical studies and case report. *J Neurosurg 23*:474–483, 1965
7. Drake CG: Subdural hematoma from arterial rupture. *J Neurosurg 18*:597–601, 1961
8. Parkinson D, Shields C: Persistent trigeminal artery: its relationship to the normal branches of the cavernous carotid. *J Neurosurg 40*:245–248, 1974
9. Serbinenko FA: Balloon catheterization and occlusion of major cerebral vessel. *J Neurosurg 41*:125–145, 1974
10. Lombardi G, Passerini A, Migliavacca F: Intracavernous aneurysms of the internal carotid artery. *AJR 89*:361–371, 1963
11. Taptas JN: Etiologie et pathogenie des exophtalmies d'origine vasculaire dites exophtalmies pusatiles. *Arch Ophtal (Paris) 10*:22–50, 1950
12. Maurer JJ, Mills M, German WJ: Triad of unilateral blindness, orbital fractures and massive epistaxis after head injury. *J Neurosurg 18*:837–840, 1961
13. Beadles CF: Aneurysms of the larger cerebral arteries. *Brain 30*:285–336, 1907
14. Bonnet P, Bonnet I: Le syndrome du trou dechire anterieur, symptomatique de l'aneurysme de la carotide intracranienne. *Rev Otoneuroophtalmol 27*:22–27, 1955
15. Davis RAD, Wetzel N, Davis L: An analysis of the results of treatment of intracranial vascular lesions by carotid artery ligation. *Ann Surg 143*:641–648, 1965
16. Jefferson G: Concerning injuries, aneurysms, and tumors involving the cavernous sinus. *Trans Ophthalmol Soc UK 73*:117–152, 1953
17. Weinberger LM, Adler FH, Grant FC: Primary pituitary adenoma and the syndrome of the cavernous sinus. A clinical and anatomic study. *Arch Ophthalmol (Chicago) 24*:1197–1236, 1940
18. Barr HWK, Blackwood W, Meadows SP: Intracavernous carotid aneurysms—a clinical pathological report. *Brain 94*:607–622, 1971
19. Bartholow R: Aneurysms of the arteries at the base of the brain: Their symptomology, diagnosis, and treatment. *Am J Med Sci 64*:375–386, 1872
20. Cogan DG, Mount HTJ: Intracranial aneurysms causing ophthalmoplegia. *Arch Ophthalmol (Chicago) 70*:757–771, 1963
21. Foix M: Syndrome de la paroi externe du sinus caverneux. Ophthalmoplegie unilaterale a marche rapidement progressive. *Bull Mem Soc Med Hop Paris 36*:1355–1361, 1920

22. Glasauer FE, Tandan PN: Trigeminal neurinoma in adolescents. *J Neurol Neurosurg Psychiatry* 32:562–568, 1969

23. Godtfredsen E, Lederman M: Studies on the cavernous sinus syndrome. 2. Diagnostic and prognostic roles of ophthalmoneurological signs and symptoms in malignant nasopharyngeal tumors. *Acta Neurol Scand* 41:51–53, 1965

24. Krayenbuhl H: Primary tumors of the fifth cranial nerve: their distinction from tumors of the Gasserian ganglion. *Brain* 49:337–352, 1936

25. Legre J, Dufour M, Debaene A, et al: Signes angiographiques des tumeurs de la region due sinus caverneux. *Neurochirurgie* 19:29–48, 1973

26. Love JG, Woltman HW: Trigeminal neuralgia and tumors of the Gasserian ganglion. *Proc Staff Meet Mayo Clin* 17:490–496, 1942

27. Malis LI: Tumors of the parasellar region. *Adv Neurol* 15:281–299, 1975

28. McGrath P: The cavernous sinus: Anatomical survey. *Aust NZ J Surg* 47:601–613, 1977

29. Sakalas R, Harbison JW, Vines FS, et al: Chronic sixth nerve palsy, initial sign of a petrous apex cavernous sinus tumor. *Arch Ophthalmol* 93:186–190, 1975

30. Trobe JD, Glaser JS, Post JD: Meningiomas and aneurysms of the cavernous sinus. Neuro-ophthalmologic features. *Arch Ophthalmol* 96:457–467, 1978

31. Trotter W: Symptoms of malignant tumors of the nasopharynx. *Lancet* 1:1277, 1911

32. Waga S, Kikuchi H, Handa J, et al.: Cavernous sinus venography. *AJR* 109:130–137, 1970

33. White JC, Ballantine HT: Intrasellar aneurysms simulating hypophyseal tumors. *J Neurosurg* 18:34–59, 1961

34. Wilson CB, Myers FK: Bilateral saccular aneurysms of the internal carotid artery in the cavernous sinus. *J Neurol Neurosurg Psychiatry* 26:174–177, 1963

35. Zuzulia YA, Romodanov SA, Patsko YV: Diagnosis and surgical treatment of benign craniobasal tumors involving the cavernous sinus. *Acta Neurochir (Suppl)* 28:287–290, 1979

36. Bronner A, Brini A, Risse JF, et al.: Painful ophthalmoplegia and syndrome of the cavernous sinus (optalmoplegie douloureuse et syndrome du sinus caverneaux d'orgine inflammatoire). *N J Fr Ophtalmol* 2:49–52, 1979

37. Hamby WB: *Carotid Cavernous Fistulae.* Springfield, IL, Charles C Thomas, 1966

38. Holmes T: Aneurysms of the internal carotid artery in the cavernous sinus. *Trans Pathol Soc London* 12:61, 1860–1861

39. Seftel DM, Kolson H, Gordon BS: Ruptured intracranial carotid artery aneurysm with fatal epistaxis. *Arch Otolaryngol* 70:52–60, 1959

40. Unsoldt R, Saffron AB, Saffron E, et al.: Metastatic infiltration of nerves on the cavernous sinus. *Arch Neurol* 37:59–61, 1980

41. Meadows SP: Intracavernous aneurysms of the carotid artery. *Arch Ophthalmol* 62:566–574, 1959

42. Jefferson G: Compression of the chiasma, optic nerves, and optic tracts by intracranial aneurysms. *Brain* 60:444–497, 1937

43. Nukui H, Imai S, Fukumachi A, et al.: Giant aneurysms of the internal carotid within the cavernous sinus associated with an aneurysm of the basilar artery. *Neurol Surg* 3:479–484, 1977

44. Jefferson G: Extrasellar extensions of pituitary adenomas. *Proc R Soc Med* 38:433–458, 1940

45. Jefferson G: On the saccular aneurysms of the internal carotid artery in the cavernous sinus. *Br J Surg* 26:267–302, 1938

46. Jefferson G: Trigeminal neurinomas with some remarks on the malignant invasion of the Gasserian ganglion. *Clin Neurosurg* 1:11–54, 1955

47. Rucker CW: The causes of paralysis of the third, fourth, and sixth cranial nerves. *Am J Ophthalmol* 61:1293–1298, 1966

48. Raeder JG: Paratrigeminal paralysis of oculo pupillary sympathetic. *Brain* 47:149–158, 1924

49. Talosa E: Periarteritic lesion of the carotid syphon with the clinical features of a carotid intraclinoid aneurysm. *J Neurol Neurosurg Psychiatry* 17:300–302, 1954

50. Johnston JA, Parkinson D: Intracranial sympathetic pathways associated with the sixth cranial nerve. *J Neurosurg* 39:236–242, 1974

51. Parkinson D: Bernard, Mitchell, Horner syndrome and others? *Surg Neurol* 11:211–233, 1979

52. Parkinson D, Johnson JA, Chaudhuri A: Sympathetic connections to the fifth and sixth cranial nerves. *Anat Rec* 191:221–226, 1978

53. Sunderland S, Hughes ESR: The pupilloconstrictor pathway and the nerves to the ocular muscles in man. *Brain* 39:301–309, 1946

54. McKinney J, Acree T, Soltz SE: Syndrome of ruptured aneurysm of intracranial portion of internal carotid artery. *Bull Neurol Inst NY* 5:247–277, 1936

55. Post M, Glaser JS, Trobe JD: Radiographic diagnosis of cavernous meningiomas and aneurysms with a review of the neurovascular anatomy of the cavernous sinus. *CRC Crit Rev Diagn Imaging* 12:1–34, 1979

56. Jefferson G: Discussion of the value of radiology in neurosurgery. *Proc R Soc Med 29*:1169–1172, 1936

57. Chase NE, Taveras JM: Carotid angiography in the diagnosis of extradural parasellar tumors. *Acta Radiol (Diagn) (Stockh) 1*:214–224, 1963

58. Laun A: Survey of traumatic aneurysms, in Pia HW, Langmaid C, Zierski J (eds): *Cerebral Aneurysms: Advances in Diagnosis and Therapy.* Berlin, Springer-Verlag, 1979, pp. 364–375

59. Lloyd GAS: The localization of lesions in the orbital apex and cavernous sinus by frontal venography. *Br J Radiol 45*:405–414, 1972

60. Demoris JV, Lana-Peixoto MA: Treatment by bilateral carotid ligation. *Surg Neurol 9*:379–381, 1978

61. Birley JL, Trotter W: Traumatic aneurysm of the intracranial portion of the internal carotid artery. *Brain 51*:184–208, 1928

62. Voris HC, Basile JXR: Recurrent epistaxis from aneurysm of the internal carotid artery. *J Neurosurg 18*:841–842, 1961

63. Adson AW: Surgical treatment of vascular diseases altering function of eyes. *Am J Ophthalmol 25*:824, 1942

64. Parkinson D: Collateral circulation of cavernous carotid artery: Anatomy. *Can J Surg 7*:251–268, 1964

65. Vandelen JR: Intercavernous traumatic aneurysms. *Surg Neurol 13*:203–207, 1980

66. Tindall GT, Goree JA, Lee JF, et al.: Effect of common carotid ligature on size of internal carotid aneurysms and distal intra carotid and retinal artery pressures. *J Neurosurg 25*:503–511, 1966

67. Tytus JS, Ward AL: The effect of cervical carotid ligation on giant intracranial aneurysms. *J Neurosurg 33*:184–190, 1970

68. Parkinson D: Transcavernous repair of carotid cavernous fistula. *J Neurosurg 26*:420–424, 1967

69. Parkinson D: Carotid cavernous fistula, in Vinken PJ, Bruyn GW (eds): *Handbook of Clinical Neurology,* vol 12. Amsterdam, North-Holland, 1972

70. Parkinson D: Carotid cavernous fistula: Direct repair with preservation of carotid artery. *J Neurosurg 38*:99–106, 1973

71. Parkinson D: Carotid cavernous fistula, direct approach with repair of fistula and preservation of the artery, in Morley TP (ed): *Current Controversies in Neurosurgery.* Philadelphia, WB Saunders, 1976, pp 237–249

72. Bedford MA: Cavernous sinus. *Br J Ophthalmol 52*:41–46, 1966

73. Solassol A, Zidane C, Slimane-Taleb S, et al: The veins of the cavernous sinus in the four month old human fetus. *C R Assoc Anat 149*:1009–1015, 1970

74. Thomas JE, Yoss RE: The parasellar syndrome. Problems in determining etiology. *Mayo Clin Proc 45*:617–623, 1970

75. Winslow JB: *Exposition Anatomique de la Structure du Corps Humain,* vol 2. London, Prevost, 1734, p 31

76. Parkinson D: Aneurysms of the cavernous sinus, in Pia HW, Langmaid C, Zierski J (eds): *Cerebral Aneurysms: Advances in Diagnosis and Therapy.* Berlin, Springer-Verlag, 1979, pp 79–82

CHAPTER 56
Surgical Treatment of Anterior Communicating Artery Aneurysms

Robert M. Crowell   Robert G. Ojemann

ANTERIOR COMMUNICATING ARTERY ANEURYSMS usually present with sub-arachnoid hemorrhage (SAH). Often the SAH is a minor "warning leak" causing severe headache and a stiff neck. Sometimes SAH produces neurologic deficits ranging from minor to profound. By virtue of its location, the anterior communicating aneurysm is liable to hemorrhage upward into the third ventricle and hypothalamic region. Damage in these areas may be associated with memory disturbance (particularly for recent events), abulia, inappropriate secretion of antidiuretic hormone, symptomatic hydrocephalus, or autonomic instability with unstable pulse and blood pressure. Alternatively, the aneurysm may rupture laterally, spilling blood into the cisterns surrounding the internal carotid and middle cerebral arteries or directly into the parenchyma including the internal capsule.

Delayed complications are common with these lesions. Bleeding into the basal cisterns and third ventricle frequently causes hydrocephalus, which may become symptomatic and require shunting. Delayed deterioration may be related to vasospasm: spasm of anterior cerebral arteries may cause lower-limb paresis or abulia; spasm of internal carotid and middle cerebral arteries may lead to hemiparesis.

In rare instances anterior communicating aneurysms reach giant size and compress visual pathways, the hypothalamus, or the internal capsule. In such instances the patient presents with visual symptoms, mental disturbance, or hemiparesis.

Preoperative Management

Initial Evaluation

When the diagnosis of SAH is suspected, the first step is to conduct a computed tomographic (CT) scan with and without contrast.[1] This test may confirm the diagnosis by establishing that blood is in the basal cisterns, interhemispheric fissure, ventricles, or adjacent brain

Department of Neurosurgery, University of Illinois, Chicago, Illinois; and Neurosurgical Service, Massachusetts General Hospital, and Department of Surgery, Harvard Medical School, Boston, Massachusetts.

We are grateful to Dr. R. S. Lees for the medical management of many of the patients discussed; to Drs. C. M. Fisher and J. P. Kistler for neurologic consultation; and Drs. P. Sundaram and F. DeBros for neuroanesthetic management. Thanks also to Mrs. Edith Tagrin for preparation of the figures and to Georgia Frederic for preparation of the manuscript.

Supported in part by the National Institute of Neurological and Communicative Diseases and Stroke through Teacher-Investigator Award NS11001 and Grant NS 17319.

Portions of this chapter are reprinted with permission from Ojemann RG, Crowell RM: Surgical Management of Cerebrovascular Disease (Baltimore, Williams and Wilkins).

tissue. In some cases the aneurysm may be seen filling with the contrast medium. Lumbar puncture may be used when the diagnosis has not been established by CT scan, but only if there is no evidence of increased intracranial pressure.

All patients with SAH should undergo screening tests of clotting function including prothrombin time (PT), partial thromboplastin time (PTT), and a platelet count. An EKG may show abnormalities related to SAH. A complete blood count and serum electrolyte and serum osmolarity should be determined as base-line values. Psychometric testing, when possible, provides a quantitative parameter so that mental status can be characterized and followed up in these cases.

Early management is guided by the clinical status and CT findings.[2] For cases of symptomatic intracranial hematoma, emergency surgical evacuation is advisable. For those patients with symptomatic hydrocephalus, emergency ventriculoperitoneal shunting may reverse the clinical symptomatology.

Medical Therapy

For stable patients without mass lesions or hydrocephalus, a standard medical regimen is instituted. This includes:

1. Bedrest.
2. Administration of fluids in an attempt to maintain normal circulating volume and central venous pressure.
3. Elastic stockings or pneumatic compression boots.
4. Epsilon aminocaproic acid (Amicar, 30 gm/day IV).
5. Anticonvulsants (diphenylhydantoin 300 mg/day).
6. Stool softeners (Colace 100 mg TID).
7. For agitation, phenobarbital (15–30 mg IM or PO Q3h).
8. For hypertension, hydralazine (5–20 mg IM q3h), to bring the systolic pressure below 150 torr without causing drowsiness. In some cases propranolol is used, and occasionally resistant hypertension requires intravenous nitroprusside for control.
9. Methylprednisolone (16–80 mg PO or IV Q6h) to reduce cerebral swelling in symptomatic patients.
10. Cimetidine (300 mg PO or IV q8h) along with antacid orally or by gastric tube every 3 hours.
11. Codeine for headache (30–60 mg PO or IM Q 3-4h).
12. Kanamycin (1 g TID) and reserpine (0.2 mg SC TID) to reduce the chance of postoperative vasospasm. These drugs are given only to grade 1 and 2 patients who do not have other contraindications.

Should a patient deteriorate, metabolic studies and CT are conducted on an emergency basis. Electrolyte imbalance may require correction. CT may reveal hydrocephalus or focal cerebral ischemia or edema. Progressive hydrocephalus requires ventriculoperitoneal shunting for relief of the symptoms. If a clear explanation for the deterioration is not found, angiography is performed. If angiography discloses a significant degree of vasospasm (grades 3–4), a program of therapy is begun, and radial arterial pressure and central venous pressure are monitored. The intravascular volume is increased with colloid or packed cells to achieve a central venous pressure of 10–12 cm of water and a hematocrit of 40 percent. A pressor is given to increase the systolic blood pressure to about 30 torr above basal levels, with a maximum of 160 torr. Phenylephrine or dopamine may be used for this purpose.

The timing of elective angiography and surgery is determined by the clinical condition as judged by the Botterell classification. For patients in good condition (grades 1–2), angiography is deferred 7 to 10 days after SAH, with surgery on the following day if no spasm is demonstrated. For patients in poor condition (grades 3–4), angiography is deferred about 2 to 3 weeks after SAH. If the patient is stable and the angiogram shows an aneurysm, surgery is performed. Whenever significant spasm is demonstrated, we defer surgery for 2 to 3 weeks and then proceed even if there is some residual spasm.

Angiography must demonstrate the sac and neck, their relation to parent arteries, and the direction in which the lesion points. Satisfactory visualization will often require oblique and base views. To assure visualization of the anterior communicating artery and both precommunal (A-1) anterior cerebral arteries, cross-compression of one carotid artery is often needed during injection of the contralateral internal carotid artery. The posterior circulation should be visualized to exclude multiple lesions. Subtraction techniques are often useful to delineate complex vascular anatomy in this area. In centers where it is available, stereoscopic views and angiotomography may be helpful for the detailed depiction of these lesions.

Anesthesia

Preoperative Medication

The night before surgery, steroids are begun if they are not already included in the regimen. We prefer methylprednisolone (Solu-medrol®) 80 mg intramuscularly at midnight and 6 A.M. In addition, propranolol (Inderol) is given, 40 mg orally at midnight. This agent appears to improve the blood pressure control intraoperatively. Blood is requested for availability during surgery. As a preoperative medication, diazepam (Valium) 10 mg intramuscularly or a neurolept agent (Innovar, 0.5 cc IM) serves nicely.

Preparation

In the induction room an intravenous route is established. This is preferably a large-bore plastic cannula, but in many patients receiving Amicar therapy, suitable veins are hard to identify. Rather than agitate such patients with repeated venipuncture efforts, it is better to place a small-gauge needle intravenously and then establish two large-bore intravenous routes after the patient is anesthetized. If necessary, the external jugular vein or a leg vein may be used. In rare cases no intravenous line can be established easily and a mask induction of anesthesia may be the best initial maneuver. A catheter is introduced into the radial artery for continuous monitoring of arterial pressure. Such monitoring is particularly important during induction, when wide swings of arterial pressure may occur. Pressor and hypotensive agents are available for infusion; phenylephrine (Neosynephrine, 10 mg in 250 cc 5% dextrose and water) and sodium nitroprusside (50 mg in 250 cc 5% dextrose in water shielded with tin foil) serve well for these needs.

Induction

Once all preparations have been made, a slow induction is carried out with preparation over 10 minutes or more before intubation. Sodium pentobarbital is given by increments (50–150 mg per increment up to 1 gm total) after initial preoxygenization. Once the patient is deeply drowsy, Halothane is given by mask (0.5 to 1.5%). Before intubation a muscle relaxant is given (curare 0.5 mg/kg). A twitch monitor is applied to the ulnar nerve to monitor the completeness of neuromuscular blockade. An additional increment of pentobarbital is given intravenously just before intratracheal intubation. Ideally the blood pressure is in the range of 100 torr systolic at this point. Laryngoscopy is carried out, and the vocal cords are sprayed with a local anesthetic solution. Further oxygenation with Halothane administered through a mask is carried out. The blood pressure response to laryngoscopy is noted; if a substantial hypertensive response occurs, an additional increment of pentobarbital is administered, or further administration of Halo-thane, or both. Finally, with the patient stable and well anesthetized, laryngoscopy is carried out with gentle endotracheal intubation. In the case of a sustained rise in blood pressure, further increments of pentobarbital are given intravenously and the concentration of Halothane may be increased temporarily. The cuff of the endotracheal tube is inflated and checked to insure that it is adequately preventing leaks. The tube is then taped in place. Controlled ventilation is preferred, with arterial PCO2 maintained in the range of 30 torr, as demonstrated by frequently sampled arterial blood gases. The arterial blood gases likewise provide a frequent check on the adequacy of oxygenation.

Reduction of Brain Tension

All patients receive 100 gm of mannitol IV while the bone flap is being turned; in many cases this is preceded by Lasix 20 mg IV. This usually relaxes the brain nicely. Solu-medrol 80 mg IV is continued every 4 hours.

In many cases of anterior communicating aneurysm, a lumbar subarachnoid spinal catheter is quite helpful. After the induction of anesthesia, such a catheter (22-gauge polyethylene tubing) may be introduced via a Touhy needle. Only a small amount of fluid is allowed to escape at the time of introduction. The catheter is led in such a fashion that further fluid may be removed by the anesthesiologist upon request.

Controlled Hypotension

Careful communication between the neuroanesthesiologist and the surgeon is crucial. Of particular importance is the pharmacologic control of blood pressure during surgery. Controlled hypotension is used to slacken the aneurysm during dissection in order to decrease the likelihood of intraoperative rupture.[3] In most patients the systolic blood pressure is maintained at about 100 torr during the initial exposure. Once the aneurysm is in view the pressure is further dropped to about 80 torr systolic. During critical dissection of the neck of the aneurysm, deep hypotension may be required (systolic blood pressure 60 torr or mean arterial blood pressure about 40 torr). Occasionally a particularly difficult portion of an aneurysm may justify a burst of very deep hypotension for 2 to 3 minutes at a mean of 20–25 torr. Most patients tolerate this type of deep hypotension without postoperative sequelae. In normal brain, autoregulation maintains local cerebral blood flow at mean arterial blood pressures of 40–45 torr. In patients with subarachnoid hemorrhage, however, autoregulation may be lost in some zones. Moreover, in some elderly patients, and those with ischemic heart disease, prolonged and deep hypotension may not be well tolerated by the brain, heart, and kidneys. In such cases, levels of controlled hypotension may be moderated. Several techniques for controlled hypotension are available. In many cases, moderate hypotension may be achieved simply by increasing the concentration of inspired Halothane. In most cases an additional agent, such as sodium nitroprusside, will be required to further diminish the blood pressure. Trimethaphan camsylate (Arfonad) or trinitroglycerine may also be used for this purpose. Another hypotensive agent that may be used for more prolonged effect is hydralazine given in increments of 5 mg intravenously. Likewise, propranolol, given preoperatively and then intraoperatively in doses as high as 1–2 mg intravenously, may be used for more prolonged hypotensive effect of a stable sort.

Vasospasm

In patients with vasospasm suspected or proved by angiography, care is taken not to lower the blood pressure as much as is normally done. Once the aneurysm is obliterated, cerebral perfusion is maximized by volume expansion with colloid and packed cells if necessary. Blood pressure is elevated to 140 torr systolic, using a pressor as necessary.

Operative Technique

Positioning and Preparation

In most cases the approach is from the right side. The head is turned to the left about 60°, with the zygoma uppermost and the vertex depressed slightly below the horizontal plane. In some cases a small roll is placed under the right shoulder of patients with limited mobility of the neck. Indications for a left subfrontal approach include: an additional left-sided aneurysm, a large anterior communicating aneurysm pointing sharply toward the right, or a large dominant left A1 feeder with no right A1 visualized on angiography.

The scalp sites are prepared with Zephiran solution, and then the Mayfield-Kees three-point headrest is applied. Additional increments of pentobarbital (50–150 mg IV) are given just before this painful stimulation.

Protective plastic shields are placed across the eyes. The proposed incision site is shaved, and steri-towels are placed to wall off the area. Either elastic bandages or pneumatic compression boots are used on the lower extremities to help prevent thrombophlebitis. The operating table then is positioned in the operating room; the anesthetist and anesthesia equipment are situated at the patient's left side below shoulder level to provide satisfactory room for the operating microscope. The scrub nurse stands on the patient's right side, and Mayo stands are attached to the table over the patient's chest and abdomen.

Incision

After the operative site has been prepared, the incision is marked with a marking pen (Fig. 56-1). In most cases an incision just behind the hairline is preferred, proceeding from the widow's peak curvilinearly to a point just above the zygoma in front of the tragus. The superficial temporal artery is palpated and marked. The incision should lie posterior to the root of the superficial temporal artery in order to preserve this structure with the flap. Occasionally in bald individuals or in cases where additional exposure is desired for another aneurysm, an alternative incision may be planned, using a wrinkle high in the forehead or a coronal incision extending across the midline. As the area is draped, the post for the Greenberg retractor is attached to the three-point headrest to the left of the patient's head.

Both surgeon and assistant use 2× loupes and headlights during the initial phases of the procedure. Local anesthesia (Marcaine 1% without epinephrine) is injected along the incision except near the superficial temporal artery. The incision is begun anteriorly and cuts down to but not through the periosteum. A scissors is inserted in the plane between the galea and the periosteum. The knife then incises down to the scissors, thus preventing injury to the underlying temporalis muscle and superficial temporal artery. Care is taken to avoid this artery, particularly near its root. The posterior branch of the superficial temporal artery is dissected free and divided between 3-0 silk ligatures, thus permitting the trunk and frontal branch of this vessel, which might be needed for later cerebral revascularization, to be reflected forward with the soft tissue flap. Hemostasis is obtained by applying Dandy hemostats to the posterior margin and Köln clips to the anterior margins of the incision. Particular care should be taken to avoid injuring the superficial temporal artery. Next the temporalis fascia is incised with a knife, and the temporalis muscle is opened with the cutting cautery. A branch of the deep temporal artery is regularly encountered within the muscle. This must be cauterized accurately to avoid pesky bleeding later. The periosteum is swept off the skull with a periosteal elevator just to the edge of the orbit, and the muscle, including the superior temporal line, is reflected from the skull with the cutting cautery until the zygomatic process of frontal bone is approached. The soft tissue flap is folded over a sponge to prevent ischemic compression and is protected with a rubber dam and a sponge soaked in bacitracin, and is held in place with silk sutures sewn into the muscle and attached by rubber bands to the drapes. A final maneuver, which permits maximum visualization beneath

FREE BONE FLAP

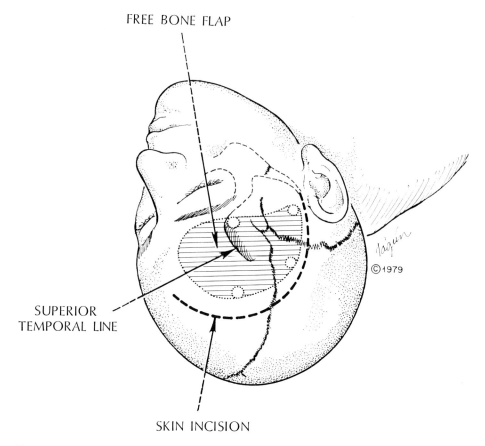

SUPERIOR
TEMPORAL LINE

©1979

SKIN INCISION

Fig. 56-1. Incision and pterional craniotomy. Skin incision is just behind hairline and the anterior branch of the superficial temporal artery. Key burr hole lies just behind the zygomatic process of the frontal bone and inferior to the superior temporal line. Often
three burr holes are sufficient.

muscle, is the application of Cushing retractors to the muscle along the zygomatic process of the
frontal bone. Tension should be applied to these retractors by attaching rubber bands and Allis
clamps to the drapes. This approach provides excellent exposure once the bone flap is removed.
We have tried the Z-formed temporalis fascia opening suggested by Yasargil and found it no better for exposure and less satisfactory from the cosmetic standpoint.

Initial Exposure

A free pterional bone flap[4] is turned with the power drill and craniotome (Fig. 56-1). The
critical burr hole is placed just behind the zygomatic process of the frontal bone and below the
end of the superior temporal line. Additional burr holes are placed in the frontal and temporal
regions, the latter just at the superior temporal line. The unsightly depression of an inferomedial
frontal burr hole can be eliminated by making a curved bony cut with the craniotome. Dura is
separated from the inner table of the skull with a No. 3 Penfield dissector. The craniotome cut is
made starting along the floor of the anterior fossa proceeding medially about 3–4 cm and then
curving in an easy arch posteriorly to the high temporal burr hole. It is advisable to angle this
saw curve slightly, beveling outward, to provide nice seating for the bone flap when it is replaced. The lateral sphenoid ridge is preserved with the bone flap, which is finally broken off by
prying with a periosteal elevator. The bone flap is carefully peeled off the dura, and the middle
meningeal artery is identified, coagulated, and cut. Bony edges are waxed for hemostasis. Addi-

tional bone is rongeured from the lateral sphenoid ridge. Care is taken at this point to avoid injury to structures in the superior orbital fissure. Frequently a small arterial branch to the dura in this region must be coagulated. These maneuvers level the sphenoid ridge effectively between the frontal and temporal lobes, thus creating unobstructed visual access to the anterior clinoid area. In some cases the inner table of bone forming the floor of the anterior fossa over the orbit will be characterized by mountainous irregularities impeding exposure. In such cases a high-speed drill may be used to smooth the area. If there is a small opening into the orbit, it should be plugged with Gelfoam or bone wax. If additional access is needed along the floor of the anterior fossa behind the supraorbital ridge, the inner table bone at the edge of the craniotomy just anterior to the key hole may also be removed with the rongeur without compromising the cosmetic appearance of the outer table. In some cases a very prominent and lateral frontal sinus may be encountered with the saw cut or bone removal. If this occurs, the mucosa should be removed, the sinus should be packed with Gelfoam soaked in bacitracin, and the opening in the bone should be covered with a flap of pericranium tissue dissected from the back of the scalp flap and then sewn to the adjacent dura. Next, the wire-pan drill is used to create holes for wires to hold the flap in place at the time of closure. Sutures of 4–0 silk, attaching the dura to the pericranial tissue, are placed around the periphery of the opening of the bone to achieve epidural hemostasis. Tiny strips of Surgicel are inserted in the epidural space as needed. Bacitracin-soaked sponges are placed over the edges of the skin and over all exposed tissue except the dura.

During this phase the surgeon can readily determine whether the brain is slack. If it is not, then measures must be taken to obtain adequate slackness; the PCO_2 may need adjustment, additional dehydration may be required, or CSF may have to be drained. Occasionally it will be necessary to puncture the ventricle to obtain a slack brain.

A linear dural incision is made approximately 6–8 mm above the inferior margin of the bony opening with inferior turning at the frontal and temporal corners. The inferior dural flap is tacked up flush with the bone edge and is held with tacking sutures under tension. Care should be taken to avoid a buckle in the center of this flap, which could interfere with intradural visualization.

The surface of the brain, under $2\times$ loupe magnification, is inspected for evidence of subdural hematoma, subarachnoid hemorrhage, or cerebral infarction. A medium-width, Teflon-coated, hand-held brain retractor is used to gently elevate the frontal lobe (Fig. 56-2). A sucker on a cottonoid can be used to gradually remove CSF that may be inferior to the frontal lobe. The retractor is advanced slowly just in front of the edge of the sphenoid wing.

The olfactory tract, an important landmark, will come into view, and following this a few millimeters posteriorly will lead to the region of the optic nerve (Fig. 56-2). Usually the arachnoid is thin and the optic nerve and carotid artery can be visualized, but at times, the arachnoid may be thicker and obscure these structures. The arachnoid is opened using a fine right-angle hook, a microdissector, or microscissors. Time should then be spent allowing further CSF to drain. It is most important that the brain be so slack that only mild retraction is needed for adequate exposure.

Next, a protective layer of rubber dam and cottonoid, precut to the proper shape, is placed like a rug over the exposed frontal lobe down to the olfactory tract. At this point the Greenberg self-retaining retractor system, holding a Teflon-coated, Dott-type posted retractor blade bent to about 60°, is placed in a position to elevate the frontal lobe. The retractor should take a low profile to give easy access to the infrafrontal cleft. Next, a narrow, hand-held retractor is used to carefully elevate the temporal lobe. Temporal tip bridging veins are divided (Fig. 57-2). Once the temporal tip is free, a covering of rubber dam and cottonoid is placed, and the lobe is held posteriorly with a slender retractor blade fixed on the Greenberg apparatus. The two retractor blades should be separated by only several millimeters at right angles to each other. Up to this point the combination of $2\times$ loupes and headlight illumination has been used for maximum mobility with adequate visualization. From this point, however, the surgical operating microscope is used to maximize illumination and visualization of critical structures.

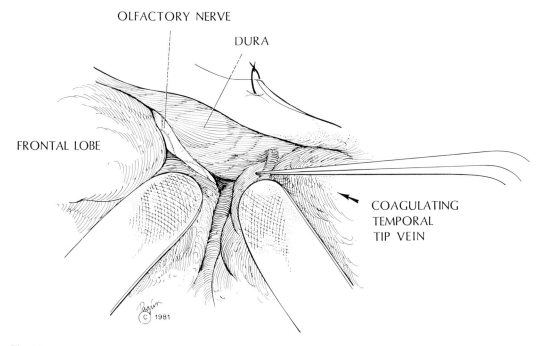

OLFACTORY NERVE

DURA

FRONTAL LOBE

COAGULATING
TEMPORAL
TIP VEIN

© 1981

Fig. 56-2.   Elevation of frontal lobe. This is done gradually with suction-removal of CSF. The olfactory tract leads back to the optic nerve. Temporal bridging veins are coagulated and cut near the cortex.

Microsurgical Dissection

We use the Zeiss operating microscope No. 1 with a 275-mm lens, 12.5 × high eye-point oculars, and angled 160-mm eyepieces.[4] The visual image is channeled via a 50:50 small beam splitter to a stereo observer tube on the left and a unified adaptor (Design for Vision) for video (Hitachi) and intermittent photography (Contax) on the right. A clear video image projected on a monitor mounted high in one corner of the operating theater provides access to the microsurgical action for all members of the microsurgical team, including the scrub nurse and anesthetist.

Dissection begins on the internal carotid artery (Fig. 56-3). The surgeon opens the cistern of the internal carotid artery further, using a 16-gauge sucker in the left hand and a fine arachnoid hook in the right, permitting free egress of CSF. With a fine dissector, the internal carotid is followed distally. In some cases the right A1 anterior cerebral artery takeoff can be visualized and the anterior edge of this vessel followed immediately toward the aneurysm (Fig. 56-4). This procedure leads right to the aneurysm and avoids an excessively large gyrus rectus corticectomy. In some cases, however, the internal carotid artery segment is long and the anterior cerebral artery takeoff high and posteriorly placed. In such instances, excessive frontal retraction would be needed to see the origin of A1, and it seems wiser to proceed directly to the gyrus rectus corticectomy. A controlled sucker device, such as the Regu-Gauge®, is helpful to provide adequate low-level suction without the danger of suction injury to critical structures. Retraction at this point involves not only elevation of the frontal lobe and olfactory tract, but also a gentle lifting of the lobe away from the interhemispheric fissure. Only when the brain is slack can this type of critical retraction be obtained and held. The direction of view at this point proceeds from temporally quite medially, facilitated by the marked leftward turning of the head. If the head is not turned far enough to the left, the surgeon will bend to the right in an awkward fashion.

A corticectomy is made in the gyrus rectus,[5] just medial to the olfactory tract, beginning at the optic nerve and extending anteriorly for about 1.5 cm (Fig. 56-5). The incision is deepened until the pia arachnoid over the A1 segment and then the interhemispheric fissure is reached. This protective layer overlying the aneurysm is left intact. The arachnoid overlying the right A1

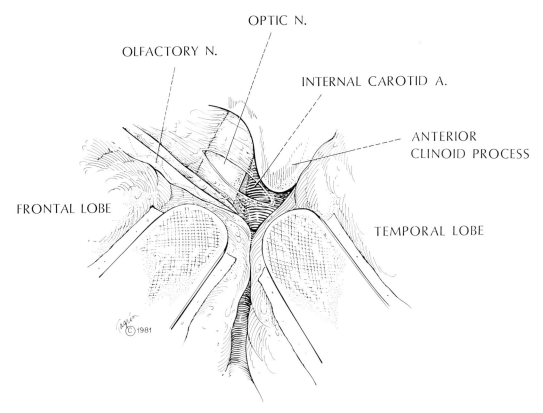

Fig. 56-3. Incision of the arachnoid. Under the microscope, a sharp hook is used to open the arachnoid over the internal carotid artery and the optic nerve. This permits further elevation of the frontal lobe.

anterior cerebral artery is opened (Fig. 56-6). Once the right A1 anterior cerebral artery is visualized, it is wise to bring the blood pressure into the range of 80 torr systolic in most patients. Branches of this vessel, which may include Heubner's artery, should be preserved. The A1 segment is followed distally to the anterior communicating artery and then to the right A2 anterior cerebral artery.[5] If possible, the aneurysm is avoided at this stage. Dissection proceeds with a combination of blunt dissection with a fine microdissector and microscissors cutting arachnoid after electrocoagulation. Next, the left A2 anterior cerebral artery is identified in the interhemispheric fissure (Fig. 56-7). Check the angiogram to determine whether the left A2 anterior cerebral artery is anterior or posterior to its right-sided counterpart. Then look in the appropriate direction to find this vessel. Once the left A2 is identified, it may be followed retrograde to the left A1 anterior cerebral artery. Careful scrutiny of the angiograms and a knowledge of the anatomic variants guide the dissection. Important normal variants include: (1) a hypoplastic A1 segment, (2) (multiple) reduplicated anterior communicating arteries, and (3) a persistent artery to the corpus callosum from the anterior communicating artery. Almost always the aneurysm arises from the junction of the larger A1 and anterior communicating arteries.

As the surgeon seeks to identify the left anterior cerebral artery segments, significant retraction of the aneurysm is often needed. This is best accomplished by leaving pia-arachnoid overlying the lesion, with retraction applied by the sucker through an intervening cottonoid. The surgeon should seek to identify and free all major arterial trunks before working on the aneurysm. Dissection then proceeds with a microdissector or the bipolar cautery and microscissors. For the typical lesion that projects straight up from the anterior communicating artery, the left A1 anterior cerebral artery may be most accessible ventrally. In this situation the anterior portion of the aneurysm and frontal lobes are gently reflected superiorly and back, permitting sharp

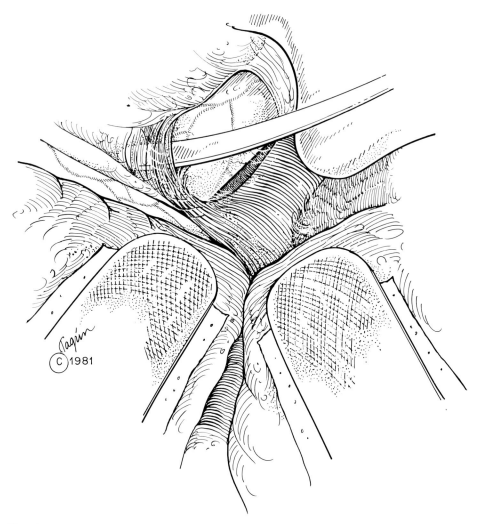

Fig. 56-4. Dissection of a right A1 artery. The anterior border of the vessel is freed of the arachnoid with a Rhoton No. 6 dissector and microscissors.

dissection of the aneurysm away from the superior surface of the chiasm and both optic nerves. In this way the ventral aspect of the anterior communicating artery and the left A1 anterior cerebral artery may be identified. When the lesion points forward, access to the left A1 is easiest from behind the lesion. In either event encirclement of the lesion is required. At this stage it is wise to leave in place any small potentially important arterial branches that are adherent to the dome of the lesion.

Dissection of the Neck of the Aneurysm

At this point, systolic blood pressure is usually in the 60–70 torr range. Brief, deep hypotension with mean arterial pressure in the 30–40 torr range is often needed. Lesions with paper-thin angry red patches near the neck will demand this adjunct to prevent rupture. In exceptional cases where the neck of the aneurysm is markedly thin, a burst of deep hypotension to the level of 20–25 torr mean may give the aneurysm the required slackness. For these maneuvers, the sucker, with or without a cottonoid, is used to reflect the lesion to one side, and a fine dissector or microscissors frees the neck from adherent structures. When visualization permits, sharp dissection is preferable. Usually the microscope provides identification of a cleavage plane right to the

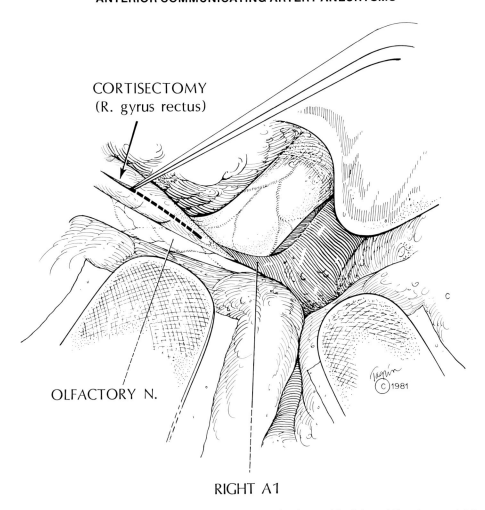

CORTISECTOMY
(R. gyrus rectus)

OLFACTORY N.

RIGHT A1

©1981

Fig. 56-5. Gyrus rectus corticectomy. Bipolar cauterization and incision of the pia over 1-1.5 cm. Care must be taken to place the corticectomy over the aneurysm site (usually near the medial edge of the optic nerve).

edge of the neck. It is wise to dissect a bit up on the dome initially in case of a tear in the neck itself, which can be disastrous. It is necessary to reflect the lesion superiorly to assure preservation of the perforating branches of the anterior communicating artery (Fig. 56-8). These vessels are often adherent to the ventral posterior wall of the aneurysm and must be carefully separated from it. In many cases direct reflection of the aneurysm anteriorly while peering over the right A2 artery will give the needed view. In some instances, however, with a posteriorly or posteroinferiorly directed lesion, reflection of the aneurysm and the right A2 artery superiorly will give a nice view of the ventral aspects of these structures and their plane of separation from the perforators. In a similar fashion, rotation/reflection of the right A1 and A2 arteries superiorly and leftward may permit satisfactory visualization of the undersurface of a down-pointing lesion. Whatever the technique, the primary aim is clear cleavage between the ventral-posterior aspect of the aneurysm and the numerous critical perforating arteries emanating from the posterior aspect of the anterior communicating artery. This is particularly important to achieve before clipping of the aneurysm because visualization of these perforators during application of the clip is frequently difficult or impossible. Finally, adherent arterial branches overlying the dome of the aneurysm may be dissected free. Such branches may yield to blunt dissection with a right-angle hook or ball dissector. In some cases where accurate visualization of the arachnoid bands is possible, sharp dissection with scissors may be preferred. If aneurysmal rupture occurs at this point,

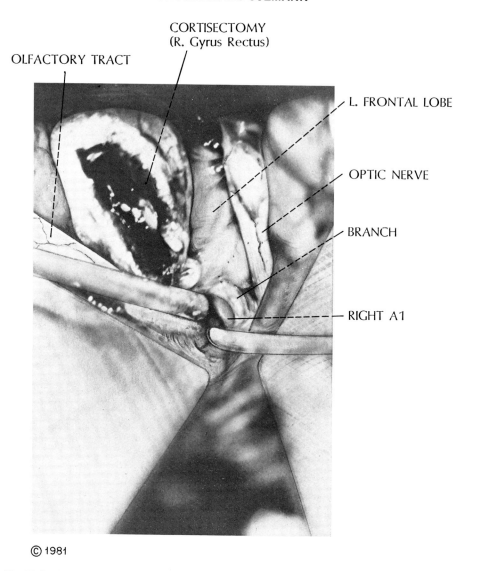

CORTISECTOMY
(R. Gyrus Rectus)

OLFACTORY TRACT

L. FRONTAL LOBE

OPTIC NERVE

BRANCH

RIGHT A1

© 1981

Fig. 56-6.   Dissection of a right A1 artery through the corticectomy. The microscope has been directed more medially. Suction and bipolar cauterization remove the cortex down to the interhemispheric pia arachnoid. With a fine dissector, the pia-arachnoid is removed from the right A1 artery and the neck of the aneurysm.

the problem can be controlled, since the aneurysm neck has been essentially completely dissected.

In case of aneurysmal rupture at any point during the dissection, deliberate action is necessary. Initially the bleeding should be controlled with suction. In some cases this can be done with a fine sucker (No. 16) or a larger sucker (No. 7 or No. 1). Very careful direction of the sucker tip to the precise point of bleeding should be attempted to clear the field of blood entirely. Then precise coagulation with the bipolar cautery or application of a bit of Surgicel or muscle with compression for a few minutes may seal a minor leak. If hemostasis can be obtained in this way, it is best to direct the dissection to another corner and return to the area of hemorrhage at a later time. In other cases bleeding is more brisk. In such circumstances, two suckers may be needed to keep the wound clear of blood. A large-bore sucker controlled by the assistant may be helpful to permit further accurate dissection by the operator. Sometimes application of a temporary clip to the dome may be helpful. This may permit continued dissection with final application of a

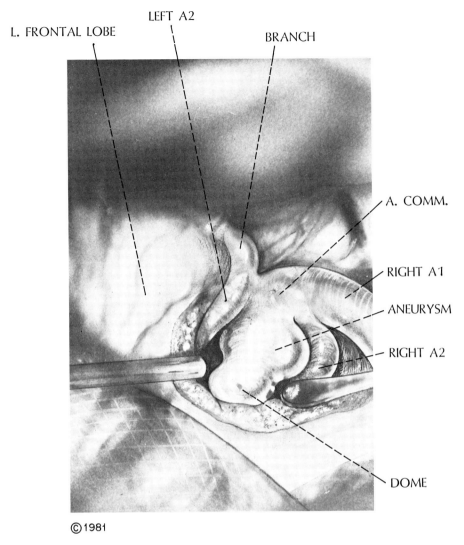

L. FRONTAL LOBE   LEFT A2   BRANCH   A. COMM.   RIGHT A1   ANEURYSM   RIGHT A2   DOME

©1981

Fig. 56-7.   Dissection of an aneurysm. Proceeding clockwise, the surgeon frees up right A1 and A2 arteries, then left A2 and A1 arteries. Finally, the aneurysm is encircled, and the dome and neck are completely dissected.

clip to the neck of the lesion. For very severe hemorrhage, intentional brief hypotension to 25 torr mean may assist in visualization of the leak and accurate hemostasis. In all events, the surgeon must proceed in an orderly fashion with temporary hemostasis, precise visualization of the source of hemorrhage and its relation to critical structures, and then accurate hemostasis. Rarely, a tear at the neck of an aneurysm will have to be repaired. This is done with either an interrupted suture technique (10–0 nylon) or tissue adhesive.

Obliteration of the Aneurysm

In the great majority of cases, a metal aneurysm clip is the best solution (Fig. 56-9). Once the lesion has been completely dissected and the relationship of its neck to surrounding critical structures including the perforating arteries is defined, the surgeon can judge what technique will best obliterate the lesion. We have usually used a Heifetz or Yasargil clip. The long, straight Heifetz clip is particularly effective for upward-pointing lesions. Because of the angle of application, the beveled clip applier frequently is most useful. This clip is also useful for lesions with a

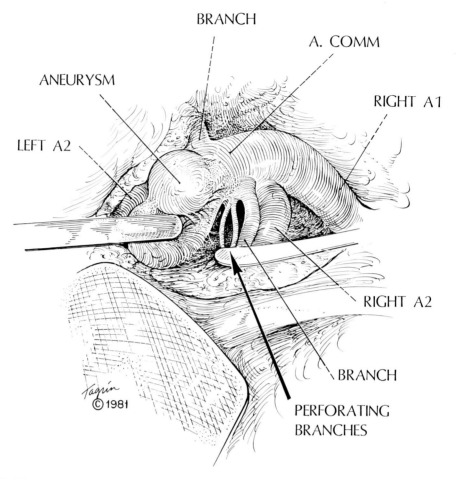

Fig. 56-8. Dissection of perforating branches. These crucial vessels emerge from the anterior communicating artery and proceed posteriorly to the hypothalamus. They must be gently freed from the aneurysm and excluded from clipping.

wide neck. In some cases the Sugita clip is used for its narrow blade and wide-opening jaws. The Yasargil clip is used for lesions with necks smaller than 5 mm. Often a projecting lobe can be gathered up with the sucker tip into the jaws of a Yasargil clip (Fig. 56-10). Release is difficult with the Yasargil and Sugita clips and may be facilitated by distracting the handle blades of the clip applier with the third and fourth fingers placed interiorly. Occasionally a Drake clip may be needed, with the aperture enclosing either the right A1 or A2 anterior cerebral artery segments (Fig. 56-11). Sometimes a slight curve or even a very abrupt curve will be handy to approximate an aneurysm neck. At times, the force of two clips may be needed to assure complete closure of a thick aneurysmal wall. In other cases, a combination of two clips is necessary for optimum obliteration of the neck of an aneurysm; we have found a straight clip may occasionally be nicely supplemented with a triangular Heifetz clip to a persistent corner, since the hubs of this pair do not mutually interfere. For giant anterior communicating aneurysms the Drake clips (up to 24 mm) may provide the only accurate and adequate clipping. Precise application of the clip is required. The clip is advanced gently, with axial rotational tiny wiggling to reduce drag. Generally it is possible to visualize one of the two blades as it advances. The clip is advanced until the tips are just beyond the opposite side of the neck, as previously calculated and in some cases actually visualized. If significant resistance is encountered, one should stop and remove the clip. Adequate dissection with freeing of arachnoid attachments will eliminate significant resistance, which could lead to perforation of the lesion with the clip. In some cases, with a paper-thin neck, a

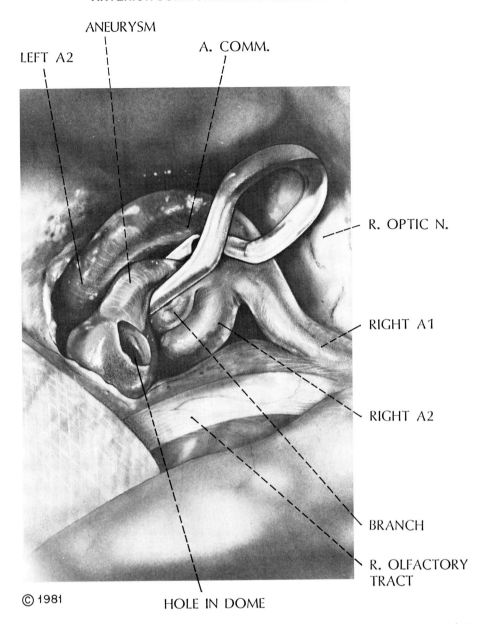

ANEURYSM

LEFT A2

A. COMM.

R. OPTIC N.

RIGHT A1

RIGHT A2

BRANCH

R. OLFACTORY TRACT

© 1981

HOLE IN DOME

Fig. 56-9. Clipping the aneurysm. The entire lesion is obliterated, with preservation of the trunk and perforating arteries. The aneurysm is opened to prove the adequacy of clipping.

burst of hypotension may be needed just at the time of clip application. After clip application, one must check the adequacy of clipping and the condition of circulation. Clip tips must be visualized beyond the opposite edge of the lesion, and the entire aneurysm should be obliterated. Both anterior cerebral arteries and the anterior communicating artery with its perforating vessels must be maintained intact. If these criteria are not satisfied, the clip may need repositioning, even multiply, to obtain a satisfactory application. If the lesion is satisfactorily clipped, this should be proved by aspirating the dome of the aneurysm with a 25-gauge needle (see Fig. 56-9). If bleeding from the aneurysm persists after the needle perforation, further obliteration will be needed. Finally, the surgeon should be satisfied that as retractors are removed the clip will not produce dangerous torque on the aneurysmal neck or compression of the optic nerve or brain.

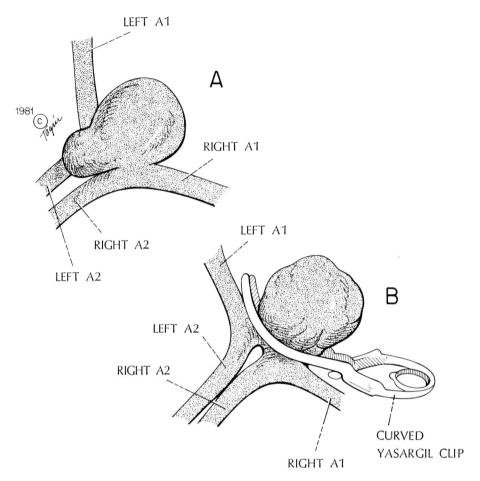

Fig. 56-10.   Problem: posterior bulge. Sucker gathers up bulge
for inclusion in curved Yasargil clip.

In some cases bipolar cauterization of the neck of the aneurysm may be helpful (Fig. 56-12). This technique, initiated by Yasargil, may narrow the neck for easier clipping. In addition, it may thicken the neck, eradicating dangerous thin spots in this critical area. The technique is helped by laboratory practice, and several technical pointers may be useful. The bipolar cautery should be set low with prior testing of its electrocautery effect. The blades of the forceps should pass completely across the neck of the lesion, for fear the points may cause electrocautery damage to the neck. As current is applied, very gentle pressure and release are applied multiply. Ideally a slow coagulation with whitening and thickening of the neck is produced without charring or sudden effects. During this time continuous irrigation of the area of coagulation should be done. In some cases, the coagulation may completely obliterate the neck; more commonly a simple thickening without total obliteration of the neck will be achieved.

Sometimes a ligature helps, particularly in lesions with a wide neck when it is difficult to define a clear area for a clip (Fig. 56-13); 3–0 silk is generally best. A variety of ligature passers are available. In some cases, where room is tight, a ligature may be placed deep to the lesion with fine forceps. Then the surgeon reflects the lesion to the opposite side, searching for the ligature beyond the lesion neck and retrieving it gently with a forceps. After the ligature is placed about the neck of the lesion, a surgeon's knot is fashioned and gently pulled taut. In other cases, the neck may be obliterated totally by these maneuvers. In other cases, the ligature narrows the neck for subsequent clipping.

Rarely, a lesion here defies clipping and ligation. In such an instance reinforcement may be

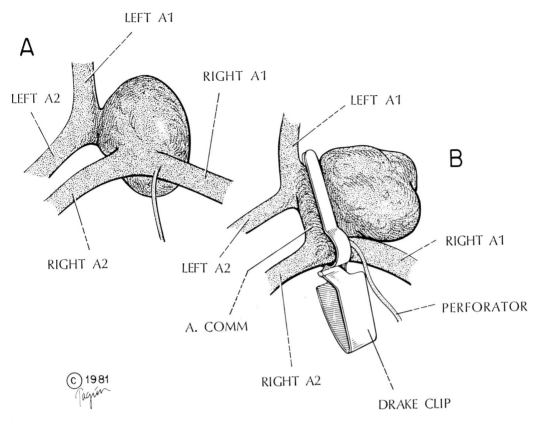

Fig. 56-11. Problem: common wall for aneurysm and right A1 artery. Drake clip spares right A1 and per-
forant arteries.

the safest technique. The classical approach is the application of muscle or acrylic, and recently
tissue adhesives have been used.

After the completion of the obliteration of the aneurysm, Surgicel is applied to the edges of
the corticectomy. At this point the neuroanesthetist gradually raises the blood pressure to the
normal level for that patient. The surgeon carefully checks to make certain that hemostasis at
the aneurysm site is adequate.

Closure

Irrigation is carried out with saline. When the brain is slack, substantial saline may be
added to fill the dead space. The dura is closed. Surgicel is placed in the epidural space for hemostasis. The bone flap is wired in place with 28-gauge stainless steel wire sutures, and the dura is
apposed to the bone flap with a central suture. The muscle, fascia, galea, and skin are closed
with appropriate sutures.

Postoperative Management

At the conclusion of the procedure, the patient is treated prophylactically against vasospasm. The central venous pressure is brought to 10 cm of water with colloid if there is no cardiac contraindication. The hematocrit is brought to 40 percent by the transfusion of packed cells
if necessary. The blood pressure is maintained in the range of 110–140 torr systolic with volume
and pressors as required. Medications include Solu-Medrol at 80 mg q6h intramuscularly, which

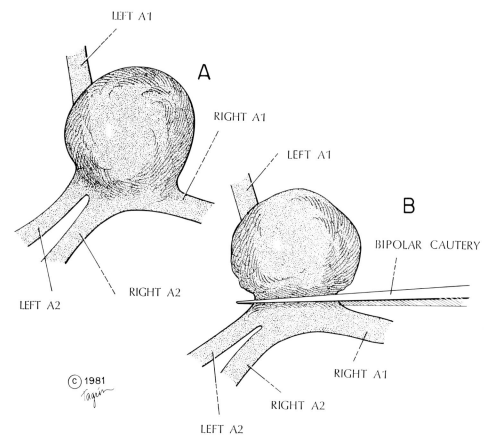

Fig. 56-12. Problem: broad base. Bipolar cauterization of the neck excludes all native arteries.

is tapered after 3 days, an antacid, and Dilantin 300 mg a day. Elastic stockings or pneumatic compression boots are continued until the patient is ambulatory.

In the case of neurologic deterioration, an immediate CT scan is performed, looking for intracranial hematoma, hydrocephalus, or cerebral edema. Appropriate treatment is instituted if these conditions are found. If the CT scan fails to disclose an adequate explanation for the deterioration, an angiogram is performed. If a vascular occlusion by the clip is disclosed, adjustment of the clip might be indicated, although we have never found this necessary. More commonly, cerebral vascular vasospasm may be demonstrated. If significant vasospasm (grade 3 + or 4 +) is seen, additional treatment is indicated. The central venous pressure should be elevated to the range of 10–12 cm with colloid and systolic blood pressure increased to 160–170 torr systolic; dopamine or neosynephrine may be used for this purpose.

In all cases postoperative angiography is recommended to ascertain the adequacy of aneurysm obliteration and maintenance of normal native vasculature.

Case Reports

Case 1: A.W. This 64-year-old right-handed female Jehovah's Witness experienced a sudden-onset severe bifrontal headache while at a religious service. Five minutes later she had a brief syncopal episode. On admission to a local hospital, a lumbar puncture showed blood in the subarachnoid. Past medical history was remarkable for hypertension and

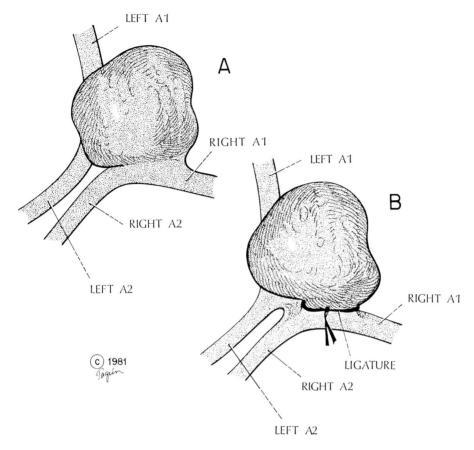

Fig. 56-13. Problem: broad base. Ligature narrows the base to permit clipping.

two myocardial infarctions. Physical examination on transfer demonstrated a blood pressure of 150/92 and a normal neurologic examination. The neck was markedly stiff. CT scan showed a small amount of blood in the basal cisterns and the interhemispheric cistern, suggesting an anterior communicating artery aneurysm. The patient was placed on a regimen of Amicar, blood pressure control, reserpine, and kanamycin. On day 8 the patient developed mild dysphasia and drift of the right upper extremity. Lumbar puncture showed no recurrence of hemorrhage. Cerebral angiography showed an anterior communicating artery aneurysm with moderate spasm of the anterior cerebral and left middle cerebral arteries. Blood pressure was elevated to the 150/70 systolic range with dopamine. The patient gradually improved but was left with a mild dysphasia. On day 14 the patient had a marked left-arm drift and probable right homonomous hemianopsia. The blood pressure was again elevated and the patient gradually improved. Pressors were tapered and the patient remained stable. On day 26 cerebral angiography showed marked improvement in vasospasm (Fig. 56-14A), and on day 27 a right frontal temporal craniotomy was carried out. Through a gyrus rectus approach, the aneurysm was dissected free and clipped with a curved Yasargil clip. A reduplicated anterior communicating artery was noted. No transfusions were needed. After surgery the patient was initially bright and awake, but gradually became drowsy and dysphasic. Dopamine was infused, with elevation of the blood pressure to the 150–170 systolic range, and the patient improved markedly with regard to mental status. She made a gradual complete recovery in speech and motor function. Repeat angiography 10 days after surgery disclosed complete obliteration of the aneurysm and no residual vasospasm (Fig. 56-14B).

Comment. The case illustrates how vasospasm may cause waxing and waning neurologic deficits. Before and after surgery, elevation of blood pressure sustained cerebral perfusion and reversed deficits. We prefer to delay operation until neurologic status is normal with improving angiographic spasm.

Case 2: M.H. This 59-year-old right-handed woman was unexpectedly given notice of termination of employment. She passed out and awoke a few minutes later. Within 1 hour she experienced the onset of bi-occipital headache

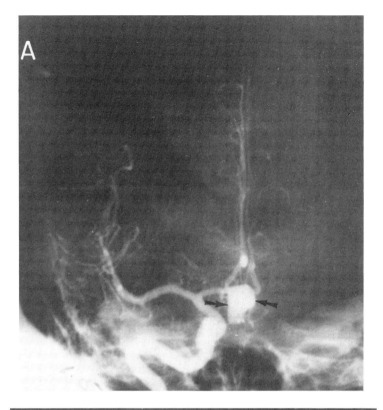

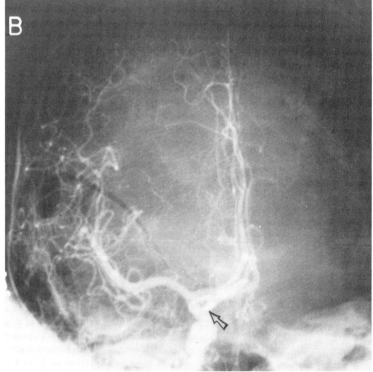

Fig. 56-14.   Case 1: typical clipping of aneurysm. A. Preoperative angiogram shows aneurysm pointing downward (closed arrows). B.
Postoperative angiogram shows Yasargil clip (open arrow) obliterating the aneurysm.

and neck pain. At a local hospital, neurologic examination showed a left Babinski sign and mild drowsiness. A lumbar puncture revealed grossly bloody cerebrospinal fluid with xanthochromia and an opening pressure of 185 mm of CSF. Neurologic examination at the time of transfer, 24 hours after the onset of illness, showed no deficits and the blood pressure was 150/88 torr. CT scan showed blood in the basal cisterns. The patient was placed on a medical program, including epsilon aminocaproic acid, blood pressure control, and sedation. There was mild intermittent confusion, progressing to marked obtundation on day 7. Angiography performed at that time showed a multi-lobular anterior communicating artery pointing forward and upward. There was severe internal carotid artery spasm bilaterally with slow distal flow. The ventricles were enlarged, and continuous spinal drainage was instituted with prompt improvement of the mental status to the point of spontaneous discussion of her own illness. On the 17th day the angiogram was repeated and diminished vasospasm was noted (Fig. 56-15A and B).

On the 18th day a right frontotemporal craniotomy was performed and an extensive subarachnoid clot was removed from around the right and left internal carotid arteries and the distal left anterior cerebral A1 segment. A Drake clip was used to obliterate the aneurysm, with the aperture encircling the right A2 segment and perforating vessels. There was moderate postoperative obtundation with return to preoperative status by 3 days postoperatively. Over the 3 weeks following operation there was waxing and waning abulia and memory abnormality, with normal gait. A lumbar puncture showed an open pressure of 88, and CT showed moderate ventricular enlargement, somewhat greater than preoperatively. The patient gradually improved spontaneously. Angiography, 1 month after surgery, showed nonfilling of the aneurysm with mild right A1 vascular narrowing (Fig. 56-15C and D). Four months after surgery the patient had returned to an entirely normal mental status.

Comment. Early CT scan showed much subarachnoid clot and predicted later serious spasm. This patient illustrates how hydrocephalus and vasospasm may together lead to deterioration. Prompt angiography confirmed both diagnoses, and spinal drainage improved the clinical status, setting the stage for surgery.

At operation, a clot was found adherent to the two arteries that were in spasm on angiography. Experience in 25 operated cases confirms that a subarachnoid clot must be present locally to cause arterial spasm.

Results

The approach described above has produced satisfactory results in our hands. Over the period 1974–1979, 52 consecutive anterior communicating artery aneurysms were treated according to this program and surgical technique. The surgical results in this series are presented in Table 56-1. Overall, 38 of the 41 patients in grade 1–2 preoperatively (92 percent) had a result that was either excellent (normal) or good (minor disability, working status unchanged). There were 2 cases in this category that were judged poor results (5 percent). One patient, despite a normal neurologic examination and extensive drug therapy over a 2-year period, had persisting disabling anxiety, which made return to work as a housepainter impossible. In 1 other case there was immediate blindness in the right eye following surgery, possibly related to intraoperative injury to the optic nerve vasculature; there was no improvement in vision over a 1-year follow-up. Among these 41 "good"-category patients, we encountered a single death, in a 47-year-old engineer who underwent uneventful clipping of anterior communicating artery and internal carotid artery aneurysms only to suffer a fatal postoperative myocardial infarction.

Results in poor-risk patients were satisfactory in a smaller percentage. Among 11 patients judged grade 3–4 preoperatively, 5 (45 percent) enjoyed a good result, with no excellent results. Five additional cases (45 percent) were judged poor results because of preoperative neurologic deficits that persisted after surgery (dementia, hemiplegia). There was a single death, a patient who presented deeply comatose with an intracerebral hematoma from a ruptured anterior communicating artery aneursym.

Postoperative angiography was performed in 48 cases. Total obliteration of the aneurysm was demonstrated in every case. "Slipped clips" were not observed. In two instances the right A1 anterior cerebral artery was narrowed and in another occluded by the clip; none of these patients was symptomatic. Otherwise, native arterial supply was intact.

We conclude that the described approach can yield satisfactory clinical results, particularly for grade 1–2 patients, although also for some grade 3–4 patients.

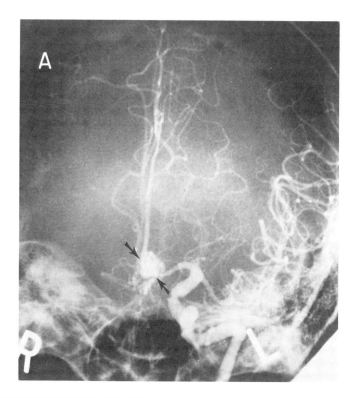

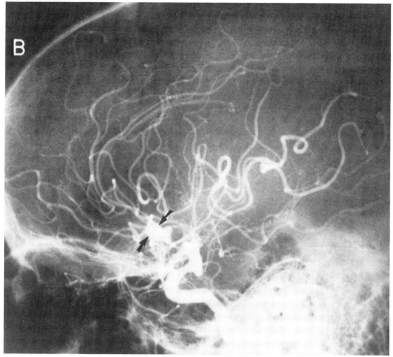

Fig. 56-15. Case 2: some unusual features. **A.** and **B.** Preoperative left-carotid angiogram shows aneurysm pointing anteriorly (closed arrows). **C.** and **D.** Postoperative left-carotid angiogram shows Drake clip (open arrows) encircling preserved right A2 artery.

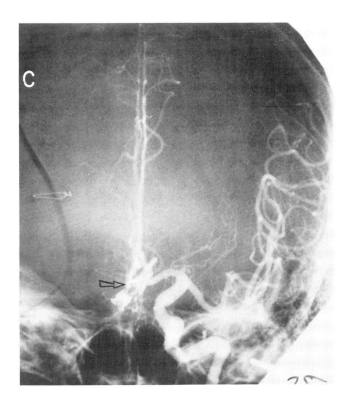

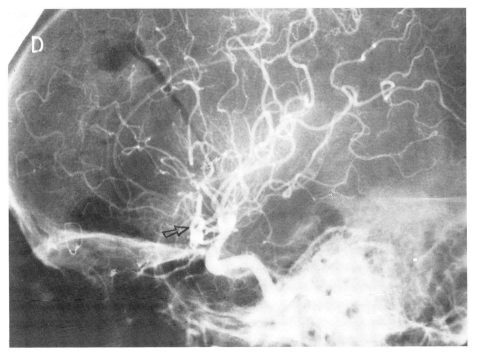

Table 56-1. Results of Surgery

	E	G	P	D	Total
Grade 1-2	28 (68%)	10(24%)	2 (5%)	1 (2%)	41
3-4		5 (45%)	5 (45%)	1 (9%)	11
Total	28 (54%)	15 (29%)	7 (14%)	2 (4%)	52

Complications

As shown in Table 56-2, microsurgical obliteration of anterior communicating artery aneurysms was associated with complications in 5 cases (9.6 percent) and death in 2 (3.8 percent).

Neurologic complications included temporary left-leg weakness due to a delayed right A2 cerebral embolus, presumably from the clip site. Multiple clip applications were required, and minimizing the number of applications probably reduces the likelihood of this problem. In another patient, unilateral blindness probably resulted from direct clip pressure or compromise of vascularity. Clip repositioning was considered too risky. In another case, disabling anxiety (without other signs) occurred after surgery, possibly related to fronto-basal irritation. Non-neurologic complications included a pulmonary embolus requiring vena cava interruption. In another patient, bilateral femoral head necrosis was noted, apparently related to high-dose steroid therapy. Bilateral total hip replacement was curative.

Death occurred in 2 patients. One patient, operated on acutely for hematoma while in deep coma, never awoke. Another patient who came through surgery without deficit suffered a fatal myocardial infarction 5 days after surgery.

Discussion

Recent technical advances now permit good surgical results in many patients with anterior communicating artery aneurysms.[4-11] CT scanning provides atraumatic diagnosis of intracranial hemorrhage and hydrocephalus.[1] Amicar decreases the rate of early recurrent hemorrhage.[9] Delay of surgery for 1 to 2 weeks allows resolution of cerebral swelling and neurologic deficits.[2] Surgery in this setting has produced good results.[4-11] Microsurgery minimizes brain damage.[4] The technique requires a smaller craniotomy and less retraction. Good illumination and precise visualization spare tiny but critical perforating arteries. Modern neuroanesthesia facilitates accurate surgical obliteration of aneurysms. Deep hypotension safely "defuses the bomb" until it can be clipped.[3] Hyperventilation and diuresis facilitate retraction and exposure.

Results gained with microsurgical direct attack[4-11] are superior to results of bedrest or indirect procedures.[12] Only rarely do special circumstances, e.g. certain giant aneurysms, require internal carotid occlusion,[13] with or without direct cerebral revascularization.[14] For most patients

Table 56-2. Complications

Morbidity		5 (9.6%)
Anxiety	1	
Blindness OD	1	
Temporary leg paresis	1	
Pulmonary embolus	1	
Bilateral femoral head necrosis	1	
Mortality		2 (3.8%)
Myocardial infarction	1	
Grade 4, never awoke	1	

who reach the operating room, a good to excellent outcome can be expected. Good surgical results broaden the indications for surgery. We recommend operation for all ruptured aneurysms in patients who achieve grade 3 status or better. In addition, surgery may be indicated for unruptured aneurysms larger than 7 mm in diameter, since these lesions probably bleed with significant frequency.[15] We recommend surgery for physiologically sound patients up to the age of 70.

Vasospasm, particularly in the preoperative period, continues to cause disability and death.[16-17] Recent studies indicate that CT done shortly after SAH can accurately predict which patients will suffer serious symptomatic vasospasm.[18] It may be that such patients warrant vigorous prophylactic management with drugs,[19-20] early surgery, or both. Recent reports of early surgery from Japan have been equivocal,[21] and a large cooperative study of the approach is under way.

The largest unsolved problem in aneurysm surgery is the patient who never reaches the operating room.[22] It has been estimated that only half of the 26,000 annual cases of SAH in the United States reach the hospital. About half of these cases reach surgery. The large remainder (as many as 18,000 cases) die before surgery, or suffer major disability. Only a diagnosis before SAH can help these patients. Perhaps the new method of digitized subtraction angiography, which can identify many aneurysms with very low risk, can diagnose some aneurysms before they rupture. Prophylactic surgery may well be warranted for some of these patients to avert major devastation from SAH.

REFERENCES

1. Davis KR, New PFJ, Ojemann RG, Crowell RM: Computed tomographic evaluation of hemorrhage secondary to intracranial aneurysm. *Am J Roentgen 127*:143–153, 1976
2. Hunt WE, Kosnik EJ: Timing and perioperative care in intracranial aneurysm surgery. *Clin Neurosurg 21*:79–87, 1974
3. Aitken RR, Drake CG: A technique of anesthesia with induced hypotension for surgical correction of intracranial aneurysms. *Clin Neurosurg 21*:107–114, 1974
4. Yasargil MG, Fox JL: The microsurgical approach to intracranial aneurysms. *Surg Neurol 3*:7–14, 1975
5. Vander Ark GD, Kempe LG, Smith DR: Anterior communicating aneurysms: the gyrus rectus approach. *Clin Neurosurg 21*:120–133, 1974
6. Crowell RM, Zervas NT: Management of intracranial aneurysm. *Med Clin North Am 63*:695–713, 1979
7. Sundt TM Jr, Whisnant JP: Subarachnoid hemorrhage from intracranial aneurysms. Surgical management and natural history of disease. *New Engl J Med 299*:116–122, 1978
8. Suzuki J (ed): *Cerebral aneurysms. Experiences with 1000 directly operated cases.* Tokyo, Neuron Publishing Co., 1979
9. Nibbelink DW, Torner K, Henderson WG: Aneurysms and subarachnoid hemorrhage. A cooperative study. Antifibrinolytic therapy in recent onset subarachnoid hemorrhage. *Stroke 6*:622–629, 1975
10. Krayenbühl HA, Yasargil MG, Flamm ES, et al: Microsurgical treatment of intracranial saccular aneurysms. *J Neurosurg 37*:678–686, 1972
11. Sengupta RP, Chin JSP, Brierley H: Quality of survival following direct surgery for anterior communicating artery aneurysms. *J Neurosurg 43*:58–64, 1975
12. Tindall GT: The treatment of anterior communicating aneurysms by proximal anterior cerebral artery ligation. *Clin Neurosurg 21*:134–150, 1974
13. Miller JR, Jawad K, Jennett B: Safety of carotid ligation and its role in the management of intracranial aneurysms. *J Neurol Neurosurg Psychiatry 40*:64–72, 1977
14. Crowell RM: Direct brain revascularization, in Schmidek H, Sweet WH (eds): *Current Techniques of Operative Neurosurgery,* New York, Grune & Stratton, 1978
15. Jane JA, Winn HR, Richardson AE: The natural history of intracranial aneurysms: rebleeding rates during the acute and long term period and implication for surgical management. *Clin Neurosurg 24*:176–184, 1977
16. Allcock JM, Drake CG: Ruptured intracranial aneurysms. The role of arterial spasm. *J Neurosurg 22*:21–29, 1965
17. Fisher CM, Roberson GJ, Ojemann RG: Cerebral vasospasm with ruptured saccular aneurysm. The clinical manifestations. *Neurosurgery 1*:245–248, 1977

18. Fisher CM, Kistler JP, Davis JM: Relation of cerebral vasospasm to subarachnoid hemorrhage visualized by computerized tomographic scanning. *Neurosurgery 6*:1–4, 1980

19. Gianotta SL, McGillicuddy JE, Kindt GW: Diagnosis and treatment of postoperative cerebral vasospasm. *Surg Neurol 8*:286–290, 1977

20. Kosnik EJ, Hunt WE: Postoperative hypertension in the management of patients with intracranial arterial aneurysms. *J Neurosurg 45*:148–154, 1976

21. Suzuki J, Onuma T, Yoshimoto T: Results of early operations on cerebral aneurysms. *Surg Neurol 11*:407–412, 1979

22. Drake CG: Perspectives on cerebral aneurysms. *Stroke 11*:124, 1980

CHAPTER 57

Surgical Management of Aneurysms of the Internal Carotid: Posterior Communicating, Anterior Choroidal, and Bifurcation Aneurysms

Henry H. Schmidek

FOLLOWING THE INTRODUCTION OF CEREBRAL ANGIOGRAPHY, which allowed the diagnosis of an intracranial aneurysm to be established and provided detailed information concerning its specific anatomic features, the era of planned surgical management of these lesions was inaugurated. It was soon discovered that aneurysms arising from the supraclinoid internal carotid artery are common and amenable to surgical treatment. In 1933, Norman Dott[1] became the first to operate on a cerebral aneurysm previously demonstrated by cerebral angiography. This aneurysm presented in a 23-year-old woman who was experiencing severe headache and progressive left oculomotor nerve palsy. The aneurysm was a 7-mm lesion attached by a narrow neck to the inferior aspect of the junction of the left internal carotid artery with its posterior communicating branch. Following cervical carotid ligation on March 24, 1933, the patient made an excellent recovery both generally and of the oculomotor nerve function. In 1936, Walter Dandy[2] began to treat aneurysms of the internal carotid artery in or near the cavernous sinus by a trapping procedure that involved ligation of the parent vessel proximal and distal to the aneurysm in the neck and within the head. He then introduced the technique of directly occluding the neck of a saccular aneurysm intracranially while preserving the parent artery. Dandy's patient, a 43-year-old chronic alcoholic, also presented with a paralysis of the oculomotor nerve. Based on these clinical findings only and without prior angiographic studies, the patient was operated on and a pea-sized aneurysm was found projecting from the outer wall of the internal carotid artery adjacent to the posterior communicating artery. The aneurysm arose by a narrow neck, projected beneath the tentorial dura, and was attached to the oculomotor nerve. A silver clip was placed across the neck of the sac flush with the wall of the internal carotid artery, obliterating the sac completely. The aneurysm as then thrombosed with electrocautery. Within 3 days, the patient's ptosis and extraocular movements began to im-

Section of Neurosurgery, University of Vermont College of Medicine, Burlington, Vermont

prove; and in 7 months there was complete return of all oculomotor nerve functions.[2] In the 50 years since these pioneering efforts, a major activity of the neurosurgical community has been directed to characterizing the natural history of cerebral aneurysms and to their perioperative and intraoperative management to reduce the morbidity associated with these phases of a patient's care. This chapter will discuss the current medical and surgical treatment of cerebral aneurysms as practiced on the Neurosurgical Service of the University of Vermont College of Medicine and address those specific factors related to ICA aneurysms arising at the level of the posterior communicating artery, anterior choroidal artery, and carotid bifurcation of which the operating surgeon should be aware.

Aneurysms of the supraclinoid carotid artery may present in patients of any age. They have been described in children within the first days of life,[3] and have been successfully operated on within the first month of age. Although uncommon in the pediatric population, cerebral aneurysms often exist in association with bacterial endocarditis, chronic lung infections, polycystic kidney disease, aortic coarctation, Marfan's or Ehler-Danlos syndrome, and familial aneurysms, so one must maintain a particular suspicion of the possibility of these lesions being present in these settings. Although 10 times less common than arteriovenous malformations, cerebral aneurysms in children are more prone to rupture and account for approximately one-third of the cases of spontaneous subarachnoid hemorrhage in children between the ages of 4 and 15 years. The vast majority of cases present with subarachnoid hemorrhage, and the clinical features are the same as those in adults. Probably less than 5 percent of the aneurysms in children present with mass effect.[4] Both adults and children may become symptomatic, however, secondary to aneurysmal expansion, which produces headache, retro-orbital or face pain, or compression of the optic pathways. It is among the aneurysms of the internal carotid artery-posterior communicating artery junction and with aneurysms at the carotid bifurcation that the highest incidence of warning signs exist before aneurysmal rupture. In a retrospective review, such warnings are described in 69.2 percent of the internal carotid artery-posterior communicating artery cases, and 60 percent of the carotid bifurcation aneurysms.[5] In these cases the complaints are related to head or face pain or mass effect on cranial nerves.

Most of the aneurysms of the internal carotid artery distal to the ophthalmic artery are discovered after they rupture. In about 40 percent of the patients with a ruptured aneurysm arising at the posterior communicating artery, an oculomotor palsy develops, sometimes immediately and sometimes within a few days of the ictus. Before subarachnoid hemorrhage, ipsilateral frontal head pain, located behind the eye and above the brow, occurs in about one-fourth of the patients. The pain may exist for months or years before the aneurysm ruptures or produces an oculomotor palsy. In 14 of 19 cases studied by Harris and Udvarhelyi,[6] oculomotor palsy appeared within 2 weeks of the onset of pain. In 4 of these patients, oculomotor palsy was the only sign of disease. These authors found that the overall incidence of oculomotor palsy was 38 percent in patients with carotid-posterior communicating artery aneurysms. Hook and Norlen[7] and Odom[8] cited 36 percent and 42 percent respectively. When the oculomotor nerve is affected by an aneurysm, paresis is usually complete with involvement of the levator, extraocular muscles, and the pupillary sphincter. A nontraumatic oculomotor palsy with pupillary involvement is, until proven otherwise, an aneurysm or tumor.[9] The oculomotor nerve is usually compressed where it enters the dura at the posterior end of the cavernous sinus. Visual defects may rarely occur in conjunction with these aneurysms and result from compression of the optic tract, thereby producing a contralateral homonymous hemianopia and pallor of the optic discs. Mental derangements may arise when the aneurysm compresses the mamillary bodies or the blood supply to the diencephalon, or pituitary insufficiency when the aneurysm grows into the sella turcica.

Aneurysms that arise at the carotid bifurcation frequently present as a subarachnoid hemorrhage in conjunction with an orbito-frontal or temporal lobe intracerebral hematoma. They may, however, grow large without rupturing and mimic a suprasellar tumor. This may produce a bitemporal field defect; or, if the aneurysm expands posteriorly and medially, it can compress an optic tract; if it expands posteriorly and inferiorly, it may compress the oculomotor nerve.

The aneurysm discovered as an incidental finding revealed during the angiographic investigation of cerebral ischemia and head trauma is an increasingly common phenomenon and its optimal management remains unresolved.[8] Taking into consideration the patient's general condition, the familial history, particularly of aneurysms or subarachnoid hemorrhage, psychologic makeup, the specific characteristics as to aneurysm site and location, and the anticipated technical ease of obliterating the lesion, the patient is presented with the option of deferring surgical intervention until a change in the size of the lesion is manifested clinically or by annual angiography or of having the operation performed electively. Given a favorable array of variables, my preference is for early surgical isolation of the aneurysm from the circulation (see Chapter 51).

Diagnostic Evaluation

After appropriate general medical and laboratory studies, all patients suspected of harboring an intracranial aneurysm are studied by computerized tomographic (CT) scanning and four-vessel cerebral angiography. In the patient without a prior subarachnoid hemorrhage, these studies are completed within 1 to 2 days of admission, whereas in a patient with a subarachnoid hemorrhage, the studies are performed within hours of hospitalization.

The CT scan performed with and without infusion of Renografin* gives evidence about intracerebral, subdural, or intraventricular hemorrhage (their location and dimensions), the extent and location of bleeding into the basal cisterns, the localization of the ruptured aneurysm in the presence of multiple aneurysms, information concerning ventricular size and hemorrhage, and the extent of cerebral edema or infarction. On occasion the aneurysm can be seen adjacent to the anterior clinoid process—particularly if it is surrounded by a rim of adjacent blood or is over 1.0 cm in diameter. Although Scotti et al.[10] concluded that the diagnosis of subarachnoid hemorrhage was possible in all cases when a CT scan was performed within 5 to 7 days after subarachnoid hemorrhage, this was not found to be the case in 12 percent of the series of Mizukami et al.[11] of 111 cases of subarachnoid hemorrhage, suggesting that it is not always possible to diagnose the subarachnoid hemorrhage with CT scanning alone. Hayward[5] reported the relationship between CT findings and the localization of ruptured aneurysms and concluded that the aneurysm could be determined in 68 percent of those arising from the internal carotid artery.

The CT scan may be of predictive value in anticipating the development of cerebral vasospasm after aneurysmal hemorrhage. In the study by Mizukami and his colleagues,[11] the presence or absence of cerebral vasospasm was judged in 75 cases in which surgical treatment was not performed before the 15th day after the hemorrhage. Cerebral angiography was repeated between days 5 and 14, this being the time frame when the presence of cerebral vasospasm was most likely to be present. When a significant collection of blood was present in the subarachnoid space, cerebral vasospasm was confirmed angiographically in 84 percent of the cases in the first 4 days after subarachnoid hemorrhage, in 75 percent of the cases in 5 to 7 days, and in 86 percent in the second week. In 8 cases where this finding was not present on CT scan after subarachnoid hemorrhage within 4 days of the ictus, no vasospasm was seen. No relationship was found between the presence of cisternal blood and cerebral vasospasm when a CT scan was performed after day 5 of the disease.

If CT scanning allows the diagnosis of subarachnoid hemorrhage to be made, and particularly if there is a mass effect and shift of brain between intracranial compartments, a lumbar puncture is not performed. If the diagnosis is in doubt, and occasionally to relieve an unremitting headache, a lumbar puncture will be performed in a patient who is awake and alert.

Cerebral angiography is usually performed under sedation and local anesthesia by the femoral route using standard catheter techniques. All four cerebral vessels are visualized, and oblique, basal, and cross-compression views are performed as indicated. The detailed anatomy of all aneurysms is further delineated with magnification angiography and subtraction studies.

*Squibb & Sons, Inc., Boston, MA

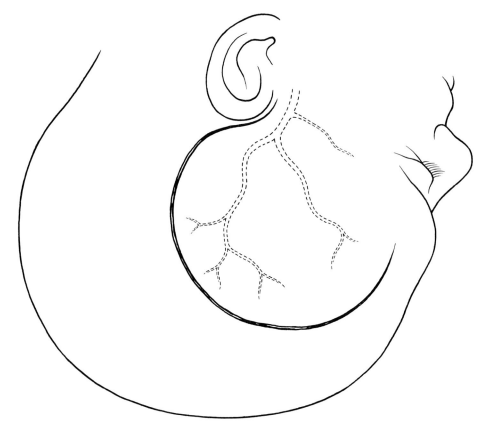

Fig. 57-1. Frequently used skin incision for the pterional approach to the internal carotid artery, posterior communicating artery, carotid bifurcation.

This allows assessment of the degree of atherosclerosis, the size, site, and configuration of the aneurysm, and the presence of other lesions, and provides a base line for evaluating the vessels for vasospasm.

In those cases in which a supraclinoid carotid aneurysm is present, the angiograms are studied specifically to assess whether the ipsilateral posterior communicating artery is an essential blood supply to the posterior cerebral artery territory and to the neck of the aneurysm, as well as the exact relationship of the posterior communicating artery. Anterior choroidal artery aneurysms usually arise from the inferior wall of the supraclinoid carotid artery and project downward. In these cases one needs an accurate assessment of the aneurysm's specific configuration since they often present as a diffuse dilatation of the wall of the carotid artery extending toward the carotid bifurcation, with the anterior choroidal artery incorporated in this dilatation. As a result the aneurysm may not be amenable to direct clipping. One should be prepared in this particular situation to reinforce rather than clip the aneurysm. Aneurysms arising at the carotid bifurcation may be extremely difficult to delineate angiographically, although these are usually small lesions with a discrete neck that can be clipped. To find and characterize these lesions, it is particularly important to have oblique views and subtraction studies to find the aneurysm among the vessels present at the termination of the carotid artery. These aneurysms also require that one perform ipsilateral carotid compression to assess the adequacy of cross-filling of the ipsilateral anterior cerebral artery from the opposite side, since it may be necessary to occlude the anterior cerebral artery with the aneurysmal neck and one needs to know whether this maneuver can be tolerated by the patient.

In patients in whom no lesion is discovered to account for the subarachnoid hemorrhage, repeat four-vessel cerebral angiography is performed 3 to 4 weeks after the first studies. Should

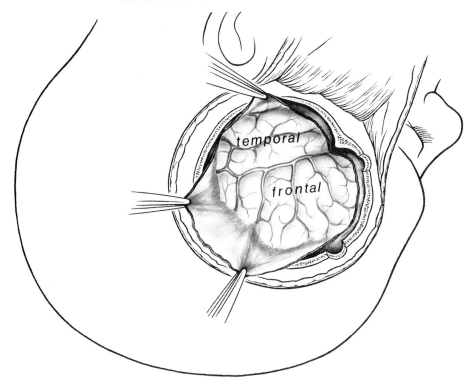

Fig. 57-2. Craniotomy after opening dura and exposing brain surface of the frontal and temporal lobes.

this study also fail to clarify the situation, a myelographic examination is performed of the entire spinal subarachnoid space in order to exclude the remote possibility that the subarachnoid hemorrhage was caused by a spinal tumor or malformation. Spinal angiography is *not* performed unless there is a strong clinical suspicion and objective data to indicate the presence of such a lesion.

Preoperative Management

The preoperative management of the patient following an aneurysmal subarachnoid hemorrhage is designed to provide symptomatic relief and reduce the tendency to rehemorrhage. The program involves bedrest, mild analgesics, anticonvulsants, steroids (dexamethasone 8–10 mg IV, six hourly), and antacids. All patients are placed on epsilon-aminocaproic acid (EACA) at a dose of 36 grams/day (i.e. 1.5 grams/hour intravenously). Although there is suggestive evidence of causal relationship between complications of thrombosis, cerebral vasospasm, hydrocephalus and myopathy, and EACA therapy in patients on the above regimen, we have not been impressed with the incidence of these problems on this service and continue to use this agent. In the absence of vasospasm, the systolic blood pressure is lowered by 20 to 30 percent to reduce wide peaks in the blood pressure, which may precipitate rebleeding. A variety of agents are used for this purpose including furosemide, hydralazine, chlorpromazine, trimethaphan camphorsulfonate, and sodium nitroprusside with progression from agents such as furosemide to sodium nitroprusside as required by the situation. These agents are used in an intensive care unit setting, allowing continuous nursing supervision and continuous arterial pressure monitoring, through an indwelling radial artery catheter.

The timing of surgical intervention depends on the patient's overall and neurologic condition and the appearance on CT scan, particularly of widespread hemorrhage in the basal cisterns. The patient in good condition, without massive cisternal blood and without angiographic evidence of vasospasm, is operated on within 1 to 2 days of admission. This delay allows the surgery to be performed under optimal circumstances with the most experienced anesthetic, surgical, and nursing team available to assist with the operation. This approach has the advantage of both preventing rehemorrhage from the aneurysm and allowing vigorous mangement of vasospasm by volume expansion and artificial hypertension in those patients who become symptomatic because of this complication. We do not yet know how the outcome with this approach compares with the outcome after waiting at least 1 to 2 weeks after the subarachnoid hemorrhage to operate on the aneurysm, and then only in patients free of vasospasm on repeat angiography. A major technical disadvantage to the approach is that the surgery can be technically more difficult and occasionally the landmarks are obliterated by extensive hemorrhage.

Patients are transferred to our neurosurgical service days or weeks after their subarachnoid hemorrhage: if the patient is obtunded and significant vasospasm is present angiographically, surgical intervention is deferred until repeat angiography no longer demonstrates the presence of such vasospasm, and the patient is maintained on the medical regimen described above.

If the patient is in good condition, without angiographic evidence of vasospasm on the contrast study performed before surgery, an operation is performed soon after admission when optimal circumstances are available to the patient.

In patients with profound neurologic deficits without an intracerebral hematoma and secondary to vasospasm an epidural pressure switch is inserted and an attempt is made to maintain the intracranial pressure under 20 torr using pentobarbital, mannitol, furosemide, and hyperventilation. Treatment is continued until the intracranial pressure remains under 20 torr without these agents; in some cases treatment has been continued for up to 14 days. Induced hypertension, systemic arterial pressure, central venous or pulmonary artery pressure, electroencephalogram, evoked responses, and blood barbiturate levels are monitored. The patients are intubated and hyperventilated to a pCO_2 of 25–30 torr and are fully supported to maintain their metabolic, cardiovascular, and respiratory function. Surgical intervention is reserved for those patients who can be weaned off this program and who have the potential for a useful existence. There is no established time frame for when surgery should be performed on this group.

In patients whose problem is complicated by an intracerebral hemorrhage: those patients who are undergoing neurologic deterioration but who are potentially salvageable and useful individuals are subjected to immediate surgery. At the time of surgery the hemorrhage is removed and the aneurysm dealt with definitively.

Surgical Anatomy

The internal carotid artery can be divided into four segments—cervical, intrapetrosal, intracavernous, and supraclinoid. The supraclinoid segment begins as the artery emerges from the cavernous sinus and passes medial to the anterior clinoid process. This portion of the artery extends upward and branches off the internal carotid artery. Originating from the supraclinoid portion, at the origins of which intracranial aneurysms often arise, are the ophthalmic, posterior communicating, and anterior choroidal arteries. The most frequent site of internal carotid artery aneurysms is at the posterior communicating artery junction, with aneurysms arising at the internal carotid artery-anterior choroidal junction and the bifurcation of the internal carotid artery being uncommon, and aneurysms arising distally on these arteries being rare, although investment of the aneurysm and the vessel by archnoid may create the impression that the aneurysm appears to arise from the artery directly.

The posterior communicating artery arises from the posteromedial surface of the internal carotid artery and runs backward for 5–10 mm to anastomose with the posterior cerebral artery. The posterior cerebral artery varies greatly in size from being rudimentary to occasionally being so large that the posterior cerebral artery appears to be arising from the internal carotid rather

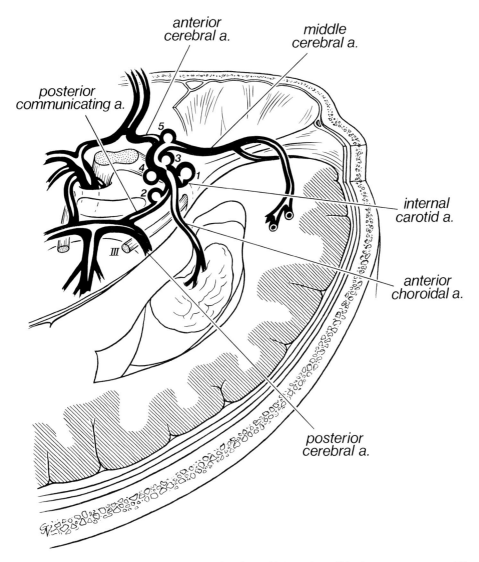

Fig. 57-3. Schematic diagram indicating the sites of internal carotid artery aneurysms and the regional anatomy of the structures surrounding these lesions.

than from the basilar artery. It is frequently larger on the left side. This vessel may constitute the main source of blood to the posterior cerebral artery. If this artery fills predominantly from the basilar artery, its occlusion is associated with little risk; whereas if the posterior communicating artery fills primarily from the posterior communicating artery, its inadvertent occlusion may result in a major cerebral infarction.

Posterior Communicating Artery

The posterior communicating artery gives rise to 4 to 12 branches. These branches enter the base of the brain and supply the genu and anterior one-third of the posterior limb of the internal capsule, the anterior one-third of the thalamus, and the walls of the third ventricle. This vessel also gives off branches to the optic tract, the optic chiasm, the cerebral peduncle, and the tuber cinereum, and terminates as the anterior thalamo-perforating artery.

Aneurysms that arise at the junction of the carotid and posterior communicating arteries may be globular, elongated, multilobular, or irregular in shape. They also may vary greatly in size, although giant cerebral aneurysms, i.e., those greater than 2.5 cm in diameter, rarely arise at this location.

The commonest type of aneurysm arising at the posterior communicating artery-internal carotid artery junction projects posterolaterally (86 percent) and involves the oculomotor nerve in about one-third of the cases. The aneurysm frequently overlies the origin of the posterior communicating artery. In the presence of multiple aneurysms, there is a 65 percent chance of one of the aneurysms being situated at this site. Since these aneurysms are most likely to bleed freely into the basal cisterns, they are also the most likely to produce a significant leptomeningeal reaction to blood and a communicating hydrocephalus. This complication is encountered in approximately one-third of patients after subarachnoid hemorrhage resulting from an aneurysm in this location.

A smaller group of cases are those directed posterolaterally and extending *above* the tentorial edge. These are a more difficult group to approach since retraction of the temporal lobe may result in premature rupture of the aneurysm. Although it is uncommon for posterior communicating arteries to be associated with an intracerebral hemorrhage, it is in this subgroup of cases that temporal lobe hemorrhages occur, which may be approached surgically through the hematoma.

Medially situated aneurysms arising at the internal carotid artery-posterior communicating artery junction occur in 3.6 percent of the cases and tend to extend beneath the optic nerve and present with visual symptoms or subarachnoid hemorrhage or both. These lesions are approached by mobilizing the frontal and temporal lobes, thereby gaining exposure of the internal carotid artery proximal and distal to the aneurysm.[6]

Anterior Choroidal Artery

The anterior choroidal artery is, next to the middle cerebral artery, the most important vascular supply to the internal capsule. The artery originates a few millimeters above the origin of the posterior communicating artery from the posterior surface of the internal carotid artery. This vessel may arise either as two separate arteries or as a single trunk that divides a short way from its origin. It is often larger on the left side, and takes a course along the optic tract, around the cerebral peduncle to the lateral geniculate body, where its main branches enter the choroid plexus of the inferior horn of the lateral ventricle and anastomoses with branches of the posterior choroidal artery. In its course it supplies branches to the optic tract, the cerebral peduncle, and the base of the brain. These branches terminate in the lateral geniculate body, the tail of the caudate nucleus, and the posterior two-thirds of the posterior limb of the internal capsule as far as the dorsal limit of the globus pollidus. The infralenticular and retrolenticular portions of the internal capsule are also vascularized by branches of the anterior choroidal artery.

Although occlusion of this artery does not invariably lead to a profound deficit, its injury may result in a contralateral hemiplegia, hemianesthesia, hemianopia, stupor, and death. Many aneurysms arising from the supraclinoid internal carotid artery involve this vessel in their wall, especially if the aneurysm is larger than 5 mm in size, and this vessel is at risk with any surgical procedure in the vicinity of the supraclinoid portion of the internal carotid artery. There is also a tendency for aneurysms to co-exist at this location, which may not be appreciated preoperatively. Clinically, these aneurysms may be indistinguishable from the internal carotid artery-posterior communicating artery aneurysm, even to involvement of the oculomotor nerve. In addition, since the anterior choroidal artery may be attached to the fundus of a posterior communicating aneurysm, this artery must be identified before the aneurysm is clipped.

The anterior choroidal aneurysm usually projects from the inferior aspect of the internal carotid artery 3–6 mm proximal to the carotid bifurcation and projects laterally, whereas the anterior choroidal artery itself curves medially. The aneurysm will often obscure the origin of the anterior choroidal aratery. There is usually an angle of separation, however, between the parent vessel and the aneurysm, which should allow a clip to be applied to the aneurysmal neck without injuring the anterior choroidal artery.

Internal carotid artery bifurcation aneurysms represent about 5 percent of intracranial aneurysms, and often present in association with a frontal intracerebral hemorrhage. The aneurysms may be difficult to delineate angiographically since they are often small and hidden by other vessels. Morphologically, the aneurysms represent either a direct continuation of the internal carotid artery trunk or possess a broad-based origin that incorporates the junction of the internal carotid artery-anterior cerebral arteries or the internal carotid artery-middle cerebral artery junction and include parts of the main trunk of the anterior or middle cerebral artery. The majority of these lesions project superiorly or superiorly and ventrally beneath the orbitofrontal lobe in the area of the anterior perforated substance. Only occasionally does the aneurysm arise from the dorsal aspect of the carotid bifurcation. Most of these aneurysms are of the same dimensions as encountered elsewhere along the carotid artery. Giant aneurysms are exceptional at this site. The dome of the aneurysm is usually covered by frontal lobe or may be located in the sylvian fissure. Among aneurysms of the supraclinoid internal carotid artery, these aneurysms are the most likely to present with an associated intracerebral hemorrhage. Exposure of these lesions requires delineation of the vessels at the bifurcation, the lenticulostriate vessels, and the anterior choroidal artery, which is best accomplished by dissection along the anterior and inferior margins of the major vessels while leaving the fundus, which is usually buried in the frontal lobe, alone.

Operative Procedure

Craniotomy is performed under general endotracheal anesthesia, usually with a "balanced technique," controlled ventilation, and continuous monitoring of electrocardiogram, blood gases, arterial pressure, and urinary output. The patient is brought to the operating room under atropine-droperidol sedation, and with a functioning intravenous, is anesthetized and gently intubated without raising the blood pressure and before insertion of the central venous pressure and arterial lines and Foley catheter. Neither spinal fluid drainage nor hypothermia is routinely used. It is important that the radial artery catheter be calibrated to reflect the blood pressure at the level of the patient's head since the operating table is flexed. The patient is in a supine position, the entire head is shaved and turned 15°–20° away from the side of the aneurysm, and then the position is maintained in the three-point headrest. The arms and legs are protected with blankets and both ends of the operating table are then flexed to facilitate the venous return from the head and lower extremities.

The operation is begun with the patient receiving mannitol (1.5 gm/kg), furosemide (20–40 mg IV), Decadron (25 mg IV), Kefsol (1.0 g IV), and Amicar (1.5 g/hour).

An aneurysm tray is available on a separate Mayo stand and consists of the entire spectrum of Yasargil, Scoville, Sugita, Drake, Mayfield, Heifetz, and Sundt clips and applicators so that the surgeon can choose the optimal configuration from this collection. The tray also includes muslin, plastics, and the Mullan instrumentation to allow alternatives to clipping the aneurysm should this tactic be preferable.

The operating microscope is draped and adjusted before it is to be used later in the operation. The preferred system is the OPMI 6 Zeiss setup on the Contraves stand, which allows the microscope to be suspended almost weightlessly and adjustments to be made effortlessly.

After the skin is cleansed with Betadine and alcohol, a scalp flap is made that extends from the zygomatic process of the temporal bone and curves anteriorly to intersect the hairline at approximately the midpoint of the superior orbital ridge, taking into account the position of the frontal branch of the facial nerve. Separate skin and muscle flaps may be reflected; however, osteoplastic bone flap is cosmetically preferable in the frontotemporal area. A frontotemporal craniotomy is fashioned flush with the anterior cranial fossa, and the dura is gradually separated to

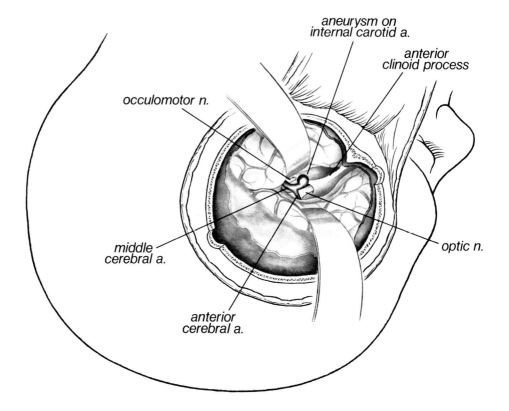

Fig. 57-4. Final exposure of the left internal carotid artery, anterior and middle cerebral arteries, optic nerve, and an aneurysm of the internal carotid artery.

allow removal of the lateral one-third of the greater wing of the sphenoid with an air drill. Before inserting the dural tenting sutures, the baseplate of the Yasargil self-retaining retractor is positioned on the superior and medial aspect of the bony opening, and microfibrillar collagen is inserted beneath the bone edges to control epidural bleeding along with the tenting sutures.

If an intracerebral hematoma is covering the frontal and temporal areas, the dura is not opened until the brain is pulsating freely. If the brain is still tense after having administered mannitol, furosemide, and hyperventilation with a PCO_2 of 25 torr, the hematoma may be gently cannulated and a few cubic centimeters of blood removed. This maneuver will often make it possible to open the dura without the brain herniating through the opening. Occasionally it is necessary to cannulate the lateral ventricle before opening the dura if the brain remains tense when there is no intracerebral hemorrhage.

The dura is opened to allow exposure to the lateral aspect of the frontal lobe and anterior temporal lobes. The exposed brain is covered with wet Gelfoam.

The initial intradural exposure of supraclinoid ICA aneurysms is along the sphenoid ridge to the anterior clinoid process. By retracting the frontal lobe or the temporal tip or both with a $^1/_2$- to 1-inch Silastic-coated retractor, dissection is carried down to the optic nerve using operating telescopes allowing 3.5–4.5× magnification in conjunction with fiberoptic headlight illumination. With gentle retraction, the optic nerve is exposed and the arachnoid is opened over the carotid artery and the optic nerve with a sharp knife, allowing aspiration of cerebrospinal fluid to provide additional exposure. The retractor then is fixed in position; if necessary, a second Silastic-coated retractor can be introduced to gain additional exposure.

It is only at this phase of the operation that the operating microscope is introduced. The microscope is used until the aneurysm is clipped. It is then removed and the operation proceeds with loupes. Further dissection is carried out at 6–16× magnification. Unless contraindicated by the patient's general condition, the patient's blood pressure may be lowered slowly to a mean of 60–80 mm Hg by deepening the level of anesthesia, infusing intravenous sodium nitroprusside or both. This technique increases the flaccidity of the aneurysm and decreases its tendency to rupture with manipulation. We do not, however, use this technique in about one-half of our cases, and often find that the aneurysm can be clipped without recourse to lowering the blood pressure.

The internal carotid artery is identified with respect to its bifurcation and inferiorly along the internal carotid artery to the aneurysm. Dissection is continued until the upper and lower borders of the aneurysmal neck and the proximal internal carotid artery can be seen. This provides proximal and distal control of the vessel in the event of bleeding. The application of temporary clips to the carotid artery is not routinely used. The arachnoid around the vessel and the aneurysmal neck is gently cut, and a passage that is free of vessels is developed on either side of the neck. Often the vessels adjacent to the aneurysm blend with the arachnoid covering the aneurysm so that it is crucial to dissect beyond this arachnoidal layer while preserving the vessels in it. Before clipping the neck, one must know the location of the anterior choroidal and posterior communicating arteries. The clip is applied and if necessary reapplied several times to ensure preservation of these vessels. The aneurysm is occluded immediately adjacent to the parent vessel to prevent recurrence of the aneurysm proximal to the clip. The majority of aneurysms can be obliterated with a suitable Yasargil or Sugita clip. Before applying a clip to the aneurysmal neck, one must test the clip and applicator to ensure that the clip can be released from its holder with minimal force.

If the aneurysm is seen to extend below the tentorium, additional exposure is achieved by coagulating and dividing the veins at the temporal tip and gradually retracting the tip of the temporal lobe posteriorly to expose the proximal internal carotid artery and the aneurysm.

If the aneurysmal sac projects above the tentorium and is buried in the temporal lobe, retraction is limited to the frontal lobe, exposing the aneurysmal neck without disturbing the lesion further.

Aneurysms arising from the carotid bifurcation are frequently encased in dense adhesions between the aneurysm, the anterior and middle cerebral arteries, and vessels entering the anterior perforated substance. One or more vessels may be incorporated in the aneurysm, and clip occlusion may compromise major arterial trunks. Dissection is carried along the internal carotid artery up toward the bifurcation, staying along the anterior and inferior margin of the anterior and middle cerebral arteries while trying to identify the lenticulostriate vessels and anterior choroidal artery.

Following clipping or reinforcement of a carotid aneurysm, the basal cisterns are irrigated of all free blood; if vasospasm is seen, a 2.5 percent papaverine solution may be applied topically on cotton pledgets to the affected vessels. If an intracerebral hemorrhage is present, enough of the clot is removed before exposing the aneurysm to carry out the dissection; it is not until after the aneurysm has been clipped, however, that the majority of the clot is removed. In the patient with an oculomotor nerve palsy, the aneurysm may be aspirated after clipping to further reduce the pressure against this nerve. No attempt is made to dissect the aneurysm from the nerve in those cases in which they are in contact. Third-nerve palsy can be expected to resolve with improvement in ptosis within a few months, followed by an increasing range of extraocular movements and the return of pupillary reactivity.

If the aneurysm cannot be obliterated with a single clip, several alternatives are available to the surgeon, including attempting to place several clips across the aneurysm; dissecting out both the neck and fundus and wrapping the entire lesion in surgical or muslin gauze, which is then impregnated with cyanoacrylate; thrombosing the aneurysm using the Mullen wiring technique; trapping the lesion by clips placed proximal and distal to the origin of the aneurysm on the parent vessel after establishing a patent intracranial-extracranial bypass; or relying on graduated cervical carotid occlusion.

If the aneurysm detaches from the parent artery during dissection, leaving a hole in the artery, this may be dealt with either by using a Sundt clip on the carotid artery or alternatively by using a Silastic T-tube, introduced through the hole in the artery to provide continued flow while the defect is repaired using standard microsurgical techniques.

Intraoperative angiography can be performed at this stage to confirm the adequacy of the clip placement while it is still possible to conveniently reapply a malpositioned clip, thus sparing the patient the experience of another angiogram under local anesthesia before discharge. This is not necessary if the aneurysm is either aspirated or opened after clipping.

Once the aneurysm is clipped, the blood pressure is brought to normotensive levels and the adequacy of hemostasis is confirmed. Amicar is discontinued. The cisterns are filled with saline, the retractors are removed, and the dura is closed. If there is any difficulty in approximating the dural edges, a lypholized dural graft* is inserted. A pressure switch is then placed in the epidural space to allow constant monitoring of the intracranial pressure, along with a medium-sized Jackson-Pratt drain,** which is emptied hourly. Postoperative antibiotics are continued until the drain and the switch are removed. The bone flap is reapproximated to assure a good cosmetic result, and the galea and skin are closed as separate layers. The incision and exit sites of the drain and switch are covered with an antibiotic ointment and a dressing is applied.

Postoperatively, the patient is maintained on much the same regimen as preoperatively, and dexamethasone, phenytoin, and codeine are continued. The intracranial pressure is kept under 20 torr and the fluid intake is restricted to 1800 cc per day for 3 to 4 days. A baseline CT scan is performed within hours of the operation to estimate the extent of cerebral edema and to establish whether there are hemorrhages or hydrocephalus. The blood pressure is maintained at normotensive levels except when cerebral vasospasm arises, and is documented angiographically. This complication is treated by the regimen described previously. Anticonvulsants are routinely continued for 6 months after surgery, and in most cases the patient is examined by postoperative angiography before discharge, unless the aneurysm has been aspirated or opened intraoperatively.

Results

The neurosurgical literature contains many reports of aneurysms managed surgically in which the morbidity and mortality in a given series was less than 10 percent, creating the impression that as a result of current anesthetic and microsurgical techniques and surgical virtuosity the problems attending the management of these lesions have to a large extent been mastered. Such, however, is not the experience of neurosurgeons functioning either at community or university hospitals. Rather, these reports reflect the results in a highly selected population of cases referred to centers of acknowledged excellence in the surgical care of aneurysms. It is my experience that the overall morbidity and mortality rate of patients admitted to our neurosurgical unit with subarachnoid hemorrhage resulting from a proven intracranial aneurysm and followed from the first day of hemorrhage to 90 days after is considerably higher, in spite of the exemplary medical and surgical care.

The dismal results attending the management of aneurysmal subarachnoid hemorrhage have been corroborated in the recent report from the Cooperative Aneurysm Study by Adams, Kassell, et al.,[12] which analyzed the experience of neurosurgeons at 11 participating institutions who managed 249 patients admitted within 3 days of subarachnoid hemorrhage and on whom surgery was not performed sooner than 12 days after the most recent subarachnoid hemorrhage. Management consisted of bedrest, anticonvulsants, sedation, analgesics, epison aminocaproic acid at 36 g per day, and steroids, as well as mannitol as indicated. One hundred fifty-eight patients were treated operatively. Among the cases in good neurologic condition, 13 were subjected to carotid ligation and 116 to intracranial operations; among the cases considered as poor

*Lyodura, Aesculap, Inc., New York, NY
**Jackson-Pratt drain, Heyerschulte, Inc., Worcester, MA

Table 57-1. Internal Carotid Artery Aneurysms
Admitted Day 0-3 after Subarachnoid Hemorrhage

14-day mortality	18% (9/50)
(preoperative)	
14-to-90-day mortality	
Nonoperated	53% (8/15)
Intracranial surgery	13% (2/16)
Carotid ligation	0% (0/8)
Both	0% (0/2)
Total mortality	38% (19/50)
(0–90 days)	

risks, 4 had carotid ligation, 20 intracranial surgery, and in the entire series 5 patients had both carotid ligation and intracranial surgery. Assessment of the overall results of the 235 cases on whom data were available shows 46 percent had a favorable outcome, 17.9 percent an unfavorable outcome, and 36.2 percent died. These results included a 55.7 percent favorable outcome and a 28.7 percent mortality among patients in good condition, although the procedure-related mortality attending intracranial surgery was only 8.8 percent.

In the Cooperative Aneurysm Study 50 patients had an aneurysm of the internal carotid artery (32 were on the middle cerebral artery, 84 were on the anterior cerebral complex, 20 were vertebrobasilar, and 63 demonstrated multiple aneurysms). The results for this group of cases are show in Table 57-1.

These results suggest, in comparison with the entire population of cases in the study, that aneurysms of the internal carotid artery are a prognostically favorable subgroup, although these cases are still associated with a 38 percent mortality within 90 days of the subarachnoid hemorrhage and a 13 percent mortality for those cases managed by intracranial surgery. Carotid ligation is not associated with any deaths in this report but has the disadvantage of about a 7 percent late rebleeding rate even when the carotid ligation was successful, and a significant morbidity that mediates against its routine use except for aneurysms within the cavernous sinus and those aneurysms whose configuration may preclude direct intracranial intervention.

REFERENCES

1. Dott NM: Intracranial aneurysms: cerebral arterio-radiography; surgical treatment. *Med J (Edinburg)* 40:219–234, 1933
2. Dandy WE: Intracranial aneurysm of the internal carotid artery cured by operation. *Ann Surg* 107:654–659, 1938
3. Okawara SH: Warning signs prior to rupture of an intracranial aneurysm. *J Neurosurg* 38:575–580, 1973
4. Gelber BR, Sundt TM Jr.: Treatment of intracavernous and giant carotid aneurysms by combined internal carotid ligation and extra to intracranial bypass. *N Neursurg* 52:1–10, 1980
5. Hayward RD, O'Reilly GV: Intracerebral haemorrhage: accuracy of CT scanning in predicing underlying aetiology. *Lancet* 1:1–4, 1976
6. Fisher CM, Kistler JP, Davis JM: Relation of cerebral vasospasm to subarachnoid hemorrhage visualized by computerized tomographic scanning. *Neurosurgery* 6:1–9, 1980
7. Hook D, Norlen G: Aneurysms of the internal carotid artery. *Acta Neurol Scand* 40:200–218, 1964
8. Odom GL: Ophthalmic involvement in neurological vascular lesions, in *Neuro-ophthalmology*, Smith JL (ed): Springfield, IL, Charles C Thomas, 1964
9. Overgaard J, Riishede J: Multiple cerebral saccular aneurysms. *Acta Neurol Scandinav* 41:363–371, 1965
10. Scotti G, Ethier R, Melancon D, et al: Computed tomography in the evaluation of intracranial aneurysms and subarachnoid hemorrhage. *Radiology* 123:85–90, 1977
11. Mizukami M, Takemae T, Tazawa T, et al: Value of computerized tomography in the prediction of cerebral vasospasm after aneurysm rupture. *Neurosurgery* 7:583–586, 1980
12. Adams HP, Kassel NF, Torner JC et al: Early mangement of aneurysmal subarachnoid hemorrhage. *J Neurosurg* 54:141–145, 1981

CHAPTER 58
Surgical Treatment of Carotid-Ophthalmic Aneurysms

Robert M. Crowell   Robert G. Ojemann

CAROTID-OPHTHALMIC ANEURYSMS usually present with subarachnoid hemorrhage (SAH).[1-6] Giant ophthalmic aneurysms may cause visual field abnormalities.[7] Rarely, an ophthalmic aneurysm may lead to transient ischemic attacks (TIAs) in the territory of the internal carotid artery, presumably on an embolic basis. We have observed 1 case in which a giant ophthalmic aneurysm produced frontal cortical irritation and the patient presented with a seizure disorder. There is a preponderance of ophthalmic aneurysms in females, and there is an unusual tendency for multiple aneurysms.[1-7]

Preoperative Management

When the diagnosis of SAH is suspected, the first step is to obtain a computed tomographic (CT) scan without and with contrast.[8] This test may establish the diagnosis by showing blood in the basal cisterns, the interhemispheric fissure, or within brain tissue. In some cases the aneurysm may be visualized. Lumbar puncture may be used to diagnose SAH if there is no evidence of increased intracranial pressure.

All patients with SAH should undergo screening tests of clotting function including prothrombin times (PT), partial thromboplastin time (PTT), and platelet count.[9] An electrocardiogram may show abnormalities related to SAH. Complete blood count, serum electrolytes, and serum osmolarity should be determined as base-line values.

Management is guided by the clinical status and by the CT findings.[10] Symptomatic intracranial hematoma may require emergency surgical evacuation. Patients with symptomatic hydrocephalus may need emergency ventriculoperitoneal shunting.

Division of Neurological Surgery, Barrow Neurological Institute, St. Joseph's Hospital and Medical Center, Phoenix, Arizona, and Neurosurgical Service, Massachusetts General Hospital, and Department of Surgery, Harvard Medical School, Boston, Massachusetts.

We are grateful to Dr. R. S. Lees for medical management of many of these patients; to Drs. C. M. Fisher and J. P. Kistler for neurologic consultation; and to Drs. P. Sundaram and F. Debros for neuroanesthesia management. Thanks also to Mrs. Edith Tagrin for preparation of the figures and Georgia Frederic for preparation of the manuscript.

Supported in part by the National Institute of Neurological and Communicative Diseases and Stroke through Teacher-Investigator Award NS11001 and Grant NS 17319.

Portions of this chapter are reprinted with permission from Ojemann RG, Crowell RM: Surgical Management of Cerebrovascular Disease (Baltimore, Williams and Wilkins).

Medical therapy

A standard medical regimen is instituted for stable patients without mass lesions. This includes:

1. Bedrest.
2. Fluid administration aimed at maintaining normal circulating volume and central venous pressure. Serum electrolytes are checked serially along with serum osmolarity and intake and output.
3. Elastic stockings or pneumatic compression boots.
4. Epsilon-aminocaproic acid (Amicar, 30 g/day intravenously).
5. Anticonvulsants (diphenylhydantoin 300 mg/day).
6. Stool softeners.
7. Phenobarbital (15–30 mg/IM/q3h), for agitation.
8. Hydralazine (5–20 mg/IM/2–3h), for hypertension, to bring the systolic pressure below 150 torr without causing drowsiness. Propanolol is used in some cases, and occasionally intravenous nitroprusside is needed for control.
9. Methylprednisolone (16–80 mg/PO or IM q6h) to reduce cerebral swelling.)
10. Cimetidine (300 mg/PO or IV q8h) along with antacid by mouth or gastric tube every 3 hours.
11. Codeine (30–60 mg/IM or PO), for headache.
12. Kanamycin (1 gm PO t.i.d.) and reserpine (0.2 mg SC t.i.d.), for patients in grades 1 and 2 to reduce the chance of postoperative vasospasm.

Metabolic studies and CT scans are rechecked on an emergency basis should a patient deteriorate. Electrolyte imbalance may require correction. The CT scan may reveal hydrocephalus or focal cerebral ischemia or edema. Progressive hydrocephalus requires ventriculoperitoneal shunting for relief of symptoms. Angiography is performed if a clear explanation of deterioration is not found. If angiography discloses a significant degree of vasospasm (grades 3 and 4), a program of therapy is begun, with monitoring of radial arterial pressure and central venous pressure. The intravascular volume is increased with colloid or packed cells to achieve a CVP of 10–12 cm H_2O and a hematocrit of 40%. A pressor is given to increase the systolic blood pressure to about 30 torr above basal levels with a maximum of 160 torr. Phenylephrine or dopamine may be used for this purpose.

The timing of elective angiography and surgery is determined by the clinical condition as judged by the Botterell classification. For patients in good condition (grades 1 and 2), angiography is deferred for 7 to 10 days after SAH, with surgery on the day following angiography if no spasm is demonstrated. For patients in poor condition (grades 3 and 4), angiography is deferred about 2 to 3 weeks after SAH. If the patient is stable and the angiogram shows an aneurysm, surgery is performed. Whenever significant spasm is demonstrated, the angiogram is repeated at weekly intervals, but after three SAHs, we usually proceed with surgery even if there is some residual spasm.

Angiography

Transfemoral selective four-vessel angiography is preferred. Studies should begin with the vessel that is suspected of harboring the bleeding lesion. If an ophthalmic artery aneurysm is disclosed, special views must be obtained for complete characterization of the sac, its neck, and the relationship to the internal carotid and the ophthalmic arteries. Standard AP and lateral projections may require supplementary views, including base, oblique, or off-lateral projections. Subtraction is often helpful in visualizing the ophthalmic artery. In case the aneurysm proves unapproachable and is best treated by an indirect procedure, views of the carotid bifurcation, external carotid, and superficial temporal arteries and collateral circulation to the carotid territory will be required. Angiotomography may be employed to obtain greater detail in representation of the aneurysm, but we have not found this technique of decisive importance.

Special tests

Transport for optional studies is not advisable when the SAH is fresh. Simple confrontation field re-examination is useful as a base line for comparison with postoperative studies. When plane skull films or angiograms suggest erosion of the anterior clinoid process, polytomographic study of this area could delineate the extent of bony erosion caused by the aneurysm.

Anesthesia

Premedication

Steroids are begun the night before surgery if they have not already been included in the regimen. We prefer methylprednisolone (Solu-medrol; 80 mg IM) at midnight and 6:00 AM. In addition, propranolol (Inderol) is given (40 mg PO) at midnight. This agent appears to improve the stability of blood pressure control intraoperatively. Blood is requested for availability during surgery. For premedication, diazepam (10 mg IM) or a neurolept agent (Innovar, 0.5 cc IM) serve nicely.

Preparation

In the induction room an intravenous route is established. This is preferably a large-bore plastic cannula, but in many patients receiving Amicar therapy, suitable veins are hard to identify. In such patients, rather than cause agitation by repeated venipuncture efforts, it is better to place a small-gauge needle intravenously, and then establish two large-bore IV routes after the patient is anesthetized. The external jugular vein or a leg vein may be used if necessary. Rarely, an intravenous line cannot be established easily and induction of anesthesia by mask may be the best initial maneuver. A catheter is introduced into the radial artery for continuous monitoring of arterial pressure. Such monitoring is particularly important during induction, when wide swings of arterial pressure may occur. Pressor and antihypertensive agents are available for infusion; phenylephrine (Neosynephrine, 10 mg in 250 cc 5% dextrose and water) and sodium nitroprusside (50 mg in 250 cc 5% dextrose in water shielded with tin foil) serve well for these needs.

Induction

Once all preparations are complete, a slow induction is carried out with preparation over 10 minutes or more before intubation. Sodium pentobarbital is given by increments (50–150 mg/ increment up to 1 g total) after initial preoxygenation. Once the patient is deeply drowsy, halothane is given by mask (0.5 to 1.5%). Before intubation a muscle relaxant is given (curare, 0.5 mg/kg). A twitch monitor is applied to the ulnar nerve to monitor the completeness of neuromuscular blockade. An additional increment of pentobarbital is given intravenously just before intratracheal intubation. Ideally, the blood pressure is in the range of 100 torr systolic at this point. Laryngoscopy is carried out, and the vocal cords are sprayed with a local anesthetic solution. The blood pressure response to laryngoscopy is noted; if a substantial hypertensive response has occurred, an additional increment of pentobarbital is administered, or further administration of halothane is carried out, or both. Finally, with the patient stable and well anesthetized, laryngoscopy is executed with gentle endotracheal intubation. In case of a sustained rise of blood pressure, further increments of pentobarbital are given intravenously and the concentration of halothane may be increased temporarily. Controlled ventilation is preferred, with arterial PCO_2 maintained in the range of 30 torr, as demonstrated by frequently sampled arterial blood gases. The arterial blood gases likewise provide a frequent check on the adequacy of oxygenation.

Reduction of brain tension

All patients receive 100 g of mannitol IV while the bone flap is being turned; in many cases this is preceded by Lasix (20 mg IV). This usually gives excellent relaxation of the brain. Solu-medrol (80 mg IV) is continued every 4 hours. For larger lesions, a spinal subarachnoid catheter may be used to withdraw cerebrospinal fluid (CSF). This was unnecessary in most of our cases.

Controlled hypotension

Careful communication between the neuroanesthesiologist and the surgeon is crucial in controlled hypotension.[11] For the pharmacologic control of blood pressure during surgery, the dialogue is of particular importance. Induced hypotension is used to slacken the aneurysm during dissection in order to decrease the likelihood of intraoperative rupture. In most patients the blood pressure is maintained at about 100 torr during the initial exposure. Once the aneurysm is in view, the pressure is dropped further to about 80 torr systolic. During critical dissection of the neck of the aneurysm deep hypotension may be required (systolic blood pressure 60 torr or mean arterial blood pressure about 40 torr). Occasionally a particularly difficult portion of an aneurysm may justify a burst of very deep hypotension for 2–3 minutes at a mean of 20–25 torr. Most patients tolerate this type of deep hypotension without postoperative sequelae. In the normal brain, autoregulation maintains local cerebral blood flow down to mean arterial blood pressures of 40–45 torr. In patients with SAH, however, autoregulation may be lost in some zones. Moreover, in some elderly patients, and in those with ischemic heart disease, prolonged and deep hypotension may not be well tolerated by the brain, heart, or kidneys. In such cases, levels of controlled hypotension may be moderated. Several techniques for controlled hypotension are available. Moderate hypotension may be achieved simply by increasing the concentration of inspired halothane in many cases. In most cases an additional agent, such as sodium nitroprusside, will be required to further diminish the blood pressure. Trimethapan camsylate (Arfonad) or trinitroglycerine also may be used for this purpose. Another agent that may be used for more prolonged hypotensive effect is hydralazine given in increments of 5 mg intravenously. Propranolol, given preoperatively and then intraoperatively in doses as high as 1–2 mg intravenously, likewise may be used for more prolonged hypotensive effect of a stable sort.

Vasospasm

Care should be taken not to lower the blood pressure as much as is normally done in patients with vasospasm, either suspected or proved by angiography. Once the aneurysm is obliterated, cerebral perfusion is maximized by volume expansion with colloid and packed cells if necessary. Blood pressure is elevated to 140 torr systolic, by use of a pressor if necessary.

Extubation

Toward the conclusion of the procedure, the anesthetic is managed in such a fashion that the muscle relaxant will have worn off and the patient may be extubated and awakened in the operating theater. This approach, which is guided by the twitch monitor, permits early assessment of neurologic function postoperatively.

Operative Technique

Positioning and Preparation

The approach in most instances is ipsilateral to the ophthalmic artery aneurysm. Occasionally, for a lesion that points medially or inferiorly from the internal carotid artery, contralateral craniotomy will provide the best visualization of the sac and its neck. In the case of bilateral ophthalmic artery aneurysms, careful selection of the most appropriate side for craniotomy may permit a direct attack on both lesions from one side.

After the induction of anesthesia, the patient is positioned supine with the head slightly elevated. The head is turned about 60°, with the zygoma uppermost and the vertex depressed slightly below the horizontal plane. In patients with limited mobility of the neck, a small roll is placed under the shoulder. The Mayfield-Kees three-point headrest is then applied after the scalp sites are prepared with Zephiran solution. Additional increments of pentobarbital (50–150 mg IV) are given just before this painful stimulation. Protective plastic shields are placed across the eyes. The proposed incision site is shaved and steri-towels are draped to wall off the area. Either elastic bandages or pneumatic compression boots are used on the lower extremities to help prevent thrombophlebitis. The scrub nurse stands on the surgeon's right side (for a right-handed surgeon) with the Mayo stands attached to the table over the patient's chest and abdomen.

Incision

In most cases an incision just behind the hairline is preferred, proceeding from the widow's peak in a curvilinear fashion to a point just above the zygoma in front of the tragus. The superficial temporal artery is palpated and marked. The incision should lie posterior to the root of the superficial temporal artery in order to preserve this structure with the flap. Occasionally in bald individuals or in cases where additional exposure is desired for another aneurysm, an alternative incision may be planned, utilizing a wrinkle high in the forehead or a coronal incision extending across the midline. As the area is draped, the post for the Greenberg retractor is attached to the three-point headrest.

Both the surgeon and assistant use 2-X loupes and headlights during the initial phases of the procedure. Local anesthesia (Marcaine 1% without epinephrine) is injected along the incision except near the superficial temporal artery. The incision is begun anteriorly and cuts to but not through the periosteum. A scissors is inserted in the plane between the galea and the periosteum, and then the knife is used to cut down to the scissors, thus preventing injury to the underlying temporalis muscle and superficial temporal artery. Care is taken to avoid this artery, particularly near its root. The posterior branch of the superficial temporal artery is dissected free and divided between 3-0 silk ligatures, thus permitting the trunk and frontal branch of this vessel, which might be needed for later cerebral revascularization, to be reflected forward with the soft tissue flap. Hemostasis is obtained by applying Dandy hemostats to the posterior margin and Köln clips to the anterior margins of the incision, with particular care being taken to avoid injury to the superficial temporal artery. Next the temporalis fascia is incised with a knife, and the temporalis muscle is opened with the cutting cautery. A branch of the deep temporal artery is regularly encountered within the muscle, and this must be cauterized accurately to avoid troublesome bleeding later. The periosteum is swept off the skull with a periosteal elevator just to the edge of the orbit, and the muscle is reflected from the skull, including the superior temporal line, with the cutting cautery until the zygomatic process of the frontal bone is approached. The soft tissue flap is folded over a sponge to prevent ischemic compression, protected with a rubber dam and a Bacitracin-soaked sponge, and held in place with silk sutures placed into the muscle and attached by rubber bands to the drapes. A final maneuver that permits maximal visualization beneath the muscle is the application of Cushing retractors to the muscle along the zygomatic process of the frontal bone, with tension applied to these retractors via rubber bands and Allis clamps attached to the drapes. This approach provides excellent exposure once the bone flap is removed. We have tried the Z-formed temporalis fascia opening suggested by Yasargil and found it no better for exposure and less satisfactory from the cosmetic standpoint.

Initial exposure

A pterional (frontotemporal) craniotomy permits satisfactory exposure of carotid-ophthalmic artery aneurysms (Fig. 58-1).[12,13] A free pterional bone flap is turned with the power drill and craniotome. The critical burr hole is placed just behind the zygomatic process of the frontal bone and below the end of the superior temporal line. Additional burr holes are placed in the low temporal and posterior frontal regions. The unsightly depression of the inferomedial frontal burr hole can be eliminated by the use of a curved bony cut with the craniotome. The dura is separated from the inner table of the skull with a No. 3 Penfield. The craniotome cut is begun along the floor of the anterior fossa, proceeding medially about 3–4 cm, and then curving in an easy arch posteriorly to the high temporal burr hole. It is well to angle this saw curve slightly, beveling outward to provide nice seating for the bone flap when it is replaced. Another saw cut with the craniotome is made between the superior and inferior temporal burr holes. Finally, the key hole and the inferior temporal burr hole are connected using rongeurs. A portion of the lateral sphenoid ridge is preserved with the bone flap, which is finally broken off by prying it with a periosteal elevator. The bone flap is carefully peeled off the dura and the middle meningeal artery is identified, coagulated, and cut. Bony edges are waxed for hemostasis. Additional bone is rongeured from the lateral sphenoid ridge. Care is taken at this point to avoid injury to structures in the superior orbital fissure. Frequently a small arterial branch to the dura in this region must be coagulated. These maneuvers effectively level the sphenoid ridge between the frontal and the temporal lobes, thus creating an unobstructed visual access to the anterior clinoid area. In some cases the inner table of bone that forms the floor of the anterior fossa over the orbit will be characterized by mountainous irregularities, impeding the view. In such cases a high-speed drill may be used to smooth the area. If a small opening into the orbit occurs, it is covered with Gelfoam. If additional access is needed along the floor of the anterior fossa behind the orbit, the inner table of bone at the edge of the craniotomy just anterior to the keyhole also may be removed with the rongeur without compromising the cosmetic appearance of the outer table. In some cases a very prominent and lateral frontal sinus may be encountered with the saw cut or bony removal. If this occurs, the mucosa should be removed, the sinus packed with Bacitracin-soaked Gelfoam, and the opening covered with a small flap of pericranium dissected from the back of the scalp flap and stitched to the adjacent dura. Next, a fine drill point is used to create holes for wires to hold the flap in place at the time of closure. Dura-to-pericranial sutures of 4-0 silk are placed around the periphery of the bony opening to achieve epidural hemostasis. Tiny strips of Surgicel are inserted in the epidural space as needed. Bacitracin-soaked sponges are placed over the skin edge and all exposed tissue except the dura.

During this phase the surgeon can readily determine whether the brain is slack. If this is not the case, measures must be taken to obtain adequate slackness; the PCO_2 may need adjustment, additional dehydration may be required, or CSF may need to be drained. Occasionally ventricular puncture will be needed to obtain a slack brain.

A linear dural incision is made approximately 6–8 mm above the inferior margin of the bony opening with inferior turning at the frontal and temporal corners. The inferior dural flap is tacked up over the bone edge, avoiding a buckle in the center of the flap, which could interfere with intradural visualization.

Under 2-X loupe magnification, a medium width, Teflon-coated, hand-held brain retractor is used to gently elevate the frontal lobe. A sucker on a cottonoid can be used to gradually re-

FREE BONE FLAP

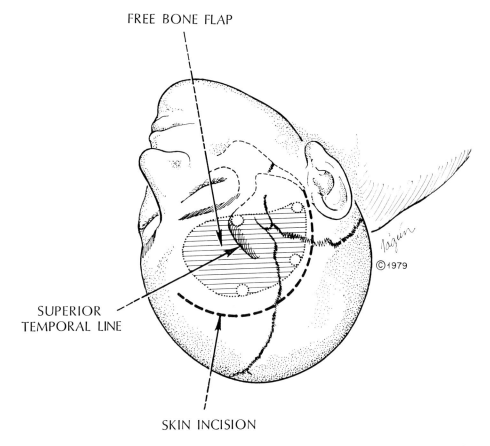

©1979

SUPERIOR
TEMPORAL LINE

SKIN INCISION

Fig. 58-1. Exposure of the lesion via a pterional craniotomy. An incision behind the hairline permits a small frontotemporal craniotomy. The frontal lobe then is gently elevated.

move any CSF that may appear inferior to the frontal lobe. The retractor is slowly advanced just in front of the edge of the sphenoid wing.

The olfactory tract, an important landmark, will come into view, and following this a few millimeters posteriorly will lead one to the region of the optic nerve. Since the frontal lobe may be adherent to the aneurysm, no effort should be made to expose the internal carotid artery at this stage. Time should be spent allowing further CSF to drain. It is most important that the brain be so slack that only mild retraction is needed for adequate exposure.

Next a protective layer of rubber dam and cottonoid, precut to the proper shape, is placed like a rug over the exposed frontal lobe down to the olfactory tract. At this point the Greenberg self-retaining retractor system holding a Teflon-coated, Dott-type posted retractor blade bent to about 60° is placed to elevate the frontal lobe. The retractor should take a low profile so as to give easy access to the infrafrontal cleft. Next a narrow hand-held retractor is used to carefully elevate the temporal lobe. Temporal-tip bridging veins are divided. Once the temporal tip is free, a covering of rubber dam and cottonoid is placed and the lobe held posteriorly with a slender retractor blade fixed on the Greenberg apparatus. The two retractor blades should be separated by only several millimeters at right angles to each other. Up to this point the combination of 2-X loupes and headlight illumination has been used for maximal mobility with adequate visualization. From this point, however, the operating microscope is used to maximize illumination and visualization of critical structures.

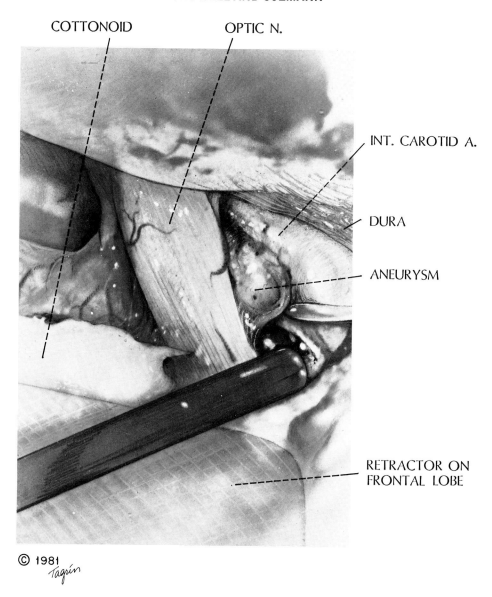

COTTONOID   OPTIC N.

INT. CAROTID A.

DURA

ANEURYSM

RETRACTOR ON
FRONTAL LOBE

© 1981

Fig. 58-2. Approach to the carotid-ophthalmic aneurysm. A right pterional craniotomy offers exposure of this right-side aneurysm. Dissection has established distal control of the internal carotid artery. The optic nerve and the anterior clinoid process hide the proximal neck of the lesion.

Microsurgical Dissection

We use the Zeiss OPMI-1 with a 275-mm objective lens, 12.5X eye pieces, and angled 160 mm binocular tubes for microsurgical dissection.[12,13] The visual image is channeled via a 50:50 small beam splitter to a stereo observer tube on one side and a unified adaptor (Designs for Vision) for video (Hitachi) and intermittent still photography (Contax) on the other side. A clear video image projected on a monitor mounted high in one corner of the operating theatre provides access to the microsurgical action for all members of the microsurgical team including the scrub nurse and anesthetist.

Under microsurgical vision, the frontal lobe is gently elevated to expose the internal carotid artery and the anterior clinoid process (Fig. 58-2). In some cases the aneurysm may need gentle dissection from the frontal lobe. Controlled hypotension is appropriate in these circumstances.

OPTIC N.   DURA

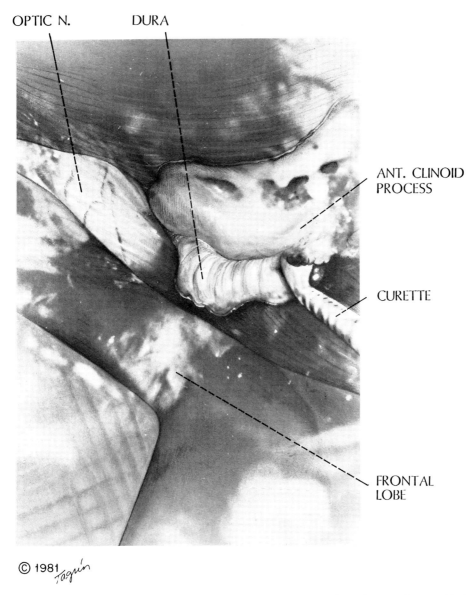

ANT. CLINOID
PROCESS

CURETTE

FRONTAL
LOBE

© 1981 Taguin

Fig. 58-3. Exposing the anterior clinoid process. After incision of the dura, a microcurette is used to dissect the dural flap off the clinoid process.

In many cases the surgical sequence involves removal of the anterior clinoid process to facilitate dissection and clipping of the aneurysm.

Removal of the anterior clinoid process.   In order to remove the anterior clinoid process,[1,6] the overlying dura must be removed (Fig. 58-3). A coated Penfield No. 4 dissector and monopolar electrocautery set at low current are used to coagulate a semicircular path over the clinoid process from medial to lateral. Great care must be exercised to avoid injury to the optic nerve, which may lie under the dura uncovered by the bone in this area. Lateral coagulation must be terminated at the edge of the cavernous sinus. This coagulated area is incised with a No. 15 knife blade. The resulting flap of dura may be conveniently elevated with a fine-angled microcurette. This flap of dura lies over the internal carotid artery, thus protecting it during subsequent drilling.

OPTIC N.   ANTERIOR
                   CLINOID PROCESS

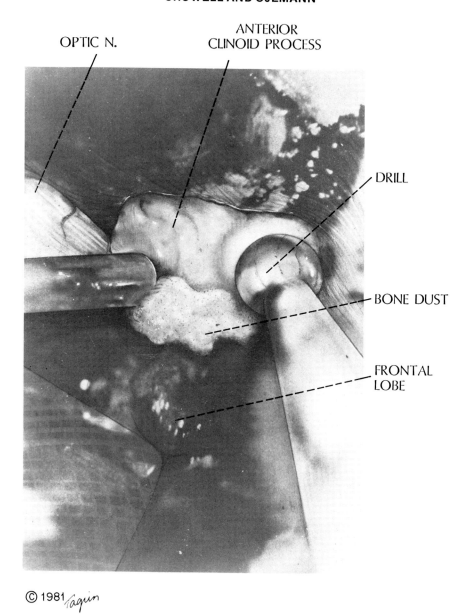

DRILL

BONE DUST

FRONTAL
LOBE

© 1981 Tagvin

Fig. 58-4. Removal of the anterior clinoid process. A high-speed drill weakens the clinoid process medially and laterally (as shown). The resulting fragment of bone is dissected free of soft tissue and removed.

The anterior clinoid process next is removed with a high-speed drill with an angled hand piece and a diamond burr (Fig. 58-4). The surgeon can conveniently control this instrument with the right hand, resting the wrist firmly while the fine sucker is held in the field with the left hand. During controlled drilling, a fine stream of irrigation is directed onto the drill point from a microirrigator held by the assistant (12-cc syringe with a 22-gauge Medicut plastic catheter). The clinoid process may be isolated by drilling its medial and lateral bony supports. Usually one drill spot accurately placed on either side of the process will achieve this goal. Once underlying soft tissue is encountered, drilling is redirected slightly superiorly or inferiorly until each buttress—lateral and medial—is weakened. Then a 5-0 straight bone currette is used to gradually fracture and mobilize the resulting anterior clinoid fragment. This is accomplished with utmost care and control to avoid abrupt movement of the fragment and possible injury to nearby structures. The

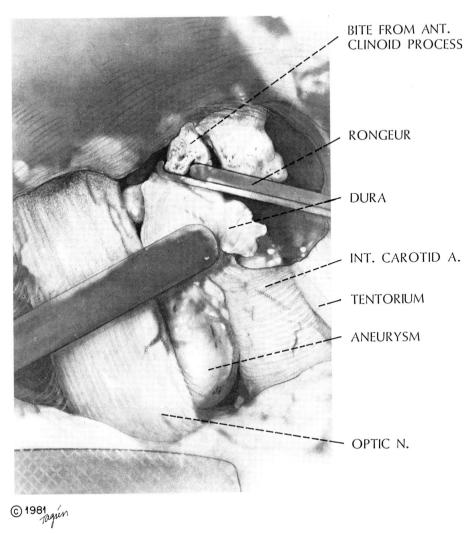

BITE FROM ANT.
CLINOID PROCESS

RONGEUR

DURA

INT. CAROTID A.

TENTORIUM

ANEURYSM

OPTIC N.

© 1981

Fig. 58-5.   Rongeuring of additional bone. A microantrostomy punch is used to gain additional access to the proximal internal carotid artery.

5-0 curette and microcurettes are used to dissect the fragment free from underlying soft tissues. If the bony exposure seems inadequate, additional drilling may be used to widen the field of view. A fine microantrostomy punch may be used for additional bony removal, if space permits (Fig. 58-5). It should be noted that paranasal sinus mucosa may in some cases extend into bone in this area. If mucosa is encountered, the overlying bony opening must be carefully waxed. If bleeding from soft tissue occurs, application of tiny amounts of Surgicel or Gelfoam may be used for hemostasis.

Dissection of the aneurysm.   Once the anterior clinoid process is removed, the protective function of the small dural flap no longer applies and it is removed. The surgeon next obtains proximal and distal control of the internal carotid artery (Fig. 58-6). In many cases distal control is straightforward. The posterior communicating and anterior choroidal arteries provide a distal boundary for dissection. Proximal control usually is a greater challenge. At this point in the procedure, because of the threat of rupture of the aneurysm, the blood pressure is lowered to about 80 torr systolic. This level of hypotension is well tolerated up to 1 hour in most patients. The internal carotid artery is freed proximal to the aneurysm. Often a microdissector serves nicely for

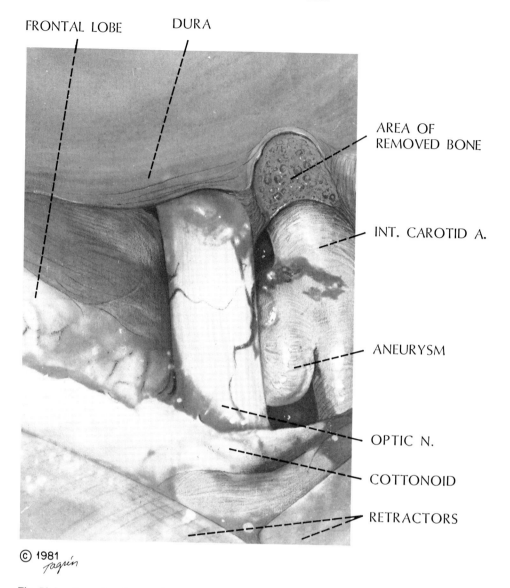

FRONTAL LOBE

DURA

AREA OF
REMOVED BONE

INT. CAROTID A.

ANEURYSM

OPTIC N.

COTTONOID

RETRACTORS

© 1981
faquin

Fig. 58-6. Exposing the proximal neck of the aneurysm. With the anterior clinoid process removed, the proximal internal carotid artery and the neck of the aneurysm can be freed. The ophthalmic artery (not seen) lies just proximal and medial to the neck of the aneurysm in this case.

this dissection. Dense arachnoid bands may be electrocoagulated with the bipolar cautery and cut sharply. Dura may be opened laterally with cauterization and sharp dissection, with the cavernous sinus as the end point. Every effort should be made to visualize and spare the ophthalmic artery, which usually arises from the internal carotid artery just proximal to the neck of the aneurysm. If the ophthalmic artery is not seen, the proximal neck of the aneurysm must be completely dissected and visualized before application of a clip in this area. In many cases where the lesion projects superiorly, gentle deflection of the lesion posteriorly with a sucker will permit passage of a fine dissector proximal to the neck and medially as far as the optic nerve or beneath it. Gentle lateral deflection of the aneurysm may permit dissection of the medial aspect of the aneurysm from the optic nerve. Lesions that point medially beneath the optic nerve will require gentle deflection of the nerve medially and superiorly to isolate the aneurysm neck.

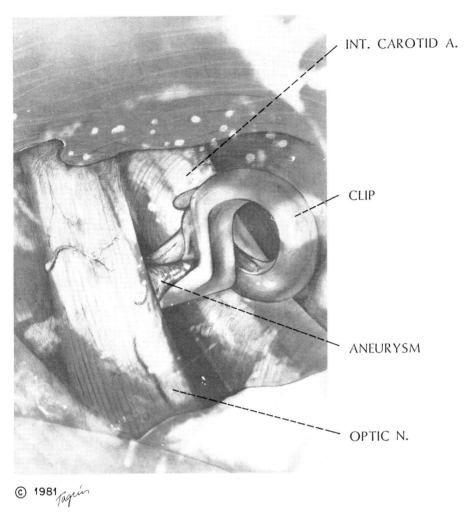

INT. CAROTID A.

CLIP

ANEURYSM

OPTIC N.

© 1981 *Tagrin*

Fig. 58-7. Clipping of the aneurysms. A narrow-bladed clip is placed cross the neck of the aneurysm and flush with the internal carotid artery. The ophthalmic artery takeoff is just lateral to the tips of the clip.

Obliteration of the aneurysm. Once the neck of the aneurysm is completely freed and the ophthalmic artery separated from it, obliteration of the aneurysm may be carried out (Fig. 58-7). This can be accomplished in many cases without substantial manipulation of the sac or neck, and thus moderate hypotension (systolic pressure 70–80 torr) provides adequate reduction of tension in the lesion. Occasionally a particularly thin-walled lesion or one requiring substantial manipulation for clipping presents a greater danger of rupture; in these circumstances a brief period of deep hypotension (2–3 minutes at systolic pressure 30–40 torr) will minimize the risk of rupture at a small risk systemically.

Various types of clips can be used to obliterate the aneurysm. The blade length is chosen to provide just enough length to fully cross the neck. Often the available space between internal carotid artery, the bony skull, and the optic nerve dictate use of the narrowest blade available. Frequently this feature favors a Yasargil clip, because of its narrow blades. The shape of the clip generally is either straight or slightly curved, with the concave aspect of the curve applied smoothly to the conforming aspect of the internal carotid artery. The angle of application generally is lateral to medial. In some cases a Heifetz clip may be applied nicely with the angled-tip applicator. In most cases the sac is deflected distally with a fine sucker in order to visualize the neck and ophthalmic artery during application of a clip. The tips of the clip are held just wide enough to encompass the neck and advanced slowly with a slight axial rotation movement to minimize friction against the lesion. Once the clip is seen to project just beyond the neck, the blades are slowly closed, with constant observation of resulting effects on the aneurysm and adjacent structures. The applicator is maintained on the clip hub, and if adverse effects are evident (incomplete neck obliteration, encroachment on the optic nerve or ophthalmic artery), then the clip is satisfactorily repositioned or removed. If the clip position seems adequate, the hub of the clip is released and the applicator removed. Occasionally this may prove difficult with the Yasargil clip, because these clips may be hard to release. It is worth testing release outside the wound before clip application. If difficulty is encountered after clip application, the clip applicator may be hyper-opened by placing the third and fourth fingers within the handle of the applicator and gently forcing the two handle components away from each other. Once the clip is place and released, the adequacy of clipping should be carefully checked. By deflecting the aneurysm dome slightly, the complete obliteration of the neck with tips of the clip extending beyond can be confirmed. Furthermore, the internal carotid artery and ophthalmic artery must be free of deformation or kinking, and the optic nerve should not be excessively deformed. Minor contact between the clip and the nerve is common. When significant displacement of the nerve is caused by the clip, further dissection of the nerve and even the chiasm may permit a gentle sloping displacement with limited infringement on the nerve. Reapplication of the clip in some cases may be necessary to avoid unsatisfactory deformation of the optic nerve.

For some aneurysms with broad necks, electrocoagulation can narrow the neck and set the stage for clipping (Fig. 58-8). For this maneuver, the bipolar catuery is set at low current, and the blades of the cautery forceps are positioned fully across the neck of the lesion. Low current is applied, and the forceps tips are gently squeezed and released repeatedly. Continuous irrigation is applied during this maneuver. The process is continued until the neck gradually shrinks, becoming whiter and thicker. If the bipolar cautery tips are only partially across the neck, perforation of the aneurysm is possible. Cauterization may thicken a reddened, thin aneurysmal neck. In situations where application of the forceps tips requires hazardous manipulation of the aneurysm, a brief burst of hypotension (systolic pressure: 30–40 torr) may slacken the lesion and diminish the hazard.

For other aneurysms with broad necks, a ligature may safely obliterate the lesion or set the stage for clipping. A fine ligature passer may facilitate postioning of a 3-0 silk ligature. Alternatively, the ligature may be placed with forceps anterior to the lesion, and then the suture is retrieved medially to the lesion with gentle deflection of the aneurysm. This latter method may minimize manipulation of the aneurysm during ligature placement. A surgeon's knot is placed and gradually tightened with two hemostats, the tips of which are applied to the sutures within 1–2 mm of the knot in order to avoid unwanted torque on the neck. Sometimes the knot may be tied down firmly, obliterating the neck. More commonly the ligature narrows the neck of the aneurysm and sets the stage for clipping.

Occasionally, unusual situations may be encountered. A Sundt clip-graft might be selected, possibly with a window for the ophthalmic artery. In some instances where obliteration cannot be achieved safely, the lesion may be reinforced with muscle or tissue adhesive.

When multiple aneurysms are present, consideration must be given to the accessibility of the remaining lesion(s) once the initial clip is placed. In general, the lesion positioned deepest in the field is dealt with first, thus retaining visualization of the more superficial lesion(s). Features of the clip employed, including size, angle, and route of application, will influence the accessibility of secondary aneurysms. In general, the smallest possible clip is used to conserve precious space in a narrow field. In the special case of bilateral ophthalmic aneurysms, the contralateral lesion is dealt with first, to permit satisfactory access for both lesions.

Clipping of contralateral ophthalmic aneurysms. Occasionally an ophthalmic aneurysm may be treated through a contralateral frontotemporal craniotomy (Fig. 58-9).[6] This approach

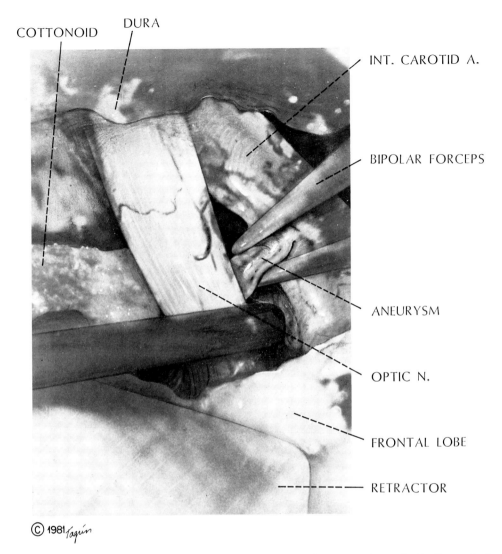

COTTONOID   DURA

INT. CAROTID A.

BIPOLAR FORCEPS

ANEURYSM

OPTIC N.

FRONTAL LOBE

RETRACTOR

© 1981 *faguín*

Fig. 58-8.   Preparation of the neck of the aneurysm. Bipolar cautery is applied to the neck of
the aneurysm to strengthen and shrink it. Forceps tips cross the neck completely
and avoid the nearby ophthalmic artery. Low current is utilized to avoid spasm to
native arteries.

may suggest itself in the case of bilateral ophthalmic aneurysms or when the aneurysm projects
inferiorly and medially. In the exposure of a contralateral lesion, retraction will be deep. Removal of CSF via a subarachnoid catheter can be useful in this circumstance. Extra care must be
taken to avoid tearing one or both olfactory tracts at the cribriform plate. As the frontal lobes
are elevated, the arachnoid attachments to the optic nerves and chiasms are severed sharply. The
contralateral proximal internal carotid artery comes into view inferior to the optic nerve. In this
area the contralateral ophthalmic aneurysm may be visualized projecting inferiorly and medially
from its origin. The neck is freed and the ophthalmic artery is preserved. A straight clip just long
enough to do the job obliterates the neck. Occasionally the bony tuberculum sella will have to be
removed to expose the proximal aneurysm neck. Coagulation and reflection of the dura for this
task will permit drilling of the obstructing bony prominence. Usually only a small amount of
bone has to be removed. Care must be taken to avoid entry into the sphenoid sinus. Careful obliteration of the opening is carried out with acrylic if such should occur.

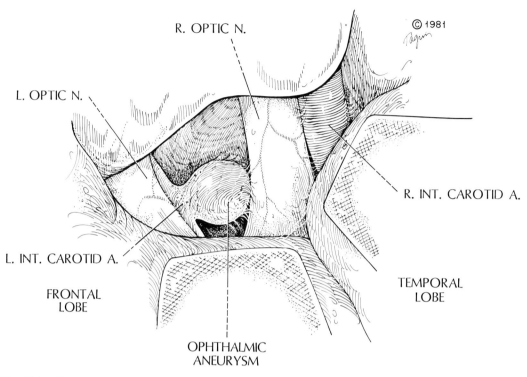

Fig. 58-9. Exposing a contralateral carotid-ophthalmic aneurysm. Through a *right* pterional craniotomy, a *left* carotid-ophthalmic aneurysm, which points medially, has been exposed. In this case an aneurysm of the right internal carotid-posterior communicating artery was clipped after the left carotid-ophthalmic lesion was obliterated.

Closure. After satisfactory clipping of the aneurysm, the blood pressure gradually is returned to the normal level for that patient, generally in the range of 125 torr systolic. The area of the aneurysm is carefully observed under the operating microscope for signs of bleeding. In the rare instance of inadequate hemostasis in the area of the aneurysm, either adjustment of the clip or application of tissue adhesive may be necessary to achieve the required hemostasis. When the field is dry, the retractors are removed and strips of Surgicel are placed over the areas of retraction. The dura is closed and tented to the bone flap. The bone is wired in place with 28-gauge stainless steel wires. Appropriate closure of the soft tissue then is done.

Indirect operation. Some lesions cannot be effectively obliterated by direct attack. This may be predicted from the angiogram if the lesion projects below the level of the ophthalmic artery into the cavernous sinus. In some cases this circumstance can be ascertained only at the time of surgery. For such aneurysms, the safest approach may be cervical carotid occlusion. Formerly, common carotid occlusion with a gradually occluding clamp was the procedure of choice. Recent reports indicate that the safest approach may be internal carotid occlusion, with cerebral revascularization.[7,14,15] Studies of cerebral blood flow may be helpful in determining the need for a bypass. STA–MCA bypass may be followed under the same anesthesia by application of the cervical internal carotid clamp. At the completion of surgery, the internal carotid is left open. If the dressings are dry on the day after surgery, aspirin (300 mg b.i.d.) and persantine (25 mg t.i.d.) are started, and gradual closure of the clamp is begun; closure is completed in 2-3 days, as tolerated. For this procedure, daily determination of the ophthalmic artery pressures may be quite useful to gauge closure of the clamp.

Postoperative Management

The patient is treated prophylactically against vasospasm at the conclusion of the procedure.[16,17] The central venous pressure is brought to 10 cm H_2O with colloid if there is no cardiac contraindication. The blood pressure is maintained in the range of 110–140 torr systolic with volume and pressors as required. Medications include Solu-medrol at 80 mg q6h IM, which is tapered after 3 days, an antacid, and Dilantin (300 mg/day). Elastic stockings or pneumatic compression boots are continued.

In the event of neurologic deterioration, an immediate CT scan is performed, looking for intracranial hematoma, hydrocephalus, or cerebral edema. Appropriate treatment is instituted if one of these conditions is found. An angiogram is performed if the CT scan fails to disclose an adequate explanation for the deterioration. If a vascular occlusion by the clip is disclosed, adjustment of the clip might be indicated (although we have never found this necessary). More commonly, cerebral vasospasms may be demonstrated. If significant vasospasm (grade 3 + or 4 +) is seen, additional treatment is indicated. The central venous pressure should be elevated to the range of 10–12 cm with colloid, and systolic blood pressure should be increased to the range of about 160–170 torr systolic; dopamine or neosynephrine may be employed for this purpose.

Postoperative angiography is recommended in all cases to ascertain the adequacy of aneurysm obliteration and maintenance of normal native vasculature.

Illustrative Case

Case 1. A 54-year-old right-handed women experienced a severe, sudden headache with brief loss of consciousness. Initial evaluation showed a normal neurologic evaluation. Her blood pressure was 180/100, and a lumbar puncture showed grossly bloody spinal fluid. On transfer, the neurologic examination was normal save for restlessness. A medical program was instituted, including Amicar and blood pressure control. The patient became slightly confused; CT scan showed moderate ventricular enlargement. Lumbar puncture on day 12 showed an opening pressure of 390 mm of CSF with clear xanthochromic fluid. Angiography on day 14 showed spasm of the right internal carotid artery with a right ophthalmic artery aneurysm and a right internal carotid-posterior communicating artery aneurysm (Fig. 58-10A). There was moderate severe hydrocephalus. On day 17 a right frontotemporal craniotomy was performed for clipping of the aneurysms (Fig. 58-10B). Postoperatively the patient was intermittently confused with gradual return to normal mentation. Angiography 10 days after surgery showed obliteration of both aneurysms (Fig. 58-10C).

Results

The approach to ophthalmic aneurysms described above has produced good results (Table 58-1). Of 15 cases treated between 1974 and 1979, 87 percent experienced excellent results (no deficit) or good results (minimal deficit). In the remaining 2 cases there was ipsilateral blindness after clipping of a giant aneurysm, and a second patient had a wound infection that required removal of an infected bone flap. These cases were listed as poor results, although in fact neither patient is expected to have restriction of activities vis-a-vis the preoperative level. In all 15 cases, obliteration of the ophthalmic artery aneurysms was possible by direct intracranial surgery.

Angiographic studies after surgery indicate total obliteration of the lesions in all 14 patients studied (1 patient refused study).

Complications

Postoperative complications were uncommon in this series of patients (Table 58-2). For a giant ophthalmic artery aneurysm, isolation, narrowing, and clipping of the neck of the lesion apparently compromised the optic nerve or the ophthalmic artery. The patient became blind in

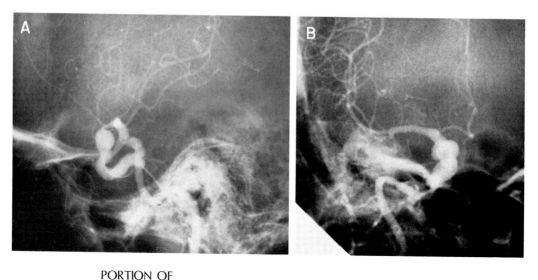

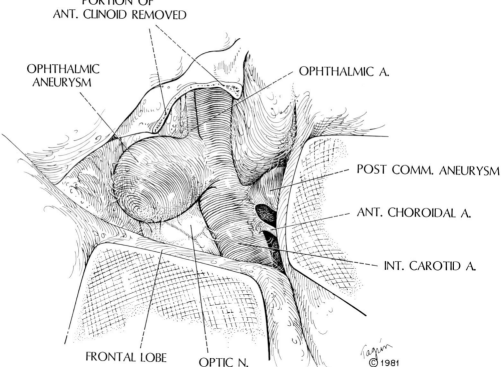

PORTION OF
ANT. CLINOID REMOVED

OPHTHALMIC
ANEURYSM

OPHTHALMIC A.

POST COMM. ANEURYSM

ANT. CHOROIDAL A.

INT. CAROTID A.

FRONTAL LOBE   OPTIC N.

©1981

Fig. 58-10.   Illustrative case: Clipping of the right carotid-ophthalmic and posterior communicating aneurysms. **A&B** Preoperative right lateral carotid angiogram demonstrates both lesions and the
ophthalmic artery. **C** Sketch depicting removal of the anterior clinoid process to expose proximal carotid-ophthalmic aneurysm. The relation of the lesion to the optic nerve and the ophthalmic artery is demonstrated. After dissection of the neck, a clip was placed across the neck
lateral to the optic nerve and sparing the ophthalmic artery. **D&E** A postoperative right lateral
carotid angiogram shows obliteration of the aneurysms and preservation of the native arteries.

the ipsilateral eye and has remained so. Despite the deficit he has returned to full activities as an
executive. In another patient, uneventful clipping of an ophthalmic aneurysm was complicated
by subgaleal infection and osteomyelitis of the bone flap. The bone flap was removed and the patient treated for 1 month with appropriate antibiotics. The neurologic status is unchanged vis-a-
vis the preoperative condition. Cranioplasty is planned in approximately 1 year.

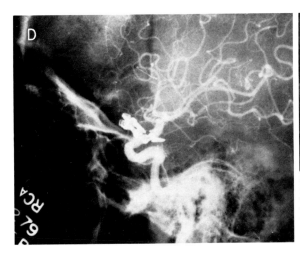
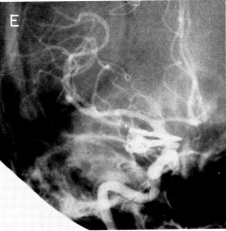

One patient experienced a transient CSF rhinorrhea. A right frontotemporal craniotomy was used for the clipping of the bilateral ophthalmic aneurysms. Drilling of the tuberculum sella was carried out in order to obtain good visualization of the origin of the contralateral ophthalmic aneurysm. Sphenoid sinus mucosa was visualized, and bone wax was used to close the small bony opening. Postoperatively there was substantial CSF rhinorrhea, which required a transsphenoidal procedure to obliterate the leak. The neurologic status of the patient was unchanged postoperatively. Despite her extended hospital stay she has made a good neurologic recovery.

Discussion

Carotid-ophthalmic aneurysms deserve separate consideration by virtue of their distinct anatomy, presentation, and surgical management.[1-7]

These lesions typically arise from the internal carotid artery just distal to the origin of the ophthalmic artery. Aneurysms of the ophthalmic artery itself are very rare. Carotid-ophthalmic aneurysms may point: (1) medially beneath the optic nerve; (2) laterally beneath the anterior clinoid process; (3) superomedially above the optic nerve; or (4) within the cavernous sinus. Complete angiography, with oblique and off-lateral views and subtraction technique, can be helpful in defining this anatomy, but often surgical exploration will be needed to determine the position of the neck of the aneurysm and its suitability for clipping.

There are several characteristic clinical features. A marked preponderance in females has been noted in several series including this one. Multiple lesions are common, particularly bilateral carotid-ophthalmic lesions. Giant lesions have been reported,[7] with optic nerve compression instead of the usual (and nonspecific) subarachnoid hemorrhage. Our 1 case of a giant carotid-ophthalmic aneurysm presenting as a seizure seems unique.

Table 58-1. Results in 15 Cases of Carotid-Ophthalmic Aneurysms Treated between 1974 and 1979 by Direct Intracranial Surgery

Aneurysm Grade	Result (%)				
	Excellent	Good	Poor	Deaths	Total
1-2	10 (67)	3 (20)	2 (13)	0	15

Table 58-2. Complications Experienced in 15 Cases of Carotid-Ophthalmic Aneurysm Treated by Direct Intracranial Surgery between 1974 and 1979

Complication*	Number of patients
Blindness (giant aneurysm)	1
CSF rhinorrhea (tuberculum drilled)	1
Infected bone flap	1
Total	3

*There were no deaths in the series.

Direct attack, with microsurgery, offers the best results.[6] For lesions of less than giant size, results are comparable to those achieved with aneurysms in other sites.[1-7] Removal of the anterior clinoid process, for most lesions, facilitates proximal control and sets the stage for clipping. Intraoperative visual-evoked responses may guide the surgical approach. It is sometimes necessary, particularly for giant aneurysms, to consider special approaches, such as cervical internal carotid occlusion with temporal-middle cerebral bypass. By virtue of their proximal location, carotid-ophthalmic aneurysms may one day be accessible to transvascular obliteration with catheter methods.

Cerebrovascular spasm may lead to cerebral infarction, either before or after surgery.[18,19] Postoperative vasospasm is minimized by delaying surgery until about 10 days after SAH, and prophylactic use of kanamycin and reserpine.[10] If proved vasospasm should become symptomatic, elevation of cardiac output and cerebral perfusion serve to restrict cerebral damage.[16,17]

The biggest problem is the SAH patient who never reaches the operating room.[20] Probably two-thirds of all SAH victims suffer devastating or fatal hemorrhage that cannot be reversed. Perhaps newer techniques, such as digital subtraction angiography can identify some of these lesions before hemorrhage. Prophylactic surgery might be justified in some asymptomatic patients to avert unheralded catastrophic bleeding.[21]

REFERENCES

1. Drake CG, Vanderlinden RG, Amacher AL: Carotid-ophthalmic aneurysms. *J Neurosurg* 29:24–31, 1968
2. Sundt TM, Jr, Murphy F: Clip grafts for aneurysm and small vessel surgery. Part 3: Clinical experience in intracranial carotid artery aneurysms. *J Neurosurg* 31:59–71, 1969
3. Guidetti B, LaTorre E: Carotid-ophthalmic aneurysms. A series of 16 cases treated by direct approach. *Acta Neurochir (Wien)* 22:289–304, 1970
4. Kothandarum P, Dawson BH, Kruyt RC: Carotid-opthalmic aneurysms: a study of 19 patients. *J Neurosurg* 34:544–548, 1971
5. Sengupta RP, Gryspeerdt GL, Hankinson J: Carotid-ophthalmic aneurysms. *J Neurol Neurosurg Psychiatry* 39:837–853, 1976
6. Yasargil MG, Gasser JC, Hodosh RM, et al: Carotid-ophthalmic aneurysms: direct microsurgical approach. *Surg Neurol* 8:155–165, 1977
7. Ferguson GG, Drake CG: Carotid-ophthalmic aneurysms—a review of 72 cases. *Clin Neurosurg* 1980, in press.
8. Davis KR, New PFJ, Ojemann RG, Crowell RM: Computed tomographic evaluation of hemorrhage secondary to intracranial aneurysm. *AJR* 127:143–153, 1976
9. Hunt WE, Kosnik EJ: Timing and perioperative care in intracranial aneurysm surgery. *Clin Neurosurg* 21:79–87, 1974
10. Crowell RM, Zervas NT: Management of intracranial aneurysm. *Med Clin N Am* 63:695–713, 1979
11. Aitken RR, Drake CG: A technique of anesthesia with induced hypotension for surgical correction of intracranial aneurysms. *Clin Neurosurg* 21:107–114, 1974
12. Krayenbühl HA, Yasargil MG, Flamm ES, et al: Microsurgical treatment of intracranial saccular aneurysms. *J Neurosurg* 37:678–686, 1972
13. Yasargil MG, Fox JL: The microsurgical approach to intracranial aneurysms. *Surg Neurol* 3:7–14, 1975
14. Crowell RM: Direct brain revascularization, in Schmidek H, Sweet WH (eds): *Current Techniques of Operative Neurosurgery*, New York, Grune & Stratton, 1978, pp 1–18

15. Miller JD, Jawad K, Jennett B: Safety of carotid ligation and its role in the management of intracranial aneurysms. *J Neurol Neurosurg Psychiatry 40*:64–72, 1977

16. Kosnik EJ, Hunt WE: Postoperative hypertension in the management of patients with intracranial arterial aneurysms. *J Neurosurg 45*:148–154, 1976

17. Gianotta SL, McGillicuddy JE, Kindt GW: Diagnosis and treatment of postoperative cerebral vasospasm. *Surg Neurol 8*:286–290, 1977

18. Allcock JM, Drake CG: Ruptured intracranial aneurysms—the role of arterial spasm. *J Neurosurg 22*:21–29, 1965

19. Fisher CM, Roberson GJ, Ojemann RG: Cerebral vasospasm with ruptured saccular aneurysm—the clinical manifestations. *Neurosurgery 1*:245–248, 1977

20. Drake CG: Perspectives on cerebral aneurysms. *Stroke 11*:124, 1980

21. Jane JA, Winn HR, Richardson AE: The natural history of intracranial aneurysms: rebleeding rates during the acute and long term period and implication for surgical management. *Clin Neurosurg 24*:176–184, 1977

CHAPTER 59
Surgical Management of Middle Cerebral Artery Aneurysms

Lindsay Symon

MIDDLE CEREBRAL ARTERY ANEURYSMS have for long had a somewhat sinister reputation. There was indeed a suggestion in the first detailed analysis of large numbers of cases presented by McKissock and his colleague[1] that female patients with middle cerebral artery aneurysms had a notably poor operative prognosis, scarcely different from conservative management. This has not proved to be the case, as with the advent of modern microsurgical methods, most surgeons would agree that direct intracranial surgical intervention on the aneurysms of the middle cerebral artery is both justified and indicated. One might suppose that because of the evocative nature of the area of the cortex that is supplied by the middle cerebral artery more of these aneurysms would fall into grades 3 or 4 of the classification of Hunt and Hess[2] than might be the case in supratentorial aneurysms as a whole. Comparison of the 62 middle cerebral artery aneurysms with the remainder of the author's personal series of 300 supratentorial aneurysms reveals that this is not the case. About a third of the middle cerebral artery aneurysms presented in grade 3, which is much the same percentage as that of the total series. About a fifth of them presented in grade 4; again, a similar statistic to the series as a whole (Table 59-1). No detectable difference in the behavior of middle cerebral artery aneurysms between male and female patients has been apparent in the author's series, nor in more recent publications. It is interesting to note that the proportion of the total series—just over 20 percent—is similar to that in Suzuki's series of 1000 supratentorial aneurysms, 174 (17.4 percent) of which were in the distribution of the middle cerebral artery.[3] It is clear that this is a less common aneurysm than the others of the anterior circle and therefore a large surgical experience has been slower to accumulate. The techniques to be described in this chapter concerning the management of these lesions have been standard in the Department of Neurological Surgery of the National Hospital, London, for many years.

Essential Investigations

Subarachnoid hemorrhage may well present in the neurosurgical unit as a surgical emergency. It is, however, essential that the general condition of the patient be investigated before any form of surgical intervention on the aneurysm is attempted. Such investigation need not be time consuming and should include a coagulation profile, a full blood count, serum electrolytes and blood urea, chest x-rays, and an evaluation of the cardiovascular status of the patient, with particular attention being given to ascertaining whether the hypertension that may well accom-

Neurological Surgery, Institute of Neurology, National Hospital, London, England

Table 59-1. Preoperative Grade in 62 Patients with Middle Cerebral Artery Aneurysms with Recent Subarachnoid Hemorrhage

Grade	No. of cases
1	10
2	19
3	20
4	12
5	1

pany subarachnoid hemorrhage is likely to have been pre-existing. These are factors that will weigh heavily in the decision for or against attempted surgical obliteration of the lesion.

It is the author's practice to proceed to computed tomographic (CT) scanning within a few hours of the patient's hospitalization. The extent of the subarachnoid hemorrhage may be judged by quantifying the amount of blood present in the basal cisterns. This finding may be of predictive value in relation to the subsequent development of cerebral vasospasm.[4,5] The presence or absence of a low-density lesion is suggestive of cerebral infarction (which, of course, will appear a few days later) or of an appreciable intracerebral hematoma, will be evident.

With a typical history and clinical findings suggestive of subarachnoid hemorrhage (stiff neck, mild hemiparesis, and blood on CT scan), the necessity for lumbar puncture may be questioned. It is the author's practice, however, to perform a lumbar puncture to confirm the subarachnoid hemorrhage unless this test has been previously performed at the referring hospital with convincing results.

Cerebral angiography is the mandatory investigation before surgery. With the advent of high-quality CT scanning, some controversy exists about the extent of angiography that is necessary. At the National Hospital angiography is performed by retrograde femoral catherization under general anesthesia, and in highly skilled hands. It is worthwhile to visualize the entire carotid circulation, to delineate both the distribution and the extent of the vasospasm and the presence of other lesions, including aneurysms. In young patients in good general condition, vertebrobasilar angiography is also performed, whereas in the elderly patient (60–70 years of age) with a convincing middle cerebral hemorrhage and a middle cerebral artery aneurysm shown at the appropriate site by carotid angiography, vertebral angiography is omitted.

Preoperative Medication

Personal preference rather than scientific analysis is an important determinant in the choice of medications used before surgery. Many surgeons place all patients with subarachnoid hemorrhage on antifibrinolytic agents. This has not been the author's practice and he has continued to prefer early surgery to a delay in preventing rehemorrhage of the aneurysm (Table 59-2). Patients with subarachnoid hemorrhage are placed on a moderate dose of steroid (e.g., 4 mg of Dexamethasone every 6 hours) as soon as they are admitted. This dosage is continued until 48 hours after surgery. Patients also are routinely placed on oxacillin (1 gm every 6 hours) beginning 24 hours before surgery and continuing for 5 days thereafter. The patients also are begun on anticonvulsants (usually Diphenylhydantoinate; 100 mg three times a day) on admission. Primidone is substituted if the patient is allergic to Dilantin. Blood levels of these agents are estimated during hospitalization, and this medication is maintained for 12 months following surgery, and then is gradually discontinued over a period of 6–8 weeks.

The Timing of Surgery

The intracranial pressure, the cerebral blood flow, and, most recently, the conduction time within the central nervous system itself[6] all have been used to attempt to select the appropriate time for surgery after a subarachnoid hemorrhage.

Although the latter technique is being developed in this clinic, the decision when to operate is still made on clinical grounds. The patient in grades 1–3 (Hunt classification) has angiography performed as soon as it is convenient. If the aneurysm neck appears difficult, arteriograms of the highest quality will be necessary, with multiple oblique views. A skilled angiographer therefore must be available. It is unlikely that the best-quality films will be obtained in the middle of the night.

The patient is allowed to recover from the angiographic session for 24 hours, and, provided the patient has been stable and there is no other major contraindication to surgery, the patient then is ready for the operation. Severe hypertension and the presence of an unstable or fluctuating neurologic condition should prompt caution.

Patients in grades 4–5 are not subjected to surgery until their condition has improved, save in the circumstances of a massive hematoma. In these instances the hematoma will have been demonstrated by CT scan, and some concern may be expressed as to the propriety of angiography in view of the serious condition of the patient. If the situation of the hematoma suggests the possibility of an underlying rupture of the middle cerebral artery aneurysm, angiography before evacuation of the hematoma is mandatory. Rupture of the aneurysm in the course of evacuation of the hematoma may prove impossible to control with safety if some prior knowledge of the regional vascular anatomy is not available. At the same time, the obliteration of the aneurysm in a patient in such poor condition is hazardous and should not be attempted unless it is forced upon the surgeon by disastrous rupture in the course of limited evacuation of the intracerebral hemorrhage. Evacuation of the hemorrhage should be made through a linear incision above and in front of the ear. This incision may be extended to a classical aneurysm flap around the outer end of the sphenoidal wing if necessary at the time, or by preference at a later date. The temporal mass is removed through a linear corticectomy. Should the hematoma lie deep within the internal capsular area, then a tentative evacuation is probably unjustified, and the patient should be treated by medical supportive measures alone. In most circumstances it is better to improve the general condition of the patient with steroids to avoid the use of dehydrating agents such as mannitol and to avoid induced hypotension. Surges of excessively high blood pressure are controlled by beta-blocking agents such as propranolol (10–20 mg t.d.s, I.M.). A seriously ill patient with a large intracerebral hematoma may improve quite remarkably over a few days and the outlook for radical surgery under these circumstances is not nearly so grave. If evacuation of the hemorrhage is unavoidable in order to save the life of the patient, the prognosis is extremely grave and must be communicated to the relatives in these terms.

The referral pattern to the National Hospital is such that the patient is seldom admitted on the day of the hemorrhage, i.e, on day 1. The patient is commonly admitted on day 2, investigated on day 3, allowed to rest on day 4, and operated upon the fifth day after hemorrhage. In some circumstances, it is possible to operate within 48 hours of the hemorrhage if the condition of the patient is excellent and recovery from angiography is prompt.

The Surgical Procedure

Planning the Approach

Two approaches to middle cerebral artery aneurysms can be employed. The approach depends on the angiographic characteristics of the aneurysm. Commonly, a middle cerebral artery aneurysm will arise in the crotch of the bifurcation or trifurcation of the middle cerebral artery (Figs. 59-1 and 59-2). These lesions are quite distal in the sylvian fissure and distal to the segment of the middle cerebral artery from which the perforating branches arise, and they are often partially embraced by the insular branches of the distal middle cerebral artery. For these aneurysms an approach through a resection of the superior temporal gyrus is preferred.

When the aneurysm arises from the more proximal part of the middle cerebral artery, often in association with a premature origin of the anterior temporal branch (Figs. 59-3 and 59-4), a

Table 59-2. The Timing of Surgery after Hospitalization in 62 Patients with Middle Cerebral Artery Aneurysms and Recent Subarachnoid Hemorrhage

Days after admission	No. of patients
0-5	15
6-10	20
11-15	10
16-21	6
21-60	11

more restricted approach through the sylvian fissure, as classically advocated by Yasargil[7] and Lougheed[8] is more appropriate and effective. These two approaches will be described in detail.

Positioning the Patient

The position of the patient for both approaches is the same. The patient is positioned on the back with the head turned well to the side opposite the aneurysm, and a frontotemporal flap is marked out around the outer end of the sphenoidal wing (Fig. 59-5). The scalp flap is turned back in a single layer, and an endeavor is made to perserve the frontalis branch of the facial nerve in the base of the flap. Although this nerve is frequently stretched in the flap resection, the exposure should not be cramped in an endeavor to avoid it. Since the healing of this flap is remarkably good, a more cosmetic flap can be attempted. If the anterior burr hole is appropriately filled in a small lateral "worry" line will be the only sign visible below the hairline. The frontalis branch of the facial nerve will recover in about 6 months even if it is severed.

The base of the scalp flap may be held down by tension sutures to allow the muscle incision

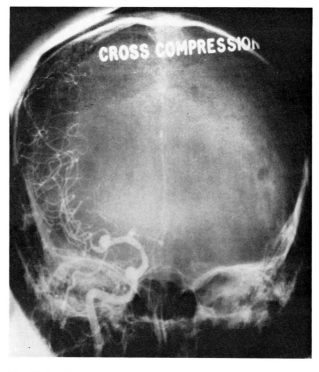

Fig. 59-1. A typical middle cerebral artery aneurysm in the crotch of the first bifurcation of the middle cerebral artery.

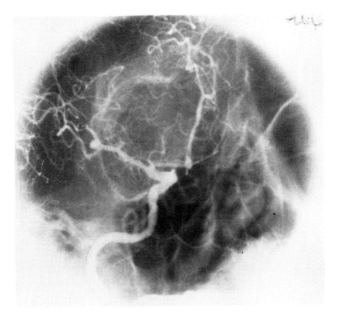

Fig. 59-2. Oblique views may help to elucidate the anatomy as in this typical bifurcation aneurysm of the middle cerebral artery.

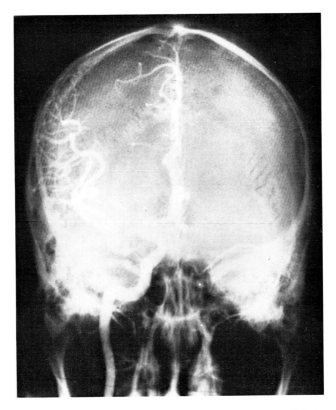

Fig. 59-3. A middle cerebral artery aneurysm that is slightly more proximal, arising at the origin of the proximal temporal branch.

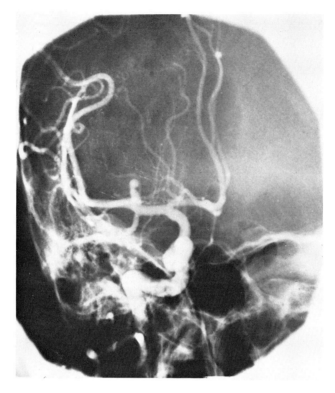

Fig. 59-4. An unusual middle cerebral aneurysm arising opposite the first very proximal bifurcation of the middle
cerebral artery, close to the segment bearing the
perforators.

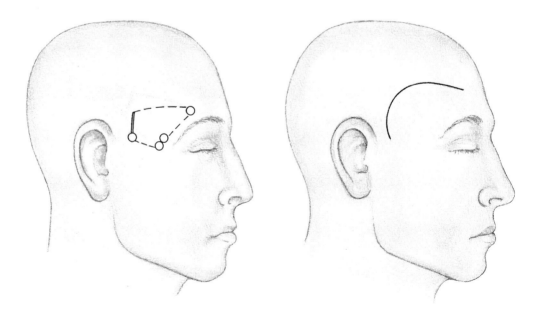

Fig. 59-5.   The position of the scalp flap and bone flap for exposure of middle cerebral artery aneurysms.

to be made close to the frontal process of the zygomatic bone. The muscle incision is carried down through the temporal fossa to expose the lateral aspect of the temporal fossa and the groove between the frontal and temporal fossae. The muscle incision is carried anteriorly to just above the superior temporal line, then sloped back to the rear of the scalp flap. The bone flap may be cut through three burr holes. One of these, which the author has referred to as a "spectacle" burr hole and which McCartney has described as a "key-hole" burr hole (personal communication), opens both the frontal and temporal fossae, and allows the outer end of the sphenoidal wing to be bitten off with sharp rongeurs. A small extension of the anterior part of the key-hole toward the floor of the frontal fossa allows the anterior saw cut to be kept low. An anterior burr hole and a burr hole fairly low posteriorly, which again may be extended with De Vilbis rongeurs to allow an adequately sized bone flap to be turned, will allow the bone flap to be broken down on the anterior part of the temporalis muscle within the temporal fossa, and avoids the necessity for subtemporal decompression. The outer end of the sphenoidal wing should be rongeured away. If the spectacle burr hole was appropriately placed, little bone removal is necessary in most cases and no great bony defect will be visible postoperatively, which means that the extensive depression in the anterior temporal fossa that is sometimes seen will not occur. The bone flap should be held back with retention sutures, duroperiosteal sutures should be inserted to preserve hemostasis, and the appropriate self-retaining retractor inserted. The post bearing a double arm for the Yasargil retractor can be placed at the posterosuperior aspect of the flap. The dura is opened through a triradiate incision that is started subfrontally and slopes down into the anterior temporal fossa. A silk suture is passed under the middle meningeal artery and is anchored to the intermuscular septum in the temporal muscle. The muscle incision commonly ends at about the level of the meningeal artery. A re-entrant incision posteriorly along the line of the sylvian fissure allows the dura to be held up in three flaps, which are sufficiently wide to ensure adequate extradural hemostasis and to prevent bleeding into the intracranial space. Continuous drainage of cerebrospinal fluid is not employed. If the intracranial tension appears to be unduly high, an attempt can be made to tap the frontal horn of the lateral ventricle. This is usually fairly straightforward; the line of the frontal horn of the lateral ventricle is continuous with the line of the curve of the anterior temporal fossa, and if the head is in the appropriate position, the floor of the frontal fossa will certainly be sloping a little away from the surgeon. Such measures to control intracranial pressure may be taken before the formal opening of the dural flap, but if the patient is in reasonable clinical condition, these measures usually are unnecessary, and adequate control of intracranial tension is commonly obtained by a fairly rapid dissection down the subfrontal region under direct vision, gentle retraction of the brain from in front of the sphenoidal wing, and opening of the arachnoid of the basal cisterns over or anterior to the optic nerve. It should be remembered that dissection of the sylvian fissure at this stage carries a risk of premature rupture of the aneurysm particularly in aneurysms that face anteriorly, and dissection to control intracranial pressure aimed at the carotid artery should stay as far away from the aneurysm as possible. At this stage subfrontal self-retaining retraction can be placed for a moment or two, and the terminal carotid artery can be defined under the operating microscope. This will usually allow a clip to be placed on the terminal carotid artery should severe rupture of the aneurysm occur before adequate control of the proximal middle cerebral artery is possible.

The route of progression from this point depends on the detailed anatomy of the aneurysm.

The Middle Cerebral Artery Aneurysm at the Trifurcation

For aneurysms of the trifurcation of the middle cerebral artery, the inner end of the sylvian fissure is opened and the terminal carotid artery is identified. The anterior $1/2$ inch of the superior temporal gyrus is resected (Fig. 59-6), the resection staying below, that is, inferior to the pia of the sylvian fissure. As the dissection deepens, hemorrhage within the sylvian fissure usually becomes apparent. The major branches of the middle cerebral artery are identified on the surface of the insula and deep to the pia with careful microscopic dissection, before the sylvian fis-

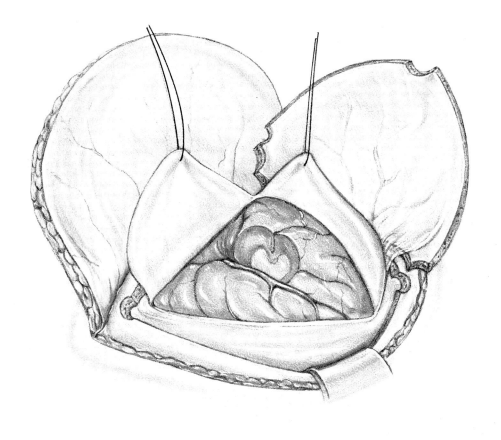

Fig. 59-6. The approach to a trifurcation aneurysm. The position of the reflected scalp and bone flap is shown, although this would normally be covered by cottonoid strips. The dural flaps are shown elevated to maintain extradural hemostasis. The proximal ½ inch or so of the superior temporal gyrus is being resected.

sure or the arachnoidal spaces of the insula are opened (Fig. 59-7). At any point, of course, a hematoma in the temporal lobe may be entered. The admitted disadvantage of this approach is that the fundus of the aneurysm is reached before its neck. Should the aneurysm bleed, temporary occlusion of the carotid artery may sufficiently reduce the hemorrhage to enable the surgeon to dissect and occlude the aneurysm. This has never been necessary in any of the author's cases, but could be contemplated if severe hemorrhage were to occur at this stage in the procedure. More commonly, the clot is entered and the branches of the middle cerebral artery embracing the aneurysm can be dissected without difficulty. It is usually wise to pass down through the temporal lobe below the aneurysm and to re-enter the fissure just proximal to the trifurcation and identify the proximal middle cerebral artery at this point, which is distal to the segment bearing the perforators. The most common potential hazard in dissection of middle cerebral artery aneurysms is damage to the segment of the middle cerebral artery that bears the perforators, and it is dissection of a difficult aneurysm embraced by the branches of the trifurcating middle cerebral artery through the fissure that is most likely to result in stretch and rupture of these vessels. With the approach through the superior temporal gyrus, the segment of the middle cerebral artery bearing the perforators is left undisturbed. With control of the proximal middle cerebral artery thus assured if necessary, more resolute dissection of the branches of the middle cerebral artery and the aneurysm embraced by these branches may continue (Fig. 59-8). Quite frequently, adhesion between the emergent branches and the fundus of the aneurysm is fairly dense over the portion of the fundus where the most recent hemorrhage has occurred, and rather

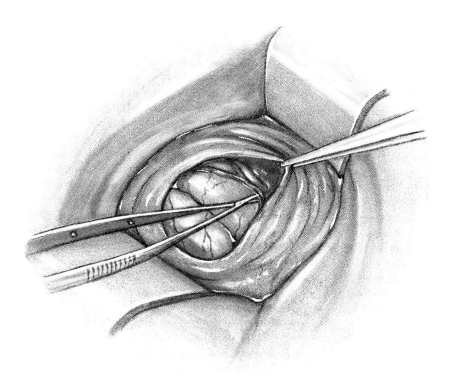

Fig. 59-7. Self-retaining retraction has been placed on the upper and lower banks of the dissection, and the view is under high magnification. The arachnoid over the insula has been opened and definition of the middle distal middle cerebral branches is under way.

curred, and rather less dense in the older part of the aneurysm close to its neck, where the wall is often rather sturdier and the main branches can be dissected from the fundus with greater ease and less risk. Rather than undergo repetitive leak and rupture of the fundus, however, a proximal clamp can be placed on the middle cerebral artery without hesitation for periods of up to 10 minutes. The author has used such proximal occlusion without evident sequelae in cases of recent subarachnoid hemorrhage for some years (Fig. 59-9). The increasing use of the electrophysiologic monitoring may well place this rule of thumb on a more eclectic basis.

Commonly, the neck of the aneurysm can be occluded with a straight or curved clip. The author's preference is for the Scoville-type clip, which is readily manipulable and easy to apply and remove. At the National Hospital, Scoville clips have been curved by the instrument makers to the appropriate degrees of curvature necessary to meet most circumstances. Unfortunately, these are not commercially available. The Suzuki-type of clip is equally good, however. The author has not found the Yasargil clips, although admittedly excellent instruments, as attractive as the Scoville clips because they are more difficult to remove and replace as a result of the design of the clip-applicator forceps. Likewise the older type of Mayfield clip applicator is now so clumsy that it obscures a good deal of the microscopic field. The attraction of the Scoville clip is that it may be placed and replaced with an artery forceps, which is a much smaller instrument.

Coagulation of the neck of the aneurysm may be practiced if it seems likely to result in a more ready application of a clip. Not infrequently a bulge of aneurysm presents on the opposite side of the trifurcation of the middle cerebral artery, and it becomes impossible to completely

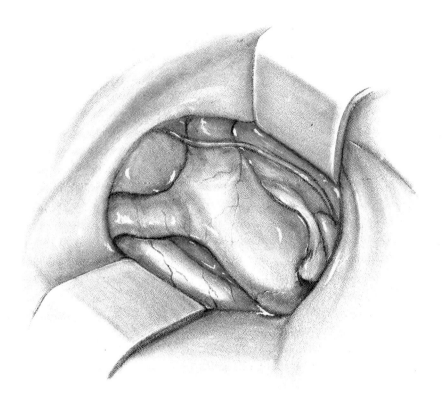

Fig. 59-8. The trifurcation of the middle cerebral artery has been exposed, the distal middle cerebral branches are shown, one on the lower bank of the insula, one running posteriorly, and the slightly unusual middle cerebral aneurysm that points posteriorly with a crossing vein is just evident. (Figures **59-8, 59-9,** and **59-10** were taken from a video tape of the actual dissection of the aneurysm shown in Figure **59-10**).

occlude the aneurysm. Under these circumstances, the major portion on one side may be clipped, and the bulge on the other side may be wrapped with gauze or muslin or reinforced with acrylic or some other suitable plastic.

The Scoville clip can be anchored in place with a drop of acrylic placed on the curved spring shank. This not only prevents the clip from coming off, but also, by expanding within the curve of the shank, tightens the force of the clip. No clip disruption has been apparent over a 10-year period using this maneuver, despite the dire warnings of electrolytic danger.[9] It is of course necessary to make absolutely certain that the position is ideal before the clip is fixed since once it is fixed, it is impossible to remove.

The Management of Giant Aneurysms of the Middle Cerebral Artery

The author's experience with giant aneurysms of the middle cerebral artery is based on six aneurysms of an inch in diameter or more, five of which qualify as giant in being space-occupying lesions, partially occupied by thrombus. Most of these patients had recently had multiple subarachnoid hemorrhages and were operated upon to prevent further bleeding. Two patients were operated upon because of recurrent episodes of hemiparesis and subarachnoid

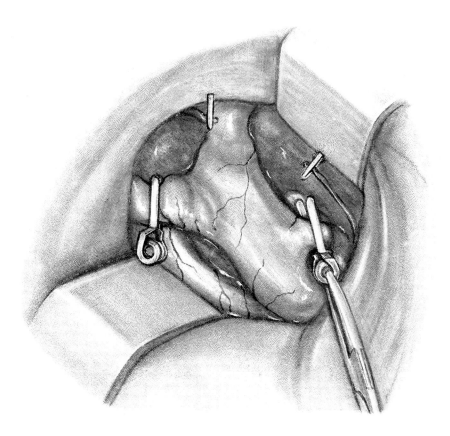

Fig. 59-9.   A further stage in dissection. A temporary clip has been placed on the proximal middle cerebral artery just proximal to the bifurcation. The definitive aneurysm clip has been placed on the neck of the aneurysm.

hemorrhage had occurred only in the remote past. One aneurysm presented with a recent subarachnoid hemorrhage and was simply a large aneurysm unoccupied by clot.

In the operative management of giant aneurysms temporary occlusion of the middle cerebral circulation is almost inevitable while the neck is defined. The apparent aneurysm that is visualized may be very much smaller than the actual aneurysm, as defined either by vascular displacement or from the CT scan, and at some stage, therefore, the aneurysm may have to be opened and the clot evacuated in order to make the wall amenable to the fashioning of a neck and the application of a ligature or clip. This is particularly true if the aneurysm is a space-occupying lesion, since occlusion of its neck alone will not relieve the mass effect. Figure 59-11 demonstrates an aneurysm that had bled recurrently over the previous 2 months, and Figure 59-12 presents an aneurysm that had bled in the remote past, and was acting as a space-occupying lesion. Many surgeons will now feel it wise to fashion a superficial temporal–middle cerebral anastomosis before tackling the aneurysm itself. The alternative method of management, which has been used in some cases, is to depend upon the collateral circulation to sustain the field of the middle cerebral artery during transient periods of middle cerebral field occlusion. In larger aneurysms, slow filling of the distal middle cerebral circulation may be seen from leptomeningeal collaterals in the preoperative angiogram, and it has therefore appeared likely that the partial obstruction of the distal middle cerebral circulation caused by the aneurysm had evoked appreciable collateral circulation. The patient whose lesion is shown in Figure 59-12 is a middle-aged female. She withstood 45 minutes of proximal and distal occlusion of the middle cerebral artery while the aneurysm neck was dissected down, the aneurysm opened, the clot evacuated, and a clip placed on the much-reduced neck of the aneurysm. The relationship of the perforating ves-

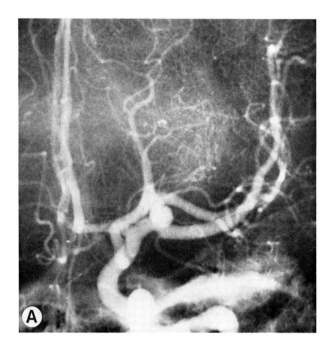

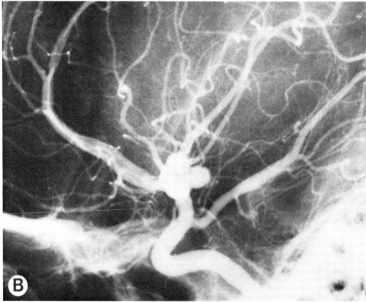

Fig. 59-10. (**A** and **B**) AP and lateral angiograms of the middle cerebral aneurysm, whose dissection is shown in the preceding figures.
This is a slightly unusual lesion, arising from a proximal bifurcation pointing backwards. Anterior dissection would have
proved extremely difficult. Above all, this is the indication for
approach through the superior temporal gyrus.

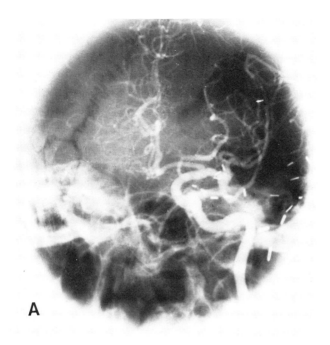

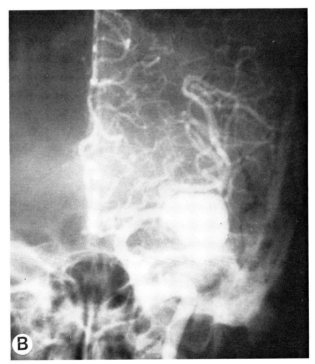

Fig. 59-11. **A.** A giant middle cerebral aneurysm that presented with subarachnoid hemorrhage. From Subarachnoid hemorrhage from intracranial aneurysm and angioma, in Ross Russell RW (ed): *Cerebral Arterial Disease.* New York, Churchill Livingstone, 1976. With permission. **B.** The giant aneurysm after ligation.

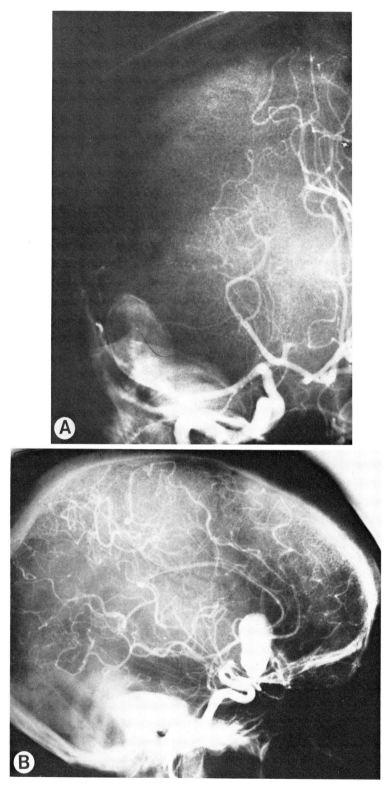

Fig. 59-12.   (**A** and **B**) AP and lateral angiograms and (**C**) a CT scan of a giant middle cerebral aneurysm that had bled in the remote past and presented with hemiparesis and raised intracranial pressure. A surrounding low density in the middle cerebral distribution is evident, and slow collateral filling of the distal middle cerebral distribution was evident on later phases of the angiogram. (**D** and **E**) AP and lateral postoperative angiograms. (**F**) A CT scan made two months postoperatively.

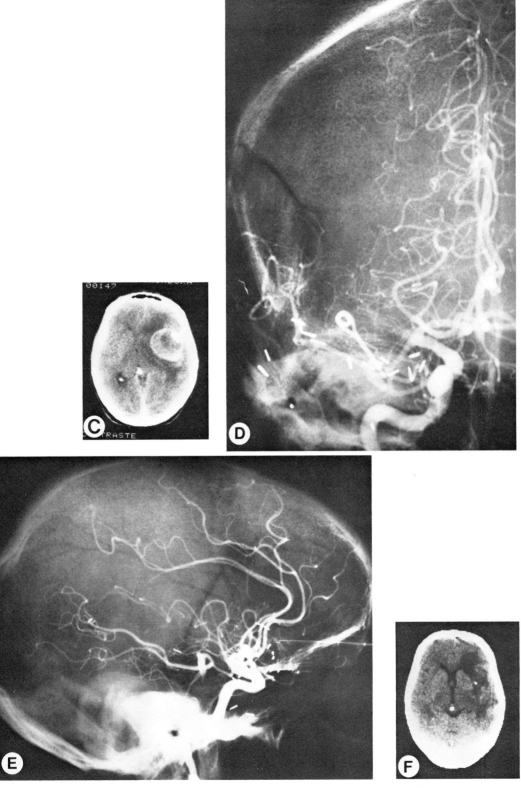

Improved filling of the distal middle cerebral field is evident, the fact that the lesion had a narrow neck is evidenced by its occlusion with a single Scoville clip, and the extent of postoperative low density is shown on the CT scan. The patient's hemiparesis had by this time disappeared, and there was no signs. Fortunately, the lesion was in the nondominant hemisphere.

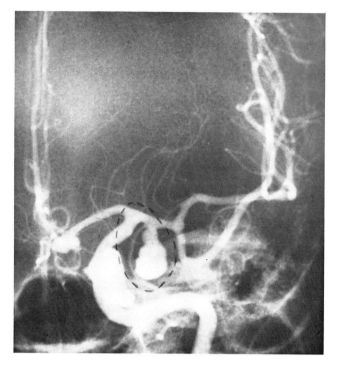

Fig. 59-13. A giant aneurysm that bled recurrently in the few months preceding surgery. The angiographic visualization was only of the center of the lesion. The approximate size of the actual aneurysm is indicated by the dotted line.

sels, as can be seen on the diagram, was elicited by preoperative angiography, and this portion of the sac was dissected with great care, although quite frequently the wall of such an aneurysm within the brain comes away very cleanly. The same cannot be said for the walls of giant aneurysms toward the base of the brain, because they become extremely adherent to structures in the subarachnoid space, other parts of the circle of Willis, the optic nerves, and so forth. Within the brain, however, they often can be dissected quite rapidly. Another giant aneurysm (Fig. 59-13) required sacrifice of the anterior temporal branch with proximal and distal occlusion of the middle cerebral artery, including the perforating segment, for 6 minutes and 30 seconds, while the neck dissection was completed. This aneurysm was occluded by a single Scoville clip once the sacrifice of the anterior temporal branch was accepted. No hemiparesis developed, and, this being a dominant hemisphere lesion, the preoperative dysphasic defect, present as a result of the last hemorrhage, was no worse, and gradually improved to normal in the postoperative period.

In the case of a third giant aneurysm (Fig. 59-11), occlusion of the proximal middle cerebral artery was maintained for 20 minutes while the sac was dissected from the distal branches and the neck was ligated. Again, some retrograde collateral filling was evident on the preoperative angiograms and no neurologic deficits resulted from the procedure.

Postoperative Care

The postoperative care of patients with aneurysms of the middle cerebral artery differs little from the general postoperative management of other aneurysm patients. These aneurysms differ from others above all because evocative hemipareses are common in the postoperative period as a result of the phenomenon of reduced perfusion (which we term "vasospasm" that afflicts the highly evocative cortex. In recent years, the induction of hypertension with metaraminol and a high fluid load (an added 500 to 1000 cc of 10% Dextran 40 in 24 hours) have been used to overcome transient postoperative deficits once the clip is safely in place.[10,11] The use of intraoperative monitoring of central conduction time has proved of increasing value while temporary clamps are in place on the middle cerebral artery. Full steroids are maintained for 48 hours postoperatively and then tapered off over the next few days. The regime of added dextran is maintained for 5 postoperative days, and the patient is allowed to get up on the fifth postoperative day.

Continuous closed subgaleal suction drainage is maintained for 2 days postoperatively, but no other attempt is made to drain cerebrospinal fluid.

A CT scan is routinely performed after surgery on all aneurysm patients on the night of the operation whether or not they are well. This will indicate whether brain swelling has occurred, and, should transient neurologic signs develop, is of value in deciding whether artificial hypertension will be used. Where transient hemiparesis develops in the postoperative period and is unattended by a shift on CT scanning, induced hypertension is certainly safe. If brain swelling already exists, however, induced hypertension should be used with caution, since transudation of fluid into an already swollen brain may occur and cause the patient's state to worsen. Under these circumstances, dehydrating agents rather than induced hypertension may be the only method open to the surgeon. Monitoring of intracranial pressure[12] may be of value in controlling a difficult situation here. For many years it was the practice in this clinic to perform postoperative angiography as a routine. With the advent of the operating microscope, this has no longer been thought necessary, and angiography is performed only rarely now following operations for middle cerebral aneurysms. Where a pouch of aneurysm has had to be left, however, postoperative angiography is of value, as it will prove to be a useful baseline should further hemorrhage occur in the future.

Results

This chapter is based on the author's personal series of operations for aneurysms of the middle cerebral artery. In a total of 300 anterior circle aneurysms with recent subarachnoid hemorrhage, there have been 62 aneurysms of the middle cerebral artery. The grade and time of surgery are shown in Table 59-2. Three of the giant aneurysms were operated upon remotely from any hemorrhage and are not included in this table.

An endeavor has been made to operate on aneurysms early, thus 35 were operated on in the first 10 days, 45 in the first 15 days, and 51 in the first 21 days. Only 15 were operated upon in the first 5 days, however, because of delay in referral.

There has been 1 death in the patients operated on in grades 1–3; an operative mortality rate of 2 percent. The total operative mortality rate, including two further deaths, one each in grades 4 and grade 5, is 4.8 percent. Unacceptable morbidity was present in one further grade 4 patient, who was confused and suffering appreciable hemiparesis preoperatively, and was densely hemiplegic postoperative. That brings the total morbidity rate (dead or unacceptably disabled) for the series to 6.4 percent. If the grade 5 case of a patient with a large clot extending to all limbs, who was subjected to angiography before the evacuation of the clot, and, since the aneurysm presented in the clot, also was subjected to clipping of the aneurysm, was excluded, the total mortality rate of 4.9 percent would be 3.2 percent and the morbidity rate, including one unacceptable result would be 4.9 percent.

There is little justification for urgent clipping of the aneurysm in patients in grade 5. It certainly will not improve the patient's prospects, and probably brings aneurysm surgery into poor repute. If the patient can be persuaded to improve by judicious evacuation of the clot or by steroid management alone, then delayed surgery presents a more attractive prospect.

REFERENCES

1. McKissock W, Richardson A, Walsh LS: Middle cerebral artery aneurysms. Further results in the controlled trial of conservative and surgical treatment of ruptured intracranial aneurysms. *Lancet* (ii):417–421, 1962
2. Hunt WE, Hess RM: Surgical risk as related to time of intervention on the repair of intracranial aneurysms. *J Neurosurg 38*:14–19, 1968
3. Suzuki J, Kodama N, Fujiwara S, et al: Surgical treatment of middle cerebral artery aneurysms: from the experience of 174 cases, in Suziki J (ed): *Cerebral Aneurysms.* Tokyo, Neuron Publishing Co., 1979, pp 278–283
4. Fisher CM, Kistler MD, Davis JM: Relation of cerebral vasospasm to subarachnoid hemorrhage visualized by computerized tomographic scanning. *Neurosurgery 6*:1–9, 1980
5. Bell BA, Kendall BE, Symon L: Computerized tomography in aneurysmal subarachnoid hemorrhage. *J Neurol Neurosurg Psychiat 43*:522–524, 1980
6. Symon L, Hargadine J, Zawirski M, et al: Central conduction time as an index of ischaemia in subarachnoid hemorrhage. *J Neurol Sci 44*:95–103, 1979
7. Yasargil MG, Fox JL: Microsurgical approach to intracranial aneurysms. *Surg Neurol 3*:7, 1975
8. Lougheed WM, Marshall BM: Measurement of the anterior circulation by intracranial procedures, Youmans, (ed): *Neurological Surgery.* Philadelphia, W.B. Saunders, 1973, pp 731–767
9. McFadden JT: Tissue reactions to standard neurosurgical metallic implants. *J Neurosurg 36*:598–603, 1972
10. Kosnick EJ, Hunt WE: Post-operative hypertension in the management of patients with intracranial aneurysms. *J Neurosurg 38*:14–19, 1976
11. Symon L: Disordered cerebrovascular physiology in aneurysmal subarachnoid hemorrhage. *Acta Neurochir 41*:7–22, 1978
12. Kassell NF, Peerless SJ, Durward QJ, et al: Neurological deterioration from cerebral vasospasm: treatment with induced arterial hypertension, in Wilkins RH (ed): *Cerebral Arterial Spasm.* (Proceedings of the 2nd International Workshop, 1979). Baltimore, Williams & Wilkins, 1979, pp 665–672

CHAPTER 60
Surgical Techniques of Posterior Cerebral Aneurysms

Sydney J. Peerless   Charles G. Drake

IT IS ONLY RECENTLY that neurosurgeons have been able to attack aneurysms of the vertebral-basilar circulation with the same safety and assurance as aneurysms arising from the carotid circulation. The reasons for this late development are many. Aneurysms arising from the posterior circulation are relatively uncommon, amounting to less than 15 percent of all aneurysms of the brain, giving few surgeons the opportunity to gain the necessary experience and confidence in exploring the confined space in front of the cerebellum. The late refinement of routine vertebral angiography resulted in only a few of these lesions being diagnosed and then only when the aneurysms had grown to giant size and presented as tumors. Before 1950, a few large masses of unknown nature were explored, found to be thrombosed aneurysms, and shelled out and secured with proximal vessel ligation by Dandy, Tonnis, Falconer, Poppen, and Logue.[1-5] Schwartz is credited with the first deliberate, direct attack on an aneurysm in the cerebellopontine angle.[6] His dramatic description of controlling the bleeding and trapping the sac that was buried in the pons is memorable—the more so when one considers the procedure was carried out without magnification, and with the crude clips and instruments available at that time. The patient did well.

At the time of Drake's original report of his own experience with 4 patients with aneurysms of the basilar bifurcation, there was considerable skepticism as to the value or safety of direct surgical attack on aneurysms of the posterior circulation. Of the 47 cases reported to that time, 14 had been treated indirectly with vertebral artery ligation and almost half of the remainder were peripheral aneurysms arising distally on branches of the vertebral or basilar artery. The 10 aneurysms arising at the basilar bifurcation proved to be technically unapproachable; less than half were clipped and the remainder were packed.[7] Jamieson emphasized his discouragement in his index report of the direct surgical treatment of 19 aneurysms of the vertebrobasilar system. Ten of his patients had died and only 4 of the survivors were employable.[8]

Although a note of optimism was evident in Drake's 1965 paper describing the treatment of aneurysms of the basilar trunk, the safe treatment of aneurysms of the basilar artery remained elusive.[9] The first 7 patients with aneurysms of the terminal basilar artery had not done well; 4 died, 1 was severely disabled, and only 2 returned to normal life. It was at this time that Drake realized the importance of identifying and sparing the tiny perforating vessels arising from the terminal basilar artery and proximal posterior cerebral arteries. It was evident that these small arteries, which were vital to the irrigation of the hypothalamus, midbrain, and pons, were often

Division of Neurosurgery, the University of Western Ontario University Hospital, London, Ontario, Canada, and Department of Surgery, the University of Western Ontario University Hospital, London, Ontario, Canada

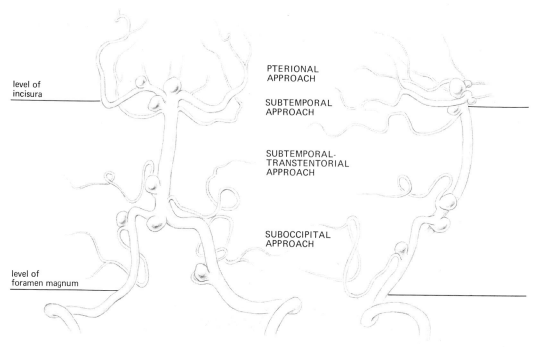

Fig. 60-1. Common sites of posterior circulation aneurysms. The level of the tentorial incisura and foramen magna are depicted at the usual site of the aneurysms relative to these fixed points noted. The surgical approaches to aneurysms of various regions is noted.

adhering to the posterior wall of the sac and were surrounded by old blood and adhesions and were frequently difficult, if not impossible, to visualize in the confined space of the exposure.

At this time, there was a dramatic improvement in the technology of neurosurgery. The operating microscope, new fine instruments and clips, and the refinements of modern neuroanesthesia including profound hypotension all were combined to bring about a remarkable improvement in results. In 1968, Drake reported 12 additional cases with no direct operative deaths and 10 good results.[10]

In the past decade, our experience has grown to more than 800 cases, and contemporary results are comparable with the results of treatment of aneurysms of the anterior circulation. Poor results today are almost entirely limited to patients harboring giant aneurysms or those who are in a poor clinical state before the operation (Fig. 60-1).

Anesthesia and Monitoring Techniques

It would be improper not to mention some of our anesthetic and monitoring techniques in that so much of the success of the actual technical procedure of approaching an aneurysm begins with the preparation of the patient and careful, moment-to-moment assessment of his condition during the procedure. Patients are brought to the operating room lightly sedated with an accurate assessment of their fluid balance. An arterial line is installed, usually with a flexible needle in the dorsalis pedis or radial artery where the arterial pressure can be continuously monitored. The patient is induced gently with pentothal, paralyzed, and then intubated with an armored tube. The anesthetic technique is basically an assisted controlled ventilation in most instances, using halothane, nitrous oxide, or a narcotic technique depending on the preference of the anesthetist; the recent tendency is toward isoflurane. The anesthetic is kept generally light with meticulous monitoring of blood gases to maintain the Pco_2 in the range of 40–45 torr and the Po_2 in excess of 100 torr.

The success of the procedure largely depends upon adequate intracranial relaxation. For this reason, we routinely give 1 g/kg of 20% mannitol, increasing this to 2 g/kg if we contemplate temporary occlusion of a major intracranial vessel. Furosemide (1 mg/kg) is given intravenously shortly after induction and the administration of mannitol. While the patient is being positioned, the anesthetist uses a Touhy needle to insert a lumbar subarachnoid catheter (PE 100) into the lumbar subarachnoid space and attaches this tubing to a closed collection bag. The lumbar subarachnoid drain is kept clamped until the dura is opened, at which time cerebrospinal fluid (CSF) drainage is commenced to add to the intracranial relaxation.

We routinely use intentional hypotension during the dissection and clipping of the aneurysm. The anesthetist prepares for this by connecting the transducer from the arterial line, at a level equal to the height of the brain, to an electronic monitor that gives systolic, diastolic, and mean pressures. Hypotension is induced by intravenous administration of sodium nitroprusside or occasionally trimethaphan camsylate (Arfrenad), or more recently by deepening the isoflurane anesthesia. Systemic arterial pressure of 50–60 torr are routinely used during the initial dissection around the aneurysm, and when manipulation of the aneurysm itself or application of the clip begins, the pressure is lowered to 40–45 torr. It has been our experience that these low pressures are routinely well tolerated for 30 to 40 minutes and have rarely been responsible for significant problems when prolonged for 60 to 90 minutes.

With the patient positioned, the anesthetist begins meticulous monitoring of fluid balance, EKG, systemic arterial blood pressure, and blood gases. Occasionally we will employ brain retractor pressure monitoring, EEG, and intraoperative cerebral blood flow (CBF) monitoring in unique situations of giant aneurysms or when we anticipate prolonged interruption of focal cerebral blood flow.[11]

Positioning

Almost all aneurysms of the basilar artery above the anterior inferior cerebellar arteries can be approached through the lateral decubitus or "park bench" position. In that we normally aim to approach the aneurysm under the nondominant temporal lobe, the patient is placed on his left side with a sandbag under the left axilla to elevate the shoulder from the table and provide free respiratory excursion of the chest. The back and chest of the patient are supported by rests attached to the table and the head is fixed in a three-point pin headrest. The alignment of the head is critical for the subtemporal approach. The anteroposterior (AP) axis should be precisely parallel to the floor, and the sagittal plane of the head tipped 15° toward the floor. The head does not move relative to the body following fixation in this position, but the whole table may be tipped head up or head down or rotated from one side to the other as necessary to gain further visual access to the upper basilar artery (Fig. 60-2).

In our initial experience with aneurysms of the upper basilar artery, we routinely turned sizeable temporal bone flaps. In our more recent 500 cases, this has proved unnecessary. As will be seen by the orientation drawings, the aim of the exposure is to get as close to the base of the skull as possible at the junction of the anterior and middle third of the temporal lobe where the temporal lobe has already begun to turn upward following the convex floor of the middle cranial fossa. Little is gained by fashioning a large bone flap up over the lateral surface of the temporal lobe or posteriorly, except in circumstances where it is necessary to divide the tentorium to gain access to the middle portions of the basilar artery (Figs. 60-3, 60-4, and 60-5).

We now routinely make a linear incision extending vertically upward, curving slightly backward at its upper extent, and originating at the zygomatic process of the temporal bone approximately one finger's width anterior to the ear. After the skin, subcutaneous tissue, and galea are divided, the temporalis fascia and muscle are divided 5 mm on either side of the vertical incision at the level of the zygomatic process. With the soft tissue held apart by a tic retractor, a single burr hole in the squamous portion of the temporal bone is enlarged with rongeurs, forming a

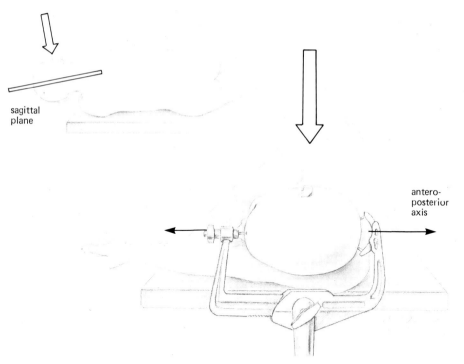

Fig. 60-2. Patient position for the subtemporal approach. Note that the anterior posterior access of the head is fixed parallel to the floor and that the sagittal plane is tipped 15° to the perpendicular. The open arrow shows the starting position of the operating microscope.

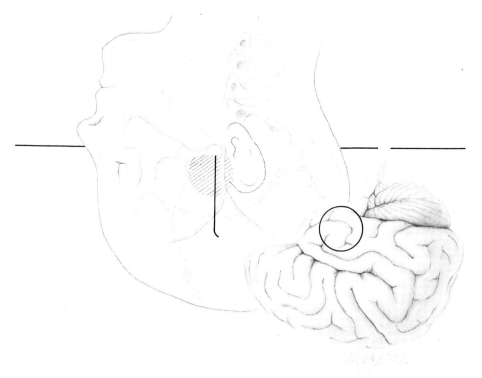

Fig. 60-3. Subtemporal approach. Relationship of scalp incision and craniectomy to skull and brain landmarks.

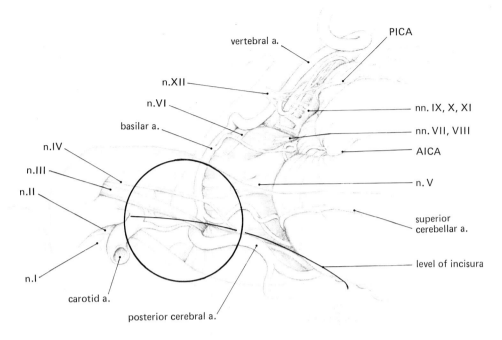

vertebral a.

PICA

n.XII

n.VI

basilar a.

n.IV

n.III

n.II

n.I

carotid a.

posterior cerebral a.

nn. IX, X, XI

nn. VII, VIII

AICA

n. V

superior
cerebellar a.

level of incisura

Fig. 60-4.   An overview of the anatomy of the vertebral basilar circulation as seen from the subtemporal approach. The circle depicts the size of the craniectomy.

somewhat pear-shaped opening that is widest at the base, with bone nibbled away down to the floor of the middle cranial fossa. The main stem and posterior branch of the superficial temporal artery are preserved in the posterior aspect of the scalp flap, but often the anterior branch of this vessel must be divided (Fig. 60-6).

The dura is opened in a triangle with the base inferior and is sutured up to the overlying soft tissue so as not to obscure the view at the base. At this point, the lumbar subarachnoid drain is opened and CSF removal is begun. A slack brain is essential. The combination of the osmotic and loop diuretic and the removal of CSF is usually sufficient to produce excellent intracranial relaxation. If the brain remains full, however, and gentle retraction of the temporal lobe does not easily expose the middle intracranial fossa, it is imperative to wait, elevate the head, remove more CSF, check to ensure that the ventilation parameters are adequate, and wait again until adequate reduction of the intracranial contents has been achieved. If, with time, the brain continues to remain full, it may be advisable to abandon the procedure and return another day. Cerebral edema is the most likely cause for a persistently swollen and tight brain. Most maneuvers on the operating table will not adequately relieve this and further retraction and manipulation run a high likelihood of aggravating the edema in the postoperative period.

With the brain relaxed, the surface of the temporal lobe should be covered with a compressed sheet of Gelfoam, and with a hand-held retractor, the undersurface of the temporal lobe is inspected for the position of bridging veins. The vein of Labbé is usually seen just beyond the posterior limits of the craniectomy. It should, when visualized, be covered with several strips of Gelfoam and protected at all costs against rupture. Similarly, bridging veins at the tip of the temporal lobe seen just beyond the anterior limits of the bony removal should also be protected. Small bridging veins from the undersurface of the temporal lobe to the tent can be coagulated and divided with impunity; the larger veins on the surface, however, should never be sacrificed for fear of producing venous swelling or infarction.

With further retraction, the uncus of the temporal lobe is gently elevated and the free edge of the tentorium comes into view. A Greenberg or Yasargil self-retaining retractor should now be fixed without excessive retractor pressure. With this retractor in place and with a 2- to 3-mm

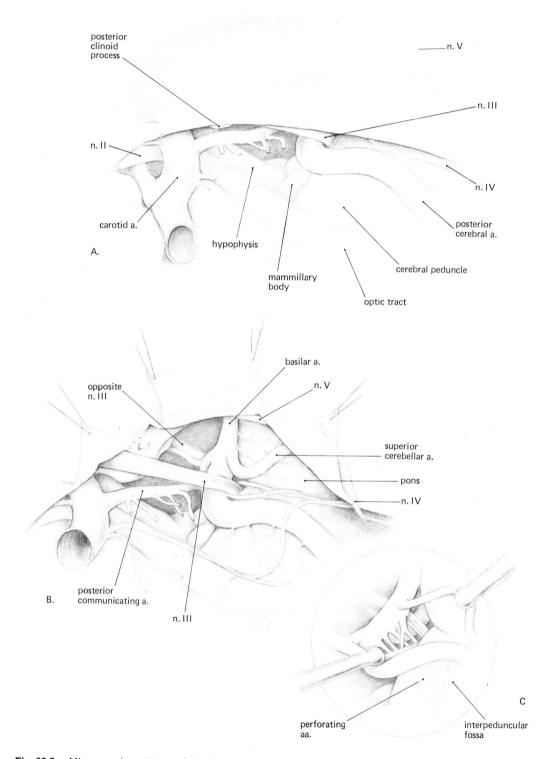

Fig. 60-5. Microscopic anatomy of the interpeduncular fossa and its contents. **A.** Uncus and hippocampal gyrus of temporal removed and tentorium intact. **B.** Tentorium divided and retracted. **C.** Terminal basilar artery drawn out of interpeduncular fossa to show perforating artery.

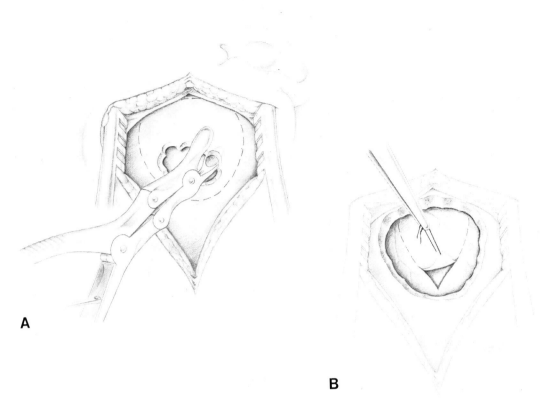

Fig. 60-6.   Subtemporal approach. Operative procedure. **A.** Exposure of dura. **B.** Dural incision.

gap visible between the uncus and the free surface of the tent, it is likely that the retractor will not need to be moved again. The position of the tip of the retractor is important. It should just touch the uncus and its overlying arachnoid and be centered at about the midpoint of the concave curve of the free edge of the tent. Positioning the retractor anterior or posterior to this will lead the surgeon forward into the interpeduncular fossa and posterior clinoid or backward onto the cerebral peduncle instead of directly medially onto the terminal basilar artery (Fig. 60-7).

It is almost always necessary at this point to pass a 4-0 silk suture through the free edge of the tentorium and tie it back into the floor of the middle cranial fossa. This maneuver provides 3–5 mm more exposure by rolling back the free edge of the tentorium. Only rarely will it be necessary to divide the tent in the exposure of aneurysms of the distal end of the basilar artery.

At this point, the operating microscope should be brought into position and, under 10–16× magnification, the operator focuses on the layer of arachnoid covering the uncus and cerebral peduncle, passing onto and under the free edge of the tentorium. It is usually possible to identify the occulomotor nerve at this point, coming up from the depths under the uncus and piercing the arachnoid in the anterior aspect of the exposure to enter its cavernous compartment. The trochlear nerve will also be seen posteriorly in the exposure, lying beneath the arachnoid and turning inferiorly underneath the tentorium. Popular textbooks of anatomy often depict the trochlear nerve passing between layers of the tentorium at this site, but it does not. It remains within its arachnoid layer, attached to the undersurface of the tentorium for about 2 cm, and swings in an arc laterally forward and then medially toward the cavernous sinus. The initial arachnoid incision should then be made by picking up the arachnoid covering the side of the peduncle superior to the trochlear nerve and inferior to the uncus. This incision is extended forward below the course of the third nerve. This arachnoid is a rather thick and complex structure, dividing anteri-

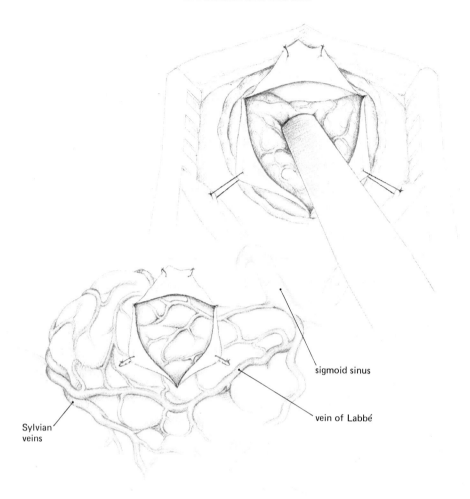

Sylvian
veins

sigmoid sinus

vein of Labbé

Fig. 60-7. Subtemporal approach. Retraction of temporal lobe and temporal lobe veins.

orly to form a band running medially across the interpeduncular fossa known as the membrane of Lilliequist. This band of arachnoid should also be sharply divided across the front of the pons to permit the removal of clot in the interpeduncular fossa and visualization of the opposite occulomotor nerve and posterior cerebral artery. (Figs. 60-8 and 60-9).

At this stage, the inexperienced surgeon will often be surprised if he is unable to see the posterior cerebral artery. This vessel, of course, follows a compound curved course, bending upward laterally, forward, and then turning backward, and is usually obscured by the third nerve, the uncus, and the mesial portion of the temporal lobe as it winds its way back around the midbrain. Branches of the superior cerebellar artery are readily apparent at this stage as they wind around the peduncle and can be followed medially to the basilar artery. The surgeon must now have a clear mental picture of the anatomy gained from knowledge of the normal anatomy and by study of the angiograms so that he or she can readily identify the structures in the depths of the exposure. It is usually best to begin removal of the blood clot in the region along the lateral aspects of the basilar artery between the superior cerebellar and the origin of P1. Once the wall of the basilar artery is in view, dissection can be carried out in that plane anteriorly and posteriorly, removing clot with suction and forceps and working from the base of the presumed neck of the aneurysm and distally toward the fundus. (Fig. 60-10)

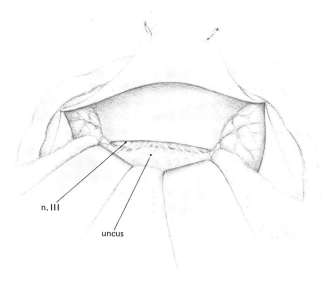

Fig. 60-8.   Subtemporal approach. Retraction of temporal lobe to expose edge of tentorium and first layer of arachnoid.

Basilar Bifurcation Aneurysms

Basilar bifurcation aneurysms may be small (up to 1.5 cm in diameter), bulbous (1.5–2.5 cm in diameter) or giant (greater than 2.5 cm in diameter). These aneurysms may point forward, directly upward, or backward. For each size and orientation, there are special problems in dissection and clipping. The position of the basilar bifurcation relative to the posterior clinoid is also an important variable to be considered in one's approach to these aneurysms. Most often, the bifurcation lies precisely at the level of the posterior clinoid, but in some cases it may be several millimeters or up to 1 cm below the clinoid, and in others, the basilar artery is elongated with the bifurcation lying some distance above the clinoid. With aneurysms arising from the basilar bifurcation located at the level of the posterior clinoid, the approach from this point will be quite straightforward. A high bifurcation will require further retraction of the uncus and, indeed, may be preferentially approached from the frontotemporal exposure after splitting the sylvian fissure. The low-lying basilar bifurcation is particularly hazardous in that the interpeduncular space narrows to the apex of a cone, making manipulation and visualization difficult around the bulging belly of the pons and, with the thin dome of the fundus, obscuring the surgeon's path to the neck.

With an aneurysm of average size and in the middle position, it is preferable at this stage to begin the dissection on the anterior surface of the aneurysm. By following the surface of the basilar artery anteriorly and superiorly, the origin of the P1 artery on the right side will be identified, as well as the anterior aspect of the neck of the sac. The neck of the sac and the termination of the basilar artery are gently retracted backward into the interpeduncular fossa and, with further removal of clot, the opposite (left) P1 artery will be exposed and visualized through a layer of arachnoid, with the left occulomotor nerve passing forward. One must use this maneuver cautiously with aneurysms pointing forward, for they are often fused to the clivus at the site of rupture; rough handling can tear away this point of junction and cause troublesome bleeding.

It is important to emphasize at this point that the termination of the basilar artery is usually widened and ectatic at the base of aneurysms arising from the bifurcation. One must have an ap-

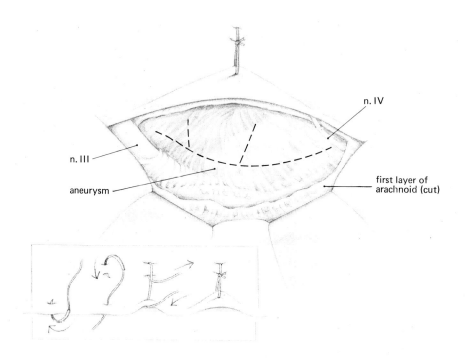

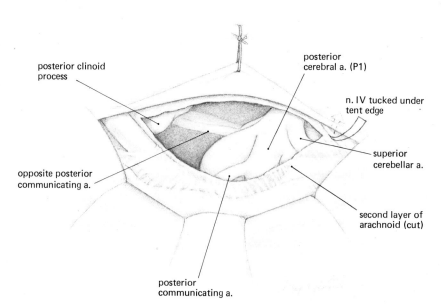

Fig. 60-9.   **A.** Subtemporal approach. First layer of arachnoid has been removed, showing the intact second layer. Tentorial edge has been sutured into the middle fossa. Inset depicts technique of suturing tentorium. **B.** Second layer of arachnoid and membrane of Lilliequist has been divided to expose the terminal basilar artery and bifurcation aneurysm. Note that the fourth cranial nerve has been tucked back under the edge of the tentorium.

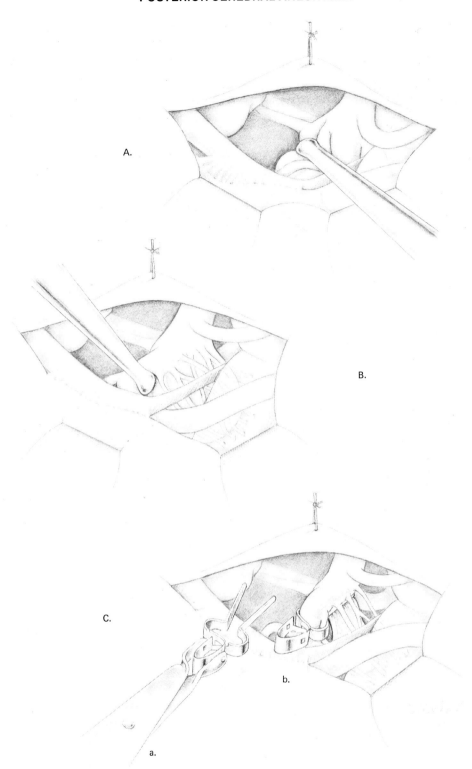

Fig. 60-10. Subtemporal approach. Exposure and clipping of a basilar bifurcation aneurysm. **A.** Dissector compressing anterior belly of aneurysm to expose opposite P1, posterior communicating artery, and oculomotor nerve. **B.** Microdissector displacing right P1 anteriorly to display perforators on side wall of aneurysm. **C.** a = Drake aperture clip. b = an aperture clip in place occluding neck of aneurysm and encircling right P1 and one perforator in the aperture.

preciation of this variation in anatomy and identify the origin of the P1 artery precisely, lest one mistake the terminal basilar artery for a portion of the sac and position the clip dangerously low, resulting in occlusion of the terminal basilar artery. Furthermore, the distal basilar artery and the origin of both posterior cerebral arteries forms a V-shaped structure as viewed from the front, making the neck of these aneurysms quite narrow. This often comes as a surprise when the aneurysm is exposed in the operating room, in that the conventional angiographic projections of this area commonly superimpose the P1 artery and the neck of the aneurysm, giving the appearance of a spuriously wide base. Bearing this in mind, care must be taken to prevent placement of a clip with blades that are too long as this would risk narrowing or occluding the opposite P1 artery. Moreover, the base of the aneurysm is narrower from front to back than from side to side, making application of the clip from the side somewhat safer, in that properly positioned clip blades are less likely to crimp the origins of the P1 artery.

After exposing the front side of the aneurysm, dissection should be directed to the right lateral and posterior aspect of the aneurysm. Here the goal is to define the posterior aspect of the sac and, more importantly, to identify and separate the perforators that arise from the proximal, posterior portion of the P1 artery and normally stream backward over the sac of the aneurysm to enter the posterior perforated substance and peduncle. These perforators are small vessels, often branching once or twice before penetrating the pia covering the brain. It is essential that each of these vital vessels be preserved and any amount of time taken to separate these vessels from the sac can be justified. Often these perforators will have to be separated with a sharp hook, or, after they have been stretched, by sharply dividing with a knife the fibrous bands fusing them to the sac. One must remember that the perforators are paired, with two to six vessels arising from each P1 artery, making it necessary to displace the terminal basilar artery and the sac away from the interpeduncular fossa and dissect across the midline to visualize the perforators on the far side, as well as those more readily seen on the near side. Displacement of the whole of the terminal basilar complex away from the interpeduncular fossa during periods of hypotension can be done using a relatively wide blade dissector.

It is important to emphasize that before any clip is placed, the origin of both of the P1 arteries must be identified on both the right and left side by looking across the front of the basilar artery and across the back, and then all the perforators arising from both of the P1 arteries passing backward and upward must be seen and separated from the sac. Occasionally, with a low or highly placed basilar bifurcation, one may momentarily confuse the opposite superior cerebellar artery with the posterior cerebral artery. To inadvertently place the clip blades proximal to the origin of the opposite P1 artery is, of course, disastrous and can be avoided by identifying the opposite occulomotor nerve and recalling that this structure always runs between the superior cerebellar and posterior cerebral arteries. The absolute confirmation of this anatomy on both the near and far sides is fundamental to the success of the procedure.

In most instances the dissection can be confined to the neck of the basilar bifurcation aneurysm and the adjacent proximal posterior cerebral arteries and their perforating branches. It is rarely necessary and, indeed, hazardous to extend the dissection up onto the body or fundus, for the wall is almost always thinner in this region and is the site of the original rupture; it will bleed again if not handled with care.

With the neck defined, the decision is now made as to the type of clip to be used, and its placement. For aneurysms that point forward or backward from the bifurcation, a simple straight clip may suffice after displacing the sac away from the P1 arteries and in the case of posterior projecting aneurysms, working the blades under the perforators. The more common aneurysm, however, projects directly upward in the line of the basilar artery and the origins of the P1 artery and cannot be secured with a simple straight or angled clip. For this reason, we have developed the aperture clip designed to enclose the P1 artery and, if necessary, adjacent perforators within the aperture, permitting the clip blades to compress only the neck of the aneurysm.

Successful use of this clip depends on precisely choosing the correct blade length, as blades that are too long will narrow or occlude the origin of the P1 segments of the posterior cerebral artery and, if too short, will permit continued filling of the aneurysm. We have frequently found it necessary to cut and file the ends of the clips to ensure the precise blade length necessary for the job. A common error is to use a clip blade that is too long.

After placing the clip, one should not breathe a sigh of relief and step back. This is perhaps the most critical part of the procedure, a time when the surgeon must quickly inspect both the anterior and posterior surfaces of the neck to ensure that the P1 segments are not kinked and that all perforators are entirely free. If there is any suspicion that a perforator is trapped or kinked by the clip or that the origins of the P1 artery are narrowed, the clip should be removed immediately, further dissection accomplished, and the clip reapplied. Commonly, the clip will have to be positioned and repositioned several times before a precise and accurate placement is achieved. Then the dome of the aneurysm should be punctured with a needle and its contents aspirated, and with the added room afforded by the collapsed sac, the whole anatomy can be reviewed and perfect positioning of the clip guaranteed.

One must recall that the height of the basilar bifurcation varies considerably. Most often, the bifurcation is at or just above the level of the dorsum sellae. Occasionally it is higher, reaching the apex of the interpeduncular cistern and tucked in behind the mamillary bodies. Rarely, the bifurcation may be higher still with the aneurysm indenting the floor of the third ventricle and posterior hypothalamus. The higher the placement of the bifurcation, the more temporal lobe retraction will be required, and retraction of the peduncle or mamillary body may even be necessary to expose the bifurcation and perforators. Retraction of these structures with a small spatula is normally well tolerated. As noted above, an aneurysm that is very high is often best approached through the so-called pterional exposure utilizing splitting and separation of the sylvian fissure.[12] With a moderately high bifurcation, it occasionally will be necessary to dissect above the oculomotor nerve in the space between the oculomotor nerve and the hippocampal gyrus. In this situation, it is sometimes necessary to enclose the oculomotor nerve along with the P1 segment in the aperture of the clip, a maneuver that is well tolerated by this hardy nerve.

If the bifurcation is unusually low (at the base of the dorsum sellae or even lower), the exposure is considerably more difficult and hazardous. The interpeduncular fossa is cone-shaped with the apex pointing downward into the groove of the pons, forcing the surgeon to gain visual access around the belly of the pons in the depths of the wound. This line of sight can be enhanced by retracting the temporal lobe somewhat more posteriorly to view the anterior aspect of the pons and the pontomesencephalic junction. Although division of the tent may be used, it frequently does not improve the exposure at this site because both the trigeminal and the trochlear nerves cross the sight line and obscure the view. Angled aperture clips are often essential for dealing with these low-placed aneurysms. It should also be remembered that the sylvian approach to basilar bifurcation aneurysms is quite unsuitable for these low-lying lesions in that it is impossible to see over the obstruction of the dorsum sellae. It should also be remembered that angiograms taken in the Townes projection usually show the P1 segments as entirely separate from the neck of the aneurysm and coming out almost straight laterally from the side of the basilar artery. The course of the posterior cerebral artery is complex, however, coursing forward and upward before it turns outward to cross above the oculomotor nerve and before swinging around the peduncle under the cover of the hippocampal gyrus. With this angiographic view in mind, the surgeon is often surprised, particularly when faced with a large or bulbous aneurysm, to see from the lateral exposure what appear to be the P1 segments and their perforators arising directly out of the sac. This is rarely if ever true but underlines the necessity of carefully dissecting between the P1 artery and the sac on both the near and far side to clearly define the lowermost portion of the neck to be clipped. This anomalous appearance of vessels arising from the side wall of the aneurysm is particularly prominent when the terminal basilar artery is ectatic.

Posterior-Projecting Aneurysms

Although the angiographic appearance of posterior-projecting aneurysms would suggest that they would be the most difficult and dangerous to expose, as a group they have proven to be quite suitable for direct surgical treatment. With these aneurysms it is usually necessary to work both above and below the third nerve to gain access to the neck. Often the perforators are more readily dissected from the neck but are densely adherent more distally on the dome, where they can and should be left untouched. With posterior-projecting aneurysms, one can readily visualize the opposite P1 artery across the front of the aneurysm and, with the position of the neck in view, it is then possible to work a fine sucker between the basilar artery and the crus with the left hand and gently draw the basilar artery forward, displacing the terminal basilar artery and the sac out of the interpeduncular fossa. Dissecting with a fine spatula in the right hand, it is then possible to see the perforators that have been stretched and to separate them from the neck on both the near and far sides. The fundus of this aneurysm is usually never seen, as it is buried high up in the interpeduncular fossa, and in that it is covered with brainstem, it is probably more secure and less likely to rupture. Because of the backward displacement of this aneurysm away from the curve of the posterior cerebral artery, one is frequently able to secure the neck with a simple straight clip, which, when placed across the neck and partially closed, allows excellent visualization across the back of the neck before final placement. A particular hazard with this aneurysm is the portion of the fundus bulging downward below the level of the neck posteriorly. This configuration makes blind application of the clip blades on the posterior aspect of the aneurysm hazardous, as the inferior blade of the clip could pierce the sac. By beginning the dissection low on the back surface of the basilar artery at the origins of the superior cerebellar arteries and working distally, however, one will usually encounter this rolled-over portion of the fundus, allowing it to be separated from the parent vessel and tipped upward before the clip blades are applied.

Anterior-Projecting Aneurysms

Anterior-projecting are the least common of the basilar bifurcation aneurysms, which is unfortunate in that they are the most straightforward to deal with. The anterior-projecting aneurysm projects upward and forward from the line of the basilar artery, with the fundus usually placed above the dorsum sellae, free of the interpeduncular fossa and mamillary bodies. In the same way, the aneurysm is usually free of the posterior cerebral arteries and perforators and only passing attention need be given to these structures in the definition of the terminal basilar anatomy. These aneurysms are, however, frequently fused to the dura of the dorsum and clivus, and care must be taken in the displacement of the aneurysm backward for fear of tearing away this attachment, which is usually at the site of rupture and, therefore, thin and friable. It is also important not to confuse this aneurysm with the bilobed bulbous sac that typically has an upward- or backward-projecting sac as well as the more obvious forward-projecting portion. In contrast, these bilobed lesions are among the most complex and difficult aneurysms to deal with because of their bulk, as well as the unusually wide and deformed terminal basilar artery.

Giant or Bulbous Basilar Bifurcation Aneurysms

Most giant or bulbous aneurysms of the basilar bifurcation project vertically and are always associated with a widened terminal basilar artery, giving the appearance that the posterior cerebral arteries are arising out of the neck and proximal fundus. As a group, these aneurysms are hazardous, in that they are difficult to expose and technically demanding to clip. The exceptional bulk of the aneurysm filling the interpeduncular cistern and deforming the parent and branch vessels makes definition of the anatomy difficult and at times impossible. It is usually necessary to firmly indent the waist of the sac anteriorly and posteriorly to visualize the neck, and often it must be held indented while the clip is being positioned. Again, it is important to clearly identify the opposite P1 artery and its perforators before the clip is finally placed. It is frequently necessary to manipulate the clip into place with the left hand while holding perforators off with a small dissector in the right hand.

Another major concern with this aneurysm is that frequently the neck of the aneurysm and the terminal ectatic basilar artery are firm and yellow with atherosclerosis. Instead of being soft and pliable, the neck and terminal basilar artery are solid and often calcified, and as the clip blades are closed, the clip tends to slide down and occlude the terminal basilar artery or the atherosclerotic plaque fractures, and fragments are driven into the P1 segments. If the clip does slip downward because of the firmness of the wall and the mass of the sac above, it may be necessary to place a clip high up across the body of the sac to occlude the fundus and permit its aspiration and then to seat a smaller clip more precisely across the neck. It is always safer, however, to clip these aneurysms somewhat more distally than at the actual neck, since considerable narrowing several millimeters proximal to the clip is the rule as the blades approximate the firm wall, and this may impede flow through the P1 segments or the proximal perforators. If the dilatation and ectasia of the terminal basilar artery are extensive, the entire vessel and its major branches will be involved in the aneurysmal dilation, making it impossible to secure the neck with a clip without occluding or seriously stenosing the orifice of one or both posterior cerebral arteries. In this situation, consideration must be given to proximal basilar artery occlusion as the only definitive form of treatment, particularly if generous posterior communicating arteries are known to be present.

Superior Cerebellar Artery Aneurysms

Super cerebellar artery aneurysms arise at the distal carina of the origin of the superior cerebellar artery. The aneurysm almost always projects laterally forward or backward, with the fundus embedded in the peduncle. As the sac enlarges, it usually occupies the whole of the length of the basilar artery between the distal carina of the superior cerebellar artery and the proximal origin of the posterior cerebral artery. The fundus frequently has an intimate association with the oculomotor nerve and often stretches this nerve above or below the sac, as well as indenting the peduncle on that side. Unless they are unusually large, these aneurysms can be dealt within a relatively straightforward manner. The subtemporal exposure gives excellent visualization of the neck and as there are no perforators arising off the segment of the basilar artery between the superior cerebellar and posterior cerebral arteries or off the superior surface of the superior cerebellar artery, the clip can be placed across the neck with concern only for preserving the integrity of the basilar artery and encompassing the whole of the neck between the blades. As noted, these aneurysms normally project laterally and, as a consequence, one is faced with approaching the left-pointing aneurysm under the dominant temporal lobe. In our experience, this represents an additional but real hazard to the patient. When this aneurysm reaches large or giant proportions, the superior and anterior surface of the sac will be in direct contact with the perforators arising off the P1 artery. These should be identified and spared as in the case of basilar bifurcation aneurysms. The larger aneurysms pointing toward the left side may be approached from the right, working across the midline and over the top of the basilar artery, for the basilar artery is usually deflected toward the right side as the sac enlarges (Fig. 60-11).

Superior cerebellar aneurysms are best dissected first on their anterior surface, again defining the plane of the basilar artery and the origins of the superior cerebellar and posterior cerebral arteries. It is then necessary to work on the distal and proximal surface of the sac to provide

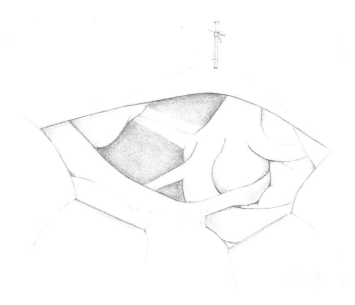

Fig. 60-11. Subtemporal approach to show superior cerebellar artery aneurysm in situ. Note that the third cranial nerve is displaced over the dome of the aneurysm.

room for the clip blades. It is preferable to work a curved clip blade from the superior and anterior surface downward, following the curve of the interior surface of the posterior cerebral artery and the lateral wall of the basilar artery as the clip blades are closed. In this way, one is able to locate the tips of the clip precisely to ensure that they are not impinging on the origin of the superior cerebellar artery. The fundus of the aneurysm can then be punctured and aspirated, and quick inspection of the posterior surface can be carried out to ensure that perforators from the P1 artery have not been picked up by the posterior blade. One must be cautious, particularly with larger aneurysms, that the clip does not slide medially and kink the basilar artery. Of course, care should always be taken to avoid injuring the third nerve by these manipulations and, indeed, it may be necessary to encircle the nerve in a curved aperture clip so that it is not deformed or compressed by the clip itself.

Posterior Cerebral Artery Aneurysms

Aneurysms arise typically at four sites along the course of the posterior cerebral artery: first, at the origin of the large perforating branches of the P1 artery; second, at the junction of the posterior communicating artery and the P1 artery; third, at the origin of the anterior and posterior occipital temporal arteries along the side of the brainstem and, finally, at the terminal branching of the vessel into its parietal and calcarine arteries. The most common sites are at the origin of the posterior communicating artery and at the first major branching at the side of the brainstem.

The more proximal aneurysms are usually dealt with in exactly the same manner as aneurysms of the terminal basilar artery. They generally are easy aneurysms to dissect in that they are somewhat more lateral and generally are situated a few millimeters away from the major perforators going to the peduncle. These perforators must be identified in the case of large or giant aneurysms, and separating these aneurysms from the neck may provide a technical challenge. The most distal aneurysms are frequently hidden under the hippocampal gyrus and require retraction somewhat more posteriorly and, occasionally, resection of a small portion of the gyrus. This is almost always necessary with those aneurysms lying in the mouth of the choroidal fissure. As with any aneurysm, the purpose is to secure the neck while maintaining normal flow through the parent and branching vessels in the region. Tiny posterior cerebral artery perforators are less of a problem, except for the segment that winds around the midbrain and normally gives rise to several circumferential vessels that must be seen and preserved. More distally (i.e., beyond the emergence of the major temporal branch of the posterior cerebral artery), it is usually acceptable and quite safe to trap a large aneurysm. In our experience, the posterior cerebral artery has perhaps the richest potential for collateralization of any of the major cerebral arteries. In 17 cases where we have deliberately or inadvertently occluded the posterior cerebral artery, we have noted only 1 case of a persistent field defect as a result of occipital infarction. One must be exceptionally cautious, however, not to occlude the vessel proximal to the posterior choroidal arteries, for ischemia and infarction in the territory of these vessels can be devastating. Deliberate occlusion of the P1 or proximal P2 segments is therefore most satisfactorily accomplished using the microtourniquet technique in an awake patient.

Basilar-Anterior Inferior Cerebellar Artery (AICA) Aneurysms

Like most aneurysms, the AICA aneurysm usually arises at the distal carina of the origin of the anterior inferior cerebellar artery and basilar artery. It is not rare, however, for these aneurysms to arise on the proximal side of this junction. This variation in the usual aneurysm anatomy should be ascertained from angiograms, for the position of the AICA may radically alter one's approach to this aneurysm. Most often the AICA aneurysm projects laterally, but it may project forward and be firmly adherent to the clivus or even point backward and be buried in the pons or pontomedullary junction. The dome of the aneurysm usually has a close relationship to the abducens nerve.

The approach to these aneurysms depends largely upon their size and configuration, for they can be reached from either above via the subtemporal transtentorial route or from below by a suboccipital craniotomy. Generally, the whole of the basilar artery down to the vertebral junctions may be exposed through the tentorium. It is the size and shape of aneurysms at the trunk of the basilar artery that determines one's approach. For example, an AICA aneurysm originating from the midpoint of the basilar artery with the dome projecting upward and the AICA arising from its proximal surface may be more safely approached by the suboccipital route. Similarly, trunk aneurysms arising from the proximal crotch of the AICA and pointing laterally and downward and buried into the medulla are often more safely visualized and clipped subtemporally through the tentorium. These aneurysms lie in a narrow and confined space some distance from either the approach from above or below. It is usually in the surgeon's (and patient's) best interest to see the aneurysm neck and the critical branch of origin first rather than be faced with the walled fundus obscuring the neck. For this reason, we prefer to plan the approach that will most readily bring the neck into view. Usually these aneurysms lie at about the junction of the middle and lower third of the clivus and close to the midline, but they may vary as much as 2 cm above or below this point and may be placed laterally as far as the cerebellopontine angle (Fig. 60-12).

When exposing this aneurysm from a subtemporal transtentorial approach, it is necessary to turn a moderately sized temporal bone flap that is centered to permit a direct line of sight down the posterior slope of the petrous bone. The vein of Labbé will be in the middle or anterior third of this exposure and must be protected and spared. With elevation of the temporal lobe the free edge of the tentorium is exposed in its posterior part and can be divided by placing a hook about 1–1.5 cm behind the attachment of the trochlear nerve. Using the hook to firmly lift the tentorium and touching it with the monopolar coagulator, the tent is divided in steps, almost to the junction of the petrosal and lateral sinuses. The anterior leaf of tentorium is then picked up with a 4-0 silk suture and stitched forward into the middle fossa. Immediately upon reflection of the tent, the arachnoidal roof in the posterior fossa will come into view. Piercing this arachnoid

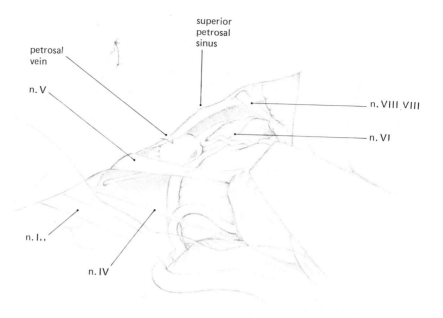

Fig. 60-12. Subtemporal transtentorial approach showing an AICA aneurysm in situ. The retractor is on the anterior edge of the cerebellum.

will be the pertrosal vein, which should be coagulated and divided immediately. Deep to the arachnoid the trochlear and trigeminal nerves will be seen. The arachnoid should be carefully opened just lateral to the trigeminal nerve and a narrow retractor blade slipped into this opening, gently elevating the anterior superior margin of the cerebellar hemisphere. With further deepening of the retractor, the pons will be gently elevated, exposing the facial and cochlear nerves just lateral to the retractor blade and crossing the cerebellopontine angle. At this point, the abducens nerve will be seen just at the tip of the retractor as a thin, slack structure coursing upward to gain the cavernous sinus. Gentle removal of clot and CSF will expose the basilar artery and the aneurysm. It is usually necessary to separate the sixth nerve from the aneurysm, but, as noted, this nerve has a lot of slack as it passes from the brain to the cavernous sinus, allowing it to be displaced either forward toward the clivus or back toward the pons to clear the neck of the aneurysm. As with the third nerve, if it is handled gently, the abducens nerve usually regains its normal function within about 3 months.

Again, it is wise to begin the dissection proximal or distal to the aneurysm on the basilar artery, removing clot and debris until the adventitia of this vessel is clearly in view. Staying within this plane, the dissection is continued toward the neck of the aneurysm, removing the clot packed into this narrow space in front of the pons. It should be recalled that the AICA usually leaves the basilar artery and then courses inferiorly in a path parallel to the main trunk of the basilar artery before turning laterally to wind around the pons. With a sizeable aneurysm, the origin of the AICA usually will not be seen initially from the transtentorial approach but obviously must be clearly identified before any attempt is made to place the clip. More often than not, its original course will be quite free of the aneurysm, but it may occasionally be firmly adherent to the inferior side and have to be dissected free from the neck and body of the sac. This maneuver can be facilitated by gently grasping the neck of the aneurysm in bipolar forceps, tipping the sac forward toward the clivus to expose the AICA, and allowing it to be sharply removed from the side wall of the aneurysm. Inasmuch as these aneurysms are frequently pointing forward and are adherent to the clivus, the identification of the basilar artery, the AICA, and clumps of perforating vessels arising from the posterior surface of the basilar artery is quite straightforward. If, however, the sac is displaced laterally or backward into the pons, then this maneuver of grasping the neck and rolling the sac out of its bed will be essential. Certainly, application of a clip in this narrow, confined space is always awkward, since the clip mechanism and applier obscure the surgeon's view at the critical moment of closure. For this reason, it is important to remove the applicator quickly and to inspect the position of the blades to ensure precision in their placement; only absolute accuracy should be accepted. Minor narrowing of the origin of the AICA, entrapment of midbasilar perforators, or partial stenosis of the basilar artery will almost always herald disaster.

Only occasionally have we encountered aneurysms arising from the trunk of the basilar artery between the AICA and the SCA, presumably at the sites of the short or long circumferential pontine vessels or even the trigeminal artery. These aneurysms usually are approached by the transtentorial route, but are difficult to expose in that they usually are partially hidden by the full belly of the pons, and more superficially the approach is guarded by the fleshy mass of the trigeminal nerve. This aneurysm usually requires gentle lateral retraction of the fifth nerve and simultaneous medial retraction of the belly of the pons for exposure. Pontine retraction should always be intermittent and all the small arterials irrigating the pons must be spared.

As a general rule, exposure of the high basilar trunk aneurysm is more safely accomplished through the subtemporal-transtentorial route, in that manipulation and retraction on the fourth, fifth, and sixth cranial nerves usually is well tolerated and has an excellent potential for full recovery. In contrast, the suboccipital exposure requires dissection between the ninth, tenth, and eleventh cranial nerves, and damage to these nerves is almost always associated with significant morbidity and not infrequently mortality secondary to aspiration and pneumonia.

Many years ago, we attempted to expose these aneurysms through the transoral-transclival approach. This exposure is always distressingly confined, usually puts the fundus of the aneurysm between the operator and the parent vessel, and runs the very real risk of postoperative meningitis. A subtemporal or suboccipital approach is much more satisfactory, making the transoral exposure unnecessary.

Vertebral Junction Aneurysms

Vertebral junction aneurysms are uncommon even in our series. They are commonly associated with anomalous development of the vertebral artery. For example, one vertebral artery terminating at the posterior inferior cerebellar artery, duplication of the proximal basilar artery, fenestration of the proximal basilar artery, or congenital absence of one vertebral artery.

Normally, the two vertebral arteries join just at or below the junction of the middle and inferior thirds of the clivus. With anomalous development, however, this point of junction may be considerably higher or lower and can be displaced well off the midline. In our experience, an equal number of these aneurysms have been approached from the subtemporal and suboccipital exposure. The decision in any one patient is therefore dependent on the size and configuration of the aneurysm more than on the absolute position of the origin of the neck. The difficulty of treating this aneurysm lies not with identification of perforating vessels, which are usually either not present or so small as to be of little consequence at this site, but rather with the extreme importance of being able to deal with the neck of the aneurysm in the very confined space of an exposure from either above or from below and ensure at the same time the patency of the basilar and vertebral artery when the clip is finally placed. One must be cautious not to choose a clip that is too long, and to identify the position of the tips of the clip with certainty once it is seated and in place. This aneurysm is always awkward and difficult to expose. Once again, great care must be taken to avoid injuring the lower cranial nerves when manipulating instruments around the front of the brainstem and to recall the importance of starting the dissection well proximal along the vertebral artery. Once the plane of the adventitial surface of the vertebral artery has been reached, it is important to stay precisely in this plane, removing a clot and debris piecemeal as one proceeds distally along the parent vessel toward the neck of the vertebral aneurysm.

These aneurysms arise from the vertebral artery usually at the distal crotch or the origin of the posterior inferior cerebellar artery and less frequently on the proximal side of the origin of this vessel. Rarely, these aneurysms arise quite separate from the PICA either proximal or distal to unnamed perforators coursing to the lateral side of the medulla and, occasionally, from the origin of the anterior spinal artery. It will be recalled that the length, caliber, and configuration of the vertebral artery as well as the site of origin of the PICA is extraordinarily variable. We have seen PICA aneurysms situated in the foramen magnum and even as low as the first denticulate ligament and as high as the middle of the clivus. We have also encountered aneurysms arising from the left vertebral artery lying in the right cerebellopontine angle. The aneurysms typically are lying quite free in the subarachnoid space, although they are intimately associated with a lower cranial nerve, but they may, particularly when they reach large or giant proportions, be buried within the medulla or inferior pons. Aneurysms of the PICA typically have an intimate association with the hypoglossal nerve, often splitting this nerve or having the nerve firmly fused to the side wall or neck of the sac. Also, these aneurysms typically originate not only from the vertebral artery but also from the proximal portion of the PICA, giving this vessel the appearance of arising out of the lateral wall of the sac, which indeed it partially does, having at least a portion of its origin involved in the aneurysmal dilatation. This configuration is important to recognize, for it is essential that the placement of the clip protect the origin of the posterior cerebellar artery.

Vertebral artery aneurysms usually are approached through a unilateral suboccipital exposure with the patient in the lateral or park bench position and with the face turned slightly toward the floor (Fig. 60-13). This position usually gives a good exposure of the aneurysm without any concern of air embolism, and it is favored by the anesthetist in that it gives good access to the endotracheal tube and is a position that ensures easy ventilation and a stable cardiovascular system. A midline or lateral paramedian incision is used with care taken to preserve the occipital nerve and to remove bone as far laterally as the mastoid air cell. The rim of the foramen magnum will be removed in most instances, but in high-lying vertebral artery aneurysms this may not be necessary. Extreme lateral or medial approaches are unnecessary as these aneurysms usually lie in close proximity to the lateral medulla, and the PICA usually projects posteriorly and upward (Fig. 60-14). After the cisterna magna is opened and CSF is removed, the retractor is placed to gently elevate the cerebellar tonsil medially and slightly upward off the medulla to expose the ninth, tenth, and eleventh nerves. With this initial retraction, the caudal loop of the PICA and the beginning intracranial course of the vertebral artery will come into view. It is at this level that the dissection should begin with magnified vision. The vertebral artery is followed distally under the emerging cranial nerve, and by staying in the plane of the vessel, one will come upon the origin of the PICA, which usually arises off the superior and slightly lateral side of the vessel and is usually placed proximal to the neck of the aneurysm. It will be remembered that the vertebral artery runs somewhat medially under the medulla, and it may therefore be necessary to gently retract the medulla to gain the necessary exposure. We have found it useful to have the patient under light general anesthesia at this stage and breathing spontaneously, so that a measure of the gentleness of medullary retraction can be gauged by the persistence of spontaneous respirations. With the vertebral artery, the origin of the PICA, and the neck of the aneurysm exposed, it is important to carry the dissection beyond the aneurysm to identify the distal vertebral artery or the origin of the basilar artery in order to gain an appreciation of the position of the structure and the total width of the aneurysm neck. The hypoglossal nerve usually is on the far side of the neck but may be on the near side or even split by the dome of the aneurysm and very frequently needs to be manipulated up off the neck to allow adequate clip placement (Fig. 60-15). We have often found it useful to narrow the neck of this type of aneurysm with bipolar cautery, taking care to avoid contact with the fibers of the vagus and spinal accessory nerve. It is also frequently useful to use aperture clips to enclose the PICA or even both PICAs and the vertebral artery, recognizing that the PICA often takes at least part of its origin from the side wall of the neck. Once again, it is important to stress that the dissection to approach this aneurysm

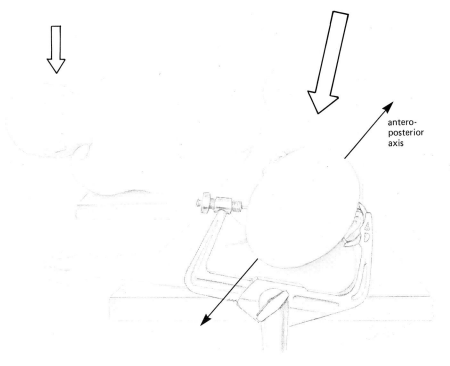

Fig. 60-13. Suboccipital approach. Note the lateral decubitus or park bench position with the face turned toward the floor. The open arrow depicts the direction of the microscope.

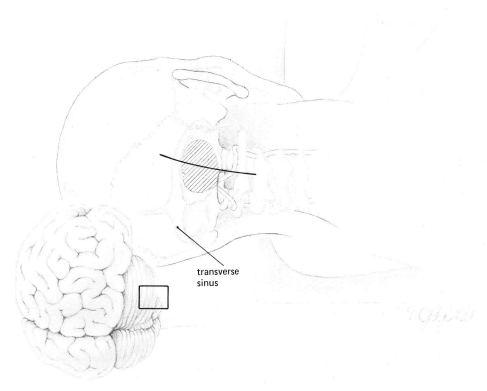

Fig. 60-14. Suboccipital approach. Relationship of incision and craniectomy to skull and brain landmarks.

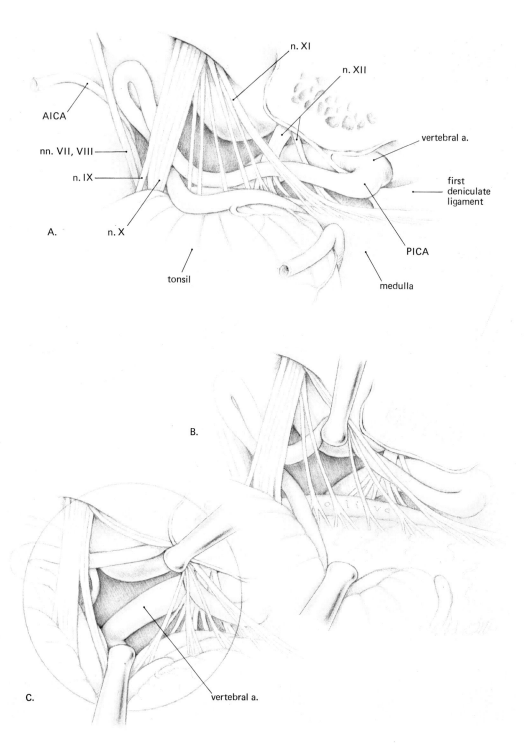

Fig. 60-15.   Suboccipital approach. To expose the right vertebral artery. **A.** Microscopic anatomy. **B.** Dissectors displacing an unusually long rostral loop of the PICA to expose the inferior olive. **C.** Filaments of lower cranial nerves displaced show distal vertebral artery.

must take place between the pharyngeal filaments of the eleventh and the lower fibers of the tenth cranial nerves and these fibers must be protected at all costs before their injury brings about distressing and dangerous postoperative complications.

Conclusions and Results

The evolution of these surgical techniques for aneurysms of the vertebral basilar system has resulted in increasingly satisfactory results as our surgical expertise has grown and has been supported by refinements in neuroradiology and neuroanesthesia. It is now possible to attack aneurysms on the vertebral basilar system and anticipate results as good as results obtained on aneurysms of the anterior circulation. In 400 cases of smaller aneurysms in the posterior circulation, we have experienced a surgical mortality of just under 4 percent, which included our earliest endeavors with these aneurysms, as well as patients in poor condition. The risks and complications of surgical attack on large aneurysms increases proportionately with the size of the lesion, but even so, in 800 of our surgical cases we have achieved excellent or good results in 81 percent, an overall surgical mortality of 6.75 percent, and an overall management morbidity of 12 percent. Overall, the basilar bifurcation is the most hazardous site for both large and small aneurysms of the posterior circulation, and it needs to be stressed again that it is the inadvertent rupture or occlusion of perforators of the P1 artery or occlusion of the terminal basilar artery by the clip or atheroma that accounts for most of the mortality and morbidity. It is essential to be completely familiar with the anatomy and accept only precise and accurate placement of the clip in every case. With technical experience and uniform excellence in neuroanesthesia most, if not all, saccular aneurysms of the vertebral basilar system will be amenable to direct surgical treatment.

REFERENCES

1. Dandy WE: *Intracranial Arterial Aneurysms.* Ithaca, Comstock, 1944
2. Tonnis W: Zur Behandlung Intrakraniellar Aneurysmen. *Arch Klin Chir 189:*474, 1937
3. Falconer MA: Surgical treatment of spontaneous intracranial hemorrhage. *Br Med J i:*790–792, 1958
4. Poppen JL: Vascular surgery of the posterior fossa. *Proc Congr Neurol Surg 6:*198, 1969
5. Logue V: Posterior fossa aneurysms, in Shillito J, Mosberg WH (eds): *Clinical Neurosurgery,* vol. 11. Baltimore, Williams and Wilkins, 1964, pp 183–207
6. Schwartz HG: Arterial aneurysms of the posterior fossa. *J Neurosurg 5:*312, 1948
7. Drake CG: Bleeding aneurysms of the basilar artery. Direct surgical management in four cases. *J Neurosurg 23:*230–238, 1961
8. Jamieson KG: Aneurysms of the vertebrobasilar system. Surgical intervention in 19 cases. *J Neurosurg 21:*781–797, 1964
9. Drake CG: Surgical treatment of ruptured aneurysms of the basilar artery. Experience with 14 cases. *J Neurosurg 23:*457–473, 1965
10. Drake CG: Further experience with surgical treatment of aneurysms of the basilar artery. *J Neurosurg 29:*372–392, 1968
11. Peerless SJ: Pre and post-operative management of intracranial aneurysms, in *Clinical Neurosurgery,* vol. 26. Baltimore, Williams & Wilkins, 1978
12. Yasargil MG, Antic J, Laciga R, et al: Microsurgical pterional approach to aneurysms of the basilar bifurcation. *Surg Neurol 6:*83, 1976

CHAPTER 61
Surgical Management of Bacterial Intracranial Aneurysms

Robert G. Ojemann

SINCE THE DESCRIPTION OF AN AORTIC ANEURYSM associated with bacterial endocarditis by William Osler in 1885,[1] the term "mycotic" aneurysm has been used to designate any aneurysm that developed following an infection in the wall of an artery. Until a few years ago almost every publication concerning intracranial "mycotic" aneurysms reported a bacterial cause for the aneurysm, usually in association with endocarditis. Reports of aneurysms related to meningitis and cavernous sinus thrombophlebitis as well as true mycotic (fungal) aneurysms now have appeared.[2] The designation "bacterial intracranial aneurysm," should be used for those aneurysms that result from bacterial infection.[3] It is suggested that all types of aneurysms caused by infection be grouped under the heading of infectious intracranial aneurysms.[2]

Several publications have reviewed the subject of bacterial intracranial aneurysms.[2-6] In one, 85 cases found at angiography, surgery, or autopsy between 1954 and 1978 were summarized.[3] In another, infectious intracranial aneurysms documented by angiography and reported in the 20 years from 1959 through 1978 were analyzed.[2] This included 53 patients with bacterial intracranial aneurysm associated with definite or probable endocarditis,[2-32] 5 cases caused by meningitis,[33-36] 7 related to cavernous sinus thrombophlebitis,[30,35,37,38] and 5 fungal aneurysms.[39-43] Subsequently, further reports of patients with bacterial aneurysms documented by angiography have appeared, bringing the total number of cases through 1980 to 81.[5,44-52]

Clinical Manifestations

The majority of bacterial intracranial aneurysms occur in patients with subacute bacterial endocarditis, some of whom have associated congenital heart disease or rheumatic heart disease. In a few patients with bacterial intracranial aneurysms, a diagnosis of endocarditis is not established. These patients usually have had a history of infection such as pharyngitis or infected laceration, or they are drug addicts.

The aneurysms are caused by infected emboli reaching the cerebral circulation and are most often located on a distal branch of an intracranial artery, usually a branch of the middle cerebral artery. This tends to differentiate this type of aneurysm from the more common developmental aneurysm that usually is found on the circle of Willis or the proximal middle cerebral artery.

Neurologic problems are frequent in patients with bacterial endocarditis and may be the presenting symptoms. Jones et al.[15] found neurologic symptoms in 29 percent (110 of 385) and

Neurosurgical Service, Massachusetts General Hospital, and Department of Surgery, Harvard Medical School, Boston, Massachusetts

Portions of this chapter are reprinted with permission from Ojemann RG, Crowell RM: Surgical Management of Cerebrovascular Disease (Baltimore, Williams and Wilkins).

Pruitt et al.[53] in 39 percent (84 of 218) of patients with bacterial endocarditis. The majority of patients have evidence of cerebral embolism with infarction, but hemorrhage (subarachnoid or intracerebral) and infarction followed by hemorrhage may occur. A few patients have had brain abscess or meningitis. Occasionally, headache has been noted without evidence of hemorrhage.[17]

Intracranial bacterial aneurysms occur in 4 to 10 percent of patients with bacterial endocarditis.[3] The incidence may be even higher since some aneurysms are asymptomatic. Multiple aneurysms occur in up to 20 percent of the patients with an aneurysm, but the true figure is unknown since very few patients have had full angiographic studies. The lesions may occur at any age.

When a patient with endocarditis develops a bacterial aneurysm it usually presents with signs and symptoms of subarachnoid or intracerebral hemorrhage. Patients without a previous diagnosis of bacterial endocarditis may have the onset of hemorrhage from a bacterial aneurysm as the first manisfestation of the disease. Another clinical group are those patients who first present with symptoms and signs of cerebral ischemia but are found to have an aneurysm when the neurologic deficit caused by the infarct is investigated by angiography, or who initially have clinical evidence of cerebral infarction and then days to weeks later develop a subarachnoid or intracerebral hemorrhage from an aneurysm.[53] Recurrent hemorrhage occurs, but the incidence is unknown.

In the reports of the 81 patients we reviewed with bacterial aneurysms caused by endocarditis and documented by angiography, 65 had enough clinical information to determine the probable initial neurologic event that led to the angiogram. This was definite or probable hemorrhage in 42, infarction in 16, infarction followed by hemorrhage in 5, and headache without hemorrhage in 2 (Table 61-1). In the 16 patients with ruptured aneurysms reported by Pruitt et al.,[53] 8 had a history suggesting embolization and infarction before the hemorrhage. At angiography an occluded vessel often was found in association with the aneurysm.

The most frequent organism cultured in patients with bacterial aneurysms caused by endocarditis has been the streptococcus (Table 61-2). Staphylococcus, however, has become a more common organism in the reports during the past few years. In some cases no organisms can be isolated from the blood culture because of effective prophylactic treatment or the use of broad-spectrum antibiotics in patients with a febrile illness. In spite of the improvement in the recovery rate from infectious endocarditis because of the effective use of antibiotics, the incidence of neurologic complications of the disease has not been significantly reduced.[17,37] It is important to note that aneurysms can develop and hemorrhage can occur in a patient who is receiving adequate antibiotic treatment.

Diagnostic Studies

When there is evidence to suggest subarachnoid hemorrhage in a patient with bacterial endocarditis, a computerized tomographic (CT) scan followed by cerebral angiography should be done. It has been suggested that the presence of cerebral embolization during the course of bacterial endocarditis is a strong indication for cerebral angiography.[23]

The CT scan should be done with and without contrast enhancement. It may localize the aneurysm either directly or by demonstrating adjacent hematoma. The extent of intracerebral or intraventricular hemorrhage is determined. Associated changes in adjacent cerebral tissue caused by edema, infarction, or abscess and the degree of hydrocephalus will be seen.

Angiography is the definitive study in outlining the location and relationship of the aneurysm to the parent vessel (Figs. 61-1A and B). If the diagnosis of associated subarachnoid hemorrhage is in doubt or if meningitis is suspected, a lumbar puncture is indicated after the CT scan has been done.

The predominant involvement of the middle cerebral artery and a distal intracranial branch when any artery is involved is striking (Table 61-3). In the 71 patients in which the site of the an-

Table 61-1. Clinical Presentation of 81 Patients with Bacterial Intracranial Aneurysms Associated with Definite or Probable Endocarditis and Documented by Angiography, 1959–1980

Finding	Number of patients
Hemorrhage	42
Infarction	16
Infarction followed by hemorrhage	5
Headache without hemorrhage	2
Not enough information	16
Total	81

giographically proven bacterial aneurysms was definitely established on the initial angiogram, 64 had at least one aneurysm on a distal branch of an intracranial artery and in 55 a middle cerebral artery branch was involved. Very few patients have had complete angiographic studies, so the true incidence of multiple aneurysms is unknown.

In 27 patients who had not had surgery, follow-up angiography was performed within a few days to 8 months after the first study, but usually within 2 to 8 weeks. A few patients had more than one follow-up study. In 8 patients a new aneurysm was found; 3 of these had a normal initial angiogram. At the time of the last angiographic study, the aneurysm was no longer visualized in 8, was smaller in 5, unchanged in 4, larger in 6, and in 4 a new aneurysm was found but no further study was reported. Seven other patients had postoperative angiography. The original aneurysm was gone in all cases, but 1 patient had a new aneurysm on the distal middle cerebral artery that had ruptured.

Treatment

A program of treatment for patients with bacterial intracranial aneurysms can be outlined based on a review of the literature.[2,3,5,11,28,53] Medical treatment should include the administration of appropriate intravenous antibiotics and the use of steroids and other medical measures to reduce cerebral edema when indicated. The use of antifibrinolytic agents has not been studied in this illness.

The place of surgical treatment has been discussed in recent reports. Bingham[11] reviewed 45 cases of bacterial intracranial aneurysms of all types where it was thought that adequate antibiotic treatment had been given and where angiography had been done. He concluded that there did not appear to be a clear-cut advantage to surgery plus antibiotics over antibiotics alone. Twenty patients received antibiotic treatment only, but 3 died from hemorrhage while under treatment. In the 25 patients who had combined antibiotic and surgical treatment, 6 died, but most of these were poor risk patients. In fact, he noted that the mortality associated with a defin

Table 61-2. Bacteria Cultured from Specimens in 81 Patients with Bacterial Intracranial Aneurysms Associated with Definite or Probable Endocarditis and Documented by Angiography, 1959–1980

Bacteria	Number of patients
Streptococcus	36
Staphylococcus	15
Pseudomonas	2
Enterococcus	1
Corynebacterium	1
Cardiobacterium	1
Multiple	4
No growth	10
No information	11

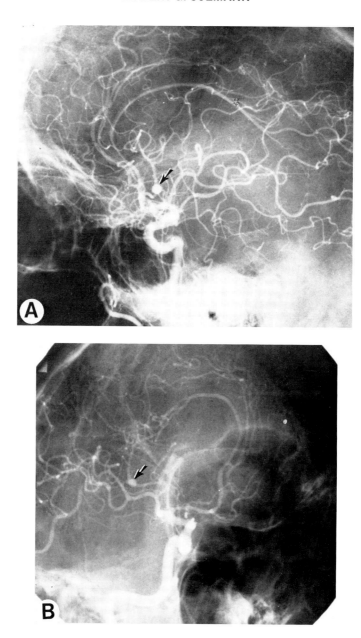

Fig. 61-1. Lateral **(A)** and oblique **(B)** angiograms showing a bacterial intracranial aneurysm (arrows) on a distal branch of the middle cere-
bral artery. Between 75 and 80 percent of these aneurysms occur
on a distal branch of the middle cerebral artery.

itive surgical procedure for a bacterial intracranial aneurysm on a distal arterial branch appears
to be quite low if one eliminates the poor risk surgical candidates. The deaths in this series were
due to cardiac or other medical problems and fatal hemorrhage from a second previously undi-
agnosed aneurysm. He recommended an operation only if the aneurysm enlarged or did not
change in size after 6 weeks of antibiotic therapy. Bohmfalk et al.[3] reviewed reports of 17 patients who had surgical removal of bacterial aneurysms of distal arterial branches. There was no
mortality. He also noted 6 patients in the literature who did not develop hemorrhage until after
completion of their antibiotic treatment for endocarditis. Cantu et al.[4] reported an autopsy se-

Table 61-3. Findings on the Initial Angiogram in 81 Patients with Bacterial Intracranial Aneurysms Associated with Definite or Probable Endocarditis, 1959–1980

Location of Aneurysm	Number of patients
Single	
Distal middle cerebral artery	44
Distal anterior cerebral artery	3
Distal posterior cerebral artery	4
Proximal intracranial artery	7
Middle cerebral artery—unspecified	3
Total	61
Multiple	
Distal middle cerebral artery only	4
Distal middle cerebral artery and other vessels	7
Combinations not including middle cerebral artery	2
Unspecified	2
Total	15
No aneurysm seen	5
Occluded artery in addition to aneurysm	13

ries of 5 patients in whom death was caused by rupture of a bacterial aneurysm; all had been receiving intensive antibiotic therapy at the time of the hemorrhage.[4] Pruitt et al.[53] reported 9 patients who were adequately treated with antibiotics before aneurysmal ruptures. Frazee et al.[5] concluded that patients with a diagnosis of bacterial endocarditis who develop sudden severe headache, focal neurologic signs, or symptoms or seizures should undergo serial angiography every 7 to 10 days throughout their hospitalization. If an aneurysm is identified, it should be excised whenever possible.

The results of a review of the literature of 81 patients who had angiography because of a neurologic symptom and were found to have a bacterial aneurysm are outlined in Table 61-4. In 30 patients treated with antibiotics where the outcome was known, 13 died. Elective surgery was done in 29 patients; 2 died, but in both instances they recovered from the surgery only to die from rupture of a second unrecognized aneurysm. As would be expected in situations where emergency surgery was required, usually because of an intracranial hematoma that had caused a serious neurologic deficit, the results were worse.

In planning the surgical treatment, it is important to remember that these aneurysms have an inflamed, friable wall that may easily fragment. In the peripheral lesions, the aneurysm can be excised with the small vessel from which it arises, usually with little or no neurologic deficit. The less common proximal or less accessible lesions may present a more serious technical problem. Treatment with antibiotics may allow the arteritis to resolve and some reparative fibrosis to take place in the wall of the aneurysm and the parent artery. The lesions then can be handled more safely at surgery.[28] If surgery is needed for a proximal lesion, a bypass graft may be required as the initial procedure.

A single aneurysm on a distal branch of the middle cerebral artery associated with subarachnoid or intracerebral hemorrhage should be excised if the medical condition of the patient is stable. For bacterial aneurysms on the proximal arterial trunks, unruptured aneurysms or those involving arteries whose excision is very likely to cause a serious neurologic deficit, a program of antibiotics and serial angiography is indicated. How often the angiogram should be done has not been established and has ranged from one to several weeks. If the aneurysm is larger at follow-up angiography, surgery is indicated. If it is the same size or smaller, the antibiotic treatment should be continued. Angiography is repeated at an appropriate interval and again when antibiotic treatment is completed. If the aneurysm does not disappear after treatment or at any time becomes larger, surgery usually is indicated.

The literature does not give a definitive answer to the question of what to do with the patient

Table 61-4. Treatment and Results in 81 Patients with Bacterial Intracranial Aneurysms Associated with Definite or Probable Endocarditis and Documented by Angiography, 1959–1980

Treatment	Results			
	Recovered*	Died	No information	Total
Antibiotics	17	13	1	31
Elective surgery**	27	2	—	29
Emergency surgery**	8	6	—	14
No treatment	1	1	1	3
No information	—	—	4	4

*Some patients who recovered from their neurologic illness subsequently died from a cardiac cause and some were left with a neurologic disability.
**Patients who had surgery also received antibiotics.

when multiple bacterial aneurysms are found. A review of 15 reported cases of multiple bacterial aneurysms caused by a variety of factors including meningitis revealed that 11 were treated non-surgically and none died as a direct result of this treatment.[5] Analysis of reports of 10 patients with multiple bacterial aneurysms seen on angiography and related to established or probable endocarditis revealed that 7 were treated by antibiotics alone with only 1 death.[2] This was a patient who also was a heroin addict and who had a brain abscess and infarction. There is no explanation for the findings of a low mortality rate with antibiotic therapy alone compared with the higher mortality rate for patients treated nonsurgically with a single aneurysm. We have already noted, however, that 2 patients who had recovered from elective surgery for removal of a single aneurysm subsequently died because of hemorrhage from a second unrecognized aneurysm. Frazee et al.[5] proposed that if multiple aneurysms are unilateral they should be excised at one operation wherever possible, and if they are bilateral, the largest aneurysm or the one presumed to have bled should be excised and the patient then followed by angiography. Another plan is to treat the patient with antibiotics and repeat the angiogram at 2-week intervals and when therapy is completed. If the lesions become larger or do not disappear after treatment, surgery may be indicated.

At the time of surgery the neurosurgeon may encounter not only an intracerebral hematoma or an area of infarction but also a brain abscess. In the series of cases reviewed 5 patients had associated brain abscess.

Conclusions

Even though there has been progress in the diagnosis and treatment of bacterial endocarditis, neurologic symptoms are frequent and bacterial aneurysms are a cause of morbidity and mortality. CT scans and angiography are indicated in patients suspected of having a bacterial intracranial aneurysm. The finding of an aneurysm on a distal intracranial arterial branch, especially of the middle cerebral artery, is strongly suggestive of an infectious etiology. A single bacterial aneurysm on a distal branch of the middle cerebral artery that has ruptured should be excised if the medical condition of the patient is stable. A bacterial aneurysm that is enlarging or does not disappear after antibiotic treatment also should be excised whenever possible. A definitive plan for treating unruptured bacterial aneurysms, those involving proximal arterial trunks, and multiple bacterial aneurysms has not been established.

REFERENCES

1. Osler W: Gulstonian lectures on malignant endocarditis. *Lancet 1*:415–418, 459–464, 505–508, 1885
2. Ojemann RG: Infectious intracranial aneurysms, in Fein J Flamm E (eds): *Cerebral Vascular Disease* (in press)

3. Bohmfalk GL, Story JL, Wissinger JP, et al.: Bacterial intracranial aneurysm. *J Neurosurg 48*:369–382, 1978

4. Cantu RC, LeMay M, Wilkinson HA: The importance of repeated angiography in the treatment of mycotic-embolic intracranial aneurysms. *J Neurosurg 25*:189–193, 1966

5. Frazee JG, Cahan LD, Winter J: Bacterial intracranial aneurysms. *J Neurosurg 53*:633–641, 1980

6. Hourihane JB: Ruptured mycotic intracranial aneurysm. A report of three cases. *Vasc Surg 4*:21–29, 1970

7. Agnoli A, Bettag W: Endokarditis und subarachnoidalblutung. *Z Neurol 199*:295–305, 1971

8. Alajouanine T, Castaigne P, Lhermitte F, et al: Cerebral arteritis of bacterial endocarditis: its late complications. *JAMA 170*:1858, 1959

9. Amine ARC: Neurosurgical complications of heroin addiction: brain abscess and mycotic aneurysm. *Surg Neurol 7*:385–386, 1977

10. Bell WE, Butler C II: Cerebral mycotic aneurysms in children. Two case reports. *Neurology 18*:81–86, 1968

11. Bingham WF: Treatment of mycotic intracranial aneurysms. *J Neurosurg 46*:428–437, 1977

12. Gilroy J, Andaya L, Thomas VJ: Intracranial mycotic aneurysms and subacute bacterial endocarditis in heroin addiction. *Neurology 23*:1193–1198, 1973

13. Harrison MJG, Hampton JR: Neurological presentation of bacterial endocarditis. *Br Med J 2*:148–151, 1967

14. Ishikawa M, Waga S, Moritake K, et al: Cerebral bacterial aneurysms: report of three cases. *Surg Neurol 2*:257–261, 1974

15. Jones HR Jr, Siekert RG, Geraci JE: Neurologic manifestations of bacterial endocarditis. *Ann Intern Med 71*:21–28, 1969

16. Katz RI, Goldberg HI, Selzer ME: Mycotic aneurysm. Case report with novel sequential angiographic findings. *Arch Intern Med 134*:939–942, 1974

17. Kaufman SL, White RI, Harrington DP, et al: Protean manifestations of mycotic aneurysm. *AJR 131*:1019–1025, 1978

18. King AB: Successful surgical treatment of an intracranial mycotic aneurysm complicated by a subdural hematoma. *J Neurosurg 17*:788–791, 1960

19. Laguna J, Derby BM, Chase R: Cardiobacterium hominis endocarditis with cerebral mycotic aneurysm. *Arch Neurol 32*:638–639, 1975

20. Matson DD: Intracranial arterial aneurysms in childhood. *J Neurosurg 23*:578–583, 1965

21. McNeel D, Evans RA, Ory EM: Angiography of cerebral mycotic aneurysms. *Acta Radiol (Diagn) 9*:407–412, 1969

22. Morin MA, Talalla A: Angiography for mycotic aneurysm (letter). *N Engl J Med 281*:1249–1250, 1969

23. Moskowitz MA, Rosenbaum AE, Tyler HR: Angiographically monitored resolution of cerebral mycotic aneurysms. *Neurology 24*:1103–1108, 1974

24. Ng KK, Wong WK, Skene-Smith H: Ruptured mycotic intracranial aneurysm. *Australas Radiol 19*:255–257, 1975

25. Noonan JA, Wilson CB, Spencer FC, et al: Cerebral and cardiac complications from bacterial endocarditis. A successfully managed case with unusual complications. *Am J Dis Child 116*:666–674, 1968

26. North-Coombes D, Schonland MM: Cerebral mycotic aneurysm. A case report. *S Afr Med J 48*:1808–1810, 1974

27. Pool JL, and Potts DG: *Aneurysm and Arteriovenous Anomalies of the Brain.* New York, Harper and Row, 1965, pp 60–62

28. Roach MR, Drake CG: Ruptured corobral aneurysms caused by micro-organisms. *N Engl J Med 273*:240–244, 1965

29. Schold C, Earnest MP: Cerebral hemorrhage from a mycotic aneurysm developing during appropriate antibiotic therapy. *Stroke 9*:267–268, 1978

30. Tanemura H, Sakai N, Yamamori T, et al: Intracranial mycotic aneurysm—report of a case. *Neurol Surg (Tokyo) 5*:871–875, 1977

31. Yarnell PR, Stears J: Intracerebral hemorrhage and occult sepsis. *Neurology 24*:870–873, 1974

32. Ziment I, Johnson BL Jr: Angiography in the management of intracranial mycotic aneurysms. *Arch Intern Med 122*:349–352, 1968

33. Harrison MJG, Hampton JR: Neurological presentation of bacterial endocarditis. *Br Med J 2*:148–151, 1967

34. Ojemann RG, New PFJ, Fleming TC: Intracranial aneurysms associated with bacterial meningitis. *Neurology 16*:1222–1226, 1966

35. Suwanwela C, Suwanwela N, Charuchinda S, et al: Intracranial mycotic aneurysms of extra-vascular origin. *J Neurosurg 36*:552–559, 1972

36. Sypert GW, Young HF: Ruptured mycotic pericallosal aneurysm with meningitis due to Neisseria meningitidis infection. Case report. *J Neurosurg 37*:467–469, 1972

37. Lansky LL, Maxwell JA: Mycotic aneurysm of the internal carotid artery in an unusual intracranial location. *Dev Med Child Neurol 17*:79–88, 1975

38. Shibuya S, Igarashi S, Amo T, et al: Mycotic aneurysms of the internal carotid artery. Case report. *J Neurosurg* 44:105–108, 1976

39. Ahuja GK, Jain N, Vijayaraghaven M, et al: Cerebral mycotic aneurysm of fungal origin. *J Neurosurg* 49:107–110, 1978

40. Davidson P, Robertson DM: A true mycotic (Aspergillus) aneurysm leading to fatal subarachnoid hemorrhage in a patient with hereditary hemorrhagic telangiectasia. Case report. *J Neurosurg* 35:71–76, 1971

41. Horten BC, Abbott GF, Porro RS: Fungal aneurysms of intracranial vessels. *Arch Neurol* 33:577–570, 1976

42. Mahaley MS, Spock A: An unusual case of intracranial aneurysm, in Smith JL (ed): *Neuro-ophthalmology,* vol 4. St. Louis, CV Mosby, 1968, pp 148–166

43. Visudhiphan P, Bunyaratavej S, Khantanaphar S: Cerebral aspergillosis. Report of 3 cases. *J Neurosurg* 38:472–476, 1973

44. Almazan V, Pulpin A, Galnan D, et al: Mycotic aneurysm secondary to bacterial endocarditis. *Arch Inst Cardiol Mex* 48:1224–32, 1978

45. Grinberg M, Lage SH, DeAlmcida GG: Infective endocarditis, cerebral mycotic aneurysm and meningeal hemorrhage. *Arq Bras Cardiol* 32:257–61, 1979

46. Jara FM, Lewis JF, Magilligan DG: Operative experience with infective endocarditis and intracerebral mycotic aneurysm. *J Thorac Cardiovasc Surg* 80:28–30, 1980

47. Maly Z: Paraventricular hemorrhage from a mycotic aneurysm. *Cesk Neurol Neurochir* 41:394–396, 1978

48. Nishimura T, Aoko N, Aruga T, et al: Case of mycotic aneurysm after open heart surgery. *No Shinkei Geka* 7:371–376, 1979

49. Sato T, Sakuta Y, Suzuki J, et al: Successful surgical treatment of intracranial mycotic aneurysm with brain abscess. *Acta Neurochir (Wien)* 47:53–61, 1979

50. Shillito J Jr: Strokes in children. *Clin Neurosurg* 23:185–219, 1976

51. Simmons KC, Sage MR, Reilly PL: CT of intracerebral hemorrhage due to mycotic aneurysm—case report. *Neuroradiology* 19:215–217, 1980

52. Valadares JB, DeSouza MT, Hankinson J, et al: Multiple intracranial mycotic aneurysms—Case report. *Arq Neuropsiquiatr* 37:311–318, 1979

53. Pruitt AA, Rubin RH, Karchmer AW, et al: Neurologic complications of bacterial endocarditis. *Medicine* 57:329–343, 1978

CHAPTER 62
Surgical Management of Traumatic Aneurysms

Dwight Parkinson

TRAUMATIC INTRACRANIAL ANEURYSMS are exceedingly rare.[1-66] Excluding intracavernous carotid aneurysms, Laun et al.[35] collected 73 cases from the world literature, including 3 from their own total of 450 aneurysms. We have collected 13 cases among our last 6,000 head injuries. In this series there were 281 extracerebral hematomas and 112 traumatic intracerebral hematomas. Considering this incidence of the intra- and extracerebral hemorrhage, it is evident that the rarity of traumatic aneurysms is not because the intracranial arteries are well protected from trauma. These aneurysms may result from blunt or penetrating head trauma,[13,14,16,20,25,39] (including iatrogenic penetrations[1,7,12,25,29,31,34,41,42,45,46,48,49,66,67]) and over 90 percent occur in association with a skull fracture.[23,26,55,56,60] Occasionally the aneurysm is partially trapped in the fracture line.[8,23,30,33] Aneurysms of the pericallosal artery probably arise after these arteries are injured by the edge of the falx.

Infratentorial traumatic aneurysms constitute no more than 5 percent of the total reported.[6,15,45,47] Saccular and arteriovenous aneurysms of the middle meningeal artery are surprisingly few considering the intimate relationship between this artery and bone.[21,27,29,30,33,35,36,41,44,45,51,64,68]

Some authors have categorized saccular traumatic aneurysms into either "true" or "false,"[8,11,23,31] and "mixed" or "dissecting" types.[54,65] Their criteria for a so-called "true" traumatic aneurysm is disruption of the arterial wall with only the adventitia left intact.[12,17,40,48] This differs from the true saccular aneurysm, which contains both intima and adventitia in its wall. Their "false" aneurysms result from full-thickness lacerations that are occluded by hematoma, which subsequently organizes and excavates to leave a saccular defect with none of the normal arterial structures in the wall.[12,19,21,46,47,52,69] "Mixed" aneurysms result from the posttraumatic rupture of a "true" aneurysm, which produces a secondary "false" aneurysm,[12] and a "dissecting" aneurysm results from the formation of a false lumen between the intima and the elastica.[54,65,70,71]

Signs and Symptoms

The cases of delayed apoplexy following head injury that were reported by Bollinger[72] may well have been due to traumatic aneurysms, although his explanation for these cases was focal brain softening and delayed hemorrhage from the unsupported and injured blood vessels. Aside from persistent headache (not always present) and the delayed deterioration following head injury, there are few clinical features that point to the diagnosis, which can only be established by angio-

Section of Neurosurgery, University of Manitoba, Winnipeg, Canada

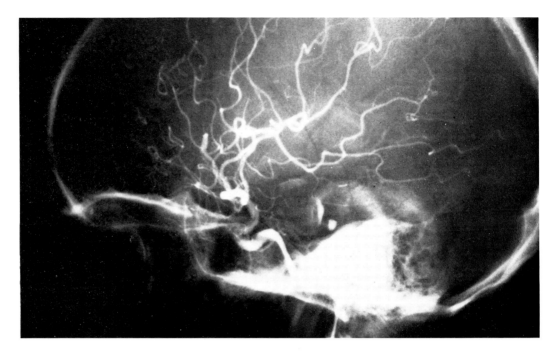

Fig. 62-1. A right carotid angiogram. The lower arrow points to a meniscus in a false aneurysm on the posterior branch of the middle meningeal artery. A second smaller globular false aneurysm can be seen behind and beneath the arrow tip. The upper arrow indicates a wide stellate temporal-parietal fracture. (Reprinted with permission from Parkinson D: Traumatic intracranial aneurysms. *J Neurosurg 52*:11–20, 1980.)

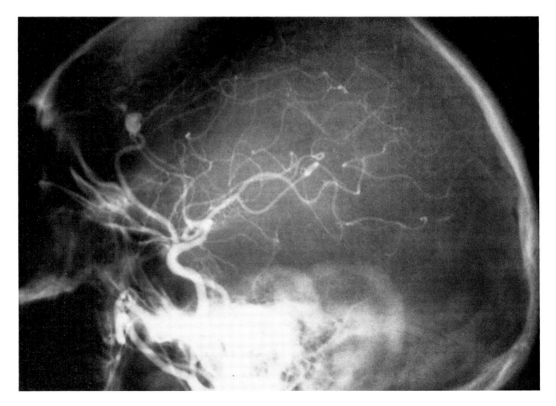

Fig. 62-2. A traumatic aneurysm on the callosal artery. The artery presumably was damaged by impingement against the edge of the falx.

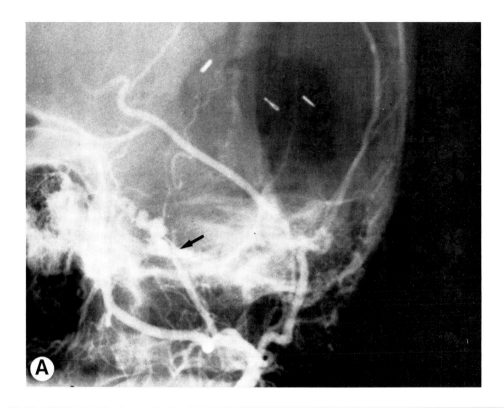

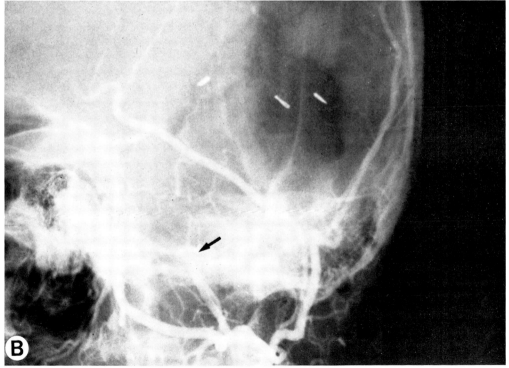

Fig. 62-3.   **A.** An intraoperative angiogram (oblique view). The black arrow points to an arteriovenous fistula coming from the middle meningeal artery. **B.** An intraoperative angiogram of the same case in Figure 62-3A showing the site of obliteration of the
arteriovenous fistula, which was accomplished by embolization and cautery. (Reprinted with permission from Parkinson D: Traumatic intracranial aneurysms. *J
Neurosurg 52*:11–20, 1980

grams of the common carotid artery.[12,17,23,34,45,46,49,61,73] These aneurysms usually enlarge progressively, but occasionally they may decrease in size or even spontaneously disappear.[6,12,17,23,34,46]

The angiographic features differentiating the traumatic from the common saccular aneurysm are: 1. Delayed filling and emptying of the aneurysmal sac (Fig. 62-1). 2. A peripheral location of the aneurysm at a site other than a branching point (Fig. 62-2). 3. Irregular contour (Fig. 62-2). 4. The absence of a neck (Fig. 62-2).[8,12,33,59,60,70] The increasing reliance on CT scanning and the decreasing use of angiography in evaluating the patient with a head injury will result in an unfortunate number of these aneurysms being missed. Early diagnosis is most important. Patients diagnosed after rupture have a mortality almost three times as high as those diagnosed before rupture.[23] The surgical mortality recorded in the literature averages 24 percent, while the untreated cases have a mortality approaching 50 percent.[45] Because of the superficial nature of these lesions, the operative mortality should be negligible and result from the extent of the associated brain damage sustained with the original trauma. Unfortunately, they are rarely recognized until their presence is heralded by delayed deterioration, by which time the salvage rate is halved. Earlier recognition can only be accomplished by a higher degree of suspicion and the increased use of angiography.

Treatment

The treatment is surgical. Although superficial, most of these lesions are frequently invisible beneath the surface, and may be difficult to find, particularly if associated with a large intracerebral hematoma. If the aneurysm is not immediately apparent, it is located very easily by placing one or two metallic clips in the suspected area for reference, and then performing an introperative angiogram, whereupon the relationship of the sac to these clips becomes immediately evident.[74] This saves time and the unnecessary destruction of tissue. The arteriovenous malformations usually are easier to find lying within the dura associated with a fracture line. Intraoperative angiography provides the surgeon with the immediate assurance that the lesion has been obliterated (Fig. 62-3).

In the future, some of the saccular lesions possibly will be amenable to excision with direct repair of the cerebral artery by graft or end-to-end anastomosis,[75] but at this time, obliteration has only been accomplished by clipping or coagulating the parent vessel as it enters the aneurysm (see Figs. 62-1 and 62-2).

The recognition of these potentially fatal lesions rose significantly during the era of angiography, with a corresponding decrease in the mortality rate. It is hoped that the trend will not be reversed as we move into the era of the CT scan, and angiography tends to be pushed aside.

REFERENCES

1. Acosta C, William PE Jr, Clark K: Traumatic aneurysms of the cerebral vessels. *J Neurosurg* *36*:531–536, 1972
2. Alexander E Jr, Adams JE, Davis CH Jr: Complications in the use of temporary intracranial arterial clip. *J Neurosurg 20*:810–811, 1963
3. Ameli NO: Aneurysms of the middle meningeal artery. *J Neurol Neurosurg Psychiatry 28*:175–178, 1965
4. Araki C, Handa H, Handa J, et al: Traumatic aneurysm of the intracranial extradural portion of the internal carotid artery. Report of a case. *J Neurosurg 23*:64–67, 1965
5. Asari S, Nakamura S, Yamada O, et al: Traumatic aneurysm of peripheral cerebral arteries. Report of two cases. *J Neurosurg 46*:795–803, 1977
6. Bank WO, Nelson PB, Drayer BP, et al: Traumatic aneurysm of the basilar artery. *AJR 130*:975–977, 1978
7. Barrett JH, Lawrence VL: Aneurysms of the internal carotid artery as a complication of mastoidectomy. *Arch Otolaryngol 72*:366–368, 1960
8. Benoit BG, Wortzman G: Traumatic cerebral aneurysms. Clinical features and natural history. *J Neurol Neurosurg Psychiatry 36*:127–138, 1973

9. Bergstrom K, Hemmingsson A: False cortical aneurysm in subdural haematoma following head injury without fracture. *Acta Radiol (Diagn) 14*:657–661, 1973

10. Birley JL, Trotter W: Traumatic aneurysm of the intracranial portion of the internal carotid artery. *Brain 51*:184–208, 1928

11. Brihaye J, Mage J, Verhiest G: Aneurysme traumatique de la carotide interne dans sa portion supraclinoidienne. *Acta Neurol Psychiatr Belg 54*:411–438, 1954

12. Burton C, Velasco F, Dorman J: Traumatic aneurysm of a peripheral cerebral artery. Review and case report. *J Neurosurg 28*:468–474, 1968

13. Carothers A: Orbitofacial wounds and cerebral artery injuries caused by umbrella tips. *JAMA 239*:1151–1152, 1978

14. Chadduck WM: Traumatic cerebral aneurysm due to speargun injury. Case report. *J Neurosurg 31*:77–79, 1969

15. Cockrill HH Jr, Jimenez JP, Goree JA: Traumatic false aneurysm of the superior cerebellar artery simulating posterior fossa tumor. Case report. *J Neurosurg 46*:377–380, 1977

16. Courville CB: Traumatic aneurysm of an intracranial artery. Description of a lesion incident to a shotgun wound of the skull and brain. *Bull Los Angeles Neurol Soc 25*:48–54, 1960

17. Cressman MR, Hayes GJ: Traumatic aneurysm of the anterior choroidal artery. Case report. *J Neurosurg 24*:102–104, 1966

18. Drake CG: Subdural haematoma from arterial rupture. *J Neurosurg 18*:597–601, 1961

19. Eichler A, Story JL, Bennett DE, et al: Traumatic aneurysm of a cerebral artery. Case report. *J Neurosurg 31*:72–76, 1969

20. Ferry DJ Jr, Kempe LG: False aneurysm secondary to penetration of the brain through orbitofacial wounds. Report of two cases. *J Neurosurg 36*:503–506, 1972

21. Fincher EF: Arteriovenous fistula between the middle meningeal artery and the greater petrosal sinus. Case report. *Ann Surg 133*:886–888, 1951

22. Finkemeyer H: Ein sackchenformiges Aneurysma der A. cerebri media als postoperative Komplikation. *Zentralbl Neurochir 15*:302–315, 1955

23. Fleischer AS, Patton JM, Tindall GT: Cerebral aneurysms of traumatic origin. *Surg Neurol 4*:233–239, 1975

24. Go KG, Penning L, Oen TS: Acute subdural haematoma in connection with angiographically demonstrated traumatic rupture of a cortical cerebral artery (presenting as false aneurysm). Report of two cases. *Neuroradiology 2*:107–110, 1971

25. Goald HJ, Ronderos A: Traumatic perforation of the intracranial portion of the internal carotid artery with eleven-day survival. Case report. *J Neurosurg 18*:401–404, 1961

26. Handa J, Shimizu Y, Matsuda M, et al: Traumatic aneurysm of the middle cerebral artery. *Am J Roentgenol Radium Ther Nucl Med 109*:127–129, 1970

27. Handa J, Shimizu Y, Sato K, et al: Traumatic aneurysm and arteriovenous fistula of the middle meningeal artery. *Clin Radiol 21*:39–41, 1970

28. Handel SF, Perpetuo FOL, Handel CH: Subdural hematomas due to ruptured cerebral aneurysms: Angiographic diagnosis and potential pitfall for CT. *AJR 130*:507–509, 1978

29. Higazi I, El-Banhawy A, El-Nady F: Importance of angiography in identifying false aneurysm of the middle meningeal artery as a cause of extradural hematoma. Case report. *J Neurosurg 30*:172–176, 1969

30. Jackson DC, du Boulay GH: Traumatic arterio-venous aneurysm of the middle meningeal artery. *Br J Radiol 37*:788–789, 1964

31. Jackson FE, Gleave JRW, Janon E: The traumatic cranial and intracranial aneurysms, in Vinken PJ, Bruyn GW (eds): *Handbook of Clinical Neurology,* vol. 24. Amsterdam, North-Holland, 1976, pp 381–398

32. Krauland W: Zur Entstehung traumatischer Aneurysmen der Schlagadern am Hirngrund. *Schweiz Z Pathol Bakt 12*:113–127, 1949

33. Kuhn RA, Kugler H: False aneurysms of the middle meningeal artery. *J Neurosurg 21*:92–96, 1964

34. Lassman LP, Ramani PS, Sengupta RP: Aneurysms of peripheral cerebral arteries due to surgical trauma. *Vasc Surg 8*:1–5, 1974

35. Laun A: Survey of traumatic aneurysms, in Pia HW, Langmaid C, Zierski J (eds): *Cerebral Aneurysms: Advances in Diagnosis and Therapy.* Berlin, Springer-Verlag, 1979, pp 364–375

36. Locksley HB: Report on the cooperative study of intracranial aneurysms and subarachnoid hemorrhage. Section V, Part 1. Natural history of subarachnoid hemorrhage, intracranial aneurysms and arteriovenous malformations. Based on 6,368 cases in the cooperative study. *J Neurosurg 25*:219–239, 1966

37. Lukin R, Chambers A: Traumatic aneurysm of peripheral cerebral artery. *Neuroradiology 8*:1–3, 1974

38. Martinez SN, Bertrand C, Thierry A: Les faux anévrismes posttraumatiques. *Can J Surg 9*:397–402, 1966

39. Maurer JJ, Mills M, German WJ: Triad of unilateral blindness, orbital fractures and massive epistaxis after head injury. *J Neurosurg 18*:837–840, 1961

40. Melvill RL, De Villiers JC: Peripheral cerebral arterial aneurysms caused by stabbing. *S Afr Med J* 51:471–473, 1977

41. Menezes AH, Graf CJ: True traumatic aneurysm of anterior cerebral artery. Case report. *J Neurosurg* 40:544–548, 1974

42. Nakamura K, Tsugane R, Ito H, et al: Traumatic arterio-venous fistula of the middle meningeal vessels. *J Neurosurg* 25:424–429, 1966

43. Overton MC III, Calvin TH Jr: Iatrogenic cerebral cortical aneurysm. Case report. *J Neurosurg* 24:672–675, 1966

44. Paillas JE, Bonnal J, Lavieille J: Angiographic images of false aneurysmal sac caused by rupture of median meningeal artery in the course of traumatic extradural hematomata. Report of 3 cases. *J Neurosurg* 21:667–671, 1964

45. Parkinson D, West M: Traumatic intracranial aneurysms. *J Neurosurg* 52:11–20, 1980

46. Perret G, Nishioka H: Report on the cooperative study of intracranial aneurysms and subarachnoid hemorrhage. Section VI. Arteriovenous malformations. An analysis of 545 cases of cranio-cerebral arteriovenous malformations and fistulae reported to the cooperative study. *J Neurosurg* 25:467–490, 1966

47. Petty JM: Epistaxis from aneurysm of the internal carotid artery due to a gunshot wound. Case report. *J Neurosurg* 30:741–743, 1969

48. Raimondi AJ, Yashon D, Reyes C, et al: Intracranial false aneurysms. *Neurochirugia* 11:219–233, 1968

49. Rumbaugh CL, Bergeron RT, Talalla A, et al: Traumatic aneurysms of the cortical cerebral arteries. Radiographic aspects. *Radiology* 96:49–54, 1970

50. Sachdev VP, Drapkin AJ, Hollin SA, et al: Subarachnoid hemorrhage following intranasal procedures. *Surg Neurol* 8:122–125, 1977

51. Sadar ES, Jane JA, Lewis LW, et al: Traumatic aneurysms of the intracranial circulation. *Surg Gynecol Obstet* 137:59–67, 1973

52. Salmon JH, Blatt ES: Aneurysm of the internal carotid artery due to closed trauma. *J Thorac Cardiovasc Surg* 56:28–32, 1968

53. Schechter MM: Angiography in head trauma. *Clin Neurosurg* 12:193–225, 1966

54. Sezimir CB, Occleshaw JV, Buxton PH: False cerebral aneurysm. Case report. *J Neurosurg* 29:636–639, 1968

55. Seftel DM, Kolson H, Gordon BS: Ruptured intracranial carotid artery aneurysm with fatal epistaxis. *Arch Otolaryngol* 70:54–60, 1959

56. Shaw CM, Foltz EL: Traumatic dissecting aneurysm of middle cerebral artery and carotid-cavernous fistula with massive intracerebral hemorrhage. Case report. *J Neurosurg* 28:475–479, 1968

57. Smith DR, Kempe LG: Cerebral false aneurysm formation in closed head trauma. Case report. *J Neurosurg* 32:357–359, 1970

58. Smith S: On the difficulties attending the diagnosis of aneurism being a contribution to surgical diagnosis and medical jurisprudence. *Am J Med Sci* 66:401–409, 1873

59. Stehbens WE: *Pathology of the Cerebral Blood Vessels.* St. Louis, CV Mosby, 1972, pp 452–455

60. Taylor PE: Delayed postoperative hemorrhage from intracranial aneurysm after craniotomy for tumor. *Neurology* 11:225–231, 1961

61. Teal JS, Bergeron RT, Rumbaugh CL, et al: Aneurysms of the petrous or cavernous portions of the internal carotid artery associated with nonpenetrating head trauma. *J Neurosurg* 38:568–574, 1973

62. Thompson JR, Harwood-Nash DC, Fitz CR: Cerebral aneurysms in children. *Am J Roentgenol Radium Ther Nucl Med* 118:163–175, 1973

63. Umebayashi Y, Kuwayama M, Handa J, et al: Traumatic aneurysm of a peripheral cerebral artery: Case report. *Clin Radiol* 21:36–38, 1970

64. Weaver DF, Gates EM, Nielsen AE: Traumatic intracranial vascular lesions producing late massive nasal hemorrhage. *Trans Am Acad Ophthalmol Otolaryngol* 65:759–774, 1961

65. White JC, Sayre GP, Whisnant JP: Experiemental destruction of the media for the production of intracranial arterial aneurysms. *J Neurosurg* 18:741–745, 1961

66. Wilson CB, Cronic F: Traumatic arteriovenous fistulas involving middle meningeal vessels. *JAMA* 188:953–957, 1964

67. Yamaura A, Makino H, Hachisu H, et al: Secondary aneurysm due to arterial injury during surgical procedures. *Surg Neurol* 10:327–333, 1978

68. Pakarinen S: Arteriovenous fistula between the middle meningeal artery and the sphenoparietal sinus. A case report. *J Neurosurg* 23:438–439, 1965

69. Voris HC, Basile JXR: Recurrent epistaxis from aneurysm of the internal carotid artery. Case report with cure by operation. *J Neurosurg* 18:841–842, 1961

70. Smith KR, Bardenheier JA III: Aneurysm of the pericallosal artery caused by closed cranial trauma. Case report. *J Neurosurg* 29:551–554, 1968

71. Wolman L: Cerebral dissecting aneurysms. *Brain* 82:276–291, 1959

72. Bollinger O: Uber traumatische Spat-Apoplexie; ein Bietrag zum Lehre von der Hirnerschutterung. *Festschr Rud Virchow* 2:457–470, 1891

73. Leslie EV, Smith BH, Zoll JG: Value of angiography in head trauma. *Radiology 78*:930–940, 1962

74. Parkinson D, Legal J, Holloway AF, et al: A new combined neurosurgical headholder and cassette changer for intraoperative serial angiography. Technical note. *J Neurosurg 48*:1038–1041, 1978

75. Dolenc V: Treatment of fusiform aneurysms of the peripheral cerebral arteries. Report of two cases. *J Neurosurg 49*:272–277, 1978

CHAPTER 63
Coating of Intracranial Aneurysms with Nontoxic Adherent Plastics

Bertram Selverstone

COATING AN INTRACRANIAL ANEURYSM in order to reinforce its wall is a highly effective technique that is applicable whenever an aneurysm cannot be safely and completely excluded from the circulation by clips or ligatures. If nontoxic adherent plastics are used, coating provides a blood-tight seal that gives immediate protection against bleeding.

Once a decision has been made to expose and deal directly with an intracranial aneurysm, it is desirable, for a number of reasons, to be prepared to coat the aneurysm: (1) Significant arterial branches may arise from the sac, especially in aneurysms of the middle cerebral and anterior communicating arteries (Figs. 63-2A and 63-3A). Coating without clipping thus permits preservation of diencephalic or capsular branches that might otherwise be excluded from the circulation (Figs. 63-2B and 63-3B). (2) Clipping or ligation of the aneurysm may deform and partially occlude the parent vessel or a major branch; this problem has been encountered in aneurysms of the vertebral artery that arose adjacent to the origin of the posterior inferior cerebellar artery (PICA). Coating without clipping was done, with preservation of the PICA. (3) In sessile aneurysms (Fig. 63-1A), it may be impossible to exclude the entire base of the sac from the arterial circulation; the liability of enlargement and rupture persists from the portion proximal to the clip (Fig. 63-1B). Effective placement of a clip may be further limited if an atheromatous plaque is present at the base of the sac. Coating will reinforce areas remaining at risk after a clip has been placed in the best available position (Fig. 63-1C). (4) If an aneurysm can be coated satisfactorily without clipping, the risk of damage to the intima by crushing with subsequent formation of an intraluminal thrombus or embolus is presumably lessened. (5) Even a well-designed and well-placed clip may be dislodged from its site, usually during the early postoperative period; routine coating of the clipped aneurysm and parent vessel will lock the clip in place. (6) Occasionally a neck of an aneurysm is so damaged in the course of dissection or clipping that hemostasis can be obtained only by means of a clip placed precariously on a torn edge or stump. Coating will lock the clip in place and seal the exposed edges of the laceration.

The use of muscle, gauze, or other material to wrap an aneurysm is qualitatively different from reinforcement by adherent plastics. The former techniques cannot be expected to provide an immediate blood-tight seal, since their efficacy depends upon the provocation of a reactive fibrosis. Protection during the high-risk period following an initial hemorrhage is incomplete at best.

Division of Neurosurgery, Brown University, and Division of Neurosurgery, Miriam and Roger Williams Hospitals, Providence, Rhode Island.
The author wishes to thank Lola-Jane Selverstone, who prepared the illustrations.

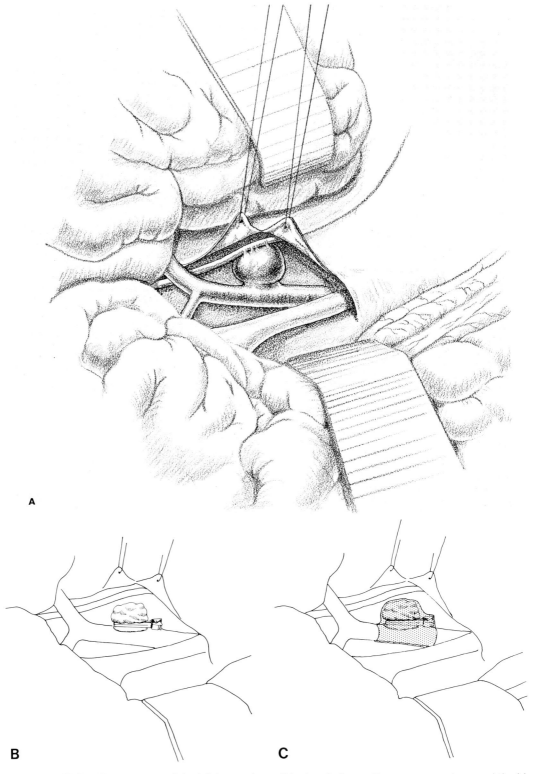

Fig. 63-1. **(A)** Sessile aneurysm of the left internal carotid artery between the cavernous sinus and the bifurcation. The temporal lobe (above) and frontal lobe have been gently displaced. The oculomotor nerve is adherent to the fundus of the aneurysm. **(B)** The aneurysm has been clipped and the oculomotor nerve dissected free. Note that the clip fails to exclude the base of the aneurysm from the arterial circulation. **(C)** The aneurysm, clip, and adjacent artery have been coated with adherent plastics. The base of the aneurysm has been reinforced and the clip secured from slipping.

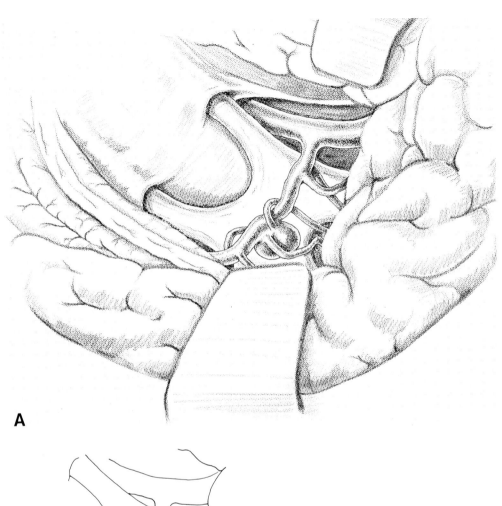

A

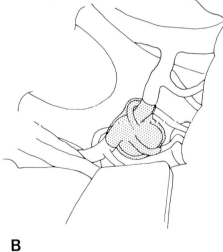

B

Fig. 63-2. **(A)** Aneurysm of the anterior communicating artery complex showing perforating branches close to the sac and A2 segments emerging from the sac. **(B)** Coating with adherent plastics has reinforced the aneurysm without disturbing the A2 branches or the perforators. Circulation through the sac is undisturbed.

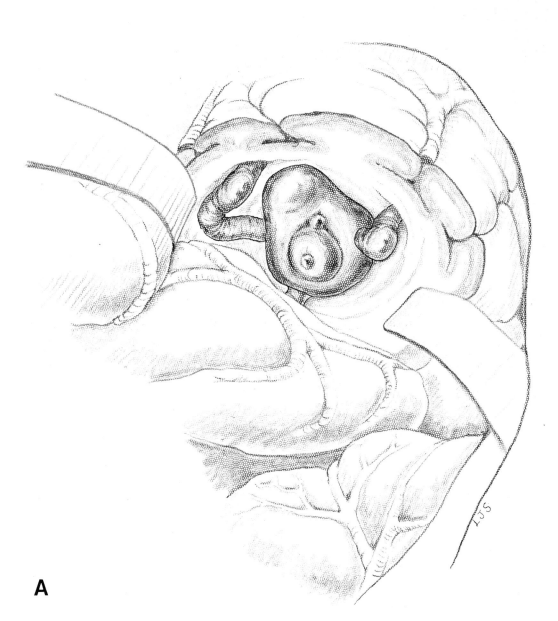

A

Fig. 63-3.   **(A)** Aneurysm of the trifurcation of the middle cerebral artery showing major branches emerging from the sac. Exposure has been obtained through a small plug of cortex near the tip of the superior temporal convolution. Overlying blood clot has been carefully sucked away, exposing the site of bleeding from a daughter aneurysm. **(B)** Coating with adherent plastics has provided adequate reinforcement of the aneurysm without disturbing flow through the sac to major arterial branches.

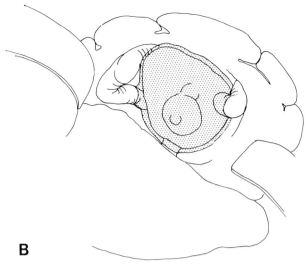

B

Fig. 63-3.   (Cont.)

Coating of Intracranial Aneurysms

The diagnosis, preoperative treatment of the patient, and surgical exposure of aneurysms that are to be coated does not differ from accepted methods employed for other techniques of obliterating these lesions (see Chapters 53–62).

Reinforcement of aneurysms with plastics was first reported in 1956 by Dutton,[3] who used methyl methacrylate to provide an investment about the lesion. Selverstone and associates reported the use of adherent plastics for a similar purpose in 1958 and subsequently.[2,4-9] This basic technique is still employed, although a number of modifications have been made that have reduced the time of polymerization of the plastic from about 45 minutes to 3 to 5 minutes.

Other authors subsequently employed a number of agents,[10,11] but none provides an adherent coating without chemically bonding to the tissue. Such a reaction must inevitably produce a zone of necrosis wherever the agent contacts the adventitia.[12] It thus may be assumed that a dead space ultimately will be present between the adhesive and the adventitia of the aneurysm.

The technique we employ uses two coats. The first layer is an artificial latex that is well tolerated by tissue and, when polymerized in situ by evaporation of its water base, becomes intimately adherent by physical coaptation rather than by chemical bonding. Necrosis and formation of a dead space thus are avoided. The latex used is a microdispersion of polyvinyl-polyvinylidene chloride copolymer. It is sprayed through a simple artist's airbrush onto the moist surface of the aneurysm and its associated vessels. Helium is used for the airbrush instead of air, since it warms rather than cools with expansion, and thus is less likely to provoke spasm in the feeding vessel. The supply of latex then is shut off, and the stream of helium used to evaporate the water base, leaving a thin, transparent coating of adherent latex.

This initial coat provides relatively little strength in itself, but it does provide a dry surface that is adherent to the aneurysm, to which is applied a second coat consisting of a mixture of two two-component epoxy resins. The second coat polymerizes in 3 to 5 minutes, producing a mild exothermia of only 2°C to 5°C; it provides a strong, resilient coating for the aneurysm. Cooling during polymerization is not necessary.

Technique of Coating

1. The aneurysm is exposed along with its parent vessels. Adherent vessels need not be dissected from the sac. Pia and arachnoid, which are adherent to the sac and usually provide a fragile seal at the site of hemorrhage, are left in place.

2.   If clips or ligatures have been placed, they are not disturbed.

3.   Insofar as possible, adjacent structures are removed from contact with the sac.

4.   If CSF collects near the sac, a narrow cottonoid strip and sucker are used to keep the field as dry as possible.

5.   Minute oozing from adventitial vessels is controlled by means of thrombin, 3% hydrogen peroxide, or Avitene.

6.   If spasm of the feeding vessels is present, it has always been possible to correct it by the application of cotton saturated with 3% papaverine, which may require as long as 10 to 15 minutes to be effective.

7.   Moistened Gelfoam is placed over adjacent structures to mask them from the coating process. No ill effects have been observed, however, when masking has been incomplete.

8.   A stream of helium then is directed at the aneurysm and feeding vessels through the airbrush, with the valve from the "color bottle," which contains the latex, closed.

9.   As soon as obvious surface moisture has evaporated, the valve is opened and the dilute artificial latex is sprayed in a fine mist about the lesion.

10. If the mist cannot be directed at all surfaces of the aneurysm, the mist of latex that floats in the air within the craniotomy opening will nevertheless be deposited on all surfaces that are not in contact with adjacent tissues or protective Gelfoam or cottonoid.

11. The valve then is closed, and the stream of helium again is directed on the aneurysm and feeding vessels. The faint, milky, thin layer of latex dries to a transparent coating.

12. Coating with the latex is repeated three or four times, the entire process requiring about 5 minutes.

13. The two syringes containing the components of the epoxy resin coating are used to inject stoichiometric amounts of the components into the barrel of a small plastic syringe, and the mixture is stirred vigorously and extruded through a plastic cannula to coat the aneurysm, a small segment of its parent vessels, and clips, if they have been used.

14. The undersurface of the aneurysm may, if necessary, be coated by extruding some of the resin on a thin piece of dry Gelfoam. This is slid into place beneath the aneurysm and brought up against its undersurface. Additional resin is added from above, until the coating is continuous. The Gelfoam is allowed to remain in place. The coating must totally surround the lesion from its tip to the parent vessel. If a clip is used, coating must be continuous from the clip to the parent vessel. Coating an aneurysm that still has a point of adhesion is inadequate unless a clip excludes this point from the base.

15. Alternatively, if desired, a single layer of medium-mesh cotton gauze may be wrapped about the sac to contain the epoxy coat.

16. The moist Gelfoam strips that were used as a protective mask for surrounding structures are removed.

17. Hardness of the resin is checked by palpation with a small dissector. When polymerized, the resin is firm but somewhat resilient.

18. The procedure is completed in routine fashion.

Postoperative Care and Complications

There are no special features in the postoperative care of these patients. A soft rubber catheter is left in the subarachnoid space near the aneurysm, draining into a rubber glove outside the dressing. Fifty to 100 ml of gradually clearing pink cerebrospinal fluid usually drains within the first 36 to 48 hours, and the catheter then is removed.

Dexamethasone is continued postoperatively in the same dose as was administered during the immediate preoperative period; it is gradually withdrawn over 6 to 8 days. Dilantin (250 mg) is given intravenously immediately after surgery and thereafter the dose is increased to 300 mg daily by mouth. It is continued for 2 years in most instances, and the dose is controlled by occasional determinations of serum concentration of Dilantin, which is kept at a low therapeutic level unless a seizure occurs. Postoperative seizures have no increased incidence with the coating technique. Meningeal imitation and fever also have shown no increased incidence with coating.

Rebleeding after an aneurysm has been fully coated has not been documented. In 1 patient in whom an aneurysm of the anterior communicating artery extended through the lamina terminalis into the third ventricle, where it was adherent to the diencephalon, the fundus of the aneurysm was not fully coated nor could a clip be applied. Rebleeding occurred in this patient postoperatively, necessitating reoperation 3 months later. During reoperation, the sac was fully freed, withdrawn from the third ventricle, and coated. This patient has no abnormal sensory or motor findings and is functioning at a reduced intellectual level.

A detailed review of 225 aneurysms that have been coated by this technique is in progress. The operative mortality rate is now under 5 percent. Our chief problem is reducing the mortality rate in those patients who, chiefly because of vascular spasm, never reach a degree of alertness sufficient to justify operation and who die of infarction or recurrent hemorrhage. Twenty-nine of the last 30 patients have resumed their former occupations. One of these who was initially demented proved to have communicating hydrocephalus; he returned to his usual business activities following a ventriculoperitoneal shunt.

REFERENCES

1. Aitken RI, Drake CG: A technique of anesthesia with induced hypotension with subsequent correction of intracranial aneurysm, in *Clinical Neurology,* Vol 21. Baltimore, Williams & Wilkins, 1974, pp 107–113
2. Selverstone B: Aneurysms at middle cerebral "trifurcation"; treatment with adherent plastics. *J Neurosurg 19*:884–888, 1962
3. Dutton JEM: Intracranial aneurysm. A new method of surgical treatment. *Br Med J 2*:585–586, 1956
4. Selverstone B, Ronis N: Coating and reinforcement of intracranial aneurysms with synthetic resins. *Bull Tufts N Engl Med Center 4*:8–12, 1958
5. Selverstone B: Vascular reinforcement with adherent plastics. *N Engl Vasc Soc Proc 19*:37, 1960–1961
6. Selverstone B: Reinforcement of intracranial aneurysms with adherent plastics. Proceedings of the British Society of Neurology and Surgery. *J Neurol Neurosurg Psychiatry 24*:92, 1961
7. Selverstone B: Treatment of intracranial aneurysms with adherent plastics. Proceedings of the Boston Society of Psychiatry and Neurology. *N Engl J Med 265*:100, 1961
8. Selverstone B, Dehghan R, Ronis N, et al: Adherent synthetic resins in experimental surgery. *Arch Surg 84*:80–84, 1962
9. Selverstone B: Treatment of intracranial aneurysm with adherent plastics, in Mosberg WH (ed): *Clinical Neurosurgery,* vol 9. Baltimore, Williams & Wilkins, 1963, pp 201–213
10. Sugar O, Tsuchiya G: Plastic coating of intracranial aneurysms with "EDH-adhesive." *J Neurosurg 21*:114–117, 1964
11. Chou S-N, Ortiz-Suarez HJ, Brown WE: Technique and material for coating aneurysms, in Wilkins RH (ed): *Clinical Neurosurgery,* Vol 21. Baltimore, Williams & Wilkins, 1974, pp 182–193
12. Sachs E, Jr, Erbinger A, Margolis G, et al: Fatality from ruptured intracranial aneurysm after coating with methyl-2-cyanoacrylate. *J Neurosurg 24*:889–891, 1966

CHAPTER 64

Intraoperative Electroencephalographic and Evoked Potential Studies in Operative Neurosurgery

J. W. McSherry

INTRAOPERATIVE MONITORING of neurophysiologic events is expanding in scope and becoming of practical clinical importance at all levels of neurosurgery. Monitoring the integrity of sensory systems during a procedure that carries a risk of inadvertent injury is feasible and practical. Historically important applications, such as thalamic localization through evoked potentials in thalamotomy cases and corticography in epilepsy surgery, were limited by the select patient population. Carotid endarterectomy and spinal reconstructions are more common procedures and can be made safer by neurophysiologic monitoring. In high-risk circumstances, electroencephalograms (EEGs) and evoked potentials (EPs) should be used.

A surge in neurophysiologic monitoring has come about because of the widespread proliferation of evoked potential hardware, which is often used with an integral computer that is capable of rapid data analysis. In the 1970s, EP monitoring achieved a leading role in diagnostic neurology because of its capacity to detect subclinical lesions in sensory systems. In the 1980s, EP monitoring, both in the intensive care setting and in the operating room, will become common. Use of the EEG, or the monitoring of the background activity of the brain, will be discussed separately from use of EPs, or the monitoring of the phasic activity of the brain induced by external events.

Evoked Potential Monitoring

Evoked potential studies evaluate the electrical events in a sensory system that result from the application of a stimulus. Nearly any sensory system can be monitored. Thus, indications for EP monitoring are (1) a desire to follow the integrity of sensory pathways during surgery, and (2) a desire to localize sensory structures during surgery.

In the first instance, there are three types of evoked response studies: visual, somatosensory, and auditory. For example, in patients undergoing procedures to straighten the spine, somatosensory evoked responses (SSEPs) are monitored to provide evidence of the integrity of the dorsal columns.[1,2,3] Using similar procedures, we have monitored the integrity of the sciatic

Clinical Neurophysiology Laboratory, Medical Center Hospital of Vermont, and the University of Vermont College of Medicine, Burlington, Vermont

nerve during hip replacement in a patient who had suffered with shortening of the leg for some time. The technique consists of stimulating a distal nerve, usually the posterior tibial nerve at the ankle or the median nerve at the wrist, and recording over the cervical cord and sensorimotor cortex. We use F_z, C_z, C_3, C_4, CP_z and C_5, C_6 of the international 10-20 system, with CP_z located halfway between C_z and P_z, and C_5 and C_6 located 2 cm posterior to C_3 and C_4. An electrode is also placed 3 cm below the inion in the midline. Amplifiers with a minimum response range of 30–3000 Hz are used and the analogue data are averaged on a computer. The recording electrodes are silver-silver chloride and are affixed with collodion. Stimulating electrodes are stainless steel and are taped over the nerve. Stimuli are produced with a Grass S-88, and are square-wave pulses of 0.2 msec duration and 60–150 volts. The stimulus delivery rate is 4–20 pulses per second.

We routinely obtain a preoperative evoked potential study when possible. We have never seen evoked responses appear during surgery that were not present in a preoperative study. Monitoring should begin before induction of anesthesia, as we have observed the disappearance of EPs after induction but before manipulations that might compromise spinal function. The choice of anesthetic is very important, as halothane isoflourane and enflurane often eliminate dependable cortical EPs. When a cervical response is obtained, the anesthetic becomes less critical as, in most cases, this potential does not appear to be affected by halothane, isoflourane, and enflurane. We did lose EPs in a patient with Charcot-Marie-Tooth disease with only NO_2 anesthesia; the EPs did not recover during a "wake up" despite the patient's return of voluntary motor function.

The evoked potentials from the cervical region are recorded with an F_z-C_{v2} montage and consist of a low-voltage negative wave at 33–35 msec following stimulation of the posterior tibial nerve. Latency variability of up to 3 msec occurs, apparently related to the use of a narcotic and other changes induced by the anesthetist. The potential is small and it cannot be recorded in all subjects, but when present it is not grossly affected by anesthetics, and allows high stimulus rates. Averages of 128 to 1024 stimuli are usually required, but it is possible to monitor responses from the right and left independently at rapid stimulus rates (e.g., 20 pulses/sec), which allows for timely observations.

If one cannot monitor cervical responses because of the location of the operative field or because of other technical factors, one must depend on cortical responses. Using the contralateral central or postcentral electrode referred to F_z, stimulation of the median nerve (or ulnar or radial) results in a negative-positive sequence of waves at 19 and 24–30-msec latency. When nerves in the legs are stimulated, the best recording electrodes vary, and we use the "best" montage for an individual patient. Either C_z or CP_z referred to F_z usually provides a sequence of positive-negative-positive waves at 41–54-msec latency. Using contralateral-central-referred-to-midline or ipsilateral-central derivations may result in more dramatic responses in some patients, and as long as the wave form is reproducible, it is suitable.

Figure 64-1 illustrates the type of averaged responses obtained during surgical procedures. The total sweep is 204.8 msec. The trace begins with the stimulation of the left posterior tibial nerve and an artifact is evident at the time of stimulation of the right posterior tibial nerve (over "R" in the figure). The vertical calibraton is 5 μV for channels 1 and 4, and 10 μV for channels 2 and 3. The horizontal calibration is for 51.2 msec. In the first channel the cervical electrode is referred to F_z (negativity at C_{v2} up) and a small potential is recorded between 28 and 35 msec following stimulation of each posterior tibial nerve. This is the cervical potential that is presumably related to dorsal column and nuclear function. When it can be recorded, monitoring can be conducted with wide latitude in the choice of anesthetics. The second and third channels are C_6 and C_5 referred to C_z (negativity in C_5 or C_6 up). Because C_z is active, a response is measured in each to stimulation of either leg, but the wave form differs depending upon the leg. The fourth channel shows the averaged activity with the C_5 derivation referred to C_6, and this channel best illustrates the difference in the cortical response following stimulation of the left-versus-right posterior tibial nerve, with an upward deviation following left stimulation and a downward deviation following right stimulation.

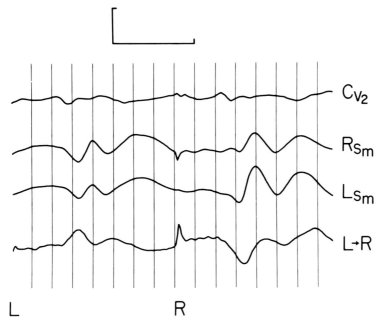

Fig. 64-1. Evoked potentials from stimulation of the right and left posterior tibial nerves. Vertical calibration 5 μV for traces C_{v2} and L→R; 10 μV for traces R_{sm} and L_{sm}. Horizontal calibration 51.2 msec. L and R below the traces mark the time of stimulation of left and right posterior tibial nerves. C_{v2} reflects electrical potentials (average) over the high cervical region. R_{sm} and L_{sm} refer to potentials arising over right and left parietal areas and L→R refers to potential in left parietal referred to right parietal regions. Average of 1024 trials at 4.9 trials/second.

In an individual patient the cortical-evoked response is consistent at a particular derivation, but among patients the best response may be encountered at differing recording sites in the centroparietal area. This may be because of variations in the location of the cortical sensory representation of the leg at the junction of the dorsal and medial aspects of the hemisphere and the anterior-posterior orientation of the evoked dipole in the rolandic sulcus. A flexible approach should be used and the derivations that best demonstrate a reproducible response selected. The high stimulus rates largely eliminate late components of the evoked response. Late components, particularly those over 100 msec in latency, are affected by levels of arousal. This property is exploited by some monitoring centers, most notably the Cleveland group.

Nash and his associates have studied a large series of patients undergoing spinal surgery and have reported their findings previously.[2] They use a variable (1–1.4 sec) interstimulus interval, which allows study of late components of the cortical-evoked potential. This provides a measure of the level of anesthesia in a paralyzed patient. Recording very small potentials like the cervical responses and using such long interstimulus intervals, is tedious, but with adequate caution in the choice of premedication and anesthetics, the larger cortical responses can be monitored with fewer stimuli. Other technical features preferred by the Cleveland group include subdermal stimulating electrodes (which permit smaller stimulating currents and, hence, less artifact) and power amplifier circuits located near the patient's head to vastly reduce the noise from other electrical and mechanical factors in the operating room.

In addition to monitoring somatosensory-evoked potentials to assess the integrity of peripheral nerves and the spinal sensory pathways, the cortical-evoked potentials may be mapped to localize the rolandic sulcus on the exposed convexity. A dipole develops across the sulcus in response to contralateral stimulation of the median nerve. Locating the dipole with a prefabricated grid of electrodes recently has been reported to be a rapid and safe procedure.[4,5] that avoids the need for awakening the patient to obtain subjective reports of sensory experience. We have, as yet, only used the technique once, and it is technically no more complex than the other monitoring technique described above. The electrode grids are not commercially available, so experience fabricating such devices from nontoxic materials is a prerequisite, and experience in localizing events from multichannel averages is also essential. Obviously, precautions regarding preanesthetic medication and anesthesia are critical.

Brainstem auditory potentials (BAPs) are a sequence of waves, a microvolt or less in amplitude, that occur within 10 msec of a click stimulus to the ear. The first wave reflects activation of the eighth cranial nerve and later potentials reflect activity in the dorsal brainstem between the eighth cranial nerve and the inferior colliculus. In performing surgery near the eighth cranial nerve it has not been feasible to know whether one compromises the eighth nerve function until the patient recovers from anesthesia. Grundy and Jannetta recently reported a series of 8 patients undergoing surgery in the cerebellopontine angle.[6] They report detecting the loss of eighth-nerve function acutely in 4 of 8 patients, and in 2 of these 4 the loss was reversible by modifying retractor pressure. In the other 2, responses were lost during induction of anesthesia. The latter 2 cases are surprising in that the BAPs are remarkably resistant to drugs and moderate hypothermia. The preoperative responses, however, were reported to be abnormal and there may have been sufficient impairment to the nerve or its vascular supply such that there was increased drug susceptibility or sensitivity to altered perfusion pressure. The technical features of BAP monitoring are similar to SSEP monitoring except that a stimulus of 0.1 msec duration, preferably 40 dB above ambient noise level and the patient's hearing threshold at 10,000 Hz, must be delivered through an earphone that is small enough to be out of the operative field and electrically shielded to avoid intolerable artifact in the first 2 msec of the recording. Very high stimulus levels may evoke a response in the contralateral ear unless masking is used. Modifying the technique, such as using 0.5 or even 1.0 msec square wave stimuli, will alter the responses but may make monitoring possible in patients with severe high-frequency loss.

Visual-evoked potentials (VEPs) to flash stimuli are rather complex in wave form and most easily used to detect dysfunction of the optic nerve (ON). The technical complexity, however, of providing flash stimulus monocularly without interfering with the operative field is an obstacle. During orbital surgery we have provided intermittent checks on ON function, but these required interruption of surgery. Reports of monitoring during intracranial surgery near the chiasm are wanting. Interpretation of changes in VEP morphology in one or the other hemisphere is particularly hazardous because many lesions can alter VEP morphology[7] but do not necessarily result in subjective field cuts.

EEG Monitoring

Electrocorticography has been employed for decades in association with cortical resections for intractable epilepsy. The number of centers performing this type of surgery has remained small because of the extensive diagnostic facilities needed to select the few patients who are likely to benefit from the procedure without unacceptable postoperative impairments. In recent years, however, EEG monitoring during carotid endarterectomy has been introduced in several centers to help reduce operative morbidity and mortality. The purpose of the monitoring is to detect physiologically significant reductions of cerebral oxygenation, particularly during periods of arterial clamping, but also during periods of hypotension throughout the procedure. Indications for the monitoring are (1) multivessel disease, or (2) a combined morbidity/mortality rate greater than 4 percent in the center performing the endarterectomies. Detection of EEG changes associated with clamping the carotid artery are reported to be 10 to 20 percent.[8,9] The incidence of detection of adverse changes is highest when there is contralateral carotid occlusion.[8] Shunt placement often reverses the changes, but transient residual dysfunction may be present postoperatively.[8,10]

The methods involved in intraoperative monitoring are essentially those of routine EEG, with electrodes placed according to the international 10-20 system. Agents such as barbiturates and diazepam derivatives are desirable in that changes in the fast activity in the EEG may be the first sign of functional hypoxia,[8] while enflurane anesthesia has been reported to be a particularly bad choice.[11] In centers equipped to perform on-line, multichannel frequency analysis, continuous monitoring of compressed spectral arrays (CSA) is desirable, particularly after the endarterectomy is complete but before the patient recovers consciousness. Thrombotic or embolic events occur on rare occasions during this interval and review of CSA will permit early detection of such adverse events. Dependence on the CSA at the time of clamping is not recommended. Some changes are episodic[10] and, as such, are readily detected by an electroencephalographer but smoothed over in a CSA. For an excellent review of a large series of monitored endarterectomies, the reader is referred to the article by Chiappa.[8] In our experience the patient with an abnormal preoperative EEG, and who has a history of previous cerebrovascular events and multivessel disease, is very difficult to evaluate from the standpoint of EEG at the time of clamping. This is also the very high-risk patient and it is not clear whether EEG monitoring will markedly alter the risk in this group. A recent review points out that, depending on the center, carotid endarterectomy is associated with a 4 to 15 percent permanent complication rate, and a 1–7 percent mortality rate.[12] Even in very high-risk patients the combined morbidity and mortality rates can be reduced below 4 percent.[13] In a center with a morbidity and mortality rate above 4 percent, especially in patients with normal or near normal base-line EEGs, intraoperative monitoring should provide timely warning of cerebral ischemia and thereby benefit patients.

Cautions and Conclusions

Several warnings are in order, especially in the area of evoked potential studies. When computer averaging techniques are used, a very powerful tool for extracting signal from noise is employed, and the signal is not necessarily what one desires. Stroboscopic flash units produce an audible click and this produces EPs in enucleated patients. Depending upon SSEPs during spinal surgery requires caution because it is not known whether compromise of the anterior spinal artery in humans will acutely impair function in the dorsal columns. We have recently studied a patient with a cervical fracture that resulted in quadraplegia and loss of pain and temperature sensation. Vibratory and position sense were normal, as were the SSEPs. This patient had stablized (1 month posttrauma) when first investigated, and the precise pathology is not known. Clearly, anterior and lateral cord function can be impaired with preserved SSEPs. Unfortunately, the most reasonable approach is to add another skilled individual to the operating room—the clinical neurophysiologist. Neither EEG nor EP monitoring is sufficiently routine to be entrusted to a technician, and errors of judgment may result in loss of sensory and motor functions. Supervision of the recording and measuring equipment is too complex a task to add to the intraoperative concerns of the surgeon and anesthesiologist. An individual who is expert in interpreting EEGs and EPs and who can adapt procedures to the case at hand is essential to intraoperative monitoring. Such monitoring will reduce the risks of carotid endarterectomy and increase the surgeon's knowledge of the imminence of destruction of sensory systems.

REFERENCES

1. Schmidek HH, Gomes FB, Seligson D, et al: Management of acute unstable thoracolumbar (T11-L1) fractures with and without neurological deficit. *Neurosurgery* 7:30–35, 1980
2. Nash CL, Lorig RA, Schatzinger LA, et al: Spinal cord monitoring during operative treatment of the spine. *Clin Orthop* 126:100–105, 1977
3. Engler GL, Spielholz NI, Bernhard WN, et al: Somatosensory evoked potentials during Harrington instrumentation for scoliosis. *J Bone Joint Surg* 60A:528–532, 1978

4. Morrell F, Hoeppner T, Whisler WW: The use of intraoperative somatosensory evoked potentials to delineate the postcentral gyrus in man. *Electroenceph clin Neurophysiol 51*:41P 1981

5. Wood C, Allison T, Goff W, et al: Localization of human sensorimotor cortex during surgery by pial surface recording of somatosensory evoked potentials. *Electroenceph clin Neurophysiol 51*:36–37, 1981

6. Grundy B, Jannetta P: BAEP monitoring during cerebellopontine angle (CPA) surgery *Electroenceph clin Neurophysiol 51*:39P, 1981

7. Kooi KA, Marshall RE: *Visual Evoked Potentials in Central Disorders of the Visual System,* Harper & Row, Hagerstown, Md 1979

8. Chiappa KH, Burke SR, Young RR: Results of electroencephalographic monitoring during 367 carotid endarterectomies. Use of a dedicated minicomputer. *Stroke 10*:381–388, 1979

9. Bracciodieta WP: Interoperative EEG monitoring during carotid endarterectomy in the community hospital. *Electroenceph clin Neurophysiol 50*:155P, 1980

10. Bracciodieta WP: EEG monitoring during carotid endarterectomy: detection of basilar artery ischemia. *Electroenceph clin Neurophysiol* (in press)

11. Bracciodieta WP: Intraoperative EEG monitoring during carotid endarterectomy: adverse effect of enflurane anaesthesia. *Electroenceph clin Neurophysiol 50*:156P, 1980

12. West H, Burton R, Roon AJ, et al: Comparative risk of operation and expectant management for carotid artery disease. *Stroke 10*:116–121, 1979

13. Ennix CL, Lawrie GM, Morris GC Jr, et al: Improved results of carotid endarterectomy in patients with symptomatic coronary disease: an analysis of 1,546 consecutive carotid operations. *Stroke 10*:122–125, 1979

Additional resource on intraoperative evoked potential studies:

Spinal Cord Monitoring Workshop Data Acquisition and Analysis, Nash, CL and Brown, RH, Ed. Cleveland, Case Western Reserve University, 1979

CHAPTER 65
Surgery of Epilepsy—Current Technique of Cortical Resection

Robert R. Hansebout

DESCRIPTIONS OF THE FALLING SICKNESS are found in the writings of man since the dawn of recorded history. Fortunately, as a result of the greater understanding of brain physiology that has developed during the past 100 years attempts at cures for epilepsy have been elevated from those forms with an aura of mysticism and superstition to forms that are more medically oriented.

Although the earliest attempts and successes at reducing seizures appear to have been surgical, the advent of modern drug therapy has allowed many epileptics to become productive. Still, current drugs may be toxic or not tolerated by some,[1] and may fail to control seizures in another 20 percent of epileptics.[2] It is estimated that about 1 in 200 persons today has epilepsy and that 10 percent of the population would be amendable to surgery.[2]

Among the surgical procedures used in the treatment of epilepsy, selective cortical resection has earned its place and has been used at an increasing number of neurosurgical centers during the past few years.[3] The following will illustrate salient features of that procedure.

Overall Conception of the Technique

In 1870, J. Hughlings Jackson first recognized that epilepsy could be the result of a sudden excessive electrical discharge of a focus in the gray matter in the brain. The experimental demonstration of functional localization in the cortex by Fritsch and associates confirmed Jackson's observations. In his book, published in 1881, William Gowers indicated that cerebral seizures either could be secondary to structural lesions of the brain or idiopathic, in which case there was no visible lesion.[4]

Otfrid Foerster, after World War I, successfully carried out a number of cortical resections in posttraumatic epileptic patients with focal lesions.[5] Wilder Penfield's scholarly elaboration of cortical function based on studies using electrical stimulation during a large series of operations for epilepsy, coupled with Herbert Jasper's neurophysiologic expertise, fully established the usefulness of cortical resection in the neurosurgical armamentarium.[6] Theodore Rasmussen's meticulous surgical technique and analytic observations have broadened the scope and safety of the procedure.[3,7]

Causes of the focal seizure discharge in both adults and children range from tumors and vascular anomalies to scars and atrophic lesions. Such an atrophic cortex was most often found in

Department of Surgery, McMaster University, Hamilton, Ontario, Canada

I wish to thank my preceptor and colleague, Dr. Theodore Rasmussen, for his helpful advice and for the use of his detailed records.

963

the medial temporal lobe.[8] This *incisural sclerosis,* as it was termed by the Montreal school, was thought to be due to birth injury, while Falconer associated this *mesial sclerosis* mainly with febrile illness and infantile seizures.[8,9] The seizures could be alleviated by removing the abnormal brain tissue.[10]

In early series discrete cicatricial lesions were surgically removed in nontumoral cases of epilepsy,[5] but subsequently, it became clear that the area of epileptogenic brain tissue usually was larger than the structural abnormality and often was composed of several areas of varying epileptogenicity. When cortex in the region of maximum electrographic abnormality is removed, seizures often cease completely. In other cases seizures then can arise from adjacent cortex, again with lower than normal thresholds for epileptogenicity. It was found that the more complete the removal of epileptogenic brain tissue, the greater the likelihood that the seizure tendency would be abolished.[3] Moreover, initial surgery abolished or reduced seizures, which later recurred or increased in frequency in a few patients. After a second operation and the removal of more epileptogenic cortex, one-half of these patients became seizure-free or had a reduced seizure tendency.[3]

Therefore, in patients with drug-refractory focal seizures the current philosophy is to localize the epileptogenic area clinically by electroencephalogram and ancillary methods. Surgery may be considered if this area is deemed to be resectable. The epileptogenic brain tissue is mapped visually, electroencephalographically, and by stimulation during surgery. As much abnormal epileptogenic cortex as possible is removed that is compatible with the least risk of causing or increasing a neurologic deficit.[3]

Criteria for Patient Selection

Seizures are a symptom of brain dysfunction, and therefore other entities, such as metabolic disturbances and brain tumor, must be excluded before it is presumed that the patient has a static lesion that requires treatment for the seizure tendency alone. Surgical treatment then is considered according to the following criteria:

1. The patient must have had an adequate trial of maximally tolerable doses of medications without a degree of control adequate to lead a fairly normal life, or must be intolerant to medications. The seizures may interfere with psychologic and intellectual development, preclude employment, or be sufficiently severe to pose a threat of mental deterioration to warrant surgical consideration. Surgery is considered only when all potentially epileptogenic areas have matured, the seizure tendency is stable, and furthermore, there is no tendency toward spontaneous regression, especially in posttraumatic epilepsy.[11,12] Surgery rarely is advisable until recurrent seizures have been present for 3 to 4 years and the patient is at least 15 to 16 years old. With the newer anesthetic techniques, however, more patients are now being operated upon in late childhood and their early teens.
2. Clinical and electroencephalographic studies should show that attacks are focal in origin and arise from a dispensible portion of brain. The more consistent the attack pattern, the better the chances that surgical extirpation will succeed. The patient must be strongly motivated to cope with an exhaustive diagnostic regimen and a lengthy operative procedure under local anesthesia.[13,14]

Investigation

Clinical

A careful history, especially regarding evidence of birth trauma, seizures early in life, and other potential causes of epilepsy, is necessary. Whether other family members have epilepsy should be known. Handedness should be ascertained. Questioning about what the patient feels at the beginning of attacks and what observers see may indicate the area of lowest seizure threshold. Phenomena such as transient dysphasia or postictal paresis are of considerable lateralizing value.

The neurologic examination, including visual fields, may be normal in temporal lobe epilepsy or show minimal to marked deficits, especially when other lobes are involved.[14]

Radiologic

Stereoscopic plain x-ray films of the skull may show smallness or asymmetry of one side, indicating brain atrophy from early life. Pneumoencephalography is the most useful method of evaluating subtle atrophic brain changes. Angiography is performed if the previous studies are normal or if a vascular malformation is suspected. A computed tomogram may show a brain tumor or an area of atrophy not demonstrated on previous studies.[14]

Electroencephalographic

The electroencephalogram gives the most useful information on the location and size of the epileptogenic area.[13] An interictal epileptiform abnormality repeated on several occasions may be significant. Recordings with pharyngeal or sphenoidal electrodes are useful in temporal lobe epilepsy.[15]

Activation procedures, such as medication withdrawal, hyperventilation, or drug-induced sleep may enhance abnormalities or even provoke a seizure, the recording of which may elucidate the focus if there is not too much muscle artifact. The intravenous injection of methohexital may enhance the epileptiform abnormality in temporal lobe epilepsy, while the intravenous injection of pentylenetetrazol may provoke the patient's habitual seizures.[15]

The intravenous injection of thiopental (the technique of Lombrosa and Erba) may permit the differentiation of primary (corticoreticular) and secondary bilaterally synchronous epileptiform abnormalities that are the result of a unilateral lesion.[16] The intracarotid injection of amobarbital and pentylenetetrazol may lateralize the unilateral lesion. In patients with bitemporal foci, stereotactic depth-electrode studies may identify the most active side when conventional recordings have failed.[15]

Telemetric recordings allow the patient freedom of movement while undergoing prolonged recording to increase the likelihood of seeing interictal epileptiform activity or to document an attack. Computer assistance may increase the effectiveness of recording using telemetry or chronic implanted depth electrodes by reducing the recording time of ictal events.[15]

Neuropsychologic

Neuropsychologic tests help to confirm the location of the focus, since they usually corroborate clinical and electroencephalographic evidence by elaborating deficits, which vary with the lobe involved and the dominance of the hemisphere. Any discrepancy between psychologic and clinical localization may indicate unusual lateralization of speech or bilateral temporal lobe lesions.[17] The intracarotid sodium amobarbital (Amytal) speech test[18] is done preoperatively when lateralization of speech is uncertain, as in left-handers, ambidextrous persons, and right-handers who have had left-hemisphere injury in infancy.[13,17] Preoperative lateralization of speech areas adds to the safety of the cortical resection, since electrical stimulation at the time of surgery may give a false-negative response.

Memory testing also is done during the intra carotid sodium amobarbital speech tests. This is especially important in temporal lobe epilepsy when there is independent epileptiform activity or evidence of injury on the side opposite that of the proposed removal. This test identifies the patient in whom surgery carries with it a risk of memory dysfunction, since only one hippocampus can be removed when the other is functional.[13,17,19]

Preoperative Preparation

When surgery is indicated and the patient accepts, it is desirable to have the epileptogenic cortex as active as possible during the operation. Thus, whenever possible, doses of most antiseizure medications are gradually reduced the week before surgery. In patients who have many attacks, an effective but short-lasting anticonvulsant may be continued until the evening before surgery, or until the patient stops all oral intake. Glucocorticoids are begun 24 hours preoperatively. Should an attack occur preoperatively, phenobarbital sodium, 240 mg may be given by intramuscular injection, or paraldehyde may be given, 10 ml orally or 20 ml rectally.[20]

Anesthesia

Whenever possible, local anesthesia, potentiated by analgesic drugs, is used so that motor, speech, and sensory areas can be mapped readily during surgery, a better electrocorticogram can be obtained, and occasionally, auras can be reproduced by stimulation. Under such conditions, motor and speech functions can be tested periodically to assure maximum safety during the removals.[10,13,21]

Atropine (0.4 mg) is given preoperatively. Uncooperative adults and children may require an endotracheal tube and general anesthesia consisting of nitrous oxide, intravenous sodium methohexital (Brietal), fentanyl, and a curariform agent.[22] The nitrous oxide is discontinued before the electrocorticogram, since it obliterates epileptiform activity.[20]

Nupercaine (dibucaine hydrochloride) has proved to be an excellent local anesthesia agent but is no longer available. Lidocaine is suggested as a substitute.[22] Unless there is a medical contraindiction, 0.5 ml of 1:1000 epinephrine is added per 125 ml of local anesthetic solution.[20] Lidocaine, 125 ml of a 1% solution, is injected into the superficial skin with a 25-gauge needle along the area of the proposed incision, with maximum saturation in the supraorbital, temporal, and occipital regions (Fig. 65-1). Then 125 ml of 0.5% lidocaine is injected down to the periosteum and in the temporalis fascia and muscle with a 20-gauge needle.[22]

This local anesthesia, fortified by intravenous injections of fentanyl and droperidol, is effective throughout the opening. Other intracranial structures are insensitive to pain, except the dura along the larger meningeal vessels. Here local anesthetic can be injected intradurally with a 27-gauge needle.[10] The patient usually is alert and comfortable throughout the procedure, and is given additional intravenous injections of fentanyl and droperidol as required. If drowsiness ensues, the patient must be roused to check motor and speech functions during cortical resection. Methohexital sodium is given intravenously should a seizure develop at any time.[22] A general anesthetic may become necessary if the patient becomes unruly, especially after a seizure. A blind transnasal intubation then may be required,[10] and followed by administration of nitrous oxide and intravenous injections of fentanyl and droperidol for balanced anesthesia.[22]

Special Aspects of the Surgical Technique

Surgical techniques for cortical resection are described in detail elsewhere.[7,8,10,20,21,23-25]

Positioning

The patient is postured comfortably on the side, with a pillow under the hip and pads protecting other bony prominences. The face is slightly inclined toward the side of the incision. The head of the table is somewhat elevated to reduce venous oozing (Fig. 65-2). The skin is sterilized, and a plastic sheet (Pliofilm) is placed around the line of incision. Towels are sutured into place in the anesthetized skin so they do not become dislodged if the patient moves. The anesthetist always has access to the patient's face.

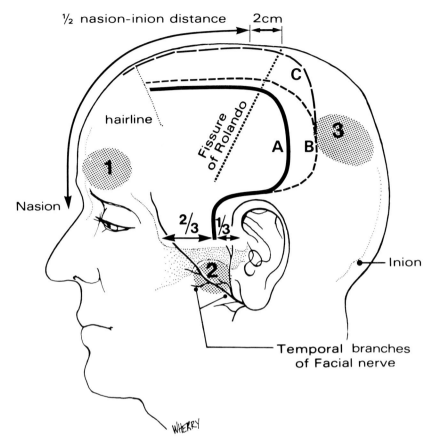

Fig. 65-1. Skin incision for (**A**) dominant, (**B**) nondominant temporal, and (**C**) frontotemporal exposures. 1, 2 and 3 denote points of maximum local anesthetic infiltration for major sensory nerves. Note external landmarks for Rolandic fissure (central sulcus).

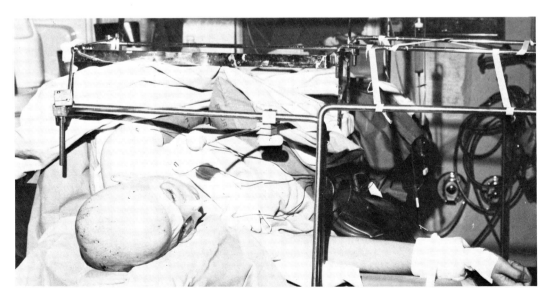

Fig. 65-2. Position for left frontotemporal exposures.

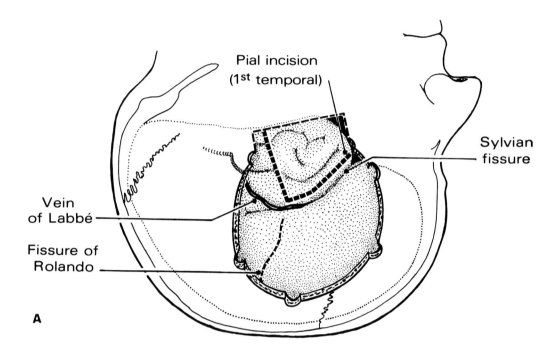

Pial incision
(1st temporal)

Sylvian
fissure

Vein
of Labbé

Fissure of
Rolando

A

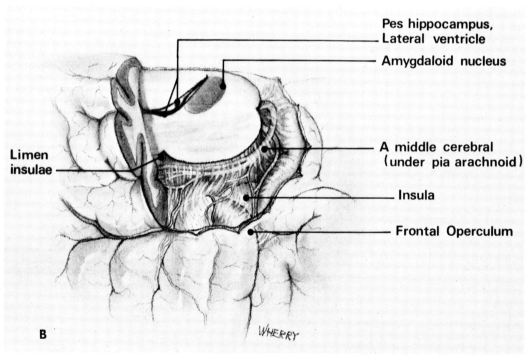

Pes hippocampus,
Lateral ventricle

Amygdaloid nucleus

A middle cerebral
(under pia arachnoid)

Insula

Frontal Operculum

Limen
insulae

B

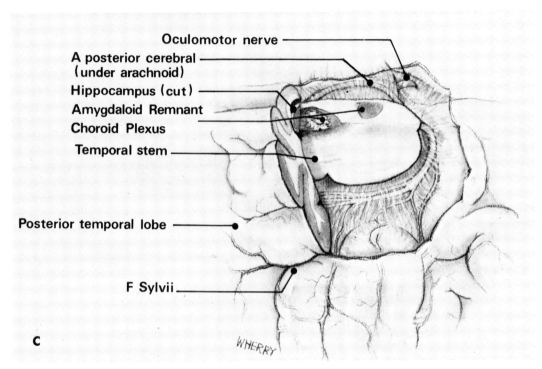

Oculomotor nerve

A posterior cerebral (under arachnoid)

Hippocampus (cut)

Amygdaloid Remnant

Choroid Plexus

Temporal stem

Posterior temporal lobe

F Sylvii

C

WHERRY

Fig. 65-3. Dominant temporal lobectomy, surgeon's view. **A.** Left temporal exposure showing line of proposed cortical resection. **B.** Superficial temporal lobe removed, exposing lateral temporal horn and lateral amygdaloid. **C.** Following removal of pes hippocampus and most of amygdaloid. Note blood vessels and third nerve protected by pia-arachnoid.

Incisions

A generous-sized opening is necessary to afford adequate exposure to map the epileptogenic area and to note its relationship to the central region on either side and the speech areas in the dominant hemisphere. A question-mark incision is the most useful for temporal lobectomy.[9] Adequate incisions for temporal and frontotemporal removals are shown in Figure 65-1. To expose the frontal lobe alone, a C-shaped incision is suggested, with the superior portion at the midline extending up to 2 cm above the frontal sinus and the posterolateral limb extending downward to the level of the zygoma.[20] If the epileptogenic focus is posterior, a C-shaped incision is made with its medial limb in the midline and the lateral limb curved downward to expose the central region.[20]

The Opening

A detailed description of the most common cortical resection—partial temporal lobectomy—will follow. The principles are easily modified for cortical resection elsewhere.

The question-mark incision is begun at the superior aspect of the zygoma at the junction of its anterior two-thirds and posterior one-third (Fig. 65-1). If the lowest part of the incision is made too anteroinferior, temporal branches of the facial nerve may be damaged, which causes a frontalis muscle palsy. The superficial temporal artery is coagulated early. The galea is separated from the temporalis fascia for the application of the skin clips. The superior portion of the incision is made down through the periosteum. The temporalis muscle and fascia are divided to the periosteum with electrocautery. With a periosteal elevator, the skin and muscle are reflected forward over a roll of gauze, and muscle *fishhooks* are applied for retraction. Burr holes are made, as in Figure 65-3A. It is important to rongeur away the sphenoid between the two burr holes to

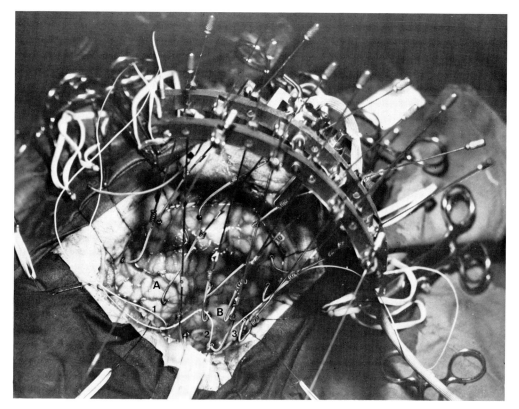

Fig. 65-4.   Electrode holder and electrodes over (**A**) left frontal, (**B**) temporal and central regions. Wire electrodes for recording from (1) undersurface of frontal and (2,3) temporal lobe.

expose the anterior temporal lobe. Moreover, if a trough is rongeured inferiorly from each of the two temporal burr holes, access to the inferior temporal region is easier and cosmetic restoration ultimately will be better. A free bone flap provides better exposure and more comfort for the patient than a hinged flap.[20] The edges of the bony opening are waxed. A hole for the electrode post is made along the superior edge of the craniotomy (see Fig. 65-7). Dural traction sutures are placed to decrease venous oozing.[7]

The middle meningeal vessels are coagulated and divided. The dura is opened a few millimeters from the bone edge. It then is pulled into a small Penrose drain and reflected anteroinferiorly over the temporalis muscle along its remaining 2 cm of attachment. The patient raises the head every 2 hours so the anesthetist can massage the downward side to prevent pressure burns.

The Electrocorticogram

Electrocorticography and depth electrode recording have proven very useful in mapping epileptogenic regions during surgery.[15,23]

A steel post is screwed into the hole at the superior edge of the craniotomy, and a 16-channel electrode holder is attached. One montage for both monopolar and bipolar recording is shown in Figure 65-4. Wire electrodes can be substituted for the usual contact electrodes for recording on the undersurface of the temporal lobe, the frontal lobe, and medial aspect of the hemisphere. Small lettered tags are placed at any site of electrographic abnormality (see Fig. 65-7).

In temporal lobe cases, the inferior eight electrodes are removed and needle depth electrodes with four contacts are inserted perpendicular to the surface of the second temporal convolution to a depth of 3.5 cm at distances of 3 and 5 cm from the tip of the temporal lobe (Fig.

65-5A). The deepest contact of the anterior depth electrode records from the amygdaloid nucleus, and the posterior electrode from the pes hippocampus. The superficial contacts record from the surface gray matter. The intermediate two contacts of the anterior depth electrode record from circuminsular cortex, and the middle two contacts of the posterior depth electrode from the gray matter in the depths of Heschl's gyri.[23] The superior eight contact electrodes retain their former position. A further electroencephalographic recording is obtained.

Electrical Stimulation Study

The brain then is electrically stimulated to determine the position of the pre- and postcentral gyri. A 2-msec square-wave pulse at 60 Hz, starting at 1 V and increasing by 0.5-V increments following each negative stimulation is used until a motor response is seen by the anesthetist, or until a sensory change is felt by the patient. Positive stimulation points are marked, using numbered tickets (see Fig. 65-7). The rolandic fissure (central sulcus) is thus identified. In the dominant hemisphere the speech areas are stimulated while the patient carries out simple verbal tasks.[23] The frontal speech area is indicated by speech arrest, while the posterior temporal area is identified by arrest or a dysphasic reaction during stimulation. A negative stimulation does not always exclude the presence of speech function in the convolution that is stimulated.[21]

Areas of after-discharge (rhythmic electroencephalographic activity different from the prestimulation activity) may develop at the stimulation site or in adjacent regions. These may indicate areas of hyperirritable cortex,[10] although the clinical significance of this has not yet been documented.[23]

Other areas of the exposed cortex and the depth electrodes then may be stimulated in an endeavor to reproduce the patient's dura. A stimulating voltage more than 3 V higher than that required to elicit motor or sensory responses is dangerous. Above such levels, a nonspecific, full-blown seizure may develop, which precludes the patient's cooperation for some time.[23]

Anatomic Considerations—Plan of Removal

The frontal (Broca) and posterior speech areas in the dominant hemisphere, as determined by stimulation studies and ablations around these areas, are shown in Figure 65-6.[26] The speech areas are indispensable and their removal is never justified.[10] The pre- and postcentral face area can be removed if pial barriers are respected so the blood supply to the rolandic and speech areas is preserved. This results in contralateral facial paresis, which subsequently improves but may leave some mild facial underaction.[25] Removal of the postcentral arm or leg area causes some persistent astereognosis and rarely is indicated unless markedly epileptogenic cortex in this area is causing a severe seizure tendency.[25] Removal of the precentral arm or leg produces contralateral spastic hemiparesis and is not indicated unless marked preoperative hemiparesis is present.[27]

Originally it was suggested that the anterior 5 to 6 cm of the dominant temporal lobe could be removed,[21] the resection being carried out along the vein of Labbé[8-10] without producing dysphasia. Because of variability in the position of this vein and the size of the temporal lobe, however, the best landmark to use is the junction of the rolandic and sylvian fissures. Removal of the dominant first and second temporal convolutions posterior to this point carries the risk of permanent dysphasia.[26]

The parietal speech zone extends superiorly 1 to 4 cm above the sylvian fissure and from 2 to 4 cm behind the postcentral sulcus. The frontal speech area occupies one or both frontal opercular convolutions anterior to the precentral gyrus.[26]

In the series from the Montreal Neurological Institute a number of epileptic patients without evidence of early damage to the left cerebral hemisphere underwent the carotid amobarbital speech test. In right-handers 96 percent had speech in the left hemisphere and 4 percent in the right hemisphere. In left-handed or ambidextrous individuals 70 percent had speech on the left,

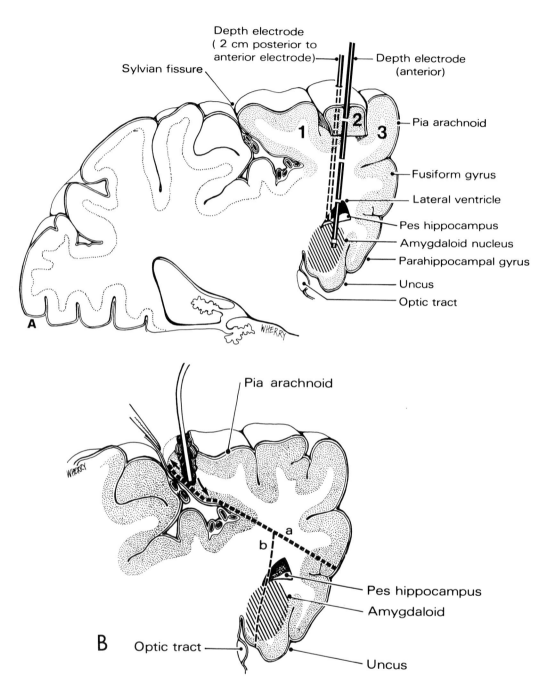

Fig. 65-5. Coronal section of left hemisphere at the tip of the temporal horn. **A.** Depth electrodes in place in amygdaloid (anterior) and hippocampus (posterior). **B.** Subpial dissection in first temporal convolution while retracting pia-arachnoid. (a) Line of superficial temporal resection. (b) Line of removal of medial temporal structures.

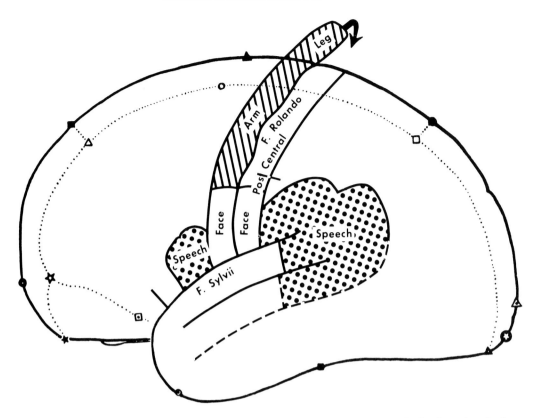

Fig. 65-6. Most common position of pre- and postcentral gyri and speech areas in dominant hemisphere.

15 percent on the right, and 15 percent had some representation of speech in each hemisphere. Similar studies of speech lateralization in individuals with early left-hemisphere damage shows more variability, with larger numbers having speech in the right hemisphere than those without early damage.[26] Thus in epileptic patients, any hemisphere is considered dominant unless the carotid amobarbital speech test provides otherwise.

When the speech and precentral regions are avoided, *unilateral* removals of frontal, parietal, and temporal cortex are possible without significant additional deficits. When possible, it is best to leave one gyrus between the cortical removal and the indispensable areas of cortex. As much white matter as practicable should be left beneath the cortical removal to reduce any neurologic deficit.

If resection is limited to the anterior 5 cm of a normal-sized temporal lobe,[8] or not posterior to the intersection of the rolandic and sylvian fissures in any temporal lobe a visual field defect is rarely seen following temporal lobectomy.[23] If the temporal horn opening is confined to the anterior 1 cm and the white matter lateral to the ventricle is preserved, geniculocalcarine tract damage is minimized, and a superior quadrantanopsia may be avoided even in removals 7 to 8 cm posterior to the temporal tip.[23]

Bilateral removal of the temporal lobes is never justified because of the profound memory loss that will result.[28]

Cortical Resection

Bearing the above principles in mind, the area of proposed cortical resection is outlined, using a piece of thread. The brain is irrigated at intervals and kept moist, especially during recordings. The thin, nonadhesive transparent plastic film is placed over cortical areas to be preserved to prevent drying of the brain and postoperative edema.[10]

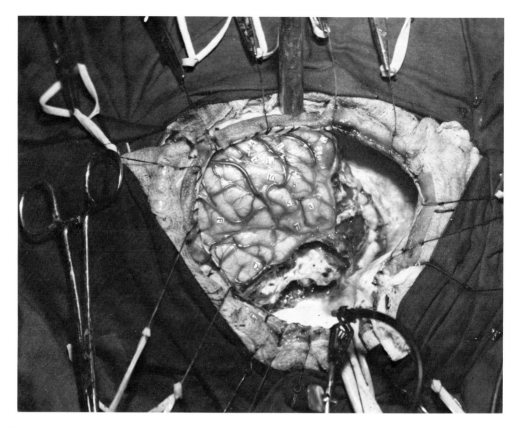

Fig. 65-7. After right frontal and temporal lobectomies with cortical incision following sulci and leaving un-traumatized convolutions at removal edge. Note steel post for electrode holder at edge of superior bone margin, and *fishhooks* retracting dura.

In temporal lobectomy, as elsewhere, subpial dissection is stressed. The pia at the summit of the first temporal gyrus is coagulated and incised with a scalpel (Fig. 65-3A). With small-bore suction, gray matter is meticulously pulled away from the pia to expose the white matter. The incision line is lengthened anteroposteriorly. The pia-arachnoid is coagulated and divided with scissors, and the incision is deepened by the suction technique. Gradually, sufficient gray matter along this gyrus is removed to expose the pia-arachnoid covering the insula (Fig. 65-5B). The superior gray matter of the first temporal convolution is suctioned away from the pia. Deeper gray matter is suctioned away from the intact pia-arachnoid, as illustrated, to expose the insula. Meticulous hemostasis is necessary and movement of the brain must be avoided. Great care must be taken not to traumatize the middle cerebral vessels situated beneath this protective pia-arachnoid in order to prevent postoperative hemiparesis[7] (Figs. 65-3B and 65-5B). At the posterior margin of the incision, in the first temporal gyrus, the line of incision is carried inferiorly toward the base of the temporal lobe (Fig. 65-3A). Cotton pledgets are placed in the incision, as dissection proceeds distally, and subsequently are removed so that the incision can be deepened using the suction. Only that brain tissue to be removed is retracted away from tissue to be preserved. Larger vessels are coagulated and divided.

When the insular surface is exposed, the incision is carried through the white matter of the temporal stem medially at an angle of about 45° to avoid deep structures in the basal temporal lobe (Figs. 65-3B and 65-5B). The posterior end of the incision then is carried forward along the fusiform gyrus and the anterior end of the first temporal gyral incision is carried anteroinferiorly until the two meet on the inferior surface of the temporal lobe. The superficial temporal lobe is lifted out, leaving white matter overlying the lateral ventricle and amygdala (Fig. 65-5B). When extremely gliotic brain is encountered, scissors may be used to incise the brain tissue.

The white matter of the anterior temporal lobe inferior to the insula is removed by suction until the ventricle is entered. The pes hippocampus then can be visualized and the amygdala is evident (Fig. 65-3B). All but the medial rim of the amygdaloid nucleus and most of the uncus are removed. The remaining portion protects the subjacent optic tract (Fig. 65-5B).[23]

If preoperative studies and depth-electrode recordings indicate hippocampal involvement and the opposite hippocampus is functional, the pes hippocampus then is removed together with the anterior parahippocampal gyrus (Fig. 65-5B).[23] Great care must be exercised to preserve the pia-arachnoid, separating these structures from the third nerve, posterior cerebral artery, and cerebral peduncle (Fig. 65-3C). Heschl's convolution on the dominant side is not removed, unless necessary, since this increases the risk of reducing the blood supply to the posterior speech area.

Postremoval Recording

Wire electrodes are placed on the undersurface of the posterior temporal lobe and orbital surface of the frontal lobe. Cortical electrodes are put on the temporal convexity, insula, amygdaloid, and hippocampal remnants. The remaining cortical electrodes are placed on the dorsolateral convexity of the hemisphere above the sylvian fissure. Persistent spiking from the hippocampus or posterior temporal lobe may require further excision, if no severe neurologic deficit will be produced. In the nondominant hemisphere, excisions are sometimes carried out to 8 cm posterior to the temporal tip. Epileptiform abnormality, recorded from the insular surface, is ignored, since further removal of cortex from that structure does not increase the success rate.[29,30] When spikes or sharp waves persist in dispensable cortex above the sylvian fissure, the subpial removal of these convolutions is carried out one by one. Preservation of the pial *barrier* protects the adjacent gyri and the sulcal blood vessels supplying those gyri and other portions of the brain.[7] Several such additional excisions may be made before a clear electroencephalographic tracing is obtained or the effort to achieve this is abandoned.[20]

Closure

A subdural drain is left beneath the bone flap. Gelatin is placed over the dural closure. The bone flap is wired into position, and burr hole covers are installed. After the galea and skin have been approximated, a wet sulfadiazine-soaked gauze is placed over the incision. A plastic sheet is placed over that and a full head dressing is used that covers the ear on the side of temporal lobectomy. The drain is removed on the first postoperative day.

Postoperative Care

An intravenous solution of glucose and saline containing 250 mg diphenylhydantoin, 240 mg phenobarbital, and 100 mg hydrocortisone per 1000 ml is given until oral intake begins. Fluids are restricted to 1500 ml daily for the first 5 postoperative days to decrease edema. Dexamethasone (6 mg every 6 hours) is given the first 5 days, and the dose then is tapered over the next 7 days. Ambulation begins on the third or fourth day. The sutures are removed on the fifth day.

Unless another medication has proven superior, diphenylhydantoin (100 mg, three times daily) and phenobarbital (60 mg, twice daily) are given for the first postoperative year.[20] If the patient then is seizure-free and has a nonepileptiform electroencephalogram, the medications gradually are reduced at 6- to 12-month intervals. Should seizures recur, the original anticonvulsant doses are restarted and reduced only after 2 seizure-free years.[20]

Complications

An aseptic meningitis, accompanied by fever up to 40°C, probably due to breakdown products of blood in the subarachnoid space, may follow large cortical resections.[31] This syndrome clears spontaneously over a 10- to 20-day period.[20]

Cerebral edema after long procedures may cause transient cortical dysfunction and seizures during the first 7 to 10 days.[10] Such *neighborhood* seizures usually originate from cortex adjacent to the removal and have no bearing on the ultimate prognosis.[20] These complications are reduced by the cortisone regime.[32]

An increasing, marked, superior quadrantanopsia occurs when the temporal lobe resection is carried progressively further behind the rolandic-sylvian junction,[13] or if care is not taken to preserve white matter lateral to the temporal horn.[23] When the occipital lobe has been removed, complete contralateral homonymous hemianopsia has resulted.[25] The memory loss that may occur when the remaining functional hippocampus is removed[33] has been avoided since 1958 by preoperative bilateral administration of the amobarbital speech and memory test, when indicated.[23] Of the 250 dominant partial temporal lobectomies done from 1958 to 1975, only 2 patients had mild persistent dysphasia.[23] Mild deficits in verbal fluency may increase after dominant temporal lobectomy,[17,33] but later, verbal fluency often improves compared with preoperative levels, if seizures are reduced.[17] Transient dysphasia may follow cortical removal from the dominant hemisphere.[24,26]

In an earlier series of dominant temporal lobectomies, especially with cortical resections above or medial to the sylvian fissure, a contralateral hemiplegia, homonymous hemianopsia, and dysphasia were sometimes noted. These were felt to be due to manipulation of the middle cerebral arteries over the insula. They can be prevented by preserving the pia-arachnoid over these vessels, avoiding arterial traction, and leaving insular cortex despite electrographic spiking.[7] Such manipulative hemiplegia has been avoided in temporal lobectomy since 1958. Cortical removals above the sylvian fissure have an incidence of hemiparesis or dysphasia of 0.5 percent unless the sensorimotor cortex is involved, in which case the risk becomes greater.[20]

Of the total 1497 operations for nontumoral lesions performed from 1928 through 1974, the operative mortality was 1 percent. From 1957 through 1975, in 820 consecutive operations there were 2 postoperative deaths, ie., 0.2 percent. In 700 temporal lobe operations from 1950 through 1973 there was no postoperative death.[20]

Results and Discussion of Experience

Histopathologic examination of specimens from 506 consecutive patients operated upon at the Montreal Neurological Institute from 1961 through 1970 showed varying etiologies for focal epilepsy. One-third had discrete lesions, a further third had essentially normal findings, while the rest had extensive lesions, such as cortical atrophy, hippocampal sclerosis, and chronic encephalitis.[34]

Cortical resection for nontumoral epilepsy was performed in 1267 patients from 1928 through 1971, with a median follow-up of 10 years in 1145 patients (Table 65-1). The seizure tendency was abolished in 36 percent, while in another 28 percent seizures were substantially, although not completely reduced. Variable results were obtained in the remaining 36 percent, with some patients experiencing a 90 percent reduction in seizures and a few essentially unchanged.[20]

In the temporal lobe series (653 patients) seizures were completely or almost completely reduced in 71 percent; in the frontal group (212 patients) in 55 percent; in the parietal group (80 patients) in 59 percent; in the central (sensorimotor) group (63 patients) in 57 percent; in the occipital lobe group (19 patients) in 68 percent; and in the group undergoing total or subtotal hemispherectomy for large destructive lesions (77 patients) in 50 percent.[20,23-25]

Up to 1971 repeat operations were performed on 129 patients who had inadequate seizure

Table 65-1. Results of Cortical Excision for Focal Epilepsy in Patients with Nontumoral Lesions Operated on During the Years 1928 Through 1971

| | Patients | | | |
| | No. | (%) | Totals No. | (%) |
Results				
Seizure-free since discharge	237	21		
Became seizure-free after some early attacks	179	15	416	36
Free of seizures 3 or more years then rare or occasional attacks	122	11		
Marked reduction in seizure tendency	198	17	320	28
Moderated or less reduction in seizure tendency			409	36
Total patients with follow-up data of 2 to 41 years: median, 10 years			1145	
Inadequate follow-up data	82			
Deaths in 2 years	22			
Postoperative deaths	15			
Total patients	1267			

Data compiled from Rasmussen.[20]

reduction. After additional epileptogenic cortex was removed 25 percent became seizure-free and 29 percent had a reduced seizure tendency.[3]

Tumors and arteriovenous malformations, the prime symptom of which was epilepsy rather than increasing neurologic deficit or increased intracranial pressure, were removed in an additional 347 patients. When the causative lesion and the surrounding epileptogenic cortex were removed as completely as possible, the reduction in seizure tendency compared favorably with the nontumor group until neoplasia recurred.[35]

The efficiency of seizure reduction thus correlates with the completeness with which the causative lesion and the epileptogenic cortex are removed rather than with the nature of the lesion or the length of time the patient had seizures.[3] About one-fourth of the patients had some postoperative seizures during the first 2 years, but these subsequently ceased. Medications were stopped after 2 years in about one-half of the patients. A further one-fifth are controlled with medication, whereas this was not possible preoperatively. In addition to the decrease in seizure tendency there may be psychologic improvement in that the patient can often hold a responsible job.[36]

In one center the temporal lobe, including hippocampal and amygdaloid regions, is removed en bloc for optimal histologic study, but the removal then is somewhat more complex than in the stages above.[9] Moreover, the contribution of the first temporal convolution to a seizure tendency has been questioned.[1,9] In the present series the best results have been obtained when as much abnormal cortex as possible is removed in addition to the hippocampus and amygdala when feasible.[36]

Although cortical resection as applied above is highly successful and safe, its application is limited to about 10 percent of epileptics in whom a focus exists in a resectable area of cortex.[2] Failures in operated cases are attributable mainly to involvement of subcortical structures by epileptogenic tissue, nondispensable areas of cortex, or a significant focus in the opposite hemisphere, particularly the temporal lobe.[3]

Stereotactic ablative procedures someday may solve the problem of dealing surgically with generalized, bilateral, or multifocal seizure disorders. To date, targets and methods are not standarized and usually these techniques have been reserved for especially intractable and complicated seizure problems.[37] Similarly, the results of commissurotomy, cerebral cooling, and cerebellar stimulation await longer follow-up.[37] The latter two procedures are of particular interest in that there is no ablation.

Although current medical management with anticonvulsants and controlled drug levels has been extremely effective, such medications may have toxic effects or may fail to control the seizures. In such instances a place remains for cortical resection in selected epileptic patients, until an ideal medication has been developed.

REFERENCES

1. Walker AE: Critique and perspective: neurosurgical management of the epilepsies in Purpura DP, Penry JK, Walter RD (eds): *Advances in Neurology,* vol. 8. New York, Raven Press, 1975, pp 333-349
2. Robb P: Focal epilepsy: the problem, prevalence, and contributing factors, in Purpura DP, Penry JK, Walter RD (eds): *Advances in Neurology,* vol. 8. New York, Raven Press, 1975, pp 11-12
3. Rasmussen TB: Surgical treatment of epilepsy: the clinical neurosciences, in Tower TB (ed): *The Nervous System,* vol. 2. New York, Raven Press, 1975, pp 277-286
4. Penfield W, Jasper H: Historical introduction, *Epilepsy and the Functional Anatomy of the Human Brain.* Boston, Little, Brown, 1954, pp 3-20
5. Foerster O, Penfield W: Structural basis of traumatic epilepsy and result of radical operation. *Brain* 53:99-120, 1930
6. Penfield W, Japser H: *Epilepsy and the Functional Anatomy of the Human Brain.* Boston, Little, Brown, 1954, pp 692-815
7. Penfield W, Lende RA, Rasmussen TB: Manipulation hemiplegia, an untoward complication in the surgery of focal epilepsy. *J Neurosurg* 18:760-776, 1961
8. Penfield W, Baldwin M: Temporal lobe seizures and technique of subtotal temporal lobectomy. *Ann Surg* 136:625-634, 1952
9. Falconer MA, Hill D, Meyer A, et al: Treatment of temporal lobe epilepsy by temporal lobectomy: Survery of findings and results, *Lancet* 1:827-835, 1955
10. Penfield W, Jasper H: Surgical Therapy. *Epilepsy and the Functional Anatomy of the Human Brain.* Boston, Little, Brown, 1954, pp 739-817
11. Caveness WF: Onset and cessation of fits following cranio-cerebral trauma. *J Neurosurg* 20:570-583, 1963
12. Walker AE, Erculei F: Post-traumatic epilepsy 15 years later. *Epilepsia* 11:17-26, 1970
13. Rasmussen TB: The role of surgery in the treatment of focal epilepsy. *Clin Neurosurg* 16:288-314, 1969
14. McNaughton FL, Rasmussen TB: Criteria for selection of patients for neurosurgical treatment: Neurosurgical management of the epilepsies, in Purpura DP, Penry JK, Walter RD (eds): *Advances in Neurology,* vol. 8. New York, Raven Press, pp 37-48
15. Gloor P: Contributions of electroencephalography and electrocorticography to the neurosurgical treatment of the epilepsies, in Purpura DP, Penry JK, Walter RD (eds): *Advances in Neurology,* vol 8. New York, Raven Press, 1975, pp 59-105
16. Lombroso CT, Erba G: Primary and secondary bilateral synchrony in epilepsy. A clinical and electroencephalographic study. *Arch Neurol* 22:321-334, 1970
17. Milner B: Psychological aspects of focal epilepsy and its neurosurgical management: Neurosurgical management of the epilepsies, in Purpura DT, Penry JK, Walter RD (eds): *Advances in Neurology,* vol. 8. New York, Raven Press, 1975, pp 299-321
18. Wada J, Rasmussen TB: Intracarotid injection of sodium amytal for the lateralization of speech dominance. Experimental and clinical observations. *J Neurosurg* 17:266-282, 1960
19. Milner B, Branch C, Rasmussen TB: Study of short-term memory after intracarotid injection of Sodium Amytal. *Trans Am Neurol Assoc* 87:224-226, 1962
20. Rasmussen TB: Cortical resection in the treatment of focal epilepsy: neurosurgical management of the epilepsies, in Purpura DP, Penry JK, Walter RD (eds): *Advances in Neurology.* vol. 8. New York, Raven Press, 1975, pp 139-154
21. Rasmussen TB, Jasper H: Temporal lobe epilepsy: indication for operation and surgical technique, in Baldwin M, Bailey P (eds): *Temporal Lobe Epilepsy.* Charles C Thomas, Springfield, IL, 1958, pp 440-460
22. Trop D: Personal communication
23. Rasmussen TB: Surgical treatment of patients with complex partial seizures, in Penry JK, Daly DD (eds): *Advances in Neurology.* vol. 11. New York, Raven Press, 1975, pp 415-449
24. Rasmussen TB: Surgery of frontal lobe epilepsy: neurosurgical management of the epilepsies, in Purpura DP, Penry JK, Walter RD (eds): *Advances in Neurology,* vol. 8. New York, Raven Press, 1975, pp 197-205

25. Rasmussen TB: Surgery for epilepsy arising in regions other than the temporal and frontal lobes, in Purpura DP, Penry JK, Walter RD (eds): *Advances in Neurology.* vol. 8. New York, Raven Press, 1975, pp 207–226

26. Rasmussen TB, Milner B: Clinical and surgical studies of the cerebral speech areas in man in Zulch KJ, Creutzfeldt O, Galbraith GC (eds): *Cerebral Localization.* New York, Springer-Verlag, 1975, pp 238–257

27. Penfield W, Rasmussen TB: Excision of cortical regions, *The Cerebral Cortex of Man.* New York, Macmillan, 1950, pp 183–201

28. Scoville WB, Milner B: Loss of recent memory after bilateral hippocampal lesions. *J Neurol Neurosurg Psychiatry* 20:11–21, 1957

29. Ajmone-Marsan C, Baldwin M: Electrocorticography, in Baldwin M, Bailey P (eds): *Temporal Lobe Epilepsy.* Springfield, IL, Charles C Thomas, 1958, pp 368–395

30. Silfvenius H, Gloor P, Rasmussen TB: Evaluation of insular ablation in surgical treatment of temporal lobe epilepsy. *Epilepsia* 5:307–320, 1964

31. Jackson IJ: Aseptic hemogenic meningitis. *Arch Neurol Psychiatr* 62:572–589, 1949

32. Rasmussen TB, Gulati DR: Cortisone in the treatment of a postoperative cerebral edema. *J Neurosurg* 19:535–544, 1962

33. Milner B: The memory deficit in bilateral hippocampal lesions. *Psychiatr Res Publ* 11:43–58, 1959

34. Mathieson G: Pathologic aspects of epilepsy with special reference to the surgical pathology of focal cerebral seizures: neurosurgical management of the epilepsies, in Purpura DP, Penry JK, Walter RD (eds): *Advances in Neurology.* vol. 8. New York, Raven Press, 1975, pp 107–138

35. Rasmussen TB: Surgery of epilepsy associated with brain tumors in Purpura DP, Penry JK, Walter RD (eds): *Advances in Neurology,* vol 8. New York, Raven Press, 1975, pp 227–239

36. Feindel W: Factors contributing to the success, or failure of surgical intervention for epilepsy, in Purpura DP, Penry JK, Walter RD (eds): *Advances in Neurology,* vol 8. New York, Raven Press, 1975, pp 281–298

37. Ojemann GA, Ward AA, Jr.: Stereotactic and other procedures for epilepsy, in Purpura DP, Pentry JK, Walter RD (eds): *Advances in Neurology,* vol 8. New York, Raven Press, 1975, pp 241–263

CHAPTER 66
Analgesia Induced by Brain Stimulation with Chronically Implanted Electrodes

Yoshio Hosobuchi

OVER THE PAST DECADE electrical stimulation has been applied in two subcortical sites to produce analgesia in humans. First, the somatosensory areas—the medial lemniscus, the sensory nuclei of the thalamus (the posterior ventralis medialis and lateralis; PVM and PVL, respectively), and the posterior limb of the internal capsule—were stimulated for the control of deafferentation pain.[1] The periaqueductal and periventricular gray matter (PAG and PVG, respectively) then were selected as the stimulation site for pain originating from peripheral noxious stimuli.[2]

The focus of this discussion is on PAG stimulation and thalamic stimulation. The following sections describe the selection of patients for the electrical stimulation procedure, the electrode implantation technique, and the final coupling of the brain electrode to a radiofrequency receiver unit after an appropriate trial of various permutations of the electrode contacts is made to achieve successful pain control.

Patient Selection

Patients who are experiencing severe and chronic intractable pain that cannot be controlled by medication, including opiates in large doses, may be considered candidates for the electrical stimulation procedure. Patients with deafferentation pain respond best to stimulation of the thalamic region, whereas those with pain of peripheral origin are candidates for stimulation of the PAG. Patients suffering from pain secondary to cancer, however, generally are poor candidates for PAG stimulation, since the efficacy of this stimulation depends greatly upon the nutritional status of the patient.

Over the past 5 years, I have used a *morphine test*: (1) to differentiate patients with pain of peripheral origin from those with deafferentation pain; and (2) to determine the presence or absence of tolerance to opiates in patients being considered for electrical stimulation of deep brain structures.[3] Making these distinctions accurately is critical for the success of subcortical stimulation for pain control, because: (1) deafferentation pain that is not responsive to opiates responds better to thalamic stimulation than to PAG stimulation, and (2) patients who have developed tolerance to the analgesic effect of opiates manifest cross-tolerance to the analgesic effect of

Department of Neurological Surgery, School of Medicine, University of California, San Francisco, California

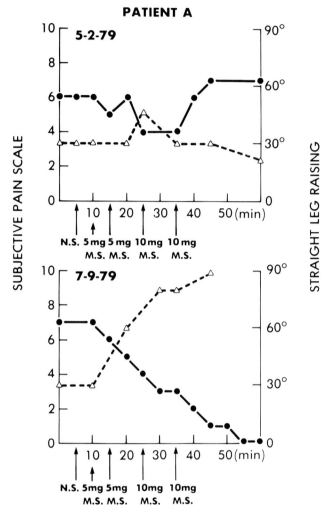

Fig. 66-1. A graph of the reactions of a patient with chronic
pain to 30 mg of morphine sulfate administered in
intravenous boluses over 35 minutes. The first test
(upper) represents the presumed opiate-tolerant
state; the later test (lower) shows the effect of tolerance reversal after several weeks of dietary loading
with L-tryptophan. The abscissas represent time in
minutes (N.S. = placebo bolus of normal saline;
M.S. = bolus or morphine sulfate); on the ordinates
are represented the patient's subjective evaluation
of pain on a scale of 0 to 10 (left) (•————•) and the
patient's tolerance of straight-leg raising in degrees from the horizontal (right) (△————△). (Reproduced with permission from Hosobuchi Y, Lamb
S, Baskin D: Tryptophan loading may reverse tolerance to opiate analgesics in humans: A preliminary
report. *Pain 9*:161–169, 1980.)

PAG stimulation.[3] Unless this tolerance is reversed before further therapy is attempted, PAG stimulation will not provide satisfactory pain control.

Morphine Test

The analgesic efficacy of opiates in the individual patient is tested in the following way: Opiate analgesics are withheld for 12 hours before the test. During the testing period, the patient lies recumbent in a hospital bed. Base-line respiration, pulse rates, and blood pressure measurements are made before testing begins and are carefully monitored from the beginning of the test until at least 2 hours afterward.

A base-line assessment of the pain level is made by the patient using a subjective visual analogue scale of 0 (no pain) to 10 (maximum pain). Morphine sulfate (up to 30 mg intravenously) is administered in divided doses over a period of 35 to 45 minutes. Administration is done in a double-blind manner; the placebo is normal saline. At intervals of 5 to 10 minutes after the first injection of morphine, the degree of pain relief is assessed by the patient using the visual analogue scale. If the patient is suffering from chronic low-back pain, his or her ability to endure straight-leg raising can be used concurrently as an objective measurement of pain relief (Fig. 66-1).

After reporting relief of pain from the morphine, or after having received 30 mg of morphine, the patient is given naloxone, an opiate antagonist. If the effect of the morphine is reversed when naloxone is administered, the probability of successfully providing analgesia by PAG stimulation.[3] Unless this tolerance is reversed before further therapy is attempted, PAG naloxone. Generally, the patient suffering from deafferentation pain caused by a neuronal lesion

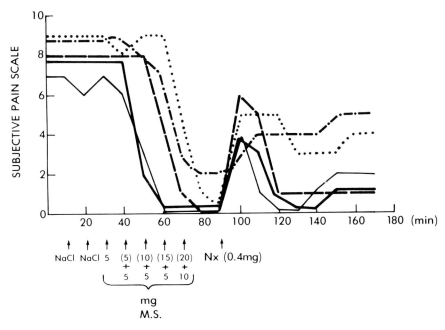

**ANALGESIC RESPONSE OF PAIN DUE TO ARACHNOIDITIS
(5 patients) TO I.V. MORPHINE**

Fig. 66-2.   A graph of the analgesic response of 5 patients with chronic pain from arachnoiditis to 30 mg of morphine sulfate administered in intravenous boluses over 70 minutes, followed at 90 minutes by an intravenous bolus of the opiate antagonist naloxone. The abscissa represents time in minutes (NaCl = placebo bolus of normal saline; M.S. = bolus of morphine sulfate; Nx = naloxone); on the ordinate are represented the patients' subjective evaluation of pain on a scale of 0 to 10.

proximal to dorsal root ganglia either experiences no relief from 30 mg of morphine or the relief mainly is due to the euphoric effect of the morphine and is not dose-dependent; it therefore requires a considerably high intravenous dose of naloxone to reverse the pain relief induced. In contrast, if the source of the patient's pain lies distal to the dorsal root ganglia (examples would include some types of deafferentation pain, such as peripheral neuropathy), then the degree of pain relief reported by the patient will reflect a more or less dose-dependent correlation with the amount of morphine administered. In this case, the analgesic effect of morphine is always reversed by a small dose of naloxone (less than 1 mg) (Fig. 66-2). If the patient undergoing the morphine test has developed tolerance to the analgesic effect of morphine, the relief from pain is partial, though it is generally dose-dependent (Fig. 66-2). Tolerance at such a stage often can be reversed by the administration of oral loading doses of the serotonin precursor, L-tryptophan (4 g daily) over a period of a few weeks (See Fig. 66-1).

Defining the tolerance of a patient to the analgesic action of opiates on the basis of responses to an intravenous 30-mg dosage of morphine is arbitrary; if a higher dose is given to these opiate-tolerant individuals, they may continue to have relief from pain. Nevertheless, if the patient shows only partial pain relief with 30 mg of morphine given intravenously within the duration of 30 to 45 minutes (that is to say, if the analgesic response is not reduced beyond the level of 3 on the visual analogue scale), withholding surgery for electrode implantation is advised until this tolerance is reversed by loading doses of L-tryptophan. After taking L-tryptophan (4 g daily) for a period of 2 to 6 weeks, patients usually report increasing analgesic efficacy of the opiate, and their demand for opiate analgesics decreases.

An obvious pitfall of the *morphine test* is that the pain may arise from mixed lesions (e.g., a chronic low-back problem concurrent with arachnoiditis and radiculopathy). In such circumstances, a second morphine test made after the period of L-tryptophan loading can differentiate between the components of the pain (e.g., patients may experience total relief from the back pain, but none or only partial relief from a burning pain in the legs or feet).

Implantation of the Electrodes

The electrode that currently is available commercially is made of pure platinum. It consists of four wires that are entwined, terminating with the individual wires separated from one another to form four 1-mm-long loops (0.8 mm in diameter). These constitute four separate contact points. They are 2 mm apart, as measured from the midpoint of each contact. The electrode contact points are labeled 0, 1, 2, and 3 by the manufacturer; 0 is the most inferior contact point. The loop of the most inferior contact (0) facilitates the insertion of the electrode into the central gray matter by encircling the tip of the special tool that is used to insert the electrode into the brain.

The implantation of the electrode is accomplished by means of a stereotactic neurosurgical procedure. Local scalp anesthesia is used. A standard stereotactic apparatus (such as the Leksell, Riechert-Mundinger, or Todd-Wells apparatuses) serves satisfactorily for this operation, although I prefer to use the Leksell apparatus.

The patient is placed in the semi-sitting position on a specially designed operating table. The head is shaved, washed with Betadine soap and water, and painted with Betadine solution. The head rests on a small suboccipital cup support. First, the stereotactic head frame is positioned and supported using calibrated ear plugs, and the midline of the apparatus (Z axis) is carefully approximated to the midsagittal plane of the head. Three entry zones on the scalp are selected for the placement of three skull pins that will be screwed into the outer table of the skull. These scalp areas are generously infiltrated with local anesthetic. The hole for the anterior skull pin is placed just behind the hairline of the forehead (for naturally bald patients, this site is approximated as closely as possible). The other two sites are positioned approximately 4 cm behind each external auditory meatus. A guiding tube that pierces the scalp is inserted at each of these three sites, and is firmly fixed to the pericranium. Then, a skull pin is inserted into each of the three guiding tubes and is screwed into the outer table of the skull using a special drill.

The surgeon must, at this point, make sure that the frame is firmly fixed to the patient's skull. The head and frame then are partially draped, leaving the patient's face exposed. The location for two separate scalp incisions are marked so as to bisect the coronal suture on each side, 2.5 cm from the midline, and the scalp is infiltrated with local anesthetic. Bilateral, paramedian, pericoronal burr holes are made 1 cm anterior to the coronal sutures and 2.5 cm from the midline. It is critical that the burr holes be made in precisely this location. (In the case of brachycephalic or dolichocephalic patients, the burr holes are moved in either an anterior or posterior direction so that the line connecting the burr holes to the posterior commissure will form an angle of 60° to 70° to the intercommissural line.) Since the target points in either the PAG or the sensory thalamic nuclei are located within 5 mm of the X and Y axis (the anteroposterior (AP) axis and ventrodorsal axis), this trajectory offers the maximum probability of the electrode contact points being placed in the region that will produce therapeutically effective stimulation.

After the burr holes are appropriately placed, the dura of the right burr hole is opened in cruciate fashion and is coagulated. The cortical surface is inspected carefully so that a major sulcus is not encountered in the trajectory. The surface of a gyrus is cauterized, a small cortical incision is made using a No. 15 blade, and the right lateral ventricle is cannulated with a Scott cannula. The tip of the cannula is aimed toward the contralateral angle of the mandible so that the catheter can be advanced to the third ventricle through the foramen of Monro. At this time 2 ml of air is introduced into the ventricle, and x-rays (AP and lateral views) are obtained to verify the location of the catheter. If necessary, the catheter positioning and x-ray exposure factors are corrected. Ventriculograms then are obtained in the AP and lateral projections using 3 ml of Conray contrast medium mixed with 7 ml of ventricular cerebrospinal fluid (CSF). These ventriculograms should delineate the foramen of Monro, the third ventricle, and the anterior and posterior commissures.

In my opinion the use of the computerized tomography (CT) scan in combination with the stereotactic apparatus for the electrode implantation procedure is unjustifiable, not only because of the expense of the CT scanning process, but more importantly because CT scanning cannot provide the surgeon with information sufficient for accurately determining the site of implantation of the electrode.

Target

Periaqueductal gray or periventricular gray.   For X and Y coordinates, the iter of the aqueduct is selected (Fig. 66-3). The laterality of the Z coordinate is therefore not influenced by the width of the third ventricle, as the target is caudal to this structure. The shape of the aqueduct is oblong in the ventral and dorsal axis at the iter, and the laterality of the target is determined by the ventral-dorsal diameter of the aqueduct at the iter, which is almost always less than 2 mm. Consequently, in most cases, the target laterality (Z coordinate) is 3 mm from the midline for the insertion tool. Since the electrode is always inserted in a position lateral to the insertion tool, the tip of the electrode usually lies 2.5 to 3.5 mm lateral from the midline of the iter of the aqueduct. The target point is marked on the ventriculogram; this point is projected perpendicularly to the reference scale of the frame, and the X, Y, and Z coordinates are calculated.

Implantation may be performed either unilaterally or bilaterally, although in my experience better analgesia is produced (by a 9 to 1 ratio) when the electrode is implanted in the left, rather than the right, PAG. Since there is no way to determine whether a patient will respond better with the electrode implanted in the left side or the right, and since bilateral implantation does not appear to produce greater morbidity, I routinely implant electrodes bilaterally to increase the chance of finding the optimal pair of contact points for stimulation that will produce the most effective analgesia.

After correct unilateral or bilateral X, Y, and Z coordinates, either unilaterally or bilater-

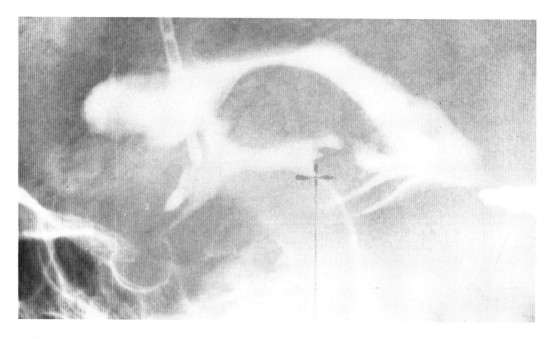

Fig. 66-3. A Conray ventriculogram, lateral view. The cross indicates the target point for the PAG electrode.

ally, for the prospective site(s) of implantation have been obtained, side bars are attached to the frame at the appropriate Y coordinate. The dura of the left burr hole is opened and the cortical surface is prepared as described earlier. The insertion tool is placed through the trajectory stage of the frame and is adjusted to ensure that the tip of the tool will hit the target point accurately. The arc is attached to the frame by clamping it to the side bar at the predetermined X and Z coordinates.

The scalp posterior to the burr holes then is infiltrated with a local anesthetic, and is penetrated with a 14-gauge needle with its stylet in place. The needle is inserted approximately 5 cm posterior to the burr holes and is passed subgaleally to each burr hole. The stylet then is removed from the needle. The percutaneous extension of the electrode is passed through the needle shaft from the site of the burr hole to the hub of the needle; as the extension appears from the needle hub, the needle is carefully withdrawn from the scalp. The connector of the electrode to the percutaneous extension is taped (with steri-strips) to the self-retaining retractor on the burr-hole incision.

The electrode now is inserted. The tip of the insertion tool is placed within the terminal loop of the electrode. The electrode always should be lateral to the insertion tool to avoid unnecessary damage to the posterior medial thalamus and hypothalamus by a leukotomy-type injury created by the angle between the insertion tool and the electrode. The surgeon holds the electrode close to the insertion tool using blunt forceps, and the assistant advances the insertion tool into the brain. It is very important to avoid excessive tension of the electrode against the insertion tool because this will uncoil the second contact point, which might alter the distance between the first contact or loop to the second contact or possibly break the loop.

When the insertion tool reaches the target point, the electrode is disengaged from the tool by very gentle clockwise and counterclockwise rotation of the tool around approximately 45°. Excessive and vigorous rotation of the tool should be avoided because it will dislodge the electrode from the target. The insertion tool is withdrawn from the brain. The electrode is temporarily fixed to the edge of the burr hole by a small ball of bone wax, and the burr hole is covered with a wet cotton ball.

Test stimulation is delivered between the most distant pair of contact points, using the most inferior contact point as the cathode. The settings for test stimulation are pulse duration—0.5 msec; frequency—50 Hz; and amplitude starting at 1 V and gradually increasing. At about 6 to 8 V, the patient invariably reports oscillopsia or an inability to initiate ocular movement. I have found that the suppression of conjugate upward gaze during stimulation is the most reliable physiologic determinant to assure correct placement of the electrode. Although pain relief is effected at a much lower amplitude, I do not use a demonstration of the analgesic efficacy of PAG stimulation in the operating room as a determinant of accurate electrode placement, since, under the stress of surgery under local anesthesia, the patient may perceive the pain to be alleviated when in fact it is not.

The same procedure is repeated to implant the electrode on the right side.

After both electrodes are implanted and after electrical stimulation induces a satisfactory ocular response, the cortex is covered with Gelfoam and the electrodes are fixed to the edge of the burr holes with cranioplastic material. A subgaleal pocket is developed and the extra length of electrode connector and percutaneous extension cable are inserted into it; the wounds then are closed in two layers. The final confirmation of electrode localization usually is made at this stage; however, if the surgeon is not certain that the electrode is situated optimally (for example, if the expected ocular response is not obtained), then confirmatory x-rays (AP and lateral views) must be made before the electrode is fixed to the burr holes by cranioplasty (Figs. 66-4A and B). Correction of the electrode position can be made by removing the electrodes, re-examining the coordinates, and reinserting the electrodes. Multiple trials of electrode insertion are unquestionably inadvisable since with each trial the risk of ocular palsy or possible intracerebral or intraventricular hemorrhage is increased.

Sensory thalamic nuclei (PVM, PVL): The basic coordinates for the sensory nuclei of the thalamus are obtained from the Schaltenbrand-Bailey stereotactic atlas. The widest coronal dimension of the nuclei is approximately 10 mm posterior to the midpoint of the line joining the anterior and posterior commissures (AC-PC line). The face area of the nucleus presents medially, starting 9 to 11 mm laterally at 2 mm below the level of the AC-PC line; the arm and leg area are located further laterally, 2 to 3 mm apart. The dimensions and location of the sensory thalamic nuclei vary considerably among individuals according to the length of the AC-PC line and the width of the third ventricle.

Exploratory stimulation of the target area with a monopolar electrode, 0.8 mm in diameter with a 2 to 3 mm exposed tip, is advised. The exploratory stimulation begins 5 mm proximal to the target point, extending perhaps 5 to 7 mm beyond the target point along the same trajectory.

The patient reports the area in which he experiences paresthesia in order to guide the surgeon in placing the stimulation electrode at the point where optimal induced paresthesia is obtained. In cases of deafferentation pain the most crisp response of induced paresthesia in the desired area of the body usually is obtained at the boundary of the gray and white matter or where the medial lemniscus enters the sensory nuclei; therefore, impedance monitoring also may be useful.

If induced paresthesia is not experienced in the desired area of the body, the surgeon must withdraw the monopolar electrode and replace it either medially or laterally, and often 2 to 3 mm posteriorly—especially in cases of pain in the lower extremity. It therefore is not unusual for the final coordinates of the target point to deviate 2 to 3 mm in any direction (X, Y, or Z) from the target initially calculated on the basis of the ventriculogram and the stereotactic atlas.

The insertion of the electrode follows essentially the same procedure as that described for the PAG target, except that the surgeon has to move the trajectory of the insertion tool 1 mm medially to ensure that the most inferior contact point of the permanent electrode rests in the correct target area. Placement of the electrode is reaffirmed by stimulation of the most distant pair of contacts, using the most inferior contact as the cathode. The stimulation settings of 0.5-msec pulse duration, 50- to 100-Hz frequency, and 1 to 3 V should induce pleasant paresthesia in

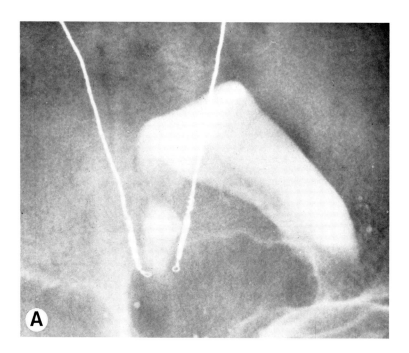

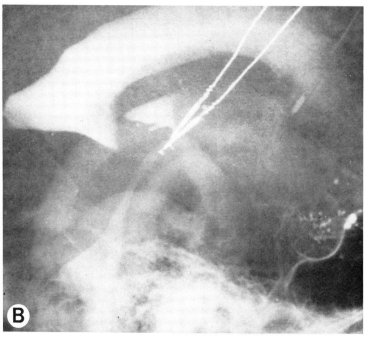

Fig. 66-4.   Bilaterally implanted PAG electrodes. Postoperative Conray ventriculograms in the (**A**) AP and (**B**) lateral views show the appropriate relationship of the electrodes to the iter of the aqueduct.

the region of the body involved with deafferentation pain. The electrodes are fixed to the burr holes by cranioplasty, and confirmatory x-rays (AP and lateral) are obtained. The wound is closed as described above.

Postimplantation Patient Care

After electrode implantation surgery, patients often complain of headache, nausea, and occasionally, in the case of PAG implantation, diplopia; in addition, they feel their original pain. To control the pain at this stage, the administration of a short-acting opiate analgesic, such as meperidine (Demerol) administered intramuscularly, is perferred in order to avoid masking an altered level of consciousness that would signify possible intracerebral or intraventricular hemorrhage. Dexamethasone (Decadron) rarely is used unless the patient complains of significant diplopia. Compazine is given intramuscularly to control nausea and vomiting if they occur.

On very rare occasions a patient may have a seizure 4 to 8 hours after surgery. This is thought to be a consequence of the circulation of potentially epileptogenic contrast medium (Conray) from the ventricular system out into the subarachnoid space over the convexities. Despite the relative infrequency of this complication (in about 2 percent to 3 percent of patients), it is wise to start the administration of Dilantin 24 hours before the implantation surgery. To ensure rapid washout of the Conray from the CSF, patients should be well hydrated. If the patient cannot maintain adequate oral fluid intake, intravenous fluid therapy is continued.

Postoperative Screening of the Contact Points

Because of the usual postoperative headache and nausea, it may not be possible to start trial stimulation through the percutaneous extension for 2 to 3 days after surgery. When the patient recovers from the acute discomfort of the operation and is able to walk, screening of the various pairs of contact points begins in order to identify the most effective pair of contact points through which stimulation best relieves the original pain.

The most inferior contact point (contact point 0) should be in the optimal anatomic position. Over 80 percent of the patients find 0 to be the most effective cathode, although the anode may vary. Occasionally 1, 2, or 3, rather than 0, is the more effective cathode. The patients are provided with a polarized cable to connect the percutaneous extension to a battery-operated stimulator for self-stimulation. They then are instructed in the use of the self-stimulation device.

Patients receiving PAG stimulation are given a timer so that the duration of their self-stimulation is strictly limited to 15 to 20 minutes for each session. The biphasic stimulation settings for PAG stimulation are 25-Hz frequency, 0.5-msec pulse duration, and one-half of the voltage that induces apparent oscillopsia in the individual patient. (For example, if the patient reports oscillopsia starting at 8 V, then 4 V should produce pain relief without causing any other neurologic or psychologic alterations.) Stimulation should be limited to no more than 15 to 20 minutes for each session, and should be used no more frequently than every 4 to 6 hours.

In the case of patients using stimulation of the sensory nuclei of the thalamus, the stimulation settings are 0.5-msec pulse duration, 50- to 100-Hz frequency; the voltage is that at which the induced paresthesia is not unpleasantly strong. The stimulation is biphasic and must be administered in ramp fashion; the optimal duration of the ramp envelope is 20 to 30 seconds. Patients must be carefully apprised of the significance of ramp stimulation, since the stimulator occasionally may malfunction and, failing to produce ramp mode, may not produce a therapeutic effect. In such a circumstance the patient should realize that the stimulator must be readjusted.

Patients are provided with a self-assessment sheet on which to rate the efficacy of the stimulation from each particular pair of contact points. The pain is assessed on a subjective scale of 0 to 10, 0 denoting "no pain" and 10 denoting pain that the patient can barely tolerate. They are instructed to note the severity of the pain before and after brain stimulation. If stimulation does not provide adequate pain relief, or if they still have postoperative headache, they are allowed to use analgesics; but they must record the time and dosage, the reason for the need of the analgesic, and the extent of the relief obtained from the medication.

In over 90 percent of patients the efficacy of brain stimulation in controlling chronic pain becomes apparent within 7 to 10 days of their initial identification of a specific pair of contact points. In some cases, however, arriving at the optimal efficacy may require more time. When the decision is delayed, it usually is because of uncertainty about whether or not the most effective pair of contact points has been selected, or because the patient's pain is related to the type or extent of his daily activities. In such situations patients are encouraged to return home while they continue the screening process. In all cases an additional 2 to 3 weeks of trial stimulation provides an answer. While the electrodes are externalized through the percutaneous extension, it is essential that the wound through which the percutaneous extension exits is kept clean by daily swabbing with hydrogen peroxide, and that local applications of antibiotic ointment are used to prevent scalp infection. If the patient is discharged from the hospital for further screening at home, a family member is fully instructed in how to care for the wound(s).

Internalization of the Electrode

When the most effective pair of contact points for analgesic brain stimulation has been identified, the patient is ready for internalization of the electrode, which will be connected to a radiofrequency receiver for transcutaneous self-stimulation.

Since this surgical procedure is primarily performed subcutaneously, it is done under general anesthesia. The percutaneous extension wires from the electrodes are cut flush with the skin before skin preparation is undertaken. The head is turned to the side opposite the site where the receiver will be placed, and is supported by a horseshoe-type of headrest. Since the percutaneous extension communicates from the skin surface to the subgaleal plane, there is a potential risk of subgaleal infection. It is therefore our custom to administer tobramycin (1.5 g/kg) and vancomycin (15 mg/kg) intravenously before making a skin incision. Antibiotic therapy every 8 hours is continued for the first 48 hours postoperatively.

After draping the patient, a 5-cm transverse subclavicular incision is made, and a subcutaneous pocket is created for the radiofrequency receiver. A 3-cm incision is made over the mastoid process, and a subcutaneous tunnel is developed from this wound to the subclavicular wound using a specially designed metal bar to which a sharp, arrowheadlike tip can be attached. Care is taken to avoid perforating the apex of the lung or tearing the anterior branch of the external jugular vein. The "arrowhead" tip then is replaced with a specially designed attachment into which the ends of the extension cable from the receiver can be secured. The extension cable connector is enclosed within this device and is delivered subcutaneously into the mastoid wound. The burr hole incision is reopened and the procedure is repeated to bring the extension connector up to the burr hole wound.

The residual cables exiting from the connector nearest to the brain electrode, which previously exited percutaneously, are cut flush with the tips of the pins of this connector and are discarded. The silicone covering on the two pins to be connected is carefully stripped. The surgeon then places a protective plastic connector boot on the lead, connects the appropriate pins and tightens the connector screws, and pulls this protective boot over the entire connection. By convention, the negative pole of the conductor is identified with a white sleeve by the manufacturer. The protective boot assembly is filled with type-A silicone medical adhesive, which is provided by the manufacturer to create a water-tight seal. The three wounds are well irrigated with saline and closed in two layers. The extra lead wire is pulled through to the subclavicular end and is placed in the subcutaneous pocket with the radiofrequency receiver.

Expected Results and Follow-up

Postoperatively, the patient starts self-stimulation within 2 or 3 days and is discharged from the hospital within 5 to 7 days. If the patients have been selected properly, the stereotactic placement of the electrodes is correct, and appropriate contact pairs of the electrodes have been identified after thorough testing, then the majority of patients should obtain good relief of pain from transcutaneous stimulation and should require no further use of opiate analgesics.[5] For patients who have PAG electrodes, it is of paramount importance that they receive L-tryptophan (4 g orally each day) to avoid their developing a tolerance to PAG stimulation. If a tolerance develops, the patient is instructed to refrain from stimulation for at least 2 weeks. By the end of this period, the analgesic efficacy of PAG stimulation usually has returned. Further details about the management of tolerance to stimulation is beyond the scope of this chapter; readers are referred to the previous publications cited below.[4-6]

REFERENCES

1. Hosobuchi Y, Adams JE, Rutkin B: Chronic thalamic stimulation for the control of facial anesthesia dolorosa. *Arch Neurol 29*:158–161, 1973
2. Hosobuchi Y, Adams JE, Linchitz R: Pain relief by electrical stimulation of the central gray matter in humans. *Science 197*:183–186, 1977
3. Hosobuchi Y, Lamb S, Baskin D: Tryptophan loading may reverse tolerance to opiate analgesics in humans: A preliminary report. *Pain 9*:161–169, 1980
4. Hosobuchi Y, Wemmer J: Disulfiram inhibition of development of tolerance to analgesia induced by central gray stimulation in humans. *Eur J Pharmacol 43*:385–387, 1977
5. Hosobuchi Y: Dietary supplementation with L-tryptophan reverses tolerance to analgesia induced by periaqueductal gray stimulation in humans, in Way EL (ed): *Endogenous and Exogenous Opiate Agonists and Antagonists*. New York, Pergamon Press, 1980, pp 375–378
6. Hosobuchi Y: The current status of analgesic brain stimulation. *Acta Neurochir (Suppl) 30*:219–227, 1980

CHAPTER 67
Functional Neurosurgery

Philip L. Gildenberg

FUNCTIONAL NEUROSURGERY is that aspect of neurosurgery that acts to change neurophysiologic function by surgical means. To discuss the indications for such procedures it is necessary to consider alternate nonsurgical treatments as well.

The usual modalities by which function of the nervous system can be changed are ablation and stimulation of specific sites. Ablation, or the production of a lesion, is accomplished by the application of heat, cold, electrical energy, or radiation. Radiation also can be used either by local insertion of a radioisotope or by focusing large amounts of radiation on a small field within the nervous system. Temporary or permanent functional changes of the nervous system also may follow application of a chemical or pharmacologic agent. This agent can be administered on a short-term basis by injection or on a long-term basis by the use of a chemode, i.e., an implanted reservoir from which minute quantities of an agent may leech over a protracted period of time. The present discussion will concentrate primarily on ablation and stimulation procedures in clinical use.

Classically, functional neurosurgery has concerned conditions in which the function of the nervous system has become defective, so that restoration of normal function or obliteration or modification of symptoms that represent an abnormal expression of nervous system function is desirable. Thus, the problems with which functional neurosurgery have been most involved have been intractable pain, movement disorders, disorders of muscle tone, affective disorders, and epilepsy.

Stereotactic Surgery

Stereotactic surgery involves techniques whereby an apparatus is employed to direct an electrode to an intracerebral target to alter the function of structures deep within the brain with minimal damage to overlying structures. Before the advent of stereotactic surgery, it was necessary to ablate a structure under direct vision.

In 1908, Horsley and Clarke[1] devised a technique that allowed an electrode to be introduced into specific subcortical structures in experimental animals. Their technique required the preparation of an atlas, which pictured brain slices in a measured relationship to landmarks on the skull of the animal, to ensure that the electrode would consistently reach a point in space that had a specific relationship to the landmarks.

To accomplish this, three planes at right angles to each other are employed to form a system of Cartesian coordinates. The horizontal or basal plane is the plane that intersects both external auditory canals and the inferior orbital ridge. The experimental apparatus is fashioned to secure the head of the animal by means of ear plugs placed in the auditory canals and tabs that rest on

Division of Neurosurgery, University of Texas Medical School, Houston, Texas

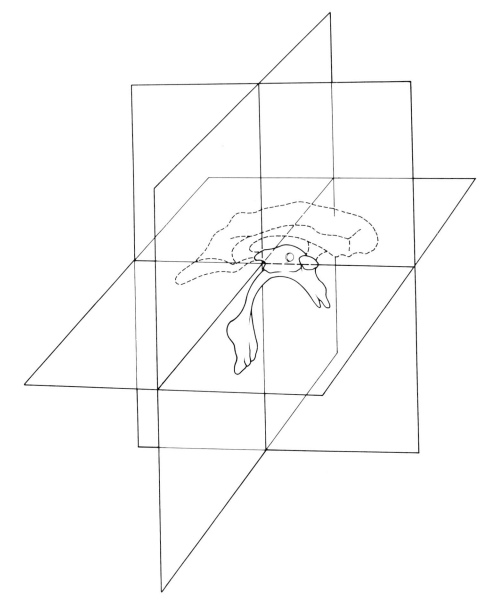

Fig. 67-1.

the inferior orbital ridges, thus aligning the head with the horizontal plane. The second plane, at right angles to the basal plane, lies in the midsagittal plane of the brain. The third plane lies at right angles to the first two, and also passes through the external auditory canals. Thus, a given point in space can be defined as lying x millimeters to the right or left of the midsagittal plane, y millimeters in front of the interaural plane, and z millimeters above the basal plane, and only one point in space can satisfy this description. It is thereby possible to identify the coordinates of a given anatomic structure from an atlas of brains sliced parallel to one of the reference planes and a measured distance from that plane; the relationship to the other planes is indicated by millimeter scales along the borders of the brain slices.

With the Horsley-Clarke apparatus it became possible to introduce an electrode into a subcortical structure with a reasonable degree of certainty, without destroying the overlying tissue. Modifications of this device are standard tools essential for neurophysiologic investigations.

Attempts to apply this system to humans were difficult. Since there is great variability between the landmarks on the skull and anatomic structures, accuracy of the system did not approach that required for clinical use.

In 1947, Spiegel et al.[2] related the coordinate system to internal landmarks within the human brain, allowing stereotactic techniques to be applied to humans. Originally, they took as their landmarks the foramen of Monro and the pineal gland.

The system currently in use is based on improved radiologic techniques. In this system the basal plane passes through a line drawn between the anterior and posterior commissures at right angles to the midsagittal plane. The third reference plane is at right angles to these two planes, and either passes through the posterior commissure or through the midpoint of the intercommissural line (Fig. 67-1). Some authors use a line between the posterior commissure and the foramen of Monro. Landmarks are visualized by a pneumoencephalogram performed just before surgery, or by instilling air or contrast material through a ventriculostomy inserted during surgery.

Stereotactic Atlas

Several atlases of the human brain have been published. The first, that of Spiegel and Wycis, published in 1952,[3] is still quite useful. One of the more widely used, however, is that of Schaltenbrand and Bailey,[4] which consists of beautifully enlarged photographs of brain slices with overlays outlining anatomic structures. The excellent atlas by Talairach et al.[5] is used by many Europeans, and recently some atlases have been specifically directed to the diencephalon[6,7,8] or the brainstem and cerebellum.[9]

A key factor in the use of stereotactic atlases is the considerable variability between brains. The coordinates obtained from a stereotactic atlas provide only approximations of where a given anatomic structure is most likely to be found. For this reason, most atlases include variability tables so that corrections in coordinates can be made for a patient whose brain does not have the same general characteristics as the representative sections appearing in the atlas.

Consequently, one must differentiate between anatomic accuracy and stereotactic or mechanical accuracy. A well-constructed stereotactic apparatus can bring the tip of an electrode to within 1 mm of a specific coordinate. Whether the desired anatomic structure lies at that coordinate is a reflection of anatomic variability, and this factor must be considered in every stereotactic procedure. Consequently, physiologic verification of the location of the electrode tip by recording or stimulation techniques is necessary whenever possible.

Types of Stereotactic Apparatus

There are three basic types of stereotactic apparatus (Fig. 67-2). The most common is the arc type (C), in which the target point lies at the center of an arc along which the electrode holder moves. The electrode approaches the brain in a direction perpendicular to the tangent of the arc, so that it is always directed toward a target point at the center of that arc. If the electrode is advanced from the arc by a distance equal to the radius of the arc, the electrode is accurately guided to the target point. If the arc is positioned so that the desired anatomic target point coincides with the mechanical target point at the center of the arc, the electrode can be advanced to the desired structure.

The three most widely used commercially available stereotactic apparatuses use the *arc principle*.[10] The *Leksell apparatus*[11] has a coordinate system radiologically indicated on a rectangular frame attached to the patient's head; the coordinate system of the frame can be related to the reference planes on the x-rays. The arc is attached to the rectangular frame so the center of the arc lies at the desired coordinate where the anatomic target is most likely located. The *Riechert apparatus*[12] has a basal ring to which the patient's head is secured, and the arc is positioned in relation to the basal ring so that the target point lies at the appropriate coordinates. The *Todd-Wells apparatus*[13] works in a reciprocal fashion. The system of arcs is in constant relation to

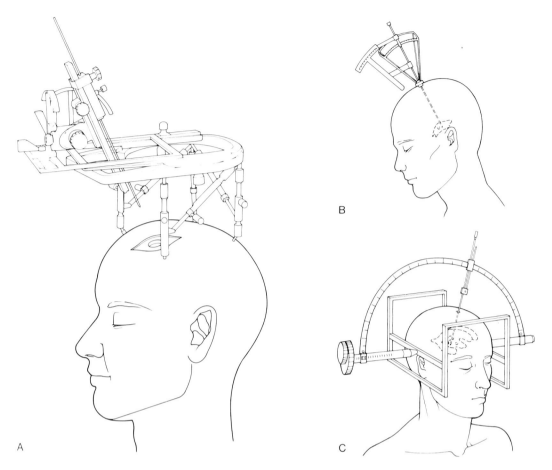

Fig. 67-2.   The three basic types of stereotactic apparatus.

the frame of the apparatus and the patient's head is moved in order to bring the anatomic structure to the mechanical target point.

The *rectilinear type* of stereotactic apparatus is based on the same principle as the Horsley-
Clarke[1] and Spiegel-Wycis[2] devices (A). It provides individually for the longitudinal and vertical
movements of the electrode by simple linear mechanical adjustments. Most of the rectilinear apparatuses that presently are available also provide for sagittal and transverse angle adjustments
so that the electrode can be aimed and advanced to the target point along a predetermined trajectory. The center of the arc of the angular adjustment, however, does not coincide with the target
point.

The *aiming type* of stereotactic apparatus consists of a ball joint screwed into a burr hole (B).
The angles of insertion of an electrode can be adjusted and the depth of insertion of the electrode
controlled so the probe can be pointed to the target and advanced into it. Since it is difficult to secure an apparatus to the edge of a burr hole, however, distortion occurs as the device is manipulated, and since angular adjustments generally are less accurate than linear adjustments, a device
that depends totally on angular adjustments tends to be less accurate.

Radiologic Considerations

Several radiologic considerations are crucial to stereotactic surgery. Since x-rays emanate
from their source in a radial fashion rather than in parallel rays, parallax and magnification may
distort the stereotactic measurements. To minimize the effects of parallax (the distortion that oc-

curs when an object is looked at obliquely), the reference planes of the stereotactic apparatus or the brain must be aligned with the central beam of the x-ray source. This is accomplished by attaching radioopaque markers to the apparatus or to the patient's head so that superimposition of those markers on the x-ray picture verifies proper alignment.

Since the x-ray beams are radial rather than parallel, x-ray images are magnified, depending on the distance between the x-ray source and the head compared to the distance between the head and the cassette. Magnification can be minimized by holding the x-ray tube at a long distance from the subject so that the rays are more nearly parallel when they reach the subject. Systems using a shorter tube-to-cassette distance require that the magnification be measured, and the actual distances can be calculated. A radiopaque centimeter scale is positioned in the midsagittal plane or plane of reference and appears on the x-ray film so that magnification can be measured. It must be remembered, however, that cerebral structures closer to the x-ray tube will have a larger magnification than those closer to the cassette, and these differences also must be corrected.

Procedure

Most functional stereotactic procedures are performed under local anesthesia so accuracy in the placement of the electrode in the proper anatomic structure can be tested and the effects of stimulation or lesion production assessed during the procedure.

After the head is shaved, the apparatus is secured to the patient's head, using local anesthesia at the contact points.

The third venticle is visualized by a pneumoencephalogram, with air instilled just before surgery, or through a burr hole with a ventricular catheter placed to instill air or contrast material. Conray, Pantopaque (metrizamide) have been used successfully, but must be used with caution. If air is used, it may be necessary to instill the air under controlled pressure to visualize the posterior commissure.

Anteroposterior (AP) and lateral x-rays are taken. The midline of the third ventricle is determined in relation to the coordinate system of the apparatus so that appropriate lateral corrections can be made.

The anterior and posterior commissures are identified on the lateral x-rays, and a line is drawn between the two. The intended target point, determined from an atlas, is measured from those reference lines and marked on the AP and lateral x-rays.

The apparatus is adjusted by a series of progressive approximations. Some arc-type apparatuses have an indicator that is visualized on the AP or lateral films to designate the mechanical target point.

With other apparatuses it is necessary to secure a probe in the electrode holder and advance that probe until it just touches the scalp or burr hole; a line is drawn on the AP and lateral x-rays through and beyond the image of the probe to indicate the trajectory. The apparatus is readjusted to bring the electrode trajectory to the intended coordinates. Another pair of AP and lateral x-rays is taken to determine whether the adjustment is accurate. Finer and finer adjustments are employed until the electrode carrier is accurately pointed to the target.

Depending on the procedure, the venticulostomy burr hole may be used to insert the electrode, or a second may be made. The dura is coagulated and incised, and the electrode is advanced to the intended target point. Anteroposterior and lateral films are taken with the electrode in position to verify the accuracy of electrode placement.

When the electrode is at the proper coordinates, it usually is necessary to employ physiologic verification to ensure that the proper anatomic structure has been impaled. If the intended target has identifiable electrical activity, such as the amygdala, depth EEG recording can provide verification. Indeed, it may be advantageous to perform such recordings as the electrode is advanced to the target point so that the appropriate change in spontaneous electrical activity can signal entrance into the desired structure. An area of abnormal electrical activity or cessation of electrical activity may characterize the target structure and may be used as a physiologic marker.

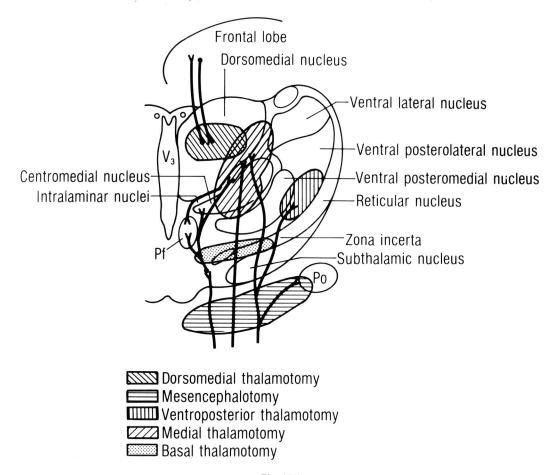

Fig. 67-3.

Single units have been successfully recorded during stereotactic surgery. This is of considerable research interest, but because the population of cells sampled is quite small, single-unit recording may not be of general clinical help during surgery, except for the recording of bursts of spontaneous activity synchronous with tremor during thalamotomy.[14] There is a great deal of extraneous electrical noise when attempts are made to record with a microelectrode or semimicroelectrode. Changes in the level of this noise can be employed to determine when the electrode is moving through the interface from one structure to another and to demonstrate that the thalamus has been entered.[14,15]

If the electrode is to be inserted into a specific somatosensory relay nucleus, such as the ventral posterolateral nucleus or the intralaminar nucleus of the thalamus, potentials evoked by stimulation of peripheral nerves are helpful indicators that these structures have been entered.

Without employing elaborate recording equipment, or in an operating room where the electrical environment is not favorable for intraoperative recording, considerable information can be obtained from stimulation. Tasker et al.[16] have produced maps based on the subjective response of patients to stimulation as an electrode is advanced within the thalamus. Contralateral motor responses can be helpful in indicating the proximity of an electrode to the internal capsule and the distribution of motor fibers therein.[17] Extraocular movements may indicate an electrode approach that is too close to oculomotor fibers.

Attempts have been made to define borders of anatomic structures by measuring electrical impedance. This can be helpful in identifying when the ventricle has been entered, but the difference of impedance between the subnuclei is not adequately specific to be helpful.

Perhaps the most gratifying physiologic test for proper electrode placement is the influence that mechanical introduction of the electrode into the proper target may have on abnormal movements. For example, patients with Parkinsonian tremor may have an abrupt cessation of tremor as the electrode reaches its target, and these patients generally have a good result when the lesion is made at that point.

If the lesion is to be made by freezing, it is possible to have a temporary cessation of activity when the area is cooled only slightly.[18] The size of the cryoprobe is large, however, and may produce suppression of activity by its insertion alone. Since brain tissue is an excellent insulator, the steep thermal gradient confines the reversibly cooled tissue to a very narrow radius.

Once the electrode is inserted to the proper target, a lesion may be produced by local ablation, or a chronic stimulating electrode may be inserted.

Several methods are used to produce lesions within the central nervous system. The most common employs a radiofrequency current, a rapidly alternating current of 50,000–2,000,000 Hz. As this current passes through the tissue adjacent to the electrode, where the current concentration is greatest, it sets ions oscillating at frequencies where the friction produces heat within the tissues. If the heat produced exceeds 45°–50°C, a permanent lesion results. A thermistor is built into the electrode tip to monitor the temperature so the strength of the radiofrequency current can be adjusted to produce a controlled lesion. The maintenance of 80°C for 60 to 90 seconds will produce a consistent and predictable lesion. The size of the lesion may be varied by using electrodes of different sizes, with larger electrodes distributing the current and heat more widely.[19]

An alternate means of producing a lesion is with a cryoprobe. Typically, the metallic probe contains several thermistors at the tip that feed back to a system of valves to allow the circulation of liquid nitrogen through the probe to cool the tissue to a predetermined level.[18] Tissue frozen at $-70°C$ for 3 minutes produces a consistent lesion.[20] The cryoprobe is less versatile than the radiofrequency electrode, precluding stimulation or recording through the probe. In addition, probes are not available to produce extremely small lesions.

Direct current now is rarely used for the production of lesions because of its inherent danger. A sudden interruption or change in current flow can cause damaging stimulation to the patient's brain and heart. Nevertheless, the use of direct current is of historical importance, since it was used both by Horsley and Clarke[1] and then by Spiegel and Wycis.[2] It is still used in research laboratories and occasionally for producing small discrete lesions in stereotactic surgery, since it is possible to produce a much smaller controlled lesion. Perhaps the best and most thorough discussion of the use of direct current to produce lesions in the brain appeared in Horsley and Clarke's original article on stereotaxis in 1908.[1]

Chronic Stimulation Techniques

To accomplish chronic stimulation, or stimulation that can be applied over weeks or months, it is necessary to control the stimulation externally with a source of sufficient power. The requirements for stimulation often are complex, so that flexibility in stimulation parameters is required. Until recently, it was only possible to stimulate the nervous system chronically through percutaneous wires directly attached to an externally powered and controlled electronic stimulator. The risk of infection and the undesirability of having wires pierce the skin make such systems impractical.

A change that revolutionized functional neurosurgery was the development of implantable electronic stimulators powered and controlled from external sources. The key was radiofrequency coupling of an external power supply and control unit with an internalized radio receiver attached by subcutaneous leads to an electrode. The internal device is activated by electronic power transmitted in the radiofrequency control signal through the skin.

The implanted radio receiver converts the radiofrequency signal to individual impulses, the

characteristics of which are dependent on the transmitted signal. The hand-held radio transmitter is connected to a disc-shaped antenna that can be taped to the skin overlying the subcutaneously implanted radio receiver. The carrier frequency is selected to minimize interference or
inadvertent stimulation from incidental radio signals.[21] Such stimulation has been applied to stereotactically implanted electrodes within the brain, or electrodes inserted over the anterior lobe
of the cerebellum,[22] or other neural structures, such as peripheral nerve or spinal cord.

Stimulation applied to nervous tissue does not mimic the physiologic activity of the stimulated structure. The stimulation parameters have been empirically determined, and may be in the
range of usual discharge frequencies of a structure, may be frequencies that block rather than
stimulate the structure, or may exert their effect by releasing regional transmitter substances.

Each type of neural tissue stimulated requires a different electrode design and a somewhat
different technique for implantation.

Implantation Technique

The radio receiver is housed in a subcutaneous pocket, usually situated below the clavicle or
on the side of the abdomen so that the patient can hold the antenna against it while using the
other hand to adjust the stimulation parameters. It is convenient to implant the stimulator just
below the clavicle in women so that the antenna can be held by the brassiere strap.[23]

A subcutaneous pocket is created through a 5–7-cm skin incision, and is packed with wet
sponges during the remainder of the dissection. A subcutaneous tunnel is made so that the leads
from the radio receiver can be passed to the electrode site. A vascular mandrell or special instrument may be used to create the tunnel from an incision over the stimulation site to the receiver
pocket. A Penrose drain is passed through the tunnel, and the electrodes or connecters are
placed in the end of the Penrose drain and secured with umbilical tape. As the drain is pulled
through the tunnel, the lead wires are drawn through the tunnel, and the Penrose drain is removed.

For *deep-brain stimulation,* the electrode consists of a multi-contact wire electrode that is
stereotactically inserted into the brain.[24] The electrode is secured to a burr hole cover specifically
designed for this purpose. Most deep-brain stimulating electrodes come with four contacts, and
the best two contacts are selected for optimal stimulation. The procedure can be done in two
stages, with expendable lead wires emerging through the scalp for a period of direct electrode
stimulation on a trial basis. When permanent internalization is desired, the electrode lead wires
are tunneled under the scalp to a site where they connect with the lead wires that are tunneled
from the radio receiver, ordinarily housed at the infraclavicular site. The connectors lie beneath
the scalp positioned so they are not uncomfortable.

Dorsal cord-stimulating electrodes were originally designed to be implanted through a one-
or two-level laminectomy.[23] Originally the electrode was sutured in the subarachnoid space
within the dura just behind the dorsal columns, following which a watertight dural closure was
attempted. There was a high incidence of cerebrospinal fluid leak and decreasing stimulation intensity, however, as presumably the electrodes became surrounded by fibrous tissue, so the electrodes were later implanted in the subdural space, without opening the arachnoid. Despite this
improvement, late electrode failure sometimes occurred within 2 years, with the development of
fibrous tissue around the electrode. The technique evolved by which a pocket was formed within
the dura in which the electrode was sutured (endodural placement), which appeared to offer a
slight advantage over the subdural or subarachnoid placement. It now appears that it is acceptable to suture the electrode epidurally, minimizing complications while still achieving adequate
stimulation.

Recent developments have facilitated implantation of dorsal cord-stimulating electrodes.
Percutaneous electrodes are available that can be passed into the epidural space under fluoroscopic guidance and local anesthesia.[25] The percutaneous electrode consists of a flexible insulated wire, usually the appropriate size to fit through an 18-gauge Tuohy needle. The distal 3–5

mm of the wire are uninsulated and form the electrode contact. The end of the wire left protruding has a bare contact to which a connector can be attached, or it may have a small extension wire that is several inches long. In the latter case the entire electrode wire is placed subcutaneously, and the extension wires are brought out through a stab wound. To convert the electrodes to a permanently implanted system, if that is desired, the extension wires are cut off, and the electrode wires themselves (which have remained in a protected subcutaneous position) are connected to the lead wires from the radio receiver.

The percutaneous electrode wires are implanted under fluoroscopic guidance. For lower extremity pain, a midthoracic placement is best. For thoracic or upper extremity pain, an upper thoracic or cervical placement may be attempted. The patient is placed in the prone position on the x-ray table. A small stab wound is made in the skin in the midline at the site of the electrode insertion. Either a monopolar system may be used with a stimulator that incorporates the indifferent electrode, or two percutaneous electrodes wires can be inserted approximately 1 level apart to form a bipolar system. The Tuohy needle is inserted into the epidural space in the midline. The electrode wires are inserted through the needle and are threaded up several segments. A stiffening wire within the electrode can be used to help guide the electrode to the proper position. When the electrode is in the correct position, the needle is removed, leaving the electrode in place.

A stimulator is attached to the lead wires so the effects of stimulation may be tested while the patient is still on the table. The electrodes are advanced, withdrawn, or repositioned until the sensation is projected to the proper area, which may take some experimentation. When the sensation is appropriate, the ends of the wire are buried in a subcutaneous pocket for later attachment under general anesthesia to a subcutaneous radio receiver.

One problem with percutaneous electrodes has been migration of the electrodes as the patient moves. If the electrode migrates to a nerve root sleeve, the sensation may be projected along the distribution of that nerve at a voltage that is too low to obtain optimal pain relief from cord stimulation. This problem has been obviated by the use of sigma-shaped percutaneous electrodes. These electrodes are straight when inserted, but when a stiffening wire is removed, they assume a curved sigma shape, which holds them in midline position in the epidural space.

Indications for Functional Neurosurgery

Pain

Types of pain. Any neurosurgeon who deals with patients with intractable pain must recognize that different types of pain require entirely different approaches. Unfortunately this all-too-obvious rule is all too frequently neglected to the disadvantage of the patient and physician. One may consider that there are three types of pain of clinical importance—acute pain, cancer pain, and chronic pain.

Acute pain is an appropriate physiologic response to tissue damage or potential tissue damage. Because acute pain is temporally self-limited, the appropriate approach is to treat the pain with analgesics and rest. The major effort is directed to treating the underlying cause of the pain. If this is done, the pain ordinarily will go away, the analgesics can be stopped, and the patient can return to his previous activities.

Cancer pain may be considered to be continually recurrent acute pain. Treatment involves the aggressive use of analgesics or narcotics. Neurosurgical management usually involves ablation or interruption of pain pathways and, occasionally, chronic stimulation.

Patients with cancer usually are anxious or depressed. Treatment also must be directed to the emotional welfare and stability of the patient in a comprehensive fashion. Tranquilizers benefit the anxiety, antidepressants may be helpful, and hypnotics may serve to secure the patient adequate rest.

Chronic pain may be defined as pain that lasts more than 3 to 6 months and that has no useful biological purpose. The original etiology may have left some residual damage or may have healed. Analgesics, particularly narcotics, may complicate the picture with a superimposed addiction, may contribute to depression, and are not appropriate for chronic pain. Patients with chronic pain frequently are depressed and regressed, and the psychologic aspects of the patient's problems often are more significant than the actual physical impairment. The pain may be perpetuated by psychiatric considerations, so that neurosurgical procedures are most often doomed to failure.

There is little use for ablative neurosurgical procedures in the management of chronic pain, and stimulation procedures are useful only in a small, well-selected group of patients.

The key to neurosurgical management of chronic pain does not lie in the technical aspects of surgical operations. The key is in patient selection. Any neurosurgeon who takes the responsibility for managing patients with pain also must take the responsibility for evaluating and attending to the multitude of psychiatric problems that surround a patient in a state of pain. It behooves the neurosurgeon dealing with chronic pain to have alternate nonsurgical methods of management available, either personally or through close colleagues.

Anatomy of pain.   Pain is a complex sensation, in contradistinction to other sensory modalities. The pathways concerning the perception of pain are multiple, and it is the interaction of these pathways that allows the sensation of pain to come to consciousness. Because of the complexity of the system, pain can be modified by numerous factors, such as mental concentration, emotional tone, and whether one anticipates feeling pain or not.

Most of the information we have about ascending pain pathways relates to acute pain. The perception of chronic pain is far more complex, and may not always involve pain pathways.

A *noxious stimulus* is defined as one that has the potential to produce tissue damage and physiologically results in the perception of acute pain in the conscious subject. The pathology that produces acute pain often is related to tissue damage, such as a laceration or fracture, inflammation, or tearing of tissue, and may produce acute pain when it reaches the threshold of the small peripheral nerve fibers. Large nerves, as a rule, have a lower threshold to natural and electrical stimulation so that stimulation strong enough to stimulate small fibers is also suprathreshold for the larger nerve fibers that relate to somatic sensations other than pain.

The sensory nerves enter the spinal cord via the segmental roots. Melzack and Wall[26] have described a gate or neurophysiologic arrangement at the dorsal root entry zone, that determines whether the pain pathways will fire. Because of this *gating mechanism,* there is competition between the large and small nerve fibers to determine whether the pain pathways fire. If the stimulus is mild or nonpainful so that the large fibers predominate, the gate will remain closed. If the intensity of the stimulus increases to the point where the small fibers predominate, the gate opens and pain is perceived.

Because pain perception depends in part on the balance between the large and small fibers, one can treat pain either by decreasing the firing of a small fiber (as with local anesthetic) or by increasing the firing of a large fiber (when you rub it, it feels better). Hence, it is possible to increase the firing of large cells by applying a nonpainful stimulus peripherally or by stimulating the dorsal columns of the spinal cord, in which case the impulse proceeds downward in a retrograde fashion (in addition to upward) to help close the gate at each spinal segment. There is further evidence that similar gating mechanisms occur higher in the nervous system, as in subthalamic levels of the brainstem.[27,28]

For the purposes of explaining ablative procedures useful in the treatment of pain, particularly cancer pain, one might consider that there are at least three ascending pain pathways that may fire when the gate is opened to conduct the sensation of pain to the brain, where it is perceived.

The *neospinothalamic tract,* or lateral spinothalamic tract, is the best known. The cells of origin lie in the posterior horn just anterior to the substantia gelatinosa, cross the midline in the anterior white commissure within a few segments, and ascend in the contralateral anterolateral quadrant of the spinal cord through the medial lemniscus to the ventral posterolateral nucleus of the thalamus. Because pain sensation running in this tract is separate from other somatosensory modalities that ascend primarily in the dorsal columns, and because the other tracts in the anterolateral quadrant of the spinal cord can be sacrificed with minimal neurologic impairment, this pathway is a convenient target for the neurosurgical treatment of cancer pain. Interruption of this pathway results in analgesia in the area of the body represented, that is, a loss of ability to perceive pain on the contralateral body below the level of the lesion. All of the sensory modalities from the body are intermingled in the ventral posterolateral (and ventral posteromedial) nucleus of the thalamus, where they synapse in a somatotopic array with neurons, which then project to the primary somatosensory area of the postcentral gyrus of the cortex. It appears that pain is brought to consciousness at thalamic levels or below, since interruption of this final neuron or the cortex may not alleviate the pain, although it may distort it or make it less localized.

The *paleospinothalamic tract* involves the same peripheral and spinal neurons as the neospinothalamic tract. The spinal neurons, however, give off collaterals to the reticular formation at the pons and midbrain levels to form the multisynaptic paleospinothalamic pathway, which ascends to those areas concerned with emotion, the hypothalamus, the intralaminar nuclei of the thalamus, the centrum medianum and parafascicularis nuclei, and the limbic lobe, which includes the cingulate gyrus, the hippocampus, and the amygdala.[29] Projection is bilateral, so that a lesion on one side may affect pain on either side of the body, but the manner in which the pain is affected is somewhat different than after a neospinothalamic tract lesion. The pain from a metastatic lesion may be gone after a lesion is made in either intralaminar nucleus, but if the patient is tested with a pin, acute pain sensation remains intact, and there is no detectable analgesia by usual methods of testing.

The *archispinothalamic system* is far less defined. There appears to be a multisynaptic pathway ascending in the spinal cord through the reticular formation to perhaps the same areas of the diencephalon and cerebrum as the paleospinothalamic tract, including the limbic system. There is no good anatomic demonstration of the location of this pathway within the spinal cord, but recent evidence suggests that, at least in some patients, this multisynaptic pathway may ascend as a relatively compact bundle somewhere near the central canal.[30] Interruption of this pathway at spinal levels may provide the same type of relief as a lesion of the paleospinothalamic pathway, that is, relief of pain without corresponding analgesia.

Curiously, a lesion in the *limbic lobe,* such as an interruption of the cingulate gyrus, may be of help in managing certain types of pain. The patient may appear to be comfortable and may no longer require narcotics; when asked, however, he may relate that the pain still exists, "but it doesn't bother me anymore." Thus, a lesion in the limbic system may relieve the suffering associated with the pain without relieving the pain itself.

In addition to the ascending pain pathways, there is a *descending pain system*, which appears to be related to the inhibition of pain. It was discovered in rats that stimulation of the area around the aqueduct at midbrain levels produced analgesia, so that the rats did not respond to noxious stimuli, so-called *stimulation-produced analgesics (SPA).*[31,32] It was verified in patients that stimulation just lateral to the posterior wall of the third ventricle and the periaqueductal gray matter may lead to relief from chronic pain or cancer pain, but not produce analgesia,[24,33,34] as discussed in Chapter 66.

Deep-brain stimulation. A number of sites have been found that produce analgesia when stimulated. The most effective are in the ventrolateral periaqueductal gray matter[35] and the gray matter just lateral to the third ventricle in the region of the posterior commissure.[34,36] In humans, the duration of pain relief may exceed the period of stimulation by hours.[34,37]

Studies suggest that opiate analgesia and stimulation-produced analgesia have so many similar characteristics that the two may operate by a common mechanism.[38,39] The most effective sites for stimulation-produced analgesia are basically those where opiate receptors have been found, particularly in the periaqueductal gray matter. There is considerable cross-tolerance between stimulation-produced analgesia and opiate analgesia, in that patients tolerant to morphine may lose the pain-relieving effects of deep-brain stimulation.[31] Also, naloxone, which is a specific narcotic antagonist, partially blocks stimulation-produced analgesia.[37,40]

It has been demonstrated that stimulation in the periventricular and periaqueductal area causes the release of endorphins into the ventricular fluid.[34] These are the same endorphins that produce analgesia when injected into certain brain sites in experimental animals, the action of which can be blocked by narcotic antagonists such as naloxone.[41] Interestingly, stimulation-produced analgesia and stimulation-produced pain relief in patients also can be blocked by naloxone, which suggests that such analgesia may depend on the release of endorphins.[31]

The procedure of chronic deep-brain stimulation of the periventricular gray matter involves the stereotactic insertion of four-contact stimulating electrodes, as elaborated in Chapter 66 and on page 1000. The usual target point (Table 67-1) lies about 1 mm posterior to the posterior commissure, 2–3 mm below the posterior commissure, and 2–3 mm lateral to the wall of the third ventricle (usually 6 mm lateral to the midline), although there is not complete agreement about those specific coordinates.[25,34] The electrode is secured to the burr hole with a special burr hole cover. The four contacts of the electrodes are connected to a special adaptor with four leads that are pulled through a needle hole in the scalp just above the ear. The incision at the burr hole is sutured. The following days or weeks can be used to test different stimulus parameters in order to determine whether the patient has pain relief from stimulation, and the optimal stimulus parameters and electrode combination to obtain such relief. When this has been accomplished, the system is internalized, usually under general anesthesia. The scalp incision is re-opened, the protruding wires are cut off, and the special adaptor is removed. A radio receiver is placed in a pocket below a clavicle and the lead wire is tunneled to emerge at the scalp incision. The two leads from the receiver are connected to the two leads of the electrode that have been selected to provide optimal stimulation, and the connection is sealed with Silastic and the incisions closed.

Denervation pain often can be managed successfully with chronic deep-brain stimulation of the somatosensory system. Electrodes are inserted into either the ventral posterior nucleus of the thalamus or the posterior limb of the internal capsule. It is hypothesized that the pain is the result of deprivation of diencephalic or cortical sensory areas from the inhibitory influences of the normally occurring sensory input. Substituting electrical stimulation for that absent sensory input may provide the patient with pain relief.

The coordinates for the somatosensory targets vary, depending upon the area of the body involved, because of the somatotopic distribution of fibers. For facial pain, the target is in the ventral posteromedial nucleus of the thalamus, and the initial coordinates are 8 mm posterior to the midpoint of the intercommissural (AC-PC) line, 8 mm lateral and 3–5 mm above the intercommissural line.[24,36] For pain in the extremities, the target is in the ventral posterolateral nucleus, and the coordinates are 9 mm posterior to the midpoint of the intercommissural line, 10–12 mm lateral and 2–5 mm above the (AC-PC) line. Alternatively, the electrode can be placed in the posterior limb of the internal capsule, in the coronal plane of the posterior commissure, 25 mm lateral and 1–2 mm above the AC-PC line.[24]

The electrodes should be inserted under local anesthesia so that stimulation can be applied and the coordinates adjusted as physiologically indicated.

Management of cancer pain.   Patients with cancer who complain of pain deserve a comprehensive program. Not only must the pain be dealt with specifically, but the emotional changes that accompany both the pain and a terminal illness must be recognized and managed.

In addition to attention to the patient's emotional welfare, the initial phase in the management of patients with cancer pain is pharmacologic. Analgesics should be given, the type and amount depending upon the amount of pain and tolerance. The patient's prognosis should be taken into account when prescribing narcotics. If the patient is expected to live for a long time, pain medications must be alternated or the dosage increased cautiously so that tolerance does not interfere prematurely with pain relief. The only narcotics that are absorbed well by mouth are codeine and methadone. If other narcotics are used orally, their dosage must be appropriate to that route of administration. For patients with severe pain who are in the advanced state of malignancy, methadone can be an extremely useful analgesic.

All narcotics are depressant drugs. This may compound significantly the emotional depression that results from the disability and the realization that an illness is terminal. Depression must be recognized and treated. Psychiatric counseling can sometimes be of help, particularly when it involves groups of cancer patients and their families. Antidepressant medication, such as the tricyclic antidepressants, may be extremely helpful, but must be given in sufficient dosage and for at least several weeks before their effect can be assessed. If the antidepressants are given at bedtime, their immediate sedative effect can also help ensure that the patient will get adequate rest.

Anxiety frequently accompanies depression in cancer patients. Again, psychiatric care or tranquilizers may be of benefit, but one must caution that the latter may increase depression, particularly when they are used in combination with narcotics. If tranquilizers are added to the patient's program, it is often possible to decrease the dose of narcotics, which may prolong their effectiveness. It is important to recognize that patients who are anxious or depressed may request narcotics for the soporific effects rather than the analgesic, and tranquilizers may be more effective and more appropriate for that use.

Patients who are fatigued tolerate pain less well, so that pain and anxiety may be considerably increased unless adequate sleep is obtained. Rather than relying solely on narcotics to ensure adequate sleep, hypnotics, especially nonbarbiturate sedatives, may be a beneficial addition to the overall program.

The principle of functional neurosurgical management of cancer pain is that interruption of the ascending pain pathways by ablative procedures may afford pain relief. The choice of procedure is determined by the distribution of the cancer pain more than its specific characteristics. The following general rules apply to the selection of procedures:

1. The most caudal or peripheral procedure that affects the entire area of pain is preferable.
2. If a patient has a minor pain in an area other than the major pain, one can anticipate an increase in the minor pain when the major pain is alleviated.
3. The less change in sensory function the better; a cordotomy usually is superior to multiple rhizotomies, since it leaves the patient with normal somatosensory sensation except for pain.
4. You should not talk a patient into having a pain procedure.
5. Be sure the patient is told of potential side-effects in detail and in advance—pain is forgotten once it is relieved, and side-effects that may have seemed minor before surgery become extremely distressing.
6. Anticipate disappointment; patients often blame all of their disability on the pain, but if the pain is alleviated and they still feel seriously ill and weak, they must acknowledge they are ill; such patients remember how they felt before the pain began, often months before, and may unrealistically expect to be returned to that vigorous state.

Various ablative procedures will be considered in ascending anatomic order.

Sensory rhizotomy involves the section of dorsal roots. Because almost every area of the body is innervated by multiple segments, it is necessary to section several roots in order to obtain relief. Consequently, almost the only indication for sensory rhizotomy in patients with cancer pain is a case in which a specific nerve or plexus of nerves is infiltrated by tumor. Before performing the surgery, it may be possible to evaluate the patient's response to a rhizotomy by blocking those nerve roots to be cut. Since sensory rhizotomy results in a loss of all modalities of sensation, the area is left insensitive, which many patients find even less tolerable than their original pain. An extremity should never be denervated completely, since the loss of proprioception feedback may cause the extremity to flail about involuntarily.

Cordotomy involves interrupting the lateral spinothalamic tract within the spinal cord. It can be done by exposing the spinal cord by laminectomy at a level above the innervation of the affected area and incising the anterolateral quadrant of the spinal cord under direct vision, or by introducing an electrode into the spinal cord at cervical levels, using a percutaneous technique as described in Chapter 73.

Cordotomy is perhaps the most widely used neurosurgical procedure for the treatment of cancer pain. It is particularly useful if the pain is unilateral, and is generally better for somatic than visceral pain. If the pain involves a lower extremity, cordotomy can be performed at either a thoracic or cervical level, but if the pain involves the upper extremity, a high cervical cordotomy must be done. Because a lesion above the C_4 level also affects fibers concerned with respiration, high cervical cordotomy can be performed only unilaterally with safety.

Cordotomy often fails to secure relief of midline pain when the spine or perineum is involved, and is particularly poor for midline pelvic pain. Risk includes weakness of the extremities ipsilateral to the lesion. If bilateral cordotomy is performed, there is a risk that bladder function will be affected, particularly if the bladder innervation is already compromised from a pelvic tumor. Some patients complain of dysesthesia in the area that become analgesic, but this does not occur often with cancer patients. Both bladder dysfunction and postcordotomy dysesthesia are less common after percutaneous cordotomy than after surgical cordotomy.[42]

Commissural myelotomy (Chapter 74) involves bisecting the spinal cord to interrupt the fibers going to the lateral spinothalamic tract as they decussate in the anterior white commissure. Classically, it is necessary to interrupt the commissural fibers throughout those dermatomes involved with the sensation of pain. Commissural myelotomy has been found to be especially valuable for bilateral or midline pain, particularly secondary to pelvic cancer, and has achieved renewed popularity recently as microneurosurgical techniques have become available.[43,44]

It has been observed many times that patients have pain relief in excess of what would be anticipated from the area of analgesia that develops after commissural myelotomy.[43-48] Indeed, it is possible to have excellent pain relief with no detectable analgesia. This observation led to the consideration that the archespinothalamic pathway may ascend in a discrete bundle near the center of the spinal cord, that it may inadvertently be interrupted by the commissural myelotomy, and that the pain relief without analgesia may be a result of the interruption of this pathway, which has not yet been described anatomically.[49] This led to the development of procedures specifically designed to interrupt this theoretical pathway. When performed stereotactically at the cervicomedullary junction, the procedure has been called extralemniscal myelotomy, and when performed under direct surgical exposure at thoracic levels it has been given the name of limited myelotomy.

In *extralemniscal myelotomy,* the electrode is inserted under stereotactic control in the midline between the posterior arch of C1 and the foramen magnum, with the patient's neck flexed.[50-52] As the electrode is advanced through the midline of the spinal cord, low-current stimulation is applied to map somatotopic distribution of the fibers in the posterior columns. As the electrode is moved progressively toward the center of the cord, the sensation is projected progressively down the legs, and when it stops, it indicates that the tip of the electrode lies anterior to the posterior columns. It is at that point that a lesion is made.[52,53]

Excellent relief of pain throughout the entire body has been reported with this procedure, especially in cancer patients, with minimal complications, even though no objective analgesia may be detected postoperatively. The procedure requires the use of a stereotactic apparatus that allows penetration of the spinal cord with the head flexed, such as the Hitchcock or Leksell apparatus.

Because of the difficulty in performing this procedure with the more commonly available stereotactic apparatuses, and because it seemed reasonable to attempt interruption of this same pathway at lower levels in the spinal cord when the pain was confined to the pelvis, the procedure of *limited myelotomy* was developed.[54,55] This procedure has been found to be particularly help-ful in patients with visceral pain of pelvic distribution, especially patients with rectal carcinoma. To date there have been no complications. There have been no posterior column symptoms, even immediately after surgery, as one often sees with extensive commissural myelotomy, and no leg weakness.

One interesting side-effect is that some of the patients with successful pain relief have great difficulty discontinuing narcotics following the procedure. They may have severe withdrawal symptoms, including sleeplessness, agitation, diarrhea, and generalized body pains, which is the opposite effect of the one seen after intralaminar thalamotomy or cingulotomy, which is charac-terized by easy discontinuation of narcotics. Overall, 75 percent of the patients have successful relief of cancer pain after limited myelotomy once they have gotten through the initial week of narcotic withdrawal, and none has demonstrated an area of analgesia.

Limited myelotomy is performed under general anesthesia with the patient in the prone po-sition. A T9 or T10 laminectomy is done in order to expose the spinal cord at approximately the twelfth thoracic dermatome. It is desirable to make the lesion above the entry of the lumbosacral segments, but to avoid the midthoracic levels where the blood supply is poorest. The midline is identified under the operating microscope and a 5-mm vertical incision is made in the pia at the midline. A small blunt microdissector is introduced until the infolded pia of the anterior median fissure is palpated, usually at a depth of 6 mm. With the blunt dissector, a mechanical lesion is made in the center of the spinal cord for a length of 5–7 mm, slightly less than one segment. Al-ternatively, the dissector may be removed and a percutaneous cervical cordotomy electrode in-serted into the center of the spinal cord and a lesion made, using the same parameters as for a percutaneous cordotomy. The intent is to interrupt a pathway that theoretically ascends near the central canal of the spinal cord, so it is not necessary to interrupt a significant number of com-missural fibers.

Splanchnicectomy (Chapter 68) can be used for abdominal visceral pain. Pain sensation from the abdominal viscera is, to a large extent, transmitted via splanchnic nerves to the sympa-thetic chains and from there through the spinal cord to join the pain-conducting systems. If the cancer is confined to the abdominal viscera and does not extend below the descending colon, ex-cellent pain relief may result from sympathetic denervation of the abdomen. Because the various abdominal sympathetic plexuses consist of a multitude of fine fibers that are extremely difficult to dissect, it is more convenient and more reliable to interrupt the sympathetic innervation just above the diaphragm.

Splanchnicectomy is perhaps the most effective procedure for pain resulting from carci-noma of the pancreas. Indeed, since pain is usually the presenting symptom and since pancreatic resection for pain relief is not usually possible, splanchnicectomy may be done at the same time as the laparotomy when tissue diagnosis is made. Under the same anesthetic, the patient is turned to the prone position and a splanchnicectomy is performed.

Medullary tractotomy involves interrupting the spinothalamic tract above spinal levels. Pain involving the head, face, or neck is obviously too high to be managed by cordotomy. The innervation of the head, however, is arranged so that pathways concerned with the perception of pain are separated from pathways involved with other modalities. Pain information that enters through the trigeminal nerve descends in the descending tract of the trigeminal nucleus as far as the upper cervical levels, where it synapses in a manner similar to that of the substantia ge-latinosa in the spinal cord. This descending trigeminal tract can be interrupted in the medulla where it lies just below the posterolateral surface. This is best done with suboccipital craniotomy and direct visualization of the medulla, although certain types of stereotactic apparatus allow electrodes to be introduced through the foramen magnum to perform medullary tractotomy.

If the procedure is done with open surgery, the landmarks are somewhat indefinite, so that it may be necessary to operate under local anesthesia and to use local electrical stimulation. The lesion is made at the level of the obex. The anterior edge of the lesion is in the line of emergence of the spinal accessory nerve rootlets. The posterior border of the cut is at the lateral edge of the nucleus cuneatus, but the small groove showing the division between the nuclei may be poorly delineated. To achieve total analgesia of the mouth area, the lesion should begin ventrally, in the spinothalamic tract, and extend dorsally well into the fasciculus cuneatus.

If medullary tractotomy is performed stereotactically, the procedure is done under local anesthetic with the patient in the prone or sitting position, depending upon which stereotactic apparatus is used.[52] The electrode is angled craniad 30° and is introduced 6 mm from the midline and 4 mm deep within the cord. It is necessary to use a fine electrode, .5–.6 mm, since the pia may be quite firm in this area and pressure on the medulla may be uncomfortable and distort the anatomy. Once the pia has been entered, verification of the position of the electrode is obtained by electrical stimulation at 50 Hz. If the electrode lies within the tract, sensation should be projected to the face at a low stimulating current. The dorsal border of the descending trigeminal tract may be defined by the homolateral responses from the fasciculus cuneatus, and the ventral border by the contralateral responses from the spinothalamic tract.

In addition to cancer pain, this procedure has been helpful to patients with postherpetic neuralgia and anesthesia dolorosa.

Because of the potential side-effects of medullary tractotomy, and because the pain may involve more than the area innervated by the trigeminal nerve, it may be preferable to use stereotactic *mesencephalotomy* for head and neck pain (Fig. 67-3). Since patients with cancer pain often have widespread pain throughout the body, mesencephalotomy is often preferred over medullary tractotomy if either is indicated.[56]

It is preferable to make the burr hole more dorsal for mesencephalotomy than for stereotactic thalamotomy. A burr hole 2 cm behind the interaural plane will allow insertion of the electrode approximately parallel to the fibers of the medial lemniscus within the brainstem to afford maximal opportunity for interrupting those fibers without affecting surrounding structures.[57] The coordinates are 5 mm posterior to the posterior commissure, 5 mm below that structure, and 5–10 mm from the midline (Table 67-1).[58]

Great care must be taken to avoid pyramidal tract fibers or oculomotor fibers. If the electrode is too low or a bit medial, stimulation at 50 Hz may produce abrupt medial deviation of the eye and pupillary constriction. If the electrode is too far lateral or anterior, stimulation at 5 Hz may cause involuntary movement of the contralateral extremities.

This suggests the two most common untoward side-effects from mesencephalotomy— diplopia and contralateral weakness. Since it is necessary to interrupt lemniscal fibers, which are the extension of the lateral spinothalamic tract, it is necessary to obtain analgesia in the area of pain in order to effect pain relief. It may be necessary to reposition the electrode by stimulating at 50 Hz and noting the patient's perception of projected sensation to the appropriate part of the body to ensure effective analgesia. It is generally inadvisable to perform mesencephalotomy bilaterally, for it can leave the patient at risk from loss of the protective influence of pain sensation throughout the body.[59]

There are several types of *thalamotomy* for pain relief. The convergence of the various pathways that relate to the different aspects of pathologic pain makes it possible to tailor the lesion within the thalamus to the needs of a given patient (Fig. 67-3). In the past, the lesions were directed to the posterior nuclei of the thalamus. A theoretical risk of producing a lesion in the ventral posterior nuclei is that it could produce a thalamic syndrome, which generally contraindicates the use of that procedure. It is more efficient, however, to interrupt the lemniscal fibers as they ascend into that nucleus through the mesencephalon, which is described as mesencephalotomy. The nonspecific fibers, concerned with the paleospinothalamic and archespinothalamic systems, ascend to the medial portion of the thalamus, where they may be interrupted without sacrificing the lemniscal pathways. Such lesions may afford pain relief without significantly altering somatic sensation.

Basal thalamotomy involves the production of a small discrete lesion to interrupt the extralemniscal fibers as they ascend toward the intralaminar nuclei, the centrum medianum, and the parafascicular nucleus. *Medial thalamotomy* involves the production of a somewhat larger lesion to interrupt these same fibers at their termination in the intralaminar nuclei and centrum

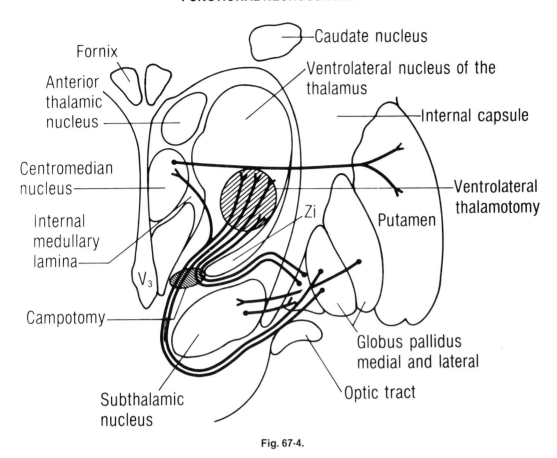

Fig. 67-4.

medianum. Although it was originally hoped that basal thalamotomy would produce longer-lasting and more complete pain relief more efficiently than intralaminar thalamotomy, the results following these two procedures are comparable. Indeed, perhaps the best chance for pain relief is produced with an intralaminar lesion extended to the same level as the basal thalamotomy, which does not appear to carry with it any greater risk.

The final type of thalamotomy for pain relief is the *dorsomedian thalamotomy,* which involves the production of a lesion in the dorsomedian nucleus to interrupt the origin of those fibers that project to the frontal lobe. This is the same thalamic lesion that has been employed for the treatment of affective disorders. Successful alleviation of pain also has been reported with bilateral lesions in the centrum medianum, the effect of which would be similar to that seen after medial thalamotomy.[58] In addition, lesions of the intralaminar nuclei have been successfully combined with lesions of the parafascicular complex for successful pain relief without analgesia.[60,61]

Stimulation at 50 Hz should be employed before production of a lesion. In basal thalamotomy, look for extraocular movements that might indicate that the electrode is too deep and encroaching on the oculomotor fibers, which lie just below the level of the basal thalamotomy lesions. Specific projection of pain sensation to the opposite side of the body may indicate that the electrode is slightly lateral and encroaching on the lemniscal fibers; although this would not compromise the result, it may cause an unnecessary sensory loss.

The medial-basal thalamotomy is done unilaterally, generally on the side opposite the greatest pain, and a dorsomedian thalamotomy may be done at the same sitting. If necessary, the second side can be done in 3 to 6 weeks. Results for cancer pain have been good; early pain relief was generally reported in 80 to 90 percent of the cases. Although medial-basal thalamotomy has also been employed for pain of benign origin, it has only a 30 to 35 percent long-term success rate for chronic pain,[62,63] so it is best avoided except for cancer pain.

Dorsomedian thalamotomy may be used alone for cancer pain.[64] The effects are similar to frontal leukotomy or cingulotomy, which have also been recognized as helpful for cancer pain. Since there is little additional risk, and conceivably potentially better results by combining the intralaminar with the dorsomedian nucleus lesion, there appears to be little advantage to performing dorsomedian thalamotomy alone for cancer pain.

Consequently, the recommended lesion for thalamotomy for treatment of cancer pain is a medial thalamotomy with a lesion in the intralaminar nuclei so that the lesion extends downward to combine with a basal thalamotomy lesion. If the patient has a great deal of emotional turmoil associated with the cancer, the lesion may be further extended medially into the dorsomedian nucleus to produce a combined dorsomedian thalamotomy as well.

The coordinates for the combined medial-basal thalamotomy (Table 67-1) require placing the burr hole somewhat more medial than usual, at approximately 2 cm from the midline, so the electrode can be introduced at an angle of 5° to the sagittal plane. The electrode should be introduced perpendicular to the intercommissural line. After the stereotactic apparatus is positioned so the electrode is directed at the proper trajectory, the electrode should be brought into contact with the skull. It may be necessary to make a second burr hole at that point or to extend the ventriculostomy burr hole, which should be done rather than compromising the angle of insertion of the electrode.

Three separate insertions should be used, with several lesions at different depths at each insertion site. A small electrode is used so the lesion is narrow. The first coordinate lies 1 mm anterior to the posterior commissure, 12 mm lateral, and at the level of the intercommissural line. After one lesion has been made at that level, the electrode is withdrawn 3–4 mm to make a second lesion, and perhaps even a third (depending upon the length of the active portion of the electrode) so that the lesions extend from the level of the intercommissural line to a point 11 mm above. The electrode then is withdrawn and reinserted 4 mm anterior to the posterior commissure, 11 mm lateral, and 2 mm above the intercommissural line, and a series of lesions is made to extend from the +2 level to the +13. The third insertion is made 9 mm anterior to the posterior commissure and 9 mm lateral, with the lesion extending from 2 mm above the intercommissural line to 13 mm above the intercommissural line.[52,63]

A lesion of the dorsomedial nucleus can be made with a somewhat larger electrode at 4 mm anterior to the posterior commissure and 4 mm lateral, so the lesion extends from 2 to 10 mm above the intercommissural line. The proximity to the insertion site for the medial-basal thalamotomy facilitates combining these two procedures.

Relief of suffering often can be obtained by interrupting the limbic system rather than interrupting or ablating the pain pathway itself. There are several areas where lesions can be conveniently made to afford pain relief for cancer patients. Such a procedure should be considered in patients with widespread metastatic disease, pain, and emotional turmoil who become drug dependent. Although these procedures may cause a slightly dulled affect in the initial postoperative period, the medication requirement is generally so much less than preoperatively that the net effect is one of reduced mental impairment.

If it is desired to make a lesion in the limbic system, *cingulotomy* may be the procedure of choice.[65,66] The technique of cingulotomy is presented in the section on surgery for affective disorders.

Although chronic stimulation techniques are more often used for chronic pain, they can be considered helpful for cancer pain as well, particularly if there is concurrent neuropathic or denervation pain.

Dorsal cord stimulation can be helpful for some patients with cancer pain, if it is not too severe. A percutaneous trial of stimulation may be helpful for patients with moderate pain from such problems as lumbosacral plexus involvement. The risks are minimal, and if satisfactory pain relief is not obtained, the percutaneous electrodes can be removed and other measures considered.

Table 67-1.

Procedure	Clinical indication	Target	Landmark	AP	Coordinates (mm) Lateral	Depth
Deep-brain stimulation	Pain	Periventricular gray	Post. comm.	A 1	6	−2 to −3
Deep-brain stimulation	Denervation pain, face	VPM	Mid AC-PC	P 8	8	+3 to +5
Deep-brain stimulation	Denervation pain, body	VPL	Mid AC-PC	P 9	10 to 12	+2 to +5
Deep-brain stimulation	Denervation pain, body	Post. limb int. capsl.	Post. comm.	0	25	+1 to +2
Mesencephalotomy	Pain	Medial lemniscus	Post. comm.	P 5	5 to 10	−5
Basal thalamotomy	Pain	Extralemniscular fibers	Post. comm.	A 1 A 4	12 11	0 to +11 +2 to +13
Medial thalamotomy	Pain	Intralaminar-CM nu.	Post. comm.	A 9	9	+2 to +13
Dorsomedian thalamotomy	Pain Affective disorders	Dorsomedial nu.	Post. comm.	A 4	4	+2 to +10
VL thalamotomy	Tremor Dystonia	VL (V.o.p) nu.	Mid AC-PC	P 2	11.5	+3
VL thalamotomy	Rigidity	VL (V.o.a) nu.	Mid AC-PC	A 2	9.5	+3
Campotomy	Tremor Rigidity Dystonia Cerebral palsy Seizures	Forel's field	Mid AC-PC	0	6	−2
Pallidotomy	Hemiballism Cerebral palsy Salaam convulsions	Globus pallidus	Ant. comm.	P 2	10	0
Cingulotomy	Pain Obsessive-compulsion Anxiety Depression	Cingulum	Ant. horn	P 30 P 30 P 18 P 18	Lat. edge 8 medial to lateral edge Lateral edge 8 medial to lateral edge	+5 +5 +5 +5
Anterior capsulotomy	Obsessive-compulsion	Ant. limb of int. capsule	Ant. clinoid	A 15 A 15 A 15	6 6 14	+10 +15 +10
Amygdalotomy	Temporal lobe seizures Salaam convulsions	Amygdala	Tip of temporal horn	A 5	5 medial to lateral edge	3 above inferior border

Deep-brain stimulation can be of value, particularly for patients with widespread pain of metastatic disease and patients with pain involving the head and neck. The contraindications would include those patients who have open and potentially infected lesions of the head, which may expose the patient to undue risk of infection from the implanted device. The details of the use of deep-brain stimulation are covered in Chapter 66.

Management of chronic pain. Chronic pain has been defined, for purposes of management, as pain that has persisted for at least 3 to 6 months, has defied attempts at treatment by ordinary means or treatment of underlying etiology, and serves no useful biologic purpose.

Although chronic pain is not primarily treated surgically, it is necessary to present an overview of its management to demonstrate the contrast in approach, instruct the surgeon about alternate means of treatment to allow better judgment for the selection of patients for surgery (or a conservative program), and to put in context those few chronic pain conditions for which a surgical procedure may be indicated.

An informal inquiry of six neurosurgeons who are leaders in the field of pain management revealed that only 1 to 15 percent of the patients referred to them for pain management were subjected to some sort of procedure. In contrast, several neurosurgeons with private general neurosurgery practices responded to this same question by indicating that 85 to 90 percent of their patients referred for the management of pain were subjected to a procedure. Even assuming that the patient population was different because more intractable pain patients were referred to neurosurgeons in a pain clinic, one must assume that many patients who had surgery at the hands of a neurosurgical generalist would not have had surgery had they been referred to neurosurgeons who were more sophisticated in the management of chronic pain. Part of this difference may be because of the availability of a chronic pain management program in their repertoire.

Several features are common to the majority of the chronic pain patients who have presented at our pain clinic.[67-69] Most stated that the current pain was similar to their initial pain, which was usually associated with an acute medical problem or injury, but worse following many medical or surgical attempts at relief. They offered medical histories of treatment failures freely and in great detail, often with considerable relish. All had tried numerous medications, and most were addicted to narcotics, but they continued to take medication that they admitted did not offer either significant or long-lasting relief, but just "to take the edge off" the pain. Significantly, all said their pain complaints were urgent or emergency problems. Not only did they describe willingness to undergo any treatment aimed at pain relief, but frequently tried to manipulate the physician into inappropriate or excessive procedures. Finally, and importantly, many claimed they had no other problem and that everything would be fine if only the doctor would take their pain away. The patient's daily life was organized around, and defined by, the pain; the pain explained all difficulties of living.

Although the chronic pain patient moved in an exaggerated, guarded fashion, on physical examination, the described disability was generally in excess of that warranted by objective physical findings.

Pervading the presentation was a sense of urgency and expectation that the physician would institute a definitive treatment in which the patient would have little responsibility, but which would make the pain suddenly and, almost magically, disappear. Such a presentation may be appropriate for acute pain but not chronic pain.

In addition to the usual chronic pain patient described above, there are several categories of pain patients the surgeon must be aware of in order to direct the program appropriate to a nonsurgical approach. Pain may be a symptom of depression. A small group of patients may have a delusional symptom of psychosis. Such patients generally are identifiable by their bizarre behavior, which can be seen only if the physician looks closely. Pain may be a symptom of anxiety, particularly anxiety about an illness, such as cardiac disease or cancer. Pain may be a symptom of hysterical neurosis, in which the pain is an attempt to resolve personal conflict that the patient cannot deal with in a healthy way; often the description of pain may relate to the underlying personal conflict, and the benefits gained by the disability may allow the patient to avoid that conflict. Patients with chronic pain frequently have unresolved grief, in which case the pain may allow identification with the lost loved one, either by the type of pain, the manner in which the pain presented, or the timing of the onset or exacerbation of the pain.

Another group of chronic pain patients is made up of those whose personality indicates a need to suffer. These patients have a life-long history of multiple surgeries of many kinds, frequent personal disasters (which always seem to occur just when everything is going well), and multiple unsuccessful doctor-patient relationships. Although this group constitutes only a moderate portion of chronic pain patients, they present repeatedly to multiple physicians, frustrating many and standing out because virtually any treatment program is doomed to failure.

Most chronic pain patients are both depressed and regressed by the time they are referred to a neurosurgeon. Depression is usual for patients who are disabled from any cause for as long as 6 months. Although it is a normal reaction to an abnormal situation, it must be managed successfully for the patient to progress from the stage of disability to that of rehabilitation.

Regression is an exaggeration of the dependency that begins during the acute phase of the patient's illness. As the patient withdraws more and more from normal activities and responsibilities, it becomes more and more difficult, both psychologically and physically, to resume these activities later. Frequently, the dependency state is reinforced by the patient's caretaker, usually the spouse, who may receive considerable psychologic gain from keeping the patient in a regressed and dependent attitude.

Most patients are addicted to inappropriate medications at the time they present for management of their chronic pain. All analgesics are designed for acute pain, virtually all produce both tolerance and addiction, most have depression as a significant side-effect, and none works for chronic pain.

Many patients are suffering from recurrent withdrawal by the time they present to the neurosurgeon. They are firmly addicted to a pain medication, usually containing a narcotic. They go through a regular cycle every few hours. They take their pain medication, but several hours later begin to go into withdrawal. As a consequence of the withdrawal, they become anxious, agitated, and, as part of the withdrawal, their pain perception becomes intensified, so their pain becomes worse. After watching the clock anxiously, they take their pain medication again at the prescribed time (or before), and find that the medication "takes the edge off the pain." They are treating the withdrawal rather than the pain, and at the same time are perpetuating the narcotic dependency. Several hours later the pattern is repeated, and the pain perception becomes intensified so that another dose of medication is taken.

The management of any patient with chronic pain should take all of these factors into account. Indeed, before making a final decision to subject a patient with chronic pain to a neurosurgical procedure, such as implantation of a stimulator, the patient should have the opportunity to participate in a chronic pain program. Many patients who may initially appear to be candidates for stimulators may find so much relief from nonsurgical means that an invasive procedure is not appropriate. Other patients may appear to be emotionally stable, but on closer inspection over time may prove to have such significant psychopathology that any procedure should be considered only with reluctance. Still other patients may be laying so much of the blame for their personal problems on their pain symptom that it becomes obvious they would neither be less disabled nor satisfied, regardless of the effectiveness of the pain-relieving procedure.

Little in the way of pain management can be accomplished unless and until both the patient and the treating physician exchange the goal of pain relief for that of rehabilitation. The attitude of the patient must be redirected from one aimed at having someone else take the pain away to one aimed at coping with the physical problem and abandoning disability as a way of life, following which, in most cases, the pain becomes significantly ameliorated.

A comprehensive *chronic pain program* should include the following:[69]

1. *Neuropsychologic evaluation,* concentrating mainly on the patient's disability and how he copes with various stresses, including pain. Neuropsychologic tests are usually worthless for identifying what proportion of the patient's pain is primarily organic and what proportion

may be primarily psychologic. Realistic goals must be set, both in regard to the patient and the place of the patient within the family.

2. *Withdrawal of medication* can usually best be accomplished abruptly, except for barbiturates and diazepam. It should be explained to the patient beforehand that he will feel lousy for several days, during which time the pain will be intensified, but that following that the pain may be significantly relieved. A period of withdrawal is also accompanied by sleeplessness, since chronic administration of pain medication may disrupt the normal diurnal sleep cycle, and many pain patients have been on sedatives. No sleep medications should be given during this stage, since they interfere with resumption of a normal sleep cycle.

3. *Treatment of depression* should include both pharmacologic and psychiatric means. Discontinuation of pain medications and tranquilizers is an important part of the treatment of depression, as is the addition of tricyclic antidepressants, which may have a direct effect on chronic pain as well.

4. *Treatment of regression* can best be managed by forcefully encouraging the patient toward self-care, generally using behavior modification techniques. Rather than always instructing the patient to do less and less, the patient should be encouraged to do more and more. It is important to involve the spouse or caretaker in the treatment of regression, since often the spouse's psychologic needs may be met by keeping the patient dependent.

5. *Resocialization* involves encouraging the patient to regain social contacts and recreational activities.

6. *Remobilization* should be done gradually and progressively. A program of progressive exercises that start at a very simple level, such as the Royal Canadian Air Force Exercise Program, will allow the patient to begin to exercise at a tolerated activity level.

7. *Physical therapy* is usually directed to the physical conditioning program. Such local modalities as heat and massage may help muscle spasm, and gentle stretching exercises can improve mobilization.

8. *Transcutaneous stimulation* can be of help, particularly in the intial phase when the patient is beginning to remobilize. It is not a pain program in itself, however, and is much more effective when incorporated into an overall program.

9. *Specific techniques* can be taught to lessen pain perception and to allow the patient to relax without the use of drugs, such as biofeedback and relaxation training.[70]

A final word of caution should be said about the manipulative patient. Many chronic pain patients have more experience than their physician in directing their program, and those patients who have a psychologic need to suffer or for the treatment to fail will often manipulate the physician into fulfilling these prophecies.

The key to managing a manipulative patient is to make it understood from the start that manipulation will not be tolerated and that the physician, not the patient, is in charge of the program. When the patient recognizes that manipulation will not accomplish its usual end, it will usually cease.

There are several procedures that are extremely helpful in the management of a few selected patients with chronic pain. The most common procedure in that category is one of *trigger point blocks,*[71] which may be a valuable adjunct to the treatment of *myofascial syndrome.* Although that syndrome has been defined variously, we can consider it to be a localized area of muscle pain and spasm secondary to a tearing injury. It commonly occurs at the origin of the back muscles at the sacral crest, the medial portion of the iliac crest and posterior iliac spine, the lower posterior cervical area, the suboccipital muscles, or the site of a laminectomy, fusion, or bone graft donor. Although the process is usually localized, the painful muscle spasm may spread to adjacent muscles and cause the pain to radiate up and down the back. In addition, the pain may be referred along the involved dermatome, but can be differentiated from radicular pain because both the radiating and local pain may be alleviated by a local trigger point block.

The trigger points of a myofascial syndrome can be identified at physical examination by a report of pain on deep muscle palpation, particularly in the locations described above, or by the palpation of localized muscle spasm or nodularity. When such a trigger point, or multiple points, are identified, the skin should be marked with a pen so the pattern can be visualized and the trigger points treated.

Treatment of trigger points may be begun by the patient with a conservative program that involves application of local heat (a bathtub or shower being preferable to a heating pad), local massage, and gentle stretching exercises. Many patients find that they can break up the pattern of muscle spasm by steady, deep, local, digital pressure several times a day.

If the patient is unable to manage the myofascial pain, physical therapy several times a week can be incorporated into the program. In addition to the modalities above, the use of a local vibrator may help break up the pattern of muscle spasm.

A series of trigger point blocks may be done for both diagnostic and therapeutic purposes. In order to identify the trigger points, 1 cc of 1% lidocaine is injected into each point. A 22-gauge $1/2$-inch needle is used, and, as the needle enters the trigger point, the physician can feel the sudden penetration of a fascial plane or the palpation of bony attachment, as the patient reports the sudden exacerbation of the pain. Alleviation of the pain on injection of a local anesthetic is diagnostic, particularly if consistent on repeated blocks.

If diagnostic blocks are successful, a series of weekly blocks with local anesthetic is undertaken. If the pain recurs promptly after each block in the series, a longer-acting local anesthetic such as bupivicaine may be substituted. If the patient still has recurrence after six or eight local anesthetic blocks but has excellent temporary relief from each series of blocks, phenol blocks may afford a long-term benefit. 500 mg of phenol crystals are dissolved in 5 cc of saline for a 10% concentration, and 1 cc of that solution is injected at each trigger point, with a maximum of 5 cc in any given weekly session.

Causalgia is treated primarily with sympathectomy (Chapter 68). If pain persists following sympathectomy, however, extralemniscal or limited myelotomy may be of benefit. Cingulotomy may also be beneficial, but experience has shown that relief of chronic pain, from whatever cause, is usually limited to 2 to 4 months.

Denervation-type pain may be treated by dorsal column stimulation or deep-brain stimulation, either in the periventricular or somatosensory areas. Since dorsal column stimulation can be evaluated percutaneously and carries less risk, that procedure should be tried first. If dorsal column stimulation is unsuccessful, or if the pain involves the face, deep-brain stimulation may be attempted (see Chapter 66). For denervation pain, electrodes should be inserted both in the periventricular area and the appropriate somatosensory area, as described above, and the appropriate leads selected by a trial of stimulation.

Postherpetic neuralgia remains an enigma. Approximately 50 percent of the patients respond to transcutaneous stimulation, however, if encouraged to persist in trying various electrode placements. If the pain is justifiably severe and relief is not obtained from transcutaneous stimulation, percutaneous dorsal column stimulation may be tried, but, again, without anticipating more than a 50 percent chance of success. It has been reported[52] that postherpetic intractable pain cases respond well to extralemniscal myelotomy. If the face is involved, it may be necessary to perform intralaminar or basal thalamotomy.

The most common chronic pain problem is that of *low back pain*. Many patients can avoid this chronic problem with appropriate management of their acute injury. It is disheartening how many patients appear at the Chronic Pain Clinic having had a laminectomy for what was described as a classic myofascial syndrome. Unless a patient presents with classic signs and symptoms of herniated lumbar or cervical disc, a myofascial syndrome should be evaluated with appropriate trigger point blocks.

The patient with chronic low back pain should undergo a chronic pain program as described above before any decision is made about a procedure. Trigger point blocks may be usefully combined with a long-term physical therapy program. After the depression, regression, and drug dependency are brought under control, the patient can be evaluated more objectively for response to transcutaneous stimulation, and later to dorsal column stimulation, if necessary. With a strict selection protocol, few patients will have dorsal column stimulators implanted, but the long-term success rate is high in those who are candidates.

I have been discouraged by the long-term effects of ablative procedures for chronic low back and leg pain. Although the short-term results are excellent with a number of procedures (such as rhizotomy, microsurgical decompression, radiofrequency rhizotomy, and interruption of pain pathways), pain relief rarely lasts longer than 2 to 4 months.

Phantom limb pain presents a particularly challenging problem. Many, if not most, patients with phantom limb pain have a great deal of emotional involvement in their physical disability, and should undergo a chronic pain clinic evaluation as the initial step in management. If the pain is actually local tenderness secondary to neuroma formation, resection of the nerve proximal to the neuroma may be helpful, whereas searching through dense scar tissue to find a neuroma is rarely rewarding. Transcutaneous stimulation can be extremely helpful for many patients with phantom limb pain, as can dorsal column stimulation or peripheral nerve stimulation.

It is of the utmost importance that the surgeon reserve the option of telling the patient that there is nothing to offer if there is nothing that stands a reasonable chance of success. Chronic pain patients are notorious for manipulating physicians into procedures against their better judgment, which, more often than not, results in an increase of the problem. When confronted directly, however, most patients accept this news gracefully. They should be admonished that there is no acceptable treatment for their problem and discouraged from traveling from physician to physician looking for a magical cure.

Movement Disorders

Anatomy of motor control. Most of the movement disorders of functional neurosurgical interest concern the extrapyramidal system, which consists of two interlocking circuits that are important from the stereotactic standpoint.

One concerns the basal ganglia and the thalamus. Fibers from the putamen enter the globus pallidus; both internal and external pallidum feed into the ventral-anterior nucleus of the thalamus by way of several pathways. The lenticular fasciculus runs above the subthalamic nucleus, and the ansa lenticularis runs below the subthalamic nucleus to join together in Forel's field H. These two pathways ascend together as the thalamic fasciculus (H1) to the ventral-anterior nucleus of the thalamus. Note that virtually the entire outflow of both the internal and external pallidum funnels together into a compact bundle as it traverses Forel's field H, where the maximum number of fibers can be interrupted with the smallest lesion (Fig. 67-4). From the thalamus, there are connections to the supplementary motor cortex. Connections within the cortex lead to fibers that project to the caudate nucleus, which in turn projects back to the putamen to complete the putamen-globus pallidus-thalamus (ventral anterior)-cortex-caudate-putamen circuit.

There is a second interlocking circuit that links the cerebellum to the basal ganglia. The major outflow from the cerebellum is via the dentate nucleus, which projects to the red nucleus. Some fibers synapse in the red nucleus and others pass directly through joining fibers that originate in the red nucleus to end in the ventro-lateral nucleus of the thalamus. The area of the thalamus involved abuts with the area that receives fibers from the globus pallidus. The ventrolateral nucleus projects to the primary and secondary motor cortex. Cortical efferent fibers descend through the internal capsule to end in the pontine nuclei. Neurons that originate in those nuclei project to the cortex of the cerebellum in a somatotopic distribution. Cerebellar cortical fibers then synapse in the dentate nucleus to complete the second cerebellum-dentate-ruber-thalamus (ventrolateral)-cortex-pontine nuclei-cerebellum motor-control circuit.

It is in the area of the thalamus where these two circuits juxtapose that stereotactic lesions are made for the treatment of involuntary movement and tremor.

Much of the stereotactic literature relates to the Hassler nomenclature of thalamic nuclei, and may be confusing to those not familiar with that system. Different criteria are used for the delineation of Hassler's nuclei and subnuclei than for the Walker terminology above, so that it is not possible to correlate them entirely, but several generalizations can be made that clarify the relationship sufficiently for the purposes of stereotactic surgery (Table 67-2).[72]

Table 67-2.

Ventral-anterior nucleus (VA)	Nucleus lateropolaris (L. po)
Ventrolateral nucleus (VL)	Nucleus ventro-oralis anterior (V.o.a)
(ventral half)	Nucleus ventro-oralis posterior (V.o.p)
	Nucleus ventrointermedius (V.im)
Ventral-posterolateral nucleus (VPL)	Nucleus ventrocaudalis externa (V.c.e)
Ventral-posteromedial nucleus (VPM)	Nucleus ventrocaudalis interna (V.c.i)

The ventral-anterior nucleus is called the nucleus lateropolaris (L.po). According to Hassler, some fibers run directly from the external lamina of the globus pallidus to the L.po, and additional fibers are carried by way of the thalamic fasciculus (H1). Cortical projections are primarily to the supplementary motor area.

The ventrolateral nucleus is divided into several subnuclei in the Hassler classification. The ventral half of the ventral-lateral nucleus is divided into the nucleus ventro-oralis anterior (V.o.a) and the nucleus ventro-oralis posterior (V.o.p), and the intermediate nucleus between these nuclei and the ventral-posteromedial and ventral-posterolateral nuclei is called the nucleus ventrointermedius (V.im).

There is evidence that the V.im receives input from the vestibular nuclei and projects to area 3a of the sensory motor cortex. It has been reported that a 5–7-Hz rhythm can be recorded from the base of the V.im. Although it has been suggested that this is the pacemaker of the tremor of Parkinson's disease, patients can get excellent relief of tremor with only minor involvement of the V.im by the lesion, suggesting that the bursting activity may be from a bundle traveling through the V.im to the V.o.p.[73,74]

The nucleus ventro-oralis anterior (V.o.a) receives axons going from the internal lamina of the globus pallidus through the thalamic fasciculus (H1) to the secondary motor cortex, so that, in some definitions, the V.o.a might actually be included in the dorsal part of the ventral-arterior nucleus. It appears to be involved in slow, specialized movements or turning of the trunk. The usual effect of stimulation of the V.o.a (as well as the V.o.p) is an increase in amplitude of the tremor of Parkinson's disease, especially at low stimulus rates (5 Hz). Tremor may be blocked by stimulation of the V.o.p, however, and if the current is sufficiently high, such a blockage may occur because of the spread of the current to the V.o.p., even though the tip of the electrode is in the V.o.a. The rate of rapidly alternating movements of the arm may be slowed by 50-Hz stimulation of the V.o.a, and stimulation of the V.o.a may cause ocular movements, with conjugate turning of the eyes to the opposite side, opening of the eyes, and possibly midriasis.

The nucleus ventro-oralis posterior (V.o.p) is the main relay of the nucleus for input from the dentato-rubro-thalamic system to the primary motor cortex, area 4. This system controls rapid, sudden movements. Since the V.o.p may be the site of the rhythmic discharges that control the 5–7-Hz tremor of Parkinson's disease, it may be possible to record bursting activity at that frequency. Stimulation at 50 Hz may block the tremor, perhaps by interfering with the generation of these burst discharges.

The ventral-posterolateral nucleus (VPL) is referred to as the nucleus ventrocaudalis externa (V.c.e), and the ventral-posteromedial nucleus (VPM) is the nucleus ventrocaudalis interna (V.c.i). The anatomic definitions of these nuclei are the same in both the Walker and Hassler nomenclature, but, according to Hassler, the nucleus ventrocaudalis is also divided into an anterior and posterior part, with duplicate somatotopic representation, with proprioception relayed to the V.c.p and a tactile homunculus in the V.c.a.[73]

Despite the appearance of an ultrascientific rationale, one must simplistically recognize that most stereotactic procedures for motor disorders involve interruption of the interlocking pathway described above, usually somewhere between the globus pallidus and the thalamus or within the thalamus, and targets have been determined empirically. Historically, the first targets for Parkinson's disease were in the globus pallidus. With more experience, the target moved to the neighborhood of the ventrolateral nucleus of the thalamus. Since fibers between these two areas must funnel through the ansa lenticularis and Forel's field, they likewise became targets. There have been many opinions about which specific coordinates are best for which symptoms, but the areas are so close and anatomic confirmation by autopsy so limited that only a few definitive statements can be made.

Autopsy confirmation indicates that improvement of rigidity of Parkinson's disease can be correlated with a lesion involving the V.o.a or H1, confirming that interruption of the pallido-thalamic connections are optimal for the improvement of rigidity.[52,75] Relief of tremor, however, correlates more closely with coagulation of the V.o.p, which involves the dentato-thalamic fibers. Both of these symptoms respond to a lesion in Forel's field, tremor responding more consistently than rigidity. Bradykinesia does not appear to be affected as much, regardless of the placement of the lesion. Gait disturbances of various types may be treated by ablation of the V.o.a.[75]

Management of movement disorders (Fig. 67-4). Coordinates may be determined by a consideration of specific symptoms. In order to produce a lesion in the ventrolateral nucleus (V.o.a) for treatment of rigidity, the electrode might be directed to the following coordinates: 2 mm anterior to the mid mid point of the intercommissural (AC-PC) line, 9.5 mm lateral, and 3 mm above the AC-PC line. If there is tremor present, it may be increased by stimulation at 5 Hz. Stimulation at 50 Hz may slow the speed of arm movements at low voltage, and at higher voltage may decrease tremor. Conjugate movement of the eyes may occur.

In order to produce a lesion in the ventrolateral nucleus (V.o.p) for treatment of tremor, insert the electrode to the coordinates 2 mm posterior to the mid AC-PC line, 11.5 lateral and 3 mm above the AC-PC line. It may be possible to record rhythmic discharges at the same frequency as the tremor, particularly with a microelectrode or semimicroelectrode. Stimulation at 50 Hz may block the tremor. There is evidence that the most effective site within the V.o.p. is that which lies just anterior to the somatosensory representation in the V.c.a of the body part affected.[74]

A lesion in Forel's field H (campus Foreli) is called campotomy, and may be used for either tremor or rigidity.[76,77] The coordinates are at the mid AC-PC line, 6 mm lateral, with the tip of the electrode 2 mm below the AC-PC line (Fig. 67-4). There is no characteristic electrical activity from that area. Stimulation at 5 Hz should assure that the pyramidal tract is not being encroached upon. Stimulation at 50 Hz may cause an increase in the tremor. If the electrode is too close to oculomotor fibers, medial deviation of the ipsilateral eye and midriasis may be seen, in which case the electrode should be raised 1 or 2 mm and tested with stimulation once again.

Parkinson's disease. Parkinson's disease is the most common motor disorder for which stereotactic surgery is used. Indeed, the popularization of stereotactic surgery occurred during the time that large numbers of patients were available, many with postencephalitic Parkinson's disease after influenza epidemics, and medical management was only marginally successful. As a large portion of the resident population was treated, and as L-dopa therapy provided relief for many other patients, the reservoir of patients for stereotactic surgery dropped.[10]

Parkinson's syndrome consists of a multitude of signs and symptoms. Although the most dramatic and obvious is the characteristic tremor, it is usually not the most disabling, since it occurs at rest and very often lessens or stops on intention. Bradykinesia, however, is usually the disabling feature of the disease. It is often associated with rigidity, and the resultant paucity of movements may make the patient "a prisoner in his own body." The postural changes that occur with Parkinson's syndrome are so characteristic that the diagnosis may be made even before the appearance of other signs. The patient stands with shoulders and head thrust forward. The kyphosis is fixed, so that the head remains suspended above the pillow when the patient is lying supine. Adding to the postural abnormality is the absence of associated movements, such that the arms no longer swing on walking, indicating that automatic arm and leg coordination is absent. Vegetative symptoms complete the characteristic picture: a masklike face, oily skin, and excessive accumulation of saliva in the mouth.

It must be recognized that although L-dopa works quite well for bradykinesia, it may have little effect on tremor, or may even make the tremor worse. In contrast, stereotactic surgery works exceedingly well against tremor and moderately well against rigidity, but may have little effect on bradykinesia. Consequently, many patients with both bradykinesia and tremor are candidates for stereotactic surgery plus L-dopa management. Also, as patients are treated with L-dopa for 3 to 5 years, many become intolerant to the medication, or the symptoms begin to break through once again, and these patients may still benefit from stereotactic surgery. Further, the response to L-dopa may be much better following a stereotactic lesion than before, and L-dopa-induced tremor and involuntary movements occur less frequently in limbs contralateral to prior stereotactic procedures.[78]

Consequently, the recommendation at present is for the following in sequence:

1. If bradykinesia is the major problem, a course of medical management should be pursued.
2. If the patient does not respond to medication or becomes intolerant to the medication, stereotactic surgery should be considered.
3. If the patient still has significant bradykinesia following stereotactic surgery, L-dopa should be tried once again in gradually escalating doses in hopes that its benefit may become enhanced.
4. If tremor is the major problem, a brief course of medical management should be tried.
5. If the patient does not respond promptly to modest doses of medication, stereotactic surgery is indicated.
6. If tremor is still a problem following stereotactic surgery, a medical program should be tried once again.
7. If the patient has symmetrical bilateral tremor, the dominant side should be operated on first to give the patient maximum rehabilitation from a unilateral procedure.
8. If it is necessary to perform stereotactic surgery on the second side, either because of bilateral tremor or because tremor on the asymptomatic side emerges afterward, a minimum of 6 to 12 weeks should elapse before the second side is done.
9. If lesions are made on both sides, every attempt should be made to make asymmetrical lesions to minimize the risk of side-effects affecting mentation or verbalization. In no case should bilateral campotomy be performed, because of a risk of mutism.

The contraindications for stereotactic surgery in patients with Parkinson's disease are related to the age and general health of the patient. The possibility of a successful result begins to decrease with patients over the age of 60, and certainly with patients over the age of 65. Older patients who have become debilitated from a long-term disability may succumb to pneumonia or other complications during the initial week following surgery, when the patient may be quite sedated from the lesion.

One can anticipate satisfactory relief of tremor in 80 to 85 percent of selected patients. The chance of neurologic complications or worsening of symptoms is approximately 4 percent, and is more likely to occur in older patients.

Essential tremor, or familial tremor, may be quite disabling, since it is a tremor of intention. The more the patient tries to stop the tremor, the worse the tremor becomes. It may not be apparent or disabling until adulthood or middle years, and may affect many members of a single family. It may respond to a medical program, particularly relaxants, but usually does not.

On the other hand, stereotactic campotomy or thalamotomy may result in immediate and dramatic relief of the tremor. The target is the same as for the tremor of Parkinson's disease, v.s. (Fig. 67-4).

Tremor may be the result of other etiologies, such as a stroke or head trauma. Because one is dealing with a nervous system that is not intact, and the damage to other parts of the motor system cannot be known, the results of stereotactic surgery are less predictable. Nevertheless, if the tremor is disabling enough and the patient is willing to risk the uncertain result, stereotactic surgery may be indicated. One must also warn the patient that the possibility of side-effects is also somewhat unpredictable and that previously resolved weakness or paralysis may return.

Stereotactic surgery can be used for selected patients with *Huntington's chorea,* and indeed this was the first use of stereotactic surgery for motor disorders.[79] Huntington's chorea is a familial disease marked by progressive mental deterioration and choreiform movements associated with degeneration of the caudate nuclei. It is important to select patients for stereotactic surgery critically, to be sure that it is the motor impairment and not the mental deterioration that is the cause of the patient's disability. Because the condition is progressive, the long-term prognosis remains poor, but it may be possible to allow the patient 6 months or a year of independence or self-care, provided his mental status is adequate. One must caution, however, that performing unilateral lesions or making a lesion in the dominant hemisphere may increase problems with mentation in patients who are functioning at a borderline level, so the procedure is not entirely without risk.

The target is either Forel's field or the ventrolateral nucleus, as it is for other nonspecific movement disorders. Symmetrical lesions should not be made bilaterally, especially in this group of patients who have impaired neurologic reserve to compensate for the lesions. Results in most patients can be gratifying, with marked decrease in choreiform movements immediately upon production of the lesion.

Hemiballism is of stereotactic interest from two standpoints. First, it has been reported as a rare complication of subthalamic stereotactic lesions, and second, hemiballism occurring after stroke may be successfully treated with stereotactic surgery.

Ballism consists of involuntary hurling, irregular, frequently violent movements of the shoulder and proximal arm, which may occur after a lesion of the subthalamic nucleus. Ordinarily, hemiballism is the result of a localized problem and consequently unilateral. There is some evidence that a partial destruction of the subthalamic nucleus may lead to ballism, but it does not occur if the nucleus is completely destroyed.

The postsurgical incidence has been reported to range from 0.3 to 9.0 percent,[80] with one series reporting 4 cases out of 4866 stereotactic surgeries.[81] This author has never seen a case following the production of a stereotactic lesion, but has participated in the treatment of several cases that occurred spontaneously, presumably following a localized stroke.

Indications for surgery in patients with spontaneous hemiballism follow the general rules for stereotactic intervention. The symptoms must be severe enough to justify the procedure, and since ballistic movements of any magnitude are invariably disabling, this criterion is often met. The patient must not be disabled from other neurologic problems, although the stroke that caused ballism may also cause other neurologic problems. Hemiballism is frequently of a transient nature so that surgery should not be contemplated unless the problem has been stable for at least 2 to 3 months.

The treatment of ballism consists of destroying the same part of the ventrolateral nucleus or Forel's field that is the general target for other movement disorders. Earlier reports also indicated successful relief of hemiballism following lesions of the medial part of the globus pallidus, and a satisfactory result can be anticipated from either target.[82]

Dystonia musculorum deformans (torsion spasm) is a progressive condition characterized by torsion of the trunk muscles with asymmetrical spasm, spasticity, and contractures of the extremities, leading to profound immobility.

The results of ventrolateral thalamotomy for dystonia musculorum deformans are somewhat unpredictable, but approximately 50 percent can be improved by stereotactic surgery. Some patients may have dramatic alleviation of virtually all symptoms, and improvement may last for many years. Others may have minimal or no improvement, even though the presenting picture may have appeared to be the same. Many patients will have a moderate or modest improvement, but become disabled once again as the progressive nature of the disease overtakes the improvement.[20]

Early treatment for dystonia musculorum deformans was pallido-ansotomy, or a lesion in the globus pallidus and associated ansa lenticularis.[83] Currently, a lesion in Forel's field or the posterior half of the ventrolateral nucleus is recommended (Fig. 67-4). A peculiarity of this condition is that the improvement may not be apparent for several weeks after the lesion is made, and may be progressive for several months thereafter. Consequently, one should initially make a generous lesion extending from Forel's field[82] into the ventrolateral nucleus,[84] and, if necessary, repeat or enlarge the lesion at 3-month intervals as long as it appears that progress is being made. Since the condition may involve primarily the trunk, it may be necessary to make bilateral lesions before any response is seen. It is recommended that the first lesion be placed on the side opposite the greater muscle spasm, particularly if extremities are affected, or, if the spasm is equal bilaterally, on the dominant side. Usually a contralateral lesion is necessary some time later, and working on the nondominant side allows the surgeon to be more generous in the size of the second lesion.

It is important that the patient recognize the unpredictability of results in this condition, and certainly a pessimistic projection should be presented. It must be recognized that there is no other available treatment, however, so many patients are desperate by the time they reach the stereotactic surgeon.

Spasmodic torticollis may be confused with the early stages of dystonia but certainly constitutes a separate disease. It may be distinguished in that it occurs more often in adults and is confined only to the neck and possibly the trapezius muscles. It may involve tilting or rotation of the head to one or the other side, or symmetrical extension (retrocollis). It may be intermittent and clonic in nature, or it may be steady and tonic.

Many patients with spasmodic torticollis have significant emotional problems, and there is considerable disagreement about what constitutes satisfactory management. The literature is loaded with single reports of a multitude of medications, but rarely do second validating reports appear. More or less mutilating procedures may be advocated.

Although there have been several reports of beneficial results from stereotactic surgery, this author has not been encouraged. Subsequent modifications may provide the key to successful alleviation of torticollis by stereotactic surgery, but it is premature to suggest that we have the answer at the present time.

Consequently, a comprehensive stepwise program has been developed for patients with spasmodic torticollis.[85] They are admitted to the Chronic Pain Unit for an evaluation period of approximately 2 weeks. The initial step is a thorough psychiatric evaluation and psychometric testing. Half of the patients who have been referred fail this initial part of the evaluation and prove to be sufficiently unstable so that major surgical procedures or the use of implanted stimulators would be contraindicated.

It is important to establish goals early in the program. Some torticollis patients have considerable neck pain and are distressed from the continual pulling sensation. Others have minimal discomfort but are self-conscious about the abnormal head position. The individual program should be directed toward alleviating the specific problem the patient finds distressing.

Patients are given training in relaxation techniques.[70] An occasional patient who has torticollis secondary to an emotional reaction to a specific psychiatric problem may benefit sufficiently from psychiatric therapy so that nothing further need be done.

Biofeedback is helpful in a very small number of patients. If the pulling sensation or muscle pain is the major problem, electromyographic biofeedback of the involved cervical muscles may be helpful. If abnormal head position is the major complaint, visual biofeedback may be employed—the patient stands in front of a mirror on which a cross has been taped and attempts to align the nose and brows with it.

All patients in the program undergo a trial of transcutaneous stimulation (TENS). Various electrode positions are tried, with both electrodes over the more involved sternocleidomastoid muscle, with one over that muscle and the other in a neutral position, with one on each side of the neck, etc. Although only a few patients respond extremely well to transcutaneous stimulation, it is such a benign procedure that a trial is warranted for every torticollis patient being considered for an invasive procedure.

Those patients who remain candidates after psychiatric evaluation, who are not sufficiently improved by a conservative program, and who can tolerate stimulation and the apparatus of TENS may be considered for dorsal cord stimulation.

The major advantage of dorsal cord stimulation is that it is possible to evaluate the patient with a percutaneously inserted subarachnoid electrode in a reasonably convenient and safe manner, and, indeed, two-thirds of the patients thus evaluated have responded satisfactorily. Another advantage of dorsal cord stimulation for the management of spasmodic torticollis is that no complications have been reported with its use.

For the percutaneous trial, the subarachnoid space is entered with a Tuohy needle introduced at the C2 level, just as in percutaneous cervical cordotomy. The electrode is threaded down to the C5 level and the needle removed, leaving the electrode in place. The patient may be up and about while a trial of stimulation is carried out over 5 to 8 days. Since only a monopolar system is employed, a transcutaneous stimulating electrode can be used as the indifferent electrode and taped to a neutral position at the base of the neck.

Stimulation frequencies up to 1500 Hz should be tried. It has been found empirically that most patients respond better to frequencies greater than 1100 Hz. It may be that the therapeutic effect is the result of depolarization of the proprioceptive nerve roots as they enter the cervical spinal cord, with resultant abolition of abnormal tonic neck reflexes.

If the patient responds to stimulation through the percutaneous electrode, the system can be converted to a permanent implanted device. Because it is difficult to obtain satisfactory placement of a percutaneous epidural electrode in patients whose neck is turning, surgically implanted electrodes have been employed. Epidural placement after a C1 laminectomy has been found to be effective. It may be necessary to order a modified transmitter to provide the stimulus frequency that has been found to be most effective. Other investigators recommend proceeding directly to a surgically implanted stimulator with no percutaneous trial.[86]

For the one-third who do not respond to dorsal cord stimulation or who are opposed to trial stimulation for any reason, the classical Dandy-Foerster operation is recommended.[87] This involves section of the anterior roots of C1, C2, and C3 bilaterally, both spinal accessory nerves, and possibly section of the anterior of root C4 on the more involved side.

A suboccipital craniectomy is performed, along with a laminectomy from C1 through C4. The dura is opened, and, under the operating microscope, the procedure is begun at the lowest root to be sectioned. The dentate ligament is cut from its attachment to the dura at each level, the anterior roots are identified, accompanying radicular arteries are dissected free and preserved, and the anterior roots are cut. It is important to identify the C1 nerve roots accurately, since failure to section all of the fibers precludes a good result. There is usually not a posterior root to C1, and the anterior root may extend in a downward direction where it may be obscured by the vertebral artery.

The usual procedure is to section the spinal accessory nerves intradurally at the same sitting, but one must recognize that that denervates the trapezius as well as the sternocleidomastoid muscle. If the patient would be disabled by shoulder weakness, it may be more desirable to section the innervation of the sternocleidomastoid muscles selectively through separate incisions in the neck.

If an intradural section of the spinal accessory nerves is done, it should be done as far laterally as possible as the nerve enters the jugular foramen. The lower-most fibers of the vagus nerve can be seen joining the spinal accessory nerve laterally, and they should be included in the section, since they are actually spinal accessory fibers. Even at that, 50 percent of the patients demonstrate some remaining innervation of sternocleidomastoid muscles if an electromyogram is done several days after surgery. This remaining innervation should be looked for routinely, and if it exists, the spinal accessory nerve should be sectioned in the neck.

The procedure to section the spinal accessory nerve peripherally is done with the patient in the supine position. A diagonal incision is made at the anterior border of the sternocleidomastoid muscle just below its attachment to the skull. Alternately, a more cosmetically satisfactory result can be obtained by allowing the skin incision to fall into a natural crease, but this compromises the exposure somewhat. Dissection is carried out on the undersurface of the sternocleido-mastoid muscle. The spinal accessory nerve can usually be found entering that muscle at the point where the lateral mass of the C2 vertebra can be palpated. The branch to the trapezius muscle usually comes off just before it enters the body of the sternocleidomastoid muscle. If not, dissection can be carried into the muscle in an attempt to separate the sternocleidomastoid fibers selectively, if that is desired. Each branch can be identified with the use of an intraoperative nerve stimulator.

The potential side-effects of the Dandy-Foerster operation involve primarily damage to the brainstem (which may follow damage to small radicular arteries) such as dysphagia, vestibular symptoms, unsteadiness, or even failure to regain consciousness after surgery. The mortality rate is reported between 1 and 4 percent. The usual potential complications of posterior fossa surgery in the sitting position must be considered, of course, such as venous air embolism or hypotension.

Eighty percent of the patients have satisfactory improvement following this procedure. There is surprisingly little loss of mobility of the neck, but loss of trapezius power may cause weakness of the shoulders.

Cerebral palsy does not lend itself readily to neurosurgical management. Although there are some aspects of the motor disorders of cerebral palsy, spasticity in particular, that may be somewhat alleviated by functional neurosurgery, the major motor disabilities involved with choreoathetosis are only minimally affected, if at all.

On the other hand, the spasticity that accompanies cerebral palsy may respond to one of several functional neurosurgical manipulations, either ablation or stimulation. A number of reports in the late 1960s encouraged the feeling that dentatotomy might be useful for the treatment of spasticity of cerebral palsy.[88,89,90] The effect decreased with long-term follow-up, however, so that it is not often used today. Nevertheless, a 30 percent improvement in spasticity was generally reported, with perhaps facilitation of nursing care in 50 percent of the patients.[89] The operation was relatively direct, with the coordinates being related to a fourth ventriculogram (although the coordinates of the dentate nucleus per se caused some disagreement). The operation was safe with surprisingly little risk of cerebellar or motor impairment.

Stereotactic thalamotomy or pallidotomy has been tried with patients with choreoathetosis, with mixed results.[91]

There is a stimulation procedure worthy of note. *Chronic cerebellar stimulation* (CCS) has been employed for spasticity of cerebral origin in cerebral palsy patients. It was observed[92] that stimulation of the anterior lobe of the cerebellum may inhibit decerebrate rigidity in experimental animals, presumably because of a descending inhibitory influence on the myotatic reflex arc. Because a similar mechanism of increase in segmental activity is involved in spasticity of cerebral palsy origin,[93,94] a technique was developed to stimulate the anterior lobe of the cerebellum in cerebral palsy patients.

The technique of implantation involves performing a small craniectomy or two craniectomies on either side of the midline just below the transverse sinus. The dura is opened parallel to the sinus and flat cerebellar electrodes are inserted; the electrodes are mounted on a Silastic pad that is the approximate length required to position the electrodes anteriorly. There are two different models, one with a single channel and the other with two separate channels requiring the implantation of two separate receivers, that seem to work equally well. The dura is closed.

The same type of radio receiver is implanted in a infraclavicular pocket for chronic cerebellar stimulation as for other implanted stimulating devices. A subcutaneous tunnel is passed to the incision overlying the suboccipital area.

Various types of stimulation have been employed, and it appears that intermittent stimulation may provide the best effect. The radio transmitter especially devised for cerebellar stimulation has the option of such duty cycles built into it so that it can be programmed to stimulate and rest at several-minute intervals. It is necessary to try various parameters for each patient to find the optimal program.

There has been considerable concern about whether the stimulation of the cerebellum causes damage, particularly to the Purkinje cells. One early report[95] indicated significant damage underlying the electrodes, but later reports[96] were not in agreement. It appears that there may have been artifacts associated with the size of the electrode and current densities in the original study, and later studies indicate there is a significant safety factor in the use of chronic cerebellar stimulation.[96] Aside from that concern, there have been no significant complications reported. One technical problem is the occasional leakage of cerebrospinal fluid along the leads, but this can be prevented by applying a purse-string suture along the tract at the time of the initial surgery.

Although chronic cerebellar stimulation was originally intended to alleviate the spasticity of cerebral palsy, there have been reports of subjective improvement in choreoathetosis as well.[93] Such improvement has not, however, been completely documented. Basically, it may be said that patients look the same but may be able to perform better. Patients who walk only with assistance may be able to walk with crutches, speech or swallowing may be significantly improved, and care may be easier. Attempts at documenting the magnitude and the mechanism of improvement have yielded inconclusive results.[94]

Nevertheless, some patients with cerebral palsy appear to have benefited from chronic cerebellar stimulation, even those whose major disability was choreoathetosis. Its use might be recommended for those patients with good mentation who could improve their motor activities with some improvement in spasticity or choreoathetosis.

It can be generalized that stereotactic lesions have a similar effect to chronic cerebellar stimulation in cerebral palsy, that is, patients look the same but may perform better. Indeed, in taking motion pictures of a number of cerebral palsy patients before and after stereotactic surgery, it was difficult to see any difference. Their performance record, however, as documented on the film, demonstrated a significant increase in motor facility.

The target point was originally defined as being in the globus pallidus, but the present recommendation is to make the primary lesion in Forel's field. If a second lesion is going to be made a lesion on the second side 3 months later, it can be made in the medial portion of the globus pallidus, at the origin of the ansa lenticularis. The target point may be 2 mm posterior to the anterior commissure, 10 mm lateral, and at the level of the intercommissural line. If stimulation produces visual sensations, the electrode should be withdrawn 1 mm. If low-frequency stimulation produces motor effects, the electrode is too close to the internal capsule and should be moved 2 mm lateral.

It is important to remember that patients with cerebral palsy have not had the opportunity to acquire a repertoire of patterned motor behavior. Even if the spasticity or abnormal movements are obviated, it is still necessary to work intensively with this group of patients to train the released muscles to do those things that would have developed automatically, an approach to "habilitation," rather than rehabilitation.

Spasticity may respond quite well to functional neurosurgery, depending on the origin of the problem. In general, one should consider whether the spasticity is of cerebral or spinal origin. Cerebral causes for spasticity include cerebral palsy, stroke, and degenerative disease. Spinal causes of spasticity include spinal cord injury, spinal cord tumor, cervical canal stenosis, and some spinal degenerative diseases. Multiple sclerosis may be a combination of cerebral and spinal spasticity, but there is generally a sufficient spinal component so that remarks concerning spinal etiology of spasticity may be taken to include multiple sclerosis.

Because the spasticity that accompanies hemiplegia after a stroke generally does not have an underlying pattern of normal motor control, functional neurosurgical procedures are not ordinarily recommended. On the other hand, spasticity of spinal origin may often be dealt with successfully, particularly the spasticity that may accompany a spinal degenerative disease such as multiple sclerosis.

Patients with *multiple sclerosis* may respond quite dramatically to dorsal cord stimulation. The mechanism for such response is not known, but one may theorize that it is the stimulation of a descending inhibitory pathway. Stimulation at relatively modest frequencies, 28–120 Hz, may allow significant improvement in function, not only of the extremities, but of the bowel and bladder as well. In fact, even though stimulation is applied to the cervical area, some patients experience improvement in speech.

Because evaluation with a percutaneous or subarachnoid electrode is quite simple, any patient with multiple sclerosis who is impaired by spasticity but still has underlying motor control and good mentation may be considered a candidate for dorsal cord stimulation.

An epidural electrode can be inserted for cervical stimulation by performing a puncture in the midline at or near the T1 level and threading the electrode upward. Because symptoms may vary from day to day, a trial of stimulation should last for at least several days. It is not uncommon for stimulation for several hours to be followed by improvement in spasticity for several days, and such an observation should not necessarily be interpreted as coincidental spontaneous remission. Stimulation is well tolerated, and it does not appear that the use of stimulators is associated with exacerbation or acceleration of the multiple sclerosis. If stimulation provides a beneficial effect, the radio receiver can be implanted and the entire system internalized.

Spasticity after partial spinal cord injury may be managed with an approach similar to that used for multiple sclerosis, but spasticity below the level of a complete spinal cord functional transection is different both in mechanism and management.

The indication for treatment of spasticity after complete spinal cord injury concerns not the injury itself but the occurrence of complications. Patients with spastic contractures of extremities for whom rehabilitation has become difficult or impossible may benefit from improved ability to position and move more advantageously. Patients whose position in bed is limited because of spastic contractures may develop decubiti, which can be managed only by resolving the spasticity to position the patient to lie off the ulcers.

One must consider the distribution of the spasticity that must be alleviated. Patients with spinal cord injury may have spasticity particularly of muscle groups on one side of a joint, leading to contracture of that joint (in contrast to patients with cerebral palsy who may have a multitude of patterns of spasticity of individual muscle groups that may prohibit full use of extremities).

Determination is made as to which muscle or groups require decreased hypertonicity, and ideally this pattern is verified by electromyography. If a single hypertonic muscle can be identified as the cause of the specific problem, treatment with 40% alcohol injection to the motor points is fairly simple and may be quite effective. If the problem involves a group of muscles with partial denervation, the nerve supplying that muscle group may be blocked with lidocaine as a temporary test, and, if effective, the lesion may be made permanent by injection of 6 to 10% phenol in saline. If the spasticity involves several muscle groups, particularly if they are unilateral, surgical or chemical rhizotomy may be considered.[97] If sensory loss already exists, a dorsal rhizotomy may be effective, without producing the atrophy of a lower motor neuron lesion. Alternatively, a rhizotomy involving some but not all of the anterior root may provide sufficient relief.

Sensory rhizotomy as an open surgical technique involves a multiple-level laminectomy to expose the spinal cord at the appropriate levels, with due attention to the discrepancy between the vertebral level and the level of the spinal nerve roots. In order to verify that the appropriate nerve roots are identified, electromyographic electrodes should be placed in the appropriate muscles, as well as adjacent muscle groups, prior to surgical draping, so the response to electrical stimulation of the exposed anterior roots can guide the surgeon to section only the appropriate spinal roots. It is necessary to separate the dentate ligament from its attachment to the dura to rotate the cord slightly to gain access to the anterior root. Care should be taken to avoid radicular arteries if preservation of spinal cord activity or segmental reflex patterns is desired.

Radiofrequency rhizotomy, as described elsewhere, may also be used to treat spasticity. It may be extremely difficult, however, to position the patient with contractures for the optimal x-ray control that this procedure requires.

One of the factors in deciding the manner in which spasticity of the lower extremities might be attacked is the function of the patient's bladder. If the patient has a contracted bladder in continual spasm, there may be an advantage to treating the spasticity of the bladder as well by one of the injection techniques. If the patient has a reflex bladder that is operating in optimal fashion with periodic evacuation, one would wish to avoid compromise of bladder function and would want to consider a longitudinal or Bischoff's myelotomy[98,99] (see Chapter 75). If the spasticity of the lower extremities is extensor and provides the patient with some weight-bearing capabilities that are best left preserved, yet problems exist with spasticity of the bladder, one might consider a presacral neurectomy or rhizotomy of the S2, S3, and S4 roots by radiofrequency current or injection.

If less selective treatment of spasticity is desired, however (either to include sacral segments or if it is not critical whether or not sacral segments are included), the simple technique of hot saline injection might be considered. This procedure can be done only on patients with complete functional transection of the spinal cord who have no sensation below the level of the injury. Saline at 80° is instilled into the subarachnoid space in order to destroy the nerve roots and possibly an isolated spinal cord segment. Because both temperature and volume are controlled, the saline cools as it mixes with cerebrospinal fluid so that the functioning cord at higher levels is protected.

The procedure can be done in the patient's room. A basin of saline with a thermometer is placed on a hot plate. Lumbar puncture is performed at L3 or L4. When a free flow of spinal fluid is obtained, a volume of saline is instilled. For a midthoracic lesion, 10 cc of saline can be rapidly injected. If spasticity persists, an additional 10–20 cc can be injected after several minutes. The spasticity may return totally or in part over the next few days, in which case the procedure is repeated. Interestingly, when two injections are performed within several days, there is much less likelihood of return of spasticity after the second injection. If spasticity persists, the volume can be adjusted accordingly.

If a more selective injection is desired, for unilateral effect only, for instance, *intrathecal phenol* can be used. The patient is placed in the lateral position on the myelogram table. A lumbar puncture is performed and 1 cc of Pantopaque is instilled. The table is tilted so that the Pantopaque is centered at the center of the roots the surgeon wants to affect. Phenol crystals are dissolved in Pantopaque, 100 mg/cc. If 2 nerve roots are to be treated, 3 ml can be used, and if 4 nerve roots, 6 ml can be used. The phenol-Pantopaque is instilled and the table readjusted as necessary to position the Pantopaque over the involved roots. The patient is allowed to remain in that position for 10 to 15 minutes, and the Pantopaque is removed.

A unique use of functional neurosurgery may be employed to break the pattern of *ankle clonus* in a patient who is otherwise ambulatory. A peripheral nerve stimulator, as used for pain treatment, can be implanted on the common peroneal nerve. Stimulation produces sufficient reciprocal inhibition between the antagonistic muscles so voluntary movement can be maintained as the pattern of clonus is broken up. The stimulus intensity and rate are adjusted to produce nonpainful sensation and sustained, slightly tonic dorsal flexion and eversion of the foot.[100,101] The frequency, duration, and amplitude of the stimulus train must be established for each patient. In general, the amplitude must be large enough to produce an H wave, the train duration must be greater than 400 msec, and the frequency must be from 30 to 50 Hz.

Development of Stereotactic Surgery

The history of the development of stereotactic surgery intimately involves surgery for affective disorders. Indeed, it was dissatisfaction with classical prefrontal lobotomy[102,103] that motivated Spiegel and Wycis[2,82] to develop the techniques for human stereotactic surgery, and the first reported stereotactic patients were treated for affective disorders. One must also put into context that the indications for psychiatric surgery of any type were much broader before the development of tranquilizers.

Historical perspective.   The original techniques of open or semiblind prefrontal lobotomy were relatively nonselective in that they interrupted the fibers to the frontal areas concerned with intellectual function, along with those fibers involved with regulation of emotions.[104-106] The original stereotactic target for affective disease was the dorsomedian nucleus of the thalamus, from which those frontal projecting fibers of emotional importance originate, but not those of intellectual function.[64,82,107] Even as techniques became more refined and selective during the 1950s and 1960s, precise interruption of only the desired tracts remained uncertain.

Although it has been more than 35 years since it has been demonstrated that psychosurgery can be performed with significantly less risk to intellect than the original nonselective procedures,[105,108] there are those who have lobbied against the use of psychosurgery, without acknowledging the progress and refinements that have occurred in that field since the introduction of stereotactic and selective techniques.

Approximately 10 years ago a movement was instigated to ban psychosurgery,[109] and a discussion of the present status of psychosurgery must examine that controversy. Four unsubstantiated allegations were made:

1. Psychosurgery was not an effective means of treatment for psychiatric conditions.
2. Psychosurgery resulted in intolerable mental deficits.
3. Psychosurgery was being used (or misused) as a social or political tool.
4. Psychosurgery was selectively used against minorities.

To investigate these allegations, the National Commission for the Protection of Human Subjects of Biomedical and Behavioral Research was formed. Not only were all four allegations proven false, but the evidence gathered to investigate these allegations demonstrated that psychosurgery was reasonably safe and effective.[110]

Despite the favorable findings of the commission, the furor provoked by this political controversy has significantly wounded the field of psychosurgery. It is estimated that the present rate of psychosurgery is only 10 percent what it was a decade ago, even though no other significant advances in psychiatric care have provided alternate forms of treatment for the group of patients that was formerly treated with psychosurgery. This low level of activity, plus perhaps the reluctance of some investigators to perform research in the area, has significantly slowed progress in the field. Nevertheless, surgery is still indicated for many patients with affective disorders, and may be their only chance of improvement.

As part of the effort to evaluate psychosurgery, the commission reviewed the extent to which psychosurgery was being practiced in the United States, and extensively reviewed the literature. Perhaps most significantly, a contract was let for a group of experts not involved with individual patients to perform a retrospective and prospective neuropsychologic examination of patients undergoing cingulotomy for a variety of psychiatric problems. This examination, representing a reasonably well-controlled and most objective review of the potential side-effects and neurologic function following cingulotomy for affective disorders (as well as pain), detected no lasting deficits in behavioral capacities from surgery,[111,112] but considerable subjective benefit.

In summary, the Commission recommended that "psychosurgery be used only to meet the health needs of individual patients and then only under strict limitations and controls, with added safeguards when the patient is a prisoner, a minor, or in a mental institution."[110] The commission also noted that the safety and efficacy of specific neurosurgical procedures for the treatment of particular disorders, however, have not been demonstrated to the degree that would permit such procedures to be considered "accepted" practice. It was recognized that degrees of expertise and ancillary psychiatric facilities varied from one neurosurgeon to another, and it was felt that the decision for psychosurgery should be in the hands of a competent team. For this reason, as well as to assure that psychosurgery would not be misused, the commission recommended that a board, similar to the institutional review boards that evaluate experimental protocols, be available at institutions where psychosurgery is contemplated, and that the composition and procedures for review of psychosurgical programs be recommended by the Department of Health, Education and Welfare (now the Deparment of Health and Human Services).[110] These recommendations were not enacted, however, partly because of the decrease in activity in the field.[113]

The commission suggested that it was still appropriate to call psychosurgery experimental, not because it did not have demonstrated safety and effectiveness, but because there were still sufficient unknowns regarding the field, and that anyone who assumed the responsibility of using this treatment should likewise assume the responsibility of maintaining available records of well-controlled observations for the further advancement of the field.

As a general rule, it should be stressed that surgery should be considered for the treatment of affective disorders only after an extensive period of psychiatric and pharmacologic management has verified that no other treatment is satisfactory. Since the indications for psychosurgery hinge on psychiatric rather than neurosurgical diagnosis, it should be considered only upon recommendation of one or preferably several psychiatrists who have personally evaluated the patient. A thorough search for underlying pathology, particularly epilepsy, should precede any psychosurgical procedure. Surgery might be considered before an extensive course of electroconvulsive therapy (ECT), since there is evidence that stereotactic procedures result in less permanent neurologic deficits than ECT.[110,111] The only exception to the recommendation for a prolonged period of psychiatric management involves those patients who are so suicidal that they would likely not survive a prolonged evaluation.

Much of the evaluation of the effectiveness of surgery for affective disorders involves the subjective impression of the examiner. Except for neuropsychologic testing to evaluate untoward side-effects, there exist few objective criteria to evaluate the efficacy of any given procedure. Nevertheless, there is some consistency in the subjective reports of both patients and physicians that allow conclusions to be drawn about the effectiveness of particular procedures for specific psychiatric problems.

There is some disagreement about the relationship between psychosurgery and surgery for chronic pain. Many patients who present with a chief complaint of intractable pain may benefit from psychosurgery, particularly cingulotomy, but the duration of benefit is often limited. Such patients ordinarily have such obvious and severe emotional problems associated with their pain that, in this group of patients, cingulotomy very often might be recommended for their affective problems alone. With this in mind, the rule otherwise stands that there is little role for ablative procedures in the management of chronic intractable pain, although it may be useful to treat cancer pain.

Anatomy of surgery for affective disorders.   The portion of the brain concerned with regulation and expression of emotions is generally referred to as the limbic system. As might be anticipated from the system that controls such a basic aspect of behavior as emotion, it consists, to a large extent, of the philogenetically old type of cortical tissue that encircles the inner part of the cerebral hemispheres—hence, the name "limbic" or border. This cortex has interconnections with other structures, such as the hypothalamus, the anterior thalamic nuclei, the cingulate gyrus, the fornix, the mamillary bodies, and the hippocampus, all of which constituted the original Papez limbic circuit.[114] This system has been expanded to include the cortex of the orbitofrontal area, the insula, and the anterior temporal lobes, along with their connections to the amygdala and the dorsomedian nucleus of the thalamus.[115]

The limbic system, as currently defined, consists of two circuits—the medial limbic circuit and the basolateral circuit[116]—and sometimes a third circuit referred to as the defense reaction circuit.[117]

The *medial limbic circuit,* or Papez circuit, is the medial frontal cortex-cingulate-hippocampal-fornix-mamillary-anterior thalamic-frontal cortex circuit and has rich connections with the reticular activating system.[118] It passes from the septal nuclei via the cingulum bundle in the cingulate gyrus to the hippocampus of the temporal lobe. Fibers pass from the hippocampal gyrus by way of the fornix to the mamillary body, and then via the mamillo-thalamic tract to the anterior nucleus of the thalamus. Fibers project from that nucleus via the anterior thalamic radiation to the orbito-frontal cortex, which projects back to the cingulum to close the circuit. Affective and autonomic responses have been obtained from stimulation of this circuit.[100,118] In addition to the involvement of this circuit with emotions, parts of the circuit are concerned with memory, such as the hippocampus, the fornix, and the mamillary bodies.[119]

The *basolateral* or *lateral limbic circuit* lies outside the brainstem and involves the orbital cortex with its cortical connections to the anterior temporal cortex, which radiates in turn to the amygdala, which serves in this case as the outflow from the temporal neocortex. Projections run from the amygdala to the dorsomedial nucleus of the thalamus, and from there to the orbital cortex to complete the orbito-frontal cortex-temporal-amygdala-dorsomedial thalamic-frontal circuit.

Thus, as in the motor-control system, we have two circuits that involve adjacent (but in this case not overlapping) areas of the thalamus, whose efferent conducting systems are comparable, forming a massive linked system.[119]

The *defense reaction circuit* connects those areas of the brain concerned with generation of emotion to the areas concerned with the visceral responses to emotion, such as fight or flight.[117] It involves connections from the hypothalamus via the stria terminalis to the amygdala, and from the amygdala back to the hypothalamus.

Since the amygdala serves as one of the major outflow tracts from the temporal cortex, it may propagate seizure activity from the temporal lobe to other areas where such abnormal activity might be expressed. If a temporal lobe seizure involves behavioral abnormalities, as is common, a lesion in the amygdala may interrupt the expression of that abnormal behavior.[120-124]

Since the limbic system is more of a functional than an anatomic unit and is defined experimentally, to a large extent, by response to stimulation, it is not surprising that simulation in humans may produce identifiable reactions that allow localization of electrode placement. Although most stereotactic surgery is performed on conscious and cooperating patients, the patient population for surgery for affective disorders sometimes makes it necessary to perform such surgery under general anesthesia. Nevertheless, awake patients are able to report the effects of stimulation,[125] which are very often emotional in nature, that is, a feeling of well-being or a feeling of anxiety and tension. Although there may be no response to stimulation in approximately half the cases, when a response docs occur, it provides good verification of electrode placement.

If there is a response on stimulation of the fibers between the thalamus and the orbital cortex within the anterior limb of the internal capsule, it is likely to be a positive response, or a feeling of well-being.[125] Likewise, as one might expect, a similar response may be obtained from stimulation of the genu of the corpus callosum. Of those patients who respond to stimulation of the cingulum, half may report a "negative" feeling, or one of dysphoria, or some other strange or ill-defined sensation, but it is uncommon for a positive response to occur.[126] Stimulation of the amygdala may produce a range of aggressive responses, such as a desire to attack the examiner, or swearing or destructive behavior.[127] One must comment, however, that the characteristic depth electroencephalogram that may be recorded from the amygdala often provides accurate localization without stimulation.

Interestingly, patients undergoing stimulation under local anesthesia rarely have autonomic or visceral responses, except perhaps secondary to a physical response. Under general anesthesia, however, stimulation of the cingulate gyrus or mesial-frontal projections usually causes apnea with less constant changes in pulse, blood pressure, and forearm blood flow.[118,128,129]

Surgical management of affective disorders. Disagreement about the technique of psychosurgery may stem from several sources, including the following:

1. Psychosurgery as originally practiced involved blind sectioning of fibers projecting to large areas of the frontal lobes. The areas affected were diffuse and inconsistent, both because of

the poor control over anatomic landmarks and the variable effect of interrupting blood supply. Although there was significant benefit to many patients, it was often at the expense of significant deterioration of mentation. At that time, however, before the advent of tranquilizers, there was often no alternate pharmacologic therapy available.[130]

2. Psychiatric diagnosis has been and remains imprecise. Even though many conditions for which there are psychosurgical indications are well defined, difference in nomenclature between countries or during different decades makes it difficult to compare ideas and results.[113]

3. Most neurosurgeons who report their experience with psychosurgery tend to report the effect of a single procedure on patients in several diagnostic categories. There is no extensive well-controlled study to compare the effects of various procedures on matched patients. Consequently, it is impossible to designate with certainty which procedure may be more effective for a particular condition, although it can generally be stated that interrupting the limbic system at any accessible point in its circuit may provide similar results. Authors who use different procedures may draw opposite conclusions.[131,132]

4. Many studies are poorly controlled and rely on such general assessments as "generally improved" or "quality of life improved." The duration of follow-up varies significantly, as does the completeness of follow-up. Often the operating surgeon may be the only one to assess the results, a problem common to many therapeutic studies. Although there are several good attempts at prospective studies with managed controls, it is difficult to obtain sufficient patients in the control groups to make meaningful comparison possible. Despite those shortcomings, however, results are generally in agreement in those studies that are well controlled.[133]

5. Early studies, before the availability of tranquilizers, concentrated on schizophrenic patients who remained management problems even though they were hospitalized. Presently, many such patients are being managed successfully by medical means, and the emphasis of psychosurgery is on specific behavioral disorders, rather than schizophrenia. In general discussions about psychiatric treatment of emotional illness, all too often there is insufficient distinction made between those early imprecise procedures and indications and the present-day procedures, which involve limited interruption of specific pathways.

Conditions that are generally agreed to be indications for psychosurgery are those characterized by a stereotyped and excessive emotional response, that is, depression,[39,134-137] chronic anxiety or tension state,[137] obsessive-compulsive states,[138] and perhaps the depressive component of manic-depressive disorder.[39]

There is considerable disagreement as to whether surgery is the appropriate treatment for aggression. The type of aggressiveness and violence for which one might consider the surgery used for epilepsy is "personal violent behavior, unwarranted and usually unprovoked acts that directly attempt to, or actually do, injure or destroy another person or thing. This does not include violence consistently organized for a political motive."[139] Most such patients have epilepsy,[140] and even those who are not classified as such have a high incidence of abnormal EEG or postoperative seizures. The implication is, of course, that the type of aggression that responds to stereotactic surgery is that associated with temporal lobe seizures, and the procedure of choice is amygdalotomy. This is in contrast to the early literature in which prefrontal lobotomy was employed in unmanageably aggressive schizophrenic patients, in which case it might have rendered the patients less aggressive or violent, but it did not have a beneficial effect on the schizophrenia itself.[104]

Some authors[141,142] attempt to interrupt the autonomic component of such aggressive behavior by producing lesions in the posterior hypothalamus. Although they report beneficial results in 80 percent or more of their patients, this procedure is not generally accepted, so that we might recommend, for the purpose of this presentation, to consider explosive aggression as a component of temporal lobe epilepsy for which amygdalotomy or temporal lobectomy would be the procedure of choice,[143] as has been found in one controlled study comparing both procedures.[144]

There has been even greater controversy concerning the use of surgery for the treatment of "hedonia," sexual delinquency, pedophilia, homosexuality, or sexual violence, with "good results" from anterior hypothalamotomy for all except homosexuality.[145-147] The indications for such surgery are both controversial and ill defined. Patients included in these series have generally been confined because of legal difficulties emanating from their behavior, but it is not always clear whether it was the sexual component of their behavior or their generally unacceptable behavior that was the problem, and whether truly voluntary consent can be given by patients so incarcerated.[148] Since the diagnoses are not defined in a standard fashion, a neurosurgeon from Sweden pointed out, when hearing of these results, "What's considered hypersexuality in Germany may be normal behavior in Sweden."

One may find it acceptable to use the same target point for obsessive-compulsive state, anxiety, and depression; that is, *cingulotomy* is the procedure most likely to give beneficial results in all three conditions with minimal chance of undesirable side-effects,[130] even though there are favorable reports on the use of anterior capsulotomy for these same conditions.[149-151]

There have been numerous cingulotomy techniques described in the literature, some with open surgery, some with relatively freehand insertion of electrodes, and some stereotactic. Since stereotactic surgery provides the best opportunity for the accurate placement of a controlled lesion with the greatest safety, that is the procedure of choice and the technique that will be presented primarily (Table 67-1).[118]

A ventriculostomy is performed as sufficient air is introduced to demonstrate the anterior horn and roof of both lateral ventricles. On the lateral x-ray, a vertical line, approximately at right angles to the intercommissural line, is drawn 3 cm behind the tip of the frontal horn. The first lesion is made on a vertical line 3 cm posterior to the tip of the frontal horn and 5 mm above the roof the ventricle at the lateral-most border of the ventricle. A second lesion is made 8 mm medial to this. Another pair of lesions are made 12 mm anterior to the first pair, for a total of four lesions on each side.[117,128] A relatively large electrode should be used, since it is desirable to interrupt as much of the cingulate bundle as possible. Lesions are made bilaterally at one sitting, since unilateral lesions are frequently not effective and bilateral lesions are well tolerated.

Alternately, target points for cingulotomy can be made 3–4 cm behind the tip of the lateral ventricle, 5 mm lateral to the midline, and both 1 and 2 cm above the roof of the ventricle.[136] Single lesions can be made at these points, if they are relatively large, that is, 1 cm in diameter. Other authors[108,152] report similar procedures, but all are designed to interrupt the cingulate bundle at various sites.

For the first 7 to 10 days postoperatively, the patient may exhibit anergia, lack of drive, and lack of initiation of conversation.[137,153] Although this initial appearance may be distressing, it is only temporary, and bears no relationship to the final clinical result. During the remainder of the first 3 weeks, the patient may show some increased irritability and verbal aggressiveness, but this gradually settles down so that many patients have achieved their final clinical results in 4 to 6 weeks.

If an adequate clinical result is not obtained after waiting a minimum of 6 to 12 weeks, lesions may also be made in the fibers extending between the thalamus and the orbital cortex as they pass through the anterior limb of the internal capsule, a so-called anterior capsulotomy or medial prefrontal leucotomy. The coordinates for these lesions are on a vertical line 1.5 cm anterior to the base of the anterior clinoid process. Three lesions are made in the form of a triangle with its apex superior. At 6 mm from the midline, one lesion is made 1 cm above the floor of the anterior fossa and a second lesion 1.5 cm above the floor of the anterior fossa. A single lateral lesion is made 14 mm from the midline and 1 cm above the floor of the anterior fossa.[118]

For those surgeons who would still prefer an open rather than a stereotactic operation, the following technique is described,[153] although others may be equally satisfactory.[154] Bilateral trephine openings are made 2.5 cm from the midline and 13 cm above the glabella. The dura is opened, and a brain needle is passed vertically until it touches the orbital plate. A core of brain tissue is dissected along the brain needle for a width of 1.5 cm. The ventricle may either be traversed or a subependymal dissection can be performed if the ependyma separates easily. Dissection continues along the tract of the brain needle through the inferior part of the cingulate gyrus, and is carried medially until the gray matter on the mesial surface of the frontal lobe is encountered and inferiorly until the subfrontal cortex is seen. The inferior portion of the dissection is entirely medial to the brain cannula, since the fibers to be interrupted are just below the mesial cortex, and the lateral fibers should be preserved.

There is some opinion[132] that obsessive-compulsive patients do better if the primary procedure is an anterior capsulotomy, but statistical comparisons suggest that cingulate lesions are preferable.[155]

It has been suggested that schizophrenic patients who are unmanageable because of a great deal of anxiety and tension may benefit from a lesion in the genu of the corpus callosum, interrupting the pathways between the two frontal lobes, a procedure called a *mesoloviotomy*.[156] Although results are encouraging, the procedure has not been widely adopted.

Epilepsy

The surgical management of epilepsy is discussed in Chapter 65. It might be appropriate, however, to review briefly the role of stereotactic surgery in the management of epilepsy.

Regardless of the surgical approach contemplated, depth electrode recording for the localization of the epileptogenic focus may be helpful, particularly when the surface electroencephalogram is inconclusive. It may be possible to obtain evidence for laterality of a temporal lobe focus, even though surface recording may show bilateral discharges,[33,157] or to identify the focus critically, so the location, shape, and extent of a resection can be tailored to an individual patient.

It is not uncommon for a seizure not to present itself during a random electroencephalographic recording session, in which case it may be necessary to perform prolonged monitoring. Since seizure activity may be particularly apparent at night or during the induction of sleep, a sleep recording may demonstrate a focus that is not otherwise apparent. There are a group of patients who fail to demonstrate sufficient interictal abnormal activity to localize the epileptogenic focus without recording an actual seizure. Other patients may not demonstrate a focus, even with prolonged sleep recording, and others still may show so much bilateral epileptogenic activity that the localization of the focus becomes obscured. In all these cases, the origin of the epileptic activity may become apparent with recording from implanted electrodes over several days or several weeks.

Epidural or subdural electrodes usually consist of several electrodes mounted on a Silastic strip, which are inserted through a small craniectomy or burr hole underneath the temporal lobe, particularly under the mesial part or at the temporal tip. The electrode wires are brought out through the scalp so direct connections can be made for recordings.

A subcortical electrode may provide more precise information about the origin of epileptic activity, particularly if prolonged recordings are made to capture the profile of a seizure. Propagation of abnormal activity from one electrode site to another can provide definite localization, particularly when the seizure activity begins in one temporal lobe and projects contralaterally or involves subcortical structures, such as the globus pallidus or thalamus.[83]

There are several types of depth electrodes for recording. The most practical are those with multiple contacts, such as Schreiber electrodes, which consist of several wires twisted together to form four separate contacts.[158] Coordinates are selected to distribute the electrode array throughout a representative portion of the temporal lobes, and four or five electrodes may be implanted on each side. Some stereotactic apparatuses, such as the Talairach apparatus, allow implantation of the electrodes from laterally, for direct access to the temporal areas.[157] If multiple electrodes are used, particularly in the temporal areas or in the area of the sylvian fissure, it is helpful to refer to an angiogram to position the electrodes to minimize the risk to vascular structures.

The electrode wires are brought out through a stab wound or scalp incision so that direct contact can be made for EEG recording. The impedance is not very dissimilar to that of scalp electrodes and remains stable for many months, so no special electronic arrangements need be made for depth recording.

Either single- or multi-contact electrodes can be used. They should be directed stereotactically to areas of suspicion, particularly the mesial temporal lobes, common sites for seizure activity where surface recordings are less accurate. Recordings can be performed directly from the amygdala or the hippocampus. Coordinates are generally determined by the configuration of the electrodes and related to a ventriculogram demonstrating the temporal horn. Ordinarily, multiple electrodes are inserted in a single session, either separately or through a single burr hole over the convexity. At least several days should be allowed before recordings are begun, since the trauma of insertion may change the electrical activity. Usually, sufficient information can be obtained from recording sessions performed over 1 to 2 weeks, but electrodes have been left for many weeks with reasonable safety.

There are some situations in which stereotactic lesions can prevent the propagation of seizure activity and consequently prevent the development of clinical seizures. Patients who cannot be satisfactorily managed with medication and whose focus is not sufficiently localized to be considered for temporal lobectomy may respond to a stereotactic subcortical lesion.

Some authors recommend stereotactic ablation as the procedure of choice over temporal lobectomy, suggesting that there is less risk of undesirable side-effects, such as amnesia, paresis, aphasia, hemianopsia, or the development of Klüver-Bucy syndrome.[82,158]

Temporal lobe seizure activity may depend on the amygdala for its propagation, and may be precipitated by stimulation of that structure,[159-161] so that stereotactic amygdalotomy may be used for temporal lobe epilepsy, especially lesions of the medial portion of that nucleus.[124,162] The amygdala can be identified readily by its characteristic electrical activity on insertion of the electrode, and relatively large lesions can be made with minor side-effects. The coordinates from which to begin the search are 5 mm anterior to the tip of the temporal horn, 5 mm medial to the lateral edge of the temporal horn, and 3 mm above a line drawn as an extension of the inferior border of the temporal horn.[163] Further confirmation of the relationship of the electrode to the amygdala may be obtained from a CT scan (v.i.).

Some authors recommend lesions in the hippocampus, which can be made most conveniently by introducing an electrode into the longitudinal axis of this gyrus,[5,164] provided the individual stereotactic apparatus allows that approach.

Because epileptogenic foci are frequently multiple, beneficial effects of such lesions may be only transient, with recurrences most frequent at about 6 months to 1 year. Success can be regained, however, by repeating the stereotactic surgery, enlarging the lesion, or interrupting a different structure within the circuit of propagation. Amygdala lesions may be combined with hippocampal lesions[157] or with unilateral interruption of the fornix[120,165] or anterior commissure.[166] A section of the fornix alone may provide specific interruption of the hippocampofugal fibers to control temporal lobe epilepsy.[167] There is interesting evidence that bilateral lesions in Forel's field H may interrupt the propagation of epileptogenic impulses originating in the cortex and basal ganglia,[168] but these effects may be only transitory and may be associated with speech disturbances if they are bilateral. Such lesions may be considered, however, in patients with seizures of diffuse origin who are intractable to other treatments.

Salaam convulsions, also called akinetic seizures, static seizures, drop seizures, nodding spasm, or propulsive petit mal, can usually be treated satisfactorily with a lesion in the globus pallidus, sometimes combined with a lesion in the amygdala.[82,169]

In resistent cases, the ventral-anterior nucleus of the thalamus may be added to the amygdala, fornix, and anterior commissure in order to obtain relief of *grand mal seizures,* if combined with temporal lobe or centrencephalic foci.[120]

Applications

CT-guided stereotactic surgery.   A new era in stereotactic surgery has just begun with the marriage of stereotaxis and computed tomographic (CT) scanning. It has become possible to insert a probe or biopsy forceps into almost any lesion that can be seen on CT scan. Although these techniques may require the use of special apparatus,[1,170-176] it is possible to calculate stereotactic coordinates directly from CT scan for use with any stereotactic apparatus (v.i.).

Swedish neurosurgeons have been leaders in this field, to the point where 45 percent of the neurosurgery being conducted at one neurosurgical center is stereotactic in nature.[164]

Stereotactic *coordinates* can be calculated directly from CT scan performed on a GE 8800 scanner with ScoutView capabilities as follows.[192]

The ScoutView produces an image that appears like an AP or a lateral skull x-ray, and can be manipulated on the console of the scanner. On the lateral ScoutView it is possible to reproduce lines that indicate the planes at which each of the slices was scanned. By relating these indicator lines to the lateral x-ray taken at the time of the stereotactic procedure, the Z axis or vertical axis can be defined. The X and Y axes can be read directly from the individual CT slices.

Although relating the ScoutView to the lateral x-ray introduces some inaccuracy, it has been calculated that the mechanical accuracy of this system is within 3 mm, and abscesses less than 1 cm have been aspirated with great reliability. Since the system does not relate to the usual stereotactic landmarks identified in various atlases, however, it has not been used for functional stereotactic surgery, but can be used to verify cingulotomy or amgydalotomy lesion placement.

A CT scan of the head is made in the usual fashion, care being taken to avoid moving the head between the CT scanning and the ScoutView.[177] The target within the lesion to be biopsied or cannulated is identified on the appropriate slice, and any number of targets in various slices may be calculated. The slice that is closest to the majority of targets is taken as the "zero slice." The zero slice is displayed on the CT console and the distance from the most anterior bone shadow to the most posterior bone shadow is measured and then bisected, and the cursor placed at that midpoint in the midline, which becomes the zero point for the measurement of the X and Y coordinates. If a target lies in the zero plane, the AP and lateral distances are measured from the zero point to the target point, and noted. If one wishes to determine the X and Y coordinates on other slices, the cursor is placed at the zero point and the display is changed to the slice demonstrating the second target point without moving the cursor. The zero point is where the cursor is displayed on the new slice, and the AP and lateral measurements can be made from that point, and all of the measurements and slice numbers noted.

The patient then is arranged for stereotactic surgery in the usual fashion, depending on which stereotactic apparatus is used. AP and lateral x-rays are taken and compared to the ScoutView. On the ScoutView, a reference plane is selected near the base of the skull, which intersects identifiable landmarks, such as the inion, the roof of the orbit, etc. A line representing this plane is then drawn on the lateral x-ray so that the identical reference plane is established.

Since the slice number of each target is known, and since the distance between slices is also known from the scanning program, lines representing the slices containing the targets are drawn on the lateral x-ray parallel to and the appropriate distance above the reference plane. The zero plane is also drawn in similar fashion; the distance between the most anterior and most posterior bony shadow is bisected on the zero plane, so that the zero point is established on the lateral x-ray. A line is drawn perpendicular to those planes through the zero point, giving the zero point on the lateral x-ray on each of the slices of interest. For each target, the line representing the appropriate slice is selected, and the previously derived anterior or posterior measurement is marked on that line the appropriate distance from the zero point, which denotes the target on the lateral x-ray. The cannula is then directed to that target, the distance from the midline already having been derived from the CT scan.

If the target is an anatomic lesion, such as a tumor or abscess, additional accuracy can be obtained by measuring impedance or electrical activity. The same device can be used to measure impedance as is used to confirm penetration of the spinal cord or ventricle, and may be particularly helpful in entering fluid-filled cavities. There may be so much fluctuation in impedance, however, as the electrode advances through the tissue that a clear demarcation of the tumor edge may not be evident, particularly if the tumor is infiltrative. In that case, the monitoring of electrical activity may be more accurate. As the edge of the tumor or mass is approached, the frequency of the spontaneous electrical activity may decrease, with the amplitude remaining the same or sometimes increasing. As the lesion is entered, electrical silence or a marked attention of amplitude may occur.

Biopsy of intracranial lesions, particularly tumors, can be both safe and diagnostic.[78-181] Although the popularity of biopsy has varied, the ability to identify on CT scan deep lesions, which invite biopsy, the recognition that biopsy of deep tumors can be safe and accurate,[180,181] and the ability to diagnose diffuse neurologic conditions by chemical or enzymatic techniques[178] has led to renewed interest in that technique. The equipment should be integrated, so that the variety of electrodes, biopsy forceps, or biopsy screws can all be inserted through the same cannula, after the cannula is advanced to the target. For most purposes the cannula need not and should not be more than 2.0–2.5 mm in diameter. If only a small amount of tissue is available, a smear preparation may provide the diagnosis of tumor.[180]

Not only can the stereotactic tissue diagnosis be helpful in anticipating the needs of an open surgical procedure, but repeated biopsies may be taken to assess the efficacy of radiation therapy or chemotherapy.

CT localization and biopsy of intracranial lesions are discussed in other chapters, as is stereotactic hypophysectomy.

Stereotactic aspiration of brain abscesses has been found to be particularly effective. With the possibility of demonstrating multiple abscesses on CT scan, each abscess in turn can be aspirated, irrigated, and, if desired, infused with antibiotic. Aspiration of an intracerebral hematoma is facilitated when an irrigating cannula is used, through which a clot can be propelled by a rotating helical mandrell.[182,183]

A colloid cyst of the third ventrical can be aspirated. Once the wall is disrupted and the normal ventricular fluid pathway is opened, the cyst usually will not recur.

Radioisotopes can be introduced through the same cannula as biopsy is taken. Sophisticated computerized techniques for selection of the appropriate radioisotope and plotting the distribution of radiation have been developed, but these techniques are so specialized that they should be attempted only in a few centers.[180,184]

There are situations in which it is desirable to combine stereotactic and open surgery, such as the retrieval of a foreign body. The patient may undergo stereotactic surgery in order to introduce a probe to the site of the foreign body along a trajectory that would be appropriate for direct surgical removal. The probe remains in place while the surgeon follows along the probe to find the target. Optionally, a section of loose-fitting Silastic tubing can be fitted around the probe before insertion, advanced to the target point, and left in place as the probe is withdrawn. The tubing can then serve as a marker for the surgeon as the foreign body or other small deep-seated target is dissected.

This technique also can be used to approach deep vascular lesions along the optimal trajectory, or to identify feeding vessels. It is necessary to transform angiographic information to CT scan or to the AP and lateral x-rays taken at the time of stereotactic surgery in order to establish the coordinate of the appropriate vessels, and a probe or Silastic marker can then be left in place in order to direct surgery to the vascular lesion.

More recent techniques have married stereotactic surgery with the use of a laser.[179] With the head secured in a stereotactic apparatus, the optimal approach to a deep-seated lesion can be made stereotactically. A core of brain tissue is removed to provide access to the lesion, at which point a laser is used under direct vision to vaporize it.

Electroneuroprostheses. An additional application of functional neurosurgery that is not readily classified with any of the above but that nevertheless represents a useful technique is that of *diaphragm pacing.* An electronic stimulator, similar to those used for dorsal cord stimulation or peripheral nerve stimulation, is implanted to stimulate the phrenic nerve to drive respiration artificially. It can be helpful in the management of high cervical quadraplegic patients, patients with failure of central regulation of ventilation, and an occasional patient with chronic obstructive pulmonary disease. It is important that the phrenic nerves and diaphragm be functional, as well as the lungs. Patients with injuries at middle levels of the cervical spinal cord may have lower motor neuron lesions of the phrenic nerve, and consequently would not benefit from phrenic nerve stimulation. A patient whose injury is confined to levels C3 or above, however, may be maintained for long periods on diaphragm pacing, obviating the need for endotracheal intubation and positive pressure respiration.

In order to assess viability of the phrenic nerve, an electrode can be inserted percutaneously along the anterior border of the scalene muscle, where the phrenic nerve will be located just medial to the brachial plexus. A brisk, contraction of the diaphragm of several centimeters on stimulation assures sufficient function of the nerve to attempt chronic stimulation.

The implanted portion of the system is similar to that used for peripheral nerve or dorsal cord stimulation. The transmitter, however, generates a coded signal that is modulated by a continuous series of pulse trains. Each train corresponds to an inspiration period and is adjustable in duration from 1.2 to 1.45 seconds in adults and from 0.5 to 0.8 seconds in infants. The respiratory rate is adjustable from 12 to 24 breaths per minute for adults and 12 to 40 breaths per minute in infants. Because smooth contraction of the diaphragm is necessary, the pulse train is tailored to provide a gradually increasing contraction. The amplitude of the first pulse in the train is relatively small, with a gradual increase until the final pulse, similar to a ramp type of stimulation. Otherwise the transmitter is essentially the same as those used for other purposes.

Unilateral stimulation generally is sufficient to provide adequate tidal volume in adults. Because of the relatively smaller volume of an infant's lung, however, and because of the mobility of the mediastinum, it is necessary to use bilateral stimulation in infants, which necessitates the installation of a second receiver and electrode. The transmitter for bilateral stimulation allows either simultaneous or alternating stimulation.[158,185]

Attempts at reproducing bladder function electrophysiologically had, until recently, been directed to the bladder or peripheral innervation. Although contraction of various bladder muscles could be obtained, coordinating contraction of various parts of the bladder with other pelvic activities that constitute normal bladder emptying was not seen. It has been well recognized that paraplegic patients may develop reflex bladder emptying, however, wherein coordinated micturition can occur through the segmental reflex patterns that exist in the isolated lower end of the spinal cord. This led Nashold[186] to investigate a manner by which reflex micturition could be initiated with electrical stimulation. It was found that in many paraplegic patients stimulation of a localized site between the S1 and S2 segments of the conus medullaris can cause a well-organized reflex bladder emptying. Such electromicturition can be applied on a chronic basis by inserting the same type of radio receiver used for other types of central nervous system stimulation, connected to a Silastic cuff bearing two electrodes that are implanted into the proper sites in the conus. Not only is excellent bladder pressure obtained by stimulation, but the pattern of contraction simulates normal micturition and results in almost complete bladder emptying. Although only a limited group of paraplegic patients are candidates for such bladder prostheses, it should be considered the best possible form of bladder management for those patients.

As a final indication for the use of functional neurosurgery, one can look to the future in which electronic circuits may substitute for entire systems that are no longer functioning. An example of that, which is not yet developed to practical application, is artificial vision for the blind by electrical stimulation of the visual cortex.[187] It has been recognized that direct stimulation of the visual cortex leads to the perception of lights at specific points in the visual field related to the area of the cortex that is stimulated, so-called phosphenes.

This led Brindley and Lewin to a pioneering experiment, in which they inserted an 81 subdural electrode array in a blind patient.[188] They could indeed produce phosphenes at specific visual field sites, although they were not sufficient to form useful images. This encouraged Dobelle[187] to pursue physiologic investigations in hopes of perfecting the technique. Since production of phosphenes can be detected only by the individual, it was necessary to use human subjects. Patients who had occipital lobes exposed for any reason, such as tumor or resection, were operated upon under local anesthesia so the area could be stimulated to map the production of phosphenes. Electrodes and stimuli were developed to stimulate over long periods with maximum safety to the underlying cortex. The consistency of the anatomic distribution of phosphene-producing points was investigated. This culminated in the implantation of electrode arrays in several blind patients.

Up to the present, stimulation is done by direct linkage to electrodes through the scalp. The television camera and computer are large and not portable, so the technique has not yet become practical. As many of the physiologic problems are solved, however, the further development of subminiature television cameras and implantable computers may provide a practical visual prosthesis. The ultimate goal is for a miniature television camera to look at the environment, convert the image by computer into a pattern, and have that pattern of phosphenes produced by selective stimulation of several of the electrodes in the area over the visual cortex, producing, in effect, artificial vision.

Perhaps even more futuristic is the auditory prosthesis described by the same group.[189] Multi-contact electrodes were threaded into the scala tympani of the cochlea of deaf volunteers. These were connected to leads that penetrated the skin over the mastoid area and led to a connector that was accessible externally. A computer-controlled stimulator was attached to the connector so that various amplitudes, frequencies, and combinations of electrodes could be stimulated to produce various sounds. The subjects could control many of the parameters of stimulation in search of stimulus characteristics that might be useful to convey information. Pitch could be controlled either by location of the activated electrode or by the frequency of stimulation. As anticipated, loudness could be controlled by the amplitude of stimulation. Various wave forms and electrode configurations change the sensation. Although simple melodies could be discriminated, speech could not be successfully simulated. Subjective sensations remained stable over a long period, and there was no problem with scar tissue or infection of the cochlea. Although these findings were preliminary, the results were encouraging from the standpoint of developing an auditory prosthesis. As additional work continues in the area it may become possible to substitute an electronic component for other end-organs that may have become damaged from injury or disease.

The history of electroneuroprostheses began as long ago as 1953, when Dr. Wendell Krieg suggested chronic stimulation of the nervous system for vision in blind patients, cochlear or auditory stimulation for deaf patients, and stimulation of motor pathways for the treatment of paralysis.[190] These "implausible" and futuristic ideas are indeed coming to pass, and the next decade will provide a significant turning point for the field of neurosurgery from one of treatment or cure to replacement of function when a cure is not possible.

REFERENCES

1. Horsley V, Clarke RH: The structure and function of the cerebellum examined by a new method. *Brain* 31:45–124, 1908
2. Spiegel EA, Wycis HT, Marks M, et al.: Stereotaxic apparatus for operations on the human brain. *Science* 106:349–350, 1947
3. Spiegel EA, Wycis HT: *Stereoencephalotomy, Part I.* New York, Grune & Stratton, 1952
4. Staltenbrand G, Bailey P: *Introduction to Stereotaxis with an Atlas of the Human Brain.* Stuttgart, Thieme, 1959
5. Talairach J, David M, Tournoux P, et al: *Atlas d'anatomie Stéréotaxique.* Paris, Masson, 1957
6. Andrew J, Watkins ES: *A Stereotaxic Atlas of the Human Thalamus.* Baltimore, Williams & Wilkins, 1969
7. Emmers R, Tasker RR: *The Human Somesthetic Thalamus.* New York, Raven Press, 1975
8. Van Buren JM, Borke RC: *Variations and Connections of the Human Thalamus. 2. Variations of the Human Diencephalon.* New York, Springer, 1972

9. Afshar F, Watkins ES, Yap JC: *Stereotaxic Atlas of the Human Brainstem and Cerebellar Nuclei.* New York, Raven Press, 1978
10. Gildenberg PL: Survey of stereotactic and functional neurosurgery in the United States and Canada. *Appl Neurophysiol 38*:31–37, 1975
11. Leksell L: *Stereotaxis and Radiosurgery. An Operative System.* Springfield, IL, Charles C. Thomas, 1971
12. Riechert T: *Stereotactic Brain Operations.* Bern, Hans Huber, 1980
13. Todd EM: *Todd-Wells Manual of Stereotaxic Procedures.* Randolph MA, Codman and Shurtleff, 1967
14. Narabayashi H, Ohye C: Importance of microstereoencephalotomy for tremor alleviation. *Appl Neurophysiol 43*:222–227, 1980
15. Fukamachi A, Ohye C, Saito Y, et al.: Estimation of the neural noise within the human thalamus. *Acta Neurochir [Suppl] 24*:121–136, 1977
16. Tasker RR, Hawrylshyn P, Rowe IH, et al.: Computerized graphic display of results of subcortical stimulation during stereotactic surgery. *Acta Neurochir [Suppl] (Wien) 24*:85–98, 1977
17. Hardy TL, Bertrand G, Thompson CJ: The position and organization of motor fibers in the internal capsule found during stereotactic surgery. *Appl Neurophysiol 42*:160–170, 1979
18. Cooper IS, Lee ASJ: Cryostatic congelation. *J Nerv Ment Dis 133*:259–263, 1961
19. Gildenberg PL (ed): Radiofrequency lesion making procedures. *Appl Neurophysiol 39*:69–132, 1976/77
20. Cooper IS: *Involuntary Movement Disorders.* New York, Hoeber, 1969
21. Gildenberg PL (ed): Safety and clinical efficacy of implanted neuroaugmentive devices. *Appl Neurophysiol 40*:69–239, 1977/78
22. Gildenberg PL: The use of pacemakers (electrical stimulation) in functional neurological disorders, in Rasmussen T, Marino R (eds.): *Functional Neurosurgery.* New York, Raven Press, 1979, pp 59–74
23. Sweet WH, Wepsic JG: Stimulation of the posterior columns of the spinal cord for pain control: Indications, technique and results. *Clin Neurosurg 21*:278–310, 1974
24. Adams JE: Technique and technical problems associated with implantation of neuroaugmentive devices. *Appl Neurophysiol 40*:111–123, 1977/78
25. North RB, Fischell TA, Long DM: Chronic dorsal column stimulation via percutaneously inserted epidural electrodes. *Appl Neurophysiol 40*:184–191, 1977/78
26. Melzack R, Wall PD: Pain mechanisms: A new theory. *Science 150*:971–979, 1965
27. Basbaum AI, Fields HL: Endogenous pain control mechanisms: Review and hypothesis. *Ann Neurol 4*:451–462, 1978
28. Gildenberg PL, Murthy KSK: Influence of dorsal column stimulation upon human thalamic somatosensory-evoked potentials. *Appl Neurophysiol 43*:8–17, 1980
29. Mehler WR: Some neurological species differences—a posteriori. *Ann NY Acad Sci 167*:424–468, 1969
30. Gildenberg PL, Hirshberg R.M.: Limited myelotomy for the treatment of intractable pain. *Neurochirur (Suppl):66*, 1981
31. Mayer DJ, Hayes RL: Stimulation-produced analgesia: Development of tolerance and cross-tolerance to morphine. *Science 188*:941–953, 1975
32. Reynolds DV: Surgery in the rat during electrical analgesia induced by focal brain stimulation. *Science 164*:445, 1969
33. Nashold BS Jr, Wilson WP, Boone E: Depth recordings and stimulation of the human brain: A twenty year experience, in Rasmussen T, Marino R (eds): *Functional Neurosurgery.* New York, Raven Press, 1979, pp 181–195
34. Richardson DE, Akil H: Pain reduction by electrical brain stimulation in man. II. Chronic self-administration in the periventricular gray matter. *J Neurosurg 47*:184–194, 1977
35. Mayer DJ, Liebeskind JC: Pain reduction by focal electrical stimulation of the brain: An anatomical and behavioral analysis. *Brain Res 68*:73–93, 1974
36. Hosobuchi Y, Adams JE, Rutkins B: Chronic thalamic stimulation for the control of facial anesthesia dolorosa. *Arch Neurol 29*:158–161, 1973
37. Hosobuchi Y, Adams JE, Linchitz R: Pain relief by electrical stimulation of the central gray matter in humans and its reversal by naloxone. *Science 197*:183–186, 1977
38. Mayer DJ, Price DD: Central nervous system mechanisms of analgesia. *Pain 2*:379–404, 1976
39. Sweet WH, Obrado S, Martín-Rodríguez JG (eds): *Neurosurgical Treatment in Psychiatry, Pain and Epilepsy.* Baltimore, University Park Press, 1977
40. Akil H, Mayer DJ, Liebeskind JC: Antagonism of stimulation-produced analgesia by naloxone, a narcotic antagonist. *Science 191*:961–962, 1976
41. Snyder SH: Opiate receptors and internal opiates. *Sci Am 236(3)*:44–48, 1977
42. Gildenberg PL: Percutaneous cervical cordotomy. *Clin Neurosurg 21*:246–256, 1974
43. Cook AW, Kawakami Y: Commissural myelotomy. *J Neurosurg 47*:1–6, 1977
44. King RG: Anterior commissurotomy for intractable pain. *J Neurosurg 47*:7–11, 1977
45. Armour D: Surgery of the spinal cord and its membranes. *Lancet 1*:691–697, 1927

46. Broager B: Commissural, sagittal myelotomy for pains in the lower half of the body of 22 patients. *Acta Neurol Scand 48*:258–259, 1972

47. Sourek K: Commissural myelotomy. *J Neurosurg 31*:524–527, 1969

48. Wertheimer P, Lecuire J: La myélotomie commissurale posteriure. A propos de 107 observations. *Acta Chir Belg 52*:568–574, 1953

49. Hitchcock ER: Stereotactic myelotomy. *J R Soc Med 67*:771–772, 1974

50. Hitchcock ER: Stereotactic cervical myelotomy. *J Neurol Neurosurg Psychiatry 33*:224–230, 1970

51. Hitchcock ER: Stereotaxis of the spinal cord. *Conf Neurol 34*:299–310, 1972

52. Schvarcz JR: Spinal cord stereotactic techniques re trigeminal nucleotomy and extralemniscal myelotomy. *Appl Neurophysiol 41*:99–112, 1978

53. Schvarcz JR: Functional exploration of the spinomedullary junction. *Acta Neurochir [Suppl] (Wien) 24*:179–185, 1977

54. Gildenberg PL, Hirshberg R: Limited myelotomy for the treatment of cancer pain. *Appl Neurophysiol* (in press)

55. Gildenberg PL, Hirshberg R: Treatment of cancer pain with limited myelotomy. *Med J of St Jos Hosp* (Houston) *16*:199–204, 1981

56. Spiegel EA, Wycis HT: Mesencephalotomy in the treatment of "intractable" facial pain. *Arch Neurol 69*:1–13, 1953

57. Nashold BS Jr: Extensive cephalic and oral pain relieved by midbrain tractotomy. *Conf Neurol 34*:382–388, 1972

58. Voris HC, Whisler WW: Results of stereotaxic surgery for intractable pain. *Conf Neurol 37*:86–96, 1975

59. Spiegel EA, Wycis HT: *Stereoencephalotomy, Part II*. New York, Grune & Stratton, 1962

60. Mark VH, Ervin FR, Hackett TP: Clinical aspects of stereotactic thalamotomy in the human. Part I. *Arch Neurol 3*:17–32, 1960

61. Mark VH, Ervin FR, Yakovlev PI: Stereotactic thalamotomy. *Arch Neurol 8*:528–538, 1963

62. Spiegel EA, Wycis HT, Szekely EG, et al: Combined dorsomedial, intralaminar and basal thalamotomy for relief of so-called intractable pain. *J Int Coll Surg 42*:160–168, 1964

63. Spiegel EA, Wycis HT, Szekely EG, et al.: Medial and basal thalamotomy in so-called intractable pain, in Knighton RS, Dumke PR (eds): *Pain*. Boston, Little, Brown, 1966, pp 503–517

64. White JC, Sweet WH: *Pain and the Neurosurgeon*. Springfield IL, Charles C Thomas, 1969

65. Foltz EL, White LE Jr: Rostral cingulotomotomy and pain "relief," in Knighton RS, Dumke PR (eds.) *Pain*. Boston, Little, Brown, 1966, pp 469–491

66. Hurt RW, Ballantine HT Jr: Stereotactic anterior cingulate lesions for persistent pain: A report of 68 cases. *Clin Neurosurg 21*:334–351, 1974

67. DeVaul RA, Faillace LA: Persistent pain and illness insistence. A medical profile of proneness to surgery. *Am J Surg 135*:828–833, 1978

68. Gildenberg PL, DeVaul RA: Management of chronic pain refractory to specific therapy, in Youmans JR (ed): *Neurological Surgery*, 2nd ed. Philadelphia, W. B. Saunders, 1981, pp 3749–3768

69. Gildenberg PL, DeVaul RA: *The Practical Management of Chronic Pain*. New York, Dekker (in press)

70. Jacobson E: *Modern Treatment of Tense Patients*. Springfield IL, Charles C Thomas, 1970

71. Travell J: Myofascial trigger points: Clinical view, in Bonica JJ, Albe-Fessard D (eds): *Advances in Pain Research and Therapy*, Vol. 1. New York, Raven Press, 1976, pp 919–926

72. Hassler R, Mundingor F, Riechert T: *Stereotaxis in Parkinson Syndrome*. Berlin, Springer-Verlag, 1979

73. Hassler R, Mundinger F, Riechert T: Pathophysiology of tremor at rest derived from the correlation of anatomical and clinical data. *Conf Neurol 32*:79–87, 1970

74. Kelly PJ: Microelectrode recording for the somatotopic placement of stereotactic thalamic lesions in the treatment of parkinsonian and cerebellar intention tremor. *Appl Neurophysiol 43*:262–266, 1980

75. Mundinger F, Riechert T: Die stereotaktischen Hirnoperationen zur Behandlung extrapyramidaler Beregungsstörungen (Parkinsonismus und Hyperkinesen) und ihre Resultate Postoperative und Langzeitergebnisse der stereotaktischen Hirnoperationen bei extrapyramidal-motorischen Bewegongsstörungen. *Teil B. Fortschr Neurol Psychiatr 31*:69–120, 1963

76. Spiegel EA, Wycis HT, Szekely EG, et al.: Campotomy in various extrapyramidal disorders. *J Neurosurg 20*:871–881, 1963

77. Spiegel EA, Wycis HT, Szekely EG, et al: Stimulation of Forel's field during stereotaxic operations in the human brain. *EEG Clin Neurophysiol 16*:537–548, 1964

78. Kelly PJ, Gillingham FJ: The long-term results of stereotaxic surgery and L-dopa therapy in patients with Parkinson's disease. A 10-year follow-up study. *J Neurosurg 53*:332–337, 1980

79. Spiegel EA, Wycis HT: Pallido-thalamotomy in chorea. *Arch Neurol Psychiatry 64*:495–496, 1950

80. Hoff A, Woringer E, Hamou I: Postoperative hemiballismus. *Neurochirurgia 11*:1–18, 1968

81. Mundinger F, Reichert T: Die stereotaktischen Hirnoperationen zur Behandlung extrapyramidaler Bewegungsstörungen und ihre Resultate. *Fortschr Neurol Psychiatr 31*:1–120, 1963

82. Spiegel EA: *Guided Brain Operations*. Basel, Karger, (in press)
83. Spiegel EA, Wycis HT: *Stereoencephalotomy, Part II* New York, Grune & Stratton, 1962
84. Cooper, IS: *Involuntary Movement Disorders*. New York, Hoeber, 1969
85. Gildenberg PL: A comprehensive program for spasmodic torticollis. *Appl Neurophysiol* (in press)
86. Waltz JM, Andreesen WH: Multiple lead spinal cord stimulation: Technique. *Appl Neurophysiol 44*(1-3), 1981 (in press)
87. Hamby WB, Schiffer S: Spasmodic torticollis: Results after cervical rhizotomy in 50 cases. *J Neurosurg 31*:323–326, 1969
88. Heimburger RF, Whitlock CC: Stereotaxic destruction of the human dentate nucleus. *Conf Neurol 26*:346–358, 1965
89. Siegfried J: Neurosurgical treatment of spasticity, in Rasmussen T, Marino R (eds): *Functional Neurosurgery*. New York, Raven Press, 1979, pp 123–128
90. Zervas N: Long term view of dentatectomy in dystonia musculorum deformans and cerebral palsy. *Acta Neurochir [Suppl] (Wien) 24*:49–51, 1977
91. Spiegel EA, Wycis HT, Baird HW: Effect of thalamic and pallidal lesions upon involuntary movements in choreoathetosis. *Trans Am Neurol Assoc 75*:234, 1950
92. Sprague JM, Chambers WW: Control of posture by reticular formation and cerebellum in the intact anesthetized and unanesthetized and in the decerebrated cat. *Am J Physiol 176*:52–64, 1954
93. Davis R, Gray E, Kudzman J: Beneficial augmentation following dorsal column stimulation in some neurological diseases. *Appl Neurophysiol 44*:37–49, 1981
94. Penn RD, Gottlieb GL, Agarwal GC: Cerebellar stimulation in man. Quantitative changes in spasticity. *J Neurosurg 48*:779–786, 1978
95. Gilman S, Dauth GW, Tennyson V, et al: Chronic cerebellar stimulation in the monkey. Preliminary observations. *Arch Neurol 32*:474–477, 1975
96. Davis R, Gray E: Technical factors important to dorsal column stimulation. *Appl Neurophysiol 44*(1-3), 1981 (in press)
97. Dimitrijevic MR, Sherwood AM: Spasticity: Medical and surgical treatment. *Neurology 30*(2):19–27, 1980
98. Bischof W: Die longitudinale myelotomie. *Zentralbl Neurochir 11*:79–88, 1951
99. Bischof W: Zür dorsalen longitudinalen myelotomie. *Zentralbl Neurochir 28*:123–126, 1967
100. Nauta, WJH: The problem of the frontal lobe: A reinterpretation. *J Psychiatr Res 8*:167–187, 1971
101. Vodovnik L, Kralj A, Stanic U, et al: Recent applications of functional electrical stimulation to stroke patients in Ljubljana. *Clin Orthop 131*:64–70, 1978
102. Freeman W: Frontal lobotomy in early schizophrenia. Long follow-up in 415 cases, in Hitchcock E, Laitinen L, Vaernet K (eds.) *Psychosurgery*. Springfield, IL, Charles C Thomas, 1972, pp 311–321
103. Freeman W: Frontal lobotomy in early schizophrenia: Long follow-up in 415 cases. *Br J Psychiatry 114*:1223–1246, 1971
104. Flor-Henry P: Progress and problems in psychosurgery. *Curr Psychiatr Ther 17*:283–298, 1977
105. Freeman W, Watts JW: *Psychosurgery*. Springfield, IL, Charles C Thomas, 1942
106. Mitchell-Heggs N, Kelly D, Richardson AE: Stereotactic limbic leucotomy: Clinical, psychological and physiological assessment at 16 months, in Sweet WH, Obrador S, Martín-Rodríguez JG (eds.): *Neurosurgical Treatment in Psychiatry, Pain and Epilepsy*. Baltimore, University Park Press, 1977, pp 367–379
107. Hackett TP, White JC, Sweet WH: Leukotomy for the relief of pain: The selection of cases and psychological hazards, in Knighton RS, Dumke PR (eds.): *Pain*. Boston, Little, Brown, 1966, pp 461–467
108. Livingston KF: The frontal lobes revisited. The case for a second look. *Arch Neurol 20*:90–95, 1969
109. Breggin PR: The return of lobotomy and psychosurgery. *Congressional Record 118*(26): Feb 24, 1972
110. National Commission for the Protection of Human Subjects of Biomedical and Behavioral Research. Report and Recommendations. Psychosurgery, Washington DC, DHEW Publications No. (05) 77-0001, 1977
111. Teuber HL, Corkin S, Twitchell TE: A study of cingulotomy in man. DHEW Publications No. (OS) 77-0002, 1977
112. Teuber JL, Corkin S, Twitchell TF: Study of cingulotomy in man: A summary, in Sweet WH, Obrador S, Martín-Rogríguez JG (eds): *Neurosurgical Treatment in Psychiatry, Pain and Epilepsy*. Baltimore, University Park Press, 1977, pp 355–362
113. Ballantine HT Jr, Giriunas IE: Advances in psychiatric surgery, in Rasmussen T, Marino R: *Functional Neurosurgery*. New York, Raven Press, 1979, pp 155–164
114. Papez JW: A proposed mechanism of emotion. *Arch Neurol Psychiatry 38*:725–743, 1937
115. Yakovlev PI: Motility behavior in the brain: Stereodynamic organization in neural coordinates of behavior. *J Nerv Ment Dis 107*:313–335, 1948
116. Livingston K: Neurosurgical aspects of primary affective disorders, in Youmans JR (ed): *Neurological Surgery*. Vol. 3, Philadelphia, Saunders, 1973, pp 1881–1900
117. Kelly D: Psychosurgery and the limbic system. *Postgrad Med J 49*:825–833, 1973
118. Richardson A: Stereotactic limbic leucotomy: Surgical technique. *Postgrad Med J 49*:860–864, 1973

119. Turner E: Custom psychosurgery. *Postgrad Med J* 49:834–844, 1973

120. Bouchard G, Kim YK, Umbach W: Stereotaxic methods in different forms of epilepsy. *Conf Neurol* 37:232–238, 1975

121. Heimburger RF, Whitlock CC, Kalsbeck JE: Stereotaxic amygdalotomy for epilepsy with aggressive behavior. *JAMA* 198:741–745, 1966

122. Mark V, Sweet WH, Ervin FR: The effect of amygdalotomy on violent behavior in patients with temporal lobe epilepsy, in Hitchcock E, Laitinen L, Vaernet K (eds): *Psychosurgery*. Springfield, IL, Charles C Thomas, 1972, pp 139–155

123. Mempel E: The effect of partial amygdalectomy on emotional disturbances and epileptic seizures. *Polish Med J* 10:969–974, 1971

124. Narabayashi H, Nagao T, Saito Y, et al.: Stereotaxic amygdalotomy for behavior disorders. *Arch Neurol* 9:1–16, 1963

125. Laitinen LV: Emotional responses to subcortical electrical stimulation in psychiatric patients. *Clin Neurol Neurosurg* 81:148–157, 1979

126. Richardson DE: Stereotaxic cingulomotomy and prefrontal lobotomy in mental disease. *South Med J* 65:1221–1224, 1972

127. Hitchcock ER, Cairns V: Amygdalotomy. *Postgrad Med J* 49:894–904, 1973

128. Kelly D, Richardson A, Mitchell-Heggs N: Stereotactic limbic leucotomy: Neurophysiological aspects and operative technique. *Br J Psychiatry* 123:133–140, 1973

129. Richardson AE, Kelly D, Mitchell-Heggs N: Lesion site determination in stereotactic limbic leukotomy, in Sweet WH, Obrador S, Martín-Rodríguez JG (eds): *Neurosurgical Treatment in Psychiatry, Pain and Epilepsy*. Baltimore, University Park Press, 1977, pp 363–365

130. Sweet WH: Treatment of medically intractable mental disease by limited frontal leucotomy—justifiable? *N Engl Med* 289:1117–1125, 1973

131. Ballantine HT Jr, Levy BS, Dagi TF, et al: Cingulotomy for psychiatric illness: Report of 13 years' experience, in Sweet, WH, Obrador S, Martín-Rodríguez JG (eds): *Neurosurgical Treatment in Psychiatry, Pain and Epilepsy*. Baltimore, University Park Press, 1977, pp 333–353

132. Kullberg G: Differences in effect of capsulotomy and cingulotomy, in Sweet WH, Obrador S, Martín-Rodríguez JG (eds): *Neurosurgical Treatment in Psychiatry, Pain and Epilepsy*. Baltimore, University Park Press, 1977, pp 301–308

133. Teuber HL, Ball J, Klett CJ, et al: Veterans Administration study of prefrontal lobotomy. *J Clin Exp Psychopath Quart Rev Psychiatr Neurol* 20:205–217, 1959

134. Bailey HE, Dowling JL, Davies E: Cingulotractotomy and related procedures for severe depressive illness (Studies in depression: IV), in Sweet WH, Obrador S, Martín-Rodríguez JG (eds): *Neurosurgical Treatment in Psychiatry, Pain and Epilepsy*. Baltimore, University Park Press, 1977, pp 229–251

135. Ballantine HT Jr, Cassidy WL, Brodeur J, et al: Frontal cingulotomy for mood disturbance, in Hitchcock E, Laitinen L, Vaernet K (eds): *Psychosurgery*. Springfield, IL, Charles C Thomas, 1972, pp 221–229

136. Ballantine HT Jr, Cassidy WL, Flanagan NB, et al.: Stereotaxic anterior cingulotomy for neuropsychiatric illness and intractable pain. *J Neurosurg* 26:488–495, 1967

137. Lopez-Ibor JJ, Lopez-Ibor A: Selection criteria for patients who should undergo psychiatric surgery, in Sweet WH, Obrador S, Martín-Rodríguez JG (eds): *Neurosurgical Treatment in Psychiatry, Pain and Epilepsy*. Baltimore, University Park Press, 1977, pp 151–162

138. Orthner H, Müller D, Roeder F: Stereotaxic psychosurgery. Techniques and results since 1955, in Hitchcock E, Laitinen L, Vaernet K (eds): *Psychosurgery*. Springfield, IL, Charles C Thomas, 1972, pp 377–390

139. Mark VH, Nevelle R: Brain surgery in aggressive epileptics. Social and ethical implications. *JAMA* 226:765–772, 1973

140. Vaernet K, Madsen A: Lesions in the amygdala and the substantia innominata in aggressive psychotic patients, in Hitchcock E, Laitinen L, Vaernet K (eds): *Psychosurgery*. Springfield, IL, Charles C Thomas, 1972, pp 187–194

141. Rubio E, Arjon V, Rodriguez-Burgos F: Stereotactic cryohypothalamotomy in aggressive behavior, in Sweet WH, Obrador S, Martín-Rodríguez JG (eds): *Neurosurgical Treatment in Psychiatry, Pain and Epilepsy*. Baltimore, University Park Press, 1977, pp 439–444

142. Schvarcz JR, Droillet R, Rios E, et al: Stereotaxic hypothalamotomy for behavior disorders. *J Neurol Neurosurg Psychiatry* 35:356–359, 1972

143. Vaernet K, Madsen AL: Stereotaxic amygdalotomy and basofrontal tractotomy in psychotics with aggressive behavior. *J Neurol Neurosurg Psychiatry* 33:858–863, 1970

144. Barcia-Salorio JL, Broseta J, Roland P, et al: Stereotactic amygdalotomy versus posteromedial hypothalamotomy in the treatment of behavioral disorders in epilepsy. *Appl Neurophysiol* (in press)

145. Dieckmann G, Hassler R: Unilateral hypothalamotomy in sexual delinquents. *Conf Neurol* 37:177–186, 1975

146. Müller D, Roeder F, Orthner H: Further results of stereotaxis in the human hypothalamus in sexual de-

viations: First use of this operation in addiction to drugs. *Neurochirurgia 16*:113–136, 1973

147. Roeder F, Orthner H, Muller D: The stereotaxic treatment of pedophilic homosexuality and other sexual deviations, in Hitchcock E, Laitinen L, Vaernet K (eds): *Psychosurgery*. Springfield, IL, Charles C Thomas, 1972, pp 87–111

148. Rieber I, Sigusch V: Psychosurgery on sex offenders and sexual "deviants" in West Germany. *Arch Sex Behav 8*:523–527, 1979

149. Crow HJ, Cooper R, Phillips DG: Controlled multifocal frontal leucotomy for psychiatric illness. *J Neurol Neurosurg Psychiatry 24*:353–360, 1961

150. Smith JS, Kiloh LG, Boots JA: Prospective evaluation of prefrontal leucotomy: Results at 30 months follow-up, in Sweet WH, Obrador S, Martín-Rodríguez JG (eds): *Neurosurgical Treatment in Psychiatry, Pain and Epilepsy*. Baltimore, University Park Press, 1977, pp 217–224

151. Ström-Olsen R, Carlisle S: Bi-frontal stereotactic tractotomy. A follow-up study of its effects of 210 patients. *Br J Psychiatry 118*:141–154, 1971

152. Martin WL, McElhaney ML, Meyer GA: Stereotactic cingulotomy: Results of psychological testing and clinical evaluation preoperatively and postoperatively, in Sweet WH, Obrador S, Martín-Rodríguez JG (eds): *Neurosurgical Treatment in Psychiatry, Pain and Epilepsy*. Baltimore, University Park Press, 1977, pp 381–386

153. Bailey HR, Dowling JL, Davies E: Studies in depression, III: The control of affective illness by cingulo-tractotomy. A review of 150 cases. *Med J Aust 2*:366–371, 1973

154. Scoville WB: Selective cortical undercutting as a means of modifying and studying frontal lobe function in man. *J Neurosurg 6*:65–73, 1949

155. Bingley T, Leksel L, Meyerson BA, et al: Long-term results of stereotactic anterior capsulotomy in chronic obsessive-compulsive neurosis, in Sweet WH, Obrador S, Martín-Rodríguez JG (eds): *Neurosurgical Treatment in Psychiatry, Pain and Epilepsy*. Baltimore, University Park Press, 1977, pp 287–299

156. Laitinen LV: Stereotactic lesions in the knee of the corpus callosum in the treatment of emotional disorders. *Lancet 1*:472–475, 1972

157. Talairach J, Bancaud J: Stereotactic approach to epilepsy. *Prog Neurol Surg 5*:297–354, 1973

158. Glenn WWL, Hogan JF, Phelps ML: Ventilatory support for the quadriplegic patient with respiratory paralysis by diaphragm pacing. *Surg Clin North Am 60*:1055–1078, 1980

159. Bancaud J, Talairach J, Morel P, et al: La corne d'Ammon et le noyau amygdalien: effets cliniques et eletriques de leur stimulation chez l'homme. *Rev Neurol 115*:329–352, 1966

160. Chapman W: Studies of the periamygdaloid area in relation to human behavior. *Res Publ Assoc Nerv Ment Dis 36*:258–277, 1958

161. Weingarten S, Charlow DG, Holmgren E: The relation of hallucination to the depth structures of the temporal lobe. *Arch Neurol [Suppl] 24*:199–216, 1977

162. Narabayashi H, Mizutani T: Epileptic seizures and stereotaxic amygdalotomy. *Conf Neurol 32*:289–297, 1970

163. Heimburger RF: Stereotaxic coordinates for amygdalotomy. *Conf Neurol 37*:202–206, 1975

164. Nádvornik P, Sramka M, Gajdosová D, et al: Longitudinal hippocampectomy. *Conf Neurol 37*:404–408, 1975

165. Mundinger F, Becker P, Groebner E, et al: Late results of stereotactic surgery of epilepsy predominantly temporal lobe type. *Acta Neurochir Suppl 23*:177–182, 1976

166. Schaltenbrand G, Spuler H, Nadjmi M, et al: Die stereotaktische behandlung der epilepsien. *Conf Neurol 27*:111–113, 1966

167. Hassler R, Riechert T: Über einen Fall von doppelseitiger Fornicotomie bei sogenannter temporaler Epilepsie. *Acta Neurochir (Wien) 5*:330–340, 1957

168. Jinnai D, Nishimoto A: Stereotaxic destruction of Forel H for treatment of epilepsy. *Neurochirurgia (Stuttg) 6*:164–176, 1963

169. Spiegel EA, Wycis HT, Baird HW: Pallidotomy and pallidoamygdalotomy in certain types of convulsive disorders. *AMA Arch Neurol Psychiatry 80*:714–728, 1958

170. Bergström M, Boëthius J, Eriksson L, et al: Head fixation device for reproducible position alignment in transmission CT and positron emission tomography. Technical note. *J Comput Assist Tomogr 5*:136–141, 1981

171. Brown R: A computerized tomography-computer graphics approach to stereotaxic localization. *J Neurosurg 50*:715–720, 1979

172. Greitz T, Bergstrom M: Stereotactic procedures in computer tomography, in Newton TH, Potts DG (eds): *Radiology of the Skull and Brain. Technical Aspects of Computer Tomography*. St. Louis, CV Mosby, 1981, pp 4286–4296

173. Jacques S, Shelden CH, McCann GD, et al: Computerized three-dimensional stereotaxic removal of small central nervous system lesions in patients. *J Neurosurg 53*:816–820, 1980

174. Koslow M, Abele MG, Griffith RC, et al: Stereotactic surgical system controlled by computed tomography. *Neurosurgery 8*:72–82, 1981

175. Rosenbaum A, Lunsford LD, Perry J: Computerized Tomography guided stereotaxis. A new approach. *Appl Neurophysiol 43*:172–173, 1980
176. Rushworth RG: Stereotactic guided biopsy in the computerized tomographic scanner. *Surg Neurol 14*:451–454, 1980
177. Kaufman HH, Gildenberg PL: New head-positioning system for use with computer tomographic scanning. *Neurosurgery 7*:147–149, 1980
178. Kaufman HH, Catalano LW: Diagnostic brain biopsy, a series. *Neurosurgery 4*:129–136, 1979
179. Kelly PJ, Alker GJ Jr: A method for stereotactic laser microsurgery in the treatment of deep seated CNS neoplasms. *Appl Neurophysiol 43*:210–215, 1980
180. Mundinger F, Ostertag C, Birg W, et al: Stereotactic treatment of brain lesions: biopsy, interstitial radiotherapy (Ir-192 and I-125) and drainage procedures. *Appl Neurophysiol* (in press)
181. Ostertag CB, Mennel HD, Kiessling M: Stereotactic biopsy of brain tumors. *Surg Neurol 14*:275–283, 1980
182. Backlund E, von Holst H: Controlled subtotal evacuation of intracerebral hematomas by stereotactic technique. *Surg Neurol 9*:99–101, 1978
183. Higgins AC, Nashold BS Jr: Modification of instrument for stereotactic evacuation of intracerebral hematoma: Technical note. *Neurosurgery 7*:604–605, 1980
184. Szikla G (ed): *Stereotactic Cerebral Irradiation.* Amsterdam, Elsevier/North Holland, 1979
185. Glenn WWL: Diaphragm pacing: Present status. *Pace 1*:357–370, 1978
186. Nashold BS Jr, Friedman H, Grimes J, et al: Electromicturition in the paraplegic: An electroneuroprosthesis to control voiding, in Fields WS (ed): *Neural Organization and Its Relevance to Prosthetics.* New York, Intercontinental Medical Book Corp, 1973, pp 349–368
187. Dobelle WH, Quest DO, Antones JL, et al: Artificial vision for the blind by electrical stimulation of the visual cortex. *Neurosurgery 5*:521–527, 1979
188. Brindley GS, Lewin WS: The sensation produced by electrical stimulation of the visual cortex. *J Physiol (Lond) 196*:479–493, 1968
189. Eddington DK, Dobelle WH, Brackmann DE, et al: Auditory prostheses research with multiple channel intracochlear stimulation in man. *Ann Otol Rhinol Laryngol [Suppl] 53*:5–39, 1978
190. Krieg WJS: Electroneuroprosthesis. History and forecast. *IMJ 136*:1–5, 1969
191. Andrew J, Edwards JMR, Rudolf N de M: The placement of stereotaxic lesions for involuntary movements other than in Parkinson's disease. *Acta Neurochir [Suppl] (Wien) 21*:39–47, 1974
192. Gildenberg PL, Kaufman HH, Murthy KSK: Calculation of stereotactic coordinates from the computed tomographic scan. *Neurosurgery 10*:580–586, 1982

CHAPTER 68
Surgery of the Sympathetic Nervous System

Russell W. Hardy, Jr.

AS DESCRIBED IN GREENWOOD'S ARTICLE, "The Origins of Sympathectomy,"[1] surgeons first employed sympathectomy during the last decade of the nineteenth century. At that time Jonnesco performed cervical ganglionectomies for the treatment of epilepsy, exophthalmic goiter, and (somewhat later) for angina pectoris. During these same years Jaboulay and later LeRiche carried out sympathectomies for the relief of trophic ulcers in the lower extremity. Further interest in the operation was stimulated by the work of Royle and Hunter, who believed sympathectomy would relieve spasticity. Although their theory was to prove erroneous, observations made on patients who had undergone sympathectomy led to increased use of the operation for vasospastic disease. Subsequently this procedure was used to treat a wide variety of conditions including angina pectoris,[2] hypertension,[3,4] and vascular disease of large and small vessels.[5-7] Currently, many of these former indications no longer exist, either because of the advent of more modern methods of treatment (as in the case of angina and hypertension) or because experience has cast doubt on the efficacy of sympathectomy (as in the treatment of claudication of vascular origin).[8]

At present the use of sympathectomy is limited to a handful of conditions, but it remains an important surgical technique, since it is uniquely effective in treating hyperhidrosis,[9] major causalgia,[10-12] and some forms of minor causalgia,[13-18] shoulder-hand syndrome,[10] and certain pain of visceral origin.[19-25] It is also used for the treatment of ischemic ulceration, Raynaud's phenomenon, rest pain, and other sequelae of vascular insufficiency.[6,7]

This chapter will discuss three separate operations. The first is upper thoracic (T2) ganglionectomy as employed to treat hyperhidrosis and causalgia in the upper extremities. The second is splanchnicectomy combined with lower thoracic sympathectomy, which is used in the treatment of pain secondary to pancreatic cancer or (rarely) for the pain of chronic pancreatitis or (even more rarely) for pain of renal origin. Third is lumbar sympathectomy, as used in the treatment of major and minor causalgia in the lower extremities.

Upper Thoracic Ganglionectomy

Anatomy

The sympathetic supply to the upper extremity is basically derived from preganglionic fibers leaving the cord from the second through the tenth anterior thoracic roots.[26] These fibers enter the paraspinal sympathetic ganglia via the white rami and synapse in the sympathetic chain. Post-

Department of Neurological Surgery, Cleveland Clinic, Cleveland, Ohio

I wish to thank my senior colleague, Donald F. Dohn, for valuable suggestions regarding the manuscript, and for permission to include his surgical data.

ganglionic fibers leave the stellate and middle cervical ganglia to join the fifth cervical through the first thoracic roots although the bulk of these fibers are found in the seventh and eighth cervical and first thoracic roots.[26,27]

According to the above schema, a resection of the second thoracic ganglion should be sufficient to denervate the upper extremity. It has been argued, however, that sympathetic efferents to the arm also are derived from the eighth cervical[28] and, more importantly, the first thoracic[29,30] roots. In addition, Kuntz has described communications between the third and second thoracic roots, and second and first thoracic roots, which might serve as an extraganglionic sympathetic pathway to the arm.[28,31] Finally, intermediate ganglia have been described in the spinal roots of C8, T1, and T2, which also might supply sympathetic fibers to the arm, independent of traditional pathways.[32]

If these various alternative pathways are viewed as significant, complete sympathetic denervation of the upper extremity would require resection of the middle cervical ganglion, the stellate ganglion, the second and third thoracic ganglia, as well as the intrathoracic nerves of Kuntz. It would also demand section of the anterior roots of T1, T2, and T3, and even then input from anterior cervical roots might persist. In fact, such an extensive procedure has been advocated in the past,[30] and a number of authors recommend at least including the inferior portion of the stellate ganglion, in addition to T2 and T3,[10,31] in order to ensure a complete sympathectomy.

It is relevant to note at this point that the sympathetic outflow to the pupil leaves the cord at T1, but that contributions also may come from T2, T3, T4, and (rarely) C8.[33] These fibers then cross the stellate ganglion and synapse with postganglionic neurons in the superior cervical ganglion. Thus, procedures that require resection of the stellate ganglion will result in a Horner's syndrome, although it has been suggested that resection of the lower half of this ganglion may be performed without risking this complication.[34]

It also should be mentioned that preganglionic sympathectomy (by division of the anterior spinal roots, white rami, and sympathetic chain but with preservation of the ganglia) was at one time recommended on the grounds that this would avoid "hypersensitivity" of end organs to circulating catecholamines.[35] Many now feel, however, that such hypersensitivity does not occur or is of minimal clinical significance following resection of the ganglia.[10,30]

In our experience, as well as in the experience of others, resection of the T2 (and possibly the T3 ganglia) has been sufficient to denervate the upper extremity and serve as adequate treatment for hyperhidrosis and causalgia.[9,36,37] By not resecting the lower portion of the stellate ganglion, the risk of a Horner's syndrome is minimized. We have not observed hypersensitivity following T2 ganglionectomy in the treatment of hyperhidrosis, and it does not occur when postganglionic sympathectomy is performed for the treatment of causalgia.[38,39]

Surgical Approaches

A variety of approaches to the cervical and upper thoracic chain have been employed. These include posterior thoracic operations via midline[5] paramedian[35] or transverse[40] incisions, cervical (with unilateral[41] or bilateral[42] incisions), and transthoracic,[43] and anterior transthoracic approaches.[44] The operation that we employ is a posterior approach through a midline incision. The anterior and lateral operations have the advantage of providing excellent visualization of the sympathetic chain, but the disadvantage of the exposure being unilateral, which means that a second procedure is required if a bilateral sympathectomy is needed. The posterior paramedian approach can afford a bilateral exposure, albeit through two separate incisions. This approach may carry the disadvantage of providing less adequate visualization of the chain, and in our experience there are occasional difficulties with the upper thoracic paramedian incision. The cervical approach can be done through either a unilateral or midline incision[42] (which affords bilateral exposure), but visualization of the upper thoracic ganglia may be difficult. The dorsal operation through a midline incision has the advantage of bilateral exposure, and we have felt that this approach afforded adequate visualization of the ganglia to be resected. Moreover, this operation can be performed readily by neurosurgeons since it is simply an extension of a standard upper thoracic laminectomy exposure.

Indications

A T2 ganglionectomy is currently used in the treatment of essential hyperhidrosis and for major causalgia (as described originally Weir Mitchell),[45] minor causalgia and certain of its variations, and occasionally for shoulder-hand syndrome. It also may be employed to treat certain conditions of vascular origin.[6]

The use of sympathectomy for the treatment of essential hyperhidrosis was first described by Kotzareff.[9] Hyperhidrosis can be a source of great embarrassment and considerable disability to the patient. It may involve the entire body including the legs and head, but symptoms are most severe and of the greatest discomfort in the upper extremities. The patients have symptoms that often date from childhood or early adolescence. Such individuals report reluctance to shake hands or touch other people, and often wear gloves to disguise their condition. The diagnosis is readily confirmed by inspection of the extremities.

Experience has confirmed the value of sympathectomy in the treatment of causalgia.[10–12] As originally described, this condition is characterized by severe burning pain, exacerbated by touch, that appears shortly after an injury to a mixed peripheral nerve,[45] most often the median or sciatic nerve. This injury occurs much more often during wartime and is relatively uncommon in civilian practice. It first may be treated by sympathetic blocks, to which a very high proportion of patients will respond. In fact, response to a block is one method of establishing the diagnosis in individuals with typical symptoms. A certain number of patients may be treated without surgery by blocks alone. If the pain recurs, however, sympathectomy may be performed, and relief of pain is obtained in a very high percentage of patients.

Sympathectomy also may be employed in the treatment of a group of ill-defined entities that are characterized by burning pain and trophic changes that may appear following peripheral nerve injury, but also are associated with a variety of other conditions including fracture, local laceration, infection, burns, subcutaneous injection, phlebitis, and arterial embolism.[13–18] A unifying mechanism has not been postulated for these conditions other than the suggestion that they may be the result of some form of sympathetic overactivity. Regardless of the etiology, certain of these conditions are said to respond to sympathectomy, although the response to surgery may well be less certain than the response of major causalgia. Favorable response to sympathetic block will select patients who may do well following surgery, but even this is no guarantee that the operation will be successful.

Operative Technique

The T2 ganglionectomy through a dorsal midline incision is most conveniently done with the patient in the sitting position, although the prone position also may be used (Figs. 68-1 through 68-8). The sitting position has the advantage that an intraoperative x-ray, confirming the level, may be obtained more conveniently than when the patient is prone. We also feel that exposure is somewhat better when the patient is erect. The principal disadvantage of the sitting position, namely air embolus, is minimal or nonexistent when surgery is carried out at this level.

An x-ray is obtained before the operation with a marker placed at the spinous process of T2. The spinous process of T2 will be opposite the lamina and medial portion of the rib of T3. These structures are exposed and confirmatory x-rays are obtained at the T3 level. Following this, the T3 transverse process and underlying rib are removed, either with a Kerrison punch or a rongeur, with care being taken to dissect free the underlying pleura. After resection of the rib and medial transverse process, the lateral border of the vertebral body is exposed by blunt dissection. The lower portion of the second rib also may need to be removed in order to expose the T2 ganglion. At this point the second intercostal nerve is elevated and the sympathetic chain vis-

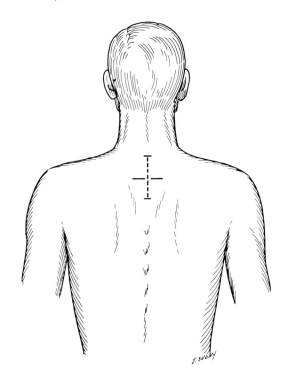

Fig. 68-1. Location of the skin incision for a T2 ganglionectomy.

ualized. The communicating rami and the chain above and below the T2 ganglion are clipped and divided, and the ganglion is removed. If convenient, the T3 ganglion also may be resected.

Following resection of the ganglion and hemostasis, the incision may be closed in layers, with care being taken to obtain a good closure of the deep fascia over the spinous process of T2 and T3. If a pleural tear has occurred during the course of the dissection, it may be managed by leaving a 12F red rubber catheter in place (within the leaves of the pleura) until a fascial closure is effected. The catheter then is removed with suction as the anesthetist applies positive pressure. This has been adequate to avoid postoperative pneumothorax in most cases.

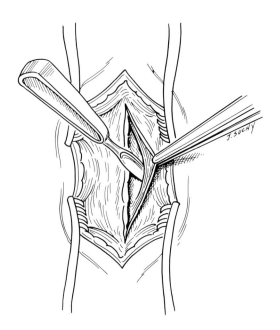

Fig. 68-2. The beginning of the exposure of the T3 lamina and transverse processes.

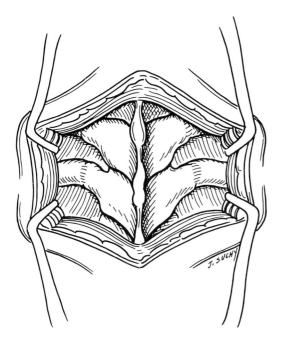

Fig. 68-3. The completed bilateral exposure of the transverse processes of T3.

Results

We have recently reviewed a series of 100 patients undergoing bilateral T2 ganglionectomy for hyperhidrosis.[9] Eighty-seven percent reported 100 percent relief of palmar hyperhidrosis; another 9 percent had incomplete (75 percent) relief or minor side effects. Four percent reported no relief, recurrent symptoms, or a major side effect. The operation was thus deemed successful in 96 percent of the patients.

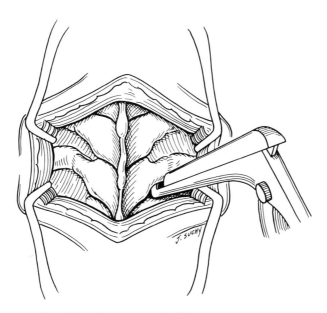

Fig. 68-4. Resection of the T3 transverse process.

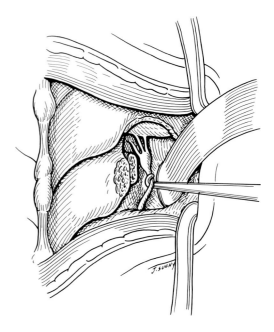

Fig. 68-5. The T3 costotransversectomy has been completed. The nerve hook is under the sympathetic chain.

Complications

Recurrent hyperhidrosis was noted in 4 patients (2 of whom underwent a second operation). Compensatory hyperhidrosis, usually transient and of a minor nature, occurred in 44 percent.

Only 1 patient in the series developed a Horner's syndrome. One developed a significant pneumothorax, and 1 an empyema. Intercostal neuralgia was seen in 6 patients. One individual developed cerebrospinal fluid drainage through the incision; this was managed conservatively. Minor wound infections appeared in 3 patients.

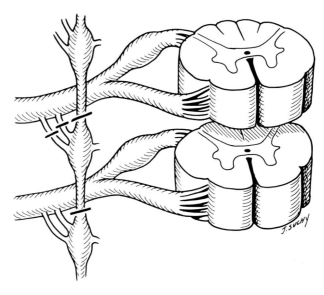

Fig. 68-6. The extent of the sympathetic resection.

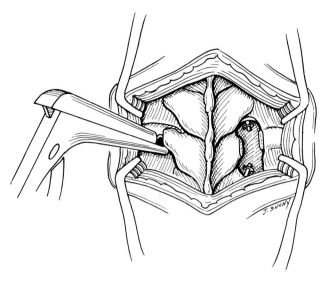

Fig. 68-7. The contralateral T3 costotransversectomy is begun.

Splanchnicectomy

Anatomy

Visceral afferents supplying the heart, pancreas, kidneys, gallbladder, and other organs have been described[37,46,47] and serve as a source of pain in various conditions affecting these structures.

Autonomic innervation to the pancreas is derived from the splanchnic nerves and from the vagus. Visceral afferents appear to travel exclusively through the splanchnic chain. These enter the cord via the greater splanchnic nerve after traversing the celiac ganglion. As described by Ray

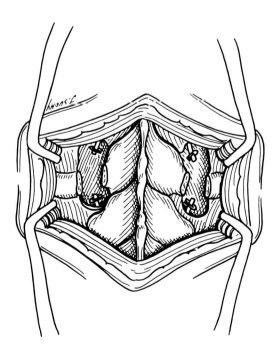

Fig. 68-8. The complete costotransversectomy and bilateral T2 ganglionectomy.

and Neill,[46] the pancreas receives bilateral innervation not only from the greater splanchnic nerves, which are derived from cord segments T4 through T9, but also from the lesser splanchnic nerves and perhaps through the lower portion of the thoracic ganglia and the upper portion of the lumbar chains. Because the pancreas receives bilateral innervation, a bilateral operation will usually be required to effect relief of pain,[22-24] although in certain instances a unilateral operation is said to be sufficient.[21,25] Innervation to the biliary tracts is supplied by the right splanchnic nerves, and the nerve supply to the kidneys is also unilateral (via the lesser and least splanchnic trunks). The minor splanchnic nerves are derived from T10 and T11 and the least splanchnic nerve from T12.[37]

It should be emphasized that while the splanchnic nerves are divided into three separate branches, in actual practice identification of these separate trunks may be difficult and there may be considerable variability from patient to patient.

Based on these anatomic considerations, the operation that we employ to denervate the pancreas is resection of the thoracic ganglia from approximately T9 through T12 together with resection of the greater, lesser, and least splanchnic nerves. Other writers have recommended a more extensive operation, including the upper lumbar ganglia,[19] but we have not found such an extensive resection to be necessary, and removal of the upper lumbar ganglia adds technical difficulty and (in the male) the risk of sexual dysfunction.[24,48]

Indications

Pain from pancreatic carcinoma may result from involvement of visceral afferent fibers or from pain secondary to the involvement of parietal somatic nerves. Any evidence of radicular pain suggests involvement of somatic nerves and is a contraindication to the procedure in the patient with pancreatic carcinoma. If doubt exists, the patient may be evaluated by means of a temporary splanchnic block. Frequently it is our practice to perform the operation in combination with diagnostic laparotomy. In a patient with upper abdominal and back pain and no evidence of somatic nerve involvement, a bilateral splanchnicectomy can be performed after closure of the abdominal incision and repositioning of the patient. Such a combined operation adds little to the overall morbidity of the laparotomy.

The operation also has been advocated for the pain of chronic pancreatitis,[15,22,25] and such pain may be relieved in certain individuals, but in our experience the operation often fails to help the patient discontinue the use of narcotics (often because the individual will develop new chronic pain at the site of operative incisions or elsewhere). Finally, a rare patient with benign pain of renal or biliary origin may be a candidate for sympathectomy,[37] although operations for these indications are rarely performed at our institution.

Operative Technique

The procedure is carried out with the patient in the prone position on a laminectomy frame or with a blanket roll beneath the hips and shoulders. (Figs. 68-9 through 68-16)[20] An incision is made four fingerbreadths lateral to the spinous process overlying the eleventh rib. Dissection is carried down until the rib is encountered. The periosteum overlying the rib is stripped with an elevator and the pleura then is separated from the underlying rib with a pigtail periosteal dissector. Approximately the lateral 4–6 cm of rib are removed with rib cutters and rongeurs. The underlying pleura then is carefully dissected from the medial portion of the rib and also from the undersurface of adjacent ribs. Normally this is not a particularly difficult maneuver and can be carried out with careful finger dissection. Some large intercostal veins may be encountered as the dissection is carried out medially. These may be easily controlled with either clips or bipolar coagulation. Final dissection of the pleura from the lateral portion of the spine and the underlying surface of the rib may be carried out with Kittner dissectors. As the pleura is being retracted, it is protected beneath an abdominal sponge.

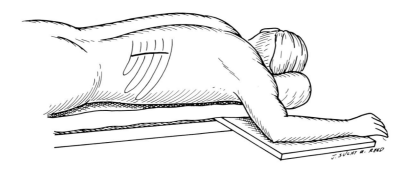

Fig. 68-9.   The location of the skin incision for lower thoracic splanchnicec-tomy–sympathectomy.

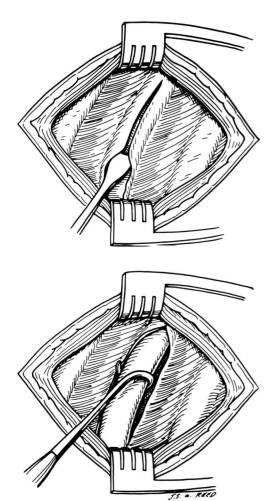

Fig. 68-10.   Subperiosteal exposure of the elev-enth rib with a periosteal elevator. The underlying periosteum then is stripped with a pigtail periosteal ele-vator.

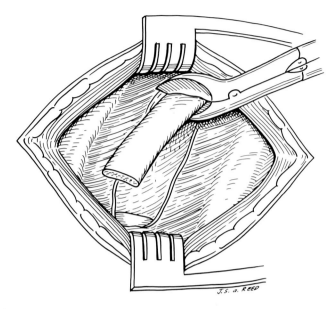

Fig. 68-11. Resection of the eleventh rib. The underlying parietal pleura then is separated from adjacent ribs by blunt dissection.

After the pleura has been swept free of the underlying surface of the rib, the remaining medial portion of the eleventh rib is removed if additional exposure is required. The exposure of the lateral portion of the adjacent vertebrae then is completed. A resection of the sympathetic ganglia and their connections, as well as the greater, lesser, and least splanchnic nerves, then is carried out. As noted above, the splanchnic nerves are not always constant structures, although the greater splanchnic nerve may be identified fairly reliably anterior to the sympathetic chain on the lateral margin of the vertebral bodies. As great a length of splanchnic nerve as possible is resected, together with any other branches of the lesser and least nerves that can be identified. In addition, resection of the ganglia, T9 through T12, together with the rami communicantes then is carried out, with the chains being divided between metal clips.

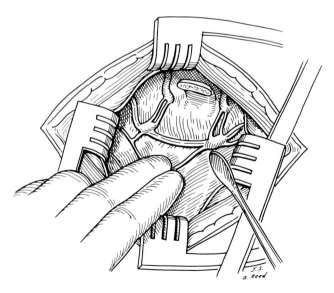

Fig. 68-12. The exposure of the sympathetic chain and splanchnic nerves.

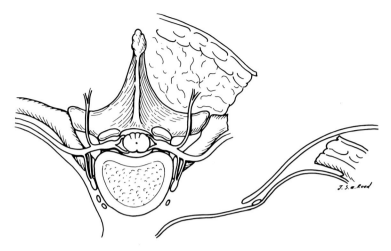

Fig. 68-13. A cross-sectional view of the exposure. The splanchnic nerves may be inadvertently retracted with the pleura.

One difficulty that is sometimes encountered is that the splanchnic nerves may be difficult to find. A common cause of this is that the nerve may be swept onto the pleura and easily can be retracted along with the parietal pleura. Careful inspection of the surface of the parietal pleura usually will identify the nerve when it cannot be found adjacent to the vertebral bodies.

If the pleura is torn during the procedure, the situation may be managed by inserting a red rubber catheter through the wound and applying suction and Valsalva's maneuver during closure. If a very large tear has occurred, a chest tube may be placed at the time of closure, or later if a substantial pneumothorax is seen on postoperative films.

The procedure is carried out bilaterally. As noted, it has not been our custom to divide the diaphragm and remove the L1 ganglia as some have advocated.

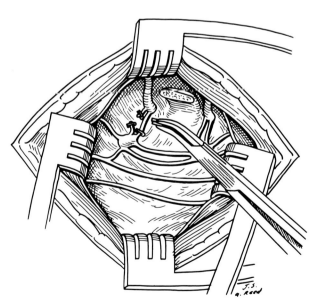

Fig. 68-14. Resection of the sympathetic chain and splanchnic nerves.

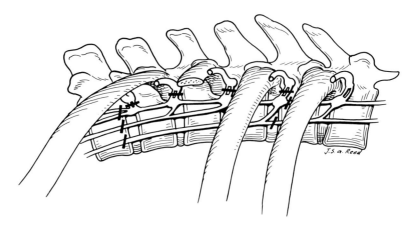

Fig. 68-15.   The ideal extent of the resection.

Results

In a series of 56 patients undergoing the procedure for pancreatic carcinoma, 70 percent had satisfactory relief of symptoms, 14 percent partial relief, and 16 percent no improvement.[23,24] Recurrence of pain was noted in 23 percent of patients, most often in those who survived for a period of several months; this recurrence of pain was partial and not regarded as a severe problem. The mortality rate in patients with cancer undergoing combined laparotomy and splanchnicectomy was 7 percent.

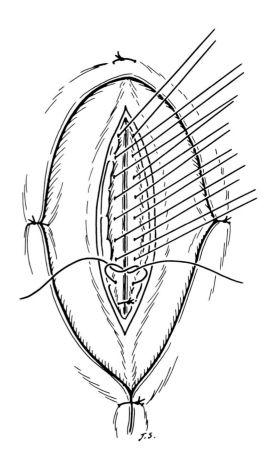

Fig. 68-16.   The layered closure of the incision.

Complications

As noted above, pleural tears occur occasionally and usually can be managed at the time of surgery or with a postoperative chest tube. Superficial wound infections, and 1 case of empyema have occurred. We have not experienced paraplegia as a complication of this procedure (caused by interference with the blood supply to the cord), but such catastrophes have been reported. In 1 patient it was speculated that the use of electrocautery initiated a vascular thrombosis with a resulting delayed paraplegia.[49]

Lumbar Sympathectomy

Anatomy

The sympathetic supply to the lower extremity is derived from the five lumbar ganglia whose efferents leave the spinal canal with the L1 and L2 roots.[26,37] Resection of the second and third lumbar ganglia should be sufficient to denervate the leg, although in a few individuals resection of the L1, L2, and T12 ganglia has been necessary to abolish the pain of causalgia completely.[12]

Indications

The major indication for lumbar sympathectomy by the neurosurgeon is either major or minor causalgia of the lower extremity. The procedure also remains useful for the treatment of ischemic rest pain and superficial ulceration secondary to arteriosclerotic vascular disease. We have not employed this operation in the treatment of hyperhidrosis of the lower extremities.

Surgical Technique

The operation may be carried out through a variety of skin incisions. We employ the transverse incision extending obliquely from beneath the costal margin to the right lower quadrant (Figs. 68-17 through 68-20). The external oblique, internal oblique, and transversus muscles are divided in the direction of their fibers. The peritoneum and renal fascia then are dissected free of the quadratus lumborum and iliac muscles with blunt finger dissection. Dissection then is carried medially over the anterior surface of the psoas muscle until the sympathetic chain is encountered between it and the vertebral body.

On the right side, the vena cava will be encountered, and bridging veins may need to be divided and clipped or coagulated. On the left, the aorta may be mobilized and will not overlie the chain.

The chain is identified and at least two ganglia are removed. The chain and rami communicantes are divided between metallic clips.

After resection of the ganglia, the muscle layers are closed separately. During this portion of the procedure the table may be straightened to facilitate closure.

In performing the operation, care should be taken to identify the ureter, which is retracted medially with the kidney, and to avoid injuring somatic nerves passing through the psoas and quadratus lumborum muscles.[41,43]

Results

Peacetime experience in the treatment of causalgia in the lower extremity is limited. Excellent results, similar to those encountered in the upper arm, are generally obtained. As noted by Ulmer and Mayfield, an incomplete result will be obtained in an occasional patient and may require an additional procedure to remove the L1 and T12 ganglia.[12]

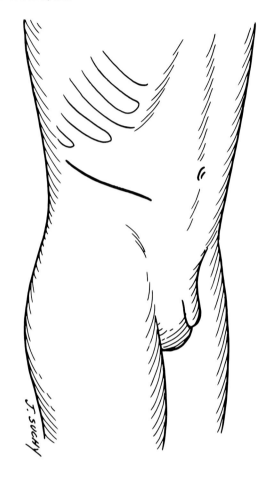

Fig. 68-17. The incision used for lumbar sympathectomy.

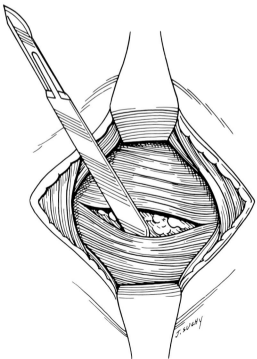

Fig. 68-18. The abdominal muscles are divided in
the direction of their fibers.

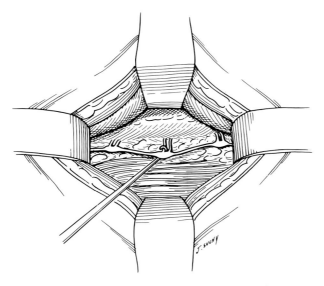

Fig. 68-19.   The sympathetic chain is identified.

Complications

The major neurologic complication is the risk of sexual dysfunction if the procedure is carried out bilaterally in the male.[48] This consideration limits its use in the treatment of hyperhidrosis and other conditions.

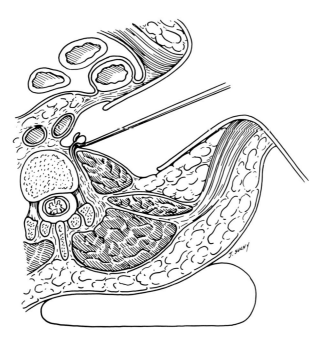

Fig. 68-20.   A cross-sectional view of the exposure following extraperitoneal retraction of the abdominal contents.

REFERENCES

1. Greenwood B: The origins of sympathectomy. *Med Hist 11*:165–169, 1967
2. White JC, Bland EF: The surgical relief of severe angina pectoris. *Medicine 27*:1–42, 1948
3. Peet MM: Splanchnic resection for hypertension. *Univ Hosp Bull, Ann Arbor Mich 1*:17–18, 1935
4. Smithwick RH: A technique for splanchnic resection for hypertension. *Surgery 7*:1–8, 1940
5. Adson AW, Brown GE: The treatment of Raynaud's disease by resection of the upper thoracic and lumbar sympathetic ganglia and trunks. *Surg Gynecol Obstet 48*:577–603, 1929
6. Dale WA, Lewis MD: Management of ischemia of the hand and fingers. *Surgery 67*:62–79, 1970
7. Myers KA, Irvine WT: An objective study of lumbar sympathectomy: II Skin ischaemia. *Br Med J 1*:943–947, 1966
8. Myers KA, Irvine WT: An objective study of lumbar sympathectomy: I Intermittent claudication. *Br Med J 1*:879–883, 1966
9. Dohn DF, Sava GM: Sympathectomy for vascular syndromes and hyperhydrosis of the upper extremities, in Keener EB (ed): *Clin Neurosurg,* vol 25. Baltimore, Williams & Wilkins, 1978, pp 637–650
10. Bergan JJ, Con J: Sympathectomy for pain relief. *Med Clin North Am 52*:147–159, 1968
11. Spurling RG: Causalgia of the upper extremity: Treatment by dorsal sympathetic ganglionectomy. *Arch Neurol Psychiatry 23*:784–788, 1930
12. Ulmer JL, Mayfield FH: Causalgia: A study of 75 cases. *Surg Gynecol Obstet 83*:789–795, 1946
13. Drucker WR, Hubay CA, Holden WD, et al: Pathogenesis of posttraumatic sympathetic dystrophy. *Am J Surg 97*:454–465, 1959
14. Echlin F, Owens FM, Wells WL: Observations on "major" and "minor" causalgia. *Arch Neurol Psychiatry 62*:183–203, 1949
15. Hardy WG, Posch JL, Webster JE, et al.: The problem of major and minor causalgias. *Am J Surg 95*:545–554, 1958
16. Homans J: Minor causalgia: A hyperesthetic neurovascular syndrome. *N Engl J Med 22*:870–874, 1940
17. McFarlane WV: Causalgic syndromes. *Aust NZ J Surg 18*:191–208, 1949
18. Wirth FP, Rutherford RB: A civilian experience with causalgia. *Arch Surg 100*:633–638, 1970
19. Connelly JE, Richards V: Bilateral splanchnicectomy and lumbodorsal sympathectomy for chronic relapsing pancreatitis. *Ann Surg 131*:58–63, 1960
20. Heisy WG, Dohn DF: Splanchnicectomy for the treatment of intractable abdominal pain. *Cleve Clin Q 34*:9–25, 1967
21. Mallet-Guy P, Beaujeu MJ: Treatment of chronic pancreatitis by unilateral splanchnicectomy. *Arch Surg 60*:233–241, 1950
22. Ray BS, Console Ad: The relief of pain in chronic (calcareous) pancreatitis by sympathectomy. *Surg Gynecol Obstet 89*:1–8, 1949
23. Sadar ES, Cooperman AM: Bilateral thoracic sympathectomy—splanchnicectomy in the treatment of intractable pain due to pancreatic carcinoma. *Cleve Clin Q 41*:185–188, 1974
24. Sadar ES, Hardy RW: Thoracic splanchnicectomy and sympathectomy for the relief of pancreatic pain. in Cooperman AM (ed): *Surgery of the Pancreas.* St. Louis, CV Mosby, 1978, pp 141–152
25. de Takats G, Walter LE, Lasner J: Splanchnic nerve section for pancreatic pain. *Ann Surg 131*:44–57, 1950
26. Pick J: *The Autonomic Nervous System.* Philadelphia, JB Lippincott, 1970
27. Sunderland S: The distribution of sympathetic fibres in the brachial plexus in man. *Brain 71*:88–102, 1948
28. Kirgis HD, Kuntz A: Inconstant sympathetic neural pathways. *Arch Surg 44*:95–102, 1942
29. Kuntz A, Dillon JB: Preganglionic components of the first thoracic nerve. *Arch Surg 44*:772–778, 1942
30. Ray BS: Sympathectomy of the upper extremity. *J Neurosurg 10*:624–633, 1953
31. Kuntz A: Distribution of the sympathetic rami to the brachial plexus. *Arch Surg 15*:871–877, 1927
32. Skoog T: Ganglia in the communicating rami of the cervical sympathetic trunk. *Lancet 28*:457–460, 1947
33. Ray BS, Hinsey JC, Geohegan WA: Observations on the distribution of the sympathetic nerves to the pupil and upper extremity as determined by stimulation of the anterior roots in man. *Ann Surg 118*:647–655, 1943
34. Palumbo LT: A new concept of the sympathetic pathways to the eye. *Surgery 42*:740–748, 1957
35. Smithwick RH: The rationale and technic of sympathectomy for the relief of vascular spasm of the extremities. *N Engl J Med 222*:699–703, 1940
36. Hyndman OR, Wolkin J: Sympathectomy of the upper extremity. *Arch Surg 45*:145–155, 1942
37. White JC: Role of sympathectomy in relief of pain, in Krayenbuhl H, Maspes PE, Sweet WH (eds): *Progress in Neurological Surgery,* vol 7. Basel, S Karger, 1976, pp 131–152
38. Mayfield FH: Personal communication
39. Nulsen FE: Personal communication
40. Love JG, Juergens JL: Second thoracic sympathetic ganglionectomy for neurologic and vascular dis-

turbances of the upper extremities. *West J Surg 72*:130–133, 1964
41. Kempe LG: *Operative Neurosurgery,* vol 2. Heidelberg, Springer-Verlag, 1970, pp 244–250
42. Lougheed WM: A simple technique for upper thoracic sympathectomy in patients requiring sympathectomy of the upper limb. *Can J Surg 8*:306–308, 1965
43. Kleinert HE, Norberg H, McDonough JJ: Surgical sympathectomy—upper and lower extremity, in Omer GE and Spinner M (eds): *Peripheral Nerve Problems.* Philadelphia, WB Saunders, 1980, pp 285–302
44. Palumbo LT: Anterior transthoracic approach for upper thoracic sympathectomy. *Arch Surg 72*:659–666, 1956
45. Richards RL: Causalgia: A centennial review. *Arch Neurol 16*:339–350, 1967
46. Ray BS, Neill CL: Abdominal visceral sensation in man. *Ann Surg 126*:709–724, 1947
47. Richins CA: The innervation of the pancreas. *J Comp Neurol 83*:223–236, 1945
48. Whitelaw GP, Smithwick RH: Some secondary effects of sympathectomy. *N Engl J Med 245*:121–130, 1951
49. Shallat RF, Klump TE: Paraplegia following thoracolumbar sympathectomy. *J Neurosurg 34*:569–571, 1971

CHAPTER 69
Surgical Management of Disorders of the Lower Cranial Nerves

Ronald I. Apfelbaum

A NUMBER OF CLINICAL SYNDROMES have been correlated with cross compression of specific cranial nerves at their exit or entrance to the brainstem. The paradigm of these syndromes is trigeminal neuralgia or tic douloureux. Dandy first observed the frequent occurrence of arterial channels, veins, or neoplasms compressing the trigeminal nerve in the posterior fossa and wrote in 1932 that these, he believed, were the cause of tic doulourex.[1] Similarly, in the motor equivalent of this problem—hemifacial spasm—Gardner and Sava[2] described vascular compressive lesions in over half of the patients they operated upon via the posterior fossa. It was not until Jannetta[3,4] applied the operating microscope to the systematic study of these problems, however, that the truly remarkable incidence of compression of the entry or exit zone of the brainstem root of these nerves was appreciated. In several large series, compressive lesions have been demonstrated in over 94 percent of the patients.[5-7] Furthermore, Jannetta has devised an operative technique to displace these vessels from the nerve without sacrificing neural integrity and has been successful in relieving the clinical syndrome in the vast majority of patients treated. In this chapter we will attempt to discuss the individual syndromes and the specific operative techniques that can be used in treating them.

Trigeminal Neuralgia

Trigeminal neuralgia is a condition characterized by a very stereotyped clinical syndrome. Patients suffering from this problem exhibit brief, extremely intense paroxysms of pain confined entirely to one or more divisions of the trigeminal nerve. These attacks may be triggered by light cutaneous stimuli, usually, but not exclusively, within the trigeminal territory. The pain typically is described as an electric shocklike sensation or an intense stabbing feeling. The most common areas of involvement are in the second and third divisions, usually anteriorly, in the region about the mouth. The dental area is especially prone to be the site of the symptoms, and for this reason many patients undergo unnecessary dental surgery without achieving satisfactory relief. The pain typically is most pronounced during the day and most patients will be pain-free or have markedly decreased episodes during the night. Patients will guard their face, refuse to allow it be touched, will avoid shaving, washing, applying makeup, eating, chewing, and brushing their teeth, since all of these maneuvers may provoke the attacks. A characteristic clinical sign is often

Leo M. Davidoff Department of Neurological Surgery, Albert Einstein College of Medicine, and Montefiore Hospital and Medical Center, Bronx, New York

made by the patient who, in describing the pain, will rapidly fling open his hand to indicate the rapid paroxysmal nature of the jolts of pain.

Approximately 50 percent of those afflicted will respond to diphenylhydantoin (Dilantin)[8] in a dose of 300 mg/day, and up to 80 percent of the patients will obtain pain relief with Tegretol.[8,9] This medication has numerous side effects and must be administered carefully. We recommend starting Tegretol at 100 mg b.i.d. and increasing it by 100 mg every other day until pain control is achieved or toxicity develops. An average dose might be 800 mg/day in four divided doses, but some patients can tolerate, and will require, two to three times as much. Our patients are instructed to take this medication on a full stomach and to have a monthly blood count made so that hematologic toxicity can be detected. In this manner, good control of the pain can be achieved in the vast majority of patients. Surgery is reserved for those who become refractory to medical treatment or who develop side effects that necessitate discounting the medication.

We have chosen to restrict this surgery to patients who have demonstrated a typical clinical picture as outlined above. Trigeminal neuralgia is an amazingly consistent disease and a similar history will be obtained from almost every patient truly suffering from this problem. A history of sustained pain that is not paroxysmal must be questioned carefully. At times, patients will describe frequent repetitive jabs of pain as one prolonged attack. This does not preclude the diagnosis of trigeminal neuralgia. A slowly developing pain that builds in intensity, lasts for variable periods of time (often hours to days), and then subsides, however, is not characteristic of this problem. The most common mistake in diagnosis in our experience has been misdiagnosing trigeminal neuralgia for chronic cluster syndrome (Horton's cephalalgia). This and other atypical facial and trigeminal neuralgias respond much less satisfactorily to this type of surgery, and its indications in these conditions is not yet clear.

In addition to meeting the specific clinical picture, patients selected for this surgery also, we feel, should have had an adequate trial of medical therapy and the syndrome proven impossible to control. At this juncture, it is our practice to explain fully the Jannetta microvascular decompressive operation as well as the procedure for selective percutaneous radiofrequency lesioning of the trigeminal nerve. The patient is asked to choose between these procedures after a clear explanation of the relative benefits and risks of each as detailed in Table 69-1 has been made. In essence then, they are asked to decide between permanent partial alteration of facial sensation and the potential for the development of dysesthetic sequelae or corneal anesthesia or both versus the Jannetta procedure, which offers the likelihood of pain relief without neural destruction and thus avoids dysesthetic sequelae and corneal anesthesia. They are cautioned, however, that the radiofrequency lesioning is a safer procedure that avoids the risks of anesthesia and surgery. It is made clear to them that these risks include potentially fatal complications. In addition, they are made aware of the risks of injury to the underlying brain or adjacent neural structures.

In Table 69-2 we have delineated the experience with these factors in our personal series. This agrees with the published literature for the most part[10-12] although we seem to have had a higher incidence of undesirable facial numbness and dysesthetic sequelae with radiofrequency lesioning than do some of the larger series in the literature. Our series, however, may be more representative of what one can expect if one does not perform a very large number of these procedures (i.e. > 25/year).

We feel that the Jannetta microvascular decompressive operation is the procedure of choice for the treatment of typical trigeminal neuralgia in an otherwise healthy patient less than 70 years of age. *The decision, however, must be made by the patient after he is fully informed about both of these procedures, since he, not the surgeon, is the one who ultimately accepts the risks and the possible sequelae.*

Preoperative Evaluation

Patients who elect to undergo this procedure are evaluated in the routine fashion used for any patient about to undergo general anesthesia, that is, routine hospital laboratory testing, a chest x-ray, and an electrocardiogram are obtained and reviewed. If the patient is older than 55

Table 69-1. The Relative Benefits and Risks of Percutaneous Trigeminal Neurolysis and Microvascular Decompression of the Trigeminal Nerve for the Treatment of Trigeminal Neuralgia

Procedure	Benefits	Risks/drawbacks
Percutaneous trigeminal neurolysis	Safe, well tolerated despite age or infirmity Brief hospitalization Repeated easily if needed	Treats symptoms, not cause Destructive; permanently alters facial sensation Risk of corneal anesthesia Dysesthetic sequellae—at times severe (denervation hyperpathia) Increased recurrences with passage of time
Microvascular decompression	Spares the nerve; patient returned to normal No numbness No dysesthesia No corneal anesthesia Treats apparent cause; may be curative	Craniectomy required; general anesthesia required Increased risk of serious, even lethal complications Should be limited to healthy patients who are younger than 70 years

years or so, or if there is any question about underlying medical problems, a complete medical evaluation also is obtained before proceeding with surgery. We obtain a computed tomographic (CT) scan with contrast augmentation before surgery to detect possibly unrecognized neoplasms or arteriovenous malformations. It has not been our practice, however, to obtain cerebral angiograms. While certainly the cerebral vessels can be delineated in this manner, the exact localization of the nerves is not determined and a difference of a few millimeters in positioning totally alters the intracranial situation. We thus feel that the information obtained by a routine angiogram is not helpful enough to warrant the small but never absent risk of angiography.

Anesthestic Considerations

A number of varied anesthetic techniques are applicable to this type of surgery and we make no attempt to influence the anesthesiologist in the choice of agents; rather, we prefer to rely upon the anesthesiologist's experience and expertise in the selection of the agent and technique that he prefers to use for each individual patient. We do feel that it is necessary, however, to

Table 69-2. The Relative Risks of Percutaneous Trigeminal Neurolysis and Microvascular Decompression of the Trigeminal Nerve for the Treatment of Trigeminal Neuralgia (Complications Noted in Our Personal Series)

Procedure	Complication	Percentage of patients affected
Percutaneous trigeminal neurolysis	Altered facial sensation	100.0
	Corneal hypesthesia	18.0
	Corneal ulceration	1.0
	Dysesthesia	22.0
	Anesthesia dolorosa	4.5
	Cranial nerve palsies	1.0
	Brain abscess	1.0
Microvascular decompression	Death	1.5
	Cerebellar hematoma	1.5
	Stroke	1.0
	Cranial nerve palsies:	
	Fourth	5.5 (transient)
	Seventh	1.5 (transient)
	Eighth	4.5

have the patient paralyzed and on controlled ventilation. This is done for two reasons: one, it minimizes motion in the field, which is greatly magnified by the operating microscope, and two, it prevents the patient from developing a gasp reflex should a small amount of air embolization occur. This reflex occurs with only a tiny entrainment of air and can rapidly result in a massive air embolism.[13]

To detect air embolization, a Doppler precordial detector and ultrasonic monitor is used. This detector must be carefully placed on the right side of the heart and its position confirmed by the intravenous injection of a small bolus of air at the beginning of the procedure. We prefer to operate with our patients in the sitting position. In this position the incidence of air embolization is higher than in the park bench or lateral decubitus position, but in any position in which the heart is higher than the head, air embolization can occur. The Doppler precordial detector is extremely sensitive[14] and will detect even the most minute amounts of air. This allows the anesthesiologist to raise the venous pressure and prevent the further entrainment of air thereby avoiding the serious sequelae of massive air embolization.

The effectiveness of the Doppler precordial detector is such that we have abandoned the use of central venous pressure (CVP) catheters for this type of surgery.[15] The CVP catheter was originally inserted to allow the aspiration of air trapped in the right atrium. The initial entrainment of small amounts of air, however, does not sequester in the atrium but rather passes through the heart into the pulmonary circulation. If it is detected at its earliest stages, raising the venous pressure to prevent further entrainment is sufficient. As such, the CVP catheter provides no useful margin of safety and rather is associated with its own set of complications, which we have chosen to avoid.

Fraser* has suggested the use of positive end-expiratory pressure (PEEP). In this manner the venous pressure can be raised almost to the level of the head thus creating the physiologic equivalent of having the patient supine while in the sitting position. This should prevent any air entrainment and add a further margin of safety. The level of the venous pressure can be adjusted to avoid seriously raising intracranial venous pressure with its associated increased intracranial pressure.

We routinely employ the use of osmotic agents (e.g., mannitol; approximately 1g/k) to minimize cerebral retraction. This is given as a rapid infusion about 15 minutes before the start of the skin incision. When using this medication it is necessary, of course, to place a Foley catheter to accommodate the diuresis that occurs intraoperatively.

As in all neurosurgical anesthesia, it is desirable for the patient to have as smooth an induction as possible, and, even more important that the termination of anesthesia be effected in such a manner that the patient is allowed to awaken gradually and not buck on the endotracheal tube.

Positioning

As indicated above, we prefer to place the patient in the sitting position for this procedure. This position offers a great many advantages to the patient and the surgeon. It can be easily achieved in patients of any physiognomy and produces a relaxed operative field with the structures in their normal anatomic relationships. It has advantages for the anesthesiologist in that it avoids chest compression, allows good ventilation, and allows good access to the patient. Cerebrospinal fluid flows out of the wound, and if any bleeding occurs, it can be washed clear with irrigation and the point of the bleeding delineated and controlled with bipolar cautery. This eliminates the need, for the most part, for using suction during this operation. Suction, we feel, is one of the most dangerous instruments that can be used in the posterior fossa because of the great potential risk of inadvertent suctioning and injury of cranial nerves, other neural structures, or small blood vessels. The positioning steps are detailed in Buchheit and Delgado's chapter on the suboccipital approach to removal of acoustic neuromas (Chapter 43). We achieve this position using a pin-fixation head holder for rigid fixation of the head. The patient is placed with

*Personal communication, Richard A. R. Fraser.

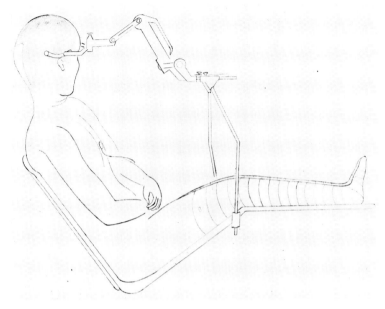

Fig. 69-1. Positioning of the patient for the semisitting position. Note the rotation of the head to the same side as the surgery (in this case to the patient's left), the support of the head in the pin-fixation holder, the use of elastic wraps on the legs and elevation of the legs to minimize venous pooling and hypotension, and the use of the Doppler precordial detector for early detection of air embolism.

his head rotated 15° to 30° to the ipsilateral side and the head flexed gently (Fig. 69-1). There should be ample room for placing one or two fingers beneath the patient's chin and at no point should the patient's neck be under tension. The elevation of the back of the table is such that the patient is actually in a semisitting or slouch position most of the time, although higher elevation of the back rest may be necessary in older patients with a stiff and less flexible neck. If the surgeon has experience and is more comfortable with other positions such as the lateral or park bench position, they certainly can be employed successfully for this procedure. Thus, the actual choice should be determined by the preference of the operating surgeon.

Operative Procedure

After the patient is satisfactorily anesthetized and positioned as described above, the operative table is also angled 15° to 20° so that the surgeon approaches the patient at an angle of approximately 45° from the midline. The hair is shaved only from the posterior quadrant of the head on the affected side and routine prepping and draping is performed. The incision is a vertical paramedian incision (Fig. 69-2) located 3 to 5 mm medial to the mastoid notch. This depression can best be identified by identifying the mastoid process and then palpating along its medial side. For exposure of the trigeminal nerve, we use a linear incision approximately 7 to 8 cm in length centered two-thirds above and one-third below the mastoid notch. *As with all microsurgery, when a limited exposure is used, the exposure must be targeted precisely.*

The scalp is routinely infiltrated with a 1:200,000 epinephrine solution if there is no anesthetic contraindications to its use. This decreases bleeding significantly. After incision of the skin, hemostasis is achieved with Dandy clamps secured to the drapes with elastic bands. Electrocautery then is used to divide the occipital muscle mass down to the occipital bone. Care is taken not to extend this incision too far inferiorly for fear of injuring the vertebral artery. The posterior auricular branch of the external carotid artery often is encountered and divided by this exposure.

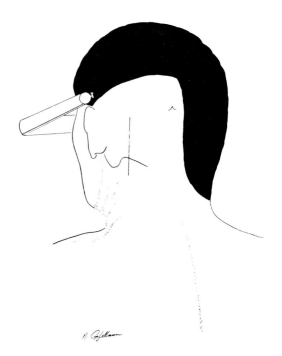

Fig. 69-2. Localization of the paramedian retromastoid incision. Note that it is placed slightly medial to the mastoid notch and centered about two-thirds above and one-third below the notch.

The muscle mass then is stripped from the posterior surface of the occipital bone. Care must be taken not to strip too far laterally in order to avoid having the incision centered too far laterally, since the degree of stripping of the muscle mass determines the localization of the exposure once the self-retaining retractor is placed. Any bridging emissary veins are coagulated and their openings in the bone sealed with bone wax.

A modified Weitlander retractor that serves as a base for a self-retaining brain retractor* then is placed (Fig. 69-3). This must be secured by placing a gauze sponge through the loops of the handle and clipping it to the drape above the patient's head in order to provide good three-point fixation and thus achieve adequate stability for the retractor arm. A burr hole then is made and enlarged into a circular craniectomy defect (Fig. 69-4). It should extend superiorly to the transverse sinus and laterally to expose the sigmoid sinus. This often carries it over mastoid air cells, which are thoroughly waxed at the completion of the craniectomy. Care is taken to displace the dura as the rongeuring proceeds in order to avoid entering the dura or the venous sinuses. Bridging veins also may be encountered and will have to be coagulated. If an opening is made into a venous emissary channel, it usually can be sealed readily with a small piece of Surgical covered with a cotton patty. A circular craniectomy defect measuring approximately 3 to 4 cm in diameter is thus created.

It cannot be emphasized too strongly that it is necessary to place this craniectomy superior and lateral enough, as determined by the venous sinuses, in order to achieve a proper exposure. The dura then is opened in an inverted L-shaped manner paralleling these channels and only a few millimeters from them (Fig. 69-4). The dura may be "teed" at the superior corner to increase the exposure. It then is secured with tenting sutures superiorly and laterally to retract the sinuses slightly and complete the exposure.

Occasionally, adhesions or bridging vessels are encountered along the superior posterior margin of the cerebellum along the transverse sinus. These must be divided sharply to free the cerebellum. The Flex-bar® retractor arm then is placed on the retractor base.* This should be positioned in such a way that a gentle arch is negotiated and sharp kinks and bends are avoided (see Fig. 69-3). Its tension is adjusted so that it remains in any position in which it is placed but can be readily moved without undo force. A specially shaped retractor blade is used.* This has an elon-

*Manufactured by Codman & Shurtleff, Inc., Randolph, MA.

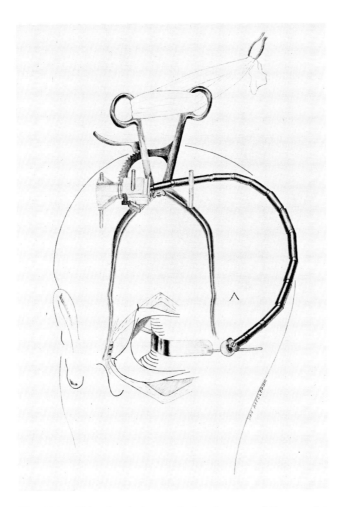

Fig. 69-3. This sketch demonstrates the use of the special cerebellar retractor. Note the fixation of the handle of the retractor with a gauze sponge looped through the rings and clamped to the drapes to provide stable three-point fixation. Note also the positioning of the flexible arm into a gentle arc that avoids sharp kinks. The dura has been opened and the cerebellum retracted to expose the petrosal vein bridging from the superior lateral margin of the cerebellum to the petrosal sinus at the junction of the tentorium and the petrous bone. This structure must be coagulated and divided.

gated finger at its superior margin. The purpose of this finger is to allow deeper retraction in the vicinity of the trigeminal nerve but avoid retracting too deeply over the seventh and eighth nerves and thus avoid injury to these structures. A narrow retractor blade could achieve the same depth of exposure superiorly but might dig into the cerebellum. The initial exposure is at the superior lateral margin of the cerebellum. This is retracted in a medial-to-inferomedial direction and the operating microscope is brought into use.

We use a 275-mm objective on the operating microscope. This allows sufficient working distance between the objective end of the microscope and the patient for the insertion of microsurgical instruments while bringing the surgeon slightly closer to the operating field than is possible with a 300-mm objective. The latter, however, can be satisfactorily employed provided the surgeon is not endowed with overly short arms. Our standard procedure is to set up the oper-

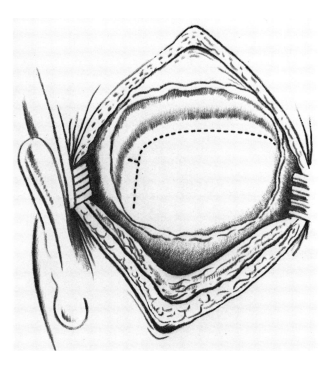

Fig. 69-4. Localization of the craniectomy defect and dural
opening. Note the lateral placement adjacent to
both the sigmoid sinus (superiorly) and the transverse sinus (laterally).

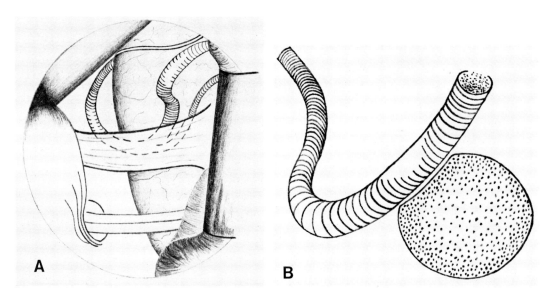

Fig. 69-5. **A.** Typical findings in trigeminal neuralgia of the left side. An elongated superior cerebellar artery is looping down and cross-compressing the root entry zone of the trigeminal nerve from an
anterior and superior direction. Note the thin fourth nerve just above the superior cerebellar artery and the relative positions of the seventh and eighth nerves below them. The arachnoid has
been opened widely to visualize these structures. **B.** Schematic lateral view showing the superior cerebellar artery coursing from the anterior (left) to the posterior (right) and impinging upon
the anterior and superior surface of the nerve at the brainstem.

Table 69-3. The Results of Percutaneous Trigeminal Neurolysis and Microvascular Decompression of the Trigeminal Nerve in the Treatment of Trigeminal Neuralgia (From the Author's Personal Series over 5 Years)

Procedure	Total no. of patients	Relieved (%)	Dysesthesia (%)	Corneal ulceration/ anesthesia (%)
Percutaneous trigeminal neurolysis	110	90	22	1
Microvascular decompression	200	94.4	0*	0*

*In patients in whom the nerve was not intentionally sectioned.

ating microscope with the stereoscopic binocular observer tube for the surgical assistant on the surgeon's left. An optical switch photo adaptor* that accommodates a 35-mm still camera and a color television camera is placed on the right side port of the beam splitter.[16] These take up little space and provide no impediment to free access between the surgeon and the surgical scrub nurse who is placed on the surgeon's right. This position is used routinely for all cases regardless of whether the exposure is on the right or left side of the patient. It allows for a standardized operative set-up and excellent access between the surgeon and the nurse. We prefer this position to the use of an overhead table with the nurse placed high because it requires less reaching by either the surgeon or the nurse and allows a freer flow of instruments and better assistance by the nurse. Parenthetically, this same position and same incision is quite satisfactory and is our preferred choice for any exposure into the cerebellopontine angle.

Before placing the microscope, an arm rest is brought into position. This is a Mayo stand, modified, as suggested by Malis, by removing the top and replacing it with a 6 × 18-inch piece of metal. This is padded, covered with a plastic sheet, and then covered with sterile drapes. Its height can be independently adjusted from the operating table to provide adequate support for the surgeon's arms.

With the microscope in place, the cerebellum is gently retracted medially and the petrosal vein identified (see Fig. 69-3). This usually is encountered approximately two-thirds of the way from the dura to the trigeminal nerve, but great variability exists and it may be absent or positioned very close to the nerve. It often consists of two channels that form a Y-type bifurcation just before entering the dura. The petrosal vein is coagulated and then divided sharply. This is best accomplished by dividing it partially to be sure that it is totally coagulated before completing the division, since once it is divided, it tends to retract out of sight, and if it is not fully coagulated, the control of bleeding could present a serious technical problem. The retractor then can be advanced, staying close to the tentorium, which should be relatively horizontal in the operative field. Variations in this view can be corrected with the use of the Trendelenburg control of the operating table. Staying high one advances above the seventh and eighth nerves without disturbing them or opening the arachnoid above them. This exposes the arachnoid overlying the trigeminal nerve. If any bleeding is encountered while retracting the cerebellum, it immediately should be suspected that a dorsal bridging vein from the cerebellum to the tentorium may have been torn. Removing the retractor and depressing the cerebellum slightly will allow inspection of this area and control of this problem before proceeding. This is an infrequent occurrence, but the surgeon must be aware of its possibility.

The arachnoid overlying the fifth nerve then must be opened sharply and widely to expose this area. This may be difficult because of the depth at which the work is being done and because of the narrow exposure. At times the arachnoid is quite thin and translucent and can be easily punctured and teased free; at other times, it is thick and opaque and must be sharply dissected. A great deal of care must be taken to avoid tugging on underlying structures. The trigeminal nerve usually will be easily identified at this point once the arachnoid is opened, and the neurovascular relationships at the brainstem then can be identified.

*Available from Designs for Vision, Inc., New York, NY.

Table 69-4. Operative Findings in 200 Consecutive Patients Undergoing Microvascular Decompression for Trigeminal Neuralgia

Operative finding	No. of patients
Arterial channels—alone or with veins	161
Venous channels only (1 with AVM)	26
Tumor (4 with arteries; 2 tumors alone)	6
Negative exploration	7
Total	200

It must be emphasized that the site of the pathology is *at* the brainstem. Vessels impinging distally on the nerve usually are not the cause of the problem. Table 69-4 details our findings. The usual situation involves the superior cerebellar artery looping down in front of the nerve and then emerging from the nerve dorsally at the point where the nerve exits from the stem (Fig. 69-5A and B). This author feels that it is quite important to open the arachnoid widely in order to allow a full inspection of the entire circumference of the nerve at the stem. Indeed, the first vessel seen may not be the only vascular channel involved in the neurovascular compression, for in a significant number of cases (19) multiple vessels have been encountered. It is also necessary to open the arachnoid anterior to the nerve to allow proper placement of the prosthesis.

The fourth nerve is a thin, delicate structure in the arachnoid above the fifth nerve, usually just below the tentorium. Great care must be taken to avoid injuring this nerve. This is one of the reasons that sharp rather than blunt dissection of the arachnoid is recommended. In addition, there may be small vascular channels traversing the subarachnoid space to the brainstem that might be injured by dissection of this arachnoid unless it is carried out quite carefully.

The Jannetta microsurgical instruments* are our preference for this procedure, but other neurosurgical instruments that are of sufficient length and properly fashioned to allow adequate vision are certainly useful. Various microsurgical scissors including the Kurze left and right pistol grip scissors* as well as straight and angled bayonetted microscissors also are employed. Once the arachnoid is opened fully and the area inspected completely, the exact nature of the compression can be determined. Occasionally we have found a microdental mirror useful in inspecting the region anterior to the nerve to be sure that channels were not being missed.* This exposure is carried out directly over the seventh and eighth nerves, and their presence must be kept in mind at all times in order to avoid traumatizing them during the dissection or when inserting or removing instruments. The arterial loops then are carefully dissected free of the nerve (Fig. 69-6).

When the superior cerebellar artery is the problem, the intent is to elevate it to a horizontal rather than a verticle loop and displace it up and away from the nerve. Small branches going to the brainstem may have been carried down with this vessel as it is gradually elongated, and normally these will not present any problem in the elevation of the vessel as long as their position is kept in mind and they are not injured. Venous channels above or below the nerve are dissected away from the nerve and are coagulated and divided. To facilitate this, small up-and-down angled bipolar forceps have been developed** and have proven their usefulness by coagulating these structures safely while avoiding the spread of current to the adjacent neural structures. In the case of vessels compressing the nerve inferiorly, they must be displaced further inferiorly away from the nerve. In all cases, it is important to avoid kinking the arterial channels as they are repositioned.

To secure these vessels free of the nerve, a small prosthesis is inserted between the artery and nerve. We have used, for this purpose Ivalon synthetic polyvinyl formyl alcohol foam sponge material that has been used as a biologic implant safely for the last 30 years.*** This mate-

*Manufactured by V. Mueller & Co., Chicago Il.
**Available from Codman & Shurtleff, Randolph, MA.
***Available from Unipoint Industries, High Point, NC.

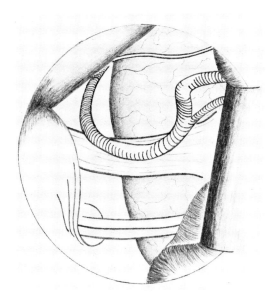

Fig. 69-6. A sketch demonstrating the view after the superior cerebellar artery has been dissected from the axilla of the trigeminal nerve.

rial comes packed in formalin and must be washed carefully to remove any trace of this preservative. It then can be cut into small blocks and autoclaved. Before its use, it must be soaked for about 10 minutes in a saline solution to rehydrate it and allow it to become soft and pliable. A small block of the material is then carved to fit between the artery and nerve. We usually fashion this as a saddle-shaped structure to fit completely over the nerve and extend both anterior and posterior to it to lock it in place (Fig. 69-7A and B). A groove cut on its superior surface then cradles the artery. In this manner, i.e., interlocked between the artery and nerve, it effectively alters the arterial force vectors and creates a satisfactory decompression. It must be wide enough to extend from the petrous bone to the brainstem but not wide enough to cause any compression. In the case of a vessel inferior to the nerve, a similar type of sponge with a longer posterior element is fashioned, and this posterior element is inserted inferior to the nerve between the artery and vein. In this manner an adequate decompression can be achieved.

On one occasion, we created a sling using a partial thickness of the tentorium that was looped down around the vessel and reattached to the tentorium with a small suture. This was effective but technically much more difficult than inserting the sponge prosthesis. If venous channels alone are encountered, no prosthesis is required. The vessels, however, are both coagulated and divided. Coagulation alone shrinks them, which creates even more tension on the nerve and allows for potential recanalization. If a tumor is encountered, it of course is removed. In most cases the tumor itself is displacing a vessel against the nerve, but tumors, as the sole etiologic agent, have been encountered on rare occasions.

If visible spasm is produced in these vessels by the surgical manipulation, a small piece of Gelfoam soaked in papaverine solution is placed on them for a few minutes to lyse the spasm. The operative field then is irrigated and the retractor removed. The cerebellum should be inspected at this point to be sure that no surface bleeding has been produced. We routinely place a piece of Gelfoam over the surface of the cerebellum and then effect a water-tight dural closure using continuous and interrupted 4-0 Nurolon* sutures. The water-tight closure minimizes the chance of a subsequent cerebrospinal fluid leak; it also promotes a smooth postoperative course. Wound closure then is effected in layers using various grades of Nurolon sutures. A small light surgical dressing is applied.

*Ethicon Inc., Somerville, NJ.

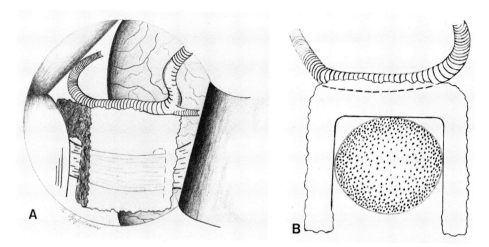

Fig. 69-7. **A.** An Ivalon sponge prosthesis is inserted as a saddle around the trigeminal nerve, which elevates the superior cerebellar artery to a more horizontal course and prevents its reapposition to the nerve. **B.** A schematic lateral view of the relationship between the artery, sponge, and nerve. Anterior is left, posterior is right.

Postoperative Considerations

Patients are nursed in the semisitting position for the first 24 hours and are observed carefully for any alterations in neural function. One must be especially alert to signs of pressure in the posterior fossa, as postoperative intracerebellar hematomas have occurred in our experience and have been responsible for patient mortality.

We routinely place our patients on dexamethasone (Decadron) before surgery and continue it for the first 24 hours. If no problems have occurred, it is discontinued at that time. Patients are allowed out of bed and begin oral intake on the first postoperative day. The Foley catheter is removed at that time, and intravenous feeding is discontinued as soon as the patient is able to achieve an adequate oral intake. The surgical dressing is removed on the second postoperative day.

Most patients have a significant postoperative headache similar to that experienced after a pneumoencephalogram. We routinely prescribe mild narcotic analgesics (such as 60 mg of codeine sulfate) and do not feel that this medication precludes adequate observation of the patient in the postoperative period. Antiemetics are used if necessary. The headache usually will subside within the first day or two, but on occasion it may persist for several weeks. Most patients convalesce rapidly from this procedure and are ready for discharge by the fifth postoperative day, following suture removal. The majority of patients will prefer another week or two at home for further convalesence. During that time their activities are not restricted; instead they are encouraged to gradually increase their activities to the limits of their tolerance. A mild oral analgesic may be prescribed during this period if required.

Operative Results and Complications

The results of this procedure, in our personal experience, correspond closely with those of Jannetta and are detailed fully as indicated in the references.[7] In summary (Table 69-3), the procedure has been effective in relieving the pain of trigeminal neuralgia in approximately 94 percent of the patients. The operative findings are detailed in Table 69-4. The majority of the patients wake up without the pain but a number will continue to have postoperative pain for a few days or even a few weeks. The pain, however, will be clearly less than that present immediately before surgery and will gradually taper off. In an occasional patient Dilantin or Tegretol may be restarted if necessary and then tapered within a few days to a few weeks.

Table 69-5. Long-Term Results in Treatment of Trigeminal Neuralgia in 200 Patients with Microvascular Decompression (5-Year Experience, Average Duration of Follow-up: 36 Months)

Result	Percentage of patients	
No pain	67	Excellent (72)
Rare pain, no medication	5	
Pain; medically controlled	20	Improved (20)
Pain; refractory	8	Failure (8)

In follow-up on 200 consecutive patients operated upon over a 5-year period (Table 69-5), with an average follow-up of 36 months, the pain has been totally controlled in 67 percent of these patients. Another 5 percent of patients have had, at some time or another, the recurrence of one or more jabs of pain. These usually have been single jabs or isolated occurrences and have not progressed on to more severe recurrences. *None* of these patients have required the reinstitution of medication. Thus, 72 percent of our patients can be considered as having an excellent result.

In another 20 percent of patients the pain has recurred to the extent that medication has been necessary but they have been able to be completely controlled with the reinstitution of medication. All of these patients were refractory to medication before surgery, and many are now being controlled on minute doses of Tegretol (such as 100 mg once or twice a day). Most of these patients (78 percent) feel that the procedure was quite beneficial to them although they obviously are a worrisome group because of the concern that they will become more severely afflicted in the future. In our experience, however, this usually has not been the case and, indeed, 37 percent of these patients have been able to discontinue the medication and remain pain-free or have so little pain that they do not feel they need medication. These 20 percent represent a satisfactory but less than perfect result. They certainly have been helped by the procedure.

In an additional 8 percent of patients severe recurrences have occurred that have been refractory to medical control. These instances indeed are failures of the procedure and have necessitated an additional, usually destructive procedure to achieve relief.

The significant complications in our series are detailed in Table 69-2. As can be seen, deaths have occurred on three occasions, emphasizing again the need for careful patient selection and information. The remainder of the other complications have for the most part been self-limited. An incidence of fourth-nerve palsy of 5.5 percent represents the most frequent complication. In each of these cases the diplopia has subsided, usually within a few days to a few weeks, but on occasion it has lasted for several months. Facial nerve palsy has occurred in 3 patients and hearing loss in 9. The facial nerve palsy has been self-limited and resulted in good to satisfactory recovery in each case, although recovery has taken up to 6 months. Hearing loss was mild in 4 patients and severe in 5. Patients who develop a hearing loss usually do not recover their hearing. This type of hearing loss must be distinguished from modest decreases in hearing that many patients experience immediately after surgery from fluid behind the eardrum (presumably tracking in through the mastoid area). This is a benign, self-limited process that will clear spontaneously within a few weeks.

Occasionally, patients will experience nonpainful twinge-like feelings in the face that are often described as a "zippy" feeling. It is not painful but often produces great anxiety in the patient who fears it is a harbinger of a return of pain. These feelings are frequent in our experience. They usually subside with the passage of time and do not appear to indicate a potential for return of pain. The patient therefore should be so reassured.

Conclusion

The Jannetta microvascular procedure, as detailed above, has proved to be an effective means of treating trigeminal neuralgia for the vast majority of patients selected for this procedure. It offers the hope of being curative by treating the apparent cause of the problem rather than just the symptoms. If offers the major advantage of sparing neural function, thereby avoiding facial sensory loss with its subsequent sequelae as well as anesthesia dolorosa or other dysesthetic sensations and corneal anesthesia, but it carries with it a small but real risk of serious sequelae including death. It therefore should not be undertaken lightly by either the patient or the surgeon. While not a terribly difficult operative technique, it requires significant microsurgical experience and skill since it is an operation in a wound of great depth through a limited exposure. *It is basically an unforgiving operation where there is little room for error in either judgment or technique.*

Trigeminal Neuralgia and Multiple Sclerosis

Trigeminal neuralgia (and glossopharyngeal neuralgia) can be a symptom of multiple sclerosis or of other demyelinating diseases. Trigeminal neuralgia will occur in 1 to 3 percent of the patients afflicted with multiple sclerosis, and 1 to 3 percent of the patients in a large series of trigeminal neuralgia will be found to suffer from multiple sclerosis. The clinical pictures are identical, and it is only the presence of neurologic dysfunction in other areas of the nervous system that alerts the surgeon to the demyelinating process. The site of pathology appears to be identical in these patients; namely, at the root entry zone of the nerve. In multiple sclerosis, however, the cause is intrinsic rather than extrinsic; namely, a demyelinating plaque in the form of a vascular channel that compresses the nerve. The Jannetta microvascular decompression operation therefore offers no benefit to these patients, and a neural destructive procedure must be employed.

Should a patient be explored and a negative exploration be encountered at the root entry zone, it is recommended that a partial section of the nerve be performed. In the case of the trigeminal nerve, the posterior inferior one-third to two-thirds of the nerve may be sectioned. This usually will provide good pain relief with only modest sensory loss. If the diagnosis is known in advance, radiofrequency lesioning is recommended.

Hemifacial Spasm

The motor analogue of trigeminal neuralgia is hemifacial spasm. Patients with this condition suffer with repetitive, painless paroxysmal twitching of the muscles of the face. Classically, this starts in the muscles about the eyes and progresses slowly and insidiously to involve the lower and midfacial musculature and, when severe, occasionally will spread to involve both the corrugator of the forehead as well as the platysma muscle on the anterior neck. At times, severe sustained contractures lasting for several seconds will occur. The patient cannot voluntarily relax, so the contractures result in a grotesque disfigurement with forced closure of the eye and a tight grimace of the mouth.

This condition is often misdiagnosed as an emotional problem and, indeed, like many neurologic problems, it will become worse during periods of emotional stress. While initially these symptoms primarily have a cosmetic impact, they can have profound influence on an individual's life by altering self-image, affecting relationships with others, and seriously altering career potential. In addition, the repetitive frequent eye closures may alter an individual's ability to read, drive a car safely, etc.

With progression of the condition, mild facial motor weakness may be noted between spasms and hearing may be moderately impaired.

Unlike trigeminal neuralgia, no medical treatment has been effective in relieving this problem. While partial division of the facial nerve has been advocated by some,[17,18] it is not a very effective procedure for hemifacial spasm, and as the condition progresses, it would involve continuous additional destruction until facial paresis and finally a facial palsy occurred.

The differential diagnosis of this condition includes several major entities. Emotional and nervous tics differ from hemifacial spasm in their multifocal presentation that involves multiple muscles, which are innervated by various nervous territories rather than being confined solely to the territory of a unilateral facial nerve. Blepharospasm is a bilateral forced contracture of the musculature about the eye. It differs from hemifacial spasm in being bilateral and involving only the musculature about the eye rather than presenting as a steady progression down the face. It appears to have a totally different etiology and is not thought to respond to this type of surgery.

More closely mimicking hemifacial spasm are the synkinetic movements that may occur following aberrant regeneration of the facial nerve after a Bell's palsy. A history of an antecedent Bell's palsy with these movements developing upon regeneration of the nerve will be most helpful in excluding it. Synkinetic movements develop with regeneration of the nerve and not as a late finding some time after adequate recovery from a Bell's palsy. Facial myokemia also must be considered in the differential. These undulating wormlike movements associated with intrinsic brainstem pathology have a distinct electromyographic pattern and can be separated by this type of evaluation. The association of other cranial nerve defects may help in the differential as well.

Indications

Patients who are in reasonably good health and less than 65 to 70 years of age are potential candidates for this type of surgery. They must be adequately informed of the potential risks, which are of the same type and magnitude as detailed above for trigeminal neuralgia. The specific cranial nerves that are at jeopardy in this type of surgery are primarily the seventh and eighth nerves and the literature[19] indicates a 5 to 8 percent incidence of either facial palsy or hearing loss or both developing after this procedure. Patients who develop facial palsy may well recover at least to a satisfactory functional degree, but patients who lose their hearing are unlikely to recover it. As with any type of surgery, the patient must be fully informed of these risks in order to be able to make an adequate decision whether to proceed.

Preoperative and anesthetic considerations as well as patient positioning are identical to that described above for trigeminal neuralgia.

Operative Procedure

The surgical incision is placed in the same location as that described for trigeminal neuralgia and is approximately the same length, but is centered slightly lower so that it is approximately half above and half below the mastoid notch. The exposure of the occipital bone and the craniectomy then are performed exactly as detailed above. The craniectomy (Fig. 69-8) is carried up close to, but does not definitely have to expose, the transverse sinus. It is important, however, that it be lateral enough to expose the sigmoid sinus and be carried down far enough to reach the floor of the posterior fossa. At this point the bone is usually fairly thin and curves to extend almost straight away from the surgeon. It is important to not leave a lip on this area that will prevent the free egrees of cerebrospinal fluid.

The dura is opened in an L-shaped or reversed-L-shaped manner parelleling the sigmoid sinus and the floor of the posterior fossa fairly close to these structures and, again, "teed" as necessary and secured with tenting sutures to widen the exposure.

The same type of self-retaining retractor system is used; however, a flat rectangular-shaped blade is used. This is placed beneath the cerebellum, and the cerebellum is elevated at its inferior lateral margin. The operating microscope, configured exactly as described above, is brought into use at this juncture. Under magnified vision, the cerebellum is gently elevated and a cottonoid strip is placed along its medial inferior edge. This acts as a wick that facilitates the drainage of cerebrospinal fluid and prevents it from welling up in the operative field. With elevation of the

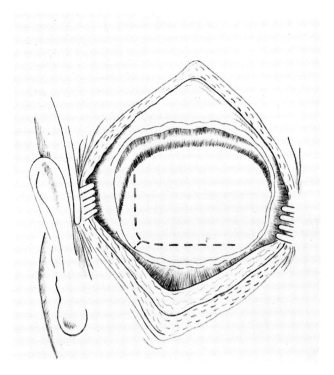

Fig. 69-8. The craniectomy defect and dural opening for exposure of the lower cranial nerves, such as for treatment of hemifacial spasm. Note that the bony
opening is carried down lower to reach the point
where the posterior fossa bone slopes directly
away from the surgeon. The dura then is opened in
an L-shaped manner close to the lateral and inferior
margins of the craniectomy.

cerebellum, the retractor can be advanced anteriorly under direct vision until the spinal part of
the eleventh cranial nerve comes into view. The arachnoid at this area is opened sharply, which
allows further elevation of the cerebellum and exposure of the remaining nerves of the jugular
foramen (Fig. 69-9). Occasionally, minute bridging veins will have to be coagulated and divided
to effect this exposure. Once the ninth cranial nerve, which is usually slightly separated from the
tenth and eleventh nerves, is identified, the exposure is carried medially by sequentially dividing
the arachnoid (using sharp dissection) between the ninth nerve and the cerebellum.

It should be noted that no attempt is made at this point to even identify the seventh and
eighth nerves at the porus acusticus, although they often may be in view at this point. They are
not followed from the porus acusticus medially to the brainstem. To do so will increase the risk
of injury to the eighth nerve. Rather, the dissection is carried out just above the ninth nerve, and
by sharply dividing the arachnoid, the cerebellum is gently elevated. Proceeding laterally to medially in this manner, the choroid plexus emanating from the lateral recess of the fourth ventricle
will soon come into view. Elevating this will expose the root entry zone of the seventh and eighth
nerves at the brainstem.

Two techniques are helpful in this visualization: to increase the exposure superiorly toward
the seventh and eighth nerves, the operating table is rotated forward using the Trendelenburg
control. This minimizes the retraction that is necessary. It also helps to replace the retractor
blade with a special retractor blade* that has an elongated process in its center. This "finger" can
be advanced up under the choroid plexus to elevate it and improve the visualization. This is a difficult area in which to work and one in which it is hard to be comfortable. The origins of the sev-

*Available from Codman & Shurtleff, Inc., Randolph, MA.

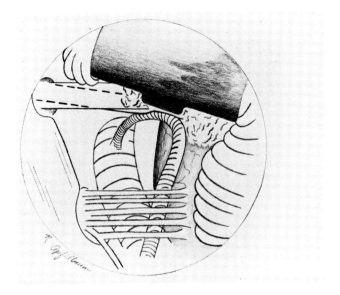

Fig. 69-9. A sketch demonstrating the view on exposure of the lower cranial nerves by *elevation* of the cerebellum. Inferiorly the spinal portion of the eleventh nerve ascends to enter the jugular foramen joined by the fibers of the ninth, tenth, and the cranial portion of the eleventh nerves. Anterior to these the vertebral artery, which gives off an elongated, tortuous posterior inferior cerebellar artery, is visible. This vessel loops cephalad before changing direction. At the apex of its loop it is indenting and cross-compressing the root entry zone of the seventh nerve, which lies slightly inferior but primarily anterior to the eighth nerve. The retractor is elevating both the cerebellum and the choroid plexus, which is emanating from the lateral recess of the fourth ventricle. This marks the root entry zone of the seventh and eighth nerves and at times obscures them.

enth and eighth nerves from the brainstem were depicted diagramatically in Chapter 43. With the alterations in this position that occur with the patient's head flexed and the table tilted forward, the facial nerve will be visible in front of the eighth nerve with its origin slightly inferior. The facial nerve usually has a slightly grayish color compared with the pure white of the eighth nerve. The individual components of the eighth nerve normally are not appreciated as separate nerves but rather run together as a compact bundle.

It is in this region where the seventh nerve leaves the brainstem that the site of cross compression will be found. Several different vessels have been encountered in our experience (Table 69-6). The anterior inferior cerebellar artery may loop up against the nerve and then extend either laterally or inferiorly. The posterior inferior cerebellar artery likewise can loop up to compress this area before taking a more inferior course. On occasion, an ectatic basilar artery will cause the same problem. On one occasion an indentation of the nerve was noted but no definite vascular channel was found. On closer inspection, however, an exostotic protruberance from the floor of the posterior fossa was noted, and when the retractor was gently released, it could be seen that this protruberance mated with the indentation on the nerve. In this instance, the protruberance was removed with a high-speed diamond drill to effect relief.

When a vessel is encountered, it must be carefully dissected free of the nerve, and a place must be found for it that will relieve the pressure on the nerve at the same time not kink or compromise the vessel. Many times small tethering branches to the brainstem limit the degree of displacement that can be achieved. One must always be aware of the possible presence of small

**Table 69-6. Operative Findings in 40 Consecutive Patients Undergoing Microvascular Decompression
for Treatment of Hemifacial Spasm**

Cause of compression of seventh nerve	No. of patients
Loop of AICA	21
Loop of PICA	11
Vertebral artery—	2
Associated with AICA origin	2
Associated with PICA origin	2
Venous channel	1
Bony exostosis	1
Total	40

branches along the medial side of the vessel going to the stem, especially at the apex of loops. After carefully dissecting the vessel free of the nerve and using the utmost in precautions not to manipulate either the seventh or eighth nerves, an Ivalon sponge prosthesis is fashioned to fit between the two. This often takes on a complicated shape because of the limited access in this area and the necessity of accommodating a number of different structures. We try to interdigitate it between the vessels and often fashion protruberances on the prosthesis to fit within the loops of the vessel to help anchor it in place.

Various prostheses have been used by surgeons employing the Jannetta procedure. Our personal experience has been primarily with Ivalon, which has proved quite satisfactory. Absorbable materials, such as Gelfoam, should be avoided because the vessel may return to its compressive position against the nerve when they are absorbed. Similarly, material such as muscle, which is easier to insert, has on occasion led to recurrences as the muscle atrophied under the continued arterial pulsations and again allowed the artery and nerve to come into contact.

Once a satisfactory decompression of the nerve is achieved, spasm is lysed with topical papaverine, the area irrigated, and the retractor removed while the effects that releasing retraction has on the vascular anatomy are carefully observed. The closure and postoperative care are identical to that used in treating patients with trigeminal neuralgia.

Operative Results and Complications

In 40 consecutive cases a cause of compression was identified in each situation. No negative explorations were encountered. The specific causes of compression are detailed in Table 69-6.

Hemifacial spasm was relieved in all of these patients. In 34 patients relief occurred immediately or within the first few days after surgery, while in a smaller subgroup of 6 patients, the hemifacial spasm was clearly improved but did not subside completely until a few weeks to as long as 6 months after surgery. We have had recurrences in 6 patients and have reoperated upon 1 patient who suffered a recurrence at 5 months and whose spasms progressively increased to their preoperative level. A technically unsatisfactory prosthesis was replaced and this effected full resolution of his facial spasms. Several of the other recurrences have been short-lived and improved spontaneously.

Complications with this procedure are detailed in Table 69-7. Hearing has been compromised in 1 patient to a moderate degree. No patients have had an immediate postoperative facial palsy, but 2 have had delayed palsies that developed about 1 week after surgery. In each case these have recovered to normal in 2 to 6 months, respectively. One moderate facial paresis developed 1 week postoperatively and resolved in 3 months. Transient trace facial weakness has been detected in 6 patients on careful examination.

Table 69-7. Complications in 40 Consecutive Patients Undergoing Microvascular Decompression
for the Treatment of Hemifacial Spasm

Complication	No. of patients
Supratentorial stroke (good recovery; some residuae)	1
Transient supratentorial dysfunction	2
Facial weakness:	
Trace (resolving)	6
Moderate (resolved fully within 3 months)	1
Severe (resolved fully within 3 months)	2
Hearing loss (moderate)	1
Focal seizures (immediately postop. in 1; at 6 months in the other)	2
Transient dysequilibrium	1

Conclusion

The Jannetta microvascular decompression as applied to the treatment of hemifacial spasm offers even more convincing results than those obtained in the treatment of trigeminal neuralgia. This is true because of the total lack of alternative forms of therapy and because of the very visible and graphic effects of the surgical procedure. The procedure, however, will always carry with it a small but significant risk of serious sequelae and, like the same procedure for trigeminal neuralgia, should not be undertaken lightly. It is a more difficult procedure than the decompression of the trigeminal nerve. Its potential benefits thus must be weighed carefully in this nonlethal, painless condition. *Again, the basically unforgiving nature of this procedure cannot be emphasized too strongly.*

Tic Convulsif

Cushing[20] described a few patients suffering from the combined clinical picture of trigeminal neuralgia and hemifacial spasm, a condition that he termed tic convulsif. These patients appear to have both entities, and it is appropriate to explore the root entry zone of both the seventh and fifth cranial nerves and to anticipate vascular channels on both nerves. It is conceivable that only one nerve will be effected because of anomolous innervation, but the safest course would be to explore both nerves.

Glossopharyngeal Neuralgia

Glossopharyngeal neuralgia is a condition that is exactly analogous to trigeminal neuralgia but occurs in the territory of the ninth cranial nerve. Patients so afflicted experience lancinating spasms of pain in the posterior tongue and throat that usually are triggered by talking and swallowing. It is a much rarer condition than trigeminal neuralgia but otherwise appears to be identical in its behavior. Like trigeminal neuralgia, it usually can be controlled medically, and surgical intervention is infrequently required.

The Jannetta microvascular decompressive technique is equally applicable to this condition as it is to trigeminal neuralgia. The preoperative considerations and alternatives are the same. The operative exposure is the same as the one detailed for the seventh cranial nerve with the modification that the root entry zone of the ninth cranial nerve is inspected and decompressed. This is accomplished by following the superior surface of the ninth nerve back to the brainstem and then visualizing this area, working between the seventh and eighth nerves above and the ninth nerve below or between the fascicles of the ninth and tenth nerves.

Because of the rarity of this condition, experience is limited, but the results appear to parallel closely that of trigeminal neuralgia.

REFERENCES

1. Dandy WE: The treatment of trigeminal neuralgia by the cerebellar route. *Ann Surg* 96:787–795, 1932
2. Gardner WJ, Sava GA: Hemifacial spasm—a reversible pathophysiologic state. *J Neurosurg* 19:240–247, 1962
3. Jannetta PJ: Arterial compression of the trigeminal nerve at the pons in patients with trigeminal neuralgia. *J Neurosurg* 26:159–162, 1967
4. Jannetta PJ: Observations on the etiology of trigeminal neuralgia, hemifacial spasm, acoustic nerve dysfunction and glossopharyngeal neuralgia. definitive microsurgical treatment and results in 117 patients. *Neurochirurgia (Stuttg)* 20:145–154, 1977
5. Jannetta PJ: Microsurgical approach to the trigeminal nerve for tic douloureux. *Prog Neurol Surg* 7:180–200, 1976
6. Apfelbaum RI, Kirk M, Terra AM: Microvascular decompression of the trigeminal nerve for the treatment of trigeminal neuralgia. *J Neurosurg Nurs* 10:77–82, 1978
7. Apfelbaum RI: The Jannetta microvascular decompressive operation for treatment of trigeminal neuralgia (in preparation)
8. White JC, Sweet WH: *Pain and the Neurosurgeon; Medical Treatment of Trigeminal Neuralgia.* Springfield, IL, Charles C Thomas, 1969, p 169
9. Rasmussen P, Riishede J: Facial pain treated with carbamazepine (Tegretol). *Acta Neurol Scand* 46:385–408, 1970
10. Tew JM, Keller JT: The treatment of trigeminal neuralgia by percutaneous radiofrequency technique. *Clin Neurosurg* 24:557–578, 1976
11. Siegfried, J: 500 percutaneous thermocoagulations of the gasserian ganglion for trigeminal pain. *Surg Neurol* 8:126–131, 1977
12. Jannetta PJ: Treatment of trigeminal neuralgia by suboccipital and transtentorial cranial operations. *Clin Neurosurg* 24:538–549, 1976
13. Adornato DC, Gildenberg PL, Ferrario CM, et al: Pathophysiology of intravenous air embolism in dogs. *Anesthesiology* 49:120–127, 1978
14. Frost EA: Anesthesia for neurosurgical procedures in the sitting position. *Weekly Anesthesiology Update,* Lesson 4, vol. 1, 1977
15. Apfelbaum RI, Duncalf D, Phillips PL: Is central venous catheterization necessary for neurosurgical procedures in the sitting position? Presented at the annual meeting of the American Association of Neurological Surgeons, New York, 1980
16. Apfelbaum RI, Neurosurgical applications of video techniques. *Clin Neurosurg* 28:246–258, 1981
17. German WJ: Surgical treatment of spasmodic facial tic. *Surgery* 11:912–914, 1942
18. Scoville WB: Partial extracranial section of seventh nerve for hemi-facial spasm. *J Neurosurg* 31:106–108, 1969
19. Jannetta PJ, Abbasy M, Maroon J, et al: Etiology and definitive microsurgical treatment of hemifacial spasm. *J Neurosurg* 47:321–328, 1977
20. Cushing H: The major trigeminal neuralgias and their surgical treatment based on experiences with 332 gasserian operations. *Amer J Med Sci* 160:157–185, 1920

CHAPTER 70

Percutaneous Rhizotomy in the Treatment of Intractable Facial Pain (Trigeminal, Glossopharyngeal, and Vagal Nerves)

John McLellan Tew, Jr.
William D. Tobler   Harry van Loveren

Trigeminal Neuralgia

THE SURGICAL TREATMENT OF TRIGEMINAL NEURALGIA continues to stimulate controversy despite the fact that this condition has been recognized and treated surgically for centuries. A totally satisfactory method of treatment has never been devised. Section of a peripheral branch of the trigeminal nerve was probably the earliest form of surgical therapy. Later, intracranial section of peripheral branches,[1,2] ganglion resection,[3] and retrogasserian rhizotomy were developed.[4-6] Some questioned the need for destructive procedures[7-10] and developed techniques for decompressing or compressing the posterior rootlets.

Peripheral procedures still are effective for the temporary control of chronic trigeminal pain, particularly as an early measure that provides the patient an opportunity to test the effect of sensory deprivation.[11,12]

Recently, the need for destructive procedures has again been questioned by Jannetta,[13] who supports Dandy's[14] observation that trigeminal neuralgia is caused, in most instances, by vascular compression at the brain stem. While this hypothesis remains an attractive suggestion for treatment, the results of its application are still being tested.

The tactic of electrocoagulation of the trigeminal nerve originally was proposed by Kirschner in 1932.[15] Despite a report of favorable results,[16] this procedure gained no practitioners in this country until Sweet refined the technique,[17,18] with the following modifications: (1) use of a short-acting anesthetic agent, which permits the patient to awaken rapidly for sensory testing during the operation; (2) use of a reliable radiofrequency current for production of the lesion; (3) use of electrical stimulation for precise localization; and (4) use of temperature monitoring for precise control of lesion configuration. This procedure has been extremely safe and has gained considerable acceptance as a method for partially destroying the sensory root.

Mayfield Neurological Institute, Cincinnati, Ohio

STEREOTAXIC TRIGEMINAL RHIZOTOMY

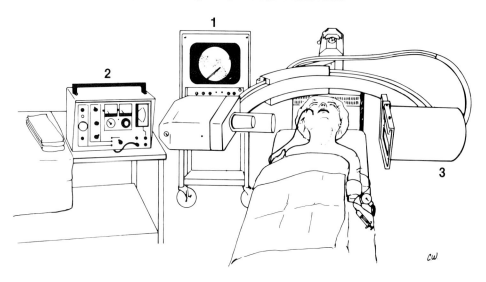

John M. Tew, Jr.,M.D.-Mayfield Neurological Institute - Cincinnati, Ohio

Fig. 70-1. The operative arrangement used for stereotactic rhizotomy of the trigeminal nerve. 1 = Image intensifer; 2 = radiofrequency generator; 3 = C-arm cine radiographic unit.

Patient Selection

Much of the enthusiasm for percutaneous trigeminal rhizotomy has been engendered by patients who were relieved from pain after many years of suffering. While the patient's acceptance of a new surgical procedure is important, its ultimate value must depend on assessments of the duration of relief and the incidence of morbidity and mortality, compared with other surgical and medical treatments.

Presently, it is our practice to consider all patients with intractable trigeminal neuralgia who have failed to obtain long-standing control with medical therapy as candidates for percutaneous rhizotomy. A person less than 50 years of age who has any indication of atypical pain is offered the alternative of posterior fossa exploration of the trigeminal root. These patients also are studied with computerized axial tomography, and selective angiographic studies.

If surgical treatment is elected, the patient and family are required to read and listen to a full explanation of current procedures available for the control of trigeminal neuralgia. Frequently the patient is advised to discuss results with others who have undergone major trigeminal surgery. This tactic reinforces the patient's understanding and appreciation of possible undesirable sensory loss. Differential sensory block enables the patient to experience the effect of sensory deprivation and may aid in the decision concerning operation for atypical facial pain.

A well educated patient is better able to accept side effects, thus greatly reducing the incidence of postoperative disappointment. It has been our policy to let the informed patient make his own decision regarding the mode of treatment. If the patient elects a destructive procedure, such as electrocoagulation, he is encouraged to indicate the degree of sensory deficit he would like to acquire. While partial sensory loss is associated with a higher incidence of recurrence, patients usually are not reluctant to undergo repeat percutaneous rhizotomy.

Technique—Percutaneous Trigeminal Rhizotomy

The rationale for electrocoagulation of the trigeminal rootlets is based on the premise that differential thermal destruction of the small, unmyelinated and finely myelinated fibers that conduct pain can be achieved.[19,20] The procedure is conducted in the radiographic suite (Fig. 70-1).

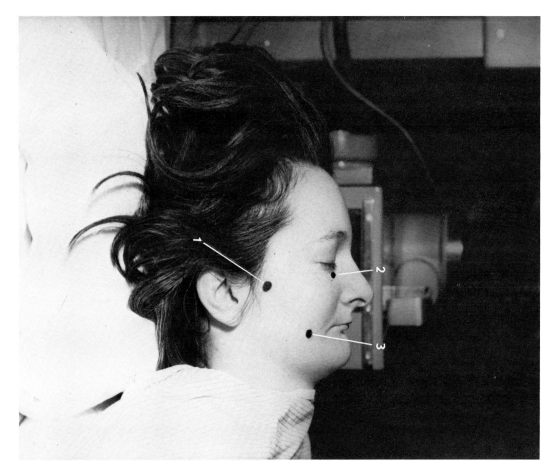

Fig. 70-2. Anatomic landmarks for electrode placement.

The patient is anesthetized with an intravenous injection of 30-50 mg of methohexital (Brevital, Eli Lilly & Co., Indianapolis, Ind.). A standard 100 mm length 20 gauge cannula and stylet are placed in the retrogasserian portion of the trigeminal nerve. Placement is by freehand manipulation but a guiding device as designed by Kirschner may be used. Three anatomic landmarks are chosen on the face (Fig 70-2): (1) point 3 cm anterior to the external auditory meatus; (2) a point beneath the medial aspect of the pupil; and (3) a point 2.5 cm lateral to the oral commisure. The first two points indicate the site of the foramen ovale and the third is the point at which the needle penetrates the skin of the jaw. The anterior approach to the foramen ovale, as advocated by Härtel,[21] is used (Fig. 70-3). Radiographic control has been reported to be of value, and we have used the image intensifier in a lateral plane as an effective method of localizing the needle.[22] Using the landmarks described, however, we have been able to penetrate the foramen ovale on the first attempt in most cases, and after a simple adjustment in all instances.

The index finger of the gloved hand is placed just inferior to the lateral pterygoid wing, and the electrode is directed into the medial portion of the foramen ovale (Fig. 70-4). If the needle enters the posterolateral aspect of the foramen, it may not lie within the dural investment of the trigeminal ganglion and, if advanced, probably will not reach the maxillary or ophthalmic divisions of the rootlet of the nerve. As the electrode is advanced, an oral airway is placed between the jaws to prevent involuntary biting of the guiding finger. Intravenous methohexital is injected as the foramen is neared. Entrance of the needle into the foramen is signaled by a wince and a brief contraction of the masseter muscle, indicating contact with the mandibular sensory and motor fibers. Before the electrode is advanced any further, a second series of radiographs is obtained to confirm proper placement of the electrode (Figs. 70-5A and B). The stylet is withdrawn

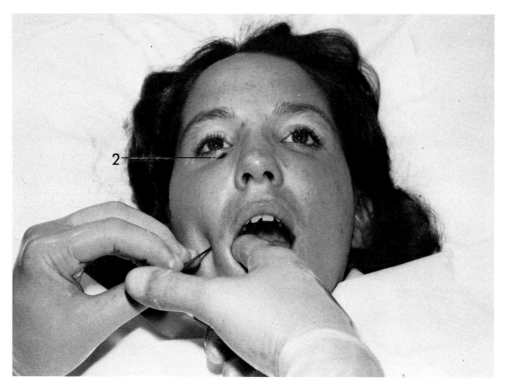

Fig. 70-3.   Illustration demonstrating needle placement according to the technique of Härtel.

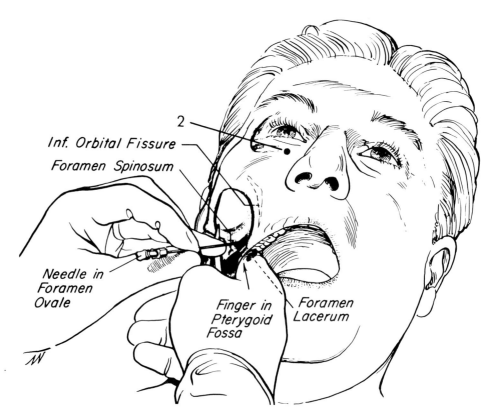

Fig. 70-4.   Freehand placement of the electrode. The guiding finger touches ptergoid wing.

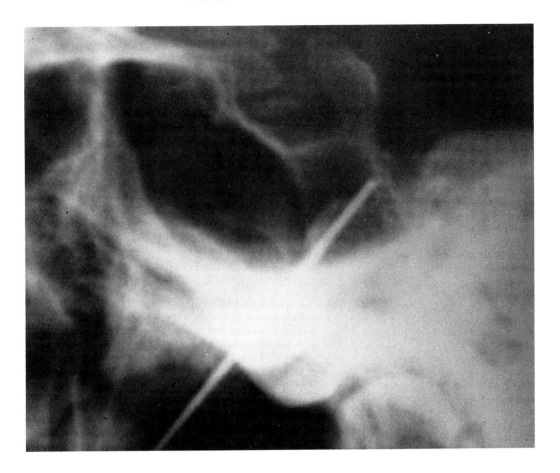

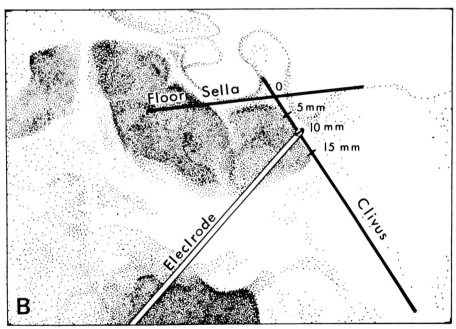

Fig. 70-5. **A.** Submento-vertex radiograph confirming electrode placement in the foramen ovale. **B.** The ideal trajectory of the electrode (5–10 mm below the intersection of a line drawn from the floor of the sella turcica to the clival line).

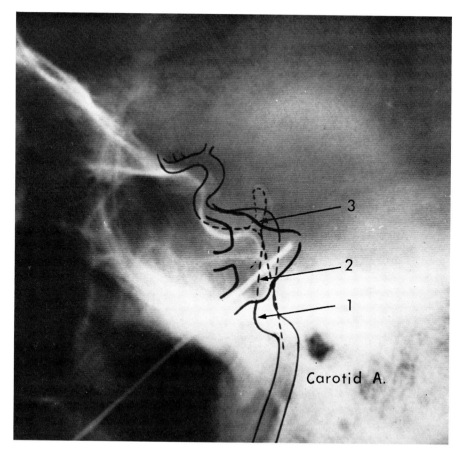

Fig. 70-6.   A composite illustration demonstrates the relationship of the carotid artery to the trigeminal ganglion and posterior rootlets. Note the location of three points of possible carotid penetration.

to determine whether the carotid artery has been penetrated. In our experience, this circumstance has occurred on only one occasion.

If the carotid artery is penetrated, the needle should be withdrawn promptly and manual pressure applied over the posterior pharyngeal space. The procedure should be discontinued for 24 to 48 hours. Ischemic complications, such as hemiparesis, have resulted from puncture of the internal carotid artery.[23] The electrode may penetrate the cartilaginous covering of the foramen lacerum, if deviated medially, and puncture the carotid artery. If the electrode is directed posterolaterally, it may pierce the carotid artery at its entrance into the petrous bone. Finally Rish[23] suggests that after the electrode passes through the foramen ovale, it may penetrate the carotid artery. This may occur if the electrode was directed anteriorly and medially into the area of the cavernous sinus (Fig. 70-6). Our anatomic studies illustrate that the carotid artery frequently is devoid of bony covering immediately ventral to Meckel's cave.

Electrode Localization.   The cannula is calibrated in order to permit extrusion of the electrode in 1 mm increments. When the electrode is fully inserted into the cannula, the curved tip extends 5 mm beyond the end of the cannula and projects 3 mm perpendicular to the axis of the electrode. The cannula is insulated so that only the extruded portion of the electrode (0-5 mm) is conductive. The electrode may be rotated through a 360° axis for stimulation and lesion production.

Final placement of the electrode tip is determined by the response to electrical stimulation.

A current of precisely 0.2 to 0.3 V at 50 to 75 cycles/sec. will reproduce the paroxysmal bouts of pain reminiscent of trigeminal neuralgia. Stimulation using higher voltage (1.0 to 2.0 V) may be required in patients who have had previous intracranial rhizotomy or repeated alcohol injections. The response evoked serves as a reliable indicator of the probe temperature required to produce a lesion.

After the cannula reaches the trigeminal cistern, stimulation should elicit a paroxysm of pain in the mandibular distribution. Lateral radiography at that time will indicate whether the tip of the electrode lies at a point 4 to 5 mm external to the profile of the clivus. If the needle is advanced 5 mm, its tip should lie at the level of the clivus, where stimulation will elicit paresthesias in the second-division rootlets. The electrode tip should not be advanced more than 8 mm deep to the profile of the clivus, since it may injure the abducens nerve in this region. Manipulation (rotation about its axis) of the curved electrode permits stimulation of different portions of the nerve (Fig. 70-7 A, B and C). Rotation of the electrode tip cephalad provides better access to the fibers of the ophthalmic division, while caudal rotation contacts the mandibular fibers. This maneuverability permits precise anatomical localization in the sensory root. If the electrode contacts the motor root, stimulation results in masseter contraction and a lateral rotation of the electrode eliminates the production of a lesion which could result in motor paresis. Although a straight electrode was used in our first 700 cases, the advantages of the curved-tip electrode described above have obviated the straight electrode technique.

Lesion Production. The geometry of the lesions varies with the medium; reproducible lesions are 5 x 5 x 4 mm and are eccentric with orientation toward the curve of the electrode. The electrode tip measures 0.5 mm in diameter. A thermocouple sensor is located at the tip of the electrode and provides calibration accuracy of $\pm$ 2° centigrade over the range of 30-100° centigrade.

Additional intravenous anesthetic is administered, and a preliminary lesion is produced at 60°C for 60 seconds. A facial blush usually appears at this point and helps to localize the region of the nerve root undergoing thermal destruction.[24] When the patient has fully awakened, careful sensory testing of the face is conducted. Repeat lesions are produced until the desired effect is achieved. Generally, sequential lesions of 60-seconds duration are made by increasing the temperature 5°C with each lesion. When analgesia is approached, great care is exercised to avoid overshooting the desired result, which includes preserving the sense of touch. After a partial lesion has been produced, it is frequently possible to complete the lesion without additional anesthetic agent. The pain associated with production of the lesion is reduced because a lower temperature is required to make an effective lesion and the curvature of the electrode avoids contact with the dura which is the principal source of pain reception in this region. This tactic is particularly valuable when partial sensation of a cornea or other trigeminal divisions are to be preserved.

Once the desired degree of sensory loss has been achieved, the patient is observed for an additional 15 minutes to determine if a fixed lesion has been produced. If the examination indicates a stable level of analgesia, the distribution and degree of deficit are determined by careful sensory testing. Touch perception is recorded in grams of pressure, using calibrated Von-Frey hairs. Masseter, pterygoid, facial, and ocular muscle function is recorded. The patient then is returned to his room and observed for 24 hours. During this period he is informed of the necessity for eye care, for avoiding jaw strain, and of the consequences of facial analgesia.

Results

At the time of this report 700 patients with typical trigeminal neuralgia were treated surgically by the percutaneous rhizotomy approach using the straight electrode. A thorough follow-up evaluation, extending over a period of 10 years, has been completed for all of these patients (Table 70-1). The average age for the group was 63 years and 60 percent were female. In 60 per-

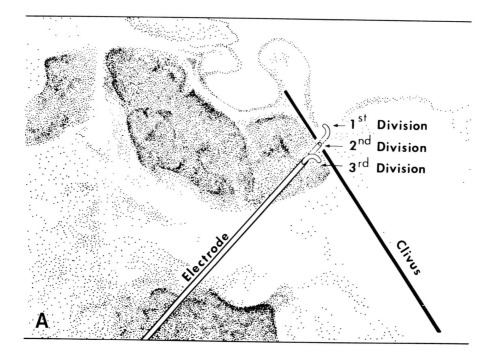

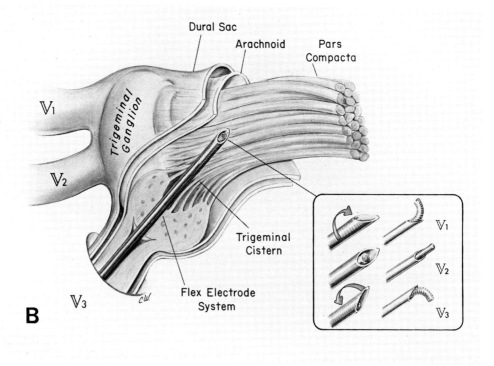

Fig. 70-7.   **A.** Composite illustration demonstrating the relationship of the trigeminal rootlets to the profile of the clivus. With the electrode tip at −5 mm, the third division is stimulated; at 0, the second division, and at +5 mm deep to the clivus, the first division fibers are stimulated. **B.** An illustration of the trigeminal rootlets and the newly developed curved electrode with thermocouple, which is capable of producing lesions in any of the three divisions from a single position. **C.** New curved electrode system, which is capable of lesion production and temperature measurement throughout the trigeminal root from a single position.

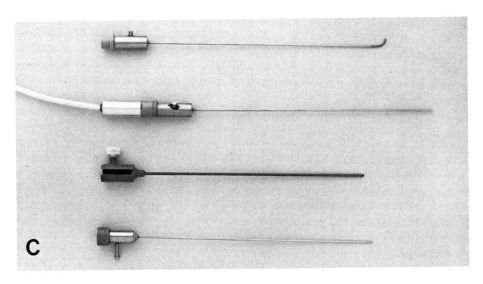

Fig. 70-7 (cont'd.)

cent the pain was located on the right, and the second and third divisions of the trigeminal nerve were commonly involved. Isolated pain in the first or third division was less frequent than in the second division. It is notable that 21 percent of patients had a significant degree of pain in the first division, although pain was isolated to this division in only 2 percent of patients.

The disease had been present for an average of 8 years and was characterized by increasingly severe episodes of paroxysmal pain and progressively shorter periods of remission. Many patients had been treated surgically, usually by nerve avulsion or alcohol injection (32 percent) while 11 percent had a prior intracranial procedure, usually subtotal rhizotomy. Nearly all patients had been treated with either diphenylhydantoin (Dilantin) or carbamazepine (Tegretol), as well as other forms of medical and physical remedies. While diphenylhydantoin was effective in over 50 percent of patients, the effect was seldom lasting or satisfactory. Carbamazepine was considered more effective: 92 percent of patients reported significant relief of a lasting nature but efficacy was limited by the tendency of most patients to develop increasing side effects to the drug as higher doses were required.

Table 70-1. Characteristics of 700 Patients Selected for Electrocoagulation

		Percent of patients
Average age	63 years	
Sex	60% female	
Side f coagulation:		
Right		60
Left		39
Bilateral		1
Division of trigeminal		
Nerve involved:		
V-1		2
V-2		20
V-3		17
V-1, V-2		14
V-2, V-3		42
V-1, V-2, V-3		5

Table 70-2. Results of Curved Electrode and Straight Electrode in the Immediate Postoperative Period

	Curved (125 Cases)	Straight (700 Cases)
Excellent	90%	76%
Good	8%	17%
Fair	2%	6%
Failure	0%	1%

A response to follow-up was obtained for all 700 patients. Many of the patients were not recalled for personal examination, however, because of advanced age, disability, distance from the examining clinic, death, or other reasons. All were contacted by questionnaire (Fig. 70-8) or phone, however, and a family member was contacted if the patient had died. At the time of evaluation 93 percent of patients reported excellent to good results. The remaining patients obtained only fair results, 6 percent because of undesirable side effects or recurrent pain. Four patients (1 percent) reported that their pain had never been relieved satisfactorily at any time after the coagulation procedure.

The curved electrode has been used to treat 125 patients over a 12 month period. All patients underwent neurological examination immediately following termination of the procedure and, again, 24 hours later. Follow-up evaluations were conducted by telephone or written inquiry 2 to 8 weeks following the procedure. At the time of evaluation 98 percent of patients reported excellent to good results. The remaining patients obtained only fair results (2 percent) because of undesirable side effects. No patient treated using the curved electrode failed to obtain relief of pain. (Table 70-2).

Side Effects

Sensory. Troublesome numbness and paresthesias from the sensory deficit proved to be the most consistent adverse side effect with both the straight and curved electrode technique. Using the curved electrode the incidence of troublesome paresthesias decreased from 27 percent to 11.2 percent (Table 70-3). Commonly, an intermittent crawling, burning, or itching sensation was described. Most patients readily adjusted to the sensory deficit, and the paresthesias usually diminished with time. The more active and mentally alert the patient, the fewer the disturbances of sensation reported. Older patients were more prone to this complication. Constant, severe dysesthesias in an anesthetic or analgesic zone (anesthesia dolorosa) rarely occurred using the straight electrode and has not occurred at all using the curved electrode technique. Three patients reported a severe burning pain that improved considerably after several months. Forty-five patients reported a significant problem with paresthesias and 11 additional patients

Table 70-3. Complications of Percutaneous Rhizotomy (Curved Electrode Compared to Straight Electrode)

	Curved Electrode (125 Cases)	Straight Electrode (700 Cases)
Masseter Weakness	8.8%	24%
Paresthesias		
Minor	11.2%	22%
Major	0%	5%
Diplopia	0%	2%
Keratitis	1.6%	4%

In preparation for writing a book on trigeminal neuralgia or tic douloureux, we are asking your cooperation in answering the following questions concerning the treatment of this condition by percutaneous electrocoagulation. We are particularly interested in knowing if the original pain for which you were treated has been controlled and if any side effects have developed as a result of this treatment. Your assistance by answering the following questions would be helpful.

1. What is the present status of your facial pain?
2. Has there been any recurrence of pain since the operative procedure?
3. To what extent is your face numb?
4. Is the numbness or loss of feeling troublesome?
5. Do you have difficulty chewing or eating food? If so, please explain.
6. Do you have double vision?
7. Do you have blurring of vision or difficulty with your eye?
8. Have you suffered any complications as a result of the procedure?
9. How do you rate the result of the operation?
   Excellent—no pain, no side effects _____
   Good—minimal pain, minimal side effects _____
   Fair—recurrence of pain, no major side effects _____
   Failure—original pain never relieved _____

Fig. 70-8. Evaluation protocol form.

complained of other symptoms related to sensory deprivation. Five patients reported a troublesome aching pain in the jaw region.

Five aged patients developed persistent excoriation of the skin about the face, nostril, or scalp. Many traumatized the skin by frequent scratching or manipulation, which could be controlled, in most cases, by applying mittens at bedtime.

Eye. Eye complications occurred in 8 percent of patients with the straight electrode; 8 (2 percent) developed neurologic keratitis. Thirty percent of this group had corneal analgesia, indicating that touch perception in the absence of pain perception does not necessarily protect against corneal ulceration. The corneal lesion was reversed in all patients by early ophthalmologic treatment. Application of a soft contact lens, meticulous eye care, and occasional tarsorrhaphy prevented permanent visual loss. Intermittent blurred vision was reported by 12 patients (4 percent). In 7 of the 12, touch perception of the cornea was preserved, although the corneal reflex was markedly diminished. Again, this finding suggests that preserving touch perception of the cornea does not necessarily protect against keratitis and visual clouding. Our experience indicates that persons with some sensory preservation of the cornea adjust more rapidly to the deficit and rarely develop ulceration. Similarly, patients with corneal anesthesia seldom develop keratitis during the later postoperative period. Patients or their relatives must be given meticulous instructions about all aspects of eye care. By carefully adhering to this practice, we suspect that serious eye complications, sometimes seen following this procedure, have been prevented. Seventy patients in this group had neuralgia involving or limited to the ophthalmic division; 72 percent achieved pain relief without losing corneal sensation, and only 6 percent developed neurolytic keratitis. In patients treated with the curved electrode the incidence of keratitis has been reduced to 1.6 percent.

Transient diplopia occurred in 7 patients (2 percent). In 5, the double vision could be explained by abducens nerve palsy and in 2 the cause was trochlear palsy. The deficit was transient in all patients. The most persistent diplopia lasted for 4 months, while in all but 1 patient it disappeared in a few weeks. This complication was seen only in patients undergoing treatment for neuralgia involving the ophthalmic division. Abducens nerve palsy may be produced if a thermal lesion is created with the tip of the electrode extending more than 5 to 8 mm past the profile of the clivus, as measured on a lateral film of the skull (Fig. 70-9). Trochlear palsy is apparently minimized if the trajectory of the electrode is not aimed toward the posterior clinoid process, where the tip may encounter the cavernous sinus.

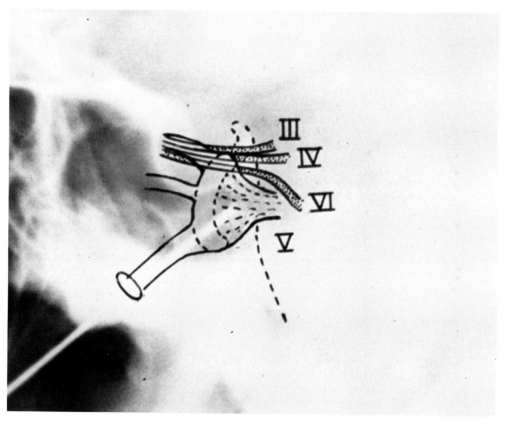

Fig. 70-9. Lateral radiograph demonstrates course of the oculomotor, abducens, and trochlear nerves and their relation to the trajectory of the electrode. The tip of the electrode should not extend more than 8 mm deep to the profile of the clivus.

The incidence of unwanted loss of corneal sensation and paresis of ocular nerves has been greatly reduced in recent years by performing electrocoagulation with the patient alert and cooperating in the evaluation during the final stage of lesion production. The occurrence of diplopia has been completely eliminated with the curved electrode technique.

Motor Paresis.   Paresis of muscles innervated by the motor root of the trigeminal nerve occurred in 24 percent of patients after treatment with the straight electrode. In most instances the deficit was partial and transient. Weakness of masseter, temporalis, and pterygoid muscles causes a mild degree of disability because of jaw deviation and loss of chewing power. Trismus was a more troublesome problem but it could be avoided or eliminated by placing the patient on a soft diet and instructing him to exercise his jaws frequently in the presence of pain or muscle weakness.

Hearing difficulties related to transient roaring, popping sounds, or fullness in the ear were reported by some patients. These symptoms are attributable to paresis of the small muscles about the eustachian tube (tensor veli palatini) and tympanic membrane (tensor tympani).

Many patients who did not have motor paresis had difficulty chewing. They related this difficulty to sensory loss in the mouth. Most did not find it significant however, since they had become accustomed to chewing on the nonpainful side.

Motor weakness of the muscles of mastication was the second most frequently occurring side effect (8.8 percent) using the curved-tip electrode. Weakness was minor in degree and involved the masseter muscle most commonly, masseter and pterygoid muscles occasionally, and unlike our experience with the straight electrode, was of no clinical significance to most patients.

Table 70-4. Comparison of Incidence of Side Effects

	Cases	Paresthesias	Anesthesia Dolorosa	Motor Root Weakness
Apfelbaum[35]	48	*	12%	2%
Burchiel[34]	78	15%	4%	*
Menzel[25]	315	93%	2%	50%
Nugent[29]	65	*	5%	43%
Sweet[32]	274	2%	1%	43%
Tew	700	22%	6%	24%

*Not reported

Herpes simplex. Lesions of herpes simplex were noted in 3 percent of patients. Since most were not examined more than 48 hours postoperatively, this figure is undoubtedly low.

Discussion

The role of percutaneous stereotaxic rhizotomy in the treatment of trigeminal neuralgia has been investigated and discussed by numerous authors.[25,28,29,30,31,32,33] Our results with 700 patients treated by stereotaxic rhizotomy using a straight electrode are compared with 125 patients recently treated with flexible curved electrodes (Table 70-2, 70-3). In spite of the extensive experience of many neurosurgeons, there continues to be a high rate of undesirable side effects in patients treated by this procedure (Table 70-4). Mild to moderate paresthesias and burning sensations were recorded in 93 percent of patients in one series.[25] Burchiel recently reported 15 percent mild paresthesias and 4 percent severe paresthesias.[34] Apfelbaum[35] reported 11 percent severe paresthesias which were sometimes as troublesome as the disease itself and for which there is no effective treatment. Sweet and Wepsic[32] reported loss of trigeminal motor function in 43 percent of patients, and in 40 percent of those, the motor loss was severe. Nugent reported motor weakness in 43 percent of his patients.[29]

In our experience the most troublesome side effects have been sensory paresthesias and trigeminal motor weakness. In comparing our results using the curved electrode with our results using the straight electrode, minor paresthesias have decreased from 22 percent to 11.2 percent and no cases of anesthesia dolorosa have been reported following the use of the curved electrode technique. Motor weakness has decreased from 24 percent to 8.8 percent, and in all cases, the weakness has been mild. Keratitis has developed in only 2 cases and diplopia has not occurred[36] (Table 70-3).

Because of the decrease in the incidence of side effects, our immediate follow-up results have improved with the curved electrode (Table 70-2). Ninety percent of patients obtained excellent results (no pain and no side effects), and 8 percent achieved good results (minimal side effects). Two percent were classified as fair results because of major side effects or failure to effectively eliminate the pain.

Recurrence of Trigeminal Neuralgia

The follow-up period varied from 1 to 10 years. Recurrent pain sufficiently severe to require repeating the procedure developed in 37 (9 percent); 13 (3 percent) had some recurrent pain that was adequately controlled with medication; and 6 (2 percent) had minor recurrent pain that did not require additional medical or surgical treatment.

Recurrent pain after percutaneous rhizotomy of the trigeminal nerve developed more frequently during the early years of our experience. At that time we tried to make minimal lesions, hoping to limit the degree of sensory deficit. The recurrence rate, however, was too high in patients with minimal sensory deficit. Subsequently we advised patients to have lesions that would

Table 70-5. Analysis of Comparative Techniques and Results in 1930 Cases

Technique	Recurrence rate (%)		Patients (%)	Complications (percent of patients)							
	Recurrence (%)	Surgical follow-up (yr)	Relief of pain (%)	Mortality	Ataxia	Corneal ulcer	Facial palsy	Ocular palsy	Motor palsy	Paresthesia	Anesthesia dolorosa
Percutaneous rhizotomy											
Tew											
700 cases	19	6	99	0	0	2	0	2	22	22	1
Sweet[17]											
274 cases	22	4	91	0	0	NR (1 pt blind)	0	0	43	2	1
Mengel[25]											
315 cases	80	12	97	0	0	0	0	NR	50	93	2
Decompression											
Svien[9]											
100 cases	84	4	24	1.0	0	0	NR	0	0	0	0
Transtemporal rhizotomy											
Peet[26]											
553 cases	14	8	95	1.6	NR	15	6	NR	NR	55	4
Posterior fossa rhizotomy											
Dandy[27]											
88 cases	NR	2	100	2.0	NR	0	1	2	0	0	0
Vascular decompression											
Jannetta[13]											
200 cases	4.5	4	98	0.5	2	0	0	1	0	0	0

NR = Not reported.

induce analgesia in the zones of pain and hypalgesia in adjacent painful zones. As a result the frequency with which pain recurred was significantly reduced, but as expected the patients complained more of numbness.

Comparisons of Percutaneous Rhizotomy with other Major Surgical Procedures

Percutaneous rhizotomy can be compared with other major surgical procedures on the basis of complications and incidence of recurrent pain. No attempt was made to compare our results with all series reported; only those that appeared to be representative were selected. Follow-up for percutaneous rhizotomy has not been as long as for intracranial rhizotomy; therefore, recurrence data may not be comparable. Data for mortality and morbidity should be significant, however (Table 70-5).

Analysis indicates that the percutaneous approach is associated with the lowest mortality and morbidity. Recurrence rates compare favorably with those following intracranial rhizotomy, if analogous portions of the root are destroyed in both operations. Facial palsy has been eliminated, but ocular palsy occurs more frequently than in any other major procedure. The incidence of troublesome numbness ranks favorably with that reported for other forms of rhizotomy. This major side effect, however, has been eliminated in decompression procedures. Temporal decompression is associated with a prohibitive recurrence rate but vascular decompression, as described by Jannetta,[13] appears to provide an attractive alternative to percutaneous rhizotomy, particularly in the young patient. As more experience is gained with this method, the incidence of successful pain relief and the freedom from recurrence can be better defined.

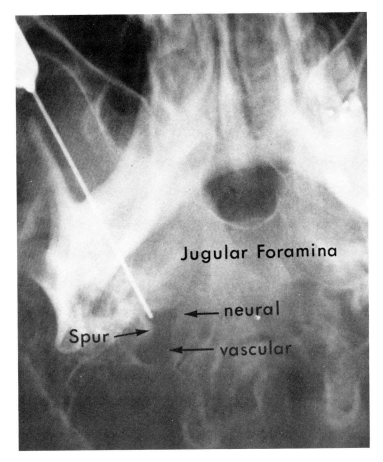

Fig. 70-10. Needle penetrating the neural portion of the jugular foramen. Note the bony spur that divides the neural from the vascular portion.

Percutaneous Coagulation in Other Painful Conditions

The percutaneous approach to the trigeminal nerve has been used to treat several other conditions. In facial pain due to multiple sclerosis (8 cases) and invasive carcinoma (14 cases) the results are promising. The technique has considerable advantages in patients with either condition. In multiple sclerosis, touch sensation and masseter function should be preserved, since pain on the opposite side may require a contralateral procedure. In the debilitated patient with invasive carcinoma, percutaneous coagulation for complete sensory denervation of the face and lasting pain relief is a simple procedure.

Atypical facial pain was treated by percutaneous rhizotomy in 22 patients. In most instances the pain resembled trigeminal neuralgia in some respects, but features of an atypical nature were noted. Several patients with dental neuralgia were included in the group. In all of these cases a preliminary differential xylocaine block was performed to familiarize the patient with sensory deprivation and to determine if pain relief could be achieved. Despite careful appraisal, the results were less satisfactory than those reported by patients treated for typical trigeminal pain.

Long-standing cluster headache (periodic migrainous neuralgia) was treated in 8 patients by denervation of the ophthalmic and maxillary zones. Six of the 8 reported satisfactory relief, and 2 failed to respond. The failures could not be predicted from the history of their disease or the preoperative differential block.

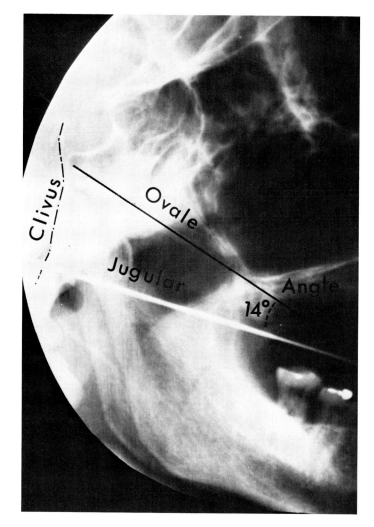

Fig. 70-11. This composite illustration demonstrates the trajectory of approaches to the foramen ovale and jugular foramen. The sagittal plane is identical for both procedures.

Postherpetic neuralgia was treated by electrocoagulation of affected rootlets in 3 patients.
The response was poor in most instances and this procedure is seldom offered in this affliction.

Pain in the Throat and Ear

Pain caused by involvement of the vagus and glossopharyngeal nerves was treated in 11 patients by percutaneous electrocoagulation of the nerve rootlets in the jugular foramen. Nine of
the 11 patients had intractable pain caused by invasive tumors and the remaining 2 had idiopathic neuralgia but were too debilitated to undergo intracranial section of the glossopharyngeal
and vagus nerves.

The technique used to place an electrode in the neural portion of the jugular foramen was
learned serendipitiously, when an electrode accidentally entered the posterior fossa through the
jugular foramen in 2 early cases being treated for trigiminal neuralgia. During subsequent studies a minor change in electrode placement was made so that the neural portion of the jugular canal (Fig. 70-10) is consistently penetrated. The needle is directed posteriorly, 14° from the angle
used to penetrate the foramen ovale; the sagittal direction is unchanged (Fig. 70-11). Stimulation

provokes pain in the ear and throat. Coughing and contraction of the sternocleidomastoid muscle may be induced.

Pain in 8 patients with invasive carcinoma was relieved until their death 4 to 11 months later. Two patients with idiopathic vagoglossopharyngeal neuralgia were relieved of pain, but vocal cord paralysis was produced in each. The procedure is not advisable in patients with intact vocal cord function, who can tolerate intracranial section of the glossopharyngeal and the upper fibers of the vagus nerves.

Conclusion

Percutaneous rhizotomy of the trigeminal nerve is a safe procedure that can produce long-standing relief from intractable trigeminal neuralgia. The incidence of recurrent pain is greater than that observed after intracranial section of posterior rootlets, but the lower morbidity rate makes the procedure more acceptable to most patients. Postoperative sensory complaints are similar to those associated with intracranial rhizotomy but can be nearly eliminated by preserving touch perception. Extratrigeminal complications are rare and reversible in most instances.

Percutaneous rhizotomy is applicable in selected types of facial pain other than typical trigeminal neuralgia. A technique for eliminating pain caused by neoplastic invasion of the trigeminal, vagus, and glossopharyngeal nerves is described.

Percutaneous rhizotomy is a destructive procedure. It is not the ideal treatment for facial pain. Therefore a more acceptable nondestructive form of therapy continues to be our goal.

REFERENCES

1. Hartley F: Intracranial neurectomy of the second and third divisions of the fifth nerve. *NY J Med* 55:317–319, 1892
2. Krause F: Resection des Trigeminus innerhalb der Schädelhöhle. *Arch Klin Chir 41*:821–832, 1892
3. Krause F: Entfernung des Ganglion Gasseri und des Central daron gelegnen trigemenusstammes. *Dtsch Med Wochenschi 19:*341, 1893
4. Horsley V: Remarks on the various surgical procedures devised for the relief or cure of trigeminal neuralgia. *Br Med J 2*:1139, 1891
5. Spiller WG, Frazier CH: The division of the sensory root of the trigeminus for the relief of tic douloureux. *Univ Pa Med Bull 14*:341, 1901
6. Spiller WG, Frazier CH: An experimental study of the regeneration of the posterior spinal root. *Univ Pa Med Bull 16*:126–128, 1903
7. Shelden CH, Pudenz RH, Freshwater D, et al: Compression rather than decompression for trigeminal neuralgia. *J Neurosurg 12*:123–126, 1955
8. Taarnhøj P: Decompression of the trigeminal root. *J Neurosurg 11*:299–305, 1954
9. Svien HS, Love JG: Results of decompression operation for trigeminal neuralgia four years plus after operation. *J Neurosurg 16*:653–663, 1959
10. Gardner WS: Concerning the mechanisms of trigeminal neuralgia and hemifacial spasm. *J Neurosurg 19*:947–958, 1962
11. Harris W: Alcohol injection of the gasserian ganglion for trigeminal neuralgia. *Lancet 1*:218–221, 1912
12. Harris W: An analysis of 1433 cases of paroxysmal trigeminal neuralgia (trigeminal-tic) and the end results of gasserian alcohol injection. *Brain 63*:209–224, 1940
13. Janetta P: Microsurgical approach to the trigeminal nerve for tic douloureux, in *Progress in Neurological Surgery,* vol. 7. Basel, Karger, 1976, pp 180–200
14. Dandy WE: Concerning the cause of trigeminal neuralgia. *Am J Surg 24*:447–455, 1934
15. Kirschner M: Elektrocoagulation des ganglion gasseri. *Zentralbl Chir 47*:2841–2843, 1932
16. Kirschner M: Zur behandlund der Trigeminusneuralgie. *Med Wochenschr 89*:235–239, 1942
17. Sweet WH, Wepsic SG: Controlled thermocoagulation of trigeminal ganglion and results for differential destruction of pain fibers. *J Neurosurg 39*:143–156, 1974
18. White JC, Sweet WH: *Pain and the Neurosurgeon.* Springfield, IL, Charles C Thomas, 1969
19. Letcher FS, Goldring S: The effect of radiofrequency current and heat on peripheral nerve action potential in the cat. *J Neurosurg 29*:42–47, 1968
20. Brodkey JS, et al: Reversible heat lesions with radiofrequency current. *J Neurosurg 27*:49–53, 1964

21. Härtel F: Ueber die intracranielle Injektionsbehandlung der Trigeminusneuralgie. *Med Klinik* *10*:582–584, 1914

22. Tator CH, Rowed DW: Fluoroscopy of foramen ovale as an aid to thermocoagulation of the gasserian ganglion. *J Neurosurg 44*:254–259, 1976

23. Rish BL: Cerebrovascular accident after percutaneous thermocoagulation of the trigeminal ganglion. *J Neurosurg 44*:376–377, 1976

24. Gonzalez G, Onofrio BM, Ken FW: Vasodilator system of the face. *J Neurosurg 42*:696–703, 1975

25. Mengel J, Piotrowsin W, Penzholz H: Long-term results of gasserian ganglion electrocoagulation. *J Neurosurg 42*:140–143, 1975

26. Peet MM, Schneider RD: Trigeminal neuralgia. *J Neurosurg 9*:367–377, 1952

27. Dandy WE: Operation for cure of tic douloureux; partial section of the sensory root at the pons. *Arch Surg 18*:687–734, 1929

28. Howe JF, Loeser JD, Black RG: Percutaneous radiofrequency trigeminal gangliolysis in the treatment of tic douloureux. *West J Med 124*:351–356, 1976

29. Nugent GR, Berry B: Trigeminal neuralgia treated by differential percutaneous radiofrequency coagulation of the gasserian ganglion. *J Neurosurg 40*:517–523, 1974

30. Onofrio BM: Radiofrequency percutaneous gasserian ganglion lesions: Results in 140 patients with trigeminal pain. *J Neurosurg 42*:132–139, 1975

31. Siegfried J: 500 percutaneous thermocoagulations of the gasserian ganglion for trigeminal pain. *Surg Neurol 8*:126–131, 1977

32. Sweet WH, Wepsic JG: Controlled thermocoagulation of trigeminal ganglion and rootlets for differential destruction of pain fibers. Part I. Trigeminal neuralgia. *J Neurosurg 40*:143–156, 1974

33. Tew JM, Keller JT: The Treatment of Trigeminal Neuralgia by Percutaneous Radiofrequency Technique. In Keener EB (ed): *Clinical Neurosurgery,* Baltimore, The Williams & Wilkins Company, 1977, pp 557–578

34. Burchiel KJ, Steege TD, Howe JF, Loeser JD: Comparison of percutaneous radiofrequency gangliolysis and microvascular decompression for the surgical management of tic douloureux. *Neurosurgery 9*:111–119, 1981

35. Apfelbaum RI: A comparison of percutaneous radiofrequency trigeminal neurolysis and microvascular decompression of the trigeminal nerve for the treatment of tic doulourex. *Neurosurgery 1*:16–21, 1977

36. van Loveren H, Tew JM, Keller JT, Nurre MA: A 10-year experience in the treatment of trigeminal neuralgia: a comparison of percutaneous stereotaxic rhizotomy and posterior fossa exploration. *J Neurosurg* (in press)

Commentary by William H. Sweet

Tew[1] as well as Lazorthes and Verdie[2] have described their method and results in the management of both idiopathic vagoglossopharyngeal neuralgia and cancer pain in the area of the ninth and tenth nerves.

It has been much more difficult for me to place an electrode tip properly for this objective than to get it into Meckel's cave for the management of trigeminal pain. The tip must lie in or just below the pars nervosa of the jugular foramen, preferably in its medial part where the upper vagal and glossopharyngeal fibers typically lie. Possibly this account may help the novice.

My principal difficulty has been in identifying with certainty the pars nervosa, and I have needed to use fluoroscopy with a standing image that my neuroradiologic colleague Dr. Paul New and I can study, as well as films for this purpose. The bony spur intruding into the jugular foramen, which separates the larger lateral opening for the jugular bulb from the smaller medial opening for the ninth, tenth, and eleventh nerves, is the key to orientation. On the way in to this destination one would prefer to miss the trigeminal third division and especially the internal carotid artery below its entrance into the petrous portion of the temporal bone. Figures 70-12A and B, views of a skull, show the black electrode shaft in proper position passing medial to both the mandibular branch and the artery. To position the electrode properly, it is best inserted only about 5 mm lateral to the labial commissure. Note that the hypoglossal foramen is further posterior in the same trajectory. In Figure 70-12B the skull is rotated a little more to the opposite side in order to make the critical bony spur more evident. I recommend deliberately aiming more medial than the pars nervosa at first, since medial to there lies a broad expanse of the undersurface of the body of the sphenoid bone, which can be struck harmlessly. Figure 70-13A illustrates the preliminary position of the electrode tip medial to the pars nervosa on bone. Figures 70-13B, C, and D are different projections in progressively increasing flexion, taken without changing the position of the electrode at the site where the successful lesions were made. They illustrate the fact that once the jugular foramen is spotted a variety of projections will show it. Viewed laterally, the electrode shaft was in line with the upper border of the tragus. Viewed in the sagittal plane, it was pointing in a line 9 mm lateral to the medial border of the lacrimal caruncle—representative of the measurements for the proper position. In this patient, who had vagoglossopharyngeal neuralgia, the electrode had to be placed in the lateral rather than the medial portion of the pars nervosa in order to secure a buzzing in the side of the throat and in front of the upper part of the pinna at 0.17 V of a square-wave signal at 50/sec. At 41°C there was burning in the ear canal. In order to go by the lateral pterygoid plate, the electrode may also have to pass below the middle of the foramen ovale. To my surprise, this usually has evoked no sensation referable to the third trigeminal division.

Because of the reports of Lazorthes[2] of 3 cases of temporary vocal cord paralysis and dysphagia and of Tew[1] of 2 cases of vocal cord paralysis, I have sought to make these lesions in smaller increments and with the patient less obtunded than for trigeminal lesions. Hoarseness and swallowing then can be checked during making of the lesion as well as after it has been produced. The patient in Figure 70-13 is an example of this. During the two hours of intermittent radiofrequency heating, the temperature of the 20-gauge electrode with a 5-mm bare tip was finally kept at 105°–107°C for 3 minutes, during which time no brevital was required. After this most unusual degree of heating, the patient had hypalgesia of the ipsilateral soft palate and oral pharynx but not of the tonsillar fossa. Not until the next day did some slight hoarseness and dysphagia develop. Some hoarseness, if she did much talking, and modest dysphagia persisted for 6 months. The pain remains relieved at $2^1/2$ years, although she has recovered normalgesia on pinprick testing. No hoarseness or dysphagia occurred in 2 other patients monitored in the same fashion during the lesions.

It may not be necessary to produce sustained hypalgesia in order to give lasting relief in

Massachusetts General Hospital, Boston, Massachusetts

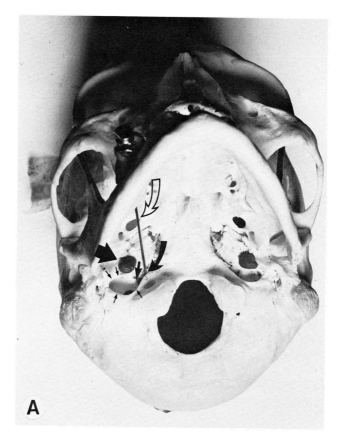

Fig. 70-12.   Basal views of the skull with an electrode tip in the
pars nervosa of the jugular foramen. **A.** Slight rotation of the skull away from the side of the electrode in the head-extended position. Open curved
arrow: electrode shaft overlying the medial corner
of the foramen ovale. Closed curved arrow: electrode tip in medial corner of the pars nervosa.
Large black arrowhead: internal carotid artery.
Small black arrowhead: bony spur separating the
pars venosa for the jugular venous bulb from the
smaller pars nervosa for the ninth, tenth, and eleventh nerves and associated ganglia. Tiny arrows:
margins of pars venosa. **B.** More marked rotation
of the skull with no extension of the head. Arrows
are as in Figure 70-12A. The bony spur is more obvious.

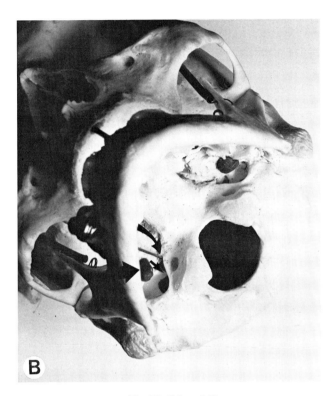

Fig. 70-12 (cont'd.)

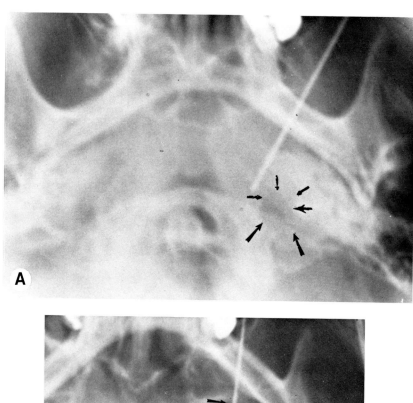

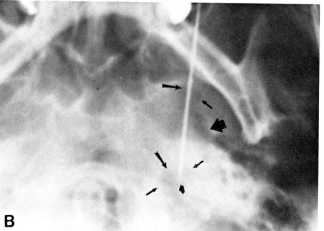

Fig. 70-13.   **A.** An electrode tip against the base of the body of the sphenoid bone medial to the pars nervosa of the foramen. **B.C.** and **D.** The electrode tip in position for lesion in the lateral part of the pars nervosa. Three projections in progressively less extension. **B.** Shaft overlies approximately the middle of the foramen ovale. Arrows in **A** and **B** outline the pars nervosa; the two anterior arrows in **B** indicate the medial and lateral margins of the foramen ovale. Large arrowhead: opening for internal carotid artery. Arrowheads in **C** and **D** outline visible margins of both the pars nervosa and the pars venosa, with small arrow pointing to bony spur that divides the two portions.

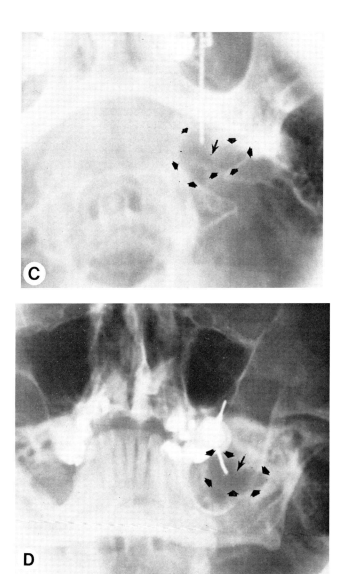

Fig. 70-13 (cont'd.)

cases of vagoglossopharyngeal neuralgia. Long-term follow-up is required to answer this question.

Isamat et al.[3] have added the logical, constant use of electrocardiography and intra-arterial blood pressure monitoring. They interpret any bradycardia or hypertension during radiofrequency heating as an undesirable vagal effect and select for their lesion the highest temperature just before the onset of that effect. Five lesion sessions with 4 of their patients with idiopathic vagoglossopharyngeal neuralgia provided relief for up to 2.8 years of follow-up in which normal phonation and swallowing were maintained in all 4.

REFERENCES

1. Tew JM: Percutaneous rhizotomy in the treatment of intractable facial pain (trigeminal, glossopharyngeal, and vagal nerves), Schmidek HH, Sweet WH: *Current Techniques in Operative Neurosurgery.* Grune & Stratton, New York, 1977
2. Lazorthes Y, Verdie J-C: Radiofrequency coagulation of the petrous ganglion in glossopharyngeal neuralgia. *Neurosurgery 4*:512–516, 1979
3. Isamat F, Ferrán E, Acebes JJ: Selective percutaneous thermocoagulation rhizotomy in essential glossopharyngeal neuralgia. *J Neurosurg* 55:575–580, 1981

CHAPTER 71

Retrogasserian Glycerol Injection as Treatment for Trigeminal Neuralgia

William H. Sweet   Charles E. Poletti

Rationale and Results of Håkanson

IN AUGUST 1975, S. Håkanson and L. Leksell sought to focus photons more precisely on the Gasserian ganglion in their trial of such therapy in the treatment of trigeminal neuralgia.[1] In order to define exactly the locus of the posterior edge of the ganglion, they injected tantalum dust into the tiny trigeminal cerebrospinal fluid (CSF) cistern (Meckel's cave), selecting the hyperbaric substance pure glycerol as the presumably innocuous agent in which to suspend the tantalum. To their surprise the patients stopped complaining of their paroxysmal provokable facial pains. Hence, instead of irradiating the Gasserian ganglion with photons, Håkanson has, in the ensuing 6-year period, developed the technique for injecting sterile 100% glycerol directly into the trigeminal cistern. This has become the treatment of choice for trigeminal neuralgia at the famous Karolinska Sjukhuset in Stockholm. He reported 130 such cases at the Third World Congress on Pain in Edinburgh on September 11, 1981.[2] For a detailed account of his first 75 cases, the reader is referred elsewhere.[3] Following an injection of 0.15–0.4 ml glycerol, which Håkanson carried out under local anesthesia, all but 4 of his first 100 patients have become free of the paroxysmal pain. In about half of them "a remarkably uniform latent period of about 5 days was required" before this occurred. In fact, in a few of them the pains at first were more severe. There is only infrequently such a latent period in a successful radiofrequency (RF) heat lesions. At his follow-up of these first 100 patients 1 to 6 years later, 65 were pain-free, 4 had incomplete relief, and *the pains had recurred in 31*. A reinjection rendered 12 of these pain-free; the recurrent symptoms were mild enough to be controlled by drugs in 19; 4 had further surgical therapy. In his first 75 cases the recurrent pains developed in those in whom an average of only 0.16 ml was injected; those who remained pain-free averaged 0.21 ml. He finds on clinical examination no significant sensory loss—indeed none even in quantitative measurements of tactile or thermal thresholds. He has seen no untoward effects such as painful dysesthesia, anesthesia dolorosa, corneal anesthesia, or involvement of other cranial nerves.

Neurosurgical Service, Massachusetts General Hospital and Harvard University Medical School, Boston, Massachusetts

We wish to thank the Neuro-Research Foundation for its support during the preparation of this manuscript.

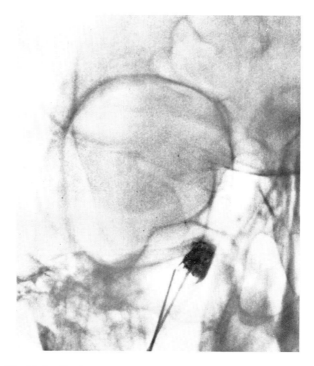

Fig. 71-1. Sagittal view of the right side of the skull with two needles through the foramen ovale, illustrating Håkanson's method of leaving in position one 22-gauge needle that has failed to yield CSF from the tirgeminal cistern. The first needle was too far lateral. Metrizamide was injected into the more medial needle within the cistern. (From Håkanson S: *Neurosurgery 9*:638–646, 1981. With permission.)

Technique of Håkanson

Håkanson's procedure for achieving these results is as follows:

The patient is seated in a rotatable chair with radiography available both by fluoroscopy and films. Premedication is with 1 ml oxicon with 1 ml scopolamine plus 5 mg droperidol (Dridol). Half this dose was used for elder or debilitated patients. Local anesthesia only was given to 74 of the first 75 patients. A 22-gauge lumbar puncture needle, outside diameter 0.7 mm, penetrates the skin well lateral to the labial commissure. Cerebrospinal fluid must be obtained. If fluoroscopy and films show the needle tip to be approximately in the correct position but no CSF appears, he leaves that needle in position and places another needle in what he thinks is a more correct spot. Figure 71-1 illustrates a position that is too lateral for the original needle. Usually the shaft must go through the medial half of the foramen ovale. This film also illustrates the next step of his procedure, in which he injects less than 1 ml of concentrated metrizamide (300 mg I/ml). Fluoroscopy shows the contrast medium filling the cistern and running back through the porus trigemini into the cerebellopontine angle. The relationship of the CSF space with the rootlets to the subdural space in the cisterna trigeminalis and to the subarachnoid space beneath the temporal lobe is illustrated by Håkanson's diagram in Figure 71-2. Films taken after the injection of the metrizamide may demonstrate that the needle is in the subarachnoid space below the temporal lobe or in the subdural space of the cistern (Fig. 71-3A). Placement in the subdural space is more evident as the metrizamide passes through the porus trigemini and lines the subarachnoid space behind the clivus (Fig. 71-3B). He found that previous open trigeminal operations in the middle cranial fossa often damaged the trigeminal cistern so that the metrizamide would leak out of it. Figure 71-4 shows the contrast medium lying medial to the needle tip in the cistern and

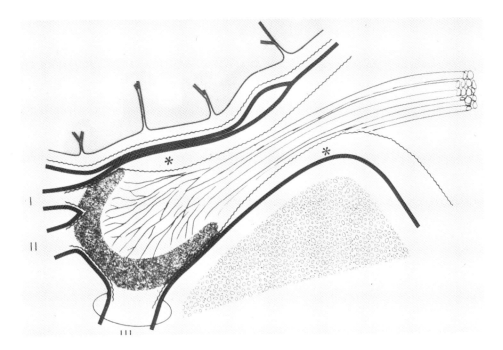

Fig. 71-2. Diagram by Håkanson illustrating the possibility of the subdural space of the trigeminal cistern being expanded by injection into it of contrast material. Asterisks
in this space above and below wavering lines indicate arachnoid membrane and
within solid lines indicate dura. Subarachnoid and subdural spaces below temporal
lobe are also indicated. (From Håkanson S:*Neurosurgery* 9:638–646, 1981. With permission.)

below one cluster of metal clips marking the site of the previous open operation. When, as occurred rarely, he is unable to enter the cistern, he makes a selective thermal lesion. Having verified the proper position of the needle tip, he then empties the metrizamide into the posterior
fossa by removing the syringe and extending the patient's head for several minutes. If the patient
has no third-division trigger zone, however, he seeks to leave a little of the heavy metrizamide
(sp gr 1.329) at the anterior end of the cistern. Then, with the patient sitting and the head markedly flexed, the metrizamide protects the third-division rootlets from the lighter glycerol (sp gr
1.242), which will in turn form a layer below the CSF (sp gr 1.007). Although he adjusts the
amount of glycerol to the volume of the cistern, he estimates from the metrizamide picture that
the total amount of glycerol that has been injected into the cistern is only 0.2–0.4 ml. Figures 71-
5A, B, and C illustrate the marked variation in size and configuration of the normal cistern. (In
one of his cases the metrizamide film revealed a small benign tumor here.) In cases with first- or
second-division neuralgia he injects up to .25 ml. The needle shaft contains about 0.05 ml. He
does not examine facial sensibility during the procedure. Once an injection is complete the patient is kept sitting in bed with the head flexed for another hour in order to keep the glycerol
mainly in the cistern. He has mixed tantalum dust with the glycerol before injection in most
cases so that later films show the exact site of the cistern in order to facilitate a future injection
therein.

Our Results

The senior author, having had the benefit of special tutorials from Håkanson in December
1978, carried out this procedure in 6 difficult patients in early 1979—3 with trigeminal neuralgia
and 3 with atypical facial neuralgia. Only 1 of the former 3 procedures was a success. A second

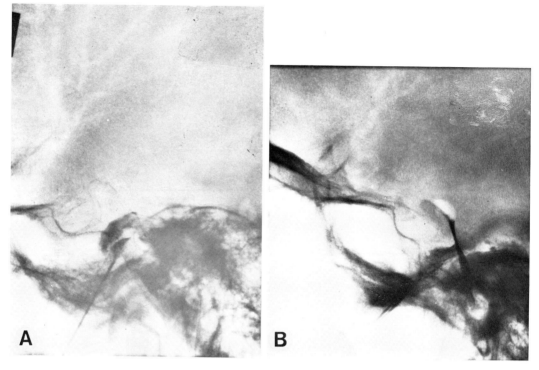

Fig. 71-3.   Lateral views of the middle third of the base of the skull. **A.** The metrizamide lies in two zones— one above and one below the rootlet zone. That this was in fact a subdural placement is more conclusively shown in Figure 71-3B in which following extension of the head the metrizamide is seen closely applied to the full length of the clivus.

patient with unusually agonizing paroxysms totally uncontrolled by his tegretol became so much worse after an injection of 0.8 cc of glycerol that we made a successful RF heat lesion on his third post-injection day. The third patient with trigeminal neuralgia remained greatly distressed by the dysesthesias in his analgesic but not anesthetic face following an RF lesion by one of us in 1972 for first- and second-division trigger zones. In March of 1979, with recurrence of his paroxysms despite patchy analgesia of V2, he was given 0.3 cc of glycerol. This produced complete analgesia of V2, and hypalgesia of V1 and V3, but gauze was localized throughout all these areas. Although the paroxysms of pain are gone, 30 months later he still has major dysesthesias along with significant depression of mood.

Only 1 of the 3 patients with atypical facial neuralgia was relieved, in her case for 6 months. An RF lesion in August 1979 has kept her pain-free for the 2 years since then.

We elected to wait for further results from Håkanson. After he kindly sent us his detailed account in December 1980, we proceeded to select another 25 patients in whom relief without dysesthesias or sensory loss would be a special boon. Trigeminal neuralgia was the diagnosis in 24, of whom 5 had long periods of constant pain as well as the more distressing provokable paroxysms. The 25th patient had the constant pain often seen with posttraumatic facial neuralgia. These 6 would have been especially likely to complain of dysesthesias after an RF lesion. Multiple sclerosis was the cause of the trigeminal pain in 7 other patients. In these patients there is an increased likelihood of bilaterality and atypical features. Attacks were occurring on the second side in 6 patients; such patients are particularly likely to be grateful for completely normal touch after a lesion on the second side.

Because we found a major though often temporary sensory loss to pin and touch after the glycerol, we were led to modify the technique. In only 5 or our 31 patients was there no significant analgesia to pin during injection or in the hour thereafter. An early analgesia rapidly faded

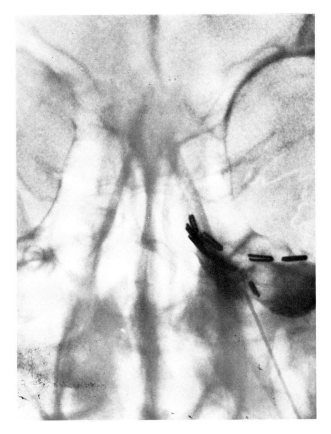

Fig. 71-4. Sagittal view of the skull near the midline. The numerous metal clips mark the site of a previous open
operation to "decompress" trigeminal rootlets. The
metrizamide has flowed medially away from the tip
of the needle (and inferior to the medial group of
clips). (Courtesy of Dr. Håkanson.)

within 24 hours in 6 other patients, but analgesia or hypalgesia of 5/10 or worse persisted for longer periods in one or more divisions of the trigger zones in 16 patients. The grading represents the patient's assessment of the intensity of pin or touch based on 10 for the corresponding contralateral normal point. This degree of loss to pin prick persisted as well in 14 patients in divisions with no trigger area. Four of these 14 patients did not have this degree of loss in the divisions of their trigger zones. We do not regard the losses to pin prick as a disadvantage, however. In fact, our only failures in the 27 patients with trigeminal neuralgia occurred in the 3 who had no analgesic areas during or shortly after injection. In the second and third patients, we observed them for 9 and 14 days respectively before proceeding to a successful RF lesion.

The loss to touch has been much less. Only 1 patient had extensive anesthesia which was in V1 and V2 and is persisting at 4½ months. Only 5 had persistent hypesthetic areas in which only finger touch could be localized.

Despite the excellent preservation of touch and the lower deficit to pin prick than we seek with RF lesions, annoying sensations or painful dysesthesia have not been entirely absent. There have been 9 such patients; 1 has already been mentioned. In 4 more the complaints remain disturbing, but in the remaining 4 they are milder or disappeared in a few weeks. In 7 of the 31 patients we had previously made a trigeminal RF lesion. In 4 the pains were recurrent on the same side after recovery of much algesic sensation to pin; in 3 there was new pain on the other side. Three of the patients found the post glycerol sensations preferable to those after the RF lesion,

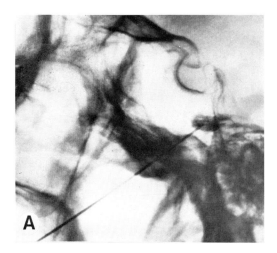
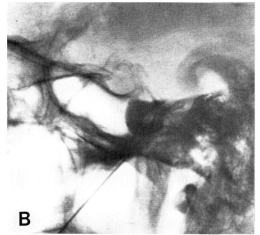
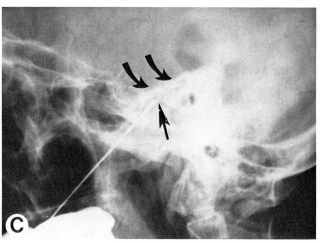

Fig. 71-5.   Lateral views of the middle one-third of the base of the skull showing **(A)** a small cistern, **(B)**, a large cistern, and **(C)** an elongated cistern with irregular borders (the straight-shafted arrow points to the tip of the needle electrode; the curved-shafted arrows point to the top of the metrizamide shadow in the trigeminal cistern). our case Ellen B. All normal variations. **A** is from Håkanson S: *Neurosurgery* 9:638–646, 1981, with permission. **B** is courtesy of Dr. Håkanson.)

but in 3 others the reverse was true. The seventh patient, whose pain was on the other side, still had a denser loss on the side of her earlier heat lesion but emphatically said that neither side bothered her at all.

A pronounced loss of corneal sensation has persisted in 5 patients; in 2 patients cotton is not felt at all at 9 and 20 weeks. The other 3 have recovered to a 1–2/10 level at 3 weeks to 3 months. The 2 with persistent corneal anesthesia both had first-division trigger zones, and one was already blind in the painful eye, so we injected her with the full 0.4 ml of glycerol. Of 5 more patients with first-division trigger zones, 4 have become pain-free after injections that reduced corneal sensation modestly to 6–8/10 upon examination weeks to 4 months later. No patient has developed keratitis. We regard the procedure as most gratifying in this difficult group.

Another encouraging feature of the results was the elimination of the constant as well as paroxysmal component in 4 of the 5 patients with both of these features. (The fifth patient, who had both components, was one of our 3 failures). It was also gratifying to have all aspects of the facial pain relieved in each of the 7 patients with multiple sclerosis.

Pains persisted briefly in 7 of the 24 patients who at once or later became virtually free of pain. These pains were usually much less severe than those before injection. They lasted for 2, 3, 5, and 17 days, 6 weeks, and "a few weeks" in 6 patients. The seventh patient continues at 6 weeks to have an occasional momentary stab on biting. This feature has, however, convinced us not to recommend the procedure for patients who have come from a distance, unless they wish to accept this hazard.

Biological Effects of Glycerol

Because of the discrepancies between our earlier results and those of Håkanson, we were led to examine in some detail the articles on the behavior of tissues exposed to glycerol. The relevant points have been developed in detail by Sweet, Poletti, and Macon.[4] In 1949 cryobiology was strikingly advanced by the discovery that cell suspensions could be successfully preserved at cryogenic temperatures over long periods if they were pretreated with glycerol.[5] Scores of articles describe the tactics for storing and restoring to effective use a great variety of cells, including spermatozoa of many species, which can then be artificially inseminated. This endocellular cryoprotectant effect, its chemical composition as half a molecule of glucose, its metabolism as a carbohydrate food, and its presence in tiny concentrations in the normal bloodstream have apparently led to the assumption that glycerol is innocuous. Thus Maher used it as the hyperbaric vehicle to aid in bringing phenol to appropriate intrathecal sites.[6]

The studies of Nathan and Sears seemed also to point to a protective rather than a toxic effect of glycerol.[7] Studying compound action potentials in the spinal roots of cats after stimulation of the relevant peripheral nerve, they found that an 0.5% aqueous solution of phenol had a more destructive effect than bathing the tissue in 7.5% or even 10% phenol dissolved in glycerol. Consequently, glycerol was a logical choice of Leksell and Håkanson when they wished to introduce tantalum dust into Meckel's cave.

This "food" injected intramuscularly or subcutaneously is amazingly toxic, however. Acute hemolytic crises are produced in rats and rabbits by as little as 0.2 cc pure glycerol/kg of body weight.[8] Its toxicity is evidenced further by its production of myoglobinuria, precipitating acute renal failure after intramuscular injection in rats. One milliliter of 50% glycerol/100 g into the muscles of the hind limb of a rat is so consistently provocative of this effect that the method has been used frequently to study acute renal failure.[9] Moreover, glycerol must be markedly diluted to be effective as a cryophylactic agent. A variety of cellular properties such as migration of neutrophils,[10] growth of chick embryo fibroblasts,[11] and conduction velocity and action potential of frog sciatic nerves[12] are all dramatically impaired upon exposure of the tissue to concentrations of glycerol above 5%. Baxter and Schacherl found that pure glycerol, 0.2 ml, injected intrathecally at the midthoracic level in cats had about the same physiologic and morphologic injurious effect on the spinal cord, nerve roots, and blood vessels as the same amount of absolute alcohol.[13] Both substances caused paralysis of the tail and slight weakness of the hind legs. The effects were, however, much less intense than those seen after injection of 7.5 % or 10% phenol in glycerol.

We cite these reports as evidence that our observations regarding the sensory loss after the introduction of glycerol into Meckel's cave may be representative of a larger series.

Our Technique

We have presented our results before our technique in order to justify the minor changes we have made in the procedure of Håkanson.

Our initial steps are identical with those we use for making a lesion by RF heating. Following an intravenous injection, usually of 2 cc of Innovar (.05 fentanyl and 2.5 mg droperidol/cc), we make our preliminary intradermal injections of 2% lidocaine 3.0 cm lateral to the labial com-

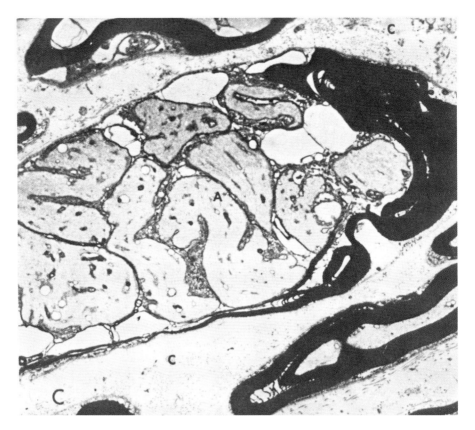

Fig. 71-6. Electron micrograph of the trigeminal root in trigeminal neuralgia (9000 X). Biopsy at retrogasserian rhizotomy in patient who had had no previous procedure on the trigeminal nerve. Note the enormously hypertrophic axis cylinder whose size and tortuosity suggest a plexiform microneuroma. Note that not only is all the myelin confined to one end of the huge fiber, but also that the Schwann cell cytoplasm between the axonal folds is degenerating. More normal myelinated fibers are depicted above and below the abnormal one. (From Beaver DL: *J Neurosurg 26*:145, 1967. With permission.)

missure and also subcutaneously in the upper temple for our ground electrode. The patient is given an injection of 20–30 mg Brevital intravenously to put him to sleep. The 20-gauge needle electrode then is inserted so that if we are unable to enter CSF in the trigeminal cistern we can make an RF lesion. We have had to make an RF lesion in only 1 patient for whom a glycerol injection was planned. By electrical stimulation at 50 cycles/sec using 1 sigma pulses usually at .08 to .2 V, and by gentle RF heating usually to 44°–50°, we elicit a reference of sensation to a small part of the face. The electrode then is adjusted so that the reference of sensation is confined to the lowest division harboring a trigger zone, i.e., the third division if both the second and third divisions contain trigger zones. (The glycerol penetrates more readily posteromedially toward first-division rootlets than it does anterolaterally toward those of the third division.) In our first cases we then injected concentrated metrizamide as described by Håkanson. Having confirmed that the metrizamide was in Meckel's cave in every one of the first 17 patients, we stopped doing this, because at this location injection of .05–0.1 cc of glycerol has given rise to some focal sensation. In the last 14 patients on whom we did not use metrizamide, every one has developed a significant sensory loss shortly after the injection of the glycerol. We conclude that the injection was into the CSF of Meckel's cave and not subdurally or into the subtemporal subarachnoid space. The focal sensation was nearly always pain, but in a few patients there were nonpainful paresthesias. In 7 patients the pain was so severe that we injected another 20–40 mg of Brevital

IV at once. One patient had such severe ipsilateral facial pain coming 14 minutes after the completion of the injection that he thought he was dying. Intense attacks of their clinical pain were provoked in 2 others by an increment of glycerol. These episodes have led us to keep the needle of a syringe loaded with Brevital lying in the sidearm of the intravenous line, ready for instant use. Utilization of the responses to electrical and chemical stimulation was helped, since in 20 patients the pain at the first glycerol injection was in the same division as that induced electrically. More importantly, analgesia resulted in 23 of the patients in the same trigeminal division as the pain on glycerol injection. The analgesia or hypalgesia spread to other divisions, as well as that or those with the trigger zones, in 19 of the 23 patients. Often the deficit was not as extensive or marked as in the division first affected. Such a spread of deficit was at times predictable because of a preceding spread of pain to these areas during the latter part of the injection. Only in 3 of our first cases did we exceed the Håkanson maximum of 0.4 cc of glycerol. In 2 patients without first-division trigger zones the first bit of glycerol produced first-division pain. Accordingly, the electrode was withdrawn so that subsequent increments did not cause pain in this division and severe corneal deficit to touch was avoided. We have had more trouble maintaining some hypalgesia in the third division than in the other two divisions, even though we have kept the patient's head well flexed and leaning to the side of the pain. Nausea has been enough of a problem with the patient sitting with the head flexed during the glycerol injection that we give them 5 to 10 mg Compazine intramuscularly before raising them to the sitting position. In 1 early patient the flabby facial tissues permitted the needle to slip clear out of the foramen ovale when she sat up with her head flexed. We now have one person maintain a grip on the needle electrode for the entire time until the injection is complete.

Sensory testing to pin prick is carried out after the first 0.2 cc or earlier if first-division pain is described. In 1 patient with only a first-division trigger zone, analgesia of skin and cornea developed after 0.2 cc. We injected no more and she had recovered much corneal sensation to cotton in a few hours, but remains pain-free at 6 months. Likewise, in other patients who develop first-division loss after 0.3 cc we terminate the injection.

In general, we prefer to place the needle tip, possibly replace it during injection, and decide how much glycerol to inject based on the responses of the conscious, cooperating patients. We keep them cooperative by administering appropriate amounts of intravenous medication.

Suggested Mechanism of Action of Glycerol

Since Håkanson's patients did not lose facial sensation, he has proposed that the glycerol preferentially destroys the abnormal large fibers that have lost their myelin in patchy fashion. The electron micrographs of Beaver (Fig. 71 6) show that the Schwann cell sheaths are also degenerated in some of these fibers, thus exposing them more directly to the toxic glycerol than even the normal unmyelinated fibers. Hellstrand, Håkanson, and Meyerson found in the nerves of the normal frog and cat that all components of the compound action potential were reduced roughly equally by glycerol.[14] We have recorded specifically from the rootlets in the divisions with trigger zones in these patients with trigeminal neuralgia. Macon, Poletti, and Sweet have found that the A-delta epsilon and the later C waves may be markedly reduced after the glycerol, coincident with development of analgesia and absence of pain on stimulation, especially in patients who tolerate kindly markedly painful as well as nonpainful stimuli to electrodes in the skin. On the other hand, the A-beta deflections may show less loss or even no reduction.[15] Figure 71-7 illustrates this feature in our most convincing tracing after glycerol.

It is our impression that both glycerol and RF heating destroy preferentially the poorly myelinated portions of the trigeminal nerve rootlets, both the normal and the abnormal. The differential destruction of the erratically demyelinated abnormal large fibers may be crucially desirable in this disorder. Such abnormal large fibers have not been described in posttraumatic, postherpetic, or atypical facial neuralgia, or in periodic migrainous neuralgia. This may be the

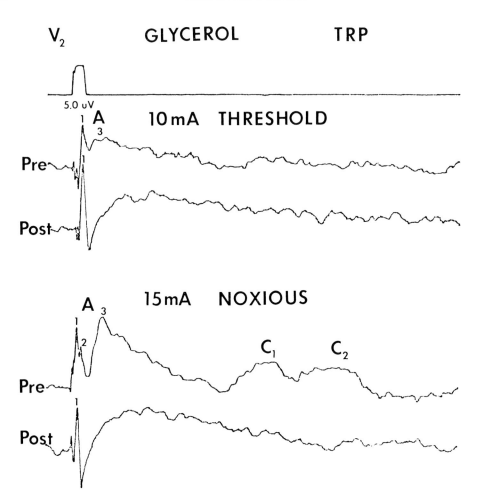

Fig. 71-7. Trigeminal root potential (TRP) in second trigeminal division obtained before and after injection of glycerol. Electrical potentials evoked in trigeminal rootlets of a pa-tient with second- and third-division typical trigeminal neuralgia. The recording electrode was a 20-gauge needle in the rootlets so placed that either a tingle or heat in the cheek occurred when either a square-wave stimulus at 50 cycles, .08V, or ra-diofrequency heat to 49° was applied at that electrode. At this site the first 0.1 cc glycerol caused pain in the cheek, nose, and around the eye. These tracings were obtained upon electrical stimulation at the stated milliamperage applied to plati-num needle electrodes about 1 cm apart penetrating the skin of the cheek. Tracings at other intensities of stimulation confirmed the results of these tracings. The post-operative tracings were made some minutes after the injection of 0.3 cc glycerol had produced dense hypalgesia to analgesia of V2 and complete analgesia of V1. A densely hypalgesic cheek at the platinum electrode sites at that time had become analgesic the following day. The deflections labeled A3 were presumed to be due to fibers in the A delta-epsilon range of diameters. We measured them to be conduct-ing at 9.9 m/sec. Those labeled C1 and C2 were conducting at 1.7 and 1.3 m/sec re-spectively. Ten mA stimuli to the platinum electrodes in the cheek were at or just below the threshold for any painful quality to the sensation. Fifteen mA was very painful, but the patient tolerated it for the 41 seconds required to average the re-sponses to 256 stimuli. At 15 mA, the A3 peak increased enormously and the new double C wave deflection was unequivocal, correlated we suggest with activation of fibers for pain in these two size ranges. Postoperatively, none of these stimuli was painful and the A3, C1, and C2 deflections disappeared while A1 remained near the original level. This was associated with preservation of localization of touch with gauze throughout the trigeminal skin, nasal mucosa, and tongue. Medication for this patient: 2 cc Innovar IV 75 minutes before the glycerol, 30 mg Brevital IV 61 minutes before the glycerol during placement of the retrogasserian needle elec-trode; no Brevital during or after the injection of glycerol. (From Sweet, W: Neuro-surgery 9:652, 1981, with permission.)

basic reason why these disorders fail to respond as well to differential destruction of the trigeminal rootlets.

Conclusion

We are continuing to recommend glycerol rather than RF lesions for patients who prefer to accept the greater risks of recurrent pain in return for the lesser likelihood of dysesthesias and severe loss of touch sensation, and for those in whom we think such dysesthesia or corneal anesthesia or both are a special hazard.

REFERENCES

1. Håkanson S: Transoval trigeminal cisternography. *Surg Neurol 10*:137–144, 1978
2. Håkanson S: Treatment of trigeminal neuralgia by injection of glycerol into the trigeminal cistern. Presented at the Third World Congress on Pain, Edinburgh, September 1981. Pain (Suppl 1):S287, 1981
3. Håkanson S: Treatment of trigeminal neuralgia by injection of glycerol into the trigeminal cistern. *Neurosurgery 9*:638–646, 1981
4. Sweet WH, Poletti CE, Macon JB: Treatment of trigeminal neuralgia and other facial pains by retrogasserian glycerol. Neurosurgery 9:647–653, 1981
5. Polge C, Smith U, Parkes AS: Revival of spermatozoa after vitrifcation and dehydration at low temperatures. *Nature 164*:666, 1949
6. Maher RM: Neurone selection in relief of pain. Further experiences with intrathecal injections. *Lancet 1*:16–19, 1957
7. Nathan PW, Sears TA: Effects of phenol on nervous conduction. *J Physiol 150*:565–580, 1960
8. Cameron GR, Finckh ES: The production of an acute haemolytic crisis by subcutaneous injection of glycerol. J Path & Bact (London) 71(1):165–172, 1956
9. Reineck HJ, O'Connor GJ, Lifschitz MD, et al: Sequential studies on the pathophysiology of glycerol-induced acute renal failure. J Lab & Clin Med 96(2):356–362, 1980
10. Yamashita T, Imaizumi N, Yuasa S: Effect of endocellular cryoprotectant upon polymorphonuclear neutrophil function during storage at low temperature. Cryobiol 16:112–117, 1979
11. Porterfield JS, Ashwood-Smith MJ: Preservation of cells in tissue culture by glycerol and dimethyl sulphoxide. *Nature 193*:548–550, 1962
12. Pribor DB, Nara, A: Toxicity and cryoprotection by dimethyl sulfoxide and by glycerol in isolated frog sciatic nerves. Crybiology 5:355–365, 1969
13. Baxter DW, Schacherl U: Experimental studies on the morphological changes produced by intrathecal phenol. Canadian Med Assoc J 86:1200–1205, 1962
14. Hellstrand E, Håkanson S, Meyerson B: In preparation
15. Macon JB, Poletti CE, Sweet WH: Human trigeminal root evoked potentials during differential thermal and chemical trigeminal rhizotomy. *Pain (Suppl 1)*:S28, 1981

CHAPTER 72
Open Cordotomy—New Techniques

Charles E. Poletti

Indications for Open Cordotomy

General: Cancer Pain Below T5

WE HAVE BECOME progressively inclined to perform cordotomy operations only on patients suffering from medically intractable cancer pain whose longevity appears limited to less than 3 years. This is because of the relatively high incidence of failures 1 to 2 years after cordotomy operations and the increasing late frequency of post cordotomy painful dysesthesias. The significant instance of unavoidable complications—including motor weakness and bladder and sexual dysfunction—are further arguments against using the operation, especially bilaterally, in patients with benign disease. Accordingly, we have been reluctant to perform cordotomies on patients with peripheral nerve or spinal cord injuries, herpetic neuralgia, or chronic calcific pancreatitis, no matter how severely afflicted. With selected cancer patients, however, the operation often relieves the patient from suffering and excessive narcotics. For these individuals the operation should be done as a priority option. If delayed too long, the operation may not arrest or reverse extensive suffering and debilitation. For patients with markedly limited life spans a percutaneous cordotomy is often selected.

The use of cordotomy operations is further limited by progressive decreases in the level of analgesia during the first 6 months following the operation. Often within 3 weeks postoperatively the level has fallen three to six segments and at 6 months the level may have lowered a total of six to eight segments. Thus, most surgeons agree that even with high cervical cordotomies many patients may have no significant hypalgesia above T2-T3. Following a T2-T3 thoracic cordotomy, the level of significant permanent hypalgesia or analgesia usually is about T10. Consequently, one can usually count on a year of analgesia six to eight levels below the operation. A further consideration is that often during these postoperative six months in which the level of analgesia is falling, the cancer is progressing to higher levels. This is an important consideration before performing the cordotomy.

More important than determining the site of the referred pain is localizing the cancerous lesion producing the pain. For instance, a recent patient with prostatic cancer and severe, deep lateral flank pain on the right side appeared to be a good candidate for unilateral open thoracic cordotomy until a body computed tomographic (CT) scan revealed a single metastasis eroding the right half of the T12 vertebra. On further direct questioning, the patient finally admitted to pain in the corresponding left lateral flank. In this case unilateral cordotomy was no longer an

Department of Neurosurgery, Massachusetts General Hospital, Boston, Massachusetts

option. We believe each cordotomy operation should be individually designed based primarily on the location of the cancerous lesion producing the pain.

Unilateral Somatic Cancer: Unilateral Cordotomy

Unilateral cordotomies are most effective for cancer not invading the viscera and for cancer located away from the midline and at or below the lower cervical region. Thus, excellent potential candidates are patients with cancer confined to the legs, the hips, the lateral retroperitoneal pelvic and abdominal space, the chest wall (e.g., breast cancer and pancoast tumor), and perhaps the lower brachial plexus. For disease below T8 we select a T2 unilateral thoracic cordotomy, which carries a lower risk than cervical cordotomy.

For the arms, as for the neck, nasopharyngeal, and facial cancer, a medullary tractomy is worth considering instead of cordotomy, although the operative mortality and incidence of postoperative dysesthesias is slightly higher. An open C2-C3 cordotomy combined with a C2, C3 and C4 dorsal rhizotomy may relieve severe pain in the brachial plexus, upper extremity, shoulder, and neck.[1] We favor open C2-C3 cordotomy, occasionally combined with rhizotomy, over a C1-C2 percutaneous cordotomy because of the marked anatomic variations at C1-C2 and the belief that consistently more complete, uncomplicated lesions with higher permanent levels of analgesia can be obtained using our open technique at C2-C3.

Unilateral Visceral pain: Bilateral Cordotomy

In general, whenever a significant component of the pain is caused by disease invading the viscera, bilateral deep cordotomies are required for satisfactory relief of suffering. Often the visceral pain from extensive cancer of the pancreas, intestine, colon, rectum, cervix, or uterus, and especially stomach and esophagus may be mediated by splanchic nerves entering the spinal cord as high as T1. Many of these visceral nociceptive afferents do not cross to the other side of the spinal cord. Accordingly, in these patients the best chance of satisfactory results rests with the highest bilateral cervical cordotomies advisable, i.e., C1-C2 percutaneous or C2-C3 open cordotomy combined with an open contralateral C5-C6 cordotomy.

Paramedian, Midline, and Bilateral Cancer: Bilateral Cordotomy

Whenever the cancer is close to the midline, unilateral cordotomy has a high probability of not securing prolonged relief. These patients very often become aware of severe contralateral pain shortly after surgery. Accordingly, it should be emphasized that even for paramedian cancers it is wise to perform a bilateral cordotomy.

When bilateral cordotomies are indicated, an open cordotomy is performed at two levels, rather than a unilateral percutaneous cordotomy followed by an open operation.

Alternatives to Bilateral Cordotomy

Whenever open bilateral cordotomies are indicated, one should seriously consider various alternative operations that are available: A midline myelotomy operation may have a higher incidence of pain relief for bilateral pain in the arms, shoulders, and neck as well as pain from bilateral visceral or extensive midline diesease. In addition, midline myelotomies, compared with bilateral cordotomies, have a significantly lower incidence of later postcordotomy dysesthesias and bladder dysfunction, sleep apnea, and motor weakness.

Recently Hitchcock[2,3] and Schvarcz[4,5,6] independently have pioneered central medullary myelotomies for high bilateral disease using stereotactic techniques. These appear promising but require special expertise.

Recently my colleagues and I developed a technically very simple nondestructive operation for intractable cancer pain in which a spinal epidural catheter is implanted for long-term admin-istration of morphine.[7] Using three administration systems, we demonstrated for the first time that direct spinal narcotics can be employed on a chronic basis for effective pain relief.

Spinal Cord Anatomic Variations and Anterolateral Cordotomy

The goal of anterolateral cordotomy is to create a lesion in fibers ascending in the spino tha-lamic tract (STT) that carry nociceptive input from one side of the body caudal to the level of the lesion. Marked anatomic variations of the spinal cord, however, frequently impede optimal le-sioning of the STT. Four major areas of anatomic variation that concern the surgeon are: (1) the course of the STT; (2) the course of the corticospinal tract (CST); (3) the position of the dentate insertion; and (4) the width of the spinal cord. Thus, in cordotomy as in aneurysm surgery, the individual patient's anatomy must be identified or analyzed. It often may be necessary to per-form a variation of the standard operation in order to maximize the probability of satisfactory results for each individual.

STT Anatomy and Variants

In some individuals the STT does not appear to decussate at all. In these patients a standard anterolateral cordotomy produces *ipsilateral* analgesia. Fortunately these cases are rare. Most individuals, however, probably have a number of uncrossed nociceptive fibers. Perhaps these permit the recovery of pain following cordotomy. In particular, the nociceptive fibers mediating visceral pain in many cases do not decussate fully, but instead ascend on both sides of the spinal cord. This should encourage the surgeon toward bilateral cordotomies when *visceral* pain is felt to be significant.

Normally the vast majority of the nociceptive fibers *do* decussate, following two predicta-ble patterns. First, the "sacral" fibers are positioned most posterolaterally and superficially. The more rostral fibers from the lumbar, thoracic, and cervical regions ascend to assume their course more anteromedially and deeper (Fig. 72-4). The sacral fibers may lie immediately anterior to the base of the normally positioned dentate (Fig. 72-4). The cordotomy lesion, therefore, should first reach as far dorsally as the equator of the spinal cord, usually at the base of the dentate in-sertion. Beginning the lesion 1–2 mm anterior to this point in some individuals results in sparing the sacral fibers.

A second relatively predictable pattern reflects the observation that pain from the superfi-cial part of the body is relayed by fibers close to the surface of the spinal cord. Progressively deeper are the fibers mediating our sense of temperature, deep pain, and, finally, visceral pain (See Fig. 73-4). Accordingly, the lesion must extend deep to the anterolateral surface of the cord, especially in patients with visceral disease. In most patients, a depth of 5 mm is required, even in the cervical region.

Perhaps most important, the lesion should include the *medial* and anterior portion of the anterior quadrant. It is often in this portion of the spinal cord that fibers from the anterior com-missure may ascend five to six segments or more before extending far enough laterally to assume their "classical" position in the "lateral" STT. In contrast, fibers from the *dorsal* horn appear to cross to the anterior commissure almost immediately, i.e., at the same level or at most within one to two segments. Yet these same fibers may then ascend for five to eight segments before "crossing" fully to form the "lateral" STT. Thus, the "anterior" STT in humans consists of as-cending fibers gradually coursing laterally to form the "lateral" STT. Accordingly, a lesion in the *lateral* anterior quadrant, albeit deep, may produce analgesia extending rostrally only eight or more segments below the lesion. In contrast, a lesion of the anterior quadrant extending to the midline may in some individuals produce analgesia to within one segment of the lesion.

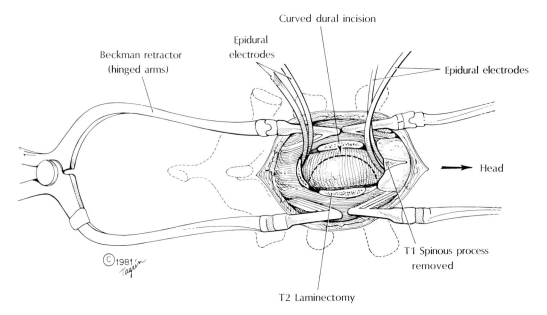

Fig. 72-1.   The spinous processes of T1, T2, and T3 are exposed. The T1 and T2 processes are removed. A complete bilateral laminectomy at T2 is shown extending far laterally on the side of the lesion. The rostral and caudal yellow ligaments are excised. The bipolar epidural electrodes are then inserted in the midline rostrally and caudally for recording sensory evoked potentials from bilateral peroneal stimulation. The projected dural incision is shown by the dotted line.

Thus, especially in cervical cordotomies where a primary goal is a high permanent level of analgesia, we recommend extending the lesion at least 1–2 mm anterior to the *most medial* exiting fibers of the ventral root, i.e., within 1–2.5 mm of the anterior spinal artery (Fig. 73-7). A lesion only as far anteriorly as the ventral root may yield a satisfactory level of analgesia in only 80 percent of patients. The technique to be described, in fact, usually permits a lesion of the entire anterior quadrant extending immediately to the midline anterior pial septum and anterior spinal artery. This lesion, we believe, produces the highest level of analgesia feasible—usually within two and occasionally within one segment.

Corticospinal Tract Anatomy and Variations

Rarely the CST does not decussate at all. Instead it descends uncrossed in the anterolateral quadrant of the cord. In these rare individuals an anterolateral cordotomy would be expected to produce contralateral plegia as these aberrant tracts are believed to finally cross near the segment of their termination on the lower motor neuron. In addition, the data of Yakovlev and Rakic[8] indicates that these abnormal patterns of the CST are probably more common than we like to believe. It seems reasonable to assume there may be associated abnormalities or displacements of the normally adjacent STT.

Frequently, however, even in normal individuals the decussating pyramidal fibers may not be fully crossed and back into the posterior aspect of the cord until the caudal half of C2. Accordingly, we are inclined to do our cervical cordotomies at C3. A C4-C5 level of analgesia, as discussed above, may still be feasible by extending the lesion to the midline. Clearly when the decussation is abnormally low, careful stimulation and monitoring —even at C3—is necessary to avoid a lesion of the CST.

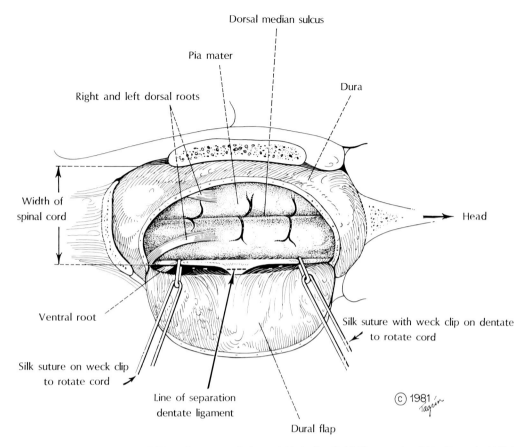

Dorsal median sulcus

Pia mater

Right and left dorsal roots

Dura

Width of
spinal cord

Head

Ventral root

Silk suture with weck clip on dentate
to rotate cord

Silk suture on weck clip
to rotate cord

Line of separation
dentate ligament

ⓒ 1981

Dural flap

Fig. 72-2. The dura is opened. The microscope is brought into the field. The arachnoid is dissected bilaterally. The dura contralaterally is retracted to permit direct measurement of the width of the spinal cord. Weck clips with silk sutures are applied to the dentate as shown. The arachnoid around the dorsal roots is dissected, freeing the roots to their exit point.

Dentate Insertion Variations

The dentate ligament is formed by the joining of a component of the ventral and dorsal spinal cord pia. Usually these join to form the dentate at the equator of the cord just anterior to the anterior extent of the CST and just posterior to the posterior extent of the sacral fibers of the SST. In a number of cases, however, as Sweet[9] has noted, the dentate origin may form anterior or posterior to this equatorial line. When it is anterior to its most common position, a lesion beginning at the dentate and extending anteriorly may not lesion nociceptive fibers from the sacrum. In cases of a posterior dentate a lesion beginning just anterior to the dentate clearly has a high probability of producing an ipsilateral motor deficit. Accordingly, the lesion should begin at the equator of the cord, irrespective of the position of the dentate. Because the equator of the rotated cord is difficult to judge we again stress physiologic stimulation and monitoring, preferably with the patient awake.

Spinal Cord Width Variations

The width of the spinal cord appears to vary as well, both in the thoracic and cervical regions. This is especially true in patients with advanced cancer. In one of our patients, for instance, extensive pelvic cancer invaded the lumbo sacral plexus bilaterally, producing significant sensory deficits and virtual paraplegia. In this patient the spinal cord at T2 under the microscope

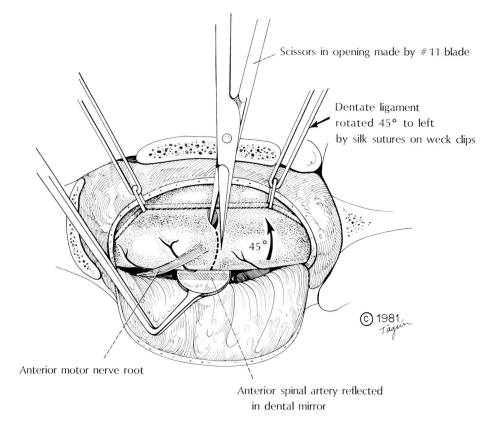

Scissors in opening made by #11 blade

Dentate ligament
rotated 45° to left
by silk sutures on weck clips

45°

© 1981
Tagein

Anterior motor nerve root

Anterior spinal artery reflected
in dental mirror

Fig. 72-3. The dentate ligament lateral attachment has been cut. Traction is applied on the silks attached by Weck clips to the dentate until the cord is rotated 45°. A small dental mirror is placed ventrolaterally to permit visualization of the anterior midline septum and the course of the anterior spinal artery. Into the hole made in the pia just anterior to the equator of the cord are placed the microsurgical scissors. These are used to cut the pia arachnoid around the anterior quadrant to within 1–2 mm of the anterior midline septum. This is usually about 2 mm anterior to the medialmost exiting ventral rootlet.

measured a total width of 5.2 mm. Obviously it would have been injudicious to try to cut the anterior quadrant to a depth of 4–5 mm, especially since at the time we were still using a cordotomy knife, not a blunt instrument capable of palpating the anterior midline septum adjacent to the anterior spinal artery. Accordingly, we recommend measuring the width of the spinal cord in each case and using that specific dimension to determine the approximate depth of the lesion.

Pre-operative Procedure

Preparations and Special Instruments

All patients are advised of the complications of cordotomy operations. When awakening the patient during the operation appears appropriate, the details and alternatives are discussed with the patient, both by the surgeon and the anesthesiologist. If there is any suspicion of impaired pulmonary function contralateral to the planned lesion, then a comprehensive series of pulmonary function tests are done. When there is impaired motion of the contralateral hemidiaphragm, a unilateral cervical cordotomy may trigger fatal postoperative respiratory complications by interrupting the exclusively ipsilateral descending projections of the ventrolateral

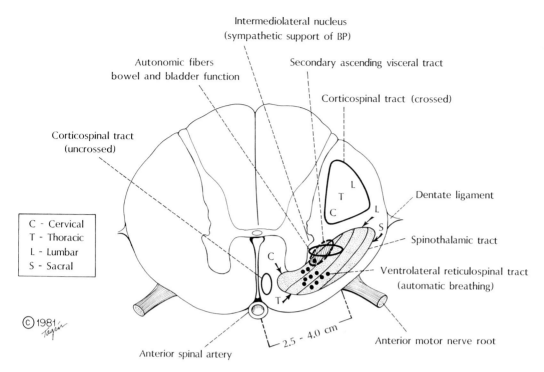

Fig. 72-4. The spinal cord at T3 with the axon tracts relevant to making lesions of the STT. Just dorsal to the equator of the cord is the descending CST. The lesion should start about 1 mm anterior to the anterior limit of the CST. The entire STT is shown, including the "anterior" and "lateral" components. It should be emphasized that intermingled within the STT fibers are other ascending and descending tracts. These of necessity must be lesioned to obtain a complete lesion of the STT. These tracts intermingled at least in part with the STT include: the ventrolateral reticulospinal tract, responsible for nonvoluntary breathing, the descending autonomic fibers for bladder and bowel sphincter control, the ascending visceral tract, and sympathetic fibers just anterolateral to their origin in the intermedolateral nucleus.

In the anteromedial aspect of the cord is the uncrossed CST adjacent to the midline septum and anterior spinal artery.

Note also that the distance from the medialmost exiting motor rootlet to the anterior spinal artery and midline septum varies from 2.0 to 3.5 mm.

reticulospinal tract (Fig. 72-4). The patient is wrapped with Ace bandages from the toes to the thigh to minimize the resulting operation-induced orthostatic hypotension. This is especially important when bilateral lesions are planned.

Electrophysiologic Monitoring Equipment (EMG)

Because of the marked potential variability in the location within the spinal cord of both the lateral spinothalamic tract and the corticospinal tracts, we conclude that intraoperative electrophysiologic stimulation of the spinal cord combined with dorsal column-evoked responses and EMG recording are useful. In order both to stimulate in the anterior quadrant to identify the STT in the awakened patient and later to stimulate while making the lesion to warn of nearby CST fibers, we use a 45° Jacobsen ball that is insulated except over the distal half of the ball and at the end of the handle. A standard stimulator is attached to the uninsulated end of the handle, preferably a simulator that is capable of constant current stimulation at 2→100 HZ. For measuring dorsal column potentials evoked by peroneal or median nerve stimulation, we use a Nicolet signal averager with bipolar epidural recording electrodes. This technique is described elsewhere.[10] Especially in cases in which wake-up anesthesia is not used, we monitor CST function by stimulating as the lesion is being made while looking for motor responses and elicited EMG

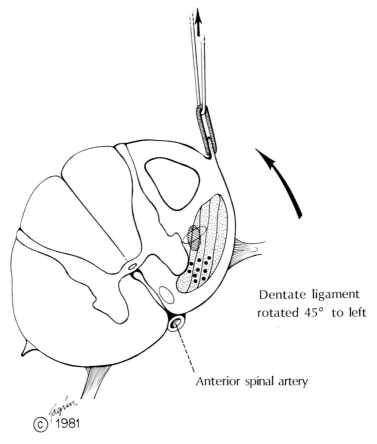

Dentate ligament
rotated 45° to left

Anterior spinal artery

© 1981

Fig. 72-5. The orientation of the relevant tracts within the cord once it has
been rotated 45°

recordings distally. A small dental mirror on a malleable shaft is used to visualize the anterior
spinal artery while making the lesion.

Operative Procedures

Anesthesia

With the improved techniques of wake-up anesthesia we have discontinued the use of local
anesthetics for cordotomy operations. Wake-up anesthesia offers the opportunity of identifying
the SST by stimulation, of monitoring bilateral motor function as the lesion is being made, and,
finally, of testing the extent of the induced sensory deficit before it is too late to enlarge the lesion. Electrophysiologic stimulation and monitoring techniques, however, are designed to maximize the probability of executing an optimal lesion even when wake-up anesthesia is not
appropriate. As a result, an increasing number of our cordotomies are done with the patient
asleep through the operation.

Position

For unilateral cordotomy with wake-up anesthesia, the patient can be placed in the swim-
mer's position with the thorax rotated 45° up from horizontal. With the spinal cord rotated 45°,
the operating microscope can be focused almost vertically and the cord viewed from a transverse

direction. When bilateral lesions are anticipated, or in cases in which wake-up anesthesia is not employed, the patient should be placed prone. Especially for cervical cordotomies the head is placed in a neutral position to decrease tethering of the cord, which may occur with too much flexion. For cervical operations, the head is held in a three-pin headrest whereas during upper thoracic operations the head is allowed to rest on a doughnut headrest. The fully bandaged legs should be elevated on blankets and the table set in moderate reverse Trendelenburg position. With the patient in this position, a decrease in blood pressure following bilateral lesions will indicate, as noted by Sindou,[11] that the depth and dorsal extent of the lesion are satisfactory.

Unilateral Cordotomy Procedure

A relatively long skin incision is made in order to provide wide lateral retraction of the skin and paraspinal muscles. This affords a view from a lateral angle of the anterior quadrant of the rotated cord.

For unilateral upper thoracic lesions the T2 and T3 laminae are exposed, while bilateral upper thoracic lesions call for exposure of the laminae of T2, T3, and T4. A complete laminectomy is done extending fully laterally on the side of the planned lesion. Next, the yellow ligament above and below the laminectomy is removed, exposing the inferior edge of the rostral lamina and the superior edge of the caudal lamina. The bipolar electrodes for recording evoked potentials from bilateral peroneal nerve stimulation are inserted in the midline epidural space rostrally and caudally (Fig. 72-1).

The dura is then opened in a semicircular fashion extending far enough laterally to allow direct visualization of the contralateral side of the spinal cord (Fig. 72-2). This permits exact measurement of the width of the spinal cord. The microscope is brought into the field. The arachnoid is opened for optimal visualization. The width of the cord is measured precisely under the microscope and a piece of bone wax is used to mark half of the cord width from the tip of the Jacobsen ball. This measurement will be used during lesioning to gauge the depth of cordotomy and to allow the tip of the Jacobsen ball to reach the midline. Once the cord width has been measured, the arachnoid opening is extended laterally over the dentate ligament.

Traction of the dorsal or ventral roots during rotation of the cord may result in painful dysesthesias postoperatively. The dorsal rootlets should therefore be freed from the cord to their point of exit or to the limit of the exposure. If necessary, the dorsal root should be cut to facilitate rotation, raher than risk a traction injury with postoperative hyperesthesia. As previously mentioned, in cervical cordotomies White and Sweet suggest performing bilateral rhizotomies of the three accessible dorsal roots in order to raise the level of analgesia and to decrease the postoperative incisional pain.

With the roots freed or cut, the cord is then rotated 45°. To rotate the cord a 4-0 silk suture is placed in two Weck clips, which are in turn placed on the dentate ligament (Fig. 3; see also Fig. 2). The silk sutures arc then used to put traction on the Weck clips and the dentate for rotating the cord. If the patient is under local anesthesia and experiences pain as the cord is rotated, the dorsal root should be cut. Alternatively, cerebrospinal fluid should be aspirated and a small cottonoid soaked in 10% cocaine applied *selectively* to the posterior root(s). If the root is sufficiently mobilized beforehand, however, pain during rotation is rarely elicited. With careful microsurgical dissection, the intact dentate insertion usually is strong enough to rotate the cord. If not, traction may be applied directly on the anterior root to rotate the cord. One should not be afraid to rotate the cord too far. If the anterior spinal artery along the anterior midline cannot be satisfactorily viewed, the dentate above and below the level of interest can be cut, permitting the cord to be rotated as much as 90° . Electrophysiologic monitoring electrodes offer additional safety features, but we have not found their use to be mandatory if the techniques above are followed as described. Once the cord is rotated 45°, a small dental mirror on a malleable handle may be used to visualize the exact course of the anterior spinal artery in the anterior midline septum, and the medial limit of the exit of the ventral rootlets (Fig. 72-3). At the most avascular part of the exposed anterior quadrant the tip of a No. 11 blade is inserted into the equator of the spinal

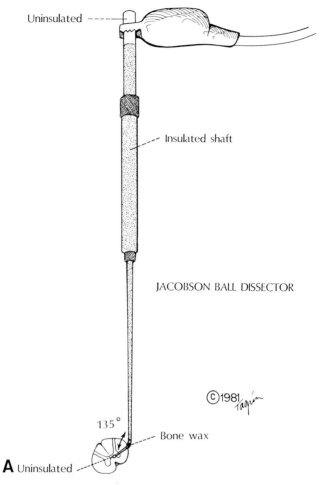

Uninsulated

Insulated shaft

JACOBSON BALL DISSECTOR

©1981 Tagrim

135°

Bone wax

A Uninsulated

Fig. 72-6.   A. The 45° Jacobsen ball tip has been inserted just anterior to the equator of the cord, and, while stimulating, is slowly advanced in the transverse axis of the cord until the tip reaches the midline (i.e., until the distal part of the bone wax marker on the tip is flush against the lateral aspect of the cord). The tip should pass far enough dorsally to include the intermedolateral nucleus and all the tracts depicted in Figure 72-4 except for the crossed CST. **B.** An enlarged view of the Jacobsen ball instrument after the initial insertion. Note that the distal half of the Jacobsen ball is uninsulated. Should this pass closer than 1 mm to the CST during its insertion into the cord, ipsilateral motor responses will be elicited. In this case the ball should be directed more anteriorly. From this position the ball is then slowly directed 90° anteriorly, palpating the midline septum.

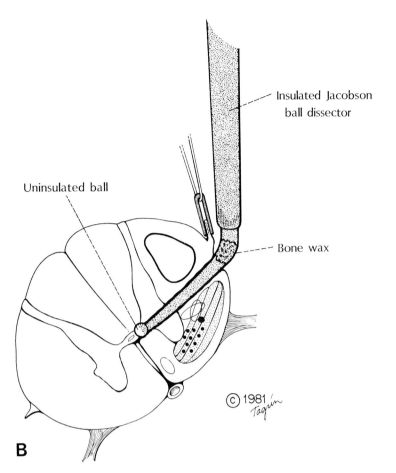

Insulated Jacobson
ball dissector

Uninsulated ball

Bone wax

© 1981
Tagrin

B

Fig. 72-6 (cont'd.)

cord. As noted, this is usually located immediately under the dentate insertion. The exact site of the dentate attachment can be established by observation and blunt palpation on the dentate insertion in a dorsal-to-ventral manner. Microsurgical scissors are placed in the small hole made in the pia by the No. 11 blade (Fig. 72-3). Only the pia arachnoid is then cut with the microscissors around the anterior quadrant of the cord. Cutting the pia with sharp scissors decreases the chance of avulsing the dentate attachment. Small pial vessels may be cauterized with bipolar microforceps. We incise the pia to a point 2 mm anterior to the medialmost exit of the ventral root, which should be at least 1 mm from the anterior spinal artery. An advantage of making the pial cut initially before lesioning the tracts is that the natural shape of the cord is subsequently preseved while the instrument is being inserted. Cutting the pia with a knife tends to distort the anatomy of the cord, making an accurate lesion difficult and placing indirect traction on adjacent vascular and neural structures.

With the incision in the pia, the cord is ready for cordotomy. Clearly, in making the spinal cord lesion the two principal cautions are to avoid transecting the cortical spinal tract, and to avoid damage to the anterior spinal artery and its main branches. The cortical spinal tract is particularly vulnerable to damage during cordotomy procedures and as mentioned previously, anatomic variations limit the surgeon's ability to execute an adequate lesion without the possibility of damaging the motor system.

In making the lesion, our operative technique is unique in that it employs the use of a blunt Jacobsen ball to simultaneously *stimulate while making the lesion*. The stimulator is attached to

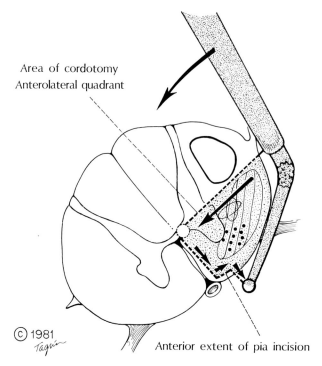

Fig. 72-7. The tip of the Jacobsen ball has been brought 90° anteriorly, palpating along the midline septum until the pia on the anterior aspect of the cord is felt. The ball is then drawn laterally along the pia until it exits from the cord at the medialmost extent of the pial incision previously made with the microscissors.

the end of the handle of the Jacobsen ball instrument. A ground electrode is inserted in the paraspinal muscles. Stimulation parameters are set for 1-msec pulses delivered at 1.5 V. This stimulus will elicit responses in the cortical spinal tract with motion in the ipsilateral arm or leg in the asleep, unparalyzed patient when the ball tip approaches within 1 mm of the CST. This blunt-tipped instrument permits a safe traverse of the anterolateral cord all the way to the medial septum while the proximity of the instrument to the cortical spinal tract dorsally is concurrently monitored by looking for stimulation-evoked motor responses. Although the Jacobsen ball is a blunt instrument, it does not distort the very soft tissue of the cord. It has been our experience, particularly with midline myelotomies, that the Jacobsen ball is fully satisfactory for transecting spinal cord tracts.

The Jacobsen ball is inserted at the equator of the cord at the dorsalmost limit of the pial opening and is directed into the transverse axis of the cord until the bone wax indicates that the ball is halfway across the width of the cord. Since the spinal cord has been rotated 45°, the tip of the Jacobsen ball is also angled 45°. Thus, during this initial motion the shaft of the instrument is held vertically (Fig. 72-6A and B). Usually the transverse diameter of the cord in the upper thoracic region is approximately 10 mm and thus initially an incision to a depth of approximately 5 mm is indicated. In the cervical region the cord may be as wide as 16 mm, in which case an incision to 8 mm is permissible. As mentioned previously, however, the size of the cord may vary. We have seen a cord width as small as 5.2 mm in the thoracic region, presumably because of atrophy of the dorsal columns and descending cortical spinal tracts. In that particular case it was necessary to insert the ball to only 2.5 mm in order to place the lesion at the center of the cord. As the ball passes near the gray of the anterior horn, an ipsilateral trapezius contraction may be obtained during cervical cordotomy and contraction of intercostal muscles during thoracic cordotomy. The presence of distal ipsilateral motor responses indicates that the stimulating Jacobsen ball is too close to the descending cortical spinal tract and must be directed more anteriorly. This is most frequently necessary when working in the cervical region, where the motor fibers may not be exclusively dorsal to the equator of the cord. Once the ball is in the center of the cord (Fig. 72-6B) it is drawn directly anteriorly along the palpable medial septum to the anteromedial corner of the anterior quadrant. The ball is then drawn laterally along the pia for about 1–2 mm until it exits from the cord at the most anteromedial extent of the pial incision (Fig. 72-7). The ball should be drawn flush against the pia of the midline septum and the anterior quadrant. The pia is firm and can be readily palpated safely from inside the cord with the Jacobsen ball. There may be marked anatomic variation in the anteromedial portion of the anterior quadrant with a large uncrossed corticospinal tract. Should this be the case, one would expect contralateral motor responses in this region from the Jacobsen ball. We have not yet encountered such a case. Should this occur, it seems prudent to skirt this tract when making the first lesion. The ball tip of the Jacobsen instrument usually can be seen as it comes out of the pia, but, if necessary, there is ususally ample room to insert the mirror in order to see exactly where the ball exits. If it exits as planned, there is a very high probability that a satisfactory lesion was performed.

It is important, as shown in Figure 72-7, to make the lesion as close as possible to the midline septum. This is especially important in the cervical region, where recently crossed fibers may lie close to the septum for many levels before assuming a more lateral and dorsal position. Hardy[12] believes that an incision extending *to* the midline can raise the level of resulting analgesia virtually to the level of the lesion.

Selective cervical cordotomies, i.e., partial lesions of the anterolateral quadrant, are not recommended for two reasons: first, cancer may spread to wider areas, and second, the topological distribution of the spinal thalamic tract does not appear to be sufficiently specific for reliable results.

It should be stressed that in the cervical region the anterior spinal artery is usually 4.5–5.0 mm from the center of the exit zone of the anterior nerve root. A lesion 2 mm from the midline will still be 2.5–3.0 mm away from the center of the exiting ventral root. Except for the danger of entry into the anterior spinal artery, there does not appear to be any disadvantage to making an incision in the medial anterior quadrant as well. We have not seen a case of contralateral motor weakness caused by transection of the uncrossed descending motor tracts.

In summary, when making the initial lesion, an attempt should be made to transect virtually the entire anterior quadrant of the cord from the equator anteriorly, extending to the midline.

Following the initial cordotomy lesion, the patient may be awakened in order to test the extent of the resulting analgesia as well as the integrity of motor function. Before awakening, Xylocaine should be injected profusely into the paraspinal muscles. When the patient awakens, pain may originate from traction on a dorsal root. This can be blocked with Xylocaine or cocaine.

With the patient awake, it is advisable to test for deep visceral pain as well as for pin-prick perception. This is especially important for patients who have a significant portion of their disease lying in deep structures of the pelvis. Both legs should also be tested for motor strength since the pyramidal tracts may not be crossed, in which case the contralateral limbs may be supplied by the spinal tract in the anterior medial quadrant with the lesion.

If the level of analgesia does not reach far enough cephalad, the lesion should be extended medially and anteriorly to include fibers adjacent to the anterior midline septum. A lesion resulting in a level of analgesia that is not sufficiently caudal, e.g., sparing the perineum and sacral distribution, should be extended closer to the equator and thus closer to the crossed cortical spinal tract. Further extensions of the initial cordotomy lesion can be made with the patient awake as transection of the spinothalamic tract is not perceived as a painful stimulus. This permits functional monitoring of the motor system as well, while extending the lesion.

Upon achieving a satisfactory distribution of analgesia, the patient is reanesthetized for closure. The Weck clips on the dentate are cut free, the cord allowed to return to normal position, and the wound closed.

Bilateral Cordotomy Procedure

Bilateral high cervical cordotomies are not performed because of the high risk of sleep apnea and other complications. If bilateral analgesia is necessary, a percutaneous or open cordotomy can be done unilaterally at C2 or C3 with a contralateral cordotomy at C5-C6 performed by the posterior or anterior approach through the C5-C6 disc space. Usually when contralateral analgesia at a high level is not mandatory, a percutaneous cordotomy will be done at C2 on one side followed by a contralateral open thoracic cordotomy at T2 or T3.

When a lower bilateral level of analgesia is satisfactory, a bilateral operation should be performed in one stage in the upper thoracic region—with one lesion at T2 and the other contralateral at T4. For this operation the laminae at T2 and T4 are each removed as well as the spinous process of T3. The rest of the procedure is as described above. If a previous unilateral cordotomy has been done at T3 and it becomes evident later that a contralateral lesion is indicated, it can be made at the lower margin of T1 as early as 5 to 7 days postoperatively.

Postoperative Precautions

Postoperative Sleep Apnea

Following C2-C3 cordotomies the patient should be placed postoperatively in the intensive care recovery room, especially because of the danger of sleep apnea. When sent back to the floor, the patient should be monitored continuously with an apnea alarm, and tidal volume should periodically be checked. The nursing staff must be alert to the potential need for prompt respiratory assistance. The potential for sleep apnea may persist for a week postoperatively, after which time these precautions can be relaxed. If sleep apnea occurs after unilateral cervical cordotomies, the patient virtually always recovers after an adequate period of assisted support.

Postoperative Weakness

At the first sign of motor weakness postoperatively, we administer high-dose steroids and maintain the blood pressure if necessary to prevent any hypotension.

Postoperative Hypotension

When bilateral lesions are done, the blood pressure must be monitored as the patient begins to mobilize—raising the head off the bed, dangling his feet, and walking. Toe-to-groin Ace wraps may be used with fluid loading and antihypotensive drugs as needed. The decrease in blood pressure—even with bilateral lesions—as well as orthostatic hypotension, gradually clears and is only a problem if unrecognized. A single episode of severe hypotension may render the blood supply significantly compromised, particularly to the upper thoracic cord. This ischemia may extend the lesion to the adjacent corticospinal tract.

Postoperative Urinary Retention

If a Foley catheter has been placed before a bilateral procedure, a cystometrogram should be done several days postoperatively before the catheter is removed.

Operative Results

The incidence of pain relief 3 months postoperatively varies from 54 to 90 percent with the average being 75 percent.[1,13,14,15] After 18 months the rate of relief falls to approximately 50 percent and stabilizes for another several years. It is generally agreed that the incidence of pain relief is greater in those patients with postoperative paresis and sphincter disturbance, suggesting a direct relation between the degree of pain relief and the extent of the lesion.

A T3 cordotomy, according to Taren et al.,[16] should be expected to produce a postoperative sensory level up to T4-T5, including postoperative loss of superficial pain, temperature, deep pain, visceral pain, and itch. The permanent level, however, usually settles at T7-T10. After cervical cordotomies, Grant and Wood[17] report an average permanent level of analgesia or hypalgesia only up to T5.

In some of our cases satisfactory and persisting relief of pain is achieved without superficial cutaneous analgesia. This dissociation between pain relief and cutaneous analgesia is seen commonly in midline myelotomies and characterizes certain thalamic lesions. Although the neurophysiologic explanation is not clear for the spinal cord, we propose that there may be two fiber systems involved, namely, in addition to the spinothalamic tract carrying acute pain perception, there also may be a midline multineuronal ascending system in the central gray matter of the spinal cord. This latter system may modulate a patient's ability to suppress chronic pain.

Operative Failures and Recurrence of Pain

Operative Failures

The most common causes of failure to achieve satisfactory analgesia following cordotomy are:

1. Failure to cut close enough to the equator of the cord so there is sparing of the sacral representation in the spinal cord.
2. Failure to cut deep in the anterior quadrant. This may produce a satisfactory level of cutaneous analgesia without adequate relief of deep and visceral pain. Accordingly, in order to make sure the deep fibers carrying deep somatic visceral pain are severed, one should test these intraoperatively with wake-up anesthesia. A satisfactory test for visceral pain is a Foley baloon inflated within the bladder.
3. Insufficient extension of the lesion anteriorly and medially. This results in a level of analgesia many segments below the level of the cordotomy.
4. Failure to cut the anterior quadrant decisively. This produces an incomplete lesion with limited and patchy analgesia.
5. Performing a unilateral cordotomy when a bilateral procedure was indicated.
6. Subsequent spread of the cancer above the level of analgesia. If this is anticipated, a higher cordotomy should be done initially.
7. Anatomic variability of the spinal cord, resulting in an unsatisfactory lesion.

Recurrence of Pain with Fading of Analgesia

If the level of analgesia falls and islands of recovered nociception occur within a few days postoperatively, the spinothalamic fibers in the periphery of the lesion have probably been bruised but not severed. The first postoperative drop in analgesic level may be caused by recovery from the direct injury of the surgery and the drop during the first week may be the result of recovery from edema and swelling. This may explain the two-to-five segment drop in the analgesic level during the first 2 postoperative weeks. In an excellent review on long-term follow-up of cordotomy patients, Grant and Wood[17] founds both islands and large areas of returned sensation commencing even within a few months. It is conceivable that this recovery of pain perception is caused by collateral regeneration of new synaptic terminals in short-chain internuncial neurons taking over the previous function of the long spinothalamic tract. Four years after cordotomy, White and Alexander[18] have found 54 percent of cordotomy patients to have recovered pain perception; subsequent higher anterolateral cordotomies generally proved unsuccessful in reinstituting analgesia. In addition to the hypothesis of collateral sprouting, long-term fading of postcordotomy analgesia may be explained by altered synaptic and membrane excitability in pre-existing potentially alternate nociceptive pathways. Indeed, in addition to first-order neurons ascending to medullary nuclei from the posterior columns, other neurons send efferent projections from the segmental gray matter. These may be partially responsible for conducting impulses concerned in the abnormal reference of pain. Partial support for this alternate pathway lies in the fact that stimulation of the dorsal column during midline myelotomy is often reported as painful by the awake patient.

Another hypothesis explaining the return of pain perception is that intrasegmental polysynaptic complexes form from collaterals of the crossing spinothalamic tract fibers. These may separate near the midline from the crossing spinothalamic tract fibers ascending in the spinal periaqueductal central gray matter to the reticular formation. Support for this hypothesis lies in the fact that relief of pain is experienced after midline commissural myelotomy or central myelotomy often not associated with cutaneous analgesia.

Accordingly, we believe that post cordotomy recovery of pain perception is less likely caused by spinal cord or thalamic axonal sprouting than by altered trans-synaptic excitability in pre-existing potentially alternate nociceptive pathways.

Operative Complications

Mortality

The mortality in various series reported in the literature varies from 3 to 21 percent.[1,13,14,15] The mortality is higher for unilateral cordotomies in the cervical region involving malignant disease and still higher for bilateral cervical cordotomies. The postoperative mortality clearly is higher in cancer patients than in patients with benign disease.

Respiratory Complications

Some authors indicate that respiratory complications are the most serious concern in high cervical cordotomies. In the past, sleep apnea has been a frequent cause of death. Voluntary control of respiration is mediated by the cortical spinal tract, but subconscious ipsilateral respiratory movements are controlled by pathways descending deep in the centrolateral part of the spinal cord. This descending unilateral respiratory pathway is called the ventrolateral reticulospinal tract. Its fibers are, at least in part, intermingled with the fibers of the lateral spinothalamic tract (See Fig. 72-4). Unilateral destruction of this pathway results in little functional respiratory loss unless contralateral respiratory function is poor. Accordingly, even for unilateral C2-C3 cordotomies, the function of the contralateral diaphragm should be evaluated preoperatively. Bilateral lesions clearly produce a high incidence of sleep apnea and death.

Postcordotomy Hypotension

Intraoperatively there may be a sudden drop in blood pressure immediately after a cordotomy lesion has been made. Sindou[11] makes the point that such a drop in pressure assures the surgeon that the lesions have been made deep enough and far enough dorsally to assure lesioning of the fibers carrying visceral pain. In unilateral thoracic cordotomies, this drop is moderate and evanescent. The blood pressure usually returns to its normal level by the end of wound closure. Following bilateral lesions it may be marked and protracted, lasting well into the postoperative period.

Blood pressure is maintained by spinal sympathetic pathways that descend partially intermingled with the ascending STT (See Fig. 72-4). Stimulation of these fibers elevates the blood pressure and the pressure within the bladder.[19] Unlike respiratory complications, blood pressure is seldom a cause of death or serious morbidity unless the patient is in a sitting position.

As noted, hypotension in the postoperative period may produce ischemia, especially in the thoracic region, thereby enlarging the surgical lesion and causing a new motor deficit.

Motor Weakness

Assuming the cortical spinal tract has a relatively normal anatomy, the two principal causes of ipsilateral motor weakness following cordotomy are a lesion extending too far posteriorly that damages the crossed cortical spinal tract, and an extension too far anteromedially that damages the anterior spinal artery with resulting ischemia. A third possible mechanism is borderline ischemia accentuated by intra- or postoperative hypotension. The fact that the upper thoracic cord is especially susceptible to such ischemic damage may explain why there is a higher incidence of paresis after thoracic cordotomy compared with the cervical procedure.

The literature indicates that the incidence of paresis or paralysis following unilateral cordotomy varies from 0 to 11 percent,[14,15,20] whereas the incidence following bilateral cordotomies can run as high as 24 percent.[15] The incidence of permanent motor deficits is clearly much higher in bilateral lesions. We believe that the implementation of stimulation techniques as described decreases the incidence of paresis.

Bladder Dysfunction

Urinary bladder dysfunction after cordotomy is frequent. Following unilateral cordotomy this complication is relatively infrequent (0 to 8 percent).[1,14,20] This disturbance usually lasts only a few days and responds well to medical management. Following bilateral cordotomies, either cervical or thoracic, the incidence of urinary dysfunction is much higher and its duration is often permanent.

When a cordotomy is done for sacral pain, sphincter disturbances are particularly likely to occur. Nathan and Smith,[21,22] having studied the physiology of micturation and defecation, have concluded that both the descending and ascending fibers responding to distention and the desire to relax sphincters are assembled in a narrow band almost crossing the equator of the cord opposite the central canal. Figure 72-4 clearly shows the high risk of bowel and bladder disturbance if a bilateral cordotomy is performed for sacral pain with the incision made close to the equator.

Sexual Dysfunction

Sweet claims that the fibers involved in sexual sensation and function lie so close to those for pain (See Fig. 72-4) that sexual function is almost always impaired after unilateral cordotomy and permanently impaired after bilateral cordotomy. Taren et al.[16] report that after section of the anterolateral tracts erection and ejaculation may still occur, but sexual sensation at the moment of orgasm is lost. Sexual potency does not seem to be disturbed with unilateral cordotomy but is almost always lost following the bilateral procedure.

Dysesthesias

The abnormal sensations that may arise immediately after cordotomy, or as long as months after the operation, are sometimes divided into two groups: (1) referred sensations; and (2) dysesthesias.

Postoperatively, soreness of the skin and pain with girdle distribution may develop at or above the level of the lesion. This usually persists only for a few weeks and may be related to undue traction of the dorsal roots when the cord was rotated.

Referred sensations may be elicited by stimulation within the analgesic area in approximately 25 percent of patients. These sensations may be felt by the patient as noxious; they are poorly localized and often referred contralaterally. After bilateral cordotomy the sensations may be referred to an area above the level of analgesia as well as to areas of escape within the analgesic zone.

More serious are the severe constant painful dysesthesias referred to levels below the cordotomy. Their onset is usually delayed, occurring with increasing frequency as the postoperative period lengthens. Post cordotomy dysesthesias become a serious problem in approximately 6 percent of patients after 2 to 3 years. As noted, cordotomy at a higher level is not effective.

REFERENCES

1. White JC, Sweet WH: *Pain and the Neurosurgeon.* Springfield, IL, Charles C Thomas, 1969
2. Hitchcock ER: Stereotactic myelotomy. *Proc R Soc Med 67:*771–772, 1964
3. Hitchcock ER: Stereotactic cervical myelotomy. *J Neurol Neurosurg Psychiatry 33:*224–230, 1970
4. Schvarcz JR: Stereotactic extralemniscal myelotomy. *J Neurol Neurosurg Psychiatry 39:*53–57, 1976
5. Schvarcz JR: Functional exploration of the spinomedullary junction. *Acta Neurochir (Suppl) 24:*179–185, 1977
6. Schvarcz JR: Spinal cord stereotactic techniques re: trigeminal nucleotomy and extralemniscal myelotomy. *Appl Neurophysiol 41:*99–112, 1978
7. Poletti CE, Cohen AM, Todd DP, et al: Clinical pain relieved by long-term epidural morphine: two case reports with permanent indwelling systems for self-administration. *J Neurosurg 55:*581–584, 1981
8. Yakovlev PI, Rakic P: Patterns of decussation of bulbar pyramidal tracts on two sides of the spinal cord. *Trans Am Neurol Assoc 91:*366–370, 1966
9. Sweet WH: Recent observations pertinent to improving anterolateral cordotomy. *Clin Neurosurg 23:*80–95, 1976
10. Macon JB, and Poletti CE: Conducted somatosensory evoked potentials during spinal surgery. Part I. Technical aspects. *J Neurosurg* (In press)
11. Sindou M: Personal communication. 1981, June.
12. Hardy D, LeClereq TA, Mercky F: Microsurgical selective cordotomy by the anterior appraoch, in Handa H (ed): *Microsurgery. International Symposium on Microsurgery,* Baltimore, University Park Press, 1973
13. Brihaye J, Retif J: Comparison of the results obtained by anterolateral cordotomy at the dorsal level and at the cervical level. *Neurochirurgie 7:*258–277, 1961
14. Diemath HE, Heppner F, Walker AE: Anterolateral chordotomy for relief of pain. *Postgrad Med 29:*485–495, 1961
15. Nathan PW: Results of antero-lateral cordotomy for pain in cancer. *J Neurol Neurosurg Psychiatry 26:*353–362, 1963
16. Taren DA, Kahn EA, Humphrey T: The surgery of pain, in Kahn EA, Crosby EC, Schneider RC, et al (eds): *Correlative Neurosurgery.* Springfield, IL, Charles C Thomas, 1969
17. Grant FC, Wood FA: Experiences with cordotomy. *Clin Neurosurg 5:*38–65, 1957
18. White JC: Anterolateral cordotomy—its effectiveness in relieving pain of non-malignant disease. *Neurochirurgia 6:*83–102, 1963
19. Kerr FW, Alexander S: Descending autonomic pathways in the spinal cord. *Arch Neurol 10:*249–261, 1964
20. McKissock W: *Second International Congress of Neurological Surgeons.* International Congress Series No. 36 E27. Amsterdam, Excerpta Medica, 1961
21. Nathan PW, Smith MC: Spinal pathways subserving defecation and sensation from the lower bowel. *J Neurol Neurosurg Psychiatry 16:*245–256, 1953
22. Nathan PW, Smith MC: The centrifugal pathway for micturition within the spinal cord. *J Neurol Neurosurg Psychiatry 21:*177–189, 1958

CHAPTER 73
Percutaneous Cordotomy—the Lateral High Cervical Technique

Ronald R. Tasker

ONE OF THE MOST IMPRESSIVE LESSONS in applied physiology was the deliberate sectioning of the human anterolateral column by Martin (at Spiller's suggestion),[1] in order to relieve intractable pain. As a result, cordotomy performed under direct vision rapidly became and remained an important neurosurgical procedure.

One of the major directions of neurosurgical exploitation, however, has been the simplification of existing techniques, particularly the substitution of percutaneous for open approaches. The introduction of percutaneous cordotomy by Mullan et al.[2] that used a radiostrontium source for lesion-making was one of the significant pioneering events in this trend. The use of radiofrequency current for lesion-making, by Rosomoff et al.,[3] assured the future of percutaneous surgery.

Just as progress in conventional stereotactic surgery depended not only upon the development of appropriate equipment for electrode guidance that incorporated suitable techniques for both radiographic localization and lesion making, but also upon physiologic means for identifying the target, so the technical elaborations of percutaneous cordotomy have followed a similar pattern with Onofrio[4] introducing the use of myelography, Gildenberg et al.[5] the use of impedance monitoring, and Sweet and White, Taren, and Hitchcock and their associates[6-10] the use of physiologic guidelines for target corroboration. The latter field has been of considerable interest to us.[11-13] As a result, it is possible to present a protocol for the percutaneous lateral high cervical technique which, if followed rigorously, makes it reliable, safe, and, with few exceptions, the procedure of choice for performing cordotomy.

Applied Anatomy and Physiology

The successful alleviation of pain by cordotomy requires the satisfaction of two basic principles: (1) the identification and section of the lateral spinothalamic tract at the appropriate segmental level; and (2) the selection of patients whose pain is dependent upon transmission of nociceptive impulses in the lateral spinothalamic tract. In other words, adequate levels of analgesia must be produced and in the right patients.

Department of Surgery, University of Toronto, and Neurosurgical Division, Toronto General Hospital, Toronto, Canada. The compilation of this data was supported by the Toronto General Hospital Foundation.

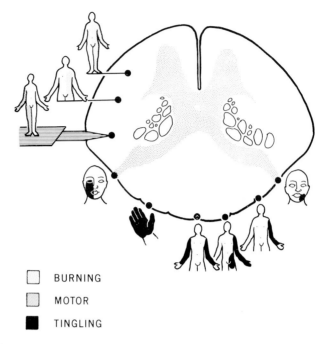

☐ BURNING

▨ MOTOR

■ TINGLING

Fig. 73-1. A diagrammatic cross-section of the human spinal cord at the level of C1 with patient supine, showing the relative positions of the dorsal and ventral horns (stippled) and the corticospinal tract (outlined bundles). The figures illustrate the actual responses elicited by 100 Hz threshold stimulation with an Owl cordotomy electrode at a variety of sites in a single patient. The electrode tip was pressed against the cord at the dorsal sites, while the cord was impaled as described in the text at the others. At the two ventral sites a feeling of contralateral burning was induced, which is typical for responses arising in the lateral spinothalamic tract whose cervical fibers lie superiorly near ventral horn and whose sacral fibers lie inferiorly adjacent to the corticospinal tract. The different bodily regions to which the responses were referred at those two sites reflect a somatotopographic arrangement within the tract. The ipsilateral motor response (tetanization) resulted from stimulation of the corticospinal tract. The array of ipsilaterally or bilaterally referred paresthetic responses obtained across the dorsum of the cord reflects stimulation of the descending tract or the cervical nucleus of trigeminal nerve and the dorsal columns. The somatotopy in the latter, with the caudal segments located nearest the midline, is well represented. (Reproduced courtesy of Chas. C. Thomas, Publisher Springfield, Ill., from Tasker RR, Organ LW, Hawrylyshyn P: *The Thalamus and Midbrain of Man: A Physiological Atlas Using Electrical Stimulation*, 1982.)

The Spinal Cord at the C1 Level

Little need be said to elaborate upon the conventional teaching that pain and temperature are perceived through receptors whose afferents synapse differentially in the dorsal horn of the spinal cord with neurons whose axons require approximately two segments to complete their decussation and to come to lie in the contralateral anterolateral columns that form the lateral spinothalamic tracts. Whatever other centripetal connections nociceptors may have, section of the lateral spinothalamic tract results in analgesia and thermanalgesia as far rostrally as two segments below the level of the section. The important immediate relations of the tract at the level of C1, shown in Figure 73-1, include the ventral horn and the corticospinal tract. The technical aim of percutaneous cordotomy is to sever all or part of this pathway without producing significant damage to neighboring structures.

Patient Selection—the Physiology of Pain: "Somatic" versus "Dysesthetic" or Deafferentation Pain

Conventional teaching has led us to try to explain all instances of nonpsychogenic pain in terms of nociceptors and peripheral nerve fibers lying within the smaller end of the dimensional spectrum. Such reasoning has led neurosurgeons to resort to cordotomy in the management of a wide variety of pain syndromes. Failure to relieve pain despite achieving analgesia in the region where the patient felt pain (unfortunately a regular observation in some of these syndromes) has led to much speculation, consternation, and uncertainty about the role of cordotomy. Although it was soon recognized that failure most often occurred in patients who suffered from pain that was not associated with malignant disease, leading to the contradictory terms "benign" and "malignant" pain, the true significance of the observations is still often overlooked.

During the 1930s and 1940s, Livingston[14] was impressed by the clinical characteristics of pain associated with certain conditions—"causalgia and reflex paralysis," "minor causalgia," "post traumatic pain syndromes," "chronic low-back disability," "facial neuralgia," and "phantom limb pain,"—characteristics that fail to conform to the concept of nociceptors that centrally transmit specific information about pain in specially coded pathways. He speculated that deafferentation was the critical feature common to all these conditions and that this deafferentation established central nervous alterations that, once established, continued to generate the sensation of pain even after exclusion of the original lesion from the nervous system.

The clearly enunciated views of Livingston have, in our opinion, been largely overlooked at the expense of ineffective approaches to the neurosurgical relief of intractable pain. For some years we have been impressed by the fact that patients may develop chronic pain of a characteristic type following lesions that produce deafferentation, such as intercostal nerve damage during thoracotomy, peripheral nerve injury, brachial plexus avulsion, postherpetic neuralgia, postcordotomy dysesthesia, spinal cord injury, and stroke.[15-17] It makes no difference whether or not the deafferentation is caused by malignant disease, as in the case of cancerous destruction of the brachial plexus. The resultant pain often appears after an interval of time, usually is causalgic (burning) or dysesthetic, bears a close distributional relationship to that of the sensory disturbance produced by the deafferentation, is frequently dramatically relieved temporarily by dosages of intravenous thiopental sodium that are insufficient to produce narcosis, but not by narcotics themselves. Despite the fact that blockade with local anesthetics at an appropriate segmental level usually relieves such pain during the duration of that blockade, neural transection at the same site seldom results in more than temporary relief. Although the precise mechanism of such pain associated with deafferentation by whatever means remains obscure, Livingston's concept remains tenable that deafferentation results in central neuronal changes, which, once established, persist by producing a "memory" for pain that further deafferentation including cordotomy cannot be expected to eradicate. Denervation neuronal hypersensitivity, either in the dorsal horn, the medial mesencephalic tegmentum, or the medial thalamus, is a possible physiologic substrate.

Indications and Contraindications for Percutaneous High Cervical Cordotomy by the Lateral Approach

Provided the technical guidelines to be outlined below are carefully followed, percutaneous high cervical cordotomy by the lateral approach is, with few exceptions, the treatment of choice for patients suffering from "somatic pain" caused by lesions below the C4 dermatome.[18] Since

Table 73-1. Indications in 244 Consecutive Cases for Percutaneous Cordotomy

Indication	Percentage
Carcinoma	
Cervix	20.0
Rectum	18.8
Lung	8.1
Breast	5.5
Colon	4.7
Other	25.2
Sarcoma	4.8
Cord Trauma	6.4
Discogenic Pain	1.3
Other, Noncancerous	5.2

the appearance of Mullan's original article, the author has performed only one open cordotomy. In the patients with deafferentation syndromes referred to above, neither percutaneous cordotomy nor deafferentation procedures by any technique usually give pain relief. Although percutaneous high cervical cordotomy by the dorsal approach has been described,[19] there appears to be no special advantage to performing the operation by this method. It is awkward for the surgeon and anesthetist alike to work with the patient in a prone position while the dorsally introduced electrode must first traverse the cord before reaching the desired target that is superficially and laterally located. Percutaneous cervical cordotomy by the low anterior approach[28] shares a similar disadvantage and yields lower levels of analgesia, and since the electrode must first traverse the disc to reach the cord, small incremental adjustments in the position of the electrode are difficult to make.

The most common conditions for which percutaneous cordotomy is performed include compressive neuralgic pain associated chiefly with cancerous involvement of the lumbosacral plexus, *but not the burning or dysesthetic pain associated with the sensory loss in such patients,* as well as cancerous involvement in the lower spine and the musculoskeletal system of the lower limbs. The procedure also is effective in relieving pain in those rare cases of chronic compressive neuralgic root pain associated with traumatic lesions of the cauda equina and also of painful skeletal lesions not associated with malignant disease. Table 73-1 lists the primary diseases for which 244 consecutive procedures were performed out of our total experience of approximately 400 cases.

Dependence for survival upon the lung ipsilateral to the proposed cord lesion is paramount among the contraindications to the procedure in otherwise apparently appropriate patients. Inadvertent unavoidable damage to the strictly ipsilaterally distributed reticulospinal pathway that lies ventrally in the cord adjacent to the lateral spinothalamic tract (Fig. 73-2) results in ipsilateral loss of involuntary respiratory excursion that progresses to respiratory arrest. Since patients with thoracic problems that led to the loss of a lung or its function in the first place usually are afflicted with pain that is located high in the chest or in the upper limb, the contemplated cordotomy must produce a high level of analgesia by severing the most ventrally located fibers of the somatotopically arranged spinothalamic tract. These fibers lie closest to the reticulospinal pathway, which makes such patients all the more susceptible to disaster.[16,18,20-27] Low cervical percutaneous cordotomy as described by Lin and his associates[28] and low anterior cervical[29,30] or high thoracic cordotomy performed by open means are not appropriate alternative procedures, since they cannot achieve the high levels of analgesia required. Other techniques of pain relief must be sought for these patients.

Because of the risk of respiratory malfunction, great caution should be exercised in performing high cervical cordotomy. In particular, high levels of analgesia should be avoided in a patient who has already undergone high cervical cordotomy on the opposite side and whose level of analgesia extends into the high thoracic or cervical dermatomes. High cervical cordotomy similarly must be carefully evaluated in any patient who has diminished respiratory function for

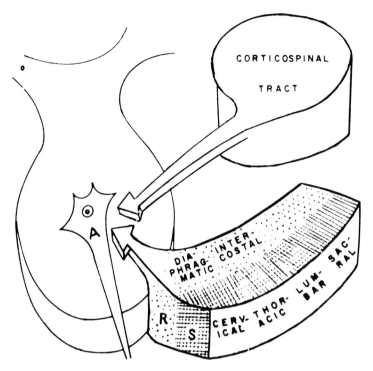

Fig. 73-2. The relative positions of the corticospinal, the reticulospinal (R), and the lateral spinothalamic tracts (S) and their somatotopic organization in the human spinal cord at C1. Note that the spinothalamic fibers that originate most rostral, lying closest to the ventral horn, are closely associated with reticulospinal fibers that provide involuntary respiratory movement. (Reproduced with permission from Hitchcock E, Leece B: Somatotopic representation of the respiratory pathways in the cervical cord of man. *J Neurosurg* 27:320–329, 1967.

whatever reason. Unfortunately, conventional respiratory functional assessment has produced no firm criteria for patient selection in such cases.[25,27] Percutaneous or open low cervical or open high thoracic cordotomy may offer a valid alternative for this rare group of patients. Since we adopted the percutaneous lateral high cervical technique we have not yet been forced to deny the procedure to a patient for these reasons.

Other theoretic contraindications to percutaneous lateral high cervical cordotomy not yet encountered by us include pathology in the high cervical area that distorts the anatomy or compromises the technical approach, or anomalies such as tract malposition or congenital rotation of the cord, the existence of which might be inferred from the failure of what was apparently a technically adequate percutaneous cordotomy.[31-36]

Percutaneous cordotomy in the uncooperative patient can be achieved safely by using general anesthesia but avoiding muscle paralysis. With the patient under general anesthesia, the surgeon is deprived of only one of the guidelines to be outlined below, i.e., the distinctive subjective sensation described by the patient when the spinothalamic tract itself is electrically stimulated. Staged bilateral percutaneous cordotomy has been used twice successfully and safely under general anesthesia.

With the passage of years we have occasionally observed falling levels of analgesia in patients in our series following cordotomy by whatever means. Although the result is difficult to explain, percutaneous cordotomy in several such patients has restored a high level of analgesia and pain relief.

Technique

Success in percutaneous cordotomy depends equally upon appropriate anesthesia, radiographic identification of the position of the electrode, monitoring of the depth of penetration of the cord by the measurement of electrical impedance, positive physiologic identification of the lateral spinothalamic tract together with avoidance of important adjacent structures, and controlled reproducible lesion-making with radiofrequency current. The procedure is greatly facilitated by the use of suitable back-up equipment such as the Owl Cordotomy System.*

Anesthesia

Although in exceptional cases percutaneous cordotomy can be performed under general anesthesia, the procedure is preferably carried out using neuroleptanalgesia. Neuroleptanalgesia enables the patient to lie comfortably still during the 45 minutes to 2 hours that the procedure requires and permits more intense levels of analgesia to be produced briefly and, repeatedly on demand while the capability for rearousing the patient repeatedly for physiologic testing is preserved.

The patient is brought to the operating room without presedation but having received his regular dose of analgesic medication. Analgesia is achieved by the intravenous administration of the short-acting narcotic fentanyl citrate, which is pushed to the limit of respiratory suppression (a rate of 12 per minute). Sedation is added as necessary by the separate intravenous administration of droperidol (2.5–5.0 mg) and diazepam (1 mg), drugs that must be used sparingly because of cumulative sedative effects they can cause if the procedure is prolonged. Alternately, small intravenous injections of thiopental sodium (75–150 mg) may be used to achieve brief narcosis, especially during introduction of the needle and lesion-making.

Positioning

Percutaneous cordotomy is facilitated by carefully positioning the patient in the supine position. The upper cervical spine should lie horizontal in order to trap contrast medium in the operative area. The patient's head and neck should be placed in a strictly anterior-posterior position and the cordotomy electrode introduced as precisely horizontal as possible in order to minimize problems in tip localization caused by parallax and to simplify interpretation of physiologic data. Biplanar radiologic control is achieved with the use of portable C-arm-type image intensifier at the head of the operating table arranged to provide a true lateral projection of the upper cervical spine while a portable x-ray unit placed beside the head of the table will provide a true AP view of the region of the odontoid. Again, rectilinear positioning minimizes errors resulting from parallax.

The Cordotomy Electrode and Back-Up System

The percutaneous cordotomy electrode used by the author and manufactured by Owl Instruments Ltd. consists of a 0.4-mm stainless steel wire insulated with shrink-fit Teflon tubing. The electrolytically sharpened tip projects 2 mm beyond the tubing. The electrode is introduced through a thin-walled 18-gauge lumber puncture (LP) needle into which it locks. Two millimeters of the insulation projects beyond the end of the needle as shown in Figure 73-3. The 2-mm length of bare tip is critical for the meaningful measurement of impedance and also corresponds to the effective depth to which the cord should be penetrated. The Teflon tubing impedes further penetration of the tip by producing a palpable sense of resistance to the fingers of the surgeon. Back-up electronics are provided by the Owl Universal RF System shown in Figure 73-4, which compactly provides controls and readings for measuring electrical impedance, providing

*Manufactured by Owl Instruments Ltd., Markham, Ontario, Canada

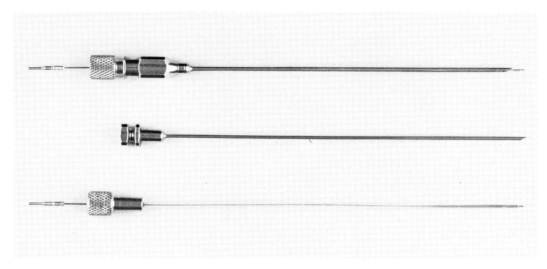

Fig. 73-3. The Owl cordotomy electrode. A 0.4-mm electrolytically sharpened stainless steel wire projects 2 mm beyond shrunk-fit Teflon tubing (bottom). A thin-walled 18 gauge LP needle (center), and the entire assembly (top) with 2 mm of the electrode projecting from the LP needle.

stimulation at 2 to 100 Hz at voltages up to 10 V and regulating the duration and strength of the radiofrequency current used in lesion-making. The electrode is used in the monopolar mode by employing a 23-gauge, 1.5 inch intramuscular needle inserted in the ipsilateral deltoid muscle as an indifferent electrode.

Radiologic Localization

Once adequate anesthesia and positioning have been achieved and the indifferent electrode inserted, the side of the neck contralateral to the patient's pain is suitably prepared and draped. The level of the cordotomy electrode holder is adjusted with the three-dimensional mechanical stage of the Owl Cordotomy System so that the lumbar puncture needle that is strictly positioned horizontally impinges on the patient's skin at the center of the C1-2 space as seen in the lateral projection on the screen of the image intensifier. After the soft tissues have been injected with local

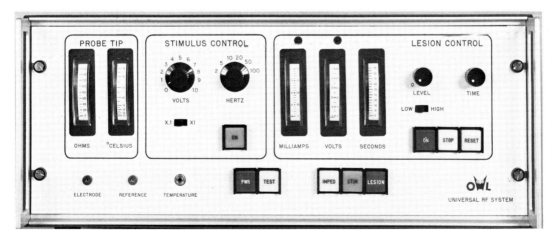

Fig. 73-4. The Owl Universal RF System for measuring electrical impedance of CSF and the spinal cord. The system provides electrical stimulation at low and high repetition rates and low and high outputs for making radiofrequency lesions. The low level of lesion control is always used for cordotomies.

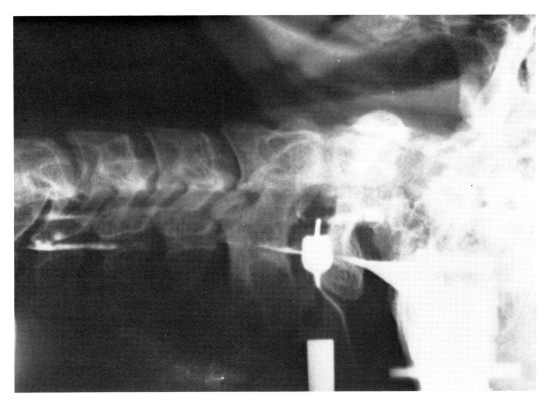

Fig. 73-5.   A lateral radiogram of the upper cervical spine showing contrast medium outlining the dorsal dura, the dentate ligament (at the tip of cordotomy electrode in the C1-2 space) and the ventral margin of the cord.

anesthetic, the needle is inserted—always horizontally. A sense of resistance is felt by the surgeon and a twinge of pain is felt by the patient as the needle penetrates first the ligamentum flavum and then the dura. To attempt to infiltrate these structures with local anesthetic is probably unwise because of the possibility of inducing high spinal anesthesia. Should this accident occur, only respiratory support need be given until the block wears off (in approximately 45 minutes), possibly with anticonvulsant coverage.

It is helpful to warn the patient in advance of the anticipated pain and to have the anesthetist increase the depth of analgesia temporarily at this stage. Keeping the needle tip centered in the C1-2 space, since this is the expected location of the dentate ligament and dorsal margin of lateral spinothalamic tract, the needle is advanced cautiously only until a flow of cerebrospinal fluid occurs when the stylet of the LP needle is removed. Several cubic centimeters of insoluble positive contrast medium (such as that used in myelography) shaken up in a 10-cc syringe with a similar quantity of cerebrospinal fluid (CSF) are now injected and, it is hoped, outline the dentate ligament as shown in Figure 73-5. The dentate ligament appears as a line of contrast medium in approximately the mid-anteroposterior plane of the spinal canal. The dentate ligament may, however, be displaced considerably either anteriorly or posteriorly and additional confusing lines of contrast medium also may be seen. The dorsal limit of the subarachnoid space nearly always is unmistakably identifiable as an appropriately placed dorsal structure, and contrast medium also may be trapped on the ventral or dorsal root line or both, or upon the ventral margin of the cord itself. If the dentate ligament is not visualized, it should first be established that the LP needle is not positioned too far dorsally and then an additional injection made. It sometimes may be necessary to forcibly inject a small volume of emulsion mixed with air to achieve suitable visualization. In a quarter or more of all patients the dentate ligament cannot be outlined despite

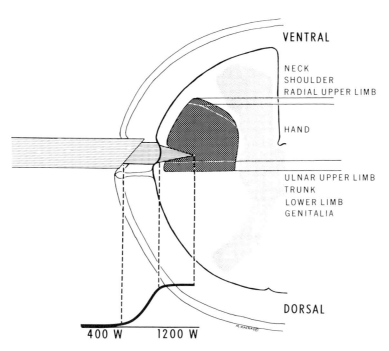

Fig. 73-6. A diagrammatic representation of the electrode penetrating the lateral spinothalamic tract (cross-hatched) during high cervical percutaneous cordotomy. The Teflon insulation restricts penetration of the tip of electrode to 2 mm. The graph illustrates typical impedance changes during penetration. Somatotopographic representation within the lateral spinothalamic tract is indicated in a ventral-to-dorsal direction.

all of the maneuvers, and the direction of the needle must be based on the other localizing criteria outlined below.

The procedure also may be performed in a similar fashion in the occipital-C1 space, although the C1-2 space is more commonly used.

Once the dentate ligament has been adequately identified, the cordotomy electrode is locked into the LP needle to minimize the loss of CSF and the whole needle-electrode assembly with 2 mm of bare tip projecting from it is advanced toward the anterior margin of the dentate ligament until:

1. A sense of gritty resistance is felt by the surgeon's fingers.
2. The patient (forewarned and supported by increased analgesia) feels a sharp pain referred to the ipsilateral side of the neck.
3. The impedance rises (see below).
4. The tip of the electrode comes to lie at or just beyond the middle of the odontoid in the AP x-ray. With increasing experience, the AP x-ray is required less often.

Impedance Monitoring

As the electrode-needle assembly is advanced, the electrical impedance about its tip is followed on the panel of the Owl Universal RF System. As the tip impales the cord, the impedance rises sharply from approximately 400 to 500 Ω in CSF to over 1000 Ω, as shown in Figure 73-6. The electrode should not be advanced further once the criteria for adequate cord penetration have been met since further penetration is unncessary and adds a third dimension to electrode localization. Furthermore, deeper penetration, i.e., forcing the Teflon tubing and LP

Table 73-2. Identification of Cord Structures at C1 by Threshold Electrical Stimulation

Structure Stimulated	Effect of Electrical Stimulation	
	2 Hz	100 Hz
Anterior horn	2-Hz twitches in C1-2 myotomes, ipsilaterally	tetanization of C1-2 myotomes
Corticospinal tract	2-Hz twitches of any ipsilateral musculature from C1 to sacral myotomes	tetanization of C1-sacral myotomes sometimes preceded by tingling, shock, or vibration in the same area as that from which the motor response arises
Descending tract or spinal nucleus of V	Usually none; occasionally ipsilateral facial throbbing or bumping	Ipsilateral facial tingling, electric shock, or vibration
Dorsal column	Usually none; occasionally ipsilateral bumping or throbbing anywhere below face	Ipsilateral tingling, vibration, or electric shock anywhere below face
Lateral spinothalamic tract	Nearly always ipsilateral 2-Hz twitches of muscles innervated by cervical roots including upper extremity. Usually no sensory effect, occasionally contralateral bumping or throbbing below neck.	No motor effect; contralateral warmth, coolness, or burning; rarely pain or tingling

needle into the cord, increases the risk of complications and usually interferes with further impedance readings. Should the cord be impaled from side to side, however, the operation should be continued in the usual way, although the patient should be monitored more closely in the postoperative period. Should the electrode-needle assembly fail to impale the cord, but rather slip dorsal or ventral to it, the proper criteria for penetration, including impedance rise, will not be met. When the electrode impinges on the opposite side of the spinal canal, the AP x-ray will disclose the faulty position and the patient will report contralateral cervical pain.

Physiologic Localization

Once the needle tip has appropriately penetrated the cord at the anterior margin of the dentate ligament, its position in the lateral spinothalamic tract must be physiologically confirmed using threshold electrical stimulation in trains of negative rectangular waves of 3 msec duration at 2 and 100 Hz. Table 73-2 lists the criteria for the identification of excitable structures found in the spinal cord at the level of C1. In practice, only responses in the anterior horn, the corticospinal tract, and the lateral spinothalamic tract are seen, because special electrode positioning is necessary to reach the more dorsally located structures. It is difficult to explain why motor effects are obtained when the spinothalamic tract is stimulated at 2 Hz. Possibly they represent activation of local cord reflexes. Similarly, the sensory effects obtained in the corticospinal tract are startling and may represent subclinical motor effects, activation of afferent pathways within the lateral columns, or, possibly, activation of muscle afferent pathways.

Identification of the Lateral Spinothalamic Tract

Table 73-3 presents in more detail the effects elicited by threshold stimulation at 2 Hz in our 244 procedures at sites at which lesions were subsequently made. Threshold averaged 3 V. The responses consisted of contractions in the ipsilateral muscles of cervical root innervation or con-

Table 73-3. Responses Elicited in 244 Procedures
with Threshold Stimulation at 2 Hz in Lateral Spinothalamic Tract at C1-2

Response	Percentage
2-Hz contractions in ipsilateral cervical myotomes	72.2
2-Hz contractions in ipsilateral cervical myotomes plus contralateral sensory	20.1
Contralateral sensory only	0.9
Contralateral motor only (significance unknown)	5.1
Ipsilateral sensory only (probably subthreshold motor)	0.9
Not specified	0.9

tralateral sensory effects or both in 93.2 percent of the sites. It is interesting that contralateral sensory effects were seen in only 21 percent of the sites with 2-Hz stimulation, while with 100-Hz stimulation such responses were seen at all sites, thus reflecting the characteristics of the stimulus that is adequate for inducing a conscious effect in the pathway. The significance of the contralateral motor and ipsilateral sensory effects is unclear, and lesions were made at sites giving rise to such effects only because all other criteria for positioning were satisfied. The ipsilateral sensory effects could have arisen either in ipsilateral spinothalamic fibers or as subthreshold responses from the corticospinal tract (see above).

Seventy-four percent of the motor responses occurring in muscles with cervical innervation observed during 2-Hz stimulation of the lateral spinothalamic tract affected the muscles of the neck, (the posterior nuchal group in 44 percent, the trapezius in 30 percent); in 24 percent the upper extremity was affected, usually along with the neck muscles.

Table 73-4 presents in more detail the types of responses elicited by threshold stimulation at 100 Hz at the lesion sites in our procedures. Thresholds averaged 0.5–1.0 V using the Owl system. They consisted of a feeling of heat or warmth in 70 percent of cases, coolness or cold in 24 percent, burning or pain in 5 percent, and isolated paresthesias in 1 percent. There appears to be no significance to the different types of effects reported. Contralateral paresthesias without temperature effects are acceptable indicators of satisfactory positioning only when all other criteria have been met. Ipsilateral sensory effects, seen in 10 percent of the cases, are acceptable only if they accompany typical temperature-coded contralateral effects, and care should be exercised to ensure that they do not represent subthreshold motor effects arising in the corticospinal tract by watching for tetanization when suprathreshold stimulation is delivered. Contralateral temperature-coded sensory effects involved the upper extremity exclusively in 41 percent of the cases, the lower extremity in 16 percent, the trunk in 14 percent, and multiples of these in 29 percent. Sixty-two percent of the latter group of responses included the upper extremity. Although the location of these sensory effects often did not closely match that of the analgesia induced by a lesion at the same site, the analgesia tended not to extend above the waist when the sensory effects were restricted to the lower limb, while extensive analgesia usually resulted when lesions were made at sites where stimulation-induced effects were perceived in the hand. Dorsoventral somatotopy within the lateral spinothalamic tract could be demonstrated readily by sequentially

Table 73-4. Contralateral Sensory Effects Produced by 100-Hz
Threshold Stimulation of the Lateral Spinothalamic Tract at C1-2 in 244 Procedures

Effect	Percentage
Warmth or heat	70
Cold or cool	24
Burning or pain	5
Tingling or vibration	1

stimulating from the dentate ligament to the ventral horn when the dermatomal level of the induced sensory effects progressed from sacral to cervical.[37] Similar progression of the levels of analgesia was seen if lesions were made progressively more ventrally (see Fig. 73-6). Contralateral sensory effects referred only to the neck or trunk, particularly centrally, are uncertain indicators of satisfactory position. Although lesions have occasionally been made at sites where such responses were obtained when other localizing criteria had been met, unsatisfactory or suspended levels of analgesia often resulted.

In summary, provided radiologic and impedance criteria have been met, it can be assumed with confidence that the electrode lies in the spinothalamic tract at a site where a lesion will be effective and safe when threshold stimulation at 2 Hz and about 3 V induces 2-Hz contractions in the ipsilateral neck muscles, and at 100 Hz at about 0.5–1.0 V contralateral sensory effects, usually of warmth. An ipsilateral motor effect induced at 2 Hz involving other than cervical myotomes or any tetanization induced at 100 Hz contraindicates lesion-making. Although unusual thresholds can be compatible with satisfactory positioning, caution must be exercised with extreme deviations, especially if other criteria have not been met.

Identification of Structures Other than the Spinothalamic Tract

Table 74-2 lists the physiologic criteria for positioning in the anterior horn, which is of little significance, and in the corticospinal tract where lesions produce paresis. It is of interest that patients who develop postoperative paresis—virtually always in the ipsilateral leg—are nearly always those in whom the contralateral sensory effect obtained during 100-Hz stimulation at the lesion site was referred to the lower extremity, which reflects the proximity of spinothalamic leg fibers of one side to corticospinal leg fibers of the other (see Fig. 73-1). This paresis is virtually always reversible provided that stimulation also did not produce tetanization in the ipsilateral leg. Such sensory effects should not contraindicate lesion-making and indeed are preferable if one seeks analgesia that is restricted to the lower parts of the body and avoids analgesia and thermanalgesia in the hand.

If criteria for suitable localization are not achieved, it must be decided whether the electrode lies dorsal or ventral to the lateral spinothalamic tract, whereupon very small appropriate positional adjustments must be made by sequentially repeating all the steps in the protocol at each new site until satisfactory position is attained.

Making the Lesion

Lesion-making using the technique described is painful because of the involvement of the pia of the cord. Once a lesion has been made, however, further enlargement at the same site is not painful. In preparation, the patient either should be briefly anesthetized with thiopental sodium or else given maximal doses of fentanyl citrate. Lesion size is determined by the duration and the level of current flow. A minimal lesion is produced by the Owl equipment if 15–20 mA flows for at least 15–20 seconds of the 30 seconds during which current is allowed to run; 30 mA is the usual level employed. A maximal lesion occurs when the current falls off abruptly after preferably 15–20 seconds in the 40–50-mA range. Pursuing a high current flow too vigorously should be avoided initially for fear of producing sudden vaporization at the lesion site, which will produce a lesion that is inadequate and prevent further lesion-making. It is best to gradually raise the current in successive 30-second runs. If lesion-making is performed with the patient conscious, ipsilateral leg power is simultaneously tested by having the patient perform straight-leg raising. No one who can hold the leg off the bed at the conclusion of the procedure has developed persistent significant paresis. Should the resulting level of analgesia be inadequate, the lesion is progressively enlarged either by increasing the current flow at the same site or by repositioning the electrode, checking the criteria for location, and making a new lesion.

Postoperative Care

No special postoperative care is required in most patients. It is best to keep the patient flat in bed for 24 hours to guard against post-lumbar puncture headache. Analgesics are necessary for postoperative headache and neck pain. Appropriate attention must be given to medications in order to conform to the patient's postoperative level of pain and to the possible problem of narcotic withdrawal. The patient should always be helped when first getting out of bed postoperatively in case of paresis. The problem of paresis usually responds to appropriate physiotherapy within a few days.

In patients who have undergone bilateral cordotomy or in those with preoperative respiratory problems, it is important to monitor vital signs and blood gases for about 3 days postoperatively in order to detect evidence of hypercapnia or hypoxia. In this way incipient failure of involuntary respiratory function can be anticipated and the patient transferred to an intensive care area where ventilation can be provided until recovery occurs.

Bilateral Cordotomy

If significant pain is present bilaterally, the procedure is repeated in identical fashion on the second side after an interval of at least 1 week. The precautions described at the outset should be observed. Of the 234 procedures completed in our study, 17.9 percent were performed on the second side.

Results

Results after cordotomy must be evaluated in terms of the following:

1. Was analgesia produced in the area of the patient's pain?
2. Was that pain relieved?
3. What, if any, complications resulted?
4. Did analgesia or pain relief change with time?
5. Were the complications temporary or permanent?

Thus we must evaluate the technical success, the physiologic success, and the precision of the procedure.

Technical Success

In a review of the 244 consecutive percutaneous cordotomies attempted which excludes 20 early cases performed by a variety of techniques but includes all other operations performed until June 1976, 10 procedures were abandoned short of lesion-making leaving 234 for postoperative assessment. In 4 of these, which were procedures being repeated because of inadequate analgesia achieved in a previous procedure, the stimulation-induced effects did not predict improvement of the status quo and therefore no additional lesion was made. The other 6 procedures were attempted in patients who proved to be too confused or uncooperative. In 4 patients in whom there were anesthetic difficulties, the procedure was successfully completed on a later occasion. One patient refused further surgery and 1 was deemed too ill to endure the procedure. Thus in 98 percent of attempted procedures and in 99 percent of patients, it was possible to complete the cordotomy.

Although a lesion was made in 99 percent of the patients, this did not necessarily imply that adequate analgesia was achieved. This feature was assessed at the time the patient was discharged from the hospital in 37.6 percent and at postdischarge follow-up as well in 62.4 percent. Only 4.3 percent of the patients were lost to follow-up and 83.8 percent of the total of these were known to be dead by June 1977. Adequate analgesia in the predetermined area of the body at the time of postdischarge followup was achieved in 92.4 percent of the patients; in 62.4 percent this was achieved with a single lesion; 2 lesions were required in 22 percent, and 3 or more lesions were required in the rest.

Physiologic Success

Despite the high incidence of analgesia in the preplanned area of the body, the incidence of pain relief was less than that for a variety of reasons. Patients with intractable pain, particularly those suffering from cancer, often have pain widely spread throughout the body; only part of the pain will fall within the potential range of the planned cordotomy. In addition, because of progressive disease, the patient may develop new pain postoperatively. Such persistent pain can hardly be construed to be a result of technical failure of cordotomy. The frequently published goal of total abolition of intractable pain for the rest of the patient's life is unrealistic. All that can expected is relief of that portion of the patient's pain that falls within the projected area of analgesia.

At the time of postdischarge follow-up, 40.7 percent of our patients complained of pain on the opposite side of the body, that is, on the side unaffected by cordotomy, and 6.2 percent complained of a new pain on the same side of the body but above the level of their analgesia; 2.5 percent complained of pain on both sides.

We have already briefly discussed deafferentation pain, which usually is not relieved by cordotomy nor, in fact, by any other deafferenting procedure, despite analgesia or even anesthesia in the area of the pain. Any coexisting "somatic" nociceptive pain will, of course, be relieved. Persistence of deafferentation pain, or its subsequent appearance following cordotomy progressing pari passu with destruction of nerve elements by cancer, also can hardly be construed as a technical failure of cordotomy. At the time of postdischarge follow-up, 13.7 percent of our patients complained of pain that was thought to be due to a deafferentation syndrome in an area rendered solidly analgic by cordotomy. Of those patients thought to suffer from pain caused by deafferentation, although 78.4 percent reported significant pain relief and 70.6 percent complete pain relief at the time of discharge from the hospital, only 50.0 percent admitted to any pain relief, and 33.3 percent to complete pain relief at the time of postdischarge follow-up.

Whereas it is difficult to understand how cordotomy could produce any relief at all of a deafferentation pain syndrome, nevertheless, most of the procedures used to treat such syndromes produce a high incidence of early relief with relapse within weeks to months until only one-fourth to one-third enjoy any lasting improvement. Whether this is a placebo effect or simply reflects the fact the deafferentation pain syndromes are not physiologically homogeneous remains to be seen.

The final problem affecting postcordotomy pain relief is postcordotomy dysesthesia. In our experience this has assumed a variety of forms. Most typically it is represented by an unpleasant dysesthetic feeling in all or part of the region of the body rendered analgesic or hypalgesic. Following cordotomy, we have seen typical nociceptive pain caused by nerve compression unassociated with clinically detectable sensory loss replaced by a burning, tingling discomfort in the same distribution despite solid analgesia. Finally, we have occasionally seen burning, tingling pain emerge postoperatively in a region of sensory loss recognized before the cordotomy. Whether this latter pain was previously masked by the somatic pain that the cordotomy relieved or whether it appears following the procedure is difficult to say. At the time of discharge from the hospital, 1.5 percent of our patients complained of some degree of postcordotomy dysesthesia, the incidence having increased by the time of postdischarge follow-up to 8.6 percent. In only one-half of these patients was the discomfort significant.

Thus, in 99 percent of the patients in whom we attempted cordotomy, the procedure was

Table 73-5. Major Complications in 234 Completed Percutaneous Cordotomies

Complication	Unilateral Procedures (N = 192)		Bilateral Procedures (N = 42)	
	Number of Patients	Percent	Number of Patients	Percent
Death	1	0.5	1	2.4
Transient respiratory failure requiring ventilation	1	0.5*	2	4.9
Permanent paresis	1	0.5*	0	
Bladder dysfunction requiring catheter or condom	7	3.7	9	22.0 7.5**
Hydrocephalus	1	0.5	0	

*Same patient.
**Permanent.

technically completed. Ninety-two and four-tenths percent had adequate analgesia in the pre-planned area of the body at the time of postdischarge follow-up. At the time of discharge from the hospital, 88 percent had complete relief, 94.4 percent had significant relief of the nociceptive or somatic pain for which the cordotomy was done, and 71.0 percent had complete relief, and 82.3 percent had significant relief at the time of postdischarge follow-up.

Bilateral Cordotomy

The overall incidence of pain relief in the 17.9 percent of our patients in whom percutaneous cordotomy was carried out bilaterally was somewhat less than it was on one side after a unilateral cordotomy. Since bilateral procedures usually were done with an interval too brief to allow full interoperative assessment, it is reasonable to estimate that if the incidence of failure to relieve pain were p on the first side, the incidence for failure on the two sides together ought to be p^2. Such a concept fits the observed 96.3 percent incidence of significant pain relief at the time of discharge from the hospital after unilateral cordotomy versus 91.5 percent for bilateral cases, and 82.7 percent significant relief at follow-up examination after unilateral cordotomy compared with 71.4 percent after bilateral operations. The incidence of pain relief after bilateral operations predicted by the p^2 rule would have been 92.7 and 68.4 percent, respectively.

Table 73-6. Percentage of Minor Complications in 234 (192 Unilateral; 42 Bilateral) Completed Percutaneous Cordotomies at Discharge and at Postdischarge Follow-Up

Complication	Unilateral Procedures (N = 192)		Bilateral Procedures (N = 42)	
	Discharge	Postdischarge	Discharge	Postdischarge
Minor respiratory problems	1.6	0.5	2.4	0
Slight paresis	21.2	8.8	22.0	2.5
Bladder dysfunction	7.3	7.7	9.5	2.5
Bowel dysfunction	1.0	3.2	9.5	0
Hypotension	1.6	0.5	9.5	5.0
Horner's syndrome	28.6	13.2	12.2	5.0
Persistent pain in head or neck	3.1	1.6	0	0
Meningismus	1.0	0	0	0
Restless leg syndrome	0.5	0.5	0	0

Complications

Tables 73-5 and 73-6 list the complications observed in the 234 out of 244 consecutive percutaneous cordotomies that we completed. The 2 deaths were the only ones encountered in our entire experience of about 400 procedures. Both were due to respiratory failure, one following unilateral cordotomy ipsilateral to a solitary lung, the other after bilateral cordotomy. Two other patients who developed respiratory distress that was severe enough to require temporary ventilation with subsequent recovery were the only ones so affected in our total experience of about 400 cases. One of these patients also was the patient who suffered permanent significant paresis. This and one other patient, operated on in 1980, who developed a progressive ataxia following bilateral cordotomy that might well have been due to cord compression by an extradural tumor rather than to the cordotomy, are the only ones in our experience who suffered permanent significant locomotor disability. One additional patient developed a postoperative hydrocephalus. This presumably was caused by a hemorrhage that blocked the cisterna magna and was successfully treated by shunting.

Impaired bladder function is, of course, a common preoperative condition in patients requiring percutaneous cordotomy. Our data indicate postoperative worsening of the status of bladder function in 3.7 percent of unilateral and 22 percent of bilateral cases that led to the necessity of catheter or condom drainage, although at the time of the latest follow-up after bilateral cordotomy, only 7.5 percent still required drainage.

Of the minor complications listed, the respiratory problems did not require ventilation, the paresis did not impair ambulation significantly, and the bladder dysfunction did not require condom or catheter drainage. Repeated cultures failed to confirm meningitis in 1 patient with meningismus and the symptoms subsided spontaneously.

Miscellaneous

We have never encountered evidence to suggest any of the anatomic anomalies of the spinal cord reported in the literature.[33-36] Neither have we encountered evidence to suggest distinctly separate pathways for the transmission of pain and temperature information. In general, levels of thermanalgesia and of analgesia have matched with, at most, a difference of a few segments. Although there may be differences in the degree of sensory loss in different modalities after cordotomy, we have never observed profound analgesia without thermanalgesia or vice versa.

Conclusions

Rigid adherence to the described technical protocol, and particularly satisfaction of the physiologic criteria, has enabled percutaneous high cervical cordotomy by the lateral approach to be completed in 99 percent of the patients in whom it was attempted. The pre-planned level of significant analgesia was achieved in 92.4 percent of the patients, and significant relief of the nociceptive pain for which the operation was planned was achieved in 82.3 percent of the patients at latest follow-up. This success was achieved at an expense of less than 1 percent mortality and an additional 1.5 percent significant morbidity.

REFERENCES

1. Spiller WG, Martin E: The treatment of persistent pain of organic origin in the lower part of the body by division of the anterolateral column of the spinal cord. *JAMA 58*:1489–1490, 1912
2. Mullan S, Harper PV, Hekmatpanah J, et al: Percutaneous interruption of spinal pain tracts by means of a strontium 90 needle. *J Neurosurg 20*:931–939, 1963
3. Rosomoff HL, Carroll F, Brown J, et al: Percutaneous radiofrequency cervical cordotomy; Technique. *J Neurosurg 23*:639–644, 1965

4. Onofrio BM: Cervical spinal cord and dentate delineation in percutaneous radiofrequency cordotomy at the level of the first to second cervical vertebrae. *Surg Gynecol Obstet 133*:30–34, 1971

5. Gildenberg PL, Zanes C, Flitter MA, et al: Impedance measuring device for detection of penetration of the spinal cord in anterior percutaneous cordotomy. Technical note. *J Neurosurg 30*:87–92, 1969

6. Sweet WH, White JC, Selverstone B, et al: Sensory responses from anterior roots and from surface and interior of spinal cord in man. *Trans Am Neurol Assoc 75*:165–169, 1950

7. Taren JA, Davis R, Crosby EC: Target physiologic corroboration in stereotactic cervical cordotomy. *J Neurosurg 30*:569–584, 1969

8. Taren JA: Physiologic corroboration in stereotactic high cervical cordotomy. *Confin Neurol 33*:285–290, 1971

9. Hitchcock E, Lewin M: Stereotactic recording from the spinal cord of man. *Br Med J 4*:44–45, 1969

10. Hitchcock ER, Tsukamoto Y: Distal and proximal sensory responses during stereotactic spinal tractotomy in man. *Ann Clin Res 5*:68–73, 1973

11. Tasker RR, Organ LW: Percutaneous cordotomy. Physiological identification of target site. *Confin Neurol 35*:110–117, 1973

12. Tasker RR, Organ LW, Smith KC: Physiological guidelines for the localization of lesions by percutaneous cordotomy. *Acta Neurochir Suppl 21*:111–117, 1974

13. Tasker RR: Percutaneous cervical cordotomy. *Appl Neurophysiol 39*:114–121, 1976/77

14. Livingston WK: *Pain mechanisms: A Physiologic Interpretation of Causalgia and its Related States.* New York, Plenum Press, 1976

15. Tasker R: Percutaneous cordotomy. *Compr Ther 1*:51–56, 1975

16. Tasker RR: The merits of percutaneous cordotomy over the open operation, in Morley TP (ed): *Current Controversies in Neurosurgery.* Philadelphia, Saunders 1976, pp 496–501

17. Tasker RR, Organ LW, Hawrylyshyn P: Deafferentation and causalgia, in Bonica JJ (ed): *Pain.* New York, Raven Press, 1980, pp 305–329, ARNMD vol. 58.

18. Tasker RR: Open cordotomy. *Prog Neurol Surg 8*:1–14, 1977

19. Crue BL, Todd EM, Carregal EJA: Posterior approach for high cervical percutaneous radiofrequency cordotomy. *Confin Neurol 30*:41–52, 1968

20. Belmusto L, Brown E, Owens G: Clinical observations on respiratory and vasomotor disturbances as related to cervical cordotomies. *J Neurosurg 20*:225–232, 1963

21. Nathan PW: The descending respiratory pathway in man. *J Neurol Neurosurg Psychiatry 26*:487–499, 1963

22. Belmusto L, Woldring S, Owens G: Localization and patterns of potentials of the respiratory pathway in the cervical spinal cord in the dog. *J Neurosurg 22*:277–283, 1965

23. Hitchcock E, Leece B: Somatotopic representation of the respiratory pathways in the cervical cord of man. *J Neurosurg 27*:320–329, 1967

24. Mullan S, Hosobuchi Y: Respiratory hazards of high cervical percutaneous cordotomy. *J Neurosurg 28*:291–297, 1968

25. Tenicela R, Rosomoff HL, Feist J, et al: Pulmonary function following percutaneous cervical cordotomy. *Anesthesiology 29*:7–16, 1968

26. Fox JL: Localization of the respiratory pathway in the upper cervical spinal cord following percutaneous cordotomy. *Neurology [Minneap] 19*:1115–1118, 1969

27. Rosomoff HL, Krieger AJ, Kuperman AJ: Effects of percutaneous cervical cordotomy on pulmonary function. *J Neurosurg 31*:620–627, 1969

28. Lin RM, Gildenberg PL, Polakoff PP: An anterior approach to percutaneous lower cervical cordotomy. *J Neurosurg 25*:553–560, 1966

29. Collis JS Jr: Anterolateral cordotomy by an anterior approach. Report of a case. *J Neurosurg 20*:445–446, 1963

30. Cloward RB: Cervical chordotomy by the anterior approach. Technique and advantages. *J Neurosurg 21*:19–25, 1964

31. French LA, Peyton WT: Ipsilateral sensory loss following cordotomy. *J Neurosurg 5*:403–404, 1948

32. Voris HC: Ipsilateral sensory loss following cordotomy: Report of a case. *Arch Neurol Psychiat 65*:95–96, 1951

33. Voris HC: Variations in the spinothalamic tract in man. *J Neurosurg 14*:55–60, 1957

34. Voris HC: Anomalies of the human spinothalamic tract, in *Proceding of the 111 International Congress Neurological Surgeons Exc. Med* Amsterdam, Excerpta Medica, 1965, pp 794–797

35. Morley TP: Congenital rotation of the spinal cord. *J Neurosurg 10*:690–692, 1953

36. Sweet WH: Percutaneous cordotomy, in Schmidek HH, Sweet WH (eds): *Current Techniques in Operative Neurosurgery.* New York, Grune & Stratton, 1977, pp 449–467

37. Tasker R: Somatotopographic representation in the human thalamus, midbrain, and spinal cord. The anatomical basis for the surgical relief of pain, in Morley TP (ed): *Current Controversies in Neurosurgery.* Philadelphia, WB Saunders, 1976, pp 485–495

CHAPTER 74
Commissural Myelotomy

John E. Adams
Robert Lippert

Yoshio Hosobuchi

COMMISSURAL OR MEDIOLONGITUDINAL MYELOTOMY was first performed for the relief of pain by Armour in 1927.[1] The rationale for this operation is obviously based upon the traditional concept that finely myelinated and unmyelinated fibers of the lateral division of the dorsal root, which subserve nociception, cross in the anterior commissure of the spinal cord at the level of or up to three segments cephalad to their point of entry into the spinal cord. Thus, by sectioning the anterior commissure over several segments, the neurosurgeon theoretically should be able to bilaterally denervate relevant segments of the body from nociceptive input. This potential ability to relieve bilateral segmental pain during a single operation without compromising the function of the descending or ascending long tracts presents obvious advantages over bilateral anterolateral spinal tractotomy at either the high thoracic or high cervical level. The naturally occurring model for spinal commissurotomy, of course, is the cystic lesion of syringomyelia, where the pathologic process interrupts the same decussating fibers as the surgeon does with a knife, producing a result that is clinically identical insofar as the segmental loss of nonciception is concerned.

The operation has enjoyed moderate popularity in European centers,[2-5] but until recently rarely has been performed in the United States.[6] It is perhaps noteworthy, however, that the introduction of the operating microscope has encouraged a revival of this operative procedure for the relief of intractable pain. This is no mere coincidence, since in spite of earlier successes achieved without benefit of the operating microscope, it is clear that both the success achieved without and prevention of postoperative complications are greatly enhanced by the microsurgical technique.

We have employed commissural myelotomy primarily to relieve intractable bilateral pain in the lower abdomen, pelvis, perineum, and lower extremities. Most patients have suffered from malignant disease, but we have employed the procedure in patients whose pain was of nonmalignant origin, such as in patients suffering from chronic adhesive arachnoiditis, trauma to the spinal column, etc. The majority of patients have had pain involving the lower segments of their body, but in a minority the pain has originated in the middle or upper thoracic region.

Technique

The position of the incision in a caudad cephalad plane is dictated by the highest segment involved in the painful process. The myelotomy must extend at least three cord segments above

Department of Neurological Surgery, University of California Medical Center, San Francisco, California

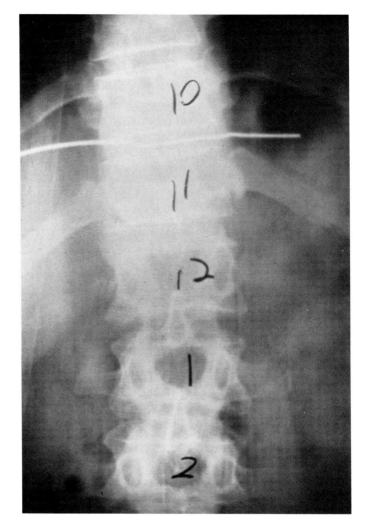

Fig. 74-1. Spinous process of T10 identified in roentgenogram by marker placed on skin.

this level. Thus, if the pain extends as high as the L1 dermatome, it will be necessary to carry the myelotomy as high as the tenth thoracic segment in the cord.

General anesthesia usually is employed, although the operation can be done under local anesthesia. The patient is placed in the prone position, since there is nothing to be gained by employing either the lateral or sitting position. A skin marker is placed over the designated spinous process, which is then verified by an intraoperative x-ray film (Fig. 74-1). After the laminectomy has been completed, if there is any doubt regarding the level, another intraoperative film can be taken.

After the appropriate laminectomy has been performed and the dura has been opened, the operating microscope is positioned and, at a magnification of four- to sixfold, the midline sulcus of the dorsal surface of the spinal cord is identified. This is accomplished by identifying the midline dorsal vein and the fine arachnoidal septum. With microdissection, the midline dorsal vein is coagulated with bipolar forceps throughout the length of proposed incision (Fig. 74-2). It also may be necessary to coagulate one or two very small arterial radicals that may cross the midline. King[7] has stressed the advisability of preserving not only the midline dorsal vein but even the smallest arterial branch. We have not, however, encountered any deleterious effects after coagu-

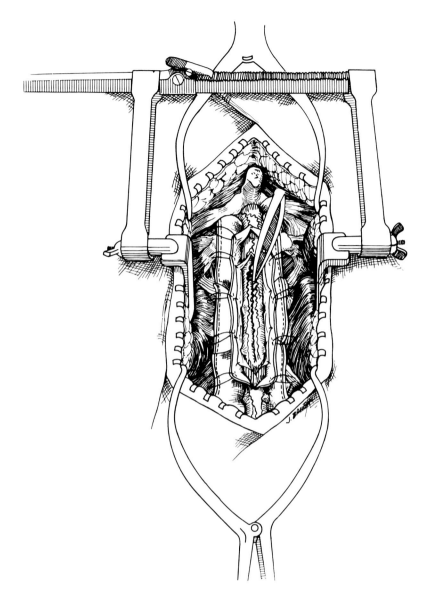

Fig. 74-2. Artist's drawing of bipolar coagulation of midline dorsal vein.

lation of these small vessels. The length of the proposed incision is thus prepared, varying from 2.5 to 4 cm, depending upon the extent of the body area involved in the painful syndrome.

Two methods have been used to carry out the section of the anterior commissure. Either an iridectomy knife or a No. 12 Bard-Parker blade held in a hemostat (Fig. 74-3) is used to penetrate the upper end of the median sulcus to a depth of 6 to 7 mm. The knife is then passed in a caudad direction, maintaining its position strictly in the midline, as viewed in the microscopic field, until the full length of the planned incision has been achieved (Fig. 74-4).

An alternative method that is sometimes employed is to develop the median incision through the pia-arachnoid with sharp section and then, with a blunt microdissector, to penetrate the midline cord through the anterior commissure, with gentle bilateral retraction of the incision to give visualization throughout.

At the present time we employ the former technique in most cases because we feel that the open technique involves more manipulation of the cord and consequently more risk of damage to the posterior columns and the lateral funiculus.

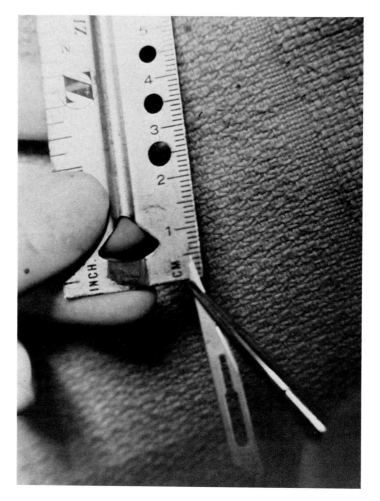

Fig. 74-3.   Desired length of cutting edge of Bard-Parker blade is measured.

King[7] prefers the open technique to ensure complete section of the anterior commissure, as well as to avoid coagulation of any blood vessels.

Postoperative Care

Postoperative mobilization and ambulation are dictated, to some extent, by the primary disease but can occur as early as the first or second postoperative day. Catheterization may be necessary, but often is not.

Results

Our results with 24 patients who have undergone this procedure are summarized in Table 74-1 and 74-2. Table 74-1 gives the results in terms of the etiology of the painful syndrome. For simplicity, the clinical result has been designated as either complete, partial, or no relief of pain. In Table 74-2 the same data are tabulated in terms of the anatomic site of pain. Since many patients had pain involving more than one area of the body, the number of pain locations represented is greater than the actual number of patients operated upon.

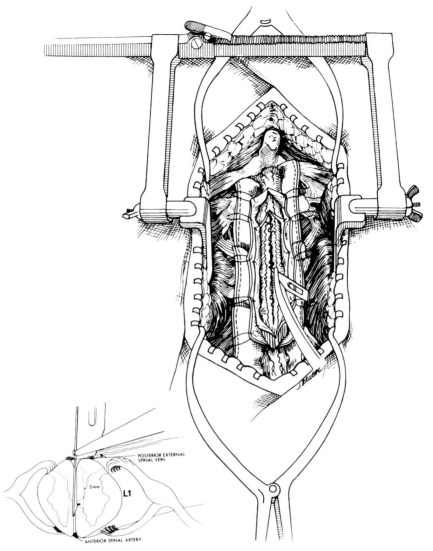

Fig. 74-4. Artist's illustration of technique of blind section through midline of spinal cord. Diagrammatic representation of the section in the coronal plane (inset).

There were no deaths in this series and complications were not serious. Bladder function that was normal preoperatively was altered in 3 patients, 2 of whom became unable to void and were discharged with a catheter in place. One patient developed partial incontinence. Weakness of the legs, present in 2 patients, appeared to be a lower motor neuron disturbance and was interpreted as being a result of damage to anterior horn cells in appropriate segments. Paresthesias or dysesthesias were temporarily encountered in most patients, but disappeared within a few days in all but 4. This complication was interpreted as being the result of trauma to posterior columns of the cord. In the 4 patients in whom these symptoms persisted, there also was a concomitant loss of position sense in the lower extremities; this did not, however, interfere significantly with ambulation.

From these results, it can be seen that commissural myelotomy should be considered in the treatment of intractable pain when that pain is primarily bilateral or involves midline structures of the body. With the advent of the operating microscope and newer microsurgical techniques, it appears to be a relatively safe procedure. In this regard the operation was abandoned after its in-

Table 74-1. Results of Commissural Myelotomy According to Etiology in 24 Patients

Diagnosis	No. of patients	Relief			Complications			Comments
		Complete	Partial	None	Bladder	Leg weakness	Persistent dysesthesia	
Carcinoma of:								
Rectum and colon	7	5	1	1	1	1	3	Pain due to pelvic extension
Cervix and uterus	4	3	1	—	—	1	—	Pain due to pelvic extension
Bladder	1	1	—	—	—	—	1	Pain due to pelvic extension
Breast	1	—	1	—	—	—	—	Metastatic to lumbar spine and pelvic mass
Prostate	3	2	1	—	—	—	—	Metastic disease to the lumbar spine
Lung	2	—	1	1	1	—	—	Metastatic to the thoracic spine and sternum
Osteogenic sarcoma	1	1	—	—	—	—	—	Metastatic to the lumbar sacral spine
Transverse myelitis	1	—	1	—	—	—	—	Girdle chest pains
Medulloblastoma	1	1	—	—	—	—	—	Metastatic to cauda equina
Paraplegia traumatic	1	1	—	—	—	—	—	Burning leg pain
Multiple sclerosis	1	1	—	—	—	—	—	Constant sacral pain plus painful flexor spasms
Sacral Chordoma	1	—	1	—	1	—	—	—
Total	24	15	7	2	3	2	4	

troduction into this country primarily because of the fear of injury to the anterior spinal artery.[8] This has not occurred in any of our cases.

In the series reported in the United States, commissural myelotomy has been performed primarily in lower segments of the cord for midline pain involving the pelvis or for bilateral lower extremity pain. In Europe and in England, however, the operation has been employed more frequently for midline or bilateral truncal pain as well as for pain involving the lower cervical areas and the upper extremities.[4]

The sensory loss following commissural myelotomy is extremely variable. In our cases no reproducible pattern was evident. The loss of awareness to pain and temperature might errati-

Table 74-2. Results of Commissural Myelotomy According to Anatomic Site of Pain

Location of pain	No. of patients	Relief			Complications		
		Complete	Partial	None	Bladder	Motor loss	Persistent dysesthesia
Chest	2	1	—	1	1	—	—
Lumbosacral spine	3	2	1	—	—	—	—
Rectum and perineum	11	7	3	1	1	1	3
Buttock	2	1	1	—	1	—	—
Legs and hips	10	7	3	—	—	1	4
Suprapubic	1	1	—	—	—	—	1
Testicular	1	—	1	—	—	—	—
Total	30	19	9	2	3	2	8

cally involve the appropriate segments, but in some instances there was only minimal loss of acute pain and temperature sensation, even though there was complete relief from chronic pain. This has been the experience of all surgeons who have performed this operation.

Discussion

As yet, there is no adequate explanation for the relief of pain obtained by this procedure. To consider that section of the decussating fibers in the anterior commissure is the sole explanation appears to be too simplistic, especially in view of the vagaries of the resultant sensory loss. Sourek[4] has hypothesized that the relief of pain is due to the involvement of two sensory systems that subserve nociception. These are the slow conducting anterolateral system and the more rapidly conducting mediodorsal system. Hitchcock[9] has produced profound and extensive analgesia following a stereotactically placed small midline lesion in the anterior commissure at either the medullary cervical junction or at the C1-2 level. He suggests that not only the pain relief but also the extensive analgesia produced by lesions at this site may be the result of interruption of decussations of both direct and crossed pain pathways ascending close to the gray matter of the spinal cord, or are possibly the result of interruption of fibers in the spinal cervical tract (Morin), which decussate in the high cervical area.

Conclusions

On the basis of our experience and a review of the literature, it would appear that spinal commissurotomy has now become a relatively safe and effective procedure. It should be seriously considered as a method to manage intractable pain related to midline structures of the body, or bilateral pain. It may well become the procedure of choice for rectal and perineal pain. At the present time, however, we still would recommend the use of other procedures for the relief of unilateral pain.

REFERENCES

1. Armour D: Surgery of the spinal cord. *Lancet* 2:691–697, 1927
2. Guillian J, Mazars G, Movillae V: La myelatomie commissurale. *Presse Med* 49:666–667, 1945
3. Neansery B, Lecuire J, Acassat L: Technique de la myelatomie commissurale posterieure. *J Chir* 60:206–213, 1944
4. Sourek K: Commissural myelotomy. *J Neurosurg* 31:524–527, 1969
5. Wertheimer P: Posterior commissural myelotomy for relief of pain. *Acta Chir Belg* 54:28–29, 1946
6. Lippert RS, Hosobuchi Y, Nielsen SL: Spinal commissurotomy. *Surg Neurol* 2:373–377, 1974
7. King RB: Anterior Commissurotomy for intractable pain. *J Neurosurg* 47:7–11, 1977
8. Putnam JJ: Myelotomy of the commissure. *Arch Neurol Psychiatry* 32:189 195, 1934
9. Hitchcock E: Stereotactic cervical myelotomy. *J Neurol Neurosurg Psychiatry* 33:224–230, 1970

CHAPTER 75
Longitudinal (Bischof's) Myelotomy

Leslie P. Ivan

THE MAIN FEATURES OF SPASTICITY arise from the exaggerated stretch reflex and the exaggerated flexor withdrawal. Any surgical procedure that can disrupt the reflex arcs participating in these two basic spinal reflexes would relieve muscle spasm and flexor withdrawal reflexes. The methods listed in Table 75-1 all relieve spasticity, but each has some disadvantage. Posterior rhizotomy has no lasting effect and produces complete sensory denervation in the segments involved, thus predisposing these areas to the development of pressure sores. Intrathecal alcohol injection gives temporary relief only and may aggravate the bladder problem. Intrathecal phenol injection is somewhat unpredictable in its effects, and even a satisfactory injection has the same disadvantage as alcohol. Cordectomy is a major procedure and its finality makes both the patient and the surgeon uneasy. Cauda equina transection, besides having the same finality as cordectomy, has the disadvantages of both anterior and posterior rhizotomy. Anterior rhizotomy is followed by severe muscle wasting and exposure of bony prominences, which increases the risk of pressure sores either in the ischial region from sitting or in the lower extremities of patients who wear braces.

Bischof's myelotomy, on the other hand, produces permanent flaccidity without loss of muscle bulk and, except for segmental analgesia, should not affect other sensory modalities. With accurate technique, all long tracts, including the pyramidal tract, should remain intact following myelotomy. An important feature of longitudinal myelotomy is that after the operation there is no late recurrence of spasticity because the short propriospinal pathways and the long collaterals were disrupted (Fig. 75-1). This disruption eliminates the influx of afferent impulses from higher and lower segments, which is the suggested cause of failure in some of the other methods.

Bischof[1] first described his procedure in 1951 and called it *longitudinal lateral myelotomy*. No response to his paper can be found in the medical literature until 1955 when Weber[2] reported the use of this technique in 2 patients, with good results. Nadvornik,[3] in 1961, reported 1 such case and commented favorably on the procedure. In 1962, Tonnis and Bischof[4] gave an account of 20 cases with a follow-up time of 2 to 8 years. Our papers with Paine and Hunt,[5,6] in 1966 and

Division of Neurosurgery, Children's Hospital of Eastern Ontario, Ottawa, Ontario, Canada

The work appearing in this chapter was supported by grants from the Medical Research Council of Canada, from the Ontario Crippled Children's Society, and from the Multiple Sclerosis Society of Canada.

Art work and photography were done by the Department of Medical Communication, Faculty of Medicine, University of Ottawa, Canada, and by the Department of Medical Illustration, Children's Hospital of Eastern Ontario.

The adjustable electrodes, the spinal cord gauges, and the special knives were developed by Mr. G. Zellerman, Accurate Surgical Instruments Company, Toronto, Ontario.

Special thanks are due to Maureen Melrose for assembling the references and editing the manuscript and to Lise Riffel for the numerous retypings.

Table 75-1. Procedures for the Relief of Spasm

Procedure	Described by
1. Posterior rhizotomy	Foerster 1910
2. Intrathecal alcohol	Dogliotti 1930
3. Intrathecal phenol	Suvansa 1931
4. Cordectomy	MacCarty 1948
5. Transsection of cauda equina	Meriowsky 1950
6. Anterior rhizotomy	Munro 1945
7. Myelotomy	Bischof 1951

1967, appear to be the first North American accounts of this operation. The procedure gained popularity in Canada, and the Canadian experience was summarized by Moyes in 1969.[7] Since then, several reports from various countries have been published,[8-12] with all authors commenting favorably on the method.

Technical Considerations and Modifications

The original Bischof's myelotomy involves separating the spinal cord longitudinally into an anterior and posterior half between the L1 and L5 segments, to which unilateral separation between S1 and S3 can be added to decrease bladder spasticity. Bischof suggested severing the cord completely into an anterior and posterior half to preserve the pyramidal tract on one side (Fig. 75-2). Later Pourpre, in 1960,[13] and Bischof, in 1967,[14] suggested an approach through the posterior median fissure (Fig. 75-3).

A further search for the ideal procedure resulted in the use of an L-shaped knife by the author, and this procedure was called *circular griseotomy* (Fig. 75-4), which worked well in animal experiments (Fig. 75-5). During laboratory trials it became obvious that both mechanical and radiofrequency destruction can be used (Fig. 75-6). It was recognized that for the relief of spasticity the effective part of the surgery is *disruption of pathways inside the gray matter. That is why the term griseotomy (cutting the gray) was proposed.*[8,15]

In experiments on 43 dogs (Table 75-2), my colleagues and I made the following observations: lateral longitudinal myelotomy, circular griseotomy, T-griseotomy, and radiofrequency lesions would all relieve spasticity; however, myelotomy on intact animals caused more paraplegia than any of the other procedures. Radiofrequency heat could reduce or eliminate spasticity, provided the lesions were made close to each other (4 mm apart), at least two lesions per segment. This would indicate that to achieve segmental relief of spasticity of the lower limbs in hu-

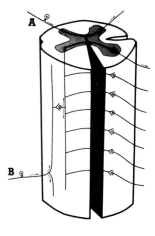

Fig. 75-1. Schematic representation of the original concept of Bischof's myelotomy. **A.** Monosynaptic reflex arc. **B.** Reflex collaterals with ascending and descending branches to motor neurons.

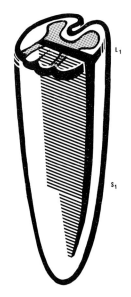

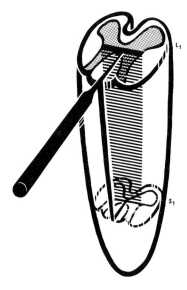

Fig. 75-2. Bischof's myelotomy. The original procedure.

Fig. 75-3. T-griseotomy.

man beings, at least 14 to 18 radiofrequency lesions should be made on each side in the equatorial line of the cord. The target area is within the gray matter in lamina 6 and 7 of Rexed (Fig. 75-7).

Indications for Myelotomy

Myelotomy can best be used for patients suffering from spasticity of the lower limbs that is of such a degree that the spasms interfere with sitting in a wheelchair or lying comfortably in bed and when there are some cord functions that are advantageous to preserve. *Without further refinement of the present technique, myelotomy should not be performed on patients who are able to walk.* In some patients the use of braces or the ability to walk may be restored following successful myelotomy, and it is possible to retain voluntary emptying of the bladder if this was preserved in the original injury or disease.

If the patient has severe pain in the lower limbs, which is not infrequent in spastic conditions, relief of this pain might be an additional indication for this type of procedure.

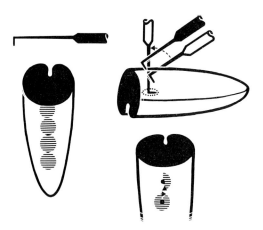

Fig. 75-4. Technique of circular griseotomy. An L-shaped instrument is inserted through the posterior midline sulcus and rotated 360° in the equatorial plane of the cord.

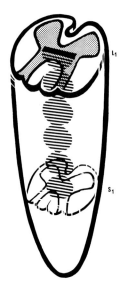

Fig. 75-5. The end result of circular griseotomy: a series of circular cuts within the gray matter.

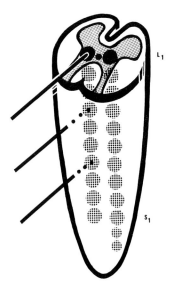

Fig. 75-6. Radiofrequency griseotomy. Radiofrequency heat microlesions within the gray matter through the posterior approach with a 0.5-mm bare-tip electrode.

Preoperative Management

Routine laboratory studies, x-ray films of the lumbosacral spine, a cystometrography, urologic assessment, exact charting of muscle strength, muscle tone, reflexes and sensory functions, and also measurement of the degree of contractures are required studies.

Most patients already have indwelling catheters. If not, a catheter should be inserted before surgery. During surgery, electrocystometrography can be performed to ascertain whether bladder tone was reduced sufficiently.

Operative Exploration

The surgery is always performed under general endotracheal anesthesia. The patient is positioned prone on the operating table, with semiflexion in hip and knee joints, and draped in such a way that an observer can report movements when nerve root stimulation is done during surgery.

The spinous processes are counted from C7 and the count double-checked by counting

Table 75-2. Segmental Relief of Spasticity

	No. of dogs	Postoperative paraplegia	Percentage
Group 1			
Lateral longitudinal myelotomy	4	4	100
Group 2			
Circular griseotomy	14	4	28
Group 3			
RF griseotomy	25	10	40
Total	43	18	

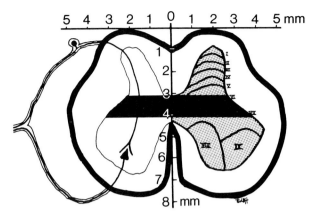

Fig. 75-7. The target area (blackened between 3 and 4 mm) within the gray matter for the relief of spasticity. The roman numbers indicate the laminar structure of the gray matter according to Rexed. The arabic numbers are reference points in millimeters.

them from the L5 vertebra. The T10 vertebra is marked, and after the patient's back is cleansed with surgical soap and Betadine scrub, the operative field is draped between the T7 and L3 spinous processes. An incision is marked between the T9 and L2 spinous processes, and the subcutaneous tissue and paraspinal muscles are infiltrated with physiologic saline. The incision is made in the midline, and, through subperiosteal dissection, the T9, T10, T11, T12, and L1 vertebrae are exposed (Fig. 75-8). A laminectomy is done on the T10, T11, T12, and L1 vertebrae. After the dura is opened, the conus medullaris should be at the caudal part of the operative field and at least 80 mm of spinal cord should be visible. Holding sutures are placed in the dura, while the operative field is kept bloodless with the usual placement of cotton pledgets (Fig. 75-9).

Using a nerve stimulator with a 2-V, 7-msec current, the T12 and S1 nerve roots should be identified. This is done by rotating the cord slightly and placing the stimulating electrode on the motor root of T12 while an observer identifies contraction of the lower abdominal muscles. Contraction can sometimes be felt by the operating surgeon through the draping. The S1 nerve root is usually the thickest of the cauda equina fibers, and when the motor root of S1 is stimulated,

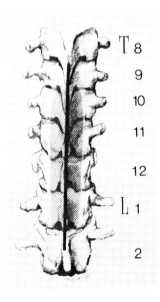

Fig. 75-8. Schematic drawing showing the extent of the incision and laminectomy.

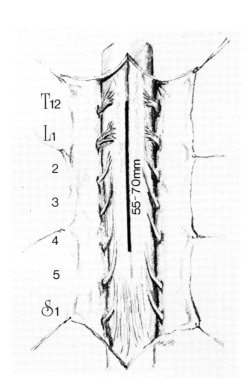

Fig. 75-9. Artist's concept of the exposed cord indicating the length of the cord between L1 and S1 segments.

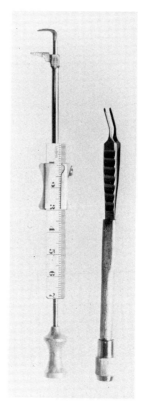

Fig. 75-10. Spinal cord gauges for measuring the width and AP diameter of the cord.

the foot should move into plantar flexion. After these two landmarks are identified (the distance between them varies between 55 to 70 mm), the surgeon should prepare the cord and instruments for the lesion-making procedure. The width and AP diameter of the cord are measured with a spinal cord gauge (Fig. 75-10). The total length of the cord subject to lesion-making is also measured (Fig. 75-9).

Lesion-Making

Four methods of lesion-making will be described. The first three depend upon mechanical instruments that are used laterally on the cord or through a posterior approach. The fourth depends upon radiofrequency heat and is done posteriorly.

Lateral Longitudinal Myelotomy

Lateral longitudinal myelotomy is the original method of Bischof (Fig. 75-11). In preparation for the myelotomy the cord is rotated sideways after the last three denticulate ligaments are cut. Some surgeons use a No. 11 blade or a keratome;[16] others, such as myself, use a slightly less sharp and smaller instrument (Fig. 75-12). If it is difficult to rotate the cord, it can be transfixed with three 20-gauge needles to make it easier to rotate and find the cutting plane. An incision then is made slowly just anterior to the attachment of the denticulate ligament in the equatorial line of the cord, in such a way that about 2.5 mm of the cord is saved on the opposite side. This

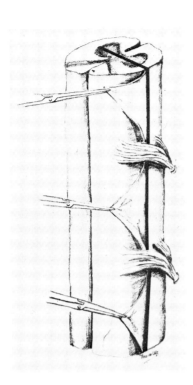

Fig. 75-11. A drawing showing the rotation of the cord and the plane of incision at the attachment of the dentate ligaments.

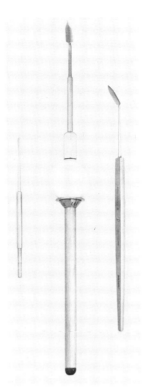

Fig. 75-12. Instruments used for the incision of the cord in lateral longitudinal myelotomy.

can be determined accurately by measuring the width of the cord (which may vary anywhere between 6 to 10 mm) and marking the knife with a hemoclip or a small piece of bone wax. The cutting (in a length of 55 to 70 mm) is done in small segments, because the space between the anterior and posterior roots prevents a continuous incision. Usually some blood begins to ooze in the line of the incision; the bleeding, however, stops when the wound is irrigated and small cotton pledgets are placed. When the oozing stops, the dura is closed with interrupted 0000 black silk sutures, and the muscle layer is closed with 0 silk or 0 chromic catgut. The fascia, subcutaneous tissue, and the skin are closed with sutures, according to the surgeon's routine. There is no need for a drain.

Posterior Longitudinal Myelotomy

Posterior longitudinal myelotomy was first described by Pourpre, in 1960,[13] who called it *Myelotomy en Croix*; the author termed it *T-griseotomy* (Fig. 75-3). After the exposure described previously and after nerve stimulation and measurements, the posterior median sulcus of the cord is identified under magnification and, avoiding injury to the dorsal vein, the posterior median fissure is entered to a depth half that of the AP diameter of the cord with an L-shaped knife (Fig. 75-13). Separation is made in the usual myelotomy plane, 3 mm on each side, sideways from the midline. The final myelotomy is reached by proceeding with the separation in small sections to avoid injuring the usually tortuous dorsal vein. At the end of this procedure a T-shaped cleavage is left in the cord for a length of 55 to 70 mm. Slight oozing is easily controlled by irrigation with physiologic saline and by placement of small cotton pledgets. The wound is closed as previously described.

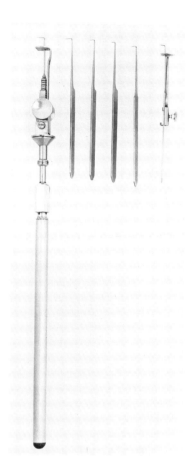

Fig. 75-13.   The L-shaped knives for T-griseotomy and the attachment for circular griseotomy.

Circular Griseotomy

Circular griseotomy (Figs. 75-4 and 75-5) was used with a stereotactic attachment in animal experiments. A freehand method with a special knife (Fig. 75-13) was used by the author in 5 patients with good results, except for 1 patient who had unilateral recurrence of spasticity. A somewhat similar method was described by Yamada et al.,[17] who reported excellent results in 14 patients, 5 of whom were able to walk following the procedure (Fig. 75-14).

Radiofrequency Griseotomy

After several years of experimentation and the development of suitable electrodes, radiofrequency griseotomy was performed on 5 adults. The technique depends upon the same exploration as the previous procedures. Special electrodes with adjustable tips are used (Fig. 75-15). Fourteen to 18 pairs of lesions are necessary to obtain satisfactory results (Fig. 75-16). The tip of the needle should be inserted 2 mm from the midline on each side, and a pair of lesions should be made at each 4-mm distance along the posterior aspect of the cord. Depending upon the measurement of the cord, the half millimeter bare tip of the electrode should reach a depth of 3 to 4 mm (Fig. 75-17). Using the Radionics lesion-maker with a test-lesion setting of 100 mA, 50-mA 10-sec-effective radiofrequency lesions are made at each insertion. Care should be taken to use a clean electrode for each lesion.

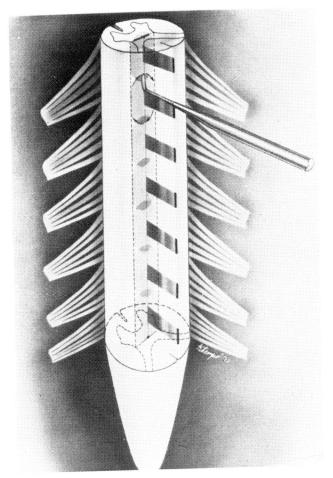

Fig. 75-14. Drawing illustrating the procedure described by Yamada et al. From Yamada S, Perot PL, Ducker TB, et al: Myelotomy for control of mass spasms in paraplegia. *J Neurosurg 45*:683–690, 1976. Reprinted with the kind permission of the author and editor.

Postoperative Care

After surgery, the patient should be turned hourly. Physiotherapy can be started on the day after surgery. Patients are able to take solid food 24 hours after surgery, although in some cases paralytic ileus may be a complicating factor. In case of pre-existing pressure sores in the sacral areas, prophylactic antibiotic treatment is justifiable to prevent wound infection. A week after surgery, wheelchair routine may start and, if the patient's condition permits, the learning of self-transfer from bed to wheelchair can be started. In case there are remaining useful functions, ambulation with long braces can be attempted 3 or 4 weeks after surgery.

Results

Most reports agree that myelotomy is one of the best available procedures for the permanent relief of spasticity. The question is, which type of myelotomy should be performed to ensure that spasticity recurs less frequently and a greater number of patients can ambulate after

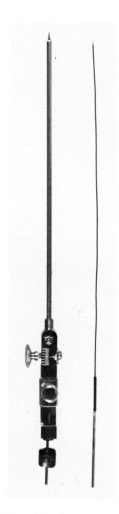

Fig. 75-15. Adjustable needle electrode with 0.5 mm bare tip. Depending on the AP diameter of the cord, the penetrating portion of the electrode can be adjusted with 0.5-mm accuracy.

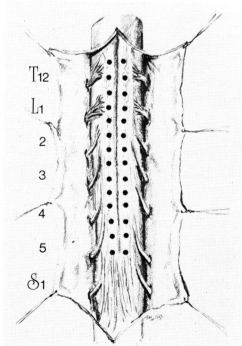

Fig. 75-16. Points of penetration on the dorsal aspect of the cord for radiofrequency griseotomy. The distance between the lesions is 4 mm, both in the craniocaudal and lateral direction.

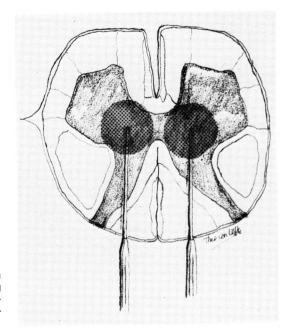

Fig. 75-17. Schematic drawing of the cord with two electrodes in position showing the approximate area of radiofrequency heat destruction in the intermediate gray matter.

surgery? Unfortunately, on the basis of the available literature, including the author's material, this question cannot be answered with certainty.

The great majority of case reports comment on the *original Bischof's method.*[7,8,10,11,18,19] It appears that with unilateral longitudinal myelotomy, spasticity recurs on the opposite side to the cord incision in about 20 percent of the cases.[20]

Posterior commissural myelotomy (myelotomy en croix or T-griseotomy), on the other hand, seems to have definite advantages compared with the original Bischof's method.[14,20] There have been only about 14 cases reported in all of the medical literature. The author's single experience showed that this was a time-consuming procedure, but the patient had good relief of spasticity; movements in the ankle joint were preserved on both sides. The paper by Laitinen and Singounas,[9] from Finland, reporting the results in 9 patients, gives a favorable impression of this method.

Circular griseotomy appeared to be a feasible procedure in animal experiments and in patients.[17] Refinement of the instrumentation and adapting it for the characteristics of the human spinal cord may make this a very valuable technique in the hands of someone who sees a large number of patients.

Radiofrequency griseotomy worked very well in animal experiments and was performed five times on patients by the author. The last 3 patients treated by this method had excellent results. One of the patients who died because of pulmonary embolism (the only fatality among 26 patients) provided us with a spinal cord specimen (Fig. 75-18). The histology showed that the lesions surprisingly were bigger than predicted from egg-white experiments. The radiofrequency lesions of the cord were entirely bloodless, but the selectivity of the method cannot be judged from the small number of cases.

My colleagues and I have frequently found that a contracture that appeared fixed clinically may disappear entirely under general anesthesia. A slight degree of contracture after myelotomy may resolve spontaneously. In a few cases we combine myelotomy with tenotomy of the hamstring muscles.

In my material, which consists of 26 cases, only 1 patient could walk with braces after surgery.

Spasticity recurs in about 20 percent of the cases. In half of these the recurrence is insignificant and not disturbing. In about 10 percent of the cases, re-operation or intrathecal alcohol injection should abolish the remaining spasticity.

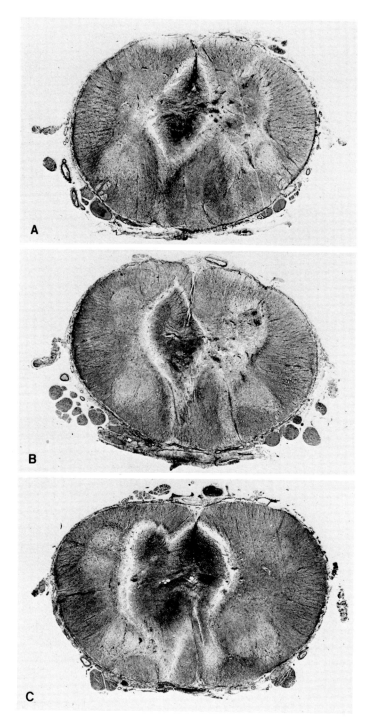

Fig. 75-18.   Histologic appearance of human spinal cord 2 days after radiofrequency griseotomy. Death was due to pulmonary embolism.
Note the lesions, which are considerably larger than expected
from egg-white experiments.

For those neurosurgeons who have an occasional case, probably the original unilateral longitudinal myelotomy is the most suitable method. For those who see many cases, a variety of modifications are available, as discussed earlier.

From the purely experimental circular griseotomy through the proved radiofrequency griseotomy to the quite well-accepted posterior commissural myelotomy, there are a variety of lesion-making methods. With the development of ultrasound and laser, a wide field of experimentation remains open. The target to be destroyed within the gray matter, corresponding roughly to lamina 6 and 7 of Rexed, is well established;[15,21] it is the intermediate gray matter around the equatorial plane of the cord.

REFERENCES

1. Bischof W: Die longitudinale myelotomie, *Zentralbl Neurochir 11*:79–88, 1951
2. Weber W: Die Behandlung der spinalen Paraspastik unter besonderer Berucksichtigung der longitudinalen Myelotomie (Bischof). *Med Monatsschr 9*:510–513, 1955
3. Nadvornik P: Effect of longitudinal myelotomy on spasticity of lower limbs and urinary bladder. *Sb Ved Pr Lek Fak Karlovy Univ 2*:77, 1959, abstracted, *Excerpta Med VIII 14*:3876, 852, 1961
4. Tonnis W, Bischof W: Ergebnisse der lumbalen Myelotomie nach Bischof. *Zentralbl Neurochir 23*:120–132, 1962
5. Ivan LP, Paine KWE, Hunt TE: Experience with Bischof's myelotomy. *Can J Surg 10*:191–195, 1967
6. Paine KW, Ivan LP, Hunt TE: The Bischof myelotomy for treatment of spasticity in paraplegics. *Proc Annu Clin Spinal Cord Inj Conf 15*:72–86, 1966
7. Moyes PD: Longitudinal myelotomy for spasticity. *J Neurosurg 31*:615–619, 1969
8. Ivan LP, Wiley JJ: Myelotomy in the management of spasticity. *Clin Orthop 108*:52–56, 1975
9. Laitinen L, Singounas E: Longitudinal myelotomy in the treatment of spasticity of the legs. *J Neurosurg 35*:536–540, 1971
10. Schirmer M, Barz D, Wenker H: Longitudinal myelotomy—indication and results. *Acta Neurochir (Vienna) 31*:308–309, 1975
11. VanderArk MC, Kempe GL: Longitudinal myelotomy in spastic paraplegia. *Milit Med 134*:608–611, 1969
12. Virozue ID, Chipko SS: Experience with 60 frontal myelotomies in treatment of spastic manifestations in patients with injuries of the spine and spinal cord. *Voprosy Neurochir 2*:21–26, 1975
13. Pourpre MH: Traitement neuro-chirurgical des contractures chez les paraplégiques post traumatiques. *Neurochirurgie 6*:229–236, 1960
14. Bischof W: Zur dorsalen longitudinalen Myelotomie. *Zentralbl Neurochir 28*:123–126, 1967
15. Ivan LP: The segmental relief of spasticity. Read before the 7th Congress of the Canadian Neurological Society, Banff, 1972
16. Asenjo A: *Neurosurgical Techniques.* Springfield, IL, Charles C Thomas, 1963
17. Yamada S, Perot PL, Ducker TB, Lockard I: Myelotomy for control of mass spasms in paraplegia. *J Neurosurg 45*:683–690, 1976
18. Galanda M, Nadvornik P, Frohlich F: Contribution to surgical treatment of spasticity in spinal cord injuries (critical remarks to longitudinal myelotomy). *Bratisl Lek List 61*:589–594, 1974
19. Dietrich J, Sonntag M: Results of treatment of leg paraspasm cases following longitudinal frontal myelotomy. *Psychiatr Neurol Med Psychol (Leipz) 31*:353–359, 1979
20. Gonsette R, André-Ballsaux G: Contribution au traitement neurochirurgical de la spasticité des membres inténeurs dans la sclérose en plaque. *Acta Neurol Psychiatr Belg 63*:460–477, 1963
21. Fever H, Horner TG, De Myer WE, Campbell RL: Anatomical and histological lesions in Bischof's myelotomy in dogs. *Surg Forum 23*:438–440, 1972

CHAPTER 76

Percutaneous Electrothermocoagulation of Spinal Nerve Trunk, Ganglion, and Rootlets

Sumio Uematsu

SELECTIVE SURGICAL INTERRUPTION OF POSTERIOR ROOTS was first carried out by both Abbe[1] and Bennett[2] in 1889. This technique was later extended to sections of anterior roots for the treatment of motor disorders. The open surgical technique limits its applicability to some debilitated patients, however. Therefore, efforts have been made to develop a less traumatic rhizotomy technique. Scoville[3] described a simplified approach for extradural spinal sensory rhizotomy. Dogliotti[4] proposed injecting ethanol alcohol via lumbar puncture into the subarachnoid space, while Maher[5] advocated the use of phenol solution. These hypobaric solutions must be injected with extreme caution, however, since their penetration is likely to be unpredictable and C-fibers as well as the larger myelinated fibers may be destroyed.[6]

Electrothermocoagulation of the Gasserian ganglion for trigeminal neuralgia was introduced by Kirschner.[7] It was later abandoned because of the high complication rate due to the uncontrolled effect of the diathermy current. In October 1965, Sweet[8] introduced an advanced technique for electrothermocoagulation of the trigeminal ganglion. Accumulated clinical experience has shown that it is possible to alleviate pain and still preserve proprioception and motor function in the trigeminal nerve.[8] Based on physiologic studies, it has been assumed that the less myelinated pain fibers were more easily destroyed by heat than were the larger fibers. A preliminary histologic study, however, revealed indiscriminate destruction of both small and large fibers rather than selective destruction of smaller, less myelinated ones. In my opinion, it is therefore logical to believe that the proportional destruction of nerve fibers increases the pain threshold but also preserves enough fibers for satisfactory proprioception and motor function (Fig. 76-1).

Our first percutaneous radiofrequency spinal rhizotomy was carried out in 1971 on an 18-year-old girl with spastic paraplegia caused by a spinal cord injury. Bilateral L1, L2, and L3 roots were denervated to reduce spasticity of the hip joints. The first successful result with this technique encouraged us to expand its use to other spinal levels to treat pain and motor disor-

Department of Neurosurgery, The Johns Hopkins University School of Medicine, Baltimore, Maryland

Gratitude is due Dr. David Bodian, Department of Anatomy, for his suggestions and for the preparation of the histologic slides used in Figure 76-1.
My thanks go to our secretarial and technical staff, Jean Arnett, Erva Baden, Debbie Gilmer, and Richard Kouba, for their careful and conscientious assistance in the completion of the manuscript.

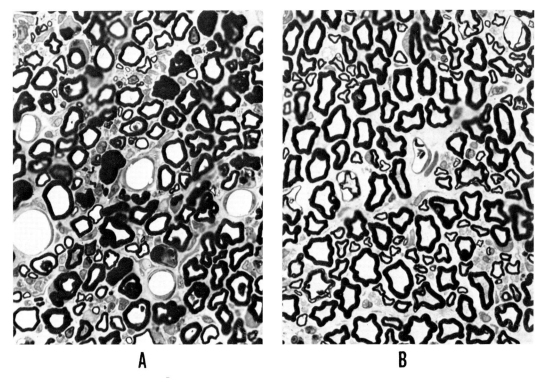

A   **B**

Fig. 76-1. Radiofrequency thermocoagulation of the sciatic nerve of a cat. **A.** Section taken at the site of the heat lesion. Note the indiscriminate effect of the heat on both the small and large myelinated fibers. The wall of the capillaries is well preserved. **B.** Control, proximal portion of same nerve, away from the heat lesion (Phosphotungstic acid hematoxylin, × 750).

ders. Possibly it also could be used to treat spasmodic torticollis[10] and cerebral palsy[11] by differential denervation of sacral rootlets.[12] The application of this technique to the release of spastic bladder was advocated in the previous chapter by this author. Young et al.[20] reported their successful results, the details of which are described in the appropriate section of this chapter.

The technique is relatively simple and definitely less invasive than surgical open rhizotomy. Its success, however, depends heavily upon the availability of a fluoroscopic x-ray monitor for precise stereotactic introduction of the probe into the intervertebral foramen. The procedure should be carried out under local anesthesia. Careful observation of the response to electrical stimulation and the assessment of sensory and motor functions during the entire period of the procedure are essential to avoid undesirable complications.

Anatomy and Physiology

Rootlets, Ganglion, and Trunk

Each spinal nerve arises from the cord through two roots: a posterior sensory and an anterior motor root. These roots traverse the subarachnoid sac, penetrate the dura, and reach the intervertebral foramen, where the posterior roots swell into the spinal ganglion, which contains the cells of origin of sensory fibers. Distal to the ganglion, the posterior and anterior roots unite and emerge from the intervertebral foramen of a mixed spinal nerve or common nerve trunk, which contains both sensory and motor fibers (Fig. 76-2).

Each nerve root has the following five parts, based upon its meningeal covering and relationship to the intervertebral foramina.

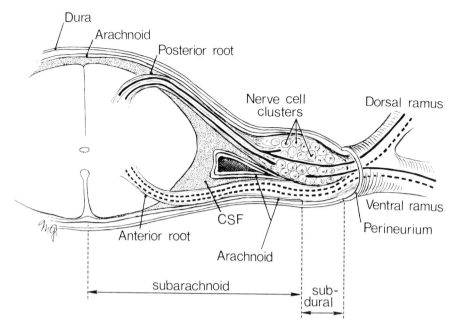

Fig. 76-2. Rootlets, ganglion, and trunk. The subarachnoidal space stops at the proximal end of the ganglion.

1. Subarachnoid
2. Subdural
3. Extra dural
4. Intraforaminal
5. Extraforaminal

Dural and arachnoid sleeves surround both the anterior and posterior nerve roots. The nerves may sometimes be separated or fused, but the arachnoid membranes are definitely separated by the dura and each root is surrounded by its own extension of the subarachnoid space. The subarachnoid space stops at the proximal end of the ganglion on the posterior roots, and in the corresponding portion on the anterior roots. At this termination, there are three meningeal layers, which blend with connective tissue of the peripheral nerves. The subarachnoid space is not believed to be continuous with either the perineural space or the lymphatic channels, but the subdural space is thought to be continuous with connective tissue of the peripheral nerves.

The posterior roots are, as a rule, thicker than the ventral ones and vary with the size of their respective ganglia. The only exception is the first cervical nerve, the dorsal root of which is greatly reduced and often missing. The largest spinal nerves are the lower cervical and the first thoracic, which form the great nerve for the upper limbs and upper sacral nerve for the lower limbs. The smallest in size are the coccygeal nerve roots. Cervical nerve roots diminish in size from below and upward.[13]

Radicular Artery

Most of the 62 embryologic radicular arteries regress during the course of development, and in the adult only six to eight functioning arteries supply the anterior while between 10 and 23 functioning arteries supply the posterior spinal artery. The radicular arteries that actually supply the spinal cord are called *radiculomedullary arteries*. They perfuse the cord via two terminal branches; the anterior and posterior radicular arteries (Fig. 76-3).

The anterior radicular arteries run in the intervertebral foramina on the anterior surface of

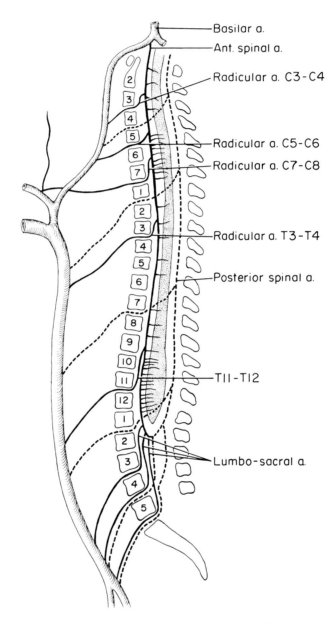

Fig. 76-3. Important arteries via the intervertebral foramens (after Djindjian R., et al. Courtesy of University Park Press, Baltimore).

the dural investment of the spinal roots, and remain extradural until they reach the lateral border of the dural sheath proper. At this point they give off short to medium dural arteries. The anterior radicular arteries then pierce the dura anterior to, and slightly below, the nerve. The arteries then run upward at an angle that depends on the spinal level, always remaining anterior to the plane of the dentate ligament. The posterior radicular arteries, in general, run along the superior border of the nerve sheath, piercing the dura through the same opening as a nerve passing between the sensory nerve filaments, to reach the posterior spinal arteries, always remaining posterior to the plane of the dentate ligament.

The blood supply of the spinal cord may be jeopardized in certain transitional regions where its arterial supply is derived from two different sources. Because the upper third of the spinal cord is supplied primarily by the anterior spinal artery, an occlusion of the C2 or C3 radicular artery, or an occlusion of the vertebral artery, can be revascularized effectively by the retrograde flow from the basilar artery. The inferior two-thirds, including the cervical enlargement, are supplied by a large artery, usually arising from the deep cervical artery, supplemented by a second artery, which is a branch of the first intercostal artery. In the presence of an obstruction of the subclavian artery, or an occlusion of the radicular artery at the interspace of C7 and C8, the only possible blood circulation comes from the contralateral subclavian system. The upper segment of the thoracic spinal cord, on the other hand, depends upon the radicular branches of the intercostal arteries. If one or more of the parent intercostal vessels is compressed, segments of the spinal cord, T1-4, cannot be adequately maintained by the small branches of the anterior spinal artery. For this reason, thoracic segment T1-4, particularly T4, is considered a vulnerable area in the distribution of the anterior spinal artery. The posterior surface of the cord most susceptible to vascular insult is also in segment T1-4. Cord segment T11 and L1, in which the blood supply depends upon the Adamkiewicz artery, is an equally vulnerable region. Any vascular injury may result in necrosis of an entire segment of the cord.[14]

Indications and Selection of Patients

The largest series of patients treated by rhizotomy suffered from pain due to various causes. When pain is limited to a relatively localized area, use of the extremities as well as bladder and bowel function are not impaired when the nerve roots are cut. Rhizotomy has long been the standard operation for relieving pain from metastatic nodes in the neck, provided the trunk of the brachial plexus is not involved.[15]

Patients are selected for rhizotomy on the basis of a detailed history and a careful physical and neurologic examination. If indicated, myelography should be performed. Routine psychometric testing and psychiatric evaluation are necessary for patients with benign chronic pain before any procedure is undertaken.

Diagnostic Paravertebral Block

As a preliminary procedure, it is generally advisable to inject a local anesthetic into the spinal nerve that is being considered for sensory root section. This procedure should be carried out under fluoroscopic control. Anesthesia equipment should be on hand to treat serious respiratory or cardiac complications, if they occur. This temporary procedure serves a dual purpose: it shows the patient what permanent sensory loss will be like, and it assures the surgeon that the given area of analgesia is likely to relieve the patient's discomfort. It does not guarantee, however, that the pain will not recur.

Table 76-1. Extent of Posterior Rhizotomy Recommended

Origin or site of pain	Involved nerves	Roots of origin	Extent of rhizotomy	Comment
Occipital scar	Greater or lesser occipital	C2-3	C2-3, C4 if present	Look for possible posterior root of first cervical
Carcinoma of cervical nodes	Superficial and deep cervical plexuses	C2-C4	C2-4, C5, and C4, if present	Eliminate cases of cranial nerve involvement. Include C5 when pain is referred to shoulder or lower neck
Epicondylar fractures and scars along medial side of forearm and hand	Ulnar	C8-T2	C8-T2	Occasional failures will result from C7 overlap
Scarring from chest wounds and thoracotomy operations	Intercostals	Variable	Generally two roots above and below nerves caught in scar	After intercostal drainage for empyema, cut 5 roots. After costectomy, cut 6 roots
Sensitive scar after herniorrhapy	Ilioinguinal and hypo-gastric	T12-L1	T11-L2	
Retroperitoneal scar and other injuries to nerve in lateral thigh	Lateral femoral Cutaneous	L2-L3	L2-L3	
Coccygodynia	S5 and coccygeal	Same	S4-Cocl	Pain following rectal resection requires additional rhizotomy of S3. This may impair detrusor activity of bladder
Angina pectoris	Thoracic cardiac rami	T1-T4	T1-T4	Bilateral rhizotomy necessary if pain radiates down both arms
Gastric, biliary, and pancreatic	Splanchnic rami	T5-T10	T5-T10	To be recommended only when splanchnicectomy fails because of involvement of somatic nerves in posterior abdominal wall
Renal	Lower splanchnic rami	T10-L1	T10-L1	Preferable to sympathectomy after previous operations on diseased kidney

From White JC, Sweet WH: *Pain and the Neurological Surgeon, A 40-year Experience*. Charles C Thomas, 1969, Springfield, Illinois, p 653

Extent of Posterior Rhizotomy

White and Sweet[6] stated that posterior rhizotomy would be effective when pain was limited to a localized area of the limb, so that an extensive rhizotomy could be avoided. With pain in the chest or abdomen, an extensive rhizotomy could be carried out (Table 76-1).

For occipital neuralgia, denervation of C2-3 is indicated. Bilateral denervation of C3-4 should be avoided, however, since it could interfere with diaphragmatic respiration.

Pain in the anterior one-third of the tongue and mandibular portion of the neck could be successfully relieved by combined rhizotomy of the fifth cranial nerve and C2-3. Pain of the ear, secondary to infiltrated cancer, could be treated in the same way. Rhizotomy may not be technically feasible, however, when pain is referred to the shoulder or lower neck. These areas are innervated by the lower half of the cervical and upper thoracic nerve (C4-T4). Denervation of C8 to T2 is required to relieve pain of ulnar nerve distribution.

To relieve intercostal neuralgia, two roots above and below the affected area must be interrupted. T11 to L2 denervation is recommended for a painful scar after herniorrhaphy. Care should be taken, however, not to injure the Adamkiewicz artery. Pain in the lateral aspect of the thigh requires denervation of L2 to L3. Motor function should be monitored carefully during electrothermocoagulation. Denervation of S4 to the coccygeal nerve is necessary to relieve coccygodynia. Bladder or bowel function is not affected by this procedure; only the dermatome between the posterior portion of the perineum and the coccyx will be denervated. Interruption of S2 and S3, particularly if bilateral, will impair bowel, bladder, and sexual function.

To alleviate pain secondary to malignancy of visceral organs, a combination of sympathectomy and rhizotomy may be required.[6]

Technique

Preparation and Anesthesia

The patient should have nothing by mouth. Heavy sedation should be avoided: the patient must be alert because patient cooperation is needed to monitor motor and sensory functions during the procedure. A few milliliters of 0.5% or 1% lidocaine are injected subcutaneously at the needle-entering point. Particular caution should be taken to avoid injecting the anesthetic into the subarachnoid space, especially in the cervical region. During electrothermocoagulation, sodium methohexital (Blevital sodium, Lilly) can be given intravenously by the anesthesiologist for C2 rhizotomy. The patient may experience extreme pain in the area of C2 during treatment. Hence, it is important to explain the procedure in detail, particularly what the patient might experience and the need for his cooperation during the procedure. This significantly reduces the amount of premedication and anesthesia required.[16,17]

Cervical Rhizotomy

The procedure is performed in a room equipped with radiologic image intensification. The patient is placed in the supine position, with the neck slightly flexed. The head and neck rest comfortably on a pillow of folded sheets. This position permits fluoroscopic examination of the lateral, oblique, and anteroposterior (AP) views of the cervical spine. The slight flexion, rather than extension, of the cervical spine moves the vertebral artery away from the intervertebral foramina. After the surgical area is prepared routinely, local anesthesia is injected at the entering point of the needle. The usual puncture site for the C2 foramen is located 1 cm below the mastoid process (Fig. 76-5).

A hollow 20-gauge needle with a short bevel and tip, completely insulated except for 5 mm of the tip,* is used. The position of the needle is adjusted and the needle advanced under fluoroscopic control in the lateral view. In this view the target posterior ganglion is the midpoint on the rostrocaudal axis and in the dorsal one-third of the foramen. On the AP view it is 0 to 2 mm medial to the medial edge of the facet (pedicle) and 2 mm caudal to the caudal margin of the inferior pedicle (Figs. 76-6 and 76-7). When the needle is placed in the target, it is gently aspirated. Occasionally, cerebrospinal fluid escapes through the needle, indicating that the tip of the needle is in the subarachnoid space. In this case the needle should be withdrawn about 1 mm and its position rechecked with the image intensifier. The stylet is then replaced with a thermocouple electrode and the nerve root electrically stimulated twice per second by a biphasic square-wave pulse 1 msec in duration at less than 1.0 V. Appropriate sensory or muscle responses should be obtained at less than 0.5 V if the probe is in direct contact with nerve fibers (Table 76-2).

Ground electrodes are placed away from the affected dermatome or myotome. If muscle contraction is observed and the pain response is reproduced, the final position of the electrode is confirmed fluoroscopically. An initial trial at 50° to 70°C is used for a period of 15 seconds, with clinical monitoring. Then a total of 90 to 120 seconds is given. The electrode is then removed and a small pressure dressing applied to the puncture site.

*Radionics, Inc., Burlington, MA.

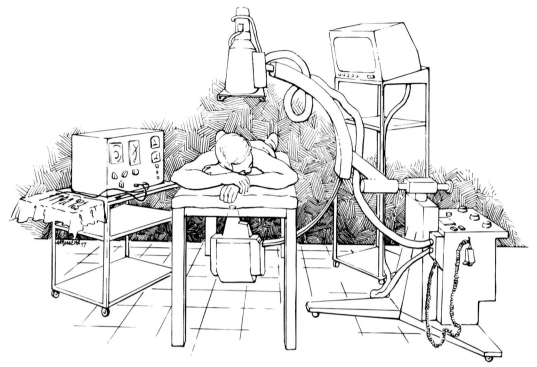

Fig. 76-4. Artist's view of set-up for the procedure. Note "C-arm fluoroscopic apparatus."

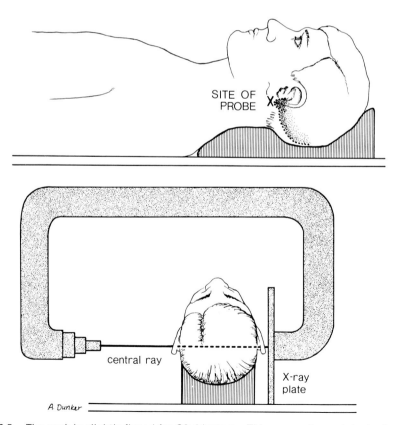

Fig. 76-5. The neck is slightly flexed for C2 rhizotomy. This moves the vertebral artery away from the intervertebral foramina.

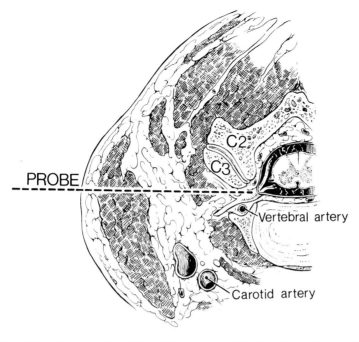

Fig. 76-6. Cross section at the C2 foramen and the direction of the needle.

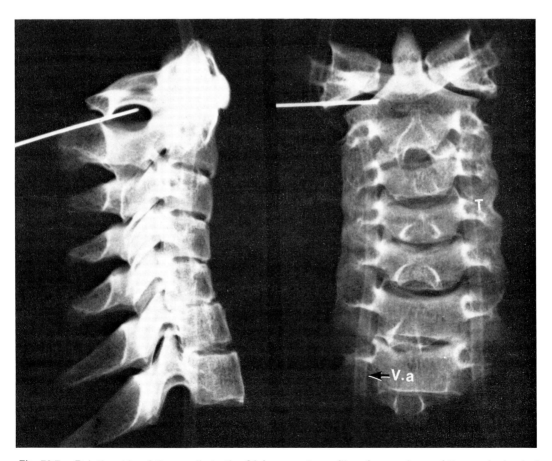

Fig. 76-7. Relationship of the needle to the C2 foramen (x-ray film of a specimen of the cervical spine). V.a = vertebral artery.

Table 76-2. Sensory and Motor Responses at Less than 0.5 V with Probe in Direct Contact with Nerve Fibers

C2	Trapezius
C3	Trapezius
C4	Supraspinatus
C5	Deltoid
C6	Biceps brachii
C7	Triceps
C8	Movement of thumb
T1	Movement of 5th finger
T2 to T5	Sensory response radiating pain to anterior chest wall at appropriate dermatome. Intercostal muscle contraction is often difficult to observe due to subcutaneous adipose tissue
T6 to T12	Abdominal muscle
L1 to L3	Iliopsoas and adductor muscle group of the thigh
L4	Hamstring, quadriceps femoris
L5	Peroneus
S1	Adductor hallucis
S2	Movement of 5th toe
S3 to S5	Sphincter ani

Modified from Raymond CT, Carpenter MB: *Human Neuroanatomy,* 6th ed., Baltimore, Williams & Wilkins, 1969, pp 196–198

When the electrode tip is in the subarachnoid space it is difficult to generate a temperature sufficient for denervation. Care should be taken not to puncture the vertebral artery when the needle is advanced into the target, as described above, under careful fluoroscopic control. This technique cannot be applied to the atlanto occipital joint because the vertebral artery takes a redundant course in this area (Fig. 76-8) and can be injured. To insert the electrode in the remaining cervical foramen, except for C2, an oblique view of the cervical spine is helpful. Electrothermocoagulation of the level below C6 and the first four thoracic roots should be car-

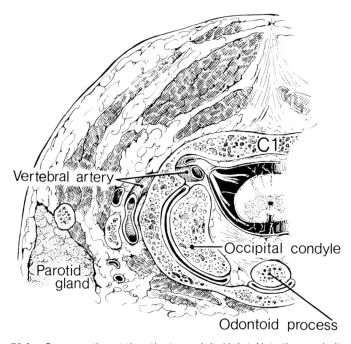

Fig. 76-8. Cross section at the atlanto-occipital joint. Note the proximity of the vertebral artery and the C1 nerve root.

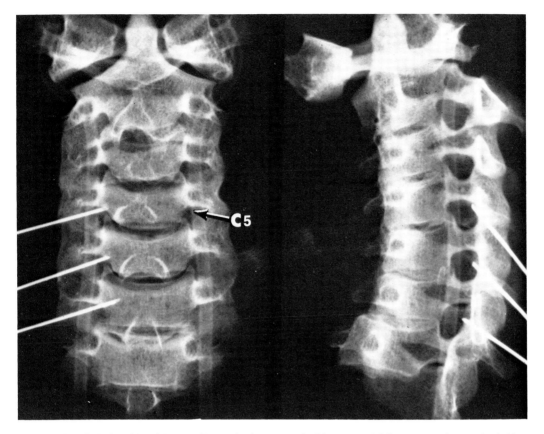

Fig. 76-9.   Relationship of the needles to the lower cervical foramens (oblique x-ray view on the left).

ried out with extreme caution to avoid injuring the important large radicular arteries. The position of the shoulder muscles and scapula may interfere with the needle puncture and make the procedure more difficult. Open surgical rhizotomy may therefore be a safer approach for this particular region (Figs. 76-9, 76-10, and 76-11).

Thoracic Rhizotomy

The patient is placed on a fluoroscopic operating table, in the prone position, with a pillow under the abdomen and the arms hanging over the table. If the upper thoracic nerves are to be blocked, a pillow should be placed under the upper chest and the patient's head should be hanging off the pillow, downward. By palpation and under the image intensifier, the anatomic relationships of the following bony landmarks are studied: (a) the spinous processes, (b) the costotransverse and facet joints on the anteroposterior view, and (c) the intervertebral foramina on the lateral view. The outline of the structure is traced on the skin with methylene blue to determine the entering point, direction, and angulation of the probe to the target foramen. It is helpful to know that in the thoracic region the spinous process of one vertebra lies in a line with those of the vertebra immediately below it. For example, the superior edge of the tip of the sixth thoracic vertebra lies in a line with the transverse processes of the seventh thoracic vertebrae (Figs. 76-12 and 76-13).

Under fluoroscopic control in the AP view, a line is traced from the head of the transverse process of the vertebra one level below the target foramen to the neck of the transverse process of the target vertebra. For example, using the sixth thoracic vertebra as the target, a line is drawn from the head of the transverse process of the seventh vertebra to the neck of the transverse

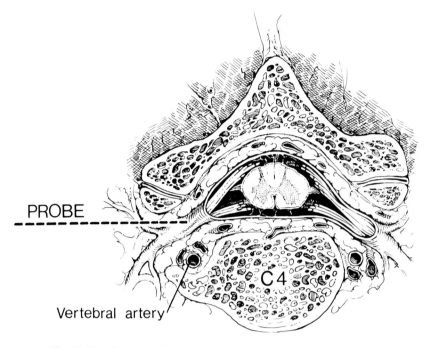

PROBE

Vertebral artery

C 4

Fig. 76-10. Cross section at the C4 and the direction of the needle.

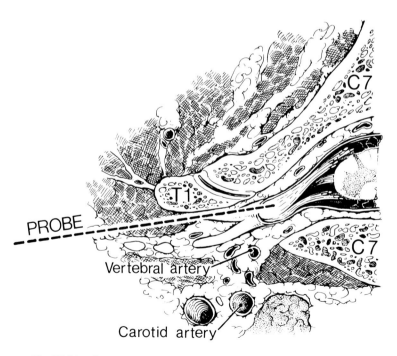

C 7

T1

PROBE

C 7

Vertebral artery

Carotid artery

Fig. 76-11. Cross section at the C7 and the direction of the needle.

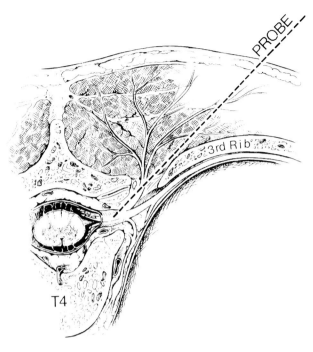

Fig. 76-12.   Cross section at the T4 foramen and the direction of the needle.

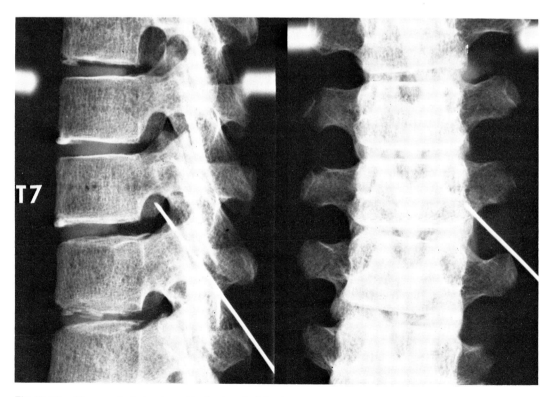

Fig. 76-13.   The needle is impinged to the head of the transverse process that is one level below the target foramen and is directed to the target foramen of the thoracic spine.

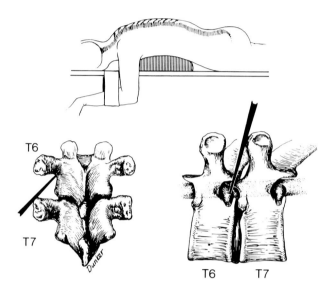

Fig. 76-14. An artist's view of the direction, angulation, and puncture site of the needle for the introduction into the thoracic intervertebral foramen.

process of the sixth thoracic vertebra. The needle entry point is approximately 3.5 to 5 cm from the midline of the vertebral body one level below the target. A local anesthetic is injected and the guiding needle advanced so that it impinges on the head of the transverse process. The needle is then angled toward the neck of the transverse process of the target foramen. Under lateral fluoroscopic control, the target foramen is identified and the needle is then carefully advanced into it. The target, in the AP view, is located 2 to 3 mm caudal to the caudal edge of the facet joint (Fig. 76-14).

After the needle is placed in the target, an attempt should always be made to gently aspirate for spinal fluid and blood. If cerebrospinal fluid is observed, the needle is withdrawn 1 to 2 mm. Often the needle tip impinges on the wall of the foramen (pedicle) before it is advanced deeply enough and multiple attempts to introduce the needle should be avoided. The patient frequently reports radiating pain along the appropriate intercostal nerve to the anterior chest or abdominal wall.

The thermoprobe is introduced after the position of the needle is confirmed. Electrode stimulation is then applied, using the same parameters described for cervical rhizotomy. After the proper location of the needle is confirmed by muscle contraction and by reproducing the pain, trial thermocoagulation is applied at a temperature of 40° to 50°C for 15 seconds, carefully observing flexion and extension movements of all toes, bilaterally, throughout the treatment period. Treatment is given in increments up to a total of 90 to 120 seconds; a maximum temperature of less than 74°C is applied for denervation of pain fibers.

If the needle enters or touches the pleura, the patient may cough while the needle is being advanced or during heating. The needle should not be inserted lateral to the transverse processes nor ventral to the foramen.

As soon as the procedure is completed, chest x-ray films are taken. Two hours after the procedure, follow-up films are taken to be certain that there is no pneumothorax. The patient should be kept under observation in the recovery room for a minimum of 2 hours. Since blood pressure may fall after multiple roots are denervated, particularly in elderly patients, blood pressure and pulse are closely monitored.

Intercostal Nerve Denervation

Intercostal nerves and vessels lie in the intercostal spaces. The nerves lie a little below the blood vessels. The intercostal nerve lies between the pleura and the posterior intercostal membrane, proximal to the angle of the ribs. In the region of the posterior axillary line, the nerves lie between the two muscle layers of the internal and external intercostal muscles. They continue forward in this relationship toward the front of the thorax. The lower six intercostal nerves, at the anterior end of the intercostal space, pass into the abdominal muscles.

The most important branch of each intercostal nerve, from the standpoint of denervation, is the lateral cutaneous. It arises from the intercostal nerve just anterior to the midaxillary line, pierces the external intercostal and anterior serratus muscles, and then divides into anterior and posterior cutaneous branches. Therefore, if the intercostal nerves are not blocked posteriorly or around the posterior axillary line, it is very easy to miss the lateral cutaneous branch and adequate analgesia will not occur. The rib, at this angle, is approximately 0.6 cm thick (Fig. 76-15).

Under local anesthesia, at the junction of the posterior axillary line and the inferior edge of the ribs, a 20-gauge needle, as described for cervical rhizotomy, impinges on the ribs at their inferior margin. Then the tip of the needle slides into the visceral aspect of the ribs, only 2 to 3 mm

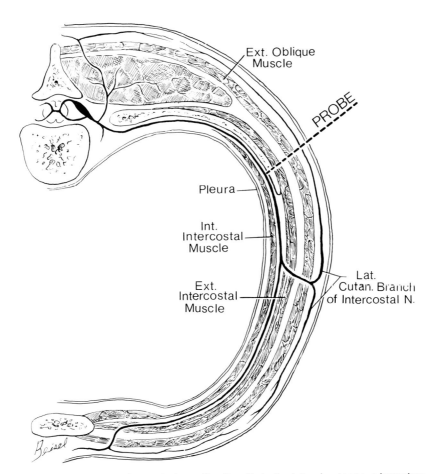

Fig. 76-15.   A probe at the posterior axillar line. Note the lateral cutaneous branches.

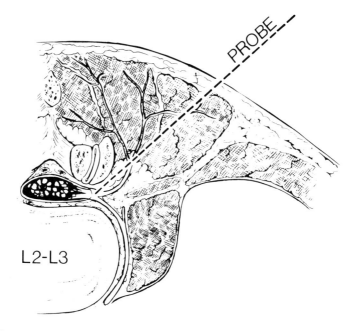

Fig. 76-16. Cross section of the L2 foramen and the direction of the needle.

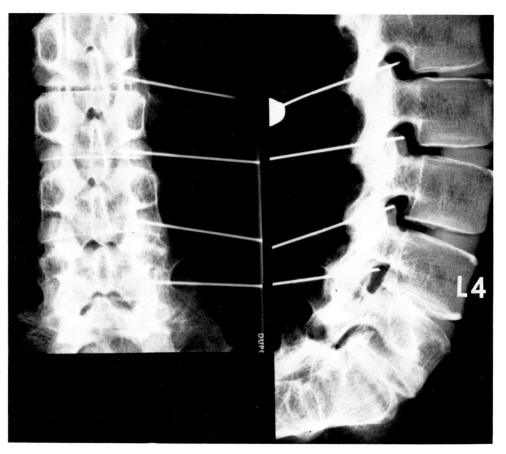

Fig. 76-17. Relationship of the needle to the first, second, third, and fourth lumbar intervertebral foramen as viewed on x-ray film.

deep from the inner aspect of the rib. At this point, stimulation by 0.2 to 0.5 V, at a rate of 2/ sec, is applied to determine the proper location of the needle. After the location is confirmed, incremental heat lesions are made, as described previously. Vital signs should be monitored for 2 hours.[18]

Lumbar Rhizotomy

The patient is placed on the operating table in the lateral recumbent position, with the affected side up. The entry point of the needle is determined by fluoroscopy in the lateral view. The foramina are easily visualized in this view. The needle entry point is usually 4 cm from the midline and the target point of the intervertebral foramen is located in the slightly rostral portion of the intervertebral disc space. The needle is advanced into the dorsal one-third of the foramen. When it is 10 mm away from the target, the x-ray tube is relocated for an anteroposterior examination to advance the needle the remaining depth. The target, in the anteroposterior view, is located 0 to 2 mm medial to the medial edge of the facet joint and 2 to 3 mm caudal to the caudal edge of the joint (Fig. 76-16 and 76-17).

When the needle is placed in the target, an attempt is always made to gently aspirate for spinal fluid or blood. If cerebrospinal fluid is observed, the needle is withdrawn 1 to 2 mm.

A thermoprobe is introduced after the position of the needle is confirmed. Electrode stimulation is then tried, using the same parameters as described for cervical rhizotomy. After proper muscle contraction and reproduction of pain, trial thermocoagulation is performed with a temperature of 40° to 50°C for 15 seconds. Flexion and extension of the toes, bilaterally, are observed during the entire treatment period. This treatment is then given in increments to a total of 90 to 120 seconds, with a maximum temperature of less than 74°C. It is more important to observe muscle contraction in the lower extremity than in the paravertebral muscles, since the latter could result from direct muscle rather than nerve-root stimulation. Particular care should be taken to avoid injuring the Adamkiewicz artery, which is in the vicinity of T11 to L1. In my opinion, rhizotomy of lumbar or lower cervical nerve roots to alleviate discogenic chronic pain should be used only in patients who already have a sensory or motor impairment, so that the procedure does not increase the degree of disability. It should not be done in patients with chronic pain who have normal sensory and motor functions of the extremity.

The Fifth Lumbar and Sacral Rhizotomy

The patient is placed in the prone position, with a large pillow under the abdomen, at the level of the iliac crest, to create flexion of the lumbosacral joint. This is particularly important for denervation of the fifth lumbar root. An anteroposterior view by fluoroscopic examination locates the fifth lumbar and sacral intervertebral foramina. The x-ray beam must be directed at a 90° angle to the longitudinal axis of the sacral spine (Fig. 76-18) to visualize the posterior and anterior sacral foramina. The same type of needle as described previously is introduced through the prepped and anesthetized skin into the posterior surface of the sacrum, just next to the target foramen. This procedure permits the operator to estimate needle depth so that it can be advanced farther through the foramen. The needle then is relocated and aimed at the center of the target foramen, under x-ray control. For fifth-lumbar denervation, the trunk of the nerve is the target. The rootlets and ganglion cannot be reached because the iliac crest and posterior superior spine of the pelvis interfere. The needle enters at the medial edge of the posterior superior iliac spine and is aimed toward the neck of the fifth lumbar transverse process. At times it is difficult to insert the needle because of lumbrosacralization or arthritic changes. The depth of the needle is determined by a lateral-view fluoroscopic examination. It is always important to aspirate for blood or spinal fluid before performing local block anesthesia or electrothermocoagulation (Figs. 76-19, 76-20, and 76-21). A sponge is placed between the gluteal folds to prevent the antiseptic solution from spilling over the perineum, which would burn the patient.

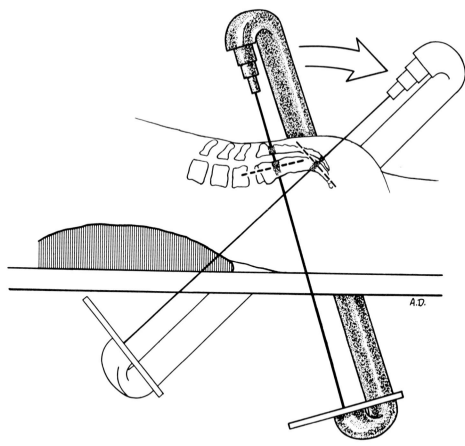

A.D.

Fig. 76-18. **A.** Artist's view of the position of the patient for a sacral rhizotomy. Note x-ray beam directed at 90° angle toward the longitudinal axis of the sacral spine. This enables fluoroscopic visualization of the sacral foramina.

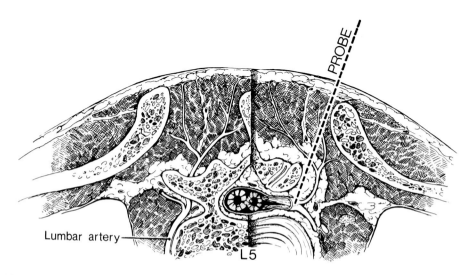

PROBE

Lumbar artery

L5

Fig. 76-19. Cross-section at the level of the L5-S1 foramen; the direction of the needle; and the relationship of the needle to the L5 root. Note that the posterior superior iliac spine interferes with the entry of the needle.

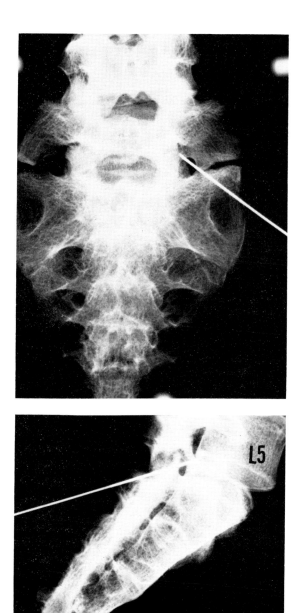

Fig. 76-20.   Direction of the needle and its relationship to the
fifth lumbar foramen as viewed on x-ray film.

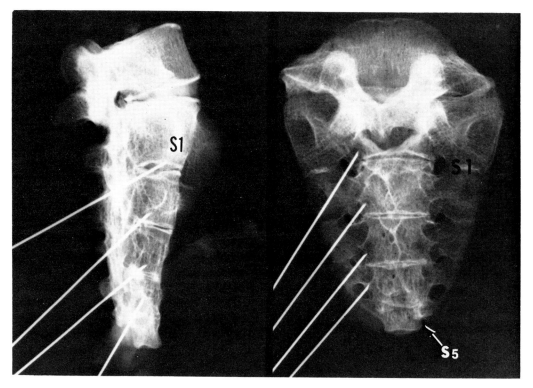

Fig. 76-21. Relationship of the needle to the first, second, third, and fourth sacral foramina as viewed on x-ray film.

The patients included in this report had neurologic disorders causing detrusor hyperreflexia. Patients were selected for evaluation if they had one or more of the following conditions: involuntary precipitous micturition, a short interval between catheterization or voiding, and autonomic hyperreflexia. Base-line urodynamic studies included cystometry, anal spincter electromyography, and a urethral pressure profile. Patients with low-threshold detrusor hyperreflexia were evaluated further with sacral blocks. Various combinations of S2, S3, and S4 nerve roots were anesthetized at the anterior sacral foramen with 1 to 2 cc of bupivacaine hydrochloride injected through the posterior sacral foramen under fluoroscopic control. The initial block included S2, S3, and S4 nerve roots bilaterally to ascertain potential maximum bladder capacity. Patients with fibrotic bladders not distensible to a capacity of 200 cc were not considered for sacral rhizotomy. Urodynometry was repeated within 1 hour of the sacral block. During the next 8 to 12 hours, the interval between catheterization or voiding, the volume of urine obtained and each occurrence of involuntary micturition and autonomic hyperreflexia were recorded. Male patients who could obtain a penile erection before the block were asked to determine the effect of the block upon erection. If the bladder capacity after the block was increased to at least 200 cc, serial blocks were performed on successive days to determine the predominant roots innervating the detrusor muscle. Percutaneous radiofrequency rhizotomy was performed at the sacral levels providing the predominant bladder nerve supply. When bladder capacity was not increased to at least 200 cc by the rhizotomy, the procedure was repeated or additional roots electrocoagulated.

The procedure was performed by inserting a No. 12 needle with stylet into the selected sacral foramen with the aid of anteroposterior and lateral fluoroscopy. An electrode (1.1 mm in diameter, with a 5-mm tip exposure and a thermistor temperature sensor) was advanced through the No. 12 needle to the anterior foramen. The radiofrequency electrocoagulation lesion was made at a temperature of 70° to 80°C for 3 minutes at each preselected level at the anterior sa-

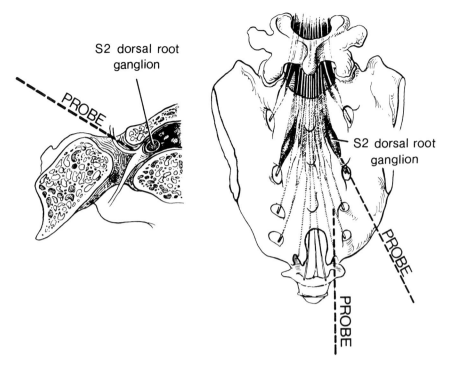

Fig. 76-22.   Left. Cross section at the level of the second sacral ganglion with probe inserted through the second sacral foramen. **Right.** Superimposed view of sacral spine with ganglia and roots. Note the probe inserted through the sacral hiatus and its tip in contact with the fifth and fourth root. A second probe is inserted through the second sacral foramen to the second ganglion.

cral foramen. Stimulation of the nerve root with cystometric monitoring to confirm the accuracy of electrode placement before making the root lesion was later added to the protocol. Frequent fluoroscopic monitoring was done during generation of the lesion to detect any change in the position of the electrode. Particular care was taken to make no lesion anterior to the anterior sacral foramen. Long-term follow-up urodynamic testing was attempted in every case.

Pain secondary to carcinoma of the rectum, with colostomy and loss of bladder control, may be treated by denervation of the second, third, and fourth sacral roots. Bladder function should be monitored cystometrically for denervation of the second, third, and fourth sacral roots when bladder and bowel function are intact.[12] The fifth, fourth, and third roots can be reached through the sacral hiatus. Electrical stimulation and fluoroscopic examination are used to guide the probe toward the target root or ganglion (Fig. 76-22).

Summary

A relatively simple technique for interrupting root, ganglion, trunk, and nerve is described as an alternative to open rhizotomy. Clinical observations of trigeminal rhizotomy support the fact that pain can be relieved and proprioception and motor function preserved with this technique. The simple technique of denervation is now available with the use of radiologic image intensification, electrical stimulation, and temperature control. The procedure can be applied to patients who are debilitated as a result of carcinoma, old age, or both, and can be repeated if necessary. Relief of flexor spasms of the hip joint secondary to traumatic paraplegia is a rewarding experience of this author.

REFERENCES

1. Abbe R: A contribution to the surgery of the spine. *Med Rec 35*:149–152, 1889
2. Bennett WH: A case in which antispasmodic pain in the left lower extremity was completely relieved by subdural division of the posterior roots of certain spinal nerves, all other treatment having proved useless. Death from sudden collapse and cerebral hemorrhage on the twelfth day after the operation, at the commencement of apparent convalescence. *Med Chir Trans (Lond) 72*:329–348, 1889
3. Scoville WB: Extradural spinal sensory rhizotomy. *J Neurosurg 25*:94–95, 1966
4. Dogliotti AM: Traitement des syndromes douloureux de la peripherie par l'alcholisation subarachnoidienne des racines posterieures a leur emergence de la moelle epiniere. *Presse Med 39*:1249–1252, 1931
5. Maher RM: Relief of pain in incurable cancer. *Lancet 1*:18–20, 1955
6. White J, Sweet W: *Pain and the Neurosurgeon, a 40-Year Experience.* Springfield, IL, Charles C Thomas, 1969, p 662
7. Kirschner M: Die Behandlung der Trigeminus Neuralgie (Nach Erfahrungen an 1113 Kranken). *Munchen Med Wochenschr 38*:235–239, 1942
8. Sweet W, Wepsic J: Controlled thermocoagulation of trigeminal ganglion and rootlets for differential destruction of pain fibers. Part 1: Trigeminal neuralgia. *J Neurosurg 40*:143–156, 1974
9. Uematsu S, Udvarhelyi G, Benson DW, et al: Percutaneous radiofrequency rhizotomy. *Surg Neurol 2*:319–325, 1974
10. Hamby WB, Schiffer: Spasmodic torticollis: Results after cervical rhizotomy in 50 cases. *J Neurosurg 31*:323–326, 1969
11. Heimburger R, Slominski O, Griswold P: Cervical posterior rhizotomy for reducing spasticity in cerebral palsy. *J Neurosurg 39*:30–34, 1973
12. Rockwold G, Bradley W, Chou S: Differential sacral rhizotomy in the treatment of neurogenic bladder dysfunction. Preliminary report of six cases. *J Neurosurg 38*:748–754, 1973
13. Vakili H: *The Spinal Cord.* New York, Intercontinental Medical Book Corp., p 20
14. Djindjian R, Hurth M, Houdart R, et al: *Angiography of the Spinal Cord.* Baltimore, University Park Press, 1970. pp 3–10
15. Onofrio BM, Campa HK: Evaluation of rhizotomy. Review of 12 years experience. *J Neurosurg 36*:751–755, 1972
16. Pawl P: Percutaneous Radiofrequency Electrocoagulation in the Control of Chronic Pain. *Surg Clin North Am 55*:167–179, 1975
17. Krayenbühl N, et al (ed): *Advances and Technical Standard in Neurosurgery,* vol 2. New York, Springer-Verlag, 1975
18. Moore DC: *Regional Block, Handbook for Use in the Clinical Practice of Medicine and Surgery.* Springfield, IL, Charles C Thomas, 1953, pp 113–150
19. White JC: Posterior rhizotomy: A possible substitute for cordotomy in otherwise intractable neuralgias of the trunk and extremities of nonmalignant origin. *Clin Neurosurg 13*:20–41, 1966
20. Young B, Mulcahy JJ: Percutaneous sacral rhizotomy. *J Neurosurg 53*:85–87, 1980

CHAPTER 77

Pain Control with Implantable Systems for the Long-Term Infusion of Intraspinal Opioids in Man

Charles E. Poletti
Henry H. Schmidek

William H. Sweet
Robert N. Pilon

THE USE OF IMPLANTABLE SYSTEMS for the long-term focal delivery of neuropharmacologic agents to the central nervous system will probably represent a major therapeutic advance. Systems are now in use to administer opiates directly to the spinal cord for the treatment of intractable pain and are being or may also be used for the delivery of hormones, neurotransmitters, antibiotics, anticoagulants, oncolytic agents, and other compounds targeted to the epidural space, cerebrospinal fluid, neuraxis, or bloodstream.[1-3] In the management of pain states this approach has the advantage of avoiding both the systemic effects associated with high-dose narcotics and of the problems associated with the surgical destruction of portions of the nervous system. The nondestructive stimulation of the dorsal columns of the cord is usually ineffective in relieving pain associated with malignant disease.[4]

Long-Term Infusion of Epidural Local Anesthetics for Intractable Pain

Attempts to control pain by means of a permanently placed subcutaneously implanted epidural system, allowing repeated intermittent injections of a local anesthetic, were first reported by Pilon and Baker in 1976.[5] The patient, a 52-year-old woman, five years after a sigmoid colectomy for adenocarcinoma, was debilitated by unilateral pain in the low back and buttock secondary to sacral metastases. The pain was largely unrelieved both by radiotherapy and unilateral thoracic cordotomy. Six months postoperatively the patient developed intractable pain on the other side, but refused a cordotomy on the second side, becoming instead dependent on large, frequent dosages of dihydromorphinone (Dilaudid) for pain relief. In order to control her pain,

The authors are grateful to the Neuro-Research Foundation for its support in the preparation of this manuscript.

Department of Neurological Science, Massachusetts General Hospital and Harvard Medical School, Boston, Massachusetts; Division of Neurological Surgery, University of Vermont College of Medicine, Burlington, Vermont

1199

an epidural catheter was placed percutaneously and threaded beneath the skin to a subcutaneous reservoir. One week following the operation, the reservoir was injected with local anesthetic. Over the next 4½ months 50 injections were delivered in this way into the reservoir, and immediate pain relief was obtained shortly thereafter. About 20 injections were performed by the patient's husband at home. By adjusting the amount and concentration of the drug, it was consistently possible to achieve pain relief while motor function was intact. No complications were associated with this mode of therapy in the 4½ month period of its use. Control of bladder and bowel function was maintained and 34 cultures of fluid aspirated before injection of the agent from the reservoir were negative for bacterial growth. Throughout this period the patient was able once again to function as a housewife.

Based on this initial experience, two of the authors (HHS and RNP) then used this technique in 3 other patients with intractable pain caused by pelvic cancer invading the lumbosacral plexus and spine. In each of these cases the epidural catheter was positioned at open operation through a semi-hemilaminectomy with intraoperative radiographic confirmation of the catheter's position. The Silastic catheter was then connected subcutaneously to a specially designed system incorporating an on-off valve and an enlarged plastic reservoir with a 20-cc volume. Bupivacaine hydrochloride (Marcaine) 0.35%, without epinephrine, was injected through the system into the epidural space. In each case it was possible to achieve consistent pain relief for 6 to 12 hours following a single injection of this agent. The system was used for 3 weeks, 1 month, and 3 months respectively in these 3 patients. In none of these cases was any problem encountered from either malfunction of the system, infections, or adverse reaction to the local anesthetic agent. The patients were freed from the use of oral or injectable narcotics, and the systems remained in continuous use until the death of the patients. Postmortem examination in two cases revealed neither evidence of epidural infection nor of epidural scar tissue formation either around the catheter or in the adjacent dura.

Long-Term Epidural Infusion of Opiates for Pain

Recently our interest has shifted from the use of local anesthetic agents in the epidural space[6] to the use of narcotics to control cancer pain. Although local anesthetics can successfully provide chronic pain relief, they block nonselectively the conduction of the nerve action potentials by reducing the amount and rate of development of the early transient increase in the permeability of the neural membranes to sodium ions normally produced by slight depolarization of the membrane.[7,8] In view of this, specific relief of pain without interference with other myelinated nerve fiber function is difficult to achieve consistently, although motor and autonomic blockade in our patients was minimal.[9] With the identification of the opiate receptors in the more posterior cells of the dorsal horns of the spinal cord[10-19] and the demonstration of pain relief using focally administered opiates, without inducing sensory, motor, or autonomic dysfunction,[15,17,18,20-23] these agents have now supplanted the use of local anesthetic agents for epidural administration in our patients.

Opiate receptors are richly distributed in laminae I & II of the dorsal horn of the spinal cord, in the peri-4th-ventricular, and in the peri-aqueductal gray matter.[14] Narcotics show both nonspecific and stereo-specific binding to tissues, i.e., the l-rotatory form binds whereas the d-rotatory form does not. Specific binding at opiate receptor sites is more tenacious, but is reversed by naloxone, which competes for the specific receptor sites.[16] The duration of action of the usual 0.4 to 0.8 mg dose of IV naloxone is limited to 1 to 4 hours and so opiates with strong binding characteristics and long durations of action may re-establish their effects some hours after a reversal dose of naloxone.[24] Radioimmunoassay studies after epidural introduction of morphine, methadone, and beta-endorphin in man reveal absorption into both the CSF and the blood stream, but the peak concentrations in CSF are 50 to 500 times greater than those in the blood plasma, and 12 hours later are 10 to 20 times those in the plasma.[25,26] The intraspinal narcotics, whether introduced intrathecally or epidurally, pass from the cerebrospinal fluid into the lipid phase of the spinal cord. The narcotics need penetrate the dorsal surface of the cord only to a depth of about 1 millimeter to reach Rexed's laminae I & II in the dorsal horn from the spinal subarachnoid space. Autoradiographs in dogs have shown that lidocaine injected in the dorsal epidural space penetrates preferentially into the dorsal periphery of the cord.[9] Because all these agents spread cephalad in the CSF, they can penetrate the floor of the fourth ventricle to reach the opiate receptors in such structures as the locus coeruleus concerned with central reflex control of respiratory and cardiovascular functions. The degree of lipid solubility of a given agent is a major determinant of the rate of transfer from cerebrospinal fluid to the substance of the spinal cord. Hence the speed of onset of neural effects, the duration of sojourn of the agent in the CSF, the distance of its travel cephalad in the CSF, the speed of its washout from the lipid neuraxis and subsequent elimination in the blood are all related to its lipid solubility. The strength of receptor binding will also determine the duration of action once the agent has diffused into the substance of the spinal cord. Thus, the clinical effects of the various narcotics can be predicted, to a large degree, by knowledge of their lipid-solubility and their specific opiate-receptor binding proclivity.[27]

In short-term studies in volunteers of thoracic and lumbar epidural injections of narcotics highly soluble in lipids, such agents as methadone and hydromorphone (Dilaudid) have been found to produce segmental pain relief with relatively little depression of respiration. Sympathetic activity is unaffected, while a segmental loss to cold and pin sensation can be detected. Lumbar epidural injections of 10 mg of morphine have produced the following effects:[28]

1. Initial segmental pain relief mainly confined to the lower limb.
2. Urinary retention.
3. Cephalad spread of pain relief—after 3 to 4 hours—to involve the upper limb.
4. Gradual depression of CO_2 response curve.
5. Persistence of pain relief and respiratory depression for 16 to 22 hours.

Our results show that the effects of rostral spread of the drug are greatly reduced by using lower doses in smaller volumes.

Likewise epidural meperidine (Demerol) 100 mg in 10 ml has relieved severe pain completely for 4 to 20 hours. Lower doses, 30 mg in 6 ml, gave similar durations of complete relief to cancer patients. None of them had any detectable change to objective sensory, motor, or sympathetic tests.[21] Larger doses of morphine, well above those required for pain relief, have produced objective analgesia to pin prick. Ten patients give 20 mg of morphine *intrathecally* in a hyperbaric solution and placed in a 40 degree head-up position did develop an analgesic level ranging from T1 to T6.[29]

Numerous clinical studies of short-term intraspinal narcotics for postoperative, obstetrical, and cancer pain have been published in the past 2 to 3 years.[3,28,30-35] Different methodologies have made it difficult to compare results, but in general the clinical results have confirmed the animal data:[37] Pain relief is dramatically profound, predominantly segmental, and prolonged when the drug exhibits strong receptor binding and low lipid solubility (e.g., morphine). Drugs with high lipid solubility and weak receptor binding, such as fentanyl, have a rapid and intense segmental effect, but as they quickly wash out the therapeutic effects are short-lived. Some severe acute pain may be more difficult to control than chronic pain. Thus, relief from cancer pain may be achieved with quite small doses of intraspinal narcotics.

The side effects of epidural opiates are common and dose-dependent and include:[38]

1. Nausea and vomiting occurring 4 to 6 hours after epidural morphine and reversed by naloxone.
2. Pruritus in 80 percent of patients after 10 mg of epidural morphine and after fentanyl. This is widespread, poorly relieved in antihistaminics, although completely relieved by naloxone.
3. Urinary retention.
4. Respiratory depression as the agent flows cephalad with CSF into the medullary subarachnoid space and ventricular systems.[39-44] The depression of respiratory sensitivity from epidu-

ral morphine follows the rostral spread of pain relief, reaching its peak at the sixth to tenth hour. A number of clinical cases have been published of delayed, profound, and prolonged respiratory depression after administration of morphine directly in the subarachnoid space. Though less frequent, this may also occur with epidural morphine, especially when applied in the cervical region.

Late respiratory depression is the most serious of the complications and may be life-threatening many hours after the patient has returned to his room; appropriate monitoring is therefore required. Intravenous naloxone promptly reverses the respiratory depression, but repeated doses may be needed. 0.4 mg is a common initial dose.

5.   The syndrome of opiate withdrawal occurred in patients whose large systemic doses of morphine were stopped when tiny doses of intraspinal morphine controlled the pain.[45]

We prefer the epidural to the intrathecal route for the administration of narcotics, since there is less chance of respiratory depression, and a possible infection is less dangerous in the epidural space than in the spinal fluid.

Preparation of Agents for Epidural Administration

Although we and others have given fentanyl, meperidine, and dilaudid epidurally, morphine sulphate is the agent with which there is the most experience. The drug should be used without preservatives. Pure morphine sulfate powder is dissolved in water, filtered, and autoclaved for 5 minutes at 121°C. We use 2 mg per cc during initial evaluation of the agents via a percutaneously placed catheter. Higher concentrations are used in the chronic systems and have the advantage that the system need be refilled less frequently.

Current Indications for Implantation of Chronic Epidural Analgetic Systems

Epidural morphine may be effective in the management of chronic pain, even in relatively low doses. The initial trials were confined to patients with cancer, and only those patients were selected in whom systemic narcotics in doses high enough to provide pain relief also left the patient obtunded and/or with other significant known side-effects of these agents. It is easier to minimize the risk of respiratory depression from a bulbar effect if the patient's cancer pain is confined to the legs, pelvis, and lower abdomen. The patients choose this approach to the control of their pain as an alternative to destructive surgical procedures such as cordotomy or myelotomy. Because of a higher incidence of respiratory depression among aged and debilitated patients, some physicians prefer to exclude these patients from this treatment; however other therapies are also more hazardous for them. Because of the relatively high risk of infection associated with these implanted foreign bodies, patients with immunosuppression may also be excluded. Some patients do not obtain relief with epidural narcotics, and hence are not candidates for a permanent surgical implant. Hence all of our patients selected for study undergo a trial of epidural morphine, often through a temporary catheter placed in the epidural space under local anesthesia. Adjacent colostomies or urethrostomies are not contraindications.

Implantable Systems Currently Available

Success of short-term clinical trials for pain control led us to the design of systems that offer the patient the benefit of long-term self-administration of epidural morphine while at home—systems 1, 2, and 3.[3] A fourth system, used more recently,[3,35,37] has been developed by the Infu-

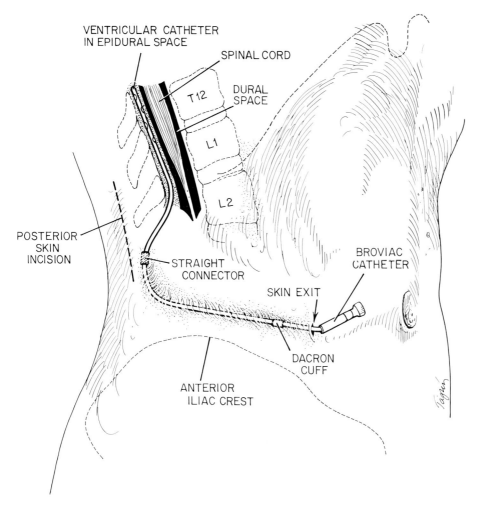

Fig. 77-1. The partially indwelling Broviac catheter system for long-term administration of morphine into the epidural space. After healing, the skin exit wound requires clean rather than sterile dressing.

said Corporation.* A fifth system, developed by NASA and just beginning clinical trials, embodies computerized telecommunication control of the pump.

Description of Four Currently Available Implantable Systems

1. A partially externalized Broviac or Hickman catheter system[34,46-53] has been used extensively in children and adults for long-term right atrial intravenous administration of chemotherapeutic agents and for hyperalimentation. Even in severely immunosuppressed patients the infection rate has been reported to be only about 8 percent. Exit tracts from the indwelling Broviac catheters tend to seal in 6 months, permitting clean rather than sterile occlusive dressing, and allow normal activity. A midlumbar injection of a large volume of fluid (10 cc rather than 2 cc) into the Broviac catheter usually carries metrizamide cephalad in the normal epidural space to the upper thoracic region. The partially indwelling system thereby offers the potential of producing pain relief at higher spinal levels with the injection of additional fluid, which acts as a vehicle to carry the morphine higher in the epidural space (Fig. 77-1).

*Infusaid Corp., Sharon, MA.

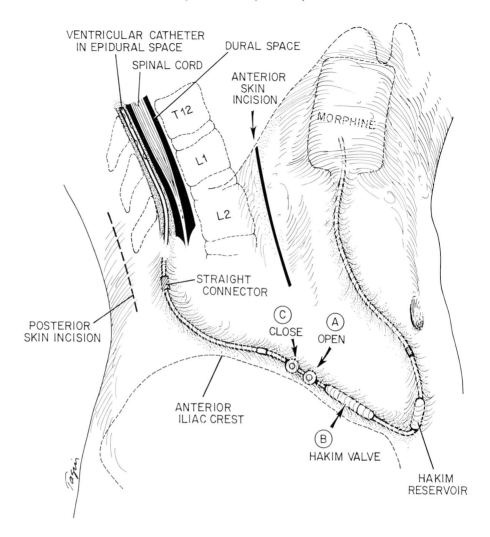

Fig. 77-2. Completely indwelling catheter system consisting of a morphine reservoir, one-way valves in tandem permitting pumping by intermittent compression of intervalvular tubing, and an on-off valve for long-term administration of morphine into the epidural space. For operation the on-off valve is opened **(A)**, the Hakim valve is pumped 20 times **(B)** delivering 2 ml of morphine, and the on-off valve is then closed **(C)**.

2. The system in the 4 patients reported here, who were maintained on chronic epidural bupivacaine, consists of a reservoir with a capacity of 20 cc, a one-way valve system, and an on-off switch.[5] This allows two doses of bupivacaine hydrochloride (Marcaine) to be given with a single percutaneous injection into the reservoir, since 16 to 20 cc of bupivacaine hydrochloride remains in the system and can subsequently be emptied by compression. A more simple tactic has been used by Lazorthes et al.,[54] who have repeatedly injected morphine directly through the skin into a subcutaneously implanted reservoir in 9 patients.

3. A completely indwelling system[3] that also allows morphine self-administration with a potentially lower risk of infection, no wound care, and reservoir refilling only every 2 to 12 months uses a Holter Silastic ventricular catheter placed through a semi-hemilaminectomy into the epidural space, and attached to a PBC-500 cc Silastic-coated blood pack (Fig. 77-2). This pack functions as a reservoir for 300 mg to 3 g of morphine in 300 cc of saline. The reservoir outlet tubing is connected to a Hakim high pressure pump valve assembly, and an on-off valve. These components are joined by subcutaneous Silastic tubing to the distal end of

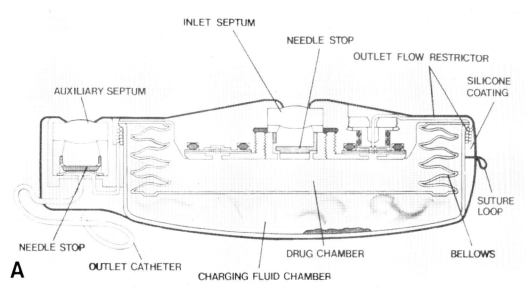

MODEL NO.	DIAMETER (mm)	THICKNESS (mm)	RESERVOIR VOLUME (ml)	EMPTY WEIGHT (gm)
100	87	28	47	187
200	87	23	32	172
400	∼	28	47	208
500	87	20	22	165

Fig. 77-3. Infusaid pump system. **A.** Model 400; **B.** Model comparisons (typical valves).

the epidural catheter and are secured in position. Postoperatively, the patient learns to self-administer the epidural morphine, pressing shut the intervalvular component of the tubing; each compression injects 0.1 cc into the epidural space. On a regimen of 2 mg of epidural morphine twice daily, one of our cases, previously reported,[3] was able to perform her chores for the seven months until her death from the progression of her malignant disease.

4. A more complicated alternative totally implantable system[1,37] consists of an implantable automatic pump reservoir that continuously infuses morphine into the epidural space at a relatively constant rate (Fig. 77-3). The Infusaid implantable infusion pump was originally developed by the University of Minnesota's Biochemical Engineering Department for the administration of heparin.[55] The system has also been used for the administration of insulin and chemotherapeutic agents. The pump is a flat, cylindrical structure, 3 cm thick, 9 cm in diameter, made of titanium, stainless steel, and silicone rubber, and weighs 180 g with a capacity of 47 cc. The infusion rate is adjustable between 0.5 and 6 cc per day. A disadvantage of the system is that the flow rate may be significantly increased by elevated body temperature or decreased atmospheric pressure. In addition, the patient might become drowsy and unaware of respiratory depression; yet the pump would automatically continue the now dangerous infusion of more morphine. This system has been demonstrated to be effective for pain control in animals,[37] and its usage for pain control in man has recently been reported by Onofrio[35] and is reported by Saunders and Coombs in this volume. The current

cost of the device is $2700. It is implanted in a subcutaneous pocket in the abdominal wall and the Silastic outlet catheter is placed in the spinal epidural space. The pump has continued to work properly for years in experimental animals. In the treatment of chronic pain states, the drug must be replenished every one to two months. This is done by injecting the agent percutaneously through a self-sealing septum. This action simultaneously recharges the pump's intrinsic energy source, allowing continued infusion at a constant and precise flow rate. The system requires no catheter flushing or dressing changes. Subsequent to implantation the patient may be able to return to a normal existence. At the present this pump has not received approval from the Federal Drug Administration for use to administer intraspinal opioids.

Initial Results of Long-Term Spinal Morphine Therapy

The first 2 patients to receive long-term epidural morphine therapy for intractable pain obtained very satisfactory relief from their cancer with 2 mg b.i.d. delivered to the lumbar epidural space.[3] On this regimen both patients stopped their high doses of systemic narcotics, became fully alert, showed no withdrawal symptoms, and returned home with markedly increased functional activity. The patient with the completely indwelling system for self-administration (see Fig. 77-2) became fully ambulatory, doing her own shopping until a month before her death 7 months later. During this period the large reservoir was refilled in the office once. The second patient, with a long-term externalized catheter (see Fig. 77-1) was less ambulatory, and, living at a distance, was cared for by his family and a visiting nurse during the 6 months until his death, without requiring return to the hospital for reservoir refills. The amount of morphine required, 2 mg b.i.d., remained constant.

In the third patient to receive long-term spinal morphine, Onofrio and colleagues[35] used continuous constant infusion of morphine into the lumbar subarachnoid space, which provided satisfactory relief of pain with only 0.62 to 1.8 mg of morphine a day. Again, this patient obtained good pain relief, even in the postoperative period, stopped systemic narcotics, showed no sedation of his mental status, and returned home able to walk again. The segmental relief of pain afforded even by intrathecal lumbar morphine is well exemplified in this patient. He experienced apparently "normal" severe pain at the dentist while maintaining very satisfactory relief from his sacral chordoma.

Intrathecal bolus injections of morphine in short-term human trials by Wang provided single dose relief for 15 hours, with the elapsed time from the instillation of the drug until its maximum effect ranging from 15 to 45 minutes; repeated injections afforded highly reproducible results.[22,36]

As the surgery required for implantation of chronic delivery systems is relatively minor, as compared with most of our neurosurgical procedures, we expect larger series to continue to show low operative mortality and morbidity.

Potential Complications

The most serious of the complications to date is respiratory depression. To minimize this possibility we recommend initial measurement of respiratory reserve whenever indicated and frequent monitoring of respiratory rate and pupil size to provide warning of depression. If intrathecal or high epidural administration is occurring, an apnea alarm and serial blood gases give added safety for the first few days of administration. In the higher risk situations, a continuing intravenous line, plus naloxone and a ventilation mask and bag near at hand, are advisable. Lazorthes et al.,[54] however, find that "bolus" administration of 1 ml of a hyperbaric (10% glucose) solution containing 3 to 7 mg morphine even into the lumbar *intrathecal* space is not hazardous if the patient is kept "semi-sitting" for 12 hours after the injection.

Common to the implantation of any foreign-body system is the increased risk of infections. This risk appears to be especially high for either partially externalized systems (see Fig. 77-1) or for systems requiring frequent percutaneous injections to refill the drug reservoir and reactivate the pump (see Fig. 77-3). Potentially, a system with a reservoir capacity of 5000 mgs (500 cc–10 mgs/cc) (see Fig. 77-2), delivering morphine into the intrathecal space, might provide pain relief for years without refilling. As sepsis may present the principal limitation to long-term usage, we believe such systems should be designed to be capable of very infrequent filling. This must be balanced against the risk of a massive dose if the reservoir were ruptured or punctured. We must weigh these factors, as we are now trying out these systems in patients with severe "benign" pain of nonlethal cause—e.g., phantom limb, post-herpetic neuralgia, postcordotomy dysesthesias, lumbar arachnoiditis, severe chronic pancreatitis, etc.

The second major limitation to the long-term usage of spinal opiates is the potential problem of tachyphylaxis and tolerance. This occurred so rapidly in 3 of our patients with benign pain that it was clearly inadvisable to implant a totally subcutaneous system. Of the 6 patients treated by Coombs et al.,[56] the daily morphine requirement to provide sustained pain relief increased in 3 of them from the initial 1 to 4 mg per day over a 28-week period to 20 to 30 mg per day. In the other 3 the increase was to 4 to 8 mg per day. Results in the initial patients reported are encouraging.[3,35,57] Of the first three patients reported from this country, only one[3] appeared to develop some tolerance: over a 6-month period the dose was increased by 0.5 mg daily every 2 months (2.0 mg b.i.d. to 3.5 mg b.i.d.). Lazorthes and colleagues,[57] after implanting reservoirs in 9 cancer patients with pain in the lower limbs and lower torso, did not encounter excessive tolerance in follow-ups from 1 to 8 months.

There may be 3 ways to reduce the tendency to develop tachyphylaxis in the spinal opiate receptors: First, as Yaksh and colleagues[58] point out, the continuous application of constant minimal doses of the opiate may reduce the tendency to tachyphylaxis by eliminating the higher peak concentrations and increased degrees of receptor activation incident to bolus injections. Secondly, there is preliminary evidence in 3 patients[20] that a single injection of epidural lidocaine may restore the opiate receptor and its associated membrane-modifying mechanism to its original sensitivity, permitting return to the originally low therapeutic morphine doses. A third possibility is offered by recent data suggesting multiple specific opiate receptors that probably have independent mechanisms and hence low cross-tolerance. Accordingly, one would hope that once one set of receptors develops tolerance to high doses of morphine, a second pain suppressor agent could be used in low doses to activate another type of receptor that has not yet developed tolerance. While this new set is being activated, the receptor set that had developed tolerance would have time to recover spontaneously its original low dose sensitivity. β-endorphine may meet these requirements, but is at present prohibitively expensive.[59] A much cheaper likely candidate has been proposed by Yaksh, namely D-ala^2-d-leu^5-enkephalin (DADL). Whereas morphine binds more to the "mu" type of opiate receptors, the enkephalins bind preferentially to such receptors of the "delta" type. Yaksh and colleagues have shown no cross-tolerance to the enkephalin analog DADL once such tolerance to intrathecal morphine has developed in rats. Moreover the DADL analog degrades much more slowly than either the natural leu- or met-enkephalin; hence it raises the threshold to noxa for longer periods. Umansky et al.[60] have shown that after 2 weeks of high daily intrathecal injections in cats, it causes no significant histologic changes in the spinal cords or nerve roots.

Another potential impediment to extended long-term usage of these implanted delivery systems—probably less of a threat, however, than sepsis or tolerance—is malfunction of the system itself. Mechanically the complicated Infusaid pump has a life expectancy of five years. Perhaps simpler systems using shunt components (see Fig. 77-2) might last even longer. Implantable pump systems with electronic battery-powered elements, such as the one currently being developed by NASA, will require surgery for battery replacement analogous to cardiac pacemakers. There again each change will increase the probability of infection. In addition to mechanical system failure, we anticipated a second possible source of system malfunction namely, scarring around the epidural catheter resulting in plugging it, or dural thickening preventing passage of morphine into the CSF and spinal cord. Neither of these occurred, however, in our patients with prolonged indwelling epidural catheters delivering xylocaine or morphine.[3,5] At autopsy, as mentioned earlier, there was no evidence of dural thickening or epidural scarring adjacent to the Silastic catheter.

These considerations of our potential ability to minimize sepsis, tolerance, and system malfunction seem encouraging. We are having an improved delivery system made, consisting of a 500-cc reservoir with two drug compartments for alternating activation of different opiate receptor sets, combined with a simple, reliable one-way valve system powered by external pressure applied by the patient himself for a long period without refilling. For people suffering from severe pain, especially those who are fully ambulatory with a variety of activities, we believe there is a great psychological value in systems that permit patient control with active self-administration. In fact, knowing that relief is readily available in some cases has decreased the usage.

The most encouraging aspect, however, of the future potential of focally applying opiates to the spinal cord rests in the remarkable specificity and efficacy of activating spinal opiate receptors. The effect is so circumscribed that pain relief is obtained without detectable interference with any other spinal cord system. There is no alteration of autonomic function such as changes in blood pressure regulation or bladder dynamics, and none in somatic motor function. In addition, not only is there no detectable alteration of proprioception, light touch, or thermal discrimination, but, most surprising, there is no apparent increase in the threshold for noxious pin pricks. These data again suggest, as do those from midline myelotomies, that the spinal cord may have two discrete neural systems, one for mediating severe chronic pain and perhaps also visceral pain, and another for mediating cutaneous acute pain perception. It is interesting that activation of the opiate receptor near threshold levels inhibits the former system but not the latter. Lastly, it is encouraging that segmental spinal opiate receptor activation rarely elicits subjective dysesthesias (except for itching) and does not depress mental alertness.

Accordingly, we envisage this application of surgically implantable systems for the chronic focal administration of pharmacologic agents to have a promising future especially for patients with intractable pain in the lower torso or lower limbs. Faced with the alternatives of systemic narcotic doses impairing their mental status or destructive major neurosurgical operations, we are finding that many patients already prefer to try this promising, relatively low-risk new therapeutic option.

REFERENCES

1. Blackshear PJ, Rohde TD, Prosl F, Buchwald H: The implantable infusion pump: A new concept in drug delivery. *Med Prog Technol* 6:149–161, 1979
2. Cohen AM, Kaufman S, Wood W, Greenfield A: Regional hepatic chemotherapy using an implantable drug infusion pump. *Am J Surg* (in press)
3. Poletti CE, Cohen AM, Todd DP, Ojemann RG, et al: Cancer pain relieved by long-term epidural morphine: Two case reports with permanent indwelling systems for self administration. *J Neurosurg* 55:581–584, 1981
4. Winkelmuller W, Dietz H, Stolke D: The clinical value of dorsal column stimulation. *Adv Neurosurg* 3:225–228, 1975
5. Pilon RN, Baker AR: Chronic pain by means of an epidural catheter. *Cancer* 37:903–905, 1976
6. Bromage PR: *Epidural Analgesia.* Philadelphia, W.B. Saunders, 1978
7. Strichartz GR: The inhibition of sodium currents in myelinated nerve by quaternary derivatives of lidocaine. *J Gen Physiol* 62:37–57, 1973
8. Taylor, RE: Effect of procaine on electrical properties of squid axon membrane. *Am J Physiol* 196:1071–1078, 1959
9. Bromage PR, Joyal AC, Binney JC: Local anesthetic drugs: Penetration from the spinal extradural space into the neuraxis. *Science* 140:392–394, 1963
10. Atweh SF, Kuhar MJ: Autroradiographic localization of opiate receptors in rat brain. I. Spinal cord and lower medulla. *Brain Res* 124:53–67, 1977
11. Cavillo O, Henry JL, Neuman RS: Effects of morphine and naloxone on dorsal horn neurones in the cat. *Can J Physiol Pharmacol* 52:1207–1211, 1974

12. Kitahata LM, Kosaka Y, Taub A, et al: Lamina-specific suppression of dorsal-horn unit activity by morphine sulfate. *Anesthesiology 41*:39–48, 1974

13. Lamotte C, Pert CB, Snyder SH: Opiate receptor binding in primate spinal cord: Distribution and changes after dorsal root section. *Brain Res 112*:407–412, 1976

14. Pert CB, Kuhar MJ, Snyder SH: Opiate receptor: Autoradiographic localization in rat brain. *Proc Natl Acad Sci USA 73*:3729–3733, 1976

15. Yaksh TL, Rudy TA: Analgesia mediated by a direct spinal action of narcotics. *Science 192*:1357–1358, 1976

16. Yaksh TL, Rudy TA: A dose ratio comparison of the interaction between morphine and cyclazocine with naloxone in rhesus monkeys on the shock titration test. *Eur J Pharmacol 46*:83–92, 1977

17. Yaksh TL, Huang SP, Rudy TA: The direct and specific opiate-like effect of met-enkephalin and analogues on spinal cord. *Neuroscience 2*:593–596, 1977

18. Yaksh TL: Analgetic actions of intrathecal opiates in cat and primate. *Brain Res 153*:205–210, 1978

19. Yaksh TL, Else RP: Release of methionine-enkephalin immunoreactivity from the rat spinal cord in vivo. *Eur J Pharmacol 63*:359–362, 1980

20. Chayen MS, Rudick V, Borvine A: Pain control with epidural injection of morphine. *Anesthesiology 53*:338–339, 1980

21. Cousins MJ, Mather LE, Glynn CJ, et al: Selective spinal analgesia. *Lancet 1*:1141–1142, 1979

22. Wang JK, Naus LA, Thomas JE: Pain relief by intrathecally applied morphine in man. *Anesthesiology 50*:149–151, 1979

23. Yaksh TL, Rudy TA: Chronic catheterization of the spinal subarachnoid space. *Physiol Behav 17*:1031–1036, 1976

24. Goodman LS, Gilman A: *The Pharmacological Basis of Therapeutics.* New York, MacMillan, 1975, p 274

25. Andersen HB, Chraemmer-Jørgenson B, Engquist A: Morphine kinetics following peridural or spinal application. *Pain* (Suppl. 1), *S250*, 1981

26. Max M, Inturris CE, Gradinski P, et al: Epidural opiates: Plasma and cerebrospinal fluid (CSF) pharmacokinetics of morphine, methadone and Beta-endorphin. *Pain* (Suppl. 1), *S122*, 1981

27. Snyder, SH: Opiate receptors and internal opiates. *Scientific American 236*:44–56, 1977

28. Bromage PR: State of art: Extradural and intrathecal narcotics. *American Society of Anesthesiologists' Refresher Course Outline 136*:1–4, 1981

29. Samii K, Feret J, Harari A, Viars P: Selective spinal analgesia. *Lancet 1*:1142, 1979

30. Baraka A, et al: Intrathecal versus epidural morphine for obstetric analgesia. *Anesthesiology 54*:136–140, 1981

31. Behar M, Magora F, Olshwang D, et al: Epidural morphine in treatment of pain. *Lancet 1*:527–528, 1979

32. Bromage PR, Camporesi E, Chestbut D: Epidural narcotics for postoperative analgesia. *Anesth Analg (Cleve) 59*:473–480, 1980

33. Ebert J, Varner PD: The effective use of epidural morphine sulfate for postoperative orthopedic pain. *Anesthesiology 53*:257–258, 1980

34. Graham JL, King R, McCaughey W: Postoperative pain relief using epidural morphine. *Anaesthesia 35*:158–160, 1980

35. Onofrio BM, Yaksh TL, Arnold PG: Continuous low-dose intrathecal morphine administration in the treatment of chronic pain of malignant origin. *Mayo Clin Proc 56*:516–520, 1981

36. Wang JK: Analgesic effect of intrathecally administered morphine. *Anesthesist 2*:3–8, 1977

37. Cohen AM, Wood WC, Bamberg BS, Risaliti A, Poletti CE: Continuous canine epidural morphine analgesia with an implanted drug infusion pump. *J Surg Res 32*:32–37, 1982

38. Boas RA: Hazards of epidural morphine. *Anaesth Intensive Care 8*:377–378, 1980

39. Baskoff JD, Watson RL, Muldoon SM: Respiratory arrest after intrathecal morphine. A case report. *Anesthesiology Rev 7*:12–15, 1980

40. Christensen V: Respiratory depression after extradural morphine. *Br J Anaesth 52*:841, 1980

41. Davies GK, Tolhurst-Cleaver CL, James TL: Respiratory depression after intrathecal narcotics. *Anaesthesia 35*:1080–1083, 1980

42. Glynn CJ, et al: Spinal narcotics and respiratory depression. *Lancet 2*:356–357, 1979

43. Liolios A, Andersen FH: Selective spinal analgesia. *Lancet 2*:357, 1979

44. Scott DB, McClure J: Selective epidural analgesia. *Lancet 1*:1410–1411, 1979

45. Tung AS, Tenicela R, Winter PM: Opiate withdrawal syndrome following intrathecal administration of morphine. *Anesthesiology 53*:340, 1980

46. Bottino J, McCredie KB, Groschel DHM, et al: Long-term intravenous therapy with peripherally inserted silicone elastomer central venous catheters in patients with malignant diseases. *Cancer 43*:1937–1943, 1979

47. Broviac JW, Cole JJ, Scribner BH: A silicone rubber arterial catheter for prolonged parenteral alimentation. *Surg Gynecol Obstet 136*:602, 1973

48. Heimbach DM, Ivey TD: Technique for placement of a permanent home hyperalimentation catheter. *Surg Gynecol Obstet 143*:634–636, 1976

49. Hickman RO, Buckner CD, Clift RA, et al: A modified right atrial catheter for access to the venous system in marrow transport recipients. *Surg Gynecol Obstet 148*:871–875, 1979

50. Hurtubise MR, Bottino JC, Lawson M, et al: Restoring patency of occluded central venous catheters. *Arch Surg 115*:212–213, 1980

51. Ponsky JL, Gauderer MWL: Expanded applications of Broviac catheter. *Arch Surg 115*:324, 1980

52. Thomas JH, MacArthur RI, Pierce GE, et al: Hickman-Broviac catheters. Indications and results. *Am J Surg 140*:791–796, 1980

53. Thomas M: The use of the Hickman catheter in the management of patients with leukaemia and other malignancies. *Br J Surg 66*:673–674, 1979

54. Lazorthes Y, Gouarderes C, Verdie JC, et al: Analgésie par injection intrathécale de morphine. *Neurochirurgie 26*:159–164, 1980

55. Chapleau CE, Robertson JJ: Spontaneous cervical carotid artery dissection: Outpatient treatment with continuous heparin infusion using a totally implantable infusion device. *Neurosurgery 8*:83–87, 1981

56. Coombs DW, Saunders RL, Gaylor MS, Colton T, Pagneau M: Continuous chronic pain relief by intraspinal narcotics infused via an implanted reservoir. (in preparation)

57. Lazorthes Y, Siegfried J, Gouarderes C, et al: PVG stimulation versus intrathecal morphine in cancer pain. *Pain* (Suppl. 1), *S29*, 1981

58. Yaksh TL: Personal communication, 1982

59. Oyama T, Matsuki A, Taneichi T, et al: β-endorphin in obstetric analgesia. *Am J Obstet Gynecol 137*:613–616, 1980

60. Umansky F, Richardson EP, Sweet WH: Histologic studies of spinal cords and roots after intrathecal injections of D-Ala^2-D-leu^5-enkephalin in cats. To be presented to the American Pain Society, Miami, October 29-31, 1982

Dartmouth-Hitchcock Medical Center Experience with Continuous Intraspinal Narcotic Analgesia by Richard L. Saunders, M.D., and Dennis W. Coombs, M.D.

In February 1981, Coombs inaugurated at a human investigation protocol to study continuous intraspinal narcotic (morphine) analgesic (CINA). To date, we have implanted 16 Infusaid reservoirs. All but 4 of the patients had pain due to malignancy. The intended route of delivery in all was epidural; however, extensive epidural metastases in 3 cases obviated this and led to a decision to use intrathecal systems. The longest period of treatment and follow-up has been 12 months. Four autopsies have been obtained, one following 9 months of continual therapy. The maximal intrathecal morphine dose used to date was 4 mg and the epidural was 30 mg. Pump flow rates of 3 cc/day are preferred. No technical malfunction of the Infusaid reservoir or infection has been identified. We now have more than 60 patient months' experience on which to base the following commentaries.

The impact of this method of managing cancer pain is best demonstrated by the virtual elimination of neural ablative procedures during the time of this protocol. The cancer patient, most commonly, although not uniformly, responds to a screening program using epidural morphine blocks. One can predict treatment response and the likelihood of side-effect (urinary retention, nausea, vomiting, and pruritis) through a series of epidural narcotic injections. These trial injections also may be used to establish the best level for ultimately placing the epidural catheter tip, assuming the analgesia is indeed segmental. We tend to agree with Neilsen et al,[1] however, that the effect is not entirely segmental. In our series, cancer patients have only rarely demonstrated the undesirable side-effects of epidural morphine, such as urinary retention, although side-effects are common with epidural morphine in the noncancer pain group. We have not used the external epidural catheter method for screening because of the expedience of an epidural spinal tap. Although it could be argued that a continual morphine effect by the external catheter is appealing, the affect of a single morphine bolus probably gives as much information with more safety. The 5 percent sepsis incidence of Zenz et al.[2] with exiting epidural catheters cannot be ignored at the screening stage. It would seem that needle blocks if effective would allow immediate placement of an implanted pump without concern for indolent contamination of the epidural space. If a chronic external catheter has been in place, we have found that it is prudent to wait before implanting the pump. This is not the case if only blocks have been used.

All patients have pre- and postimplantation assessment with a Zung self-rating depression scale, a self-esteem scale, Melzacks's McGill pain questionnaire, and Scotts's visual pain analogue scale. Further psychiatric pain unit observations include bimonthly patient/spouse interviews with behavioral checklists on to the number of hours the patient has been active, the extent of socializing, and avocational pursuits. Finally, two measures of psychomotor and cognitive function are obtained, using Trails "B" and the cognitive-capacity screening examination. Uniformly these patients' postimplantation assessments demonstrated significantly reduced pain recording with significant improvements in all psychometric parameters without cognitive changes. It was difficult with these dying cancer patients to make comparisons beyond the short term. A significant decrease in narcotic analgesic use was still present at 3 months postimplantation. Most but not all patients required increases in their morphine delivery over time. The older patient seemed to develop less tolerance in general.

The two important clinical observations are first the significance of prior major narcotic exposure. All patients in our group had been addicted. Although this may be a contraindication to ablative procedures, it is probably a prerequisite for intraspinal narcotic usage in our view. It may be that a further safety factor is created by prior narcotic usage. Second, as noted by Poletti et al.,[3] we find the elderly patient to be a good candidate for this method. Indeed the elderly patient does not handle systemic narcotics well, and a picture of obtundation reasonably attributed to the primary disease actually may be due to overmedication with systemic drugs. With the miniscule morphine doses by continuous pump, 1 patient in this series (78 years old) became an active member of her household for 9 months before her painless death.

The concerns for respiratory depression are compelling; however, it is reassuring to note that in our series this complication has not been experienced as long as the pump has been handled properly. One patient did experience respiratory effect when his pump was improperly refilled and a small amount of morphine was injected subcutaneously. Because of this abiding concern, we have chosen to treat primarily those cases with lower body pain to avoid drug levels at the brainstem of a magnitude that would cause respiratory depression. One patient with C8 pain has been uneventfully managed, and one other patient was found to have the epidural catheter at the C7 level inadvertently with no respiratory effects. It is probable, however, that levels of drug in the continuous mode high enough to cause depression simply do not occur. Indeed our preliminary measures of cisternal cerebrospinal fluid morphine levels during CINA (epidural) in both sheep and humans demonstrate a range of morphine levels inadequate to cause severe respiratory depression in the clinical doses used to date, regardless of catheter level. The capability for measuring drug levels in spinal fluid would seem an essential component of any program adopting this method of pain management and certainly when attempts are made to extend the range of intraspinal therapeutics with other agents.

This brings us to one final major point: the surgical exercise of placing continuous pumps is not really unusual. The procedure is actually quite simple. We are just beginning to scratch the surface of the possible neuropharmacologic permutations with both intermittent and continuous intraspinal pump therapy. The method used to deliver these agents will be relatively unimportant in contrast to the neuropharmacokinetic and toxicologic observations possible with intraspinal agent investigation. There is a unique appeal in the feasibility of manipulating pain with a system that the scientist totally controls on a day-to-day basis with no irreversible effects.

REFERENCES

1. Neilsen CH, Camporesi EM, Bromage PR, et al: CO2 sensitivity after epidural and IV morphine. *Anesthesiology 55*:372, 1981
2. Zenz M, Schappler-Scheele B, Neuhaus R, et al: Long-term peridural morphine analgesia in cancer pain. *Lancet 1*:91, 1981
3. Poletti, C.E., Cohen, A.M., Todd, D.P., et al. *Neurosurgery 55*:581–584, 1981

CHAPTER 78
Approaches to the Cervical Spine C1-T1

Robert A. Robinson

THERE ARE THREE SURGICAL APPROACHES to the cervical spine:

1. The posterior approach
2. The anterior and anterolateral approaches
3. The lateral approach

The posterior approach to the spine dates to 700AD, when Paul of Aegina,[1] after warning of the danger, advised that if the spine were broken, fragments should be removed by an incision through the skin and the wound closed with sutures. As early as 1549, Ambrose Paré,[2] the redoubtable French army surgeon, operated through a posterior incision for depressed splinters of bone impinging on the spinal cord and nerve roots. Therefore, since it is the oldest, the posterior approach to the cervical spine will be considered first.

Exposure of Posterior Elements of the Cervical Spine

The posterior exposure can be used to perform a variety of procedures.[3-12] It is performed with the patient in the prone, lateral, or sitting position. In general, adjustable but secure fixation of the patient's head, with resulting control of the cervical spine during the surgical procedure, is mandatory. Proper positioning of the patient for surgery requires that (a) the cervical spine be maintained in optimum position for the procedure to be undertaken; (b) the head be fixed so that gross motion of the cervical spine during the operative procedure is not allowed, but the position of the neck can be adjusted, (c) pressure on the eyes be prevented during the procedure, and (d) adequate ventilatory exchange and cardiac function be monitored throughout the procedure.

The Halo cast was developed in 1959.[5] If the skeletal stability of a neck has been compromised by poliomyelitis, dysplasia (such as a deficient odontoid), infection, tumor, or injury, it can be stabilized for surgery in such a device, or by skull tong traction on a Stryker frame, or, occasionally, in a full-length plaster bed. These external devices are applied before anterior, lateral, and posterior spine surgery to avoid damage to the spinal cord, vertebral arteries, and nerve roots by unguarded motion, since spinal instability is markedly increased under anesthesia.

The skin overlying the occipital portion of the skull, the posterior portion of the neck, the shoulders, and the upper back is included in the prepared operative field. If a bone graft is to be used, the relevant skin area also is prepped and draped. A midline incision over the cervical

Department of Orthopaedic Surgery, The Johns Hopkins University School of Medicine and the Johns Hopkins Hospital, Baltimore, Maryland

spine, with "Y" extensions superiorly if needed, is made in the skin overlying the palpable tips of the spinous processes.

After the skin incision has been made, a dilute solution of saline and adrenalin (usually less than 1:100,000) may be injected into the subcutaneous and muscular tissues through which the incision will be carried. If the injection is administered before the skin incision is made, bony landmarks may be obliterated and the midline obscured. The incision is carried through the subcutaneous tissue until the tips of the spinous processes of the cervical spine are identified. The spinous processes and laminae of the appropriate cervical vertebrae then are exposed subperiosteally.

X-ray control should be used to confirm the vertebral levels of the cervical spine during surgery. Very often the posterior spinous process of C3 is completely hidden under that of C2 and the posterior spinous processes of C7 and T1 can be confused.

If the posterior arch of the first cervical vertebra is to be exposed, the posterior elements of the second cervical vertebra are first exposed subperiosteally, the occipital portion of the skull then is exposed, and dissection is carried into the midline between these two structures until the posterior tubercle of the arch of the first cervical vertebra is identified. Dissection then is carried laterally to each side of the midline for a distance of 0.5 inch, thus exposing the posterior arch of the first cervical vertebra. Care must be taken to expose no more than 1 inch of the posterior arch of the first cervical vertebra in order to prevent inadvertent damage to the vertebral artery or the surrounding plexus of veins. It must be emphasized that subperiosteal exposure of the posterior elements of the cervical spine must be carried out with a sharp periosteal elevator. At no time should decortication of the posterior elements of the cervical spine be attempted with a mallet and an osteotome or gouge; that is, only manual subperiosteal elevation or decortication should be carried out. A mallet should never be used in the posterior portion of the cervical spine. If the spine appears to be very unstable, a Kocher clamp placed on the spinous process of the unstable segment may be used to steady it during subperiosteal dissection.

It should be pointed out that the ligamentum flavum runs from the posterior arch of one vertebra to another, except at C1. Normally its attachment to the laminae of C1 is relatively slight, and it is continuous from the posterior arch of C2 up to and through the posterior rim of the foramen magnum. The sagittal cross section of the posterior arch of C1 is triangular, however, with its apex pointing toward the spinal canal. Therefore, if it appears that attempts to loosen the ligamentum flavum from the arch of C1 may cause pressure on the spinal contents, as, for instance, when an attempt is made to loosen it in order to pass a wire loop around the posterior arch of C1, it might be better to drill holes vertically through the arch of C1 posteriorly to its anterior leading edge. A wire can be passed through these holes to fix a posterior bone graft between C1 and C2. If the posterior arch of C1 is absent, or the quality of the bone is poor, as it may be in rheumatoid disease, such C1-2 stabilization procedures probably should be extended upward to the base of the skull and downward to the posterior spinous processes of both C2 and C3.[3,13]

In general, the bone need be exposed only subperiosteally in the cervical spine in order to create a biologically efficient bed for a bone graft. Some surgeons prefer to roughen the periosteal bone surfaces with a burr preparatory to fusion, but, as pointed out some years ago by William Rogers, this is not necessary.[39]

The idea that a wire loop alone will cause an injured cervical motion segment to fuse solidly with bone without a bone graft is fallacious. Therefore, bone grafts and 12 weeks of postoperative immobilization are advised. In posterior fusion wire is used to stabilize the graft, while in anterior fusions braided silk now is used, if necessary, to stabilize the bone graft instead of wire.[10,14]

Once the posterior part of the cervical spine is exposed and the exact *geography* is determined by x-ray, various types of surgery can be carried out. If extensive laminectomies, sometimes including facetectomies, are carried out in a spine that is unstable before surgery, or if instability has been created during surgery, then there are surgical methods for reestablishing spinal stability in the same operation through the same posterior exposure of the cervical spine. When fusion of the cervical spine if *critical,* both an anterior and posterior fusion of the same motion segments are recommended.[8]

Anterolateral Approaches to the Cervical Spine

Anterolateral approaches to the cervical spine became popular shortly after 1950.[15-21] Aseptic surgery, general anesthesia with controlled pressure, gaseous anesthesia with endotracheal inbutation, readily available stored blood for transfusions, antibiotics (particularly streptomycin and penicillin), and intraoperaive x-ray control all had been developed during the 100 years preceding 1950. In fact, the antituberculous drug streptomycin was developed approximately 5 years before that time.

As in so many advances in surgery of the spine, however, there has long been a human desire to help those afflicted with spinal tuberculosis. In order to directly approach the usual site of tuberculous lesions in the spine, the vertebral bodies had to be approached anteriorly. Therefore, although anterior approaches to the cervical spine were used only rarely by surgeons before about 1950, they were used nevertheless. According to Verbiest,[22] Boudot,[23] who based his thesis on an operation of Professor Michel, is probably the first to have pointed out the possibility of a retromastoid approach that permitted one to expose the transverse cervical apophyses. Chien,[24] Cheyne,[25] Burckhardt,[26] and Auffret[27] all drained retropharyngeal abscesses, most of which were probably tuberculous, by an anterolateral approach, either just anterior to or posterior to the sternocleidomastoid muscle.

Küttner[22,28] treated aneurysms of vertebral arteries through a lateral approach about 1917.

According to Verbiest,[22] Auffret, in 1896, was the first to use the transbuccal, direct anterior approach to the C2, C3, and C4 vertebral bodies. He preferred the anterolateral approach, however, for the transverse processes of C2 through C7 and for the bodies of C5, C6, and C7. He stated: "The fact that I originated the direct exposure of the anterior aspect of the first three cervical vertebrae does not totally blind me from recognizing that it is possible when necessary, that is from extreme necessity, to approach these vertebral bodies laterally." He judged that the lateral approach was still full of problems.

Burckhardt[26] preferred to drain retropharyngeal abscesses by an approach medial to the sternocleidomastoid muscle and the neurovascular bundle.

Lahey[29] used a parasternocleidomastoid approach to marsupialize and eventually remove esophageal diverticulae. (It interests me that Dr. Lahey does not mention the anterior cervical spine, which must have been visible to him; obviously his chief interest was anterior to the spine.)

In any event, anterior approaches to the cervical spine are at least 100 years old and probably much older. For instance, retropharyngeal abscesses that interfered with breathing sometimes may have drained spontaneously, or they may have been incised through the back of the throat via the mouth and not reported for as long as surgery has been practiced, as were peritonsillar abscesses. Recently Fang et al.[30] electively used this direct anterior approach to the cervical spine through the mouth to fuse the lateral masses of C1 and C2.

Anterolateral Exposure from the First Cervical Vertebra to the First or Second Thoracic Vertebra

The technique used for anterolateral exposure of the cervical spine has been described in detail previously.[9,31] As I do it, the patient is supine on an operating table with a radiolucent top. The neck is at first stablized by 5 lb of traction applied through a head halter. The shoulders are gently pulled caudally with adhesive tape, and the table then is placed in about a 5° Trendelenburg position. A cylindrical pneumatic support is placed transversely under the neck, the shoulders are slightly elevated by a folded sheet, and the occiput, after traction is applied, just clears the table. As the cervical spine is exposed, traction is usually increased to 20 lb.

The procedure often is performed through a transverse skin incision, which should be centered over the anterior border of the sternomastoid muscle and placed over the segment of the spine to be exposed. When the platysma muscle has been exposed, it is grasped between forceps and sharply incised at the lateral limb of the transverse incision, just anterior to the external jugular vein, bluntly separated from the underlying structures, and sharply incised in the line of the skin incision. The underlying sternomastoid muscle then is visible. The anterior border of the sternomastoid muscle must be clearly identified and mobilized throughout the limits of the exposure so that its medial border can be retracted laterally to expose the middle layer of the cervical fascia. The omohyoid muscle can be seen crossing the field at about the level of C5-6 and may be mobilized and retracted inferiorly or superiorly, or transected in its midtendinous segment. The carotid sheath then is identified, and the middle layer of cervical fascia is incised just medial and parallel to the carotid sheath, which allows retraction of the carotid sheath and sternomastoid muscle laterally. Usually very little traction is necessary once the esophagus and trachea are retracted medially. At first, however, the neurovascular bundle is retracted slightly and the anterior surface of the cervical spine is visualized, as is the esophagus, which lies just posterior to the trachea, or, in the superior portion of the neck, the larynx. The prevertebral and alar fascias are incised longitudinally in the midline of the neck and retreated medially and laterally. The prevertebral fascias are easily retracted laterally over the underlying anterior longitudinal ligament of the cervical spine. The longus colli muscles then may be elevated sharply from the intervertebral discs and vertebral bodies and retracted laterally. Just before this is done, the vein and artery that emerge on either side of each spinal segment and enter the vertebral body just superior to their point of emergence laterally from under the longus colli muscles should be cauterized. Cauterization helps keep the wound relatively bloodless.

At this point in the exposure a lateral x-ray of the cervical spine can be obtained after a needle is placed into a disc for exact localization. A very excellent anatomic landmark, however, is the bony promontory on the transverse processes of C6, the *carotid tubercle,* which is opposite the vertebral body of C6. The intervertebral disc between the vertebral bodies of C5 and 6 thus can be spotted for placement of the needle.

When many motion segments of the cervical spine from C1-2 through T1-2 are to be exposed anteriorly, a more vertical incision may be used, which extends from near the tip of the mastoid process to the suprasternal notch along the anterior border of the underlying sternocleidomastoid muscle. Through such an incision, different types of anterior and lateral operations can be done on cervical vertebral bodies and intervertebral discs, transverse processes, and vertebral arteries. In general, after the initial exposure is made through the superficial layer of the deep fascia surrounding the sternocleidomastoid muscle, I proceed to the front of the spine at C5-6 and then, layer by fascial layer, proceed upward toward the tip of the mastoid process. Through such an incision, I have removed the bulk of a plasma cell myeloma in C2 and replaced it with an inverted clothespin-shaped graft, and I have drained an acute pyogenic abscess involving the C1 odontoid joint.

More Extensive Exposure of the Cervical
Spine Anterolaterally

The exposure that has just been described is known to head-and-neck surgeons as the Lincoln Highway to the neck. In its unmodified form it usually is adequate for disc surgery and for draining abscesses, and for the removal and replacement of vertebral bodies. It was extended upward and developed for microsurgery of clivus tumors by Stevenson et al.[34] Verbiest, with modifications of his own, uses the extensive anterolateral approach for his "lateral" approach to the cervical spine.[37]

In 1973 and 1975, however, we presented a description and anatomic drawings of an exposure to the front and side of the cervical spine that allows visualization of the anterior arch of the first cervical vertebra, the anterior structures of the remainder of the cervical spine, and the base of the skull. It was demonstrated to Dr. Lee Riley and myself[32,33] by Dr. Robert Chambers, a head and neck surgeon, and has been used to achieve the exposure necessary to perform the excision of lesions of the upper cervical spine and fusion of the first, second, and third vertebral segments.[17]

A tracheotomy must be performed and anesthesia maintained through the tracheotomy. The incision is begun just to the left of the midline in the submandibular area, carried posteriorly to the angle of the mandible, then gently curved lateral to the posterior border of the sternomastoid muscle to the base of the neck, and finally curved anteriorly and inferiorly, crossing the clavicle and ending in the suprasternal space. The incision is developed through the platysma muscle, and the skin and muscle flap so outlined is retracted medially to expose the sternomastoid and strap muscles, the pharynx, the thyroid gland, the edge of the mandible, and the submaxillary triangle. The anterior surface of the lower cervical spine is identified by reflecting the sternomastoid muscle and carotid sheath laterally, transecting the omohyoid muscle in its tendinous portion, incising the prevertebral fasciae in the midline, and retracting the prevertebral fasciae, the thyroid gland, the esophagus, and the trachea medially. Development of this plane superiorly, however, is impeded by the superior thyroid artery, the superior laryngeal neurovascular bundle, the hypoglossal nerve, the stylohyoid muscle, and the digastric muscle. The superior thyroid artery should be ligated and divided, the stylohyoid muscle and the digastric muscle divided and reflected, and the superior laryngeal nerve and the hypoglossal nerve identified and protected. When this has been done, the larynx and pharynx may be retracted medially, the external carotid artery retracted laterally, and the floor of the submaxillary triangle retracted superiorly, so that the base of the skull and the anterior arch of the first cervical vertebra can be visualized. If further exposure is required, it is provided by excising the submaxillary gland and anteriorly dislocating the temporal mandibular joint. This is easily performed manually with the patient anesthetized, which permits rotation of the mandible superiorly and to the right side of the patient. Complete exposure of the anterior arch of the first cervical vertebra, the odontoid process, and both vertebral arteries now may be obtained.

Anterior fusion at C1-3 is accomplished by cutting a trough in the anterior aspect of the second and third vertebral bodies to the level of the posterior cortex of the odontoid process and removing the cancellous bone from the odontoid process with a small curette, which converts it into a hollow shell surrounded by cortical bone. A bone graft then is cut from the anterior iliac crest and shaped to the dimensions of the previously constructed trough in the anterior aspects of the vertebral bodies of the second and third cervical vertebrae. The superior end of the bone graft is shaped to resemble a saddle or clothespin, with one protrusion of the *clothespin* being fitted into the odontoid process and the other protrusion cradling the anterior arch of the first cervical vertebra. The distal end is locked into the trough in the bodies of the second and third cervical vertebrae. A loop of heavy, braided silk suture is placed through the caudal portion of the bone graft and through the cortex of the second and third vertebral bodies. The graft is tied into place to prevent anterior displacement of its caudal portion.

Exposure of the Transverse Processes, Pedicles, and Vertebral Artery from the Third through the Seventh Cervical Segments

Exposure of the transverse processes, the pedicles, and the vertebral artery from the C3 through the C7 segments is achieved through a skin incision that begins behind the junction of the upper and middle third of the sternocleidomastoid muscle, runs down to the junction of the middle and lower thirds of that muscle along the posterior border of the sternomastoid muscle, and then swings anteriorly to the suprasternal notch.[32] The incision is deepened to the platysma muscle, which then is grasped between forceps at the lateral limb of the incision, bluntly elevated from the underlying structures, and divided in line with the skin incision. The anterior and posterior borders of the sternomastoid muscle must be clearly demonstrated. The deep surface of the sternomastoid muscle is freed from the underlying structures so that it is possible to pass a finger under the sternomastoid muscle, which then is sharply divided and retracted superiorly and inferiorly. The omohyoid muscle, lying deep to the sternomastoid, is divided and retracted in a similar fashion. This brings into view the anterior scalene muscle, the phrenic nerve lying on the anterior surface of the anterior scalene muscle, and the cords of the brachial plexus emerging from under the lateral border of the anterior scalene muscle. The phrenic nerve is mobilized throughout the limits of the incision and may be gently retracted anteriorly. Great care must be exercised at this stage of the exposure to prevent damage to the cords of the brachial plexus as they emerge from under the lateral border of the anterior scalene muscle. The brachial plexus must be identified and protected. The anterior scalene muscle then is sharply divided, approximately 1 inch inferior to the site of desired exposure, and the entire superior portion of the muscle is excised. Care must be taken to avoid damage to the vertebral artery as it passes between the bony foramen and the transverse processes of the second through sixth cervical vertebrae, as the slips of origin of the anterior scalene muscle are dissected from the anterior tubercles of the transverse processes. If the pedicles are to be exposed, the vertebral artery should be identified and controlled with tapes placed about it proximal and distal to the site of desired exposure. With sharp dissection, the longus colli muscle is reflected medially, and any remaining fibers of the scalene muscle are reflected distally and laterally to expose the transverse processes in their entirety as well as the uncovertebral joint, the pedicle, the neural foramen, and the emerging nerve root.

Closure is effected by leaving a drain at the level of the resected portion of the anterior scalene muscle and reapproximating the omohyoid, the sternomastoid, and the platysma muscles. The skin edges should be approximated with fine interrupted sutures, which may be removed on the third postoperative day.

There also are lateral approaches to the cervical spine. One approach was described by Barbour.[35] It is a lateral approach to the joint between C1 and C2 through an incision below the mastoid process on either side of the neck. E. Simmons[36] et al. of Toronto reported their experience with this lateral approach for fusion of C1 to C2.

Another lateral approach to C2-3 through C6-7 is one reported by Verbiest.[14,22,37] It actually is one that involves the deep rather than the superficial (e.g., skin incision) approach to the intervertebral foramina of the cervical spine and the posterior aspects of the vertebral bodies through the intervertebral foramina—procedures that can be carried out through the exposures reported by Robinson and Riley[9,33] and by Riley.[32]

Verbiest discusses such lateral transforaminal surgery through this approach for a variety of clinical problems.[14,37] He specifically discusses the advantages and dangers of direct lateral removal of bony spurs and disc protrusions by mobilizing the vertebral artery from the transverse process of the cervical vertebrae as described by Henry.[38] Part or all of the transverse process was removed, on occasion,[22] and then osseous and discal material protrusions that may have been compressing the vascular and neural tissue in the intervertebral foramina and more medially on the anterior and anterolateral face of the spinal canal through the intervertebral foramen were removed, as recommended by Jung.

Remarks

Throughout the literature concerning indications for neck surgery that has appeared during the past 25 years, there has been some basic disagreement among authors. This is due to a lack of understanding of one outstanding feature of the biology of living bone—its ability to constantly remodel.

In the approach to bony protrusions (actually osseous-cartilaginous protrusions) that irritate vascular and neural tissue when they move (e.g., lateral spurs from the edges of vertebral bodies), or neural tissue, it appears that two etiologic factors are responsible for the development of such osseocartilaginous protrusions or spurs: (a) a degenerated disc, and (b) residual motion at the motion level of that disc.

The attack on the problem is very simple. The degenerated disc (that is whatever is left of it) should be removed and then the height of the disc cavity should be increased with a bone graft to take any buckling out of the posterior longitudinal ligament, and the ligamentum flavum. The vertical dimension of the intervertebral foramen also should be increased. In this way motion will be stopped.

The patient should be advised to limit activity until there is true osseous fusion between the two vertebrae in the motion segment that has had the fusion surgery. Once solid bone fusion is achieved, the remodeling process takes over and the spurs are resorbed in 9 to 18 months.

Therefore I have seldom used the intraforaminal approaches used by Jung and by Verbiest[22] to remove spurs. Neither do I use Cloward's[16] method to remove bone spurs from the edges of vertebral bodies contiguous to a degenerated intervertebral disc. I am more interested in the effect of immobilization of bone spurs by solid osseous interbody fusion and the subsequent effect of the bone remodeling process on those osseous cartilaginous-protrusions called *bone spurs.*

On the other hand, to remove malignant or benign tumors of the cervical spine that constantly compress neural or vascular tissue, any and all combinations of the approaches discussed above and listed in the bibliography of this chapter are important.

REFERENCES

1. Jung A: Resection de l'articulation unco-vertebrale et ouverture de trou de conjugaison par voie auterieure dons le traitement de la neuralgie cervico brachiale. Technique operatoire. *Mem Acad Chir* 89:361, 1963
2. Walker AE: *A History of Neurological Surgery.* (Facsimile of 1951 edition) New York, Hafner, 1967, p 366
3. Forsyth HF, Alexander ED, Davis C, et al: The advantages of early spine fusion in the treatment of fracture dislocation of the cervical spine. *J Bone Surg* 41A:17–36, 1959
4. McGraw RW, Rusch RM: Atlanto-axial arthrodesis. *J Bone Joint Surg* 55B:482–489, 1973
5. Perry J, Nickel VL, Downey MD: Total cervical spine fusion for neck paralysis. *J Bone Joint Surg* 41A:37–59, 1959
6. Rogers WA: Treatment of fracture-dislocation of the cervical spine. *J Bone Joint Surg* 24:245–258, 1942
7. Rogers WA: Fractures and dislocations of the cervical spine. *J Bone Joint Surg* 39A:341–376, 1957
8. Robinson RA: Anterior and posterior cervical spine fusions. *Clin Orthop* 35:34–62, 1964
9. Robinson RA, Riley LH: Techniques of exposure and fusion of the cervical spine. *Clin Orthop* 109:78–84, 1975
10. Robinson RA, Southwick WO: Indications and techniques for early stabilization of the neck in some fracture dislocations of the cervical spine. *South Med J* 53:565–579, 1960
11. Scoville WB: Discussion: The anterior approach for removal of ruptured disks. *J Neurosurg* 15:615, 1958
12. Scoville, WD: Types of cervical disk lesions and their surgical approaches. *JAMA* 196:49–481, 1966
13. Robinson RA, Southwick WO: Surgical Approaches to the Cervical Spine: Instruction Course Lectures of the American Academy of Orthopedic Surgeons, vol. 17. St Louis, CV Mosby, 1960, pp 299–330
14. Verbiest H: Anterolateral operations for fractures and dislocations in the middle and lower parts of the cervical spine. *J Bone Joint Surg* 51A:1489–1531, 1969
15. Bailey RW, Badgley CE: Stabilization of the cervical spine by anterior fusion. *J Bone Joint Surg* 42A:565–594, 1960
16. Cloward RB: The anterior approach for ruptured cervical disks. *J Neurosurg* 15:602–614, 1958
17. Dereymaeker A, Mulier J: Nouvelle cure neurochirurgicale des discopathies cervicales. *Neurochirurgie* 2:233–234, 1956
18. Robinson RA, Smith GW: Antero-lateral cervical disc removal and interbody fusion for the cervical disc syndrome. *Bull Johns Hopkins Hosp* 96:223–224, 1955
19. Robinson RA, Walker AE, Ferlic DC, et al: The results of anterior interbody fusion of the cervical spine. *J Bone Joint Surg* 44A:1569–1587, 1962

20. Smith GW, Robinson RA: The treatment of certain cervical spine disorders by anterior removal of the intervertebral disc and interbody fusion. *J Bone Joint Surg 40A*:607–624, 1958

21. Southwick WO, Robinson RA: Surgical approaches to the vertebral bodies in the cervical and lumbar regions. *J Bone Joint Surg 39A*: 631–643, 1957

22. Verbiest H: La chirurgia anterieure et laterale du rachis cervical, Suppl. 2, Tome 16, *Neuro-Chirurgie*. Paris, Masson et cie, 1970

23. Boudot L: Des resections des apophyses transverses des vertebres. Strasbourg, These, No. 812, 1964

24. Chien J: Retropharyngeal abscess. *Br Med J 2*:255–256, 1877

25. Cheyne WW: Case of retropharyngeal abscess pointing in the pharynx but opened by an incision behind the sternomastoid cure. *Med Times Gaz 2*:254, 1881

26. Burckhardt H: Ueber die eroffnung der retropharyngealen abscesse. Zentralblatt Chir *15*:57–60, 1888

27. Auffret C: Intervention dans les lesions du rachis. *Arch Med Navale 66*:435–450, 1896

28. Küttner H: Die verletzungen und traumatischen aneurysmen der vertebralisgefässe am halse und ihre operative behandlung. *Beit Klin Chir 108*:1–60, 1917

29. Lahey FH: The technique of the two stage operation for Pulsion Oesophageal diverticulum. *Surg Gynecol Obstet 43*:359–365, 1926

30. Fang HSY, Ong GB: Direct anterior approach to the upper cervical spine. *J Bone Joint Surg 44A*:1588–1604, 1962

31. Riley LH: Cervical disc surgery: its role and indications. *Symposium on Disease of the Intervertebral Disc*, Orthopaedic Clinics of North America. Philadelphia, WB Saunders, 1971, pp 443–452

32. Riley LH: Surgical approaches to the anterior structures of the cervical spine. *Clin Orthop 91*:16–20, 1973

33. Robinson RA, Riley LH: Anterior interbody fusion of the cervical spine, chap. 144. *The Craft of Surgery.* 2nd ed. Boston, Little Brown 1971, pp 1873–1881

34. Stevenson GC, Stoney RJ, Perkins RK, et al: A transcervical transclival approach to the ventral surface of the brain stem for removal of a clivus chordoma. *J Neurosurg 24*:544–551, 1966

35. Barbour JR: Screw fixation in fractures of the odontoid process. *S Aust Clin 5*:20–24, 1971

36. Simmons EH, Dutoit G Jr.: Lateral atlantoaxial arthrodesis. *Orthop Clin N Am 9*:1101–1114, 1978

37. Verbiest, H: A lateral approach to the cervical spine: technique and indications. *J Neurosurg 28*:191–203, 1968

38. Henry AK: *Extensile Exposure.* 2nd ed. Baltimore, Williams & Wilkins, 1957, pp 58–72

39. Rogers WA: In Crenshaw AH (ed): *Campbell's Operative Orthopaedics, Vol. 1* (5th ed). St. Louis, C.V. Mosby, 1971, p 624

CHAPTER 79
Craniovertebral Abnormalities and Their Treatment

John C. VanGilder   Arnold H. Menezes

CRANIOVERTEBRAL JUNCTION ABNORMALITIES may be congenital, inflammatory, developmental, or traumatic in origin (Table 79-1).[1-8] To effectively treat these disorders when symptomatic, a knowledge of the embryology and the functional anatomy of the area is necessary. A myriad of abnormal neurologic findings may be present that are secondary to compression or ischemia of neural tissue. The surgical management of these disorders is dependent upon precise identification of the underlying pathophysiology as determined by appropriate radiologic studies. The operative treatment includes anterior and/or posterior approaches to the craniovertebral junction with or without bony fusion. Our experience with 45 patients treated surgically who had neurologic symptoms from craniovertebral abnormalities is the basis for management of these complex disorders.

History

Subsequent to the first description of spontaneous atlantoaxial dislocation in 1830 by Bell,[9] lesions of the cervicomedullary junction have emerged from a state of being medical curiosities into an era where they can be effectively managed. Except for acute dislocations, the treatment of occipitoatlantoaxial-joint pathology was marked with failure before the era of skeletal traction.[4] Subsequently, it was apparent that the majority of both acute and chronic dislocations could be reduced even years after the initial injury.

The early operative procedures were posterior decompressions of the cervicomedullary junction with and without fusion for stabilization. Posterior decompression in those patients with irreducible compression of neural tissue at the craniovertebral area often is associated with a high operative risk and a low incidence of improvement. The majority of patients are unchanged or have increased neurologic deficit, especially when the cervicomedullary compromise is ventrally situated.[2,4,5,10-12]

More recently, transpalatine-transoral[2,5,6,11,13-20] and extrapharyngeal[5,21,22] ventral operations were described for fractures, tumors, congenital abnormalities, infection, and inflammatory conditions at the cervicomedullary junction. Stabilization of the atlanto-occipital joint usually has been done by fusing the spinal column posteriorly. The transpharyngeal route for anterior fusion has met with limited success, and further refinement of the technique may result in its future use.

No single anterior or posterior surgical procedure can be used for all of the patients with craniovertebral abnormalities. It is necessary to select the operation or combination of opera-

Division of Neurosurgery, University of Iowa Hospitals and Clinics, Iowa City, Iowa

Table 79-1. Pathological States in 45 Patients with Abnormalities of the Craniovertebral Junction

Pathology	No. of patients
Rheumatoid arthritis	7
(Down's syndrome)	(3)
Odontoid dysgenesis	3
Basilar impression	11
(rheumatoid arthritis)	(1)
Unfused odontoid with	
upward migration	2
Klippel-Feil	9
(Chiari malformation)	(4)
Rickets	2
Spondylo-epiphyseal dysplasia	2
Abnormal condyles and occiput	6
Traumatic (dislocation with posterior	
compression at occiput, C1, C2)	3

tions for each patient on an individual basis to correct the pathologic process responsible for the neurologic deficit.[2,5,6,20]

Embyrology-Anatomy

By definition, the craniovertebral junction includes the foramen magnum, the atlas, and the axis vertebrae. The occipital bone is formed by fusion of four sclerotomes. The proatlas is the most caudal of these sclerotomes and loses its identity in humans. The neural arch of the primitive proatlas divides into anterior and posterior segments.[23] The former gives rise to the occipital condyles and the latter fuses with the atlas to help form its rostral articular facets. If the posterior segment of the proatlas remains separate, the atlas has bipartite cranial articular facets—a rare anomaly that may result in horizontal instability of this joint. The proatlas also forms the dorsal portion of the C1 lateral masses and gives rise to the distal ossification center of the dens.[24]

The atlas is derived from the first cervical sclerotome as well as the proatlas. The body of the atlas as such disappears and gives origin to the dens. The anterior arch of the atlas has one center of ossification, and at times two centers may be present. The posterior arches of the atlas ossify by the age of 3 to 4 years.

The axis is developed from four primary ossification centers. The dens is formed by the C1 sclerotome, the two neural arches and the body of the axis from the C2 sclerotomes, and the tip of the dens develops from the proatlas. The tip of the dens is fused with the body by the age of 12 years. The remainder of the segments ossify and are fused by the age of 3 years.

Dysgenesis of the odontoid process may encompass a variety of congenital anomalies. Failure of the proatlas and the dens to fuse results in *ossiculum terminale*. An *os odontoideum* represents failure of the odontoid process and the axis body to fuse. Hypoplasia and agenesis of the dens is the result of developmental failure of the distal ossification centers. The common pathophysiology that produces neurologic deficit with agenesis or hypoplasia of the dens is instability between the first and second cervical vertebrae because of incompetence of the cruciate ligament.

An occipital vertebra is a bony structure that is separate from the foramen magnum and incorporates the occipital condyles. The anterior arch may be partially or completely fused to the anterior margin of the foramen magnum, and the transverse process, if present, does not have a foramen for the vertebral artery. In contrast, an atlanto-occipital fusion is characterized by ankylosis between the atlas and the skull base, usually with persistence of the normal joints. The transverse process of the atlas has foramina for the vertebral arteries.

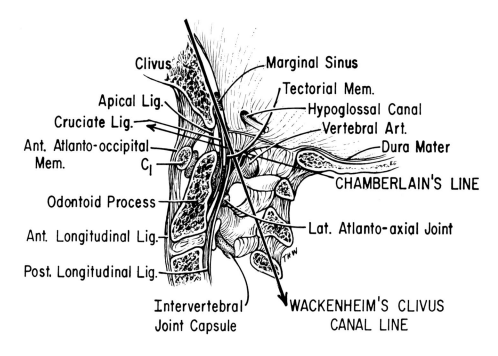

Clivus
Apical Lig.
Cruciate Lig.
Ant. Atlanto-occipital Mem. C₁
Odontoid Process
Ant. Longitudinal Lig.
Post. Longitudinal Lig.
Intervertebral Joint Capsule

Marginal Sinus
Tectorial Mem.
Hypoglossal Canal
Vertebral Art.
Dura Mater
CHAMBERLAIN'S LINE
Lat. Atlanto-axial Joint
WACKENHEIM'S CLIVUS CANAL LINE

RELATIONSHIP AT THE CRANIOVERTEBRAL JUNCTION

Fig. 79-1. A drawing of the anatomic relationships of the bone and soft tissue in the midsagittal plane of the craniovertebral junction.

The occipitoatlantoaxial joints are complex, both anatomically and kinematically (Fig. 79-1)[25,26] In addition to the two occipito-atlantal articulations, there are four atlanto-axial joints with a common synovial lining between the dens and the anterior arch of the atlas, the dens and the transverse ligament, and between the lateral masses. The second cervical nerve passes through the capsule of each atlanto-axial joint.

The dens is approximated to the anterior arch of the atlas by the transverse ligament, which is anchored to the tubercle on the mesial aspect of each lateral mass of the atlas. This ligament is responsible for the stability of the atlanto-axial joint. The axis is connected to the occiput by the alar ligaments that course obliquely upward from the posterior lateral surface of the dens to the anterior medial aspect of the occipital condyles; the apical dens ligament continues from the medial aspect of the foramen magnum to the tip of the dens, the tentorial membrane (an extension of the deep layer of the posterior longitudinal ligament) the cruciate ligament consisting of the transverse ligament plus triangular ascending and descending slips to the anterior rim of the foramen magnum and the axis, respectively.

The atlantoaxial joints have convex articular surfaces with a horizontal orientation.[24] Because these convex surfaces are not exactly reciprocal, a telescoping effect occurs during rotation of the head. There is limited movement in the atlantoaxial joint and head-spine motion is basically between the occipital condyles and C2. Because of the intervening C1–C2 convex joint, there is potential decreased stability at the craniovertebral junction with extension, flexion, and rotation. Hypermobility of the occipito-atlantal joint may progressively increase in patients with congenital high cervical fusion. This may be the etiology of basilar invagination associated with the Klippel-Feil abnormality.

The development of the neck musculature is inadequate to supplement joint stability until the age of 8.[6,27] Before this age, laxity of the ligamentous tissue permits excessive movement of

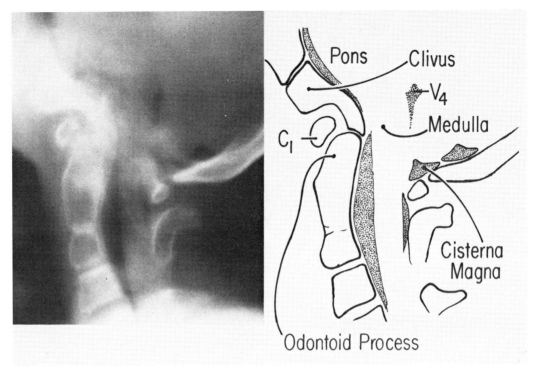

Fig. 79-2. A lateral midline polytome of an air myelogram, demonstrating ventral compression of the cervicomedullary junction (left). The air column is obliterated at the distal clivus and dens. The schematic drawing (right) illustrates the structures that can be identified.

the occipito-atlanto-axial articulations.[25,26,28] Forward gliding of the skull in relation to the spine occurs if hypoplastic occipital condyles are present. This is the mechanism for the development of neurologic deficit in children who have spondylo-epiphyseal dysplasia, Conradi's syndrome, and Morquio's syndrome. These syndromes are often associated with ossiculum terminale.[6]

The lymphatic drainage of the occipito-atlanto-axial joints is through retropharyngeal glands to the deep cervical lymphatic chain. In children, since the neck musculature is not fully developed, C1–C2 subluxation may develop secondary to nasopharyngeal infections.[6,29]

In the osseoligamentous destruction caused by rheumatoid arthritis, the synovial bursae and associated ligaments that surround the odontoid process are damaged, with a resulting loss of stability.[30] Subluxation may occur secondary to the atlas moving anteriorly on the axis (caused by insufficiency of the cruciate ligament or fracture of the odontoid process), the atlas moving posteriorly on the axis (from erosion or fracture of the odontoid process), or by telescoping of the skull on the axis (from destruction of the lateral atlantoaxial-apophyseal joints). Chronic subluxation often results in ligamentous hypertrophy and the accumulation of granulation tissue behind the odontoid process from the hypertrophied soft tissue. Even though bone alignment is present on roentgenograms there may be ventral compression of the cervicomedullary junction by soft tissue.

Signs and Symptoms

Cervicomedullary junction abnormalities present with a myriad of symptoms and signs including myelopathy; brainstem, cranial nerve, and cervical root dysfunction; or vascular insufficiency, or any combination of these.[4,5,7,8,31] In our series, evidence of myelopathy was present in all but 1 patient; each presented with variable weakness in the upper and lower extremities. The extent of neurologic motor deficit was a spectrum from easy fatigability to quadriparesis. Both motor and sensory abnormalities were frequently poorly localized, e.g., 5 patients presented with paraparesis. A myelopathy mimicking the central cord syndrome usually was present in patients having basilar invagination. The pathophysiology of motor myelopathy has been attributed to repetitive trauma to the pyramidal tracts secondary to chronic compression. The false localizing signs have been attributed to stagnant hypoxia of the cervical spinal cord from venous stasis.[32]

Cervical root symptoms usually are manifested by suboccipital headaches in the sensory distribution of the second cervical nerve. The paresthesias are from irritation of the nerve as it transverses through the lateral atlantoaxial joint capsule.[24]

Brainstem signs include nystagmus to lateral gaze, and in 3 patients downbeat nystagmus was present. This latter finding has been well documented with cervicomedullary pathology.[5,33] Respiratory arrest and sleep apnea were associated with both anterior and posterior compression of the cervicomedullary junction in 2 patients, resolving in each instance after decompression. Dysfunction of the trigeminal, glossopharyngeal, vagus, and accessory cranial nerves has been identified in this patient population, with sparing of the hypoglossal nerve in all patients. Tinnitus or diminished hearing or both was present in about 25 percent of the patients, but was an infrequent complaint.

Symptoms attributed to vascular compromise included syncope, vertigo, episodic hemiparesis, altered level of consciousness, and transient loss of visual fields. These symptoms may be secondary to repetitive trauma to spinal cord vessels, intermittent obstruction by angulation, or stretching of the vertebral or anterior spinal arteries or both from excessive mobility of an unstable atlantoaxial joint. Although several patients exhibited vascular symptoms, only 1 case demonstrated angiographic evidence of vascular compromise at the occipito-atlas junction.

Diagnostic Investigations

To assess the cervicobasilar relationships, there are several reference lines used to evaluate the plain roentgenograms. McRae's line measures the sagittal diameter of the foramen magnum from its anterior margin to its posterior margin (average: 35 mm). The Towne's projection is useful for determining the transverse diameter of the foramen magnum (35 mm ± 4 mm). Chamberlain's line is a diagonal from the hard palate to the posterior margin of the foramen magnum (Fig. 79-1). The odontoid process should not extend more than one-third of its length above this line. Wackenheim's clivus–canal line is drawn along the posterior surface of the clivus (Fig. 79-1). Basilar invagination results in intersection of this line by the odontoid process. Fishgold's digastric line is measured on the frontal projections and connects the digastric grooves. The line is normally 11 mm ± 4 mm above the atlanto-occipital junction. The digastric line is the upper limit in position for the odontoid tip. Patients with abnormalities of the craniovertebral junction become symptomatic when the effective diameter of the canal at the foramen magnum (from the posterior surface of the odontoid process to the posterior margin of foramen magnum) is less than 19 mm.[35]

Special radiologic procedures are necessary to clarify the etiology and the pathophysiology of the abnormality.[5,6,20] These include pleuri-directional tomography of the craniovertebral junction. Flexion and extension views are made to determine stability and to identify the "irreducible" lesion.

Gas or metrizamide myelography with pleuri-directional tomography is employed once a diagnosis is suspected on the plain roentgenograms. The procedure is done in the lateral position and should include extension and flexion positions. This will demonstrate the size of the spinal cord, the subarachnoid spaces, and the brainstem. Anomalies such as the Chiari malformation and hydromyelia can be identified, the latter by the "collapsing cord sign." An example of ventral compression at the cervicomedullary junction is illustrated in Figure 79-2.

Vertebral angiography may identify stretched or occluded vessels of the posterior cerebral circulation. We have demonstrated appreciable differences in vessel caliber by comparing flexion and extension roentgenograms by using angiography.

Computerized axial tomograms with horizontal and sagittal reconstructions have been used to identify the bony abnormalites as well as the position of neural structures in relation to bone and soft tissue. This equipment is not generally available at all institutions.

Operative Technique

Anterior Transoral-Transpharyngeal Approach

The transoral-transpharyngeal route is used to relieve ventral irreducible compression on the cervicomedullary junction. Nasal and pharyngeal cultures are obtained 3 days before the proposed operation. No antibiotics are given if normal flora are present. It is prudent to have the patient's nutritional status in the best possible condition before surgery.

The patient is placed supine on the operating table and maintained in skeletal traction. We prefer either Crutchfield or Gardner-Wells tongs, and traction between 5 and 10 pounds is sufficient to maintain satisfactory alignment of the cervico-occipital junction. After positioning, the patient is intubated while awake using regional block and topical anesthesia to the pharynx and larynx. Following intubation and before administration of general anesthesia, the neurologic examination is repeated to ensure that no significant change has occurred subsequent to positioning the patient for surgery. We perform a tracheostomy in each patient to provide for better exposure during the operation and to ensure an adequate airway postoperatively, since lingual edema is common.

The mouth is retracted open using a self-retaining Dingman mouth retractor with careful attention to placement of the rubber guard over the teeth. This instrument has the advantage of allowing self-retaining retractors to be attached to the frame to depress the tongue and to allow for lateral exposure of the oral cavity. It is wise to loosen the tongue retractor intermittently during the operation to relieve lingual congestion.

A gauze packing is used to occlude the laryngopharynx to prevent blood leakage into the stomach. After infiltration of the soft palate with 1% Xylocaine with 1:200,000 epinephrine or normal saline, a midline incision is made extending from the hard palate, diverting from the midline only at the base of the uvula (Fig. 79-3). This incision ensures both minimal bleeding and unrestricted healing of the soft palate, for the palatine artery with its accompanying palatine nerve enters the soft palate laterally and terminates in the midline. Retraction stay sutures are placed in both soft palate flaps to allow maximum exposure of the pharynx rostral to the caudal portion of the clivus.

The surgeon can visualize and palpate the body of the dens, the arch of the atlas, and the caudal extent of the clivus through the retropharyngeal musculature. A linear midline incision is made through the posterior pharyngeal wall, which can be easily separated from the underlying anterior longitudinal ligament and its rostral anterior atlanto-occipital extension. Stay sutures or a self-retaining retractor are used to maintain lateral retraction of the muscle (Fig. 79-4).

Following exposure of the anterior longitudinal ligament, the operating microscope is used to provide magnification and a concentrated light source. The anterior longitudinal ligament is coagulated to reduce bleeding, and the anterior body of the axis and the anterior arch of the atlas are exposed in the subperiosteal plane with a periosteal elevator. The ventral atlanto-axial articulation is separated and the anterior arch of the atlas is removed using a 1.5-mm foot plate, 45° angled punch rongeur to expose the anterior atlanto-occipital membrane (Fig. 79-5). This latter structure is resected, including the apical ligament of the dens, to expose the caudal portion of the clivus. It is often necessary to resect a portion of the caudal clivus if the odontoid invagination is severe in order to expose the rostral tip of the odontoid process. If such a maneuver is nec-

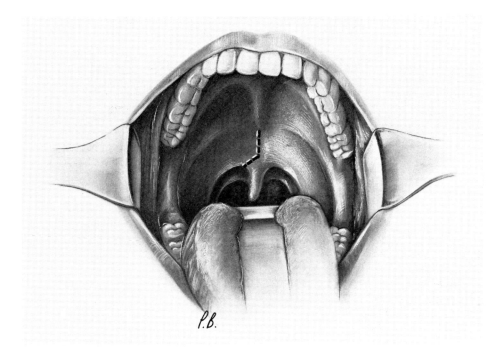

Fig. 79-3.   A drawing of the oral cavity to illustrate the incision in the midline of the soft palate (broken line).

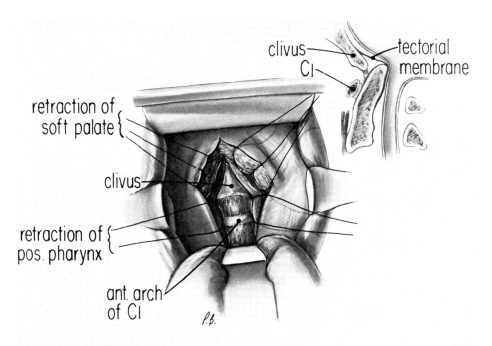

Fig. 79-4.   A drawing illustrating exposure of the clivus, the anterior arch of the atlas, and the odontoid process with placement of stay sutures in the soft palate and pharynx. The corresponding midline sagittal drawing is inset in the upper right.

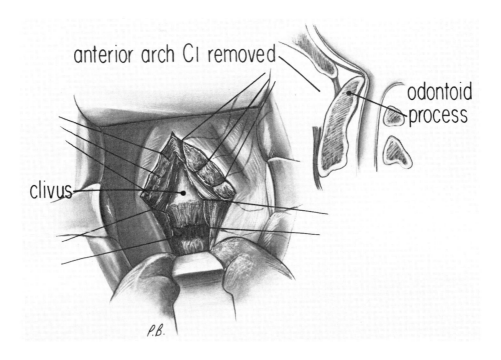

anterior arch CI removed

odontoid process

clivus

P.B.

Fig. 79-5. A drawing illustrating the operative site after excision of the anterior arch of C1 with the apical ligament still intact. The corresponding midline sagittal drawing is inset in the upper right.

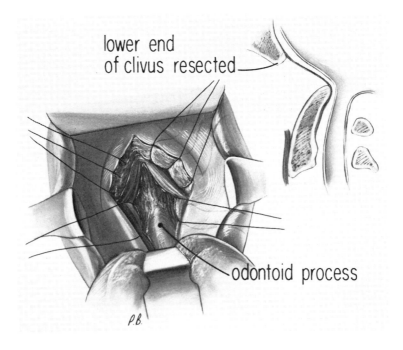

lower end of clivus resected

odontoid process

P.B.

Fig. 79-6. A drawing illustrating the operative site after excision of the apical ligament and the caudal clivus to expose the odontoid tip. The corresponding midline sagittal drawing is inset in the upper right.

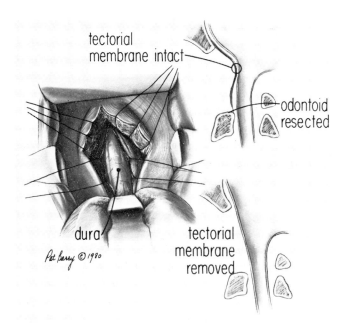

tectorial
membrane intact

odontoid
resected

dura

tectorial
membrane
removed

Pat Berry ©1980

Fig. 79-7.   A drawing of the cervicomedullary junction after removal of the dens. After adequate decompression,
the dura should protrude into the decompression
site. The drawing in the upper right illustrates failure of decompression because of a hypertrophied
tentorial membrane. The drawing of the sagittal reconstruction in the lower right demonstrates adequate ventral decompression following removal of
the hypertrophied tissue.

essary, the tissue posterior to the clivus must be carefully separated from the bone, as the dura
can easily be penetrated and bleeding from the marginal sinus may be troublesome (Fig. 79-6).

The surgeon should next identify the distal tip of the odontoid process by stripping ligamentous tissue free from its osseous ventral surface. The distal portion of the dens is removed with
an air drill and the steel cutting burr to thin the bone. A diamond burr then is substituted to remove the thin dorsal bony shell and avoid tearing of the posterior soft tissue. We prefer a 45° angled drill hand-piece attachment, which enables unrestricted visualization of the surgical field.
After identifying the tissue plane posterior to the rostral dens, the remaining odontoid process
and body of the axis is removed in a rostral-caudal direction for decompression of the cervicomedullary junction (Fig. 79-7). In children it is important to preserve the cruciate ligament and
tentorial membrane. If the periosteum is not violated, this will allow for further new bone formation and spontaneous ventral fusion. This has occurred in several of our cases.

In those patients with inflammatory disorders, particularly rheumatoid arthritis, hypertrophy and thickening of the ligamentous tissue is extensive. Adequate ventral decompression will
not be accomplished until this tissue is removed adjacent to the dura (Fig. 79-7). This soft tissue
decompression is best done after identification of the dura rostrally. The dura-ligamentous plane
then is developed with sharp and blunt dissection in a caudal direction. The surgeon can be assured that adequate cervicomedullary decompression has been accomplished when the pulsatile
dura protrudes ventrally into the surgical decompression site.

If the dura is inadvertently torn or cerebrospinal fluid is identified, repair of the fistula can
be accomplished by placing two to three layers of fascia over the rent. The fascia is harvested
from the external oblique aponeurosis or from the anterior lateral thigh. In this situation a lumbar cerebrospinal fluid drain is maintained for 7 days postoperatively. In our experience, closing

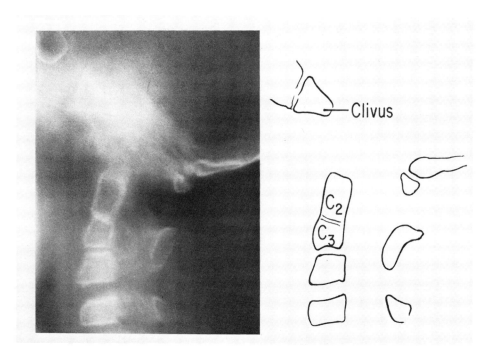

Fig. 79-8. A midline tomogram (left) following transoral-transpharyngeal resection of the caudal clivus and odontoid process. The postoperative roentgenogram is of the same
patient illustrated in Figure 79-2. The schematic drawing on the right identifies the
bone structures.

the dura with sutures has not been successful and resulted in persistent cerebrospinal fluid leak in
1 case. The leak was repaired successfully with a fascia graft.

The pharyngeal musculature and aponeurosis is closed with interrupted 3-0 polyglycolic absorbable sutures in two layers. The soft palate is approximated by closing the nasal mucosa with
interrupted polyglycolic sutures. Vertical mattress sutures placed through the oral mucosa include the muscle to ensure snug approximation.

In the postoperative period the patient is maintained in 5-pound skeletal traction. Intravenous fluids are administered for 6 days, followed by graduated feeding to a regular diet by the
fourteenth day after surgery. Flexion-extension roentgenograms are obtained between 7 and 10
days after surgery to determine occipito-cervical stability. If instability is present, a posterior fusion is done when the patient is in satisfactory condition, usually between 10 and 14 days following the initial surgery. If intravenous antibiotics are used, they are discontinued 48 hours after
surgery if the dura has not been violated. If the dura is not intact and a fascia graft has been used
for repair, intravenous antibiotics are continued for 14 days after surgery. The tracheostomy is
discontinued as soon as the patient's status permits. An example of resection of the caudal clivus
and anterior odontoid is illustrated in Figure 79-8.

Posterior Fusion

The basic principles of positioning for posterior operations as described previously with the
transoral-transpharyngeal operation are adhered to. The patient is intubated while awake,
maintained in skeletal traction, and positioned on the operating table in the prone position. The
head is placed on a cerebellar headrest, which ensures that no inadvertent pressure is placed
about the eyes. A lateral roentgenogram is obtained to confirm that proper cervical alignment
has been established. After repeating the neurologic examination, the patient is anesthetized.

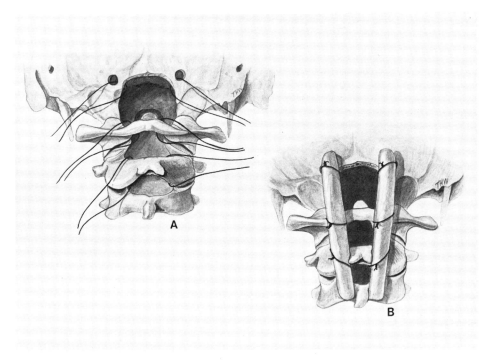

Fig. 79-9.   A drawing illustrating placement of the wires under the laminae and through the occipital bone **(A)**. The bone graft is secured to the occiput and the laminae with wire
(B).

A midline incision is made to the deep cervical fascia from the inion to C4. The spinous
processes are exposed by incising through the avascular ligamentum nuchae. The paracervical
musculature is dissected off the spinous processes and laminae in the subperiosteal plane. We
prefer to use a combination of cutting current and a two-periosteal-elevator technique (one elevator is used to retract the muscle and the other is used for the subperiosteal dissection) with precautions to avoid excessive vertebral manipulation. The suboccipital musculature is dissected
from the squamous occipital bone in a subperiosteal plane with both cutting current and sharp-
blunt dissection.

   In those patients with unstable occipito-atlanto-axial articulation, fusion includes the occiput. A notch is placed inferiorly and superiorly in each laminae and a hole is drilled through each
side of the suboccipital bone lateral to the foramen magnum. Twisted No. 26 stainless steel wire
is placed under each laminae and passed through the occipital bone (Fig. 79-9A). The twisted wire
is prepared by bending the material into two equal lengths, securing the bent end into a hand
drill where the bit is placed, and grasping the free ends with needle holders. The wire is twisted
using the drill by keeping equal tension on the ends. This maneuver increases the tensile strength
of the wire approximately 16 X.

   Bone donor sites are either the rib or ileum. The bone graft is notched similar to the laminae
and a hole is placed in the distal end for the occipital wire. The graft then is secured to the opposing laminar surface and suboccipital bone by twisting the end of the wires together (Fig. 79-
9B). Bone chips may be placed along the fusion area for additional strength.

   The patient is maintained in skeletal traction for 7 days after surgery and immobilized in
Halo traction for 6 months or until the fusion is solid. The plastic vest to anchor the Halo that is
commercially available has the advantages of less weight and improved patient comfort compared with the body cast. Infection has been avoided by cleansing the skull-fixation pins with alcohol twice a day. The lateral roentgenograms of a patient before and after posterior fusion are
shown in Figure 79-10.

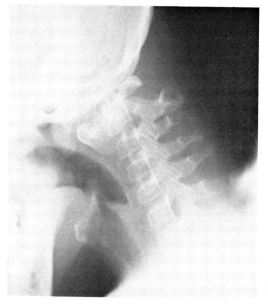
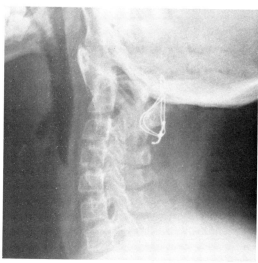

Fig. 79-10. A lateral preoperative roentgenogram (left) showing anterior subluxation of C1 to the occiput and atlantoaxial dislocation. The postoperative roentgenogram (right) illustrates posterior C2-occipital fusion and C1 laminectomy. Note the spontaneous fusion between the clivus, atlas, and odontoid complex after posterior fixation.

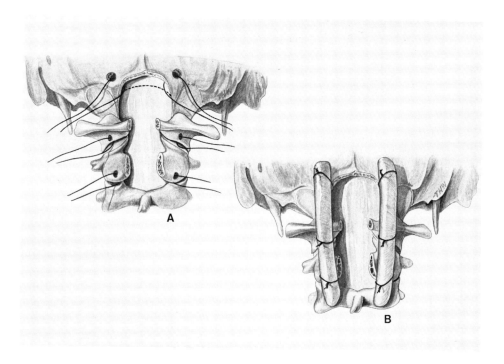

Fig. 79-11. **A.** A drawing illustrating placement of holes and wire through the occipital bone and the C1-C2 inferior facets after laminectomy. **B.** The graft is secured to the occiput and facets.

Table 79-2. Surgical Management of 45 Patients with Abnormalities of the Craniovertebral Junction

Preoperative stability	Site of compression	Decompression approach	Postoperative stability	Posterior fusion
Reducible* (9)	—	—	—	+ (9)
Irreducible (36)	Ventral (13)	Transoral Trans-palatine clivus odontoid resection	Stable (9)	—
			Unstable (4)	+ (4)
	Dorsal (23)	Posterior decompression	Stable (7)	—
			Unstable (16)	+ (16)

*Reducible = Restoration of CVJ anatomic relationships, relieving compression on the cervicomedullary junction.

Posterior Decompression with and without Fusion

The procedure of positioning the patient on the operating table before anesthesia, outlined previously, is followed. The spinous processes and laminae are exposed by the same operative technique described under posterior fusion. For decompression, a suboccipital craniectomy is done to include the posterior and lateral bone surrounding the foramen magnum. The laminae and spinous processes of C1–C2–C3 are removed in a rostral-caudal direction. The laminectomy should extend laterally to the mesial portion of the facets.

For stabilization subsequent to laminectomy, the lateral interfacet fusion is used. The muscle and capsular ligaments are removed from the C1–C2 or C3 posterior facets with cutting current, periosteal elevators, and sharp bone curettes. Holes are drilled through the inferior facet into the interfacet joint of each vertebra incorporated in the fusion, and in the suboccipital bone if occipital fusion is desired. A No. 26 stainless steel twisted wire as prepared in the previous description is passed through the openings (Fig. 79-11A). This is facilitated by spreading the interfacet joint with a Freer elevator. Either rib or split-thickness iliac bone is placed adjacent to the facets or occiput or both, and the grafts are secured by the wire (Fig. 79-11B).

The postoperative management of lateral fusion is identical to that described for posterior fusion without laminectomy except that it is often necessary to maintain Halo traction for a longer period.

Results

The type and incidence of operative procedure in our series of 45 consecutive patients with symptomatic craniovertebral junction abnormalities is outlined in Table 79-2.

Forty-four patients recovered or improved neurologically after surgery. The only death was a 66-year-old woman who presented with a rapidly progressive quadriparesis and respiratory arrest. She had severe basilar invagination and underwent anterior removal of the odontoid process, the rostral one-third of the C2 body, and posterior fusion. The patient was ambulatory after surgery, but died from sepsis of urinary tract origin. A delayed cerebrospinal fluid fistula developed in 1 patient after a transoral operation. The fistula was closed with fascia, as described in the section on the operative technique. One child with spondylo-epiphyseal dysplasia and occipito-atlantoaxial instability with ossiculum terminale had a posterior decompression with fusion of the occiput to C1–C2. She had resorption of the bone grafts and required another operation for refusion.

Three patients presented to us with continued progression of neurologic deficit after posterior decompression for irreducible ventral pathology. Each improved after anterior odontoidectomy.

REFERENCES

1. Bharucha EP, Dastur HM: Craniovertebral anomalies. (A report on 40 cases.) *Brain 87*:469–480, 1964
2. Greenberg AD: Atlanto-axial dislocations. *Brain 91*:655–684, 1968
3. Kopits SE, Perovic MN, McKusick V, et al: Congenital atlantoaxial dislocations in various forms of dwarfism. (Abstract) *J Bone Joint Surg 54*:1349–1350, 1972
4. List CF: Neurologic syndromes accompanying developmental anomalies of occipital bone, atlas and axis. *Arch Neurol Psychiatry 45*:577–616, 1941
5. Menezes AH, VanGilder JC, Graf CJ, et al: Craniocervical abnormalities. *J Neurosurg 53*:444–455, 1980
6. Menezes AH, Graf CJ, Hibri N: Abnormalities of the cranio-vertebral junction with cervico-medullary compression. *Childs Brain 7*:15–30, 1980
7. Michie I, Clark M: Neurological syndromes associated with cervical and craniocervical anomalies. *Arch Neurol 18*:241–247, 1968
8. Spillane JD, Pallis C, Jones AM: Developmental abnormalities in the region of the foramen magnum. *Brain 80*:11–48, 1957
9. Bell C: *The Nervous System of the Human Body.* London, Longman, Rees, Orme, Brown and Green, 1830
10. Dastur DK, Wadia NH, Desai AD, et al: Medullo-spinal compression due to atlanto-axial dislocation and sudden haematomyelia during decompression. Pathology, pathogenesis and clinical correlations. *Brain 88*:897–924, 1965
11. Greenberg AD, Scoville WB, Davey LM: Transoral decompression of the atlantoaxial dislocation due to odontoid hypoplasia. Report of two cases. *J Neurosurg 28*:266–269, 1968
12. Symonds CP, Meadows SP: Compression of the spinal cord in the neighbourhood of the foramen magnum. With a note on the surgical approach, by Julian Taylor. *Brain 60*:52–84, 1937
13. Cannoni M: La voi trans-orale dans l'abord des lesions de la region du clivus. *J Fr Otorhinolaryngol 27*:81–85, 1978
14. Delandsheer JM, Caron JP, Jomin M: (The transbucco-pharyngeal approach and malformations of the cervico-occipital joint.) *Neurochirurgie 23*:276–281, 1977
15. Estridge MN, Smith RA: Transoral fusion of odontoid fracture. Case report. *J Neurosurg 27*:462–465, 1967
16. Fang HSY, Ong GB: Direct anterior approach to the upper cervical spine. *J Bone Joint Surg 44*:1588–1604, 1962
17. Mullan S, Naunton R, Hekmatpanah J, et al: The use of an anterior approach to ventrally placed tumors in the foramen magnum and vertebral column. *J Neurosurg 24*:536–543, 1966
18. Pech A, Cannoni M, Magnan J, et al: (The trans-oral approach in oto-neurosurgery.) *Ann Otolaryngol Chir Cervicofac 91*:281–292, 1974
19. Sukoff MH, Kadin MM, Moran T: Transoral decompression for myelopathy caused by rheumatoid arthritis of the cervical apine. Case report. *J Neurosurg 37*:451–464, 1949
20. VanGilder JC, Menezes AH: Craniovertebral abnormalities. Symptoms, etiology and treatment. *Contemporary NeuroSurgery,* Vol. 3, Lesson 7, 1981
21. Bonney G: Stabilization of the upper cervical spine by the transpharyngeal route. *Proc R Soc Med 63*:896–897, 1970
22. DeAndrade JR, MacNab I: Anterior occipito-cervical fusion using an extra-pharyngeal exposure. *J Bone Joint Surg 51*:1621–1626, 1969
23. Ganguly DN, Roy KK: A study on the cranio-vertebral joint in the man. *Anat Anz 114*:433–452, 1964
24. Shapiro R, Youngberg AS, Rothman SLG: The differential diagnosis of traumatic lesions of the occipito-atlanto-axial segment. *Radiol Clin North Am 11*:505–526, 1973
25. White AA III, Panjabi MM: The clinical biomechanics of the occipitoatlantoaxial complex. *Orthop Clin North Am 9*:867–878, 1978
26. Holmes JC, Hall JE: Fusion for instability and potential instability of the cervical spine in children and adolescents. *Orthop Clin North Am 9*:923–943, 1978
27. Alexander E Jr, Forsyth HF, Davis CH Jr, et al: Dislocation of the atlas on the axis. *J Neurosurg 15*:353–371, 1958

28. Gilles RH, Bina M, Sotrel A: Infantile atlantoccipital instability. The potential danger of extreme extension. *Am J Dis Child 133*:30–37, 1979
29. Hess JH, Bronstein IP, Abelson SM: Atlanto-axial dislocations. Unassociated with trauma and secondary to inflammatory foci in the neck. *Am J Dis Child 49*:1137–1147, 1935
30. O'Leary P, Ranawat CS, Pellicci PM: The cervical spine in rheumatoid arthritis. *Contemp Surg 7*:13–17, 1975
31. Schneider RC, Schemm GW: Vertebral artery insufficiency in acute and chronic spinal trauma. *J Neurosurg 18*:348–360, 1961
32. Taylor AR, Byrnes DP: Foramen magnum and high cervical cord compression. *Brain 97*:473–480, 1974
33. Cogan DG, Barrows LJ: Platybasia and Arnold-Chiari malformation. *Arch Ophthalmol 52*:13–29, 1954
34. Dolan KD: Cervicobasilar relationships. *Radiol Clin North Am 15*:155–166, 1977
35. McRae DL: The significance of abnormalities of the cervical spine. *Am J Roentgenol Radium Ther 84*:3–25, 1960
36. Apuzzo MLJ, Weiss MH, Heiden J: Transoral exposure of the atlantoaxial region. *Neurosurgery 3*:201–207, 1978

CHAPTER 80
Anterior Cervical Disc Excision in Cervical Spondylosis

Henry H. Schmidek

OVER THE PAST TWO DECADES operations have been devised in which a direct anterior or anterolateral approach has been used to gain access to the spine from the base of the skull to the sacrum. This inventiveness has been particularly apparent with regard to the surgical management of disorders of the cervical spine.[1] In the neck, anterior approaches have undergone constant redevelopment and reassessment so that they could be used to treat cervical disc disease, cervical fractures, tumors, and infections of the bodies of the vertebrae. At the present time at least a half dozen variations of the anterior approach have been fashioned.[2-9] All allow access to the ventral aspect of the dura, the nerve root sheaths, and the vertebral arteries, and all provide for considerable flexibility in the approach available to remove lesions that impinge on these structures or are associated with spinal instability. Not only do they allow for the removal of extruded cartilage or bony overgrowth, but they also can be used with the supine position during surgery and with dissection in avascular planes. Their associated low morbidity has resulted in their widespread acceptance in the treatment of sequelae of cervical spondylosis.

The anterolateral approaches to the cervical spine originated in order to explore those afflicted with tuberculosis of the spine. In order to reach the site of these lesions, the vertebral bodies had to be approached anteriorly. This approach then was applied to the treatment of cervical disc disease associated with radiculopathy and myelopathy. This application began with the reports of Robinson[7,10,11] and of Cloward[5,6,12] in the 1960s and has since become a standard part of the neurosurgical armamentarium. This is easy to understand, since the predominant changes associated with cervical spondylosis are situated ventral to neurovascular structures within the spine. The anterolateral approach allows these structures to be decompressed directly.

Surgical Indications

Cervical Radiculopathy

Cervical disc disease often involves several levels of the spine, although it is seen most often at the levels of C4-5, C5-6, and C6-7. These herniations, both of the "hard" or "soft" type, are situated centrally, laterally, or anterolaterally. The lateral and anterolateral herniations project into the intervertebral foramina, whereas the central disc herniations may be limited to the mid-

Division of Neurosurgery, University of Vermont College of Medicine, Burlington, Vermont

line. As the disc degenerates, its nucleus is affected first and begins to bulge transversely. The patient may then experience neck and arm pain, occipital headache, and, occasionally, anterior chest pain. The *painful disc syndrome* has been defined as a mechanical pain in the neck, shoulders, and arm, often with subjective numbness in a dermatome. In the early stages of the deterioration of the disc, pain may develop when the fibers of the annulus or adjacent structures, such as the anterior and posterior ligaments, become stretched. In these cases, standard radiographic studies remain normal, but discography may help to identify the particular disc responsible for the patient's symptoms.

Further degeneration leads to cracking and fissuring of the disc. These may extend into the joints of Luschka, and nuclear material may be extruded into these joints beneath or through the posterior longitudinal ligament or through the cartilaginous plates into the vertebral bodies. Changes in the cartilage further interfere with nutrition of the disc, contributing to its degeneration. Radiographically, the disc space now is narrowed and the spine is slightly shortened. Sliding movements between the vertebrae and alterations in the bone adjacent to the disc develop. The end of the vertebral body mushrooms and expands, and bony outgrowths develop around the periphery because of periosteal activity provoked by the abnormal direction and stresses on lamellar fibers. Osteophytes develop around the lateral margins of the vertebrae. The "hard" disc is a degenerative spur mainly associated with outgrowth from the uncovertebral joint, but it may be accompanied by spur formation in the immediate adjacent posterior portion of the disc. The radicular symptoms and signs associated with either "hard" or "soft" discs are probably due to a combination of neural compression and perineural inflammation which results.

Surgical decompression is appropriate in cervical radiculopathy with subjective and objective evidence of nerve root compression in which conservative treatment, involving adequate sedation and analgesics, traction, and physical therapy, fails. As mentioned by Scoville,[13] unrelenting symptoms usually should be present for a 3- to 4-week period, although some patients who experience severe pain and neurologic deficit require surgery almost immediately after their symptoms begin. In these patients cervical traction often accentuates their discomfort, and, inevitably, a large disc fragment is found to be responsible for their discomfort (Fig. 80-1).

Cervical Spondylotic Myelopathy

Cervical spondylotic myelopathy often occurs in patients who have a canal that is narrower than normal (normal: 17 ± 5 mm with a 6 ft tube-to-film distance), and in whom osteophytes and ligamentous hypertrophy further compromise the size of the canal.[1] The pathogenesis of the disease remains uncertain. Compression of the cord by disc material or traction of the cord against osteophytes is etiologically important, particularly in the case of an acute myelopathy, e.g., one associated with traumatic disc protrusion. In chronic myelopathy, however, the factors of disc degeneration, spur formation, foraminal encroachment, and a congenitally narrow canal are probably potentiated by motion at the involved levels. It may be that the motion results in the progression of signs and symptoms.

Studies of the vascular supply of the spinal cord[14] have shown a large radicular artery analogous to Adamkiewicz from C6 to C7, and in some cases a watershed area may exist in the cord at C4. Zulch has noted in a few cases that following a fracture dislocation at C5-6 there may be extensive necrosis from C4 to T4, corresponding to the vascular supply in the cord. Whether or not compromise of this radicular vessel is important in some cases of myelopathy is not known. Acute myelopathy secondary to thrombosis of the anterior spinal artery is very rare and does not explain the progression seen in chronic myelopathy. It may be that, secondary to the spondylotic changes and the distortion and flattening of the cord, there is distortion of its intrinsic arterioles and the subsequent compromise of the feeding and intrinsic vessels of the cord, leading to vascular insufficiency of the cord. It has been suggested by Robinson[15] that the stepwise progression of neurologic deficit characteristically seen in certain cases with cervical spondylotic myelopathy actually represents repeated small infarctions within the cord substance.

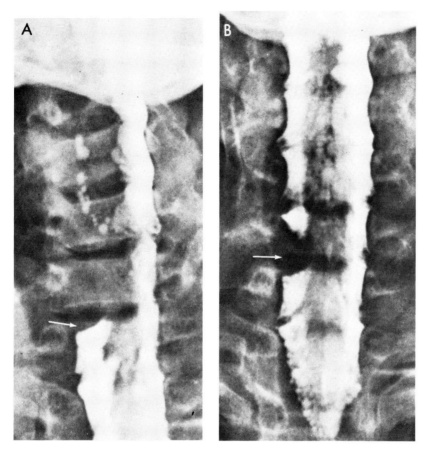

Fig. 80-1. A cervical myelogram showing a laterally situated free disc fragment in a patient with intractable radiculopathy.

Cervical spondylotic myelopathy was identified and characterized as a distinct entity in the classic paper by Clarke,[16] who reviewed the case histories of 120 patients with myclopathy and evidence of spinal cord compression on myelopathy, and was further defined by Gregorius[17] as consisting of five distinct syndromes within this overall group of patients, including (1) a transverse lesion syndrome with corticospinal, spinothalamic, and dorsal column involvement; (2) a motor system syndrome with corticospinal tract and anterior horn cell dysfunction; (3) a mixed syndrome with root and cord findings presenting with radicular pain and long tract involvement; (4) a partial Brown-Séquard syndrome; and (5) an antral cord syndrome with distal arm weakness. They noted that although complete remission was never seen, regression occurred in 2 patients. Of their 120 cases, 75 percent had a series of episodes with progression, 20 percent were steadily and slowly progressing, and 5 percent had a rapid onset of findings, with plateauing before further deterioration at a later date. It also was noted that of 22 patients managed nonoperatively, 16 were treated with a neck brace alone. In 8 of the 16 patients, walking, the ability to dress, and radicular signs in the arms improved; this improvement was striking in 2. Although the remaining patients did not improve, neither did their disease progress.

At a later date, Lees and Turner[18] and Balla et al.[19] also attempted to define the natural history of cervical myelopathy. In Lees' series deterioration often ceased after the first few years; other patients experienced remissions lasting for years and then became worse. Progression and recurrence were particularly evident in patients with a congenitally narrow canal. Balla et al.,[19] in a series of 123 patients followed for up to 10 years, found that without treatment 52 percent improved, 35 percent remained unchanged, and 13 percent became worse.

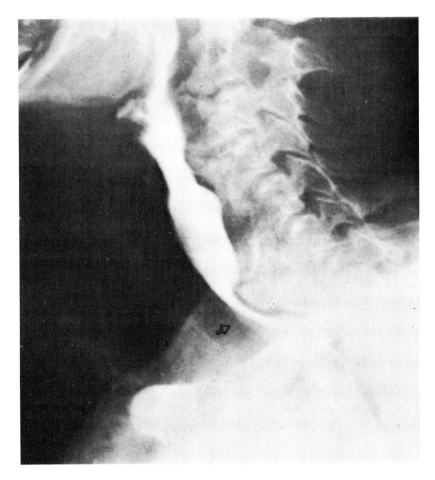

Fig. 80-2. A cervical osteophyte (arrow) in a patient with dysphagia. (Reproduced with permission from Meeks LW, Renshaw TS: Vertebral osteophytosis and dysphagia. *J Bone Joint Surg 55A*:197–201, 1973.)

Dysphagia Associated with Cervical Spondylosis

Compression of the esophagus or hypopharynx by osteophytes had been reported in the literature since 1926. A review, in 1960, reported 36 cases of dysphagia associated with osteophytes.[20] In 1971, Maran and Jacobson[21] reported the tenth case treated surgically. These authors also advocated interbody fusion in addition to excision of the osteophyte to prevent recurrent spur formation at the involved level.[22,23]

Compression of the hypopharynx is not experienced as dysphagia but as a lump in the throat and is seen with osteophytic compression above C6. Cervical osteophytes have been reported along the entire cervical spine, with C5-6 being the most common site. In two-thirds of the cases, one level is involved, and in the remaining one-third, osteophytes at several levels contribute to the symptoms. Surgical removal of the exostosis usually is not indicated, although with persistent symptomatology the lesion can be excised by the anterolateral approach with consideration given at that time to the removal of the involved degenerate disc.

Vertebral Artery Compression Associated with Cervical Spondylosis

Osteophytes projecting from the uncovertebral joints can intrude into the foramina transversaria and cause vertebral artery compression. To be clinically significant, this compression must impair the flow of blood to the brainstem. Hutchinson and Yates[24] have shown that the effect of vertebral artery compression by osteophytes can be enhanced by rotating the head or extending the neck, which may result in giddiness or drop attacks. These symptoms, however, also may occur in the absence of head movement. Disease of this kind is exceedingly rare, and in his experience Fisher[25] has seen a single case in which it may have been appropriate to remove an osteophyte that compressed the vertebral artery. This was not done, however, since the patient suffered a major stroke at the time of angiography.

Primary or secondary lateral extraspinal extrusions may indent or occlude the vertebral artery in its second portion. In 2 patients with traumatic lateral disc rupture, angiograms showed compression and displacement of the vertebral artery. These patients presented with radicular pains and motor deficit. Both, however, had normal cervical myelograms, so that this investigation sometimes is useful in delineating ruptured cervical disc.[26]

Diagnostic Evaluation

Investigations of cervical spondylosis involve not only standard roentgenograms but also flexion and extension views of the spine to obtain evidence of spinal stability. The musculature of the cervical region, the ligamentous structures, especially the ligamentum nuchae and posterior longitudinal ligament, and the bond between the vertebral bodies because of the discs are major factors responsible for the stability of the cervical spine. White et al.[27] (Figs. 80-3 and 80-4), in a recent biomechanical study of adult cadaver spines, have shown that the ligaments normally permit very little motion between vertebrae and that horizontal motions (greater than 3.5 mm) of one vertebral body on another, as seen on plain lateral roentgenograms, indicate instability. If the angulation of one vertebral body with respect to another is 11° greater than the angulation of adjacent vertebrae and the vertebral body is not compressed, the spine is relatively unstable. A major number of ligaments must be injured to permit motion exceeding these limits and most spines begin to fail under physiologic loads when these displacements are exceeded. The instability causes the spine to lose its ability to move without further deformity, excessive pain, and potential neurologic worsening.

Cervical myelography is performed preoperatively in all cases of cervical myelopathy or radiculopathy. The neurologic examination alone does not provide all the information required to plan an appropriate operation. With severe myelopathy, a lateral C1-2 puncture is preferable to instilling contrast medium by the lumbar route, since the study will not require hyperextension of the cervical spine, which results in maximal impingement on the cord and has been associated with neurologic worsening following standard myelography. Although air myelography was used extensively to study the myelopathic case, we now preferentially use metrizamide (Squibb) in conjunction with polytomography and computerized tomographic (CT) scanning to outline the cervical cord and establish its relationship to the spinal canal. This agent may be introduced by cervical or lumbar puncture and is considerably less stressful on the patient than air myelography.

Electromyography and nerve conduction studies provide additional *objective* evidence of root compression in patients with relatively minor neurologic findings. It is also important in differentiating root, plexus, peripheral nerve, and muscle disorders, which, in early stages, may mimic cervical radiculopathy. This study also may help to uncover a second problem that may co-exist with radiculopathy, e.g., carpal tunnel syndrome or ulnar neuropathy.

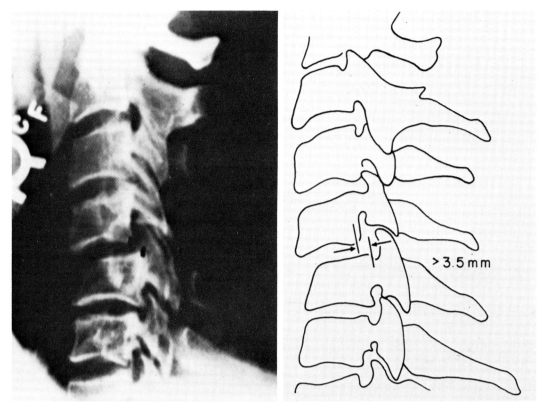

Fig. 80-3. Biomechanical studies have shown that horizontal motion in excess of 3.5 mm as demonstrated on plain roentgenograms indicates instability. (Reprinted from White AA, Johnson RM, Panjabi MM, et al: Biomechanical analysis of clinical stability in the cervical spine. *Clin Orthop 109*:85–96, 1975. With permission of J.B. Lippincott.)

Angiography to demonstrate cerebral vasculature is occasionally warranted and should include a survey of both intra- and extracranial vessels for a comprehensive evaluation of cerebral circulation. This should be done in conjunction with head turning to determine whether this maneuver further compromises flow in the vertebral artery and reproduces the symptoms.

Computerized tomography of the cervical spine with sagittal reconstruction has been found to be extraordinarily helpful in assessing the cervical spine by delineating irregular spurs and the canal topography, and flattening or displacement of the spinal cord. The CT techniques are used to complement the other studies listed above. However, pantopaque myelography remains the mainstay in the investigation of cases of cervical spondylosis.

Surgical Anatomy

Even though the anterolateral exposure to the cervical spine has been described previously, it is worth reviewing the following anatomic points. The anterior approach is the easiest along the anterior margin of the sternomastoid and medial to the carotid sheath (Fig. 80-5). The incision may be centered by noting the hyoid bone at the level of C3, the thyroid cartilage opposite C4, and the cricoid opposite the level of C6 (Fig. 80-6).

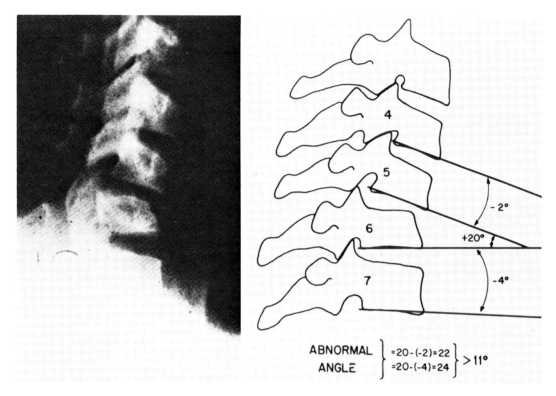

Fig. 80-4. Biomechanical studies have shown that angulation of one vertebral body of more than 11° with respect to another indicates an unstable spine. (Reprinted from White AA, Johnson RM, Panjabi MM, et al: Biomechanical analysis of clinical stability in the cervical spine. *Clin Orthop* 109:85–96, 1975. With permission of J.B. Lippincott.)

Dissection is carried out in avascular planes, passing through the pretracheal fascia first and then the prevertebral fascia. The longus colli muscles, covering the lateral parts of the vertebral body, the vertebral canal, and the transverse processes, then can be seen (Fig. 80-7). These muscles extend from the atlas to the body of T3 and are a major factor in the stability of the cervical spine. There is no muscle covering the anterior aspect of the vertebrae in the midline (Fig. 80-8). The cervical sympathetic chain lies on the longus colli muscles and extends from C2 to T1 (Fig. 80-8). Since a Horner's syndrome will result from damage to the sympathetic nerve fibers, it is important to retract the longus colli, starting at its medial edge.

The anterior longitudinal ligament is a strong band that extends from the base of the skull to the sacrum (Fig. 80-9). It is thickest in its midportion, tapers laterally, and is bound to the anterior annulus, functioning to limit the extension of the spine. The posterior longitudinal ligament also extends as a thick band from the skull to the sacrum, between the posterior annulus and the dura. Since the ligament does not extend laterally over the nerve roots, its normally thick portion, which prevents disc material from extruding into the spinal canal, is absent, permitting disc material to enter the foramen. Functionally, this ligament limits flexion of the spine.

Physiologically, the ligamentum flavum does not compress the dura or spinal cord; however, as elasticity is lost, the ligamentum buckles, compressing the spinal cord.

The left recurrent laryngeal branch of the vagus nerve arises at the level of the aortic arch, loops beneath the arch, and then passes between the trachea and the esophagus to reach the larynx. On the right side, the recurrent laryngeal nerve has an inconstant course. It usually descends within the carotid sheath, looping beneath the subclavian artery to reach the larynx between the trachea and the esophagus. The nerve may follow one of several aberrant courses,

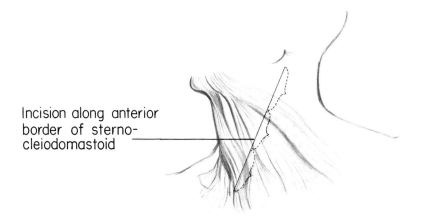

Incision along anterior
border of sterno-
cleiodomastoid

Fig. 80-5. The line of incision for the anterior approach.

leaving the carotid sheath at a higher level. To avoid injury to an aberrant right recurrent laryngeal nerve, it is preferable to operate on the left side of the neck, irrespective of the side of the radicular symptoms.

Surgical Procedure

Prophylactic antibiotic coverage is begun immediately preoperatively. The patient is placed in the supine position on an operating table and is placed under general anesthesia. The neck is moderately hyperextended by placing a roll beneath the shoulder blades, and the head is turned about 10° to the right. After the patient is draped, but before dissection is started, a lateral cervical scout roentgenogram is taken to ensure adequate radiographic technique, and a needle is placed on the spine to localize the interspace to be operated upon. Dissection then is carried out with headlight illumination and magnifying loupes of 3.5–4.5 X. The operating microscope may be used instead of the loupes.

The procedure is routinely performed through a longitudinal skin incision on the *left* side, centered over the anterior border of the sternomastoid muscle and the segment of spine to be exposed (see Figs. 80-4 and 80-5). This vertical incision is preferred since different types of anterior and lateral operations on cervical vertebral bodies and intervertebral discs, transverse processes, and vertebral arteries can be carried out without undue traction.

When the platysma has been exposed, it is grasped with forceps and incised parallel to the anterior margin of the sternomastoid. The underlying sternomastoid muscle then is visible (Fig. 80-10). The anterior border of the sternomastoid must be clearly indentified and mobilized throughout the limits of the exposure so that the medial border of the sternomastoid muscle can be retracted laterally to expose the middle layer of the cervical fascia. The omohyoid muscle can be seen crossing the field at about the level of C5–6 and may be retracted or transected at its mid-tendinous segment. The carotid sheath then is identified. An avascular plane is developed through the cervical fascia medial and parallel to the carotid sheath. The carotid sheath and the sternomastoid muscle are retracted laterally (Fig. 80-11). As this is done, the anterior surface of the cervical spine is seen. The esophagus and trachea are retracted medially. The prevertebral fascia is cauterized with Malis bipolar cautery and incised longitudinally in the midline, exposing the anterior longitudinal ligament. The medial aspect of the longus colli muscles are identified and cauterized for a length corresponding to the discs to be exposed (Fig. 80-12). This helps to keep the wound essentially bloodless. Cloward blades are placed beneath the medial edges of the longus colli muscles (Fig. 80-13). This is probably the single most important maneuver in the operation; failure to correctly position the blades is responsible for most of the complications associated with this operation. When the vertical incision is used, a single set of blades placed

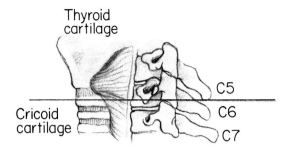

Fig. 80-6. Points for centering the incision opposite C5 and C6.

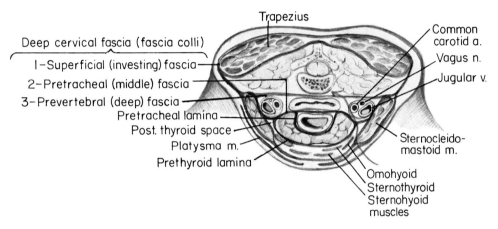

Fig. 80-7. Cross-section representation at the C5 level of the spine indicating the fascial planes and the avascular surgical approach to the anterior spine.

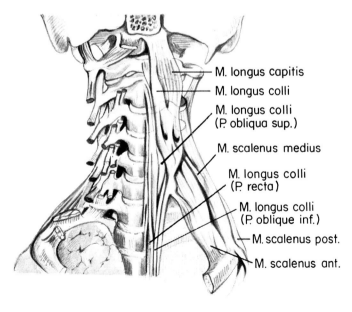

Fig. 80-8. Relationships of the anterior cervical musculature to the cervical spine.

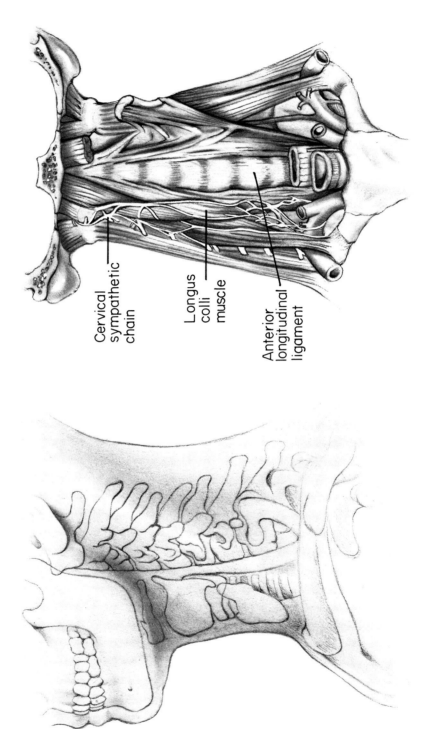

Fig. 80-9. An illustration showing the relationship of the cervical sympathetic chain, anterior spinal musculature, and anterior longitudinal ligament to the spine.

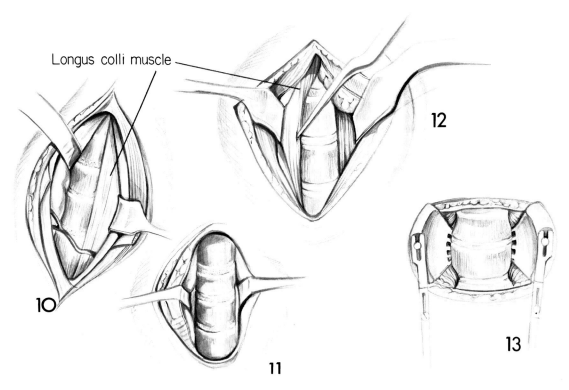

Longus colli muscle

10 11 12 13

Figs. 80-10 and 11. View of the anterior spine after medial retraction of the trachea and esophagus and lateral retraction of the carotid sheath and its contents.

Fig. 80-12. Cauterization of the medial aspects of the longus colli muscles before placement of Cloward retractor blades.

Fig. 80-13. Position of the Cloward blades beneath longus colli muscles.

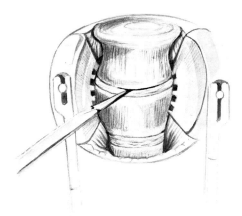

Fig. 80-14. Incision of the disc space.

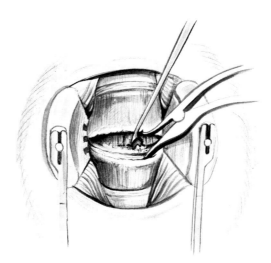

Fig. 80-15. Removal of the contents of the interspace and placement of the intervertebral spreader.

beneath the muscle edges will suffice to give adequate exposure. A fine needle then is placed in the disc space, leaving the blades in position, and a cross-table, cervical-spine roentgenogram is obtained to confirm the disc level.

The margins of the disc to be entered are cauterized and the disc is incised (Fig. 80-14). It is often necessary to remove the bony spurs overhanging the disc space from the upper vertebra before significant amounts of intervertebral disc can be removed. Once the anterior one-half to two-thirds of the disc and the cartilaginous plates have been removed, the disc-space spreader is introduced between the bodies (Fig. 80-15). Dissection up to this point is continued under 3.5–4.5X loupes or the procedure may be completed at 6-15X magnification using the operating microscope.

Under magnification, the remainder of the disc is excised to the posterior longitudinal ligament, which appears as a structure with glistening white fibers that are vertically aligned (Figs. 80-16A, B, and C). The remaining cartilage and disc are removed with fine curettes. The posterior ligament is removed when there is an otherwise inaccessible large fragment beneath it or in the presence of severe cord compression. The defect often can be seen in the posterior ligament through which a fragment of disc is extruding. Lateral dissection will expose the uncovertebral joints and the dura, which are no longer covered by the posterior longitudinal ligament (Figs. 80-17A and B).

Using a 20° angled drill, the osteophytes above and below the disc space are carefully removed, particularly if one decides to perform an anterior discectomy without fusion, to prevent subsequent nerve root compression.

If a fusion is to be performed, a horseshoe-shaped plug of bone with three cortical edges is taken from the ilium using a reciprocating saw with blades 8–10 mm apart. The graft is countersunk in the disc space, and a lateral cervical film is taken to check its position (Fig. 80-18). The wound is irrigated and a drain is placed above the anterior aspect of the spine, bringing it out through the lower end of the incision. The platysma and skin are closed with fine suture and the drain is removed in 12 hours. Relief following surgery for radiculopathy is apparent to many patients soon after they awaken from anesthesia. Codeine suffices for any pain. The patient is allowed to get out of bed within a day, often in a molded plastic cervical collar, and is discharged within 3 to 4 days. The patient remains immobilized in the Philadelphia collar until there is radiologic evidence of bony fusion. Antibiotics are discontinued after a single postoperative dose.

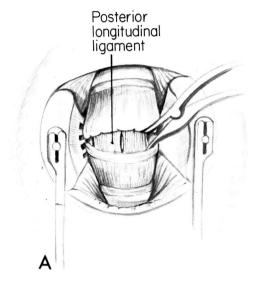

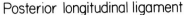

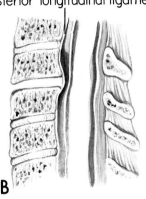

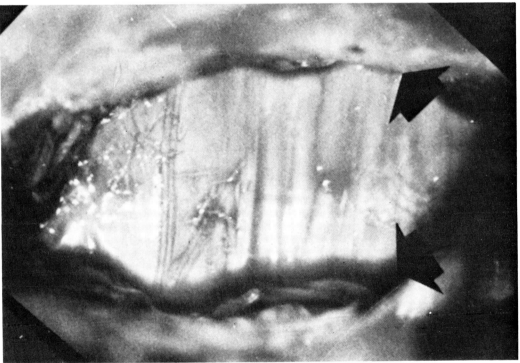

Fig. 80-16. **A.** Appearance of the dura following removal of disc material, the cartilaginous plates, and posterior longitudinal ligament. **B.** Relationship of the posterior longitudinal ligament to the intervertebral disc and cervical dura. **C.** Appearance of the posterior longitudinal ligament under magnification, as seen through the disc space in the cervical region. (Reproduced with permission from Kosary IZ, et al: Microsurgery in anterior approach to cervical discs, in *Surgical Neurology,* vol. 6, No. 5, Tryon, N.C., Paul C Bucy & Associates, 1976, p 276.)

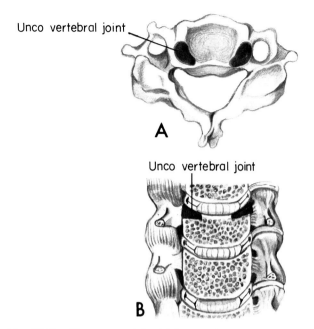

Fig. 80-17. The uncovertebral joints and their local relationships.

Complications

Tew[28] has recently summarized a combined experience of possible complications of this operation and they appear formidable. Lunsford[29] also quotes a complication rate of 13 percent for discectomy alone and a rate of 23 percent overall in their series. In reality, however, the complication rate of the procedure in experienced hands is very modest, and serious neurologic injury is extremely rare. There may be a transient exacerbation of pain, however, after the surgery. The exception lies in the re-operative case in which re-exploration of the neck can be extremely difficult. In this group of patients serious problems can and do arise.

Retraction-related problems are the most common form of postoperative morbidity, and result in laryngeal edema, hoarseness, dysphagia, or a sensation of lump in the throat.[30] These can be avoided by a generous vertical incision, preferably in the *left* side; meticulous placement, under magnification, of the blades of the Cloward retractor beneath the medial aspect of the longus colli muscles; a gentle degree of retraction; and a drain placed prevertebrally at the end of the operation. Should these retraction-related problems arise, a short course of steroid therapy has been found useful. Occasionally, emergency tracheostomy has been necessary because of upper airway obstruction secondary to extensive retraction on it.

Profuse bleeding from the disc space is unusual but disconcerting when it does occur. The bleeding is due either to injury to the bone as the cartilaginous plates are removed, injury to the vertebral body with the disc-space spreader, or a small dural tear with a cerebrospinal fluid (CSF) leak, which decompresses epidural veins and can result in profuse venous bleeding. In the majority of these cases the bleeding can be controlled with gentle pressure and Avitene in the disc space. Injury to the carotid artery has been reported with resultant cerebral ischemia secondary to excessive compression of the vessel by retraction, and to the vertebral artery by dissection carried into the vertebral canal. The complications that result from excessive bleeding can be reduced by ensuring that if a graft is used there is adequate room to each side of the graft to allow blood to extravasate away from the canal. This is accomplished by fashioning a graft that does not fill that interspace completely in the coronal plane, but leaves a tunnel on each side of the graft extending from the prevertebral area to the spinal canal. In addition, a Jackson-Pratt

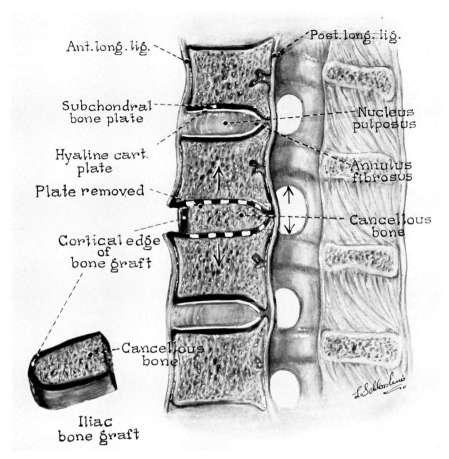

Fig. 80-18. The appearance and positioning of the iliac-crest bone graft in a Smith-Robinson-type anterior cervical fusion. (Reproduced with permission from Arthrodesis, in Crenshaw AH (ed): *Campbell's Operative Orthopedics,* 5th ed. St. Louis, C.V. Mosby, 1971, as modified from Robinson RA, Walker AE, Ferlic DC, et al: The results of anterior interbody fusion of the cervical spine. *J Bone Joint Surg 44A:*1569–1587, 1962.)

drain is placed anterior to the spine to remove blood and irrigating fluid for 24 hours postoperatively.

Esophageal perforation is a retraction-related complication that can be prevented by using the blades properly and which, if it occurs and is recognized, should be repaired immediately. Interrupted nonabsorbable sutures are used to repair the rupture, and the area is drained. Fusion under these circumstances is contraindicated.

Fusion-related problems are the main reason for the enthusiasm for anterior discectomy without fusion. Graft extrusion and donor-site problems occur in about 2 percent to 4 percent of cases, and with the interbody technique, fusion failed in 10 percent of Tew's cases.[28] The incidence of failures was even higher with the Cloward technique. On the other hand, the significant postoperative discomfort that followed discectomy without fusion in over one third of our cases, characterized by a nagging neck, shoulder, and intrascapular pain often lasting several months after surgery but subsiding eventually, is a significant consideration when deciding the merit of this modification of the anterolateral operation in the treatment of spondylosis. Although a recent report[29] claims no difference in results following disc excision with or without fusion, it does not address the very real set of complaints seen in patients on our service in whom fusion has not been performed. Many of the complaints are related to donor-site pain or infection, and this can be minimized by using either cadaver or freeze-dried bone. This same report also finds no difference in results between the Cloward and the Smith-Robinson fusion techniques; however, this does not correspond with other reported experiences and we prefer the Robinson technique on this service. The reason for this is based on the biomechanical study of Simmons,[31] which demonstrated that the surface area of the rectangular graft is approximately 30 percent more than the surface area of the cylindrical graft of comparable size, that stability studies show the keystone graft to be more stable than the dowel graft, and that the fusion rate in the keystone graft is 100 percent.

The second consideration is the effect eliminating the graft will have on the stability of the cervical spine. Although interbody fusion is often unnecessary and spontaneous fusion occurs within 6 months after one-, two-, or three-level disc excision in which the disc, cartilaginous plates, and osteophytes have been removed, the overall results depend on the number of variables responsible for maintaining stability altered by the spondylotic processes before surgery. In a patient with a disc degeneration alone, the stability may well be maintained by various muscular and ligamentous structures, and the disc can be removed and fusion occur without a graft. In patients with advanced spondylosis, however, degenerative changes affect most of the supporting structures of the spine, and subluxation often is seen even before surgery. This latter situation, particularly if it is associated with myelopathy and buckling of the ligamentum flavum, would not favor eliminating the graft. The significant degrees of angulation seen in up to 20 percent of the cases in recently reported series according to the criteria discussed earlier represent spinal instability. This instability may eventually escalate into a series of problems significantly worse than the reticulopathy for which the operation was originally performed.

Results of Anterolateral Disc Excision:
I. Cervical Radiculopathy

The results of surgery for cervical radiculopathy have been consistently reported as excellent in many series,[4,6,7,10,13,16,29,32-38] irrespective of whether an anterior or posterior approach was used to decompress the nerve root. Improvement is seen in approximately 90 percent of the cases, an observation I have reconfirmed with my own and with another 350 cases performed by the staff of Massachusetts General Hospital in Boston, which I reviewed. The advantages of the anterior approach for the treatment of this condition have been enumerated, and for these reasons this operation should be standard for the management of cervical radiculopathy due to disc disease at one or many levels.

Radiculopathy associated with evidence of disc degeneration at more than one, two, or three levels may be managed without fusion, following disc excision. Following discectomy without fusion, intrascapular, neck, and shoulder pain are considerably more frequent than with fusion, although the complaints usually subside within 6 to 12 weeks. Later secondary fusion may be required in some patients with persistent symptoms. If fusion is not performed, however, one may anticipate further narrowing of the interspace and one must therefore remove posterior osteophytes to prevent subsequent nerve root compression.

When radiographic findings are extensive and suggest alterations, not only in the disc but also of ligamentous and bony structures, then disc excision with coincident removal of the annulus, anterior longitudinal ligament, and possibly, the posterior longitudinal ligament may potentiate the area's instability.

It has, by now, been repeatedly shown that it is possible to excise the discs from between several contiguous cervical vertebrae without fusion and without instability,[35,38,39] and without a difference in the complication rate from excision of one or of several discs.[29]

II. Cervical Myelopathy

The results of decompressive surgery for myelopathy associated with cervical spondylosis have been reviewed several times.[40-45] When cervical spondylosis was first recognized as a cause of myelopathy, it appeared that favorable results should be produced by removing the mechanical impingement. Allen[46] attempted to remove the protusions extradurally through a posterior laminectomy, with disastrous results. Subsequently, posterior laminectomies and foraminotomies were fashioned to allow the cord to migrate away from the spondylotic projections along the anterior aspect of the spine. Collating the various reports, and in my own review of 45 cases, good to excellent results were obtained in approximately 60 percent of patients; another 10 to 15 percent became worse immediately after the surgery. Long-term follow-up revealed that none of the patients ever completely returned to normal. Stoops and King[47] reported 42 patients treated by extensive laminectomy without opening the dura. These patients were followed for up to 6 years. Even though 80 percent were said to show improvement, no prognostic factor could be identified.

Crandall,[28] reporting on his long-term study of 55 patients with cervical myelopathy followed from 2 to 25 years, felt that a history of deficit for less than 1 year was associated with a better prognosis. In contrast, a poor outcome is predictable among patients with preoperative sphinteric disturbances shown to be due to the myelopathy. Among these cases, none improved, irrespective of the type of operation.

The debate concerning the appropriate surgical procedure(s) in the management of cervical myelopathy continues. The operative procedure needs to be tailored to the particulars of the case. Posterior cervical laminectomy has a specific indication in patients with prominent dorsal encroachment on the cord due either to bony or ligamentous structures[48] (Figs. 80-19A, B, C, and D). Excessive cervical lordosis may be seen in patients with spondylotic myelopathy; overlapping of the lamina, referred to as *shingling*, may contribute to the myelopathy. Vertebral subluxation also may be seen and may lead to pinching of the cord, from the posterior, by the laminae and infolded ligamentum flavum.[49]

Inaccessibility to a disc space, e.g., C2-3 or C3-4 in some cases, is an indication for posterior decompressive cervical laminectomy, as is a secondary procedure in the presence of neurologic progression, particularly with posterior column signs, and in some cases with widespread bony changes and spontaneous fusions anterior to the spinal cord. I do not believe it should be used routinely in the management of myelopathy. It has been reported in several series that even in the presence of technically faultless surgery, up to 20 percent of cases treated by laminectomy had an increased deficit after surgery. In our experience this is particularly true if the dura is opened and the dentate ligaments are sectioned. Also, following laminectomy, cervical instability is a risk, particularly when there has been a generous decompression, both rostrocaudally and laterally.

Dereymaeker et al.[50] analyzed two groups of patients with spondylotic myelopathy operated upon either by the anterior or posterior approach and followed for 2 to 6 years. Clinical and radiographic findings showed that of 31 patients with anterior fusion, 20 were improved; of 12 who had laminectomy with excision of the disc, 4 were improved.

Crandall and Batzdorf[42] reported that of 28 cases of myelopathy treated by anterior discectomy and fusion, 71 percent were improved when posterior projections were removed from the floor of the canal, and the involved interspaces were stabilized. In no case was the patient made worse by the operation. This experience was reaffirmed in Crandall's latest report,[28] showing that none of his cases treated by the Cloward operation was worse postoperatively, but postoperative disability again was increased following decompressive laminectomy. Bohlman[48] has reported his experience with anterior discectomy and interbody arthrodesis in 17 cases of myelopathy. In most no attempt was made to remove the posterior longitudinal ligament or osteophytes. Cartilaginous plates and disc material were removed, under magnification, up to the posterior longitudinal ligament. Neural function was not lost in any of the 17 cases treated, and of the 17, 14 improved over their preoperative condition. Bone remodeling occurred at the fused levels and the size of the osteophytes decreased with time.

In a series based on 32 cases of myelopathy published by Lunsford,[29] among these patients, 92 percent had anterior spondylotic deficits and 13 had a sagittal canal width of under 13 mm at one or more levels. Fifty-nine percent had a myelopathy only and 41 percent had a myeloradiculopathy. Eight cases had a previous posterior cervical decompressive procedure,

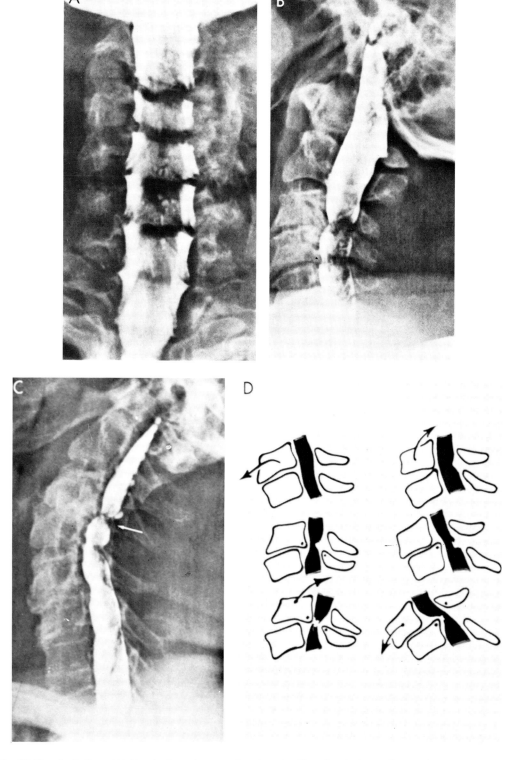

Fig. 80-19.   **A, B, C,** and **D.** Cervical myelogram showing significant anterior and posterior compression of the spinal cord. (Reproduced with permission from Epstein JA, et al: Myelopathy in cervical spondylosis with vertebral subluxation and hyperlordosis. *J Neurosurg 32*:423. Copyright 1970 American Association of Neurological Surgeons.)

and 1 case a previous anterior operation—so that actually only 24 of the cases reported address the merits of the anterior approach alone. Surgery involved removal of ventral osteophytes at one or more levels, with 2 patients having four levels operated upon in two separate stages. In this study, one-half of the patients improved, and one-half of the patients were either unimproved or worse. No predictive indices could be identified, although it was the authors' impression that patients over 60 years of age and those symptomatic for more than 2 years tended to have unsatisfactory results. There was no difference in outcome based on the severity of the myelopathy, the number of levels operated upon, or the presence of canal stenosis.

A recent comparative study[51] reviews the experience with 50 cases treated by means of extensive laminectomy, foraminotomy, and excision of osteophytes for cervical myeloradiculopathy. In this study Epstein again emphasizes the importance of careful patient selection, adequate laminectomy including two levels above and below areas of significant canal encroachment, and foraminal decompression with removal of only the inner third of the foramen. In this series 85 percent of patients improved and 15 percent were not improved following this operation. In a comparison with other forms of posterior operation, this yielded the best results, and compared to a 73 percent improved category following anterior cervical discectomy.

The anterior approach has evolved into an operative procedure for most cases of cervical spondylotic myelopathy, provided that the major compressive elements are situated anterior to the spinal cord. Whether the osteophytes require radical removal in this situation is problematic, however we attempt radical removal of the osteophytes. It is possible with the operating microscope and diamond drills to remove them without substantial risk, and on our service this is done in conjunction with fusion of the involved interspaces in cases of myelopathy. If a fusion is not performed, increased movement at the operated levels and the possibility that the function of the spinal cord will be made worse are the risks.

REFERENCES

1. Adams CBT, Logue V: Studies in cervical spondylotic myelopathy. 3. Some functional effects of operations for cervical spondylotic myelopathy. *Brain* 94:587–594, 1971
2. Aronson NI: The management of soft cervical disc protrusions using the Smith-Robinson approach. *Clin Neurosurg* 20:253–258, 1973
3. Bailey RW, Badjley CE: Stabilization of the cervical spine by anterior fusion. *J Bone Joint Surg* 42A:565–594, 1960
4. Bailey RW: *The Cervical Spine*. Philadelphia, Lea and Febiger, 1974
5. Cloward RB: New method of diagnosis and treatment of cervical disc disease. *Clin Neurosurg* 8:93–132, 1962
6. Cloward RB: Lesions of the intervertebral disc and their treatment by interbody fusion methods. *Clin Orthop* 27:51–77, 1963
7. Smith GW, Robinson RA: The treatment of certain cervical spine disorders by anterior removal of the intervertebral disc and interbody fusion. *J Bone Joint Surg* 40A:607–624, 1958
8. Murphy MB, Bado M: Anterior cervical discectomy without interbody bone graft. *J Neurosurg* 37:71–74, 1972
9. Robertson JT: Anterior operations for herniated cervical disc and for myelopathy. *Clin Neurosurg* 25:245–250, 1978
10. Robinson RA, Walker AE, Ferlick DE: The results of anterior interbody fusion of the cervical spine. *J Bone Joint Surg* 44A:1569–1587, 1962
11. Robinson RA: Anterior and posterior cervical fusions. *Clin Orthop* 35:34–62, 1964
12. Cloward RB: Treatment of acute fractures and fracture-dislocations of the cervical spine by vertebral body fusion. *J Neurosurg* 18:201–209, 1961

13. Scoville WB, Dohrmann AM, Corkill AR: Late results of cervical disc surgery. *J Neurosurg* 45:203–310, 1976

14. Zulch KJ: Personal communications, 1976

15. Robinson RA: Personal communication, 1976

16. Clarke E, Robinson PK: Cervical myelopathy: Complication of cervical spondylosis. *Brain* 79:483–510, 1956

17. Gregorius FK, Estrin T, Crandall PH: Cervical spondylotic radiculopathy and myelopathy: A long-term follow-up study. *Arch Neurol* 33:618–625, 1976

18. Lees F, Turner JWA: Natural history and prognosis of cervical spondylosis. *Br Med J* 2:1607–1610, 1963

19. Roth DA: Cervical analgesic discography: a new test for the definitive diagnosis of the painful disc syndrome. *JAMA* 235:1713, 1976

20. Hilding DA, Tachdjian MO: Dysphagia and hypertrophic spurring of the cervical spine. *N Engl J Med* 263:11, 1960

21. Maran A, Jacobson I: Cervical osteophytes presenting with pharyngeal symptoms. *Laryngoscope* 81:412, 1971

22. Facer JA: Osteophytes of the cervical spine causing dysphagia. *Arch Otolaryngol* 86:341, 1967

23. Meeks LW, Renshaw TS: Ankylosing vertebral hyperostosis and dysphagia, in Bailey RW (ed): *The Cervical Spine.* Philadelphia, Lea and Febiger, 1974, pp 242–249

24. Hutchinson EC, Yates PO: The cervical portion of the vertebral artery. A clinicopathological study. *Brain* 79:319–330, 1956

25. Fisher CM: Personal communication, 1976

26. Verbiest H: From anterior to lateral operations on the cervical spine. *Neurosurg Rev* 1:47–67, 1978

27. White AA, Johnson RM, Panjabi MM, et al: Biomechanical analysis of clinical stability in the cervical spine. *Clin Orthop* 109:85–96, 1975

28. Tew JM Jr, Mayfield FH: Complications of surgery of the anterior cervical spine. *Clin Neurosurg* 23:424–434, 1976

29. Lunsford LD, Bissonette DJ, Jannetta PJ, et al: Anterior surgery for cervical disc disease. *J Neurosurg* 53:1–19, 1980

30. Heeneman H: Vocal cord paralysis following approaches to the anterior cervical spine. *Laryngoscope* 83:17–21, 1973

31. Simmons EH, Bhalla SK: Anterior cervical discectomy and fusion: A clinical and biomechanical study with eight year follow-up. *J Bone Joint Surg* 51B:225–237, 1969

32. Aronson N, Bagan N, Filtzer DL: Results of using the Smith-Robinson approach for herniated and extruded cervical discs. *J Neurosurg* 32:721–722, 1970

33. Aronson N, Filtzer DL: Treatment concepts of cervical spine disease using the anterior approach, in *American Academy of Orthopedic Surgeons Instructional Course Lectures,* vol. 21, St. Louis, CV Mosby

34. Hirsch C: Cervical disc rupture: Diagnosis and therapy. *Acta Orthop Scand* 30:172–186, 1960

35. Martins AN: AC discectomy with/without interbody bone graft. *J Neurosurg* 44:290–295, 1976

36. Riley LH Jr, Robinson RA, Johnson DA: The results of anterior interbody fusion of the cervical spine. Review of 93 consecutive cases. *J Neurosurg* 30:127–133, 1969

37. Rothman RH, Simeone FA: *The Spine.* Philadelphia, WB Saunders, 1975

38. Robertson JT: Anterior cervical disc removal with and without fusion. Presented at the 33rd Annual Meeting of the American Academy of Neurological Surgery, Lake Tahoe, Nevada, September 29, 1971

39. Hankinson HL, Wilson CB: Use of the operating microscope in anterior cervical discectomy without fusion. *J Neurosurg* 43:452–456, 1975

40. Bishara SN: The posterior operation in the treatment of cervical spondylosis with myelopathy: A long-term follow-up study. *J Neurol Neurosurg Psychiatry* 34:393–398, 1971

41. Brain WR: Some unsolved problems of cervical spondylosis. *Br Med J* 1:711–773, 1963

42. Brain WR, Northfield DWC, Wilkinson M: Neurological manifestations of cervical spondylosis. *Brain* 75:187, 1952

43. Brain L, Wilkinson M: *Cervical Spondylosis.* Philadelphia, WB Saunders, 1967

44. Northfield AC: *The Surgery of the Central Nervous System.* Oxford, Blackwell, 1973, pp 711–752

45. Robinson RA, Afeiche N: Cervical spondylotic myelopathy: Etiology and treatment concepts. Cervical Spine Research Society, Philadelphia, Pennsylvania, November 19, 1976

46. Allen KL: Neuropathies caused by bony spurs in the cervical spine with special reference to surgical treatment. *J Neurol Neurosurg Psychiatry* 15:20–36, 1952

47. Stoops WL, King RB: Neural complications of cervical spondylosis: their response to laminectomy and foraminotomy. *J Neurosurg* 19:986–999, 1962

48. Bohlman HH: Cervical spondylosis with moderate to severe myelopathy: Treatment of anterior cervical discectomy and fusion. Presented at Cervical Spine Research Society, Philadelphia, November 20, 1976

49. Epstein JA, Carras LA, Epstein BS, et al: Myelopathy in cervical spondylosis with vertebral subluxation and hyperlordosis. *J Neurosurg 32*:421–426, 1970
50. Cleveland D: Interspace reconstruction and spinal stabilization after disc removal. *Lancet 76*:327–331, 1956
51. Epstein JA, Janin Y, Carras R, Lavine LS: A comparative study of the treatment of cervical spondylotic myeloradiculopathy. *Acta Neurochirurgica 61*: 89–104, 1982

CHAPTER 81
Transthoracic Disc Excision

Frederick A. Simeone   Ralph Rashbaum

SYMPTOMATIC HERNIATIONS OF THORACIC INTERVERTEBRAL DISCS are the rarest yet most devastating of all disc lesions. They present problems in diagnosis, and, historically, treatment by ordinary laminectomy has been attended with appalling results. Of Mueller's 4 cases, 3 were paraplegic after surgery.[1] Perot and Munro reviewed 91 cases from various sources in 1969.[2] Forty of these patients were not improved by surgery, and 16 were rendered paraplegic as a result of the operation. The results were most unfavorable in cases of *central* disc herniations, particularly those with advanced preoperative neurologic deficits. As might be expected, patients with lateral disc herniations and minimal neurologic deficit fared better postoperatively. All patients treated by ordinary laminectomy were characterized by the same discouraging conclusions.[3-9]

In 1960, Hulme[10] treated 4 cases through a lateral (costotransversectomy) approach with encouraging results; 3 were cured and 1 showed improvement. Perot and Munro,[2] 9 years later, described the transpleural approach through an ordinary thoracotomy incision in 2 patients, both of whom made a complete recovery. During the same year, Ransohoff and coworkers[9] described a similar procedure. These two approaches will be described in detail below, with additional comments about the use of the operating microscope when dissection near the spinal cord begins. In most of the series of symptomatic disc lesions described, thoracic disc herniations represent 0.25 percent to 0.75 percent of all symptomatic disc lesions. They are seen between the fourth to twelfth thoracic interspaces, with the greatest percentage occurring between T8 and T11. Patients may present with pain in a radicular distribution, acute or chronic in nature, with laterally placed lesions. Patients with central herniations develop paraparesis, with or without sensory complaints, and with an acute or chronic onset. There is nothing characteristic about chronic thoracic disc herniations that can lead to a clinical distinction among other causes of thoracic spinal cord compression.

On radiologic examination the offending disc is often calcified, although calcification in thoracic discs is sufficiently common that this finding itself normally just increases the suspicion of thoracic disc protrusion. Accurate myelography, particularly with painstaking efforts to achieve optimum lateral views, is absolutely necessary. No operation for thoracic disc herniation should be undertaken without myelograms that clearly outline the lesion; contrast medium may have to be instilled cisternally. When the offending lesion is identified, great care must be taken to develop criteria for localizing the proper disc intraoperatively. The thoracic spine is approached by the alternative routes described below; it is most difficult to find the appropriate level during surgery. Consequently, we often will insert a sterile needle into a spinous process on the morning of surgery (with radiologic control) and retain this marker throughout the operation.

Division of Neurosurgery, University of Pennsylvania School of Medicine, and Pennsylvania Hospital, Philadelphia, Pennsylvania

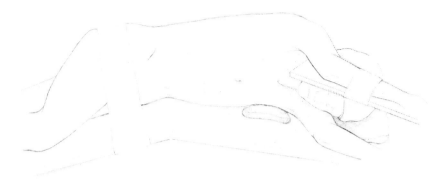

Fig. 81-1.

Surgical Technique

Costotransversectomy and Disc Excision

This procedure is carried out with the patient under general anesthesia and intubated with a cuffed endotracheal tube. The anesthesiologist must be able to inflate the patient's lungs should the pleural cavity be entered inadvertently.

The patient lies in a modified lateral decubitus position, elevated 30° from the straight prone, so that the surgeon may stand opposite the abdomen (Fig. 81-1). A pad is placed in the axilla and below the shoulders. To avoid increased venous pressure the abdomen must be kept free by carefully placed supports under the chest and iliac crest. The uppermost knee is flexed, and a pillow is placed between the legs. The approach may be made from either side; the choice depends upon the presence of lateralizing features in the clinical presentation. If unilateral root pain is the principal symptom, then the interspace should be approached from the same side. With central disc herniations, or in the absence of lateralizing findings, the right-sided approach has been used because, statistically, the important artery of Adamkiewicz usually originates from the left lower intercostal vessels (roughly T8 to L2).

It is essential to localize the lesion at this point, either with a needle that previously has been inserted into the spinous process, as mentioned earlier, or by marking the rib to be removed by injecting indigocarmine onto it subcutaneously.

The skin incision follows a long semilunar course, extending the length of at least three vertebral bodies above and below the disc space in question (Fig. 81-2). The incision extends at least

325

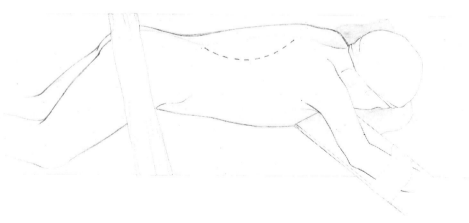

Fig. 81-2.

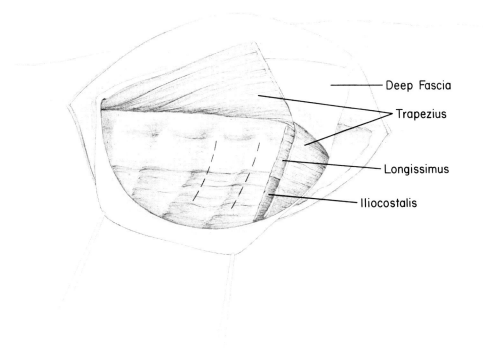

Fig. 81-3.

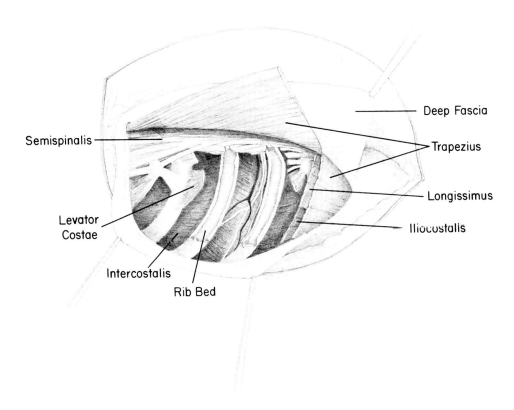

Fig. 81-4.

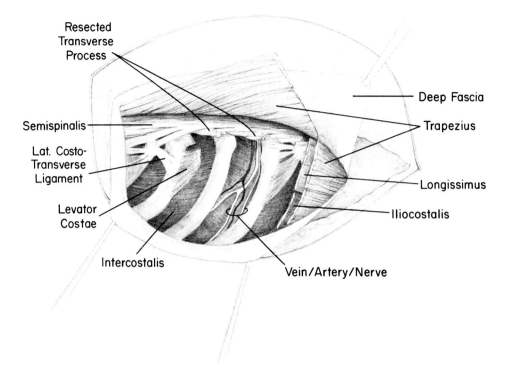

Fig. 81-5.

20 cm laterally from the midline at the apex of the curve. Dissection proceeds through the skin and subcutaneous tissue to the deep fascia, all of which are elevated and retracted medially to the spinous processes (Fig. 81-3). The trapezius muscle can be incised in line with the skin incision and retracted medially. This exposes the erector spinae muscle mass (semispinalis longissimus, and iliocostalis muscles), which is reflected medially by stripping the muscles from their attachments. Alternatively, the muscle mass can be transected over the rib to be removed and the

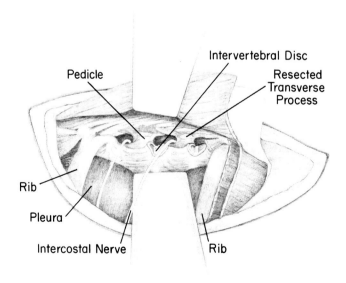

Fig. 81-6.

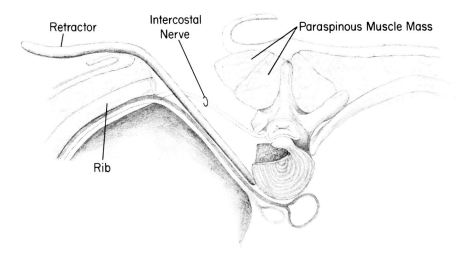

Retractor   Intercostal Nerve   Paraspinous Muscle Mass

Rib

Fig. 81-7.

muscles retracted in a cephalic and caudal direction, for easier access to the lamina as well as to the rib to be removed. This rib is identified and the intercostal neurovascular complex is separated from its inferior surface. The periosteum is stripped from the rib, about the width of the incision, with a Doyen separator (Fig. 81-4).

Attention then is directed to the attachment of the rib with the vertebral bodies. The transverse process is removed with a rongeur so that the articulation of the rib head and its costotransverse and capsular ligaments can be identified and sectioned. The rib is cut at the most lateral portion of the incision (approximately 20 cm of rib are removed), and it is disarticulated from the vertebral body (Fig. 81-5).

When the rib is removed, the intercostal vein, artery, and nerve can be followed through their entrance into the spinal canal. It is not necessary to sacrifice any of these structures, although the muscular branches of the intercostal artery can be cauterized as needed (Fig. 81-6). The parietal pleura is separated from the ribs, above and below, as well as from the spinal column, and it is depressed with a malleable ribbon or large Deaver retractor. The segmental vessels along the side of the vertebrae are identified. They should not be damaged; if bleeding develops, however, it may be controlled by silver clips or coagulation.

The intervertebral foramen is identified by tracing the intracostal nerve medially. The nerve enters the spinal canal between two pedicles. The latter structures are cleaned with a periosteal elevator and then removed piecemeal with a Kerrison rongeur. A high-speed air drill may facilitate removal of the pedicle. If we use an air drill, we also prefer to use an operating microscope at that time, because it provides excellent illumination and magnification of important neural structures underlying the bone that is to be removed. The microscope is used throughout the rest

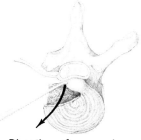

Direction of removal

Fig. 81-8.

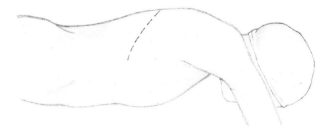

Fig. 81-9.

of the procedure on the vertebra and discs. When the pedicle is removed, the lateral aspect of the dural sac and the intrusion of the disc into the canal can be appreciated (Fig. 81-7). An incision is made into the midportion of the disc space, well away from the spinal cord, and the space is emptied by curettage and the use of pituitary rongeurs. A small portion of the opposing margins of the vertebral bodies, nearest the spinal canal, can be curetted away to ease access to the disc space (Fig. 81-8). Through this opening, fragments closer to the dural canal may be separated and pushed into the emptied disc space for later removal. A Penfield dissector can be used to palpate the posterior longitudinal ligament for sequestered disc material. This instrument also can depress the annulus fibrosis into the intervertebral disc space to determine if the spinal canal is really fully decompressed.

The interspace is irrigated thoroughly and meticulous hemostasis is achieved. Through positive pressure ventilation, the pleura is checked for leaks. If it has been violated, an extrapleural chest tube may be placed before completing the closure. The wound is closed in layers. A chest x-ray film taken in the recovery room will help if there are concerns about a pneumothorax.

Transthoracic (Transpleural) Disc Excision

This procedure is considerably more formidable than costotransversectomy, but it provides direct access to the anterior and lateral portions of the disc. A thoracic surgeon is required, at least in the early experiences with this approach. The patient's general medical and pulmonary status must be checked preoperatively. A postoperative unit for the management of thoracotomy patients is required. The degree of postoperative pain is greater, as is the possibility of significant intraoperative bleeding.

The operation is carried out with the patient under general anesthesia and intubated with a cuffed endotracheal tube. A Carlens tube should be used so that each lung may be ventilated separately if the surgical situation requires this.

The chest is entered through a standard right posterior thoracotomy incision (Fig. 81-9).

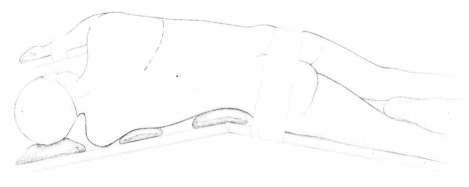

Fig. 81-10.

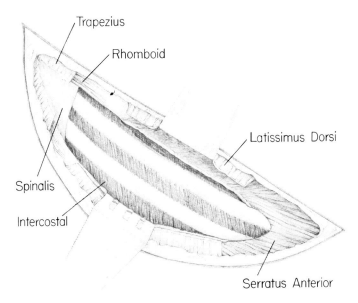

Fig. 81-11.

The right side is chosen because the artery of Adamkiewicz usually enters on the left side (80 percent of cases) and because the heart and great vessels pose a problem through a left transthoracic incision. The patient is positioned in the straight lateral posture, leaning somewhat toward his abdomen so that the chest contents (with the exception of the azygius vein) will gravitate out of the operative field. The surgeon stands on the spinal side of the patient, and a better view is obtained if the patient is tilted slightly toward him (Fig. 81-10). Careful positioning of the patient over the table break or kidney rest will enable the anesthesiologist, at the appropriate time, to flex the thoracic spine laterally, thereby opening the interspace. In younger patients, there will be sufficient elasticity of the rib ligaments so that the rib spreader will provide sufficient exposure.

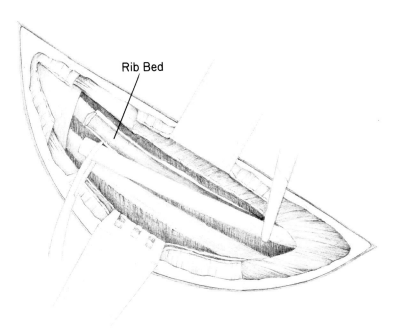

Fig. 81-12.

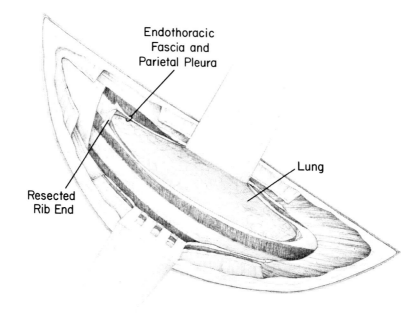

Endothoracic
Fascia and
Parietal Pleura

Lung

Resected
Rib End

Fig. 81-13.

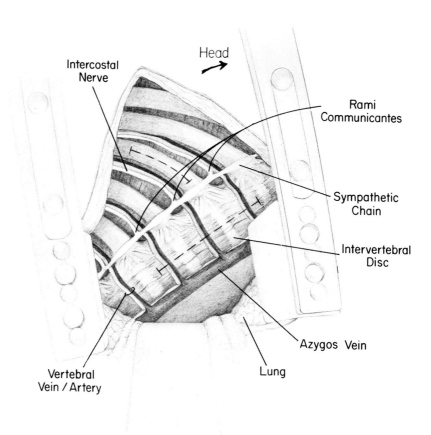

Head

Intercostal
Nerve

Rami
Communicantes

Sympathetic
Chain

Intervertebral
Disc

Azygos Vein

Lung

Vertebral
Vein / Artery

Fig. 81-14.

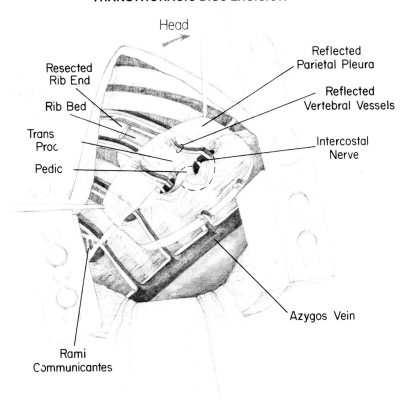

Fig. 81-15.

If such is not the case, the rib opposite that offending intervertebral disc may be removed (Fig. 81-11). The lateral aspect of the rib is sectioned first, and the head of the rib can be removed through the endothoracic fascia (Fig. 81-12). At least 15 cm of rib, including the rib head, must be removed in order to gain complete exposure to the lateral-most portion of the spinal canal (Fig. 81-13). Prior to disarticulation of the rib, identification of the intercostal nerve and vessels is important. The vessels should be preserved and the intercostal nerve may be followed to the appropriate intervertebral foramen. A specifically numbered rib will articulate with a posterior-superior margin of the vertebral body whose number it shares, as well as the posterior-inferior margin of the vertebra above. For example, the T8 rib will articulate with the body of T8 and T7, and it will cross the T7-8 interspace.

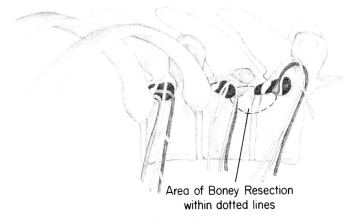

Area of Boney Resection
within dotted lines

Fig. 81-16.

Attention now is directed to the lateral aspect of the vertebral body above and below the offending disc. A linear incision is made in the parietal pleura extending from the middle of each vertebral body. The incision is extended at its ends, and the pleura is reflected laterally (Fig. 81-14). Careful dissection of the parietal pleura from the vertebral body will expose the intervertebral vessels, as well as the sympathetic chain. It is necessary to ligate the segmental artery and vein above and below the disc lesion to gain adequate exposure. The intercostal nerve is followed to its foramen and gently retracted to expose the pedicles above and below (Fig. 81-15). The Kerrison rongeur or high-speed air drill is used to remove the pedicles so that the dural sac above and below the disc lesion is readily demonstrated. With the use of an operating microscope, disc protrusion into the canal is readily seen. The intervertebral disc is incised in its anterior two-thirds and its contents are emptied with pituitary rongeurs and curettes. No attempt is made to remove the extruded fragment initially. With flexion of the table or alteration of the kidney rest, the interspace may be opened and a lamina spreader introduced. When the space is emptied, the surgeon may use an air drill to remove a small segment of the vertebral body at the opposing margins (Fig. 81-16). A larger window into the spinal canal made in this fashion will enable disc fragments to be picked away from beneath the dural sac with small curettes. The dura is not retracted, but the floor of the spinal canal is palpated repeatedly with flat instruments (Penfield dissectors) to retrieve sequestered fragments and to ascertain the effectiveness of decompression. The annulus fibrosis and its associated ligaments may be forced into the interspace and subsequently retrieved, and the area is irrigated thoroughly when the surgeon is confident that the spinal cord has been decompressed.

The parietal pleura now may be sutured over the vertebral bodies with running sutures of chromic catgut. Following the placement of an apical dependent chest tube through separate stab wounds, the chest is closed in routine fashion. The chest tubes are subsequently placed to underwater suction drainage, which can be removed when no further air leaks or drainage are present (usually 2 to 4 days). Repeated chest x-rays are used to follow the size of the pneumothorax if one persists during the immediate postoperative period.

Conclusion

Costotransversectomy and the transthoracic approach to thoracic disc herniations have offered patients new hope for cure without great fear of postoperative paraplegia. The costotransversectomy approach is a less formidable operation, and with the operating microscope, provides an adequate exposure to the lateral spinal canal. This approach is probably satisfactory for most symptomatic thoracic disc herniations. Where a more aggressive attack on the anterior surface of the spinal canal is required, transthoracic disc excision provides excellent visualization of the ventral surface of the spinal cord.

REFERENCES

1. Mueller R: Prolapse of thoracic intervertebral discs. *Acta Med Scand* 139:99, 1951
2. Perot PL, Munro OD: Transthoracic removal of midline thoracic disc protrusions causing spinal cord compression. *J Neurosurg* 31:452–462, 1969
3. Arseni C, Nash F: Protrusion of thoracic intervertebral discs. *Acta Neurochir 11*:1–33, 1963
4. Logue V: Thoracic intervertebral disc prolapse with spinal cord compression. *J Neurol Neurosurg Psychiatry* 15:227–241, 1952
5. Love JG, Schorn VG: Thoracic disc protrusions. *JAMA* 191:627–631, 1965
6. Reeves DL, Brown, HA: Thoracic intervertebral disc protrusion with cord compression. *J Neurosurg* 28:24–28, 1968
7. Svein HJ, Karavitis AL: Multiple protrusions of intervertebral discs in the upper thoracic region: Report of case. *Proc Staff Meet Mayo Clin* 29:375–378, 1954
8. Tovi D, Strang RR: Thoracic intervertebral disc protrusions. *Acta Chir Scand Suppl 267*: 1960
9. Ransohoff J, Spencer F, Slew F, et al: Transthoracic removal of thoracic disc. Report of three cases. *J Neurosurg* 31:459–461, 1969
10. Hulme A: The surgical approach to thoracic intervertebral disc protrusions. *J Neurol Neurosurg Psychiatry 23*:133–137, 1960

CHAPTER 82

The Anterior Anterolateral Approach to the Thoracic and Thoracolumbar Spine

Henry H. Schmidek
David Seligson

Laurence H. Coffin
Francisco B. Gomes

THE SURGICAL APPROACH to the fractured, unstable thoracic and thoracolumbar space dates to the early nineteenth century when Cline[1] resected the injured spinous processes and laminae of a paraplegic patient with a thoracic fracture-dislocation within 24 hours of injury. He was unable to reduce the dislocation and the patient subsequently died. For years thereafter, this case was cited in medical circles as a glaring example of the futility of performing surgery in patients with spinal injuries. In 1827, Tyrrell[2] reported the unsuccessful results of decompressive laminectomy in several cases of spinal dislocation with compression of the spinal cord. Both Cline and Tyrrell used an operation that dates to about 650 AD in which the spinous processes and laminae are removed through a vertical midline incision centered over the injured portion of the spine.

In 1829, Smith[3] operated on a man who fell from a horse and was rendered paraplegic. The spinous processes and depressed laminae of three thoracic vertebrae were removed, the dura inspected, and the incision closed. This patient survived the operation and his neurologic condition improved.

Beginning with these early operations, posterior laminectomy has remained the mainstay procedure for decompression of the spinal cord and nerve roots. In the fractured spine, however, removal of the posterior elements may further contribute to the instability of the spine and may be attended by a worsening of the neurologic and orthopedic condition of the patient. The use of surgical alternatives to this operation has evolved slowly among neurosurgeons except in the specific case of the herniated thoracic disc. In this situation, costotransversectomy gained wide acceptance after it was appreciated that attempts to remove the disc protrusion via laminectomy were attended by an unacceptably high incidence of postoperative neurologic deterioration.

Until recently, thoracic and thoracolumbar fractures have been treated by combinations of decompressive laminectomy and posterior spinal fusion. Only in the last decade have neurologic and orthopedic surgeons regularly employed alternative surgical approaches that allow explora-

Divisions of Neurosurgery, Thoracic and Cardiac Surgery, and Orthopedics, Medical Center Hospital of Vermont, Burlington, Vermont

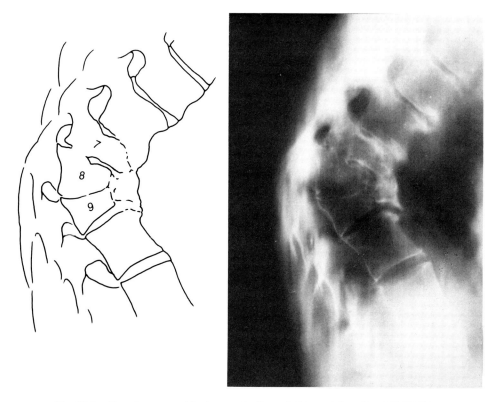

Fig. 82-1. Roentgenographic demonstration of gibbus deformity at T7-T8-T9.

tion of the spine by an anterior, anterolateral, posterolateral, or posterior approach, thereby allowing the procedure to be tailored to the particulars of a specific case.[4-8]

The surgical management of the thoracic and thoracolumbar regions of the spine may require alternative approaches depending upon the situation. In the thoracic spine, ventrally situated lesions can be exposed either by a costotransversectomy, by a transthoracic-extrapleural approach, or by a transthoracic-transpleural route. The costotransversectomy and the extrapleural approaches are described in Chapter 81. The transthoracic-transpleural approach is described in this chapter. The virtue of this technique is that it allows removal, in one stage, of pathologic material situated ventral to the dura over several spinal segments and concurrent stabilization of the spine with autogenous bone and fixateurs inserted into the intact vertebral bodies in those cases in which it may not be possible to instrument the spine posteriorly. This operation is useful both when dealing with cases of acute thoracic fractures and with cases treated by decompressive laminectomy for trauma or tumor who then develop postlaminectomy kyphosis and progressive neurologic deficit (Fig. 82-1). These patients present with an increasing sharp angular kyphosis, usually between T3 and T8 over the apex where the spinal cord is stretched and attenuated (Fig. 82-2). A progressive neurologic deficit then will become manifest and evolve as the deformity increases. Since the posterior elements have been removed, the angulation of the spine makes posterior instrumentation either biomechanically unsound or technically impossible, and there are limited surgical options to arrest the progression of the process. We have found one-stage transthoracic-transpleural decompression and stabilization a particularly useful operation for this situation. In the past year, 6 patients with this presentation were operated upon, all of whom presented with progressive paraparesis. Among these patients a marked neurologic improvement and alleviation of all (except their immediate, operatively induced) pain occurred within *days* of surgery, even though the problem had been of longstanding duration. The mechanism of this improvement is unclear and may be related to either improved axo-

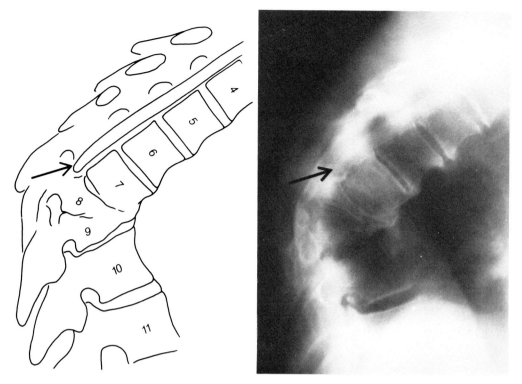

Fig. 82-2.   Air myelography and sagittal tomography indicating cord compression over extent of gibbus deformity between T7-T8-T9.

plasmic flow within the compressed portion of the spinal cord or relief of chronic vascular insufficiency in this segment of the spinal cord. The gratifying experience obtained with these techniques in these cases, in the absence of an increased morbidity associated with their use, has encouraged our advocating them to our colleagues.

Fractures of the thoracolumbar region with ventrally situated retropulsed disc and bone arising from the vertebral body may be exposed through a posterior midline incision with retraction providing exposure lateral to the facet joints. It is not necessary to approach the spine in these patients transabdominally or transperitoneally. Subsequent to removal of the transverse process, it is possible to identify the neural foramen, to remove the ipsilateral pedicle, and then to undermine the retropulsed bone from the body above to that below the level of injury. The entire piece of bone then is removed from the vertebral canal. Following this decompression, stabilization is accomplished by bone grafts placed anteriorly between vertebral bodies and Harrington-rod or Weiss-spring instrumentation in conjunction with a spinal fusion placed over the laminae posteriorly. Those patients either neurologically intact or with partial lesions are not instrumented until their decompression has been accomplished. Both decompression and stabilization are carried out as a single operative procedure and not staged.

Preoperative Assessment in Acute Spinal Injuries

All patients suspected of having sustained a significant spinal injury are assessed in the emergency department by the neurosurgical and orthopedic representatives of the Spinal Cord Injury Group. Over the next hours, the other members of this group *automatically* review the patient's situation from a respiratory, urologic, psychiatric, rehabilitation, and social-service viewpoint and plan the care that the patient and his family require during and subsequent to the acute hospitalization. At the initial examination, the patient's neurologic function is categorized using the classification of Frankel et al.[10] In addition to general, physical, and neurologic assessment, all patients with a major thoracic spine injury undergo pulmonary function tests including arterial blood gas determinations.

The patients with thoracic or thoracolumbar fractures whose intellectual function is not markedly impaired invariably complain of severe posterior or dorsal midline back pain, and a palpable deformity is often present. Significant associated injuries involving rib fractures often in conjunction with injury to the spleen or liver, head injuries, neck injuries, and extremity fractures are present in approximately 60 percent of patients. After stabilizing the patient's overall condition, anteroposterior and lateral x-ray films of the spine are obtained to define the area of injury, following which the area of injury also is examined by CT scanning, occasionally supplemented by polytomography and stress studies of the spine in flexion and extension, to assess stability. Spinal instability, however, often is obvious from gross malalignment on the plain roentgenograms of the spine. Comminution of the vertebral body, sharply wedged (50 percent) compression of the vertebral body, fractures involving both anterior and posterior elements, widening of the interspinous distance, or dislocation of one vertebra on another greater than 2.0 mm also indicate instability.

Although plain roentgenograms of the spine help to localize the level of injury and demonstrate gross fractures and dislocations, the best appreciation of the extent of bony injury and deformity is obtained by horizontal and sagittal CT reconstructions of the fracture site. These studies often reveal an almost stereotyped group of findings in these cases,[11] with destruction and retropulsion of a portion of the body into the spinal canal, solitary fracture of a pedicle, and fracture of one or both laminae. These findings may be associated with the dislocation of one vertebra on another and sagittal rotation of vertebrae.[11]

The findings of the CT scan allow one to forego routine preoperative myelography in these cases. Myelography is now reserved for the unusual case exhibiting a significant neurologic deficit in conjunction with roentgenograms and CT scans that do not provide an adequate explanation of the clinical findings. Because the delineation of the herniated "soft" thoracolumbar discs by CT scan alone is marginal, metrizamide is instilled intrathecally and myelography is performed, followed by CT scanning of the appropriate section of the spine. The demonstration of nonrelief of dural compression in cases with retropulsed bone fragments subjected to vertebral distraction and alignment with the Harrington apparatus alone in about one-half of our cases in which this tactic was used has caused us to adopt the combined approach to these cases in which an anterolateral decompression is performed *before* Harrington rod fixation.

Decompression using the anterolateral approach has been used in all cases with a partial neurologic deficit and the "standard" CT abnormality, and occasionally in paraplegic patients in the hope that by decompressing the cauda equina some nerve root function may return, a result with important implications regarding the patient's rehabilitation. The last patient in whom this approach was used showed return of function of the L2 and L3 roots and now has crude pin and touch reception in one leg. There has been no recovery of spinal cord function in any of the 9 paraplegic patients after surgery.

Spinal cord angiography has been advocated to evaluate dorsolumbar fractures in order to identify the artery of Adamkiewicz and to avoid intraoperative iatrogenic injury to this vessel.[12] Chou[13] has indicated, however, that the intercostal arteries can be ligated at multiple levels without producing spinal cord ischemia, since the radicular arteries originate proximal to the point of ligation of the intercostal arteries at the time of thoracotomy (Fig. 82-3). Radicular arteries, however, can be injured by the removal of the head of the rib or by dissection adjacent to the neural foramen. Although not used in our service, spinal angiography may be useful with fractures between T8 and L1, particularly if an approach is planned from the left side. We have been unable to find any cases in the literature of neurologic deficit following proximal ligation of a single thoracic radicular artery. It should not be necessary to sacrifice more than one artery in carrying out this operation.

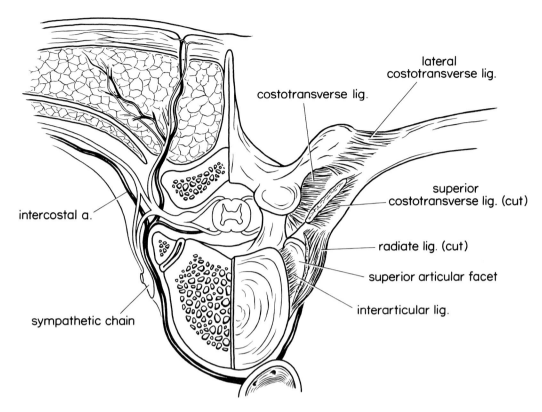

Fig. 82-3. Relationships of intercostal arteries and nerves to musculoskeletal structures at midthoracic level.

Following these radiographic studies, patients are transferred to an operating-type Stryker frame and remain on this device until they are mobilzed in a period of weeks. All surgical procedures are performed with the patient on this frame, thereby avoiding the need to move the patient on several occasions from bed to operating table.

Base-line somatosensory evoked potentials from the lower extremities are obtained on all patients shortly after hospitalization.[14] When responses can be recorded from the cortical electrodes, this technique is used intraoperatively to continuously monitor spinal cord function, particularly during distraction of or manipulation of structures adjacent to the spinal cord or nerve roots.

The technique for recording the SSERs involves stimulation of the posterior tibial nerve at the ankle with an intensity sufficient to obtain a motor response. The cathode is switched to the proximal electrode position. Stimuli are produced by a Grass stimulator* with a stimulus isolation unit and pulse duration of 0.2 msec with voltages of 70–150 V. During operation the voltage is often increased to 150 V to ensure an adequate stimulus. Responses are measured at the second cervical vertebra (3 cm below the union), and at CZ and CPZ (halfway between CZ and PZ in the international 10-20 system) with a reference at F2 and the ground electrode on the leg or head, selected to minimize stimulus artifact. Electrodes for recording are silver-silver chloride held in place with collodion. Amplification is provided by a Grass 8 electroencephalograph with a frequency response of 0.3–10,000 Hz. The data are averaged on a Nicolet 1062 averager** and photographed from an oscilloscope screen. Stimuli are presented at H3 and a 200-msec epoch, following which the stimulus is averaged.

In none of the paraplegic patients was it possible to record a response from the somatosensory cortex, whereas in all other cases these responses were present. Intraoperative monitoring is used in all but paraplegic patients during decompression of the dural contents and during spinal

*Grass Instrument Co., Quincy, Massachusetts.
**Nicolet Instrument Corp., Madison, Wisconsin.

instrumentation. In 2 cases, a qualitative improvement in the wave-form pattern occurred almost immediately after decompression, and these patients made an excellent neurologic recovery.

Surgery normally is performed within 5 to 7 days after injury unless the neurologic deficit increases. This problem has been encountered in only 1 patient. During exploration, the dura along the anterior aspect of the spine was seen to have ruptured at the level of the fracture, allowing blood from the fracture to track intradurally to compress neural elements. By separating the edges of the torn dura, the hematoma was easily evacuated, and the patient regained his previous neurologic function. Our review of the literature indicates that, except in cases of neurologic worsening, emergent operation does not have an effect on the extent of neurologic recovery,[15] and in these patients the associated injuries often are a major contraindication to immediate surgical intervention. Although this seems to be a good general rule, one exception is the patient presenting with a total thoracolumbar dislocation. In these cases the surgeon must be conversant with each of the techniques described in this chapter since it may be impossible to accomplish adequate alignment with the anterolateral approach combined with Harrington instrumentation. A direct anterior approach to the spine with excision of a major portion of the involved body, anterior fusion, and instrumentation may be preferable.

Operative Procedures

Transthoracic Approach to the Thoracic Spine for Decompression and Sterilization

In the patient undergoing transthoracic or thoracoabdominal exploration, the spine at the level of maximal deformity or injury is marked radiographically. The patient is anesthetized with a double-lumen endotracheal tube, and the proper position of the endotracheal tube is confirmed radiographically. An approach via a right-sided thoracotomy is preferred. The patient is carefully positioned in a three-quarter prone position for thoracotomy, and the draping is done to allow access to the iliac crest so that additional amounts of bone can be harvested and used with the fusion if this is needed. In order to minimize blood loss and to ensure the gentlest possible handling of tissues, the operation is performed using standard microsurgical techniques, $4.5 \times$ magnifying loupes, and headlight illumination. Controlled hypotension has not been necessary.

The skin incision is carried from the posterior midline overlying the area of deformity to the anterior axillary line (Fig. 82-4). The subcutaneous tissues are divided in the line of the incision, and the latissimus dorsi is sectioned. A plane of dissection is developed by running two fingers behind the muscle and dividing the muscle with cutting current. Posteriorly, the trapezius and the rhomboid major muscles are divided in the line of the incision. Some fibers of the sacrospinalis also may require division. Anteriorly, the serratus anterior is divided over the selected rib.

The ribs may be counted externally anteriorly from the second rib, which is prominent at its junction with the sternum. In the posterolateral position the horizontal border of the first rib may be palpated and used for counting. In lower incisions the ribs may be counted upward from the twelfth rib, which is palpated externally. The intercostal muscles are divided in the same way. The entire rib is resected subperiosteally, and this bone is reserved for bone graft. The pleural space is entered through the periosteal bed. After placement of a conventional Finochietto rib spreader and collapse of the lung, the sympathetic chain is identified and the intercostal nerve traced into the neural foramen. Depending upon the level chosen for decompression, the azygos vein may require division between secure suture ligatures in order to gain access to the anterior aspect of the vertebral column (Fig. 82-5). The overlying pleura, endothoracic fascia, and fibrous tissue is dissected off the vertebral bodies, care being taken to avoid injury to the thoracic duct, which lies on the vertebral bodies between the level of the aortic hiatus and T5, and to con-

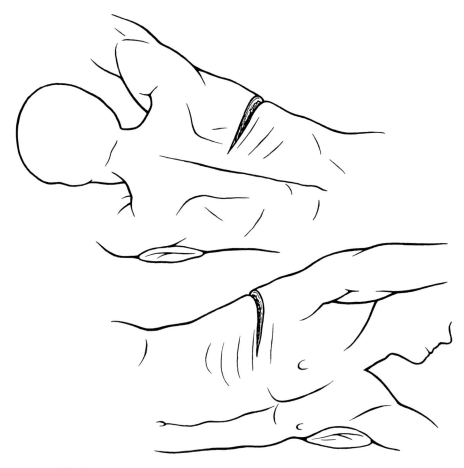

Fig. 82-4.   Positioning for transthoracic approach to the thoracic spine.

trol bleeding from the intercostal arteries coursing from the aorta. If the thoracic duct is known to be injured, it should be ligated with nonabsorbable suture and not clipped. Prior administration of colored cream through a nasogastric tube will help identify this structure.

After identification of the fractures, the bone that has been destroyed or retropulsed is removed under magnification using loupes or the operating microscope, curettes, and a high-speed air drill (Fig. 82-6). The intervertebral discs and cartilaginous end plates on the ends of the vertebrae are removed to facilitate subsequent incorporation of the bone placed between the remaining vertebral bodies. *Usually decompression can be accomplished without resorting to removal of the entire vertebral body.* Only the bone that is impinging into the spinal canal is removed, and this bone is removed over at least the height of the vertebral body, thereby reconstituting the normal cross-sectional diameter of the spinal canal. To accomplish this it is necessary first to undermine the bone projecting into the spinal canal with the air drill, which thereby provides adequate space to allow the retropulsed bone fragment to be depressed away from the ventral aspect of the dural sac. This approach is analogous to the technique described in Chapter 81 for the removal of a herniated thoracic disc; however, the extent of the defect created in the vertebral body or bodies when dealing with a fracture is greater and necessitates removal of one-third to one-half of the vertebral body adjacent to the spinal canal to achieve an adequate decompression (Fig. 82-7).

Following thoracotomy and microneurosurgical removal of the discs, retropulsed vertebral bone fragments, epidural hematoma, and repair of dural tears, the levels for a fusion are selected to the nearest intact vertebral bodies above and below the level of fracture-dislocation.

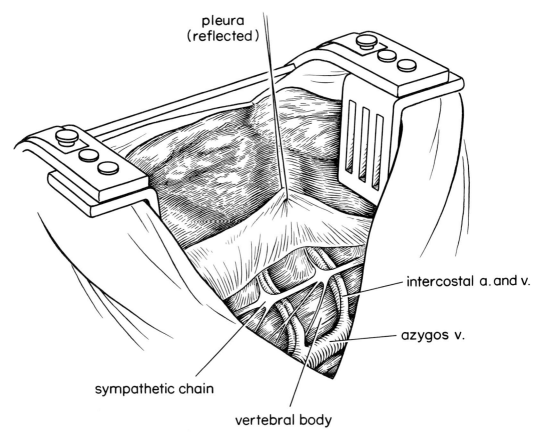

pleura
(reflected)

intercostal a. and v.

azygos v.

sympathetic chain

vertebral body

Fig. 82-5. Surgical anatomy: Collapse of the lung, exposing parietal pleura and strictures on the anterolateral aspect of the thoracic spine.

Screws must be placed in intact vertebral bodies, but the longer the lever arms, the less secure the fixation. The segmental vessels must be suture ligated on the vertebral bodies to be instrumented. The vertebral body is exposed subperiosteally, and it is necessary to be able to feel the surface of the vertebral body from the distal side so that screws can be properly aimed and seated and thoracic injury avoided. Rib struts are used for fusion. Disc spaces included in the fusion have been previously curetted. Correction of deformity is reserved for those cases without a rigid deficit, and is made by extending the thoracic spine on the operating table. The Santa Casa distractors (DePuy Co.) are useful if marked kyphosis is present over several levels (Fig. 82-8). Slots are cut in the vertebral bodies above and below the site of decompression to receive grafts fashioned from sections of rib removed during thoracotomy. These grafts are cut and tapped into prepared recesses in the vertebral body with a bone set. The bone graft must be placed before application of the fixation device.

Stabilization then is performed. Anterior and posterior titanium rods are fitted to the Dwyer screws. Either single or double staples are used depending upon the configuration present. With a small degree of kyphosis and a solid vertebral body, it is possible to seat a double staple into the vertebral body, while with small vertebral bodies and marked deformity it is safer to use two single staples. Screw and staple size are measured and the proper size selected. Care must be taken that the end of the screw penetrates the distal cortex of the vertebra. Portions of Keith needles inserted in the disc are helpful in guiding the screws so they lie transversely in the vertebral bodies. Staples are measured and set into the disc space, and the screws are turned through the staples so they lie firmly and flush with the vertebral body. Then the titanium rods are cut and guided through the holes in the screws, one anterior and one posterior, to control

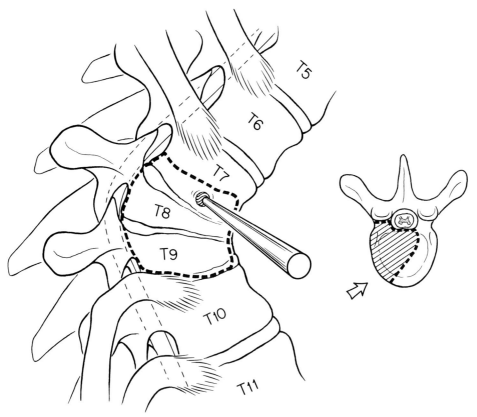

Fig. 82-6. Extent of bone removal in this case involving three spinal segments, leaving a shell of vertebral body to allow some lateral stability for rib grafts while removing the apex of the gibbus.

bending at the level of the fracture. The rods are secured in place in the screws by crimping the screw head. A single chest tube is brought through the anterior axillary line and the collapsed lung is re-expanded with the drainage tube to the posterior paravertebral gutter.

At the time of closure the pleura must be reapproximated with chromic catgut, and a rib approximator is used to appose the ribs above and below the bed from which a rib has been removed. The trapezius, rhomboids, serratus anterior, and latissimus dorsi are reapproximated anatomically with nonabsorbable suture material. The subcutaneous tissue is closed with fine, synthetic absorbent suture material and the skin is closed with a running nylon suture.

Postoperatively, the patient is nursed on a Stryker frame. The chest tube is removed in 24 to 48 hours if it is adynamic. The patients are kept on the Stryker for 6 to 8 weeks following decompression fusion and then are mobilized in a molded plastic orthosis. If the patient is not unstable, ambulation is begun at approximately 2 weeks. Intraoperative evoked responses and myelography are performed as described in the section on thoracolumbar fractures.

When a thoracoabdominal incision is required to provide exposure of the vertebral bodies of T11-T12, and L1, an incision is planned that extends from the posterior axillary line, in the selected interspace (usually T7-8), and moves forward to the midline of the abdomen. The serratus anterior is split as are the fibers of the external oblique muscle. The anterior rectus sheath, the ipsilateral rectus muscle, the intercostal muscles, and the pleura are cut, thereby entering the chest cavity. In the abdomen, the incision divides the posterior rectus sheath, exposing, but not entering through, the peritoneum. The diaphragm is divided peripherally along its insertion to the spine. This muscle is subsequently repaired with interrupted nonabsorbable sutures.

These approaches provide excellent access from approximately T3 to L2 anteriorly. Exposure of T1 to T3 is best accomplished by a posteriorly oriented thoracotomy from midline to the

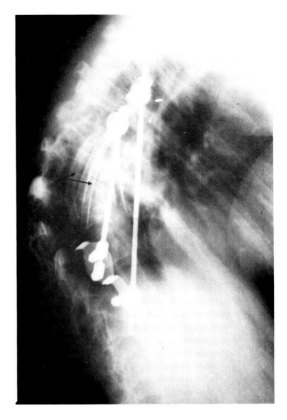

Fig. 82-7.   Anterior instrumentation and rib graft stabilization after anterolateral decompression as a one-stage procedure.

anterior axillary line with lateral displacement of the scapula and its attached musculature. This exposure allows for both neural decompression of these segments and anterior stabilization.

Anterolateral Approach to the Thoracolumbar Spine Injuries

In those cases in which there is a major compromise of the spinal canal width, usually secondary to a retropulsed fragment of the body of the vertebra, and the patient is either neurologically intact (Frankel Grade E) or has a partial injury (Grades B, C, or D), the patient is placed in a three-quarter prone position, and a long vertical midline incision is made and exploration is carried out lateral to the facet joint. This approach allows removal of a pedicle, undermining of the retropulsed fragment of bone with an air drill and diamond burrs, and decompressing the dura without pressure being exerted against the intradural structures (Fig. 82-6).

Harrington instrumentation is performed to the second intact vertebra above and below the level of injury, and the superior and inferior hooks are seated on the side opposite the anterolateral decompression. If spinal asymmetry is present, it is most convenient to perform the decompression on the convexity of the scoliosis; the distraction then is made on the concavity of the curve. The Harrington distraction is placed, and reduction is performed both manually and using the distractor. Preoperative halofemoral traction is not employed. Decortication and excision of the facet joints are performed, and the side opposite the distractor is instrumented with a distraction rod. If severe rotation is present, such that distraction would increase the deformity, compression is applied to the convexity. The distractor is reversed and the fusion then is completed. Fusion is carried out in the area spanned by the rods, omitting the vertebra where the

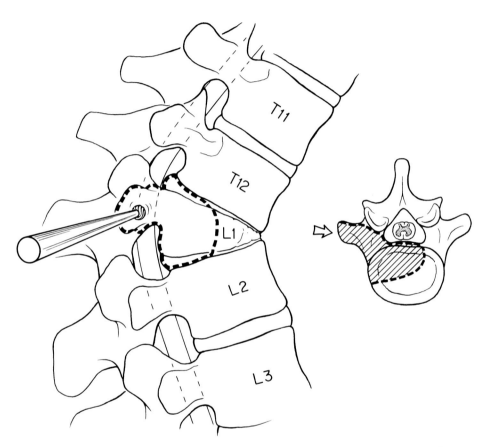

Fig. 82-8.   Extent of decompression for one-level anterolateral spinal decompression.

hooks were seated to preserve motion in as many normal segments as possible. In all patients a bone graft is placed in addition to the Harrington instrumentation.

In the paraplegic patient, a full anterolateral decompression usually is *not* performed; the injured area is examined by distracting the spinous processes at the fracture site. The interspinous and yellow ligaments are often damaged by the accident and, with the removal of minimal amounts of bone in conjunction with the removal of these ligaments, the presence of a large herniated disc fragment can be excluded without removing significant amounts of bone, which could further contribute to the spine's instability. After limited exploration, the spine is stabilized with Harrington rods and bone taken from the iliac crest placed over the laminae and transverse process. Intraoperative myelography is performed to make sure contrast medium freely flows past the fracture, since it is hoped that by providing neural decompression, nerve root function may be regained for some of the nerves of the cauda equina and the problem of chronic pain arising from compression of neural structures at the level of the fracture site avoided.

Postoperatively, the patient remains on the Stryker frame and is then mobilized in a body jacket or brace. The timing of initial bracing and transfer to a regular bed depends on the security of instrumentation at the time of operation. Patients with significant neurologic deficit are placed in molded plastic body jackets that can be removed for skin care; patients without neurologic deficits are treated in plaster of Paris body jackets. Spinal bracing is continued for 1 year— the last 6 months with support being provided by a Jewett brace. Patients are seen at monthly intervals for examination by x-ray films. Spinal stability is studied with computer-assisted stereoradiography before rod removal in symptomatic patients.[12]

The complication rate attending both the transthoracic-transpleural operation and the anterolateral approach to the thoracolumbar spine has been low. These procedures require 3 to 4 hours to accomplish. When microsurgical techniques are used, blood loss from the neurosurgical portion of the operation is approximately 350 cc. It is during the fusion that 750–1000 cc of blood is lost and usually is replaced, since extensive areas of bone are denuded to assure an adequate fusion. Compression neuropathy of the brachial plexus has been noted on one occasion, resulting from positioning on the operating Stryker frame. One case of dislodged Harrington rod has occurred to date in the entire series. There has not been an increased incidence of pulmonary complications with these operations. This probably is largely a matter of patient selection; the patients were predominately young, otherwise healthy persons.[16]

REFERENCES

1. Cline HJ Jr, cited by Hayward G: An account of a case of fractures and dislocation of the spine. *N Engl J Med Surg 4*:1–3, 1815
2. Tyrrell F: Compression of the spinal marrow from displacement of the vertebrae, consequent upon injury. Operation of removing the arch and spinous processes of the twelfth dorsal vertebra. *Lancet 11*:658–688, 1827
3. Smith AG: An account of a case in which portions of three dorsal vertebrae were removed for the relief of paralysis from fracture, with partial success. *North Am MESJ 8*:94–97, 1829
4. Cook WA: Transthoracic vertebral surgery. *Ann Thorac Surg 12*:54–68, 1971
5. Erickson DL, Leider LL, Browne W: One-stage decompression-stabilization for thoracolumbar fractures. *Spine 2*:53–56, 1977
6. Flesch JR, Leider LL, Erickson DL, et al: Harrington instrumentation and spine fusion for unstable fractures and fracture-dislocations of the thoracic and lumbar spine. *J Bone Joint Surg 59A*:143–153, 1977
7. Norrell H: The treatment of unstable spinal fractures and dislocations. *Clin Neurosurg 25*:193–208, 1978
8. Riseborough EJ: The anterior approach to the spine for the correction of deformities of the axial skeleton. *Clin Orthop 9*:207, 1973
9. De Oliviera JC: A new type of fracture-dislocation of the thoracolumbar spine. *J Bone Joint Surg 60A*:481–488, 1978
10. Frankel HL, Hancock DO, Hyslop G, et al: The value of postural reduction in the initial management of closed injuries of the spine with paraplegia and tetraplegia. *Paraplegia 7*:179–192, 1969

11. Schmidek HH, Gomes FB, Seligson D, et al: Management of acute unstable thoracolumbar (T11-L1) fractures with and without neurological deficit. *Neurosurgery 7*:30–35, 1980
12. Böhler J: Operative treatment of fractures of the dorsal and lumbar spine. *J Trauma 10*:1119–1122, 1970
13. Chou SN: Alternative surgical approaches to the thoracic spine. *Clin Neurosurg 20*:306–321, 1973
14. Cusick JD, Myklebust JB, Larson SJ, et al: Spinal cord evaluation by cortical evoked responses. *Arch Neurol 36*:140–143, 1979
15. Larson SJ, Holst RA, Hemmy DC, et al: Lateral extracavitary approach to traumatic lesions of the thoracic and lumbar spine. *J Neurosurg 45*:628–637, 1976
16. Gertzbein SD, Offierski C: Complete fracture-dislocation of the thoracic spine without spinal cord injury. A case report. *J Bone Joint Surg 61A*:449–451, 1979

CHAPTER 83
Lumbar Disc Excision

Bernard E. Finneson

Caveat Disc Surgeon

THE FIRST DISC OPERATION is relatively easy. The repeat operative procedure, however, presents a problem both in technique and, even more, in satisfactory outcome. The recommended solution to this problem is to avoid the first operation that is apt to lead to a less than satisfactory result, and thus not create a clinical condition that requires repeat disc surgery.

Patient Selection

The most important single consideration affecting the outcome of lumbar disc surgery is patient selection. What factors help predict whether a patient will improve from surgery? The surgeon who can select a patient who will benefit from surgical intervention has won half the battle before the incision is made. It is perhaps even more important for the surgeon to be able to predict those individuals who will not benefit from surgery. The surgeon who operates on this type of patient is handicapped before he starts; a satisfactory clinical result is not likely even with the finest, most meticulous surgical technique. The most that can reasonably be expected is that the patient will not be too discernibly worse after surgery. It should be emphasized that the lack of response to nonsurgical treatment is not in itself, an indication for surgery. All too often the patient with low back pain who is not readily cured with nonsurgical management is brought to the operating room under the banner of "we must do something for this poor suffering patient." This "something" is often a variety of new, and sometimes irrversible, surgically produced signs and symptoms, which are superimposed upon the original complaints. The surgeon should remember that no matter how severe and intractable the pain is, it can always be made worse with surgery.

Fallibility of the Neurologic Examination

Neurosurgeons, in comparison to their orthopedic colleagues, are perhaps a bit more prone to rely upon the neurologic examination to identify the level of disc protrusion. There are, of course, certain general findings, such as severe paraspinal muscle spasm in the lumbar area or poor mobility of the lumbar spine that are common to most disc syndromes at any level and that are not considered of localizing value. The classic findings of a diminished or absent Achilles reflex and numbness along the lateral aspect of the foot in the presence of sciatic pain generally would

Low Back Pain Clinic, Crozer-Chester Medical Center, Chester, Pennsylvania, and Department of Neurosurgery, Hahnemann Medical College and Hospital, Philadelphia, Pennsylvania

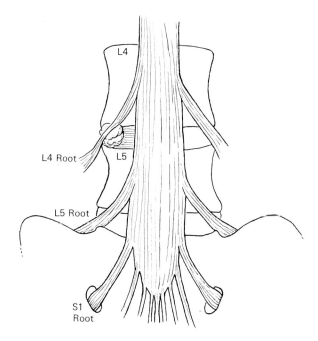

Fig. 83-1. Foraminal root compressive syndrome. The laterally situated L4-5 disc protrusion will extend into
the intervertebral foramen impinging upon the L4
root and simulate an L3-4 syndrome. (Reprinted
from Finneson BE: *Low Back Pain.* 2nd ed. Philadelphia, Lippincott, 1981, with permission.)

be accepted as representing an L5-S1 disc protrusion. If the lumbar spine films demonstrate a
narrow disc space at the level of L5-S1, some disc surgeons might forego the myelogram and
proceed with surgery. In most cases they would be right, and a surgically treatable lesion would
be found at the L5-S1 level. Three factors can be responsible for neurologic changes, however,
that may mislead the surgeon as to the involved interspace.

1. *Location of the disc protrusion (Fig. 83-1).* The disc fragment may extrude laterally into the
   foramen so that it compresses the exiting root from the interspace above. Such a laterally located fragment at the L5-S1 foramen may produce an L4-5 syndrome.
2. *Neuroanatomic changes (Fig. 83-2).* A partially lumbarized first sacral segment, which may
   be dismissed as being of no clinical significance, might be associated with a *postfixed* plexus.
   In such a situation an L5-S1 disc protrusion may produce weakness of the great toe and
   numbness over the dorsum of the foot within the L5 dermatome and might be identified as a
   L4-5 protrusion at the level of L4-5 on the basis of the neurologic examination.
3. *Temporal changes.* As the patient grows older, degenerative changes within the discs occur
   in a progressively cephalad direction. This is well documented by discography, which demonstrates that degenerative changes usually occur first at the L5-S1 level; some years later
   they advance to the L4-5 interspace, and with advancing age, they advance progressively
   cephalad. For this reason, an individual over the age of 50 who has severe sciatica associated
   with an Achilles reflex and a narrow L5-S1 disc space could be suffering from an acute lesion
   at the level of L4-5. The absent Achilles reflex may be a residual finding from a previously
   protruded lesion at the level of L5-S1 that has long since fibrosed, leaving less mobility at
   that level, and that is no longer a source of pain. The new painful disc lesion at the level of
   L4-5 may not have been present long enough to establish hard neurologic findings.

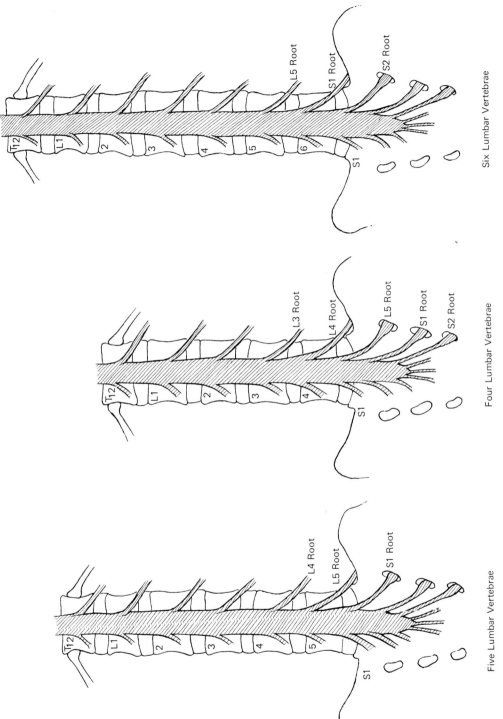

Five Lumbar Vertebrae

Four Lumbar Vertebrae

Six Lumbar Vertebrae

Fig. 83-2. Transitional lumbosacral vertebral and root function. (Reprinted from Finneson BE: *Low Back Pain.* 2nd Ed. Philadelphia, Lippincott, 1981, with permission.)

Myelography

Lumbar myelograms should be done on all patients before lumbar disc surgery. These myelograms are used principally to confirm clinical localization and to determine if more than one disc herniation is present. They also help to rule out possible lumbar spinal tumors, which very easily can simulate herniated lumbar discs. Although used mainly as a preoperative test, myelography is occasionally performed on patients who have not fared well with an adequate course of conservative management and in whom there is significant uncertainty regarding the nature of their complaints. The myelogram is not infallible and is associated with a significant incidence of both false negatives and false positives. Most false negatives are noted at the L5-S1 level, where there is a large space between the anterior dural edge and the posterior bony spine. This space is less wide above the L5-S1 level, so the incidence of false negatives is much less from the level of L4-5 upward. The incidence of false positives is greater in patients over the age of 55 because of the hypertrophic osteoarthritic degenerative changes associated with advancing years.

Lumbar Disc Surgery Predictive Score Card

It must be recognized that any surgical judgment that is based primarily on such a subjective symptom as pain can have as many variables as there are surgeons. All medical judgments relating to therapy are made by assigning positive and negative relative values to various aspects of the clinical picture, with the final decision being made by mentally balancing out these relative values. A numerical value system is not commonly used, but such a system may allow surgeons to communicate more easily about this complex problem.

A review of the various clinical factors that play a role in surgical decision making was carried out in 200 postsurgical patients who had a good result and was compared with 96 postsurgical patients who had a poor result.[1] This clinical review was employed as a base on which to list the major positive and negative factors involved in preoperative selection and to assign these factors positive and negative numerical values. Employment of such a system provides a "predictive number" indicating the likely outcome of surgery. In an effort to make the system useable by almost all physicians who are involved in lumbar disc surgery, only those criteria that have broad acceptance and that are generally employed were included. Studies that have less widespread use, such as electromyography, discography, lumbar venography, computerized tomographic (CT) scanning, and special psychologic studies, were purposely excluded. The result of this study was a Lumbar Disc Surgery Predictive Score Card (Fig. 83-3).

Positive Score Card Factors

The predictive score card lists 7 positive factors with a total of 115 possible points.

Factor 1. The key word is incapacitating. If pain is not severe enough to hamper activities of daily living, the patient often is likely to be unsatisfied with the results of surgery.

Factor 2. Excision of a herniated lumbar disc usually will relieve nerve root pain. If sciatica is not the major symptom, and surgery provides relief of sciatica but no improvement of the back pain, the unhappy patient may well ignore the disappearance of the minor sciatica and concentrate on the persisting predominant back pain.

Factor 3. Body position should affect a lumbar disc syndrome if it is indeed a mechanical problem. Sciatic syndromes that are unaffected by changes in body position are often nonmechanical in nature and will not be alleviated by the mechanical removal of pressure.

Factor 4. A neurologic examination that demonstrates a single root syndrome indicating a specific interspace obviously increases the possibility of a successful outcome.

Factor 5. It is important that the myelographic defect corroborate the neurologic examina-

LUMBAR DISC SURGERY PREDICTIVE SCORE CARD

This questionnaire is of predictive value when limited to candidates for excision of a herniated lumbar disc who have not previously undergone lumbar spine surgery. It is not designed to encompass candidates for other types of lumbar spine surgery such as decompressive laminectomy or fusion.

Positive Points	POSITIVE FACTORS	NEGATIVE FACTORS	Negative Points
5	1. Low back and sciatic pain severe enough to be incapacitating.	1. **Back pain primarily**	15
15	2. Sciatica is more severe than back pain.	2. **Gross obesity**	10
5	3. Weight bearing (sitting or standing) aggravates the pain; bedrest (in some position) eases the pain.	3. **Nonorganic signs and symptoms** —entire leg numb; simultaneous weakness of flexion and extension of toes; extension of pain into areas not explainable by an organic lesion.	10
25	4. Neurologic examination demonstrates a single root syndrome indicating a specific interspace.		
25	5. Myelographic defect corroborating the neurologic examination.	4. **Poor psychologic background**— attempted suicide, unrealistically high expectations from surgery; previous admissions for nonorganic symptoms—hyperventilation—unexplainable chest pains and abdominal pains—intractable incisional pain; alcoholic; not happy with job; physical demands of present occupation excessive; hostility to environment–employer–spouse; much time off from work for medical reasons (man out of work 6 months—woman out of work 16 months).	15
10	6. Positive straight-leg-raising test.		
20	Crossed-straight-leg-raising test.		
10	7. Patient's realistic self-appraisal of future life style.		
		5. **Secondary gain**—work-connected accident; vehicular accident; medico-legal adversary situation; near retirement age—eligible for disability pension if symptoms persist.	20
		6. **History of previous lawsuits** for medico-legal problems.	10

Positive Total

Negative Total

Subtract negative total from positive total [ ] **for predictive number.**

SCORING
75 & over . . . . good
65—75 . . . . fair
55—65. . . . . marginal
below 55. poor

Fig. 83-3. A sample Lumbar Disc Surgery Predictive Score Card.

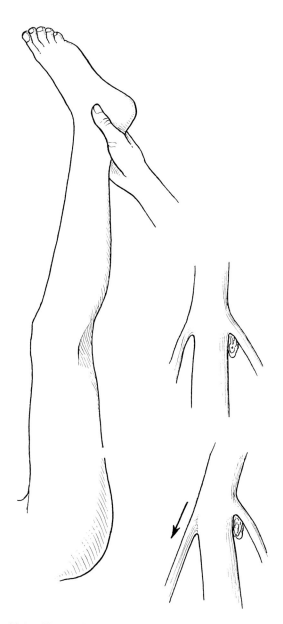

Fig. 83-4. The well leg-raising test of Fajerstajn. (Reprinted from Finneson BE: *Low Back Pain.* 2nd ed. Philadelphia, Lippincott, 1981, with permission.)

tion. It must be kept in mind that various reports indicate abnormal lumbar myelographs in (low back) symptom-free patients in percentages varying from 25 percent to 30 percent.

Factor 6. The straight-leg-raising test is a good predictive factor. The crossed-straight-leg-raising test (the nonpainful leg is raised, which produces aggravation of pain radiating into the painful leg) is twice as effective (Fig. 83-4).

Factor 7. The patient's realistic appraisal of future life style is an important factor that easily may be ignored by the surgeon. The only way to appreciate the patient's postoperative expectations is to spend some time listening to the patient.

Negative Score Card Factors

The score card lists 6 negative factors with a total of 80 possible points.

Factor 1. Back pain primarily is the reverse of positive factor 2.

Factor 2. Although grossly obese people initially seem to do about the same as those patients with a more normal habitus, after 1 or 2 years the recurrence rate is somewhat higher.

Factor 3. Simultaneous weakness in flexion and extension of the great toe cannot be explained by pressure on a single root, and unless some neurologic explanation can be offered for this finding, it should be considered nonorganic.

Factor 4. Poor psychologic background is a "mixed bag," but any of these factors should cause the surgeon to be cautious. The alcoholic, for example, may have demonstrated a very steady work history in the past and may never have been hospitalized previously. It should be recognized, however, that alcoholics arise every morning and set about their tasks only with great effort and difficulty. Any break in their routine may produce a behavior reversal.

Factor 5, secondary gain, and *Factor 6,* history of lawsuits, are self-explanatory.

By adding the positive scores and adding the negative scores and subtracting the negative total from the positive total, the surgeon can derive a predictive number and compare it against the scoring table (see Fig. 83-3) to determine the likely outcome of disc surgery.

Predictive Factors

The four most important factors in determining a satisfactory outcome for surgery are:

1. Sciatic pain more severe than the back pain.
2. An abnormal myelogram that correlates with the clinical picture.
3. Positive Leségue sign.
4. Neurologic deficit.

The crossed Leségue sign is probably the most specific test for lumbar disc herniation. If all four of the above factors are present, technically adequate surgery is likely to produce a satisfactory result. If one of them is absent, the surgeon should be very satisfied with the accuracy of the other three factors before proceeding. Surgery considered when only one or two of these factors is positive is likely to be associated with a high incidence of less than satisfactory results. With these factors in mind, there are four indications for surgery:

1. Intractable pain.
2. Progressively worsening neurologic deficit.
3. Intractable recurrence of pain.
4. Cauda equina syndrome.

With the exception of the cauda equina syndrome, each of these indications is relative and will depend on how well the patient tolerates the symptoms, on the extent of the neurologic deficit, and on the psychologic and sociologic background of the patient.

Contraindications to Surgery

There are five important contraindications to surgery:

1. A first episode of low back and sciatic pain without an adequate trial of conservative management.
2. Intermittent low back pain associated with occasional pains of an equivocal nature, extending into one or the other lower extremity, and an equivocal myelogram.

3. A prolonged history of intermittent low back pain and an equivocal myelogram.

4. Low back and intermittent sciatic pain with a myelogram demonstrating a lesion on the "wrong" or pain-free side. (I have seen 2 patients on whom disc surgery was performed with "a contralateral myelogram," and the two surgeons who elected to proceed on the basis of this information were divided in choosing the side of surgery upon which to operate. The one who operated upon the painful side used as his justification myelographic evidence of disc dysfunction at a specific interspace; since the pain was on the opposite side, he decided it would be best to decompress the nerve root on the side of the pain rather than on the side of the myelographic defect. The surgeon who elected to operate on the side of the myelographic defect rather than on the side of the pain felt that the disc protrusion might cause a shift of the cauda equina enclosed within its dural sac, which would press the opposite root against the lamina and produce radicular symptoms. Both patients did poorly after surgery.)

5. Improvement of the patient. In the presence of significant motor weakness, if some slight improvement in the pain occurs, it may be justifiable to proceed with surgery. If pain is the primary symptom, however, improvement is an indication to cancel surgery. (I adhere to this principle and have canceled many scheduled cases on the day of surgery upon being told that the patient no longer had pain or that the pain was markedly improved.) Pain surgery performed during an interval of improvement may result in patient dissatisfaction, despite an adequate postoperative result. The patient may be less willing to accept residual symptoms, even of a relatively minor nature, and is more apt to question in retrospect how pressing and indispensable the need was for surgery. If, in the face of improvement, the patient is discharged and subsequently readmitted for surgery with an exacerbation of pain, occasional residual symptoms may be tolerated more kindly. When contemplating lumbar disc surgery, the indications must be clear to the patient as well as to the surgeon.

Exploratory Lumbar Disc Surgery

Ten years ago the patient who presented with persisting sciatica and a normal myelogram and who failed to respond to conservative treatment efforts often was considered by many surgeons as a suitable candidate for exploratory lumbar disc surgery. Usually the L5-S1 and L4-5 levels were explored on the symptomatic side. Although some patients possibly benefited by this approach, a significant group either were not improved or were worse after surgery. At this time, with the additional diagnostic help provided by lumbar epidural venography and computerized tomography of the lumbar spine, surgeons are able to assess those intraspinal areas that previously may have been hidden. Given these new diagnostic tools, a suitable indication for a blind exploration based purely on the persistence of pain is inconceivable. The likelihood of finding a surgically treatable lesion if a myelogram, epidural venogram, and CT scan are all normal is so poor that the era of exploratory lumbar disc surgery is best brought to a close.

Surgery

Historical Development

Fifty years ago an occasional laminectomy was performed for lumbar disc disease and the extruded disc fragments were identified as "chondromata." There was some question regarding the exact nature of these lesions, although many surgeons did recognize them as consisting of displaced intervertebral disc material. The surgical technique used in the removal of such lesions invariably involved an extensive bilateral laminectomy. This usually was followed by opening the dura in the midline, separating the nerve roots to either side, and palpating the anterior spinal canal by means of a narrow probe until the underlying protrusion was identified. The anterior dura then was incised over the most eminent portion of the protrusion, and, through this very limited anterior dural opening, the protruding portion of the disc was exposed and removed.

The entire concept of ruptured intervertebral discs changed after the classic paper of Mixter and Barr.[2] They conclusively and unequivocally demonstrated the origin of these lesions, laid to rest any lingering doubt that they were neoplasms, and documented their etiology as protrusions of the nucleus of an intervertebral disc. They delineated the lumbar disc syndrome and the indications for surgical treatment of this condition. Shortly after the appearance of this paper, the surgical technique for protruding lumbar intervertebral discs underwent an important change, with the dura being left intact and the protruding disc being removed extradurally, although the extensive bilateral laminectomy was continued. Further surgical refinements followed, including the hemilaminectomy, which leaves the spinous process and lamina intact on the pain-free side. Twenty-five or 30 years ago it became common practice to carry out lumbar disc surgery in most cases by means of the unilateral interlaminar approach.

In the past 6 or 7 years the combined use of a fiberoptic headlight and $2^{1}/_{2}$–$4^{1}/_{2} \times$ operating loupes has been accepted by an increasing number of disc surgeons. The fiberoptic lighting is helpful, not only in providing dependable illumination to the depths of the incision, but in eliminating the technical necessity for the rather long laminectomy incision that extends over three interspaces (although the actual disc surgery was confined to an interlaminar space measuring approximately $^{1}/_{2}$ inch). The lengthy skin and muscle incision was required to allow the standard overhead operating room lighting to illuminate the apex or depth of the operative field. With the brighter beam of light made available with fiberoptic techniques, a much smaller incision is possible. The magnification provided by the operating loupes aids greatly in assuring delicate handling of tissue and helps prevent nerve root damage. Increasing the magnification to $25 \times$ with the use of an operating microscope has led to the development of a specific microsurgical discectomy technique involving a distinct departure from prior surgical concepts. A much more limited removal of disc material is performed. This technique avoids laminectomy, curettement of the disc space, and removal of epidural fat, and it avoids incision of the annulus fibrosis with a scalpel; instead, it employs a blunt probe to perforate this surface.

With advances in knowledge and equipment, continued technical changes can be anticipated.

Choice of Operative Procedure

Once the decision has been made that surgery is indicated, the surgeon must determine which operative procedure is most suitable for the patient's particular low back dysfunction.

Is a disc herniation producing a clear single-root syndrome? If so, interlaminar disc excision is the procedure of choice.

Is it primarily a stenotic lumbar spinal canal syndrome associated with sciatica produced by foraminal impingement and secondary to a bony spur? Attempting to treat this condition with an interlaminar disc excision often is technically difficult and is likely to have a disappointing clinical result. The operation of choice for a stenotic lumbar spinal canal is decompressive laminectomy and foraminotomy at the appropriate level.

If the symptoms are unilateral and the myelographic defect is bilateral, should surgery be confined to the side of the pain or should a bilateral interlaminar disc excision be performed? This is often a gray area and may be open to controversy. As a basic principle, performing the minimal amount of surgery that can adequately relieve the symptoms is preferred rather than attempting prophylactic surgery of symptoms that have not yet developed. Whichever decision is made in this situation can be wrong. Following a bilateral interlaminar operation, the patient may awaken from the anesthesia with postoperative pain in the previously painless leg. Surgery can be confined to the painful side, and in the near or distant future, pain may develop on the nonoperated side.

Should disc excision be followed by a fusion? We do not routinely perform a combined disc excision and spinal fusion, but reserve this combined procedure for the unusual situation.

Double-checking the Side of Lesion

Performing an operative procedure on the "wrong side" is not a common mishap, but it can occur when surgery is performed on any structure that is paired. Patients who have undergone herniorrhaphies, hip surgery, cataract surgery, or carpal tunnel decompressions occasionally have awakened from anesthesia and have been surprised to find the surgical dressing and the incisional discomfort at an unanticipated site. Because the patient undergoing lumbar disc surgery is in the prone position with his "sides reversed," this error may occur with greater frequency than is likely to happen in the supine position. The best way to preclude this blunder is for the surgeon to remain alert to such a possibility and to establish a preventive behavior pattern.

When reviewing spine x-ray films, the surgeon should make a point of placing the films on the view box as though the patient were in the prone position, with the left marker on the left side. Radiologists, who are trained to visualize films as though the patient is in the anatomic position, may look with mild disfavor at this heresy. It is not the radiologist, however, who will be sued for operating on the wrong side. This practice reinforces a mental image of the spine patient in the prone position.

Another helpful aid to lateralization is the small tatoo that is routinely made at the completion of a myelogram. This permanent mark is radiologically localized at the level of the lesion and is placed laterally on the side of the pain.

Prior to the induction of anesthesia, the patient should always be asked to indicate the painful leg. Of course, the painful side is noted on the chart and the myelograms also are labeled appropriately.

Anesthesia

Many surgeons prefer the use of spinal anesthesia, employing a hypobaric solution; epidural anesthesia also has some advocates. Intravenous sodium pentothal supplemented with halo-

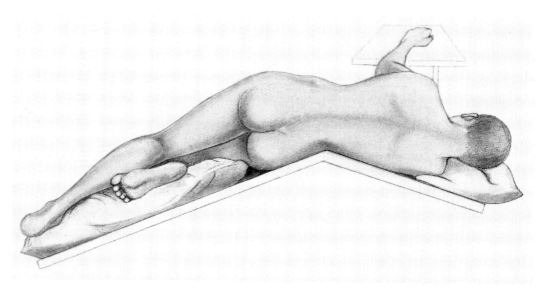

Fig. 83-5.   Lateral position for lumbar disc surgery. (Reprinted from Finneson BE: *Low Back Pain.* 2nd ed. Philadelphia, Lippincott, 1981, with permission.)

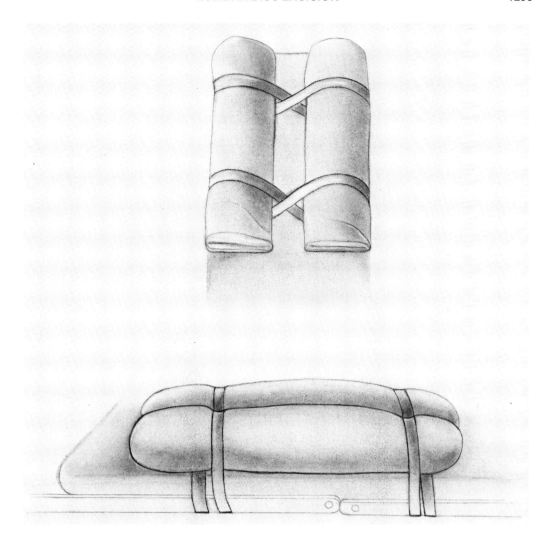

Fig. 83-6.   Blanket rolls taped in place. (Reprinted from Finneson BE: *Low Back Pain.* 2nd ed. Philadelphia, Lippincott, 1981, with permission.)

thane, nitrous oxide, and oxygen administered through an endotracheal tube is the anesthesia of personal choice and is probably used by the majority of clinics in lumbar disc surgery.

Position

A variety of positions have been used for operating upon patients with protruded lumbar discs.

For the unilateral disc excision, many surgeons prefer the lateral position (Fig. 83-5). This is the position of choice from the point of view of anesthesia, because it does not hamper respiratory excursions as much as the prone position. The principal surgical advantage is that the lateral position allows the abdomen to be relatively free, which reduces pressure on the great veins and, in turn, reduces epidural venous distention and bleeding. This position does not allow blood to pool within the depths of the wound, and it promotes posterior lumbar flexion. Another technical advantage is that the surgeon can spread the uppermost interlaminar space laterally by positioning the patient on the table so that the disc space involved is above the flexion break in the table and then flexing the table.

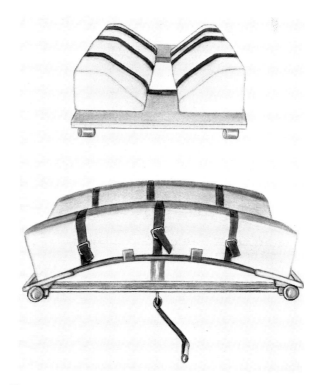

Fig. 83-7. Prone position frame. (Reprinted from Finneson BE: *Low Back Pain.* 2nd ed. Philadelphia, Lippincott, 1981, with permission.)

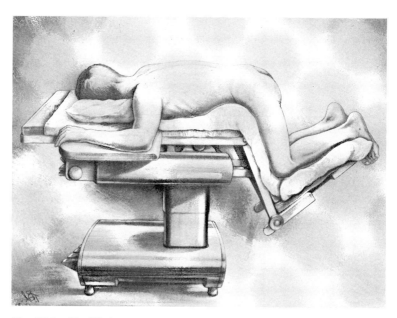

Fig. 83-8. Modified prone position. (Reprinted from Finneson BE: *Low Back Pain.* 2nd ed. Philadelphia, Lippincott, 1981, with permission.)

The disadvantage of this position is more increased difficulty on the part of the assistant in holding the root retractor or in performing other necessary functions. Those who are not experienced with this position may find it technically unsatisfactory.

Most lumbar disc surgeons prefer the prone position, in which the patient is intubated on a litter. After the endotracheal tube has been taped securely in place, the patient is rolled onto the operating table, which has previously been prepared either with blanket rolls or a "prone position frame" (Figs. 83-6 and 83-7).

A modification of the prone position can be obtained by flexing the hips and knees 90°, with no effort made to flex the lumbar spine itself. Flexing the hip affords satisfactory flexion of the lumbar spine comparable to the other positions, and it may be associated with somewhat less abdominal pressure. To achieve this position, a minor adjustment of the operating table is accomplished by removing the adjustable headrest and fitting it to the footrest so that it will provide adequate support for the legs (Fig. 84-8).

The thin patient with a flat belly will do well either with the prone position frame or with blanket rolls. Such a position, however, is poorly tolerated by the obese individual, since neither the frame nor the blanket rolls will adequately accommodate a large, protuberant abdomen. Abdominal compression is apt to increase lumbar epidural venous distention, and the resulting hemorrhage will be an impediment to satisfactory visualization. In the presence of copious epidural bleeding, the surgeon may have difficulty concentrating on the prime objective of disc excision and adequate nerve root decompression, since the major efforts will be directed at controlling the hemorrhage. Such an irritating environment may lead to a mishap and is not conducive to the calm and deliberate atmosphere so helpful to safe and smooth surgery.

Several positions have evolved in which the abdomen is completely free and unencumbered. Usually some sort of operating table attachment is required to secure and immobilize the hips and thighs. This support is usually assembled by a friendly hospital maintenance machinist or a handy surgeon.

Surface Landmarks

After the patient is draped, the iliac crests and other bony landmarks that provide approximate relationships to spinal level are obscured. For this reason, it is necessary to prepare a surface guide to interspace identification before draping. Personal preference is the cutaneous tatoo, which is made at the level of the disc protrusion using fluoroscopic guidance after completion of the myelogram. If this is not part of the surgeon's routine, other aids can be employed.

If a myelogram has been done recently, the lumbar puncture mark on the skin can be used as a landmark for the spinal level. For example, if the lumbar puncture needle is seen on the myelogram films to be at the L3-4 interspace, this will serve as an excellent surface guide for identification of the underlying vertebrae. If a myelogram has not been carried out recently, the first interspace at or immediately below the iliac crest can be considered L3-4 (Fig. 83-9). Using this as a starting site, one may count down to the involved interspace and scratch a "crosshatch" in the skin at that level with a sterile hypodermic needle subsequent to cleansing the skin with an alcohol sponge (Fig. 83-10).

When using surface guides, the elasticity of the skin must be kept in mind, particularly with obese patients. This elasticity may permit a surface marking to shift to the extent of an interspace from the distortion caused by the use of retractors and alterations in the degree of lumbar flexion during surgery.

Incisions

For many years my routine incision extended over approximately three spinous processes to allow for interspace localization and for adequate illumination, with the ends of the incision permitting overhead lighting to funnel in. I considered the short incision an ego trip on the part of

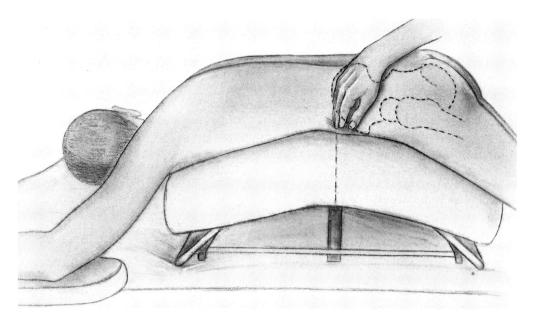

Fig. 83-9. Flexion "break" in table or frame at level of iliac crest. (Reprinted from Finneson BE: *Low Back Pain.* 2nd ed. Philadelphia, Lippincott, 1981, with permission.)

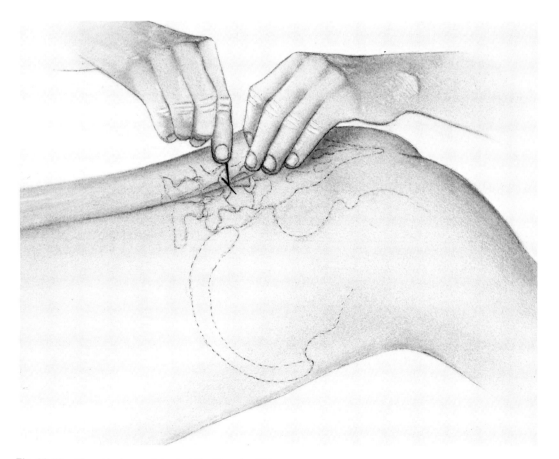

Fig. 83-10. The skin is scratched at the "involved" interspinous space. (Reprinted from Finneson BE: *Low Back Pain.* 2nd ed. Philadelphia, Lippincott, 1981, with permission.)

the surgeon. Further experience has changed my opinion, and I presently believe that the short incision is beneficial to the patient's postoperative recovery.

There is no question that patients feel immeasurably better in the immediate interval after a short-incision operation than after a large or standard-incision operation. Of greater importance is the fact that the long incision, which extends over several spinous processes, produces a band of scar that extends from the skin and attaches to the spinous processes and laminae along the length of the incision. This scar tissue is not as supple as nonscarred muscle and fascia. The lack of elasticity and suppleness is not conducive to a nicely distributed lumbar curvature after the wound has healed. This nonsupple lumbar spine probably makes the patient more vulnerable to recurrent low back dysfunction in the future.

When a small incision is made, the precise location of the involved interspace is crucial, as described under the section "Surface Landmarks."

When the small incision is used, fiberoptic lighting and magnification are a necessity. The fiberoptic lighting and operating loupes or the operating microscope are of great advantage. These instruments aid greatly in assuring that tissue is handled delicately and they help to prevent nerve root damage. I consider them an integral and essential aid to the surgery.

There are a variety of methods used to control skin bleeding, including Michel clips, Kolodney clamps, and mosquitoes. Weitlaner self-retaining retractors, which place the skin under tension, will stop most of the minor skin bleeding; the several remaining subcutaneous vessels are easily controlled by cautery. Blood vessel cauterization should not be performed with a hemostat, since it invariably results in considerable tissue destruction. When carried out near the surface of the skin, hemostat cauterization may result in a full-thickness skin burn, and the resulting skin slough or necrosis may eventuate into a wound infection. To properly control skin bleeding with cautery, an assistant should use fine-toothed forceps to evert the skin edge, while the surgeon employs suction to locate the bleeding vessel precisely, and then uses a fine-tipped Cushing forceps to cauterize only the vessel, taking care to avoid cautery spread to surrounding tissue.

A second knife ("clean knife") should be used to incise through fat to the fascia. If the patient is extremely obese, the Weitlaner retractors may have to be reset more deeply. Additional bleeding can be controlled with the use of the cautery. When performing the initial incision, the surgeon should not be obsessive about sweeping the fat cleanly away from the fascia. He must remember that a surgical procedure is being carried out, not an anatomic exposure. This step can only serve to increase the blood loss and, even more serious, to create a false space that may fill with blood in the postoperative period.

Subperiosteal Dissection

The subperiosteal muscles can be dissected by a variety of methods (Fig. 83-11). I prefer to use a periosteal elevator pressed against the edge of the spinous process and to cut directly against the lateral edge of the spine. In this manner the posterior spinous ligament or supraspinal ligament, which is a strong fibrous cord that extends without interruption along the tips of the spinous processes from C7 to the median sacral crest and which is continuous with the interspinal ligaments, is preserved. It is valuable to preserve this structure and so to avoid unnecessary weakening of the spinal supporting ligaments. To prevent unnecessary tissue destruction and scarring, a scalpel should be used to incise the fascia rather than a cutting cautery. The muscles are best stripped from the spinous processes and lamina with the bimanual two-periosteal-elevator method. One periosteal elevator is used to retract the muscle mass laterally, while the other is used to perform a careful subperiosteal dissection. The periosteum should be peeled as cleanly as possible from the spinous process and lamina without penetrating the muscle which, if torn, may be a source of troublesome bleeding.

After the subperiosteal dissection has been accomplished under direct vision, a sponge extended to its full length is used to strip the bone of any remaining fragments of muscle and fas-

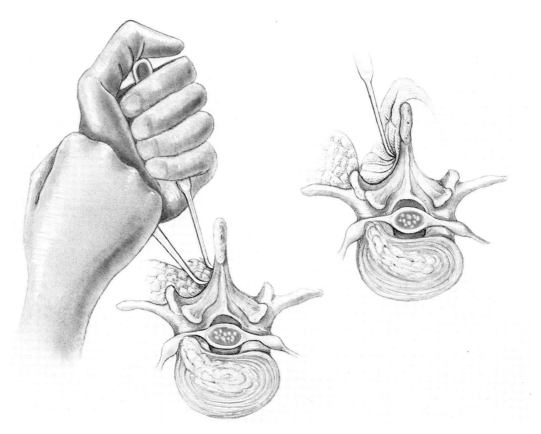

Fig. 83-11. Subperiosteal dissection technique. (Reprinted from Finneson BE: *Low Back Pain.* 2nd ed. Philadelphia, Lippincott, 1981 with permission.)

cia. As bone is cleaned with the sponge, it should be allowed to accumulate within the incision to act as a tamponade and prevent muscle bleeding. Any bleeding occurring from the cut edge of the fascia is controlled with cautery. The subperiosteal muscle dissection is carried out laterally to expose the articulation between the superior and inferior articular processes.

After all surface bleeding has been controlled, the sponges are removed and the desired interspace is localized by the time-honored method of palpating the sacrum and then counting up from it. This localization should be checked with the plain x-ray films of the spine to be sure that the patient does not have a lumbarized first sacral segment or sacralized fifth lumbar segment. Skeletal localization then should be correlated with the myelographic defect.

If the sacrum cannot be adequately palpated, or if for some other reason the surgeon is not totally satisfied with the identification of the anatomic level, surgery should be stopped at this point and a definite interspace confirmation obtained with a lateral lumbar spine roentgenogram.

One topic not likely to be discussed at length in the medical literature is the frequency of interspace misidentification at surgery. I occasionally find such an error in a referred patient, and I am aware of two occasions when I myself made such a mistake. Both of my mishaps occurred in the 1950s, when I was less aware of my fallibility and much too decisive to slow up my surgery for an "unnecessary x-ray film." This error is most likely to occur in either grossly obese patients or patients whose partial lumbarization of the first sacral segment dorsal element confuses the surgeon.

When in doubt, it is important to obtain a roentgenogram, not only for the surgeon's peace of mind but also so that he can be absolutely certain that the interspace being worked on is the proper one. When pathology is not apparent at first inspection, such knowledge may provide additional incentive for a most thorough and meticulous interspace exploration and decompression, including a generous foraminal decompression.

Once the surgeon is completely satisfied that proper localization has been established, he can place the hemilaminectomy retractors in position (Fig. 83-12A). A variety of hemilaminectomy retractors is available, the simplest being the Taylor spinal retractor, which consists of a right-angled metal ribbon with a slightly hooked tip that can be inserted laterally and cephalad to the articular facet. The great disadvantage is that it has to be either hand-held by the assistant or tied to the base of the operating table or to the foot of the surgeon. Also, it has the unfortunate propensity to slip out of place occasionally—invariably at the worst possible moment of the procedure.

Most surgeons prefer a self-retaining hemilaminectomy retractor based on the many modifications of the Hoen hemilaminectomy retractor (Fig. 83-12B).

When positioning the hemilaminectomy retractors, the shortest blades possible should be used to achieve adequate exposure, so that the flange of the blades will rest flush with the skin surface. If the flange projects above the skin, it increases the depth through which the surgeon must work. The spinous process blade of the retractor should fit between the spinous interspaces, with the hook or hooks embedded into the interspinous ligaments. The muscle blade should rise above the hump of the articular facet (Fig. 83-12C). An occasional error is made by impinging the tip of the muscle blade against the facet; this causes the exposure to be needlessly narrow. By placing the paraspinal muscles under tension, the retractors will stop most muscle bleeding. After the retractors are in place and the exposure is deemed satisfactory, any remaining muscle bleeding is controlled with cautery.

It must be emphasized that the remainder of the surgery takes place in that small keyhole of interlaminar space, and any skin, fascia, or muscle bleeding will funnel directly into the work area. If the assistant has to provide suction to remove the blood, either his head will be in the way, which will obstruct the surgeon's vision, or the assistant will be poking the suction tip into the wound blindly, which also has its disadvantages. The other alternative is for the surgeon to hold the suction in one hand and operate with the other; this also is not really satisfactory. Control of bleeding at this stage is therefore a must for smooth, safe surgery.

Developing the Interspace

The laminae vary greatly in width, in angulation, and in position relative to each other, so that occasionally the interlaminar space is sufficiently wide to permit exposure and removal of a protruding intervertebral disc without removal of any, or very little, bone. This widened interlaminar space is seen most commonly between the L_5-S_1 levels and less frequently above the interspace.

The more strenuous bone work of the operation is followed by relatively delicate dissection of the soft tissue interspace involving yellow ligament, nerve root, and dura. This strenuous manual work tends to create a hand tremor that is distressingly obvious when the surgery is being performed with magnification techniques such as loupes or an operating microscope. Air-powered rongeurs can be used for much of the bone work in the hope of reducing a postexertion tremor that may develop while manipulating the nerve root and other soft tissues within the interspace.

When dealing with an interspace of normal dimensions, any rongeur, including duckbilled, Leksell, or Kerrison, can be used to remove the overhanging, inferior edge of the superior vertebrae (Fig. 83-13). If working on the L_5-S_1 interspace, this would be the inferior edge of the L5 lamina. Some surgeons prefer rongeuring away the inferior half of the superior lamina, which exposes the superior border of the yellow ligament. This can be grasped with an Allis tissue forceps and the remainder of the ligament excised by sharp dissection with a scalpel. I prefer to remove only the inferior one-third of the superior lamina so that the edge of the yellow ligament is not exposed. Bone wax is used to control all bone bleeding from the rongeured edge of the

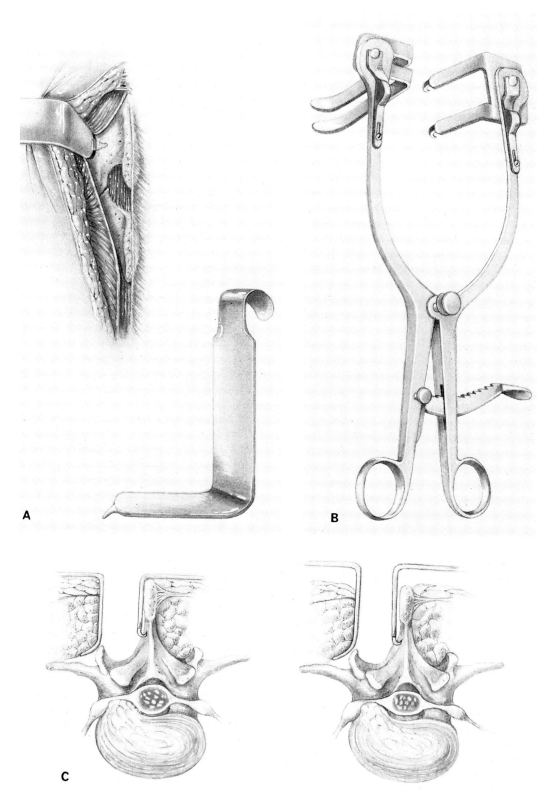

Fig. 83-12. **A.** Taylor hemilaminectomy retractor. **B.** Hoen hemilaminectomy retractor. **C.** If the hemilaminectomy retractor blades are longer than necessary, the depth through which the surgeon must work is increased. (Reprinted from Finneson BE: *Low Back Pain.* 2nd ed. Philadelphia, Lippincott, 1981, with permission.)

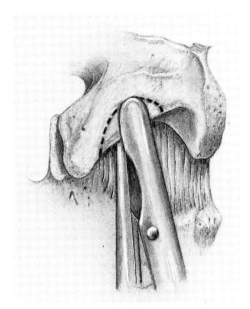

Fig. 83-13. The overhanging edge of the superior lamina is rongeured. (Reprinted from Finneson BE: *Low Back Pain.* 2nd ed. Philadelphia, Lippincott, 1981, with permission.)

lamina. After the one-third overhang of the superior lamina has been removed, an ample area of the ligamentum flavum will be exposed to view. A No. 11 blade on a long handle then is used to make a shallow incision in the ligamentum flavum along the direction of its fibers. The edge of the incision is grasped with an Allis forceps and tugged laterally in order to spread the incision. This allows the No. 11 blade to be used to incise the entire thickness of the yellow ligament down to the epidural fat (Fig. 83-14). After a small, moistened cotton patty has been introduced beneath the ligamentum flavum to separate it from the dura, this incision is extended from the superior lamina to the inferior lamina. Care should be taken to insert merely the tip of the blade beneath the ligament to avoid accidentally cutting into the dura. A second Allis forceps is used to get a firmer grasp on the full thickness of yellow ligament. A curette is introduced below the yellow ligament against the inferior surface of the superior vertebra, which permits a flap of yellow ligament to be curetted laterally while the remainder is left attached to the dorsal surface of the inferior lamina. This attachment then can be safely excised with a scalpel or scissors (Fig. 83-15).

Epidural Fat and Nerve Root Damage

Once the yellow ligament has been excised, the epidural fat can be clearly visualized. Treatment of the epidural fat recently has developed into a conjectural issue. It is now generally agreed that preservation of a layer of epidural fat, especially around the nerve root, will be helpful in preventing subsequent encasement of the root within the dense epidural scar tissue that forms following an interspace exploration. For this reason, surgeons attempt to carry out disc excision without disturbing the epidural fat. This fatty layer, however, almost always obscures the dura and nerve root. In this laudable effort to prevent future damage of the root by postoperative scar tissue, the surgeon may create immediate and possibly persisting injury to the root during surgery because of his inability to visualize this structure adequately.

Frequently, a flap of epidural fat can be retracted so that good visualization of the root and dura is obtained. After completion of this procedure, the epidural fat can be tucked back into position around the root. If satisfactory root identification and visualization are not possible with

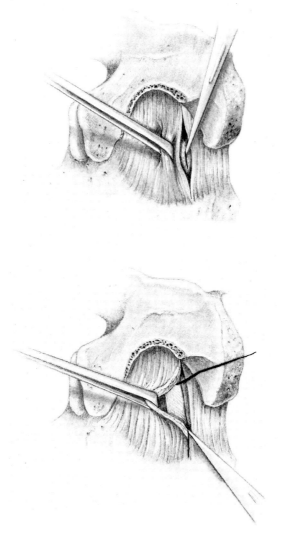

Fig. 83-14. The yellow ligament is cut. (Reprinted from Finneson BE: *Low Back Pain.* 2nd ed. Philadelphia, Lippincott, 1981, with permission.)

preservation of the fat, however, it should be excised. A surgeon is not able to protect a structure that cannot be adequately visualized, and I am aware of two recent postoperative nerve root injuries that two separate surgeons attributed to their desire to preserve the epidural fat. If the epidural fat has been removed, a small stamp of subcutaneous fat can be placed over the dura and nerve root as a free fat graft. Subsequent dissections and explorations have demonstrated a reasonably high rate of "take" of this type of graft.

It is important to remember that the goal of surgery is adequate decompression of the root, while at the same time gently and safely handling the root. At this stage of the surgery, nerve root damage may occur in two ways. One occasional error is to mistake the lateral reflection of the yellow ligament immediately over the root for the root itself. Sometimes after excision of the medial portion of the yellow ligament, the lateral portion rolls up on itself, creating a cylindrical appearance that may be quite deceptive (Fig. 83-16). If this cylinder is retracted medially, the underlying root may be mistakenly identified as a bulging disc, which is then attacked with vigor. Another error may occur when the interlaminar exposure is extended laterally and the lateral re-

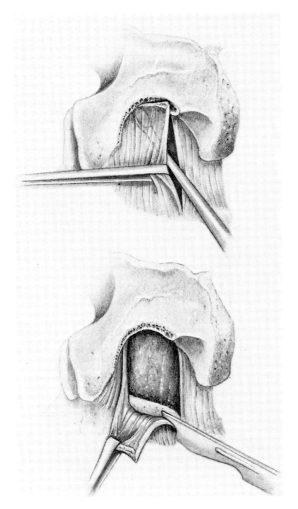

Fig. 83-15. The yellow ligament is curetted. (Reprinted from Finneson BE: *Low Back Pain.* 2nd ed. Philadelphia, Lippincott, 1981, with permission.)

flection of yellow ligament and bone is trimmed. This portion of the exposure must be performed under good visualization, with care being taken to hug the inferior bony and ligamentous surface with the jaws of the Schlesinger punch. If the tip of this rongeur is inserted too deeply, it may grasp a bit of the root along with the edge of the yellow ligament and bone. As the surgeon tugs on the instrument, a fairly long, glistening piece of tissue, resembling spaghetti, comes out, followed by bloody spinal fluid. These errors are classifiable as surgical tragedies and usually can be avoided by proper hemostasis, good visualization, and a cautious pace at this point in the operation.

A thin edge of bone is removed from the superior edge of the inferior lamina using a laminectomy punch that is not angled downward. The 40° angled jaw is helpful in working on the superior lamina and laterally, but may produce a dural tear at the inferior lamina (Fig. 83-17). A slight fold of dura may bulge and be pinched and torn in the jaws of the bone-biting instrument. Most of the fibers in the dura are longitudinal (running up and down); if the instrument catches a fiber and the surgeon pulls without adequate visualization, to quote that outstanding spinal surgeon George Ehni, "The dura will rip open like a seam." Just a small bit of bone easily can cause a tear an inch long in the dura. If the dura is opened inadvertently, a small hole is usually easier to close than a large one. Dissection should therefore proceed cautiously on the inferior lamina. A

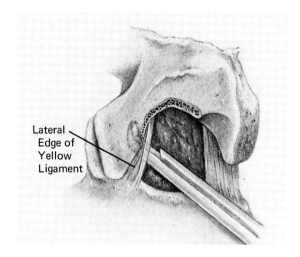

Fig. 83-16. In widening the interspace, do not mistake the roll-up lateral edge of yellow ligament for the root. (Reprinted from Finneson BE: *Low Back Pain.* 2nd ed. Philadelphia, Lippincott, 1981, with permission.)

bite of bone should not be taken with the rongeur and ripped out. The instrument should be closed carefully and the bone eased out very slowly, so that if the dura is tugged even slightly, the surgeon will be able to visualize the tenting of the dura and can then release the instrument and inspect the area carefully before proceeding further. This type of complication always occurs before an adequate exposure has been obtained. Cerebrospinal fluid may fill the wound suddenly, becoming tinged with blood, so that it is impossible to see the damaged area. There is a tendency to try to close this opening immediately, but this is a mistake. It is also a mistake to try to visualize the damage by putting a sucker directly into the wound, because the roots may float out of the dural tear with the escaping spinal fluid, catch on the tip of the sucker, and sometimes be severely damaged. Instead of direct suction, a cottonoid should be inserted into the opening, and

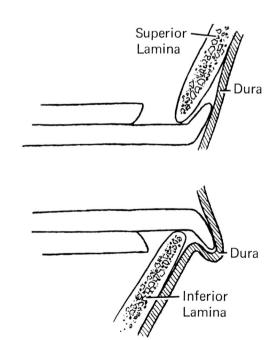

Fig. 83-17. The laminectomy punch with a 40° angled jaw is helpful when working on the superior lamina, but is not suited for the slope of the inferior lamina and may produce a dural tear. (Reprinted from Finneson BE: *Low Back Pain.* 2nd ed. Philadelphia, Lippincott, 1981, with permission.)

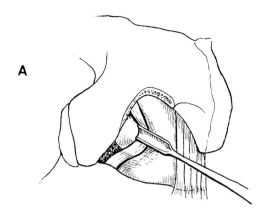

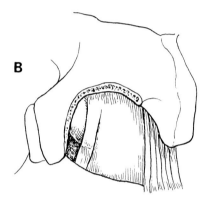

Fig. 83-18. **A.** Overstretched root and dural sac with an inadequate lateral bony exposure. **B.** Very little root retraction is necessary with adequate lateral bony exposure. (Reprinted from Finneson BE: *Low Back Pain.* 2nd ed. Philadelphia, Lippincott, 1981, with permission.)

suction should be applied only on the cottonoid until the structures can be seen. Then a square of Gelfoam can be placed over the dural tear and a cottonoid can be placed on top of the Gelfoam square. The table should be tilted head down so that spinal fluid pressure will decrease in the lumbar region. If the table or laminectomy frame is flexed, it should be flattened. The surgeon then can proceed as though the dura had not been opened. After the disc has been excised and the root has been decompressed, full attention can be given to the torn dura. Before closing the dural tear, it is necessary to expose both sides and both ends of the tear. Dural closure must be watertight; 4-0 or 5-0 suture material should be used.

In carrying out a lateral bony exposure, a partial excision of the facet may be necessary for exposure of the lateral margin of the nerve root. This does not cause pain or an unstable spine when performed unilaterally. Bilateral facet excision and disc excision at that level may produce spinal instability and pain.

An adequate intervertebral lateral exposure may be of value for three reasons:

1. It facilitates satisfactory disc excision because there is less danger of overstretching the nerve root and dural sac as these structures are retracted medially. With an adequate lateral exposure, much less root retraction is necessary to afford good access to the disc (Figs. 83-18 A and B).
2. A satisfactory lateral exposure is the first step of a foraminotomy that provides bony decompression of the involved root, and almost always manifests some degree of edema and swelling.
3. In the years after surgery, hypertrophic osteoarthritic bony spurring, in association with postoperative epidural and perineural scarring, will be less likely to lead to root compression symptoms in the presence of a generous lateral exposure and foraminotomy.

Following an adequate bony exposure, the epidural fat will be visible. If the nerve root is obscured by the fat, two Cushing forceps can be used to separate the fat from the underlying dura and nerve root. In order to preserve the fat, it should be peeled medially to form a retractable flap that can be tucked back into place around the root after disc excision. Only after exposure of the nerve root can blood vessels within the epidural fat be safely cauterized without danger of damage to the root by cautery current. The Malis bipolar coagulator with bipolar forceps allows current to flow only from one forceps tip to the other. This isolated current, which produces much less heat, reduces the likelihood of inadvertent nerve root irritation or damage.

Interlaminar Surgery

Although the interlaminar space is rather small, the minute anatomy of this area does vary considerably. It is always amazing to see how much can be hidden within this tiny space. An orderly and systematic approach to the area is paramount to successful disc surgery.

Inspection

The field should be dry at this stage. If bleeding remains a problem, decreasing lumbar flexion to a flatter position may reduce abdominal pressure and so reduce engorgement of the lumbar epidural veins. If this change in position is effective in controlling epidural venous bleeding, the surgeon should proceed with surgery in the flatter position.

Is the root elevated or is it flat? Does the root appear swollen or hyperemic, or is it the same color as the rest of the dura?

In patients who have had long-standing symptoms, adhesions between the nerve root and the posterior longitudinal ligament are occasionally quite dense. Very careful dissection of the root and the dura may be necessary to allow free retraction and exposure of the protruding disc.

Root Tension

It should be possible to retract medially, without resistance, a root that is under no pressure, using a narrow blunt retractor. As a rule, the typical protruding disc will be quite apparent when the root is retracted medially and manifests itself by slight elevation of the root and by increased pressure on medial retraction. It is at this stage of the procedure that considerable care must be taken to avoid stretching a compromised root. When the disc protrusion is extensive, it is best not to retract the root too vigorously over it in order to avoid excessive stretching of the root. When the root is under too much pressure to be retracted medially with ease, the root should not be retracted but should be decompressed by working laterally to it.

If extruded disc fragments are free within the canal, they usually can be manipulated laterally, grasped with the pituitary forceps, and gently removed. If the disc is not extruded but is bulging so much that the nerve cannot be moved medially easily, the surgeon should work lateral to the disc, introduce the pituitary forceps into the intervertebral disc space, and remove disc fragments piecemeal until the root can be retracted more easily over the partially decompressed annular shell.

The major error at this point comes under the heading of "grandstanding." There is a temptation to demonstrate the pathology to any and all present in the operating room. The root is retracted medially and maintained in an overstretched position while residents, interns, nurses, and visitors are invited to inspect the protruding disc. This is not the time to "entertain the troops," and a herniated disc is not a very spectacular sight in any event. Retraction of such a swollen, inflamed nerve is best kept to a minimum to avoid adding to the irreversible damage already caused by the disc protrusion.

Sometimes a disc protrusion is a bit more medial, and the nerve root does not appear ele-

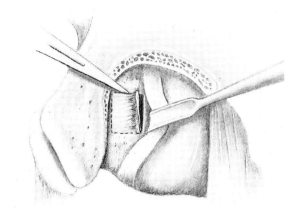

Fig. 83-19. Incision of rectangular window through the annulus fibrosus. (Reprinted from Finneson BE: *Low Back Pain.* 2nd ed. Philadelphia, Lippincott, 1981, with permission.)

vated or under pressure. On attempting to retract the nerve root medially, however, an obstruction is encountered. The surgeon then must be careful to lift the root and dura to determine whether a medially protruding disc is present.

Intervertebral Disc Excision

Once the disc has been partially excised, there is little difficulty in retracting the root medially. A nerve root retractor then can be used to expose the disc space more completely. A No. 11 blade is used to make a rectangular slab-shaped window through the annulus, and through this opening an adequate subtotal excision of disc contents is performed. This window extends from the most medial exposure of the annulus to the lateral limits of the bony exposure and comprises the entire width of the intervertebral disc, which is bounded by the bodies of the superior and inferior vertebrae (Fig. 83-19). Pituitary forceps of various sizes and shapes, as well as a curette, can be used to free up loose fragments of disc material. Excision of a rectangular slab of annulus may prevent the remaining shell of annulus from buckling as the disc space narrows. This buckling is to be prevented because it may fibrose and provide a source of root compression a year or two postoperatively. It is generally accepted that some reduction of the intervertebral space will occur. This seems likely in view of the fact that patients with long-standing disc disease who have not had surgery will often demonstrate interspace narrowing.

In using intervertebral disc rongeur forceps within the intervertebral space, great care is necessary to avoid penetrating the instrument through the anterior annulus fibrosus and the anterior longitudinal ligament. Such penetration is precarious and may result in laceration of one of the great vessels located anterior to the vertebral space (Fig. 83-20). Experienced and competent lumbar disc surgeons have suffered this calamity, and when working deep within the intervertebral space, the surgeon must remain alert to the possibility of this mishap. Degenerative changes affecting an intervertebral disc are generalized and may cause softening of the anterior annular fibers and anterior longitudinal ligament. These structures, when reasonably firm, will usually offer resistance to instrument penetration; but when softened, the surgeon may unknowingly poke through the anterior annular fibers with disc rongeur forceps. After such inadvertent penetration, the iliac artery may be grasped and torn by the forceps. Various methods

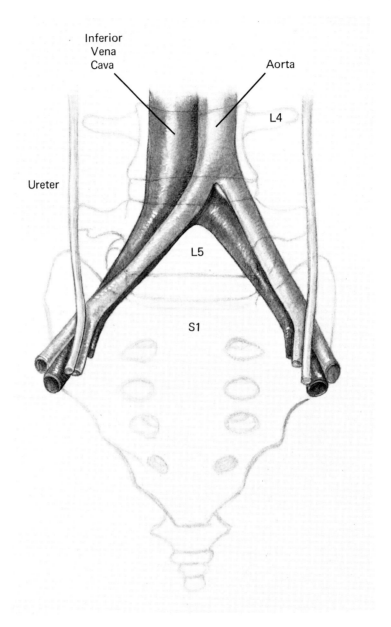

Fig. 83-20. The major vessels and ureters and their relationship to the anterior lumbar spine. (Reprinted from Finneson BE: *Low Back Pain,* 2nd ed. Philadelphia, Lippincott, 1981, with permission.)

have been advocated to avoid this problem, including marking the instruments 1¹/₂ inches from the tip as a visual reminder of depth penetration. Good lighting and magnification aid in depth perception and in visualization of the interior of the disc space.

Free Disc Fragments

Occasionally the protruded disc is in the "axilla" between the dural sac and the nerve root. A most meticulous dissection of this extruded fragment is necessary, and care should be taken when this fragment is grasped with an intervertebral disc rongeur forceps to avoid damage to the adjacent laterally displaced nerve root. It is occasionally difficult to recognize a completely free

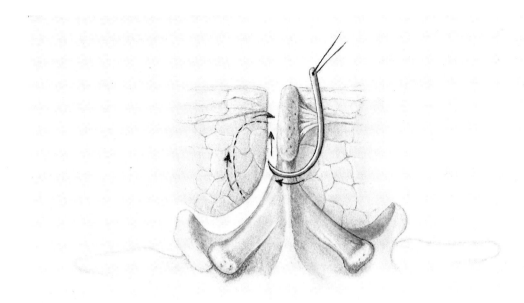

Fig. 83-21. Muscle closure to eliminate "dead space." (Reprinted from Finneson BE: *Low Back Pain.* 2nd ed. Philadelpia, Lippincott, 1981, with permission.)

extruded fragment within the axilla. It may resemble epidural fat, and in some cases, only the tip of the extruded fragment presents dorsally, with the bulk of it not being visible and indenting the inferior portion of the dural sac medially. The surgeon, unaware of this large extrusion, may retract the nerve root and dural sac medially together with the free fragment and expose a bulging or protruding annulus. The disc protrusion will be excised and the interspace evacuated as thoroughly as possible by the usual methods, including curettage and the use of the intervertebral disc forceps. The offending free fragment that is causing root pressure, however, will inadvertently be left untouched. The lack of free nerve root mobility may be an indication that such a fragment is present. When the nerve root is not free, further inspection is necessary.

A free disc fragment may extrude beneath the posterior spinal ligament. It occasionally will produce a sizable mass that is capable of producing symptoms that will not be evident to casual inspection. Palpation over the posterior spinal ligament with a thin elevator will disclose this extrusion, and it can be "milked" laterally to expose an amount of disc tissue sufficient enough to be grasped with the intervertebral disc forceps and removed.

Surgical Judgment

In those patients in whom there is no gross protrusion of the disc but rather a slightly humped-up annulus, the surgeon must use judgment in deciding whether to excise the high annulus and curette the intervertebral disc space, or to be content with posterior bony decompression of the nerve root by means of a foraminotomy.

A disc should not be violated unless it can be seen to be causing nerve root pressure. Once the disc is violated, however, thorough disc excision is probably advisable. A bulging annulus does not have to be removed, particularly if the nerve root can be adequately decompressed. The root can easily go over a slight hump as long as there is no bony counterpressure above it. Sometimes a generous foraminotomy alone is adequate. In equivocal cases, injection of saline into the disc with a 10-ml syringe may be helpful. If the bulging disc does not take more than 1 or 2 ml of saline without a great deal of pressure, it might be tempting to limit the approach to a decompressive foraminotomy. On the other hand, if the entire 10 ml of the saline can be injected into the intervertebral disc space without a great deal of difficulty, the disc could be considered more pathologic.

Nerve Root Anomalies

Occasionally the nerve root exiting from the foramen above the surgically exposed interspace will descend medially beneath the facets of the next lower interspace. This minor deviation is not significant unless the surgeon happens to carry out a rather extensive lateral interlaminar exposure. Because the surgeon's attention is focused on the nerve root under direct vision, he may be unaware of an equally vital neural structure that is partially hidden by the lateral reflection of the yellow ligament. Even more rarely, two nerve roots may exit from the same foramen. When the dura and its nerve root is exposed, there is a second root just lateral to the first root. If it is recognized as a nerve root, there is no problem, but occasionally the laterally positioned root is mistaken for a bulging disc, and attempts are made to excise it. In doing so the root may be injured beyond repair. There is no substitute for good lighting and magnification. In addition, the operation should always be done questioningly, since the surgeon is working through a "keyhole," and identification of structures is extremely important.

After the protruded intervertebral disc has been adequately excised, the operating room table or spinal rest is flattened, so that the original flexed position is now a relatively straight one. This change is position places the root under less tension, narrows the posterior intervertebral disc space, and increases the depth between the skin surface and the interlaminar space. The interspace then is re-explored, and occasionally several additional fragments of disc material can be removed with the posterior vertebral bodies closer together. At the termination of the procedure, the nerve root should be under no pressure whatsoever, either anteriorly from the intervertebral disc or from bony constriction within the intervertebral foramen, which should have been partially opened during the bony dissection.

Bleeding from epidural veins should be carefully controlled before closure of the wound. Occasionally, a small pledget of Gelfoam is required to control venous bleeding.

Wound Closure

The suture material of personal preference is 2-0 chromic gut for muscle and fascia, 3-0 plain gut for subcutaneous tissue, and monofilament nylon for skin.

An important, but often overlooked, hemilaminectomy closure technique is the elimination of the dead space, which may fill with clot and contribute to postoperative discomfort (Fig. 83-21). This is accomplished with 2-0 chromic suture passed through the interspinous ligament and then into the paraspinal muscles to approximate the paraspinal muscles against the laminae and spinous processes. This hemostatic suture should not be tied so tight that it causes muscle necrosis.

REFERENCES

1. Finneson BE: A lumbar disc surgery predictive score card, *Spine 3*:186–188, 1978
2. Barr JS, Mixter WJ: Posterior protrusion of the lumbar intervertebral discs. *J Bone Jt Surg 23*:444–456, 1941

CHAPTER 84
Microsurgical Lumbar Disc Excision

Donald H. Wilson   Robert Harbaugh

IN 1934, MIXTER AND BARR[1] reported that a protruded lumbar disc was a common cause of sciatica and that the pain could be relieved by removing the offending disc. At that time, the clinical and radiologic features of such a protrusion were imprecise, so the operation had to be exploratory as well as therapeutic. Total laminectomies often were performed at several levels in order to discover a single protruded disc, which was eventually removed *through* the dura. The mortality rate exceeded 20 percent.

The standard discectomy of today represents a considerable refinement of the procedure performed by Mixter and Barr less than 50 years ago. But there is still room for improvement. The "failed disc" syndrome[2] remains a common cause of disability. This syndrome may be defined as the recurrence of sciatica some time after an apparently successful lumbar discectomy, and is due to two factors, either singly or in combination: poor selection of the patient and excessive trauma to the contents of the epidural space.

The ligamentum flavum is the protective cover of the spinal canal. If it is not replaced by an equally effective barrier, scar tissue may proliferate from torn muscle and bind the dura and nerve root to the walls of the canal. A free fat graft[3] has been shown to be the most effective replacement for ligamentum flavum.

The nerve roots within the lumbar canal move several millimeters with each stride, and their lubrication is provided by the abundant fat that encases them.[4-6] Destruction of epidural fat by hemorrhage or manipulation diminishes the ability of the nerve roots to slide, and replacement of fat by scar tissue further binds the roots to the walls of the lumbar canal. The result is a traction neuropathy as severe as the pressure neuropathy from the disc protrusion. When direct trauma to a nerve root is superimposed upon the indirect damage from hemorrhage and loss of epidural fat, all the factors necessary for the "failed disc" syndrome are present.

By defining the weaknesses of the standard discectomy operation, criteria for improvement of the procedure can be established: smaller incisions with less dissection of muscle, preservation of the ligamentum flavum, preservation of epidural fat by gentle manipulation of the contents of the epidural space, meticulous hemostasis, and, of course, adequate removal of the disc.

If means become available to fulfill these criteria, the operation evolves. But it must be shown through the results that the newer operation is equal to the *best* results obtainable from the older technique.

The means for refining standard lumbar discectomy may be present in microsurgical technique. Microneurosurgery is an evolving field that requires proficiency in the use of a microscope for operations within the cranial cavity and spinal canal. Magnification and brilliant illumina-

Section of Neurosurgery, Dartmouth-Hitchcock Medical Center, Hanover, New Hampshire

tion have allowed neurosurgeons to refine many standard operations and to devise new ones for problems in hitherto inaccessible areas. The contributions microsurgery makes to an operation are small incisions, meticulous hemostasis, and precise removal of diseased tissue.

Within the spinal canal, the use of microsurgical technique has become necessary for the removal of angiomatous malformations[7,8] and intramedullary tumors,[9] and is recommended for the removal of cervical and thoracic disc protrusion.[10,11] It is therefore surprising that there have been so few reports of its use in the most frequently performed neurosurgical operation, lumbar discectomy.

Microsurgical Lumbar Discectomy

Many of the protocols and procedures used in standard lumbar discectomy are the same for microsurgical lumbar discectomy.

Selection of Patients

Patients should be admitted to the hospital after a reasonable trial of bedrest has failed to relieve their sciatica. Back pain alone is not a reason for admission. Physical examination and plain x-rays of the chest and lumbar vertebrae should precede myelography (metrizimide was substituted for Pantopaque in our department when that dye was introduced in 1977).

An abnormal myelogram with abnormal signs, or abnormal signs with an equivocal myelogram, are indications for surgery. A normal or equivocal myelogram without abnormal signs, however, indicates a need for further conservative treatment or an epidural venogram. In our experience venography has revealed hidden protrusions on several occasions.

Operative Technique

On the night before surgery the patient is instructed to take a shower using povidone-iodine detergent. In the operating room the patient is placed under endotracheal, or preferably, epidural anesthesia, and is placed prone and slightly flexed at the waist on the operating table. "Vacuum" bolsters* positioned on either side of the body allow the abdomen and chest to sag between them. The back is shaved with an electric razor then cleansed with povidone-iodine detergent. This is followed by the application of 10% povidone-iodine solution. A spinal needle is inserted between the two appropriate spinous processes, and a lateral x-ray is taken to mark the correct interspace.

A 1-inch incision is made between the two appropriate spinous processes. Dissection proceeds through the connective tissue and fat to the lumbodorsal fascia. This is incised to one side of the midline crossing fibers, which assures support for placement of the self-retaining Williams retractor. This paramedian incision, which spares the interspinous ligament, is continued close to the spine until it is long enough to allow easy insertion of a finger. The lateral extension of the interspinous ligament is divided down to the interlaminar space. When this ligament gives way, the index finger is used to probe down to the interlaminar space. A periosteal elevator then is used to push an open 4 × 6-inch sponge ahead of it with a downward, then lateral sweeping motion, which cleans all tissue from the ligamentum flavum. The sponge is removed and replaced with the narrow Williams retractor (Fig. 84-1).

An operating microscope e.g., a Zeiss OPMI I-H equipped with 12.5× eyepieces, inclined binocular tubes, and a 300-mm objective is brought into use. Magnification changer settings range from 0.4 to 1 as the dissection proceeds deeper.

The ligamentum flavum is incised along the border of the inferior lamina from the midline laterally with a No. 11 blade. When epidural fat is seen, a small cottonoid patty is stuffed into the

*Olympia Vac-Pac #30, Olympia Medical Corp., Seattle, Washington.

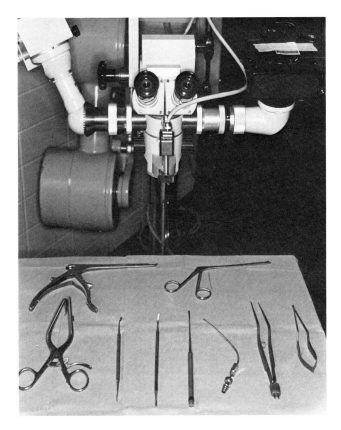

Fig. 84-1. Instruments required for microsurgical lumbar disc excision (clockwise from upper left): angled Kerrison rongeur, small pituitary forceps, microscissors, bipolar cautery forceps, thin sucker, Penfield dissector, dental probe (long end), dental probe (shovel-tip), Retractor (Williams).

epidural space under the ligamentum. Incision of this structure continues close to the facets then medially along the border of the upper lamina. This forms a flap of ligamentum flavum that is hinged on the midline. The edge of the flap is folded back and sutured to the periosteum with a 4-0 silk suture swadged to a semicircular needle. The retracted flap will not interfere with access to the lateral aspect of the epidural space. There is a falciform edge to the ligamentum flavum where it ends and attaches itself to the facets. This edge lies directly over the lateral edge of the nerve root, which is a good landmark. This falciform edge is removed with a small, angled Kerrison rongeur.

At the large L5-S1 interlaminar space it is never necessary to remove the medial borders of the facets. Above this level, however, the interlaminar spaces become smaller and the disc spaces more superior to them, which requires the removal of bone. A high-speed, low-torque air drill* wears away the medial borders of the facets. The drill leaves no sharp edges and stops bleeding from the bone by its eburnating quality. A cutting burr is employed at first, but the edge of the inferior facet is removed with a diamond burr. These maneuvers open a corridor to the disc that runs lateral to the root and through Batson's plexus, which is enmeshed in fat. A channel is formed through these structures with bipolar coagulating forceps and microscissors. The dominant hand uses these instruments while the other hand holds a small-bore silver sucker. At this point the lateral edge of the nerve root may be visible, but often it is hidden in fat.

When the floor of the epidural canal is reached, the protruded disc often may be felt before

*Minos Hi-Speed, 3M Co., St. Paul, Minnesota.

it is seen. It is wise to push away any fat and veins over the disc before removing disc material. Also, decompression may result in bleeding at a distance from the herniation.

A Penfield dissector or septal elevator pierces the posterior longitudinal ligament and annulus. A Williams "microdisc" forceps is inserted through the opening and is used to remove the degenerated nucleus. As the removal proceeds, larger forceps are used to enlarge the hole and extract more disc. Curettes are not used. Injury to the cartilaginous endplates should be avoided.

The space beneath the root is probed gently for any remaining fragments of the disc before the operation is concluded.

The empty interspace and the wound then are filled with a 10% povidone-iodine solution, which is gradually diluted with saline and then sucked away. The flap of ligamentum flavum is brought down and the edge tied laterally to residual connective tissue with one 4-0 silk suture. Above the L5 level, the interlaminar space may have too little ligamentum flavum to allow a hinged flap to be fashioned. In this case, only the very lateral aspect of the ligament is removed.

Two or three 3-0 silk sutures are placed to approximate the lumbodorsal fascia. The more superficial tissue is closed with one to two 3-0 silk sutures, which allows the skin to be apposed gently with a single, running subcuticular suture of 4-0 Prolene. A 2 × 2-inch dressing is applied over the wound and sealed with paper tapes. This dressing is removed on the following morning.

The patient may go to the bathroom on the evening of the surgery. He may require a paraenteral narcotic for 1 day, although oral codeine usually suffices. The patient is encouraged to take short walks on the day after surgery, but this is not insisted upon. A program of physiotherapy begins and continues for 1 week or less, depending upon the well-being of the patient. The Prolene sutures are removed when the patient is sent home. During the next 4 weeks of convalescence the patient is instructed not to drive, to rest frequently, and to be patient with the needs of his body. If the patient's energy has returned at the end of that time, he is allowed to resume normal activities.

Analysis of Cases

As stated above, the rationale behind microsurgical lumbar discectomy is improvement of the procedure. In an effort to determine the extent of the improvement (if any) offered by the microsurgical technique over the standard discectomy procedure, we analyzed and compared two series of patients who underwent standard and microsurgical discectomy. From August 1976 to December 1979, 400 patients have undergone microsurgical lumbar discectomy (MSD) in our center. We analyzed the results of 100 MSDs and compared them to the results obtained after 100 standard discectomies.

All operations were performed by the same surgeon (D.W.) and were analyzed by another (R.H.). One hundred standard operations were chosen from the years 1971 and 1972 and 100 microsurgical discectomies were chosen from the years 1977 and 1978. This selection assured us that all of the patients were followed for a minimum of 2 years and that the standard discectomies were the last to be performed with the naked eye. The patient profiles (Table 84-1) were similar to those of Schramm and his colleagues[12] in their statistical survery of 3238 lumbar discectomies.

Patient Profile

Protrusions occurred at the usual levels in an average ratio of men to women (Table 84-1). Most patients in this rural community were engaged in moderate to heavy work. Few expected disability compensation after a reasonable period of convalescence. Most were anxious to resume their jobs. If they were not well, they returned to us promptly. These factors suggested that the results of this sampling represented our "disc" population.

Table 84-1. Patient Profile

	Standard discectomy	Microdiscectomy
No. of patients	100 (76 males)	100 (63 males)
Disc herniations	103	101
Positive myelogram	99	98
Positive venogram	0	2
Spinal level involved		
L2-3	2	1
L3-4	3	2
L4-5	51	65
L5-S1	47	33
Type of work		
Heavy	51	34
Moderate	40	58
Light	9	8

Results of the Operations

Fewer patients required a second operation after the MSD procedure, although as much disc material as possible was removed in both procedures (Table 84-2). Herniations at two levels were rare, a fact confirmed by the statistical analysis of Schramm et al.[12] It would seem to be unnecessary and harmful to explore two levels routinely or on the evidence of a slight myelographic abnormality.

Hemorrhage was mild in both techniques, but even less so in MSD. None of the patients required a transfusion.

Complications from either technique were few, indicating that standard discectomy was performed well and that MSD could equal it. An excessive number of dural tears from MSD reflected the initial difficulty of refining a new technique.

Postoperative Results

In all phases of convalescence microsurgical discectomy was superior to the standard operation; patients returned to work (which was moderate to heavy) in less than half the time (Table 84-3). The figures suggested that their general well-being was present on the day after surgery and that well-being was sustained; few were incapacitated and few required further surgery. More patients required a second operation for recurrent protrusion after the standard operation. It is noteworthy that most recurrences occurred within 2 years of the first operation, indicating that our follow-up of 2 years was enough to show the true incidence of recurrence. Incidence of the "failed disc" syndrome was low for both techniques, corresponding to the minimal blood loss during surgery. Following microsurgical discectomy, however, the syndrome was reduced to one-half of that occurring after the standard operation.

These data showed that only 1 patient had "discitis" following a microsurgical operation. We believed that this was not a true incidence, so we reviewed all microsurgical discectomies, and found 9 cases of diagnosed "discitis" in 400 MSDs. Microsurgical technique did not seem to protect the patient against this complication.

Discussion

Williams[13] was the first to design and implement a microsurgical operation for the removal of a lumbar disc. He had an unusual incentive: Lumbar disc protrusion was an occupational hazard for the chorus girls who danced in the casinos of Las Vegas, and many required surgery.

Table 84-2. Operative Results

	Standard discectomy	Microdiscectomy
Patients with previous discectomy	11	5
Mean time for procedure (minutes)	90	85
Mean blood loss per operation (cc)	110	50
No. of patients requiring transfusion	0	0
Operative complications		
Dural tears		
(none with persistent CSF leak)	1	5
Root damage	1 (S1 anesthesia)	0
	1 (foot drop)	
Miscellaneous	3 patients presented with herniations at 2 levels	1 patient presented with herniation at 2 levels
		2 patients required laminectomy at time of microdiscectomy

Visible scars and a long convalescence were causes for dismissal from their jobs. They could not appeal the decision and there was no lack of healthier young women to fill the vacancies.

Between 1972 and 1977 Williams performed 532 "microlumbar" discectomies and reported his results, which were excellent. We were inspired by his work, but from the beginning our views differed—in the requirements for hemostasis and in the amount of disc to be removed. The results of our first 83 cases, beginning in 1976, approximated his. The comparison was made in a preliminary report,[14] and is confirmed in the present one: Patient profile, operative, and postoperative results were good, and similar. But the differences have widened.

Williams believed that coagulation within the epidural space was unnecessary and unwarranted, whereas we found the bipolar coagulating forceps to be indispensable. He did not calculate blood loss during his operations beyond saying that it was "minimal," and "if rupture of the veins does occur, bleeding will stop spontaneously when the herniated disc has been decompressed." This has not been our experience. When bleeding occurred it did so *at the time of* decompression and did not stop spontaneously.

He also held the opinion that lumbar disc protrusion was not a disease of the whole disc but of the annulus alone. If he reduced the pressure on the annulus by removing a minimal amount of nucleus, the structure and function of the disc would be restored. He separated the fibers of the annulus with a Penfield dissector, which allowed them to close like a "sphincter" after decompression. Williams also believed that by retaining much of the nucleus, the "kissing-bone" syndrome would not occur. He defined this syndrome as postoperative collapse of the interspace, which caused the apposing vertebrae to rub together and produce intractable back pain.

We were not persuaded by these arguments. Analysis of our operations revealed that no complications occurred from the use of bipolar coagulation within the spinal canal and that hemostasis was excellent. We have rarely, if ever, seen apposing vertebrae "kiss" each other after subtotal removal of disc material either by MSD or by the standard operation. Some interspaces became narrower, but endplates did not touch or rub.

Only 4 patients in this series of MSDs required a second operation for recurrent disc protrusion or a new protrusion, a total of 4 percent. Williams reoperated on 48 such patients for a total of 9.1 percent.

From these comparisons it would seem that lumbar disc protrusion is a disorder of the whole disc, and that subtotal removal of the nucleus remains the better treatment. It is also a reasonable deduction that the good results obtained in this series and Williams's series did not depend so much upon the amount of disc removed as upon the preservation of structure and function of normal tissue.

Table 84-3. Postoperative Results

	Standard discectomy	Microdiscectomy
Mean time to ambulation (days)	2.51	1.03
Mean time to discharge (days)	6.75	4.12
Mean time until return to work (weeks)	11.76	4.80
Recurrent disc	8 (6 in first 2 yrs)	2
New disc	3	2
Failed disc*	7	3
Postoperative complications	0	2
Postoperative infections	0	1 discitis 1 wound infection with meningitis

*Had not returned to work 1 year after operation or required analgesics and/or muscle relaxants.

Williams's hesitation to invade the disc space may, however, have had one decided, inadvertent advantage. He had no infections of any kind, whereas we had 9 cases of "discitis" in 400 microsurgical discectomies, a disturbing figure. In several large series of standard discectomies, the incidence of "discitis" ranged from 0.3 to 3 percent: Our incidence was 2.3 percent and all were in the category of "aseptic" discitis, i.e., no overt wound infection, normal temperature, normal WBC, elevated sedimentation rate, severe paravertebral muscle spasm, and eventual endplate sclerosis that ranged from none to marked. All these cases were in Teng's[15] Grade I: "A narrowing interspace with or without minimal erosion of the endplates in the early stage" and healing in approximately 3 months.

The final pieces of disc removed from our patients were sent routinely for culture. The report invariably came back "no growth."

The cause of "aseptic" discitis remains obscure. In most cases the evidence is against its being a bacterial infection. Both Teng and Williams suggested that trauma to the cartilaginous endplates of the vertebrae may be responsible for severe pain, or "aseptic" discitis. Although we have never employed curettement of the endplates, the rongeurs unquestionably flaked off pieces of cartilage during a radical disc removal. Perhaps we should be more meticulous in our preservation of endplate cartilage.

Conclusions

In this series the standard operation was of good quality, with few complications. Microsurgical discectomy was able to equal the results of standard discectomy in all areas, and to surpass it in the convalescent phase; patients returned to their usual activity in half the time. By diminishing trauma to the normal anatomy, microsurgical discectomy enhanced the well-being of patients and prepared them for a swifter return to normal health.

Most of the disc was removed in both the standard and the microsurgical operations, which was probably responsible for the smaller number of recurrences than Williams reported with his minimal discectomy. Our invasion of the disc space, however, produced a 2.3 percent incidence of "aseptic" discitis, much the same as has been reported in other series, while Williams reported no infections of any kind. Rigorous attention to sparing the cartilaginous endplates may reduce this complication.

REFERENCES

1. Mixter WJ, Barr JS: Rupture of the intervertebral disc with involvement of the spinal canal. *N Engl J Med 211*:210-215, 1934
2. Fager CA, Freidberg SR: Analysis of failures and poor results of lumbar spine surgery. *Spine 5*:84-94, 1980

 3. Langenskiold A, Kiviluoto O: Prevention of epidural scar formation after operations on the lumbar spine by means of free fat transplants. *Clin Orthop 115*:92–95, 1976

 4. Gardner WJ, Goebert HW, Sehgal AD: Intraspinal corticosteroids in the treatment of sciatica. *Trans Am Neurol Assoc 86*:214–215, 1961

 5. Gardner WJ: Backache and soft living. *Arch Environ Health 5*:96–99, 1962

 6. Goebert HW, Jallo SJ, Gardner WJ, et al: Sciatica: Treatment with epidural injections of procaine and hydrocortisone. *Cleve Clin Quart 27*:191–197, 1960

 7. DaPian R, Pasqualin A, Scienza R, et al: Microsurgical treatment of ten arteriovenous malformations in critical areas of the cerebrum. *J Microsurg 1*:305–320, 1980

 8. Yasargil MG, Delong WB, Guarnaschelli JJ: Complete microsurgical excision of cervical extramedullary and intramedullary vascular malformations. *Surg Neurol 4*:211–224, 1975

 9. Greenwood J Jr: Surgical removal of intramedullary tumors. *J Neurosurg 26*:276–282, 1967

10. Harkinson HL, Wilson CB: Use of the operating microscope in anterior cervical discectomy without fusion. *J Neurosurg 43*:452–456, 1975

11. Patterson RH Jr, Arbit EA: A surgical approach through the pedicle to protruded thoracic discs. *J Neurosurg 48*:768–772, 1978

12. Schramm J, Oppel F, Umbach W, et al.: Complications after lumbar operation on intervertebral discs: Results of a statistical survery. *Nervenarzt 49*:26–33, 1978

13. Williams RW: Microlumbar discectomy: A conservative surgical approach to the virgin herniated lumbar disc. *Spine 3*:175–182, 1978

14. Wilson DH, Kenning J: Microsurgical lumbar discectomy: Preliminary report of 83 consecutive cases. *Neurosurgery 4*:137–139, 1979

15. Teng P: Postoperative lumbar diskitis. *Bull Los Angeles Neurol Soc 37*:114–123, 1972

Microsurgical Lumbar Discectomy: A Dissenting View by Richard L. Saunders

The substance of my criticism of Dr. Wilson's procedure is not in his case analysis or opinions, but in the application of the operating microscope, which I believe to be excessive. Having worked with Dr. Wilson throughout the development of this operation, I know his dedication and enthusiasm. This dissenting comment is not from a skeptic. I fully endorse the value of the operating microscope for added precision in the handling of nervous tissue. The brilliant light and magnification are the inescapable contributions of the operating microscope. In particular, the ease with which Batson's venous plexus can be controlled is a gratifying delight. Whether the management of Batson's plexus and the handling of epidural fat is critical to the outcome of lumbar discectomy may yet be proved, but as Dr. Wilson rightfully points out, this respect for tissue is unlikely to be bad. The additional dividend from this operation is the commonality of lumbar discs, which allows much technical microsurgical exercise so important to training programs.

My dissent stems from two concerns: the restricted access to the interlaminar space and the compromised epidural exposure. The poor results in disc surgery are not usually the residual from incisional morbidity as much as persisting neural symptoms. The least significant contribution of the operating microscope to neurosurgery in general has been in the change in the size of incisions in most procedures. Excessively small incisions and soft tissue restriction is not synonymous with minimizing neural tissue exposure and retraction. Using the microscope for restrictive exposure of the interlaminar space is to be a slave to the instrument. Williams's bandaid surgery for belly dancers probably developed more from the need for good cosmetics than any other factor. Eliminating the gimmickry of the tiny soft tissue exposure is my primary recommendation.

My second criticism, related to the first, is perhaps of more substance than simply an objection to gimmickry. I think the generous exposure of the epidural space is of utmost importance for adequate disc surgery.

The critical area of disc surgery lies in the epidural space; the goals are the precise removal of all offending disc pathology, the avoidance of excessive arachnoidal inflammation, and the elimination of foraminal compromise by spondylotic spur. The microscope facilitates all of these goals. If the epidural space is the critical feature, then adequate exposure of the lateral annulus and the foramen by removal of lamina along the medial edge of the pedicle is important. To omit this minor aspect of epidural exposure simply ignores the possibility of foraminal fragment and spondylotic ridge, which myelography simply cannot always define. These have been the admonitions of such acknowledged experts as MacNab[1] and Fager[2].

To overuse a surgical instrument such as the operating microscope and thereby purposefully compromise exposure both of the interlaminar and the epidural space risk unnecessary failure. A surgical tool should refine the accomplishments of the past and not contrive a new exercise.

REFERENCES

1. MacNab I: Negative disc exploration: an analysis of the causes of nerve-root involvement in sixty-eight patients. *J Bone Joint Surg* 53A:891–903, 1971
2. Fager CA, Freidberg SR: Analysis of failures and poor results of lumbar spine surgery. *Spine* 5:87–94, 1980

CHAPTER 85
Techniques of Fusion in the Cervical, Thoracic, and Lumbar Spine

Robert C. Cantu

WHILE AN ASSORTMENT of wire, silk, rods, screws, and, more recently, plastics have been employed individually and in combination to stabilize the vertebral column, spinal fusion refers to a surgical procedure performed on adjacent vertebrae that leads to an immobilized bony continuity. Using this definition, Russell A. Hibbs and Fred H. Albee in New York City ushered in the history of spinal fusion in 1911.[1] For Hibbs, intervertebral fusion was the natural end result of his interest in arthrodesing techniques that commenced some 29 years earlier in 1882 with Albert in Vienna. Among the earliest to popularize arthrodesis in the United States, Hibbs carried out the first recorded operation of fusion of the spine at the New York Orthopedic Hospital on January 9, 1911.[2] The fusion was achieved by overlapping osseous elements locally derived. Eventually this included spinous processes, laminae, and intervertebral articulations (facet joints). It was reported on May 28, 1911 in the *New York State Medical Journal*,[3] and it became known throughout the orthopedic world as the Hibbs fusion operation. With only minor modifications, it has remained the standard for over half a century.

Fred H. Albee, also of New York City, was primarily interested in improving bone graft operations. After exposing the spinous processes and laminae, he split the former in the sagittal plane and inserted a tibial cortical graft into the cleft thus formed. He first performed such a fusion in 1909, and he reported his work before the American Orthopedic Association in 1911.[1] His paper was subsequently published in the *Journal of the American Medical Association*.[4] Albee's fusion had considerable acceptance during his lifetime because of his worldwide travels, but eventually lost popularity to the Hibbs procedure.

Other major contributions to spinal fusion include a report by MacKenzie-Forbes of Montreal in 1920 of denuding the cortical surfaces of the spinous processes and laminae, leaving the cortical slivers overlapping adjacent counterparts.[5] In 1922, Samuel Kleinberg first reported the use of beef-bone grafts and continued to use beef bone until his death in 1957.[6]

Ralph Ghormley of the Mayo Clinic in 1933 recognized the easily accessible abundant supply of autogenous bone from the iliac crest.[7] His report led to a flood of reports regarding the relative merits of cancellous bone versus the stiffer bracing factor offered by the rigid cortical bone. A third minor voice advocated specially prepared beef bone, but cancellous bone from the ilium won the most adherents.

The first two anterior approaches to the lumbar spine both appeared in British journals in 1936. Walter Mercer of Edinburgh described using bone from the iliac crest as an anterior bone

Neurosurgical Service, Department of Surgery, Emerson Hospital, Concord, Masachusetts

graft between the fifth lumbar vertebra and the sacrum.[8] J. A. Jenkins reported in the *British Journal of Surgery* on an abdominal approach for exposing the fifth lumbar vertebra and the sacrum. A bone drill was passed from L5 into S1, and a cortical tibial graft was inserted into the hole.[9] Both of these reports were on cases of spondylolisthesis.

Interfacet screws—metal screws placed across denuded articular facets—were suggested in an effort to improve the efficiency of spinal fusion by James W. Toumey of the Lahey Clinic in Boston in 1943[10] and by Don King of San Francisco in 1944.[11]

Posterior interbody fusion through a laminectomy exposure following disc excision was first reported in *Surgery, Gynecology, and Obstetrics* in 1946 by Irwin A. Jaslow, an orthopedic surgeon in New Bedford, Massachusetts.[12] Ralph B. Cloward of Honolulu in 1952 reported the first large series of his variation of this procedure.[13]

Anterior cervical spine fusion was reported by Robinson and Smith in 1955[14] and by Ralph Cloward in 1958.[15]

Having presented a sketch of the salient milestones in the history of spine fusion, I wish now to be very practical regarding the indications and recommended types of spinal fusion for conditions of the cervical, thoracic, and lumbar regions.

Fusion of the Cervical Spine

Robert A. Robinson in Chapter 78 covers the posterior, anterior, anterolateral, and lateral approaches to the cervical spine. He discusses posterior fusions including both the standard wire and bone C1-C2 or C1-C2-C3 fusions for odontoid instability, as well as the anterior approach to fusing C1-C3. Robinson also discusses the role of skull traction and Halo-cast cervical traction and immobilization.

Schmidek in Chapter 80 recounts in detail the anterolateral approach to the cervical spine and the use of either the Cloward or Smith-Robinson anterior spinal fusion in cervical spondylosis. With these excellent descriptions of the indications for and various approaches to the cervical spine, my remarks will be confined to posterior cervical spinal fusion below C2 whether for instability secondary to fracture-dislocation, traumatic subluxation, or instability following extensive laminectomy. Yashon in Chapter 88 discusses the surgical management of spinal trauma per se. The modified posterior fusion of Robinson and Southwick discussed here is equally applicable to stabilizing iatrogenic extensive instability following decompressive laminectomy as that following fracture-dislocation.

After the laminectomy has been completed, the last exposed facet joint at the cranial end is slightly opened with an osteotome, and either a suction tip or a No. 4 Penfield dissector then is inserted and the osteotome removed. Using a Hall air drill, a hole is drilled through the inferior facet into the joint space (Fig. 85-1). A No. 20 wire then is passed through the hole. Bilaterally, this is carried out from the cranial-most exposed facet to the level below of the first intact spinous process. A corticocancellous graft 2 cm wide by whatever length is required is taken from the outer table of the posterior iliac crest. Cancellous side down, the graft is securely wired to the facets (Fig. 85-2). Additional cancellous bone may be tucked laterally. The careful wiring of the graft at each facet ensures the most rapid and secure union.

Comments. I would like to express certain personal biases regarding cervical spinal fusion gleaned from more than 15 years of practice and reflection. The comments of Robinson regarding the remodeling of bone are certainly true. Since the central nervous system is unforgiving of transgressions, the major charge to the neurosurgeon must be not to harm or inflict neurologic deficit on the patient. The simplest, safest, successful procedure should be the one employed. It has been my experience with cervical spondylotic disease that if 2–3 mm of disc space and resultant neuroforamen distraction can be accomplished, that there is no need to attempt the more risky osteophyte removal in the neuroforamen. With distraction, there will be room for the nerves to exit, and with firm fusion, the osteophytes will be largely absorbed within 18 months.

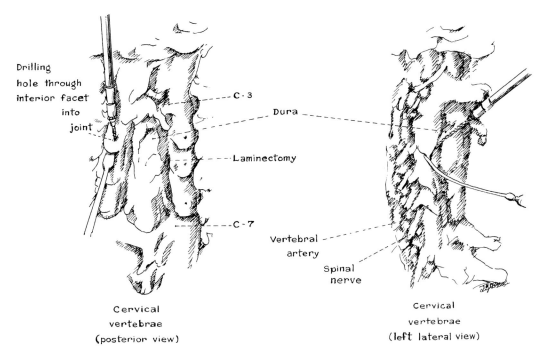

Drilling
hole through
interior facet
into
joint

C-3

Dura

Laminectomy

C-7

Vertebral
artery

Spinal
nerve

Cervical
vertebrae
(posterior view)

Cervical
vertebrae
(left lateral view)

Fig. 85-1.

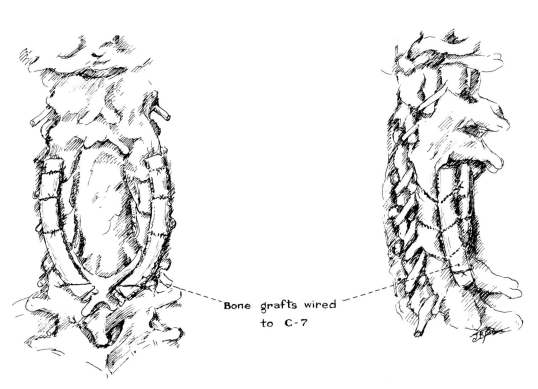

Bone grafts wired
to C-7

Fig. 85-2.

It has been said that in posterior cervical fusion all that has to be done is clean the lamina and lay on the bone. In my experience, I have found that roughening the bed, i.e., lamina, facets, and spinous processes, with a Hall burr, using wire fixation, employing corticocancellous grafts from the posterior iliac crest with the cancellous side down and using many additional slivers of cancellous bone obtained with gouges maximally ensures the rapidity and solidarity of the fusion.

Fusion of the Thoracic and Lumbar Spine

Today, the indication for fusion of the thoracic and lumbar spine is primarily instability resulting from traumatic, congenital, degenerative, or neoplastic disease. Unlike the situation shortly after the turn of the century, tuberculosis is now rarely an indication for spinal fusion. The indications for fusion in the minds of most spine surgeons, be they orthopedists or neurosurgeons, are currently more limited than in the past. Among the common anomalies once considered as indications for spinal fusion that are generally no longer thought to be such are cases of laminectomy with marked disc-space narrowing, transitional vertebrae, tropism, degenerative spondylolisthesis, increased lumbar lordosis, and lumbosacral tilt. Because of the low rate of solid fusion, except when internal fixation is used, such as with the Harrington technique, lumbar three-level fusions now are rarely done.

Paul Lin in Chapter 86 comprehensively covers the technique of posterior lumbar interbody fusion while Goldner, Wood, and Urbaniak accomplish the same for anterior lumbar interbody fusion in Chapter 87. While neither technique is as widely used as the standard posterior and posterolateral fusions I will discuss, each still has special indications, and the reader is referred to Lin and Goldner's chapters for their discussion.

Techniques of Thoracic and Lumbar Spine Fusion—Hibbs Fusion

Initially described in 1911, the most popular technique for posterior spinal fusion remains, with minor variations, the Hibbs fusion. By this technique, bony union is attempted at two points bilaterally—the laminae and the articular processes (facet joints). The skin, subcutaneous tissues, deep fascia, and supraspinous ligaments are incised in the midline. With Cobb or other periosteal elevators, the periosteum is stripped from the sides of the spinous processes and the dorsal surface of the laminae. Bleeding is controlled by electrocautery of frank arterial sources and packing for the ooze. Interspinous ligaments are incised, muscles are elevated from the ligamentum flavum, and the fossa distal to the articular facet joint is exposed. The fat pad in this fossa is removed with a scalpel or curette. The spinous process is removed with rongeurs. The posterior layer (about two-thirds) of the ligamentum flavum is freed with a curette from the proximal and distal laminae. The articular cartilage and cortical bone are removed with osteotomes, either straight or curved, from the facet joints. Then additional small cuts into the articular processes are made parallel with the joint line so these thin slivers of bone fill the joint space (Fig. 85-3). All cortical bone of the lateral fossa, facet joint, and lamina is cut into chips with a gouge. Additional chips of cortical bone and especially cancellous bone taken from the iliac crest may be added to the lamina slivers. The periosteum, ligaments, and muscles then are snugly sutured over the bone chips with interrupted O Dexon sutures. The subcutaneous tissues are closed with 3-0 Dexon and the skin with nylon or subcuticular suture.

While King in 1940 inserted metal screws across the articular facets after removal of the articular cartilage (Fig. 85-4), this author agrees with Bosworth, who believes that screw fixation is not of value when evaluated relative to the difficulties encountered by its use. Another popular modification of the Hibbs technique is to use a solid "clothespin" graft between the spinous

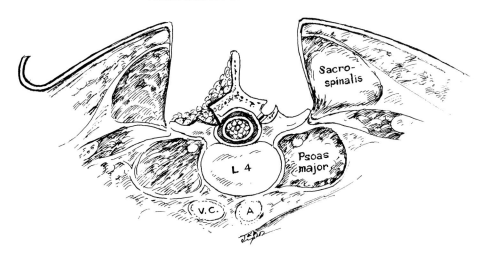

Skin incision is midline and all tissues are stripped from spinous processes, laminae, and transverse processes. Anterior two-thirds of facets are excised.

Fig. 85-3.

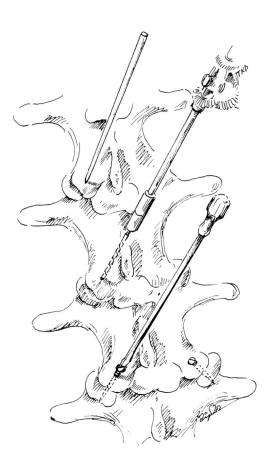

Technique of inserting screws across apophyseal joints.

Fig. 85-4.

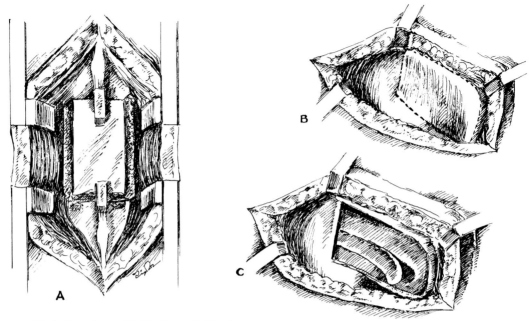

(A) clothespin graft firmly seated between spinous processes.
(B) graft fashioned from posterior crest of ilium.
(C) reinforcing cancellous iliac grafts.

Fig. 85-5.

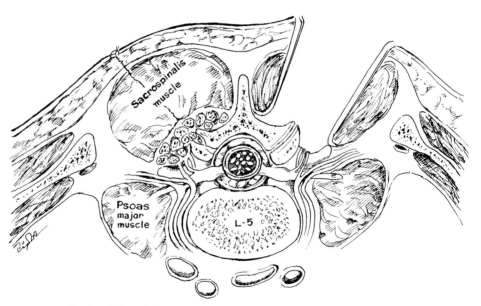

Posterolateral fusion sacrospinalis muscle is split longitudinally and laminae, articular facets, and transverse processes are all included in fusion.

Fig. 85-6.

processes of the fifth lumbar and first sacral vertebra. The cancellous side is placed down against the roughened lamina and the cortical side is dorsal (Fig. 85-5).

Posterolateral or Intertransverse Fusion

Initially described by Cleveland, Bosworth, and F. R. Thompson in 1948[16] as a technique for pseudoarthrosis repair, the lateral fusion was quickly adopted for use in congenital or surgical laminal defects, spondylolisthesis, and postlaminectomy patients with chronic pain that was thought to be due to instability. The operation may be unilateral or bilateral and cover one or more levels.

The skin may be incised either along the lateral border of the paraspinal muscles or in the midline. The distal end curves across the posterior crest of the ilium. The lumbodorsal fascia is incised an inch or more lateral to the midline and the sacrospinalis muscle is split longitudinally. The lamina, articular facets, and transverse processes are exposed, and the cortical surfaces are removed with osteotomes (Fig. 85-6). Cartilage is removed from the facets with an osteotome. Bone now is taken from the iliac crest. One long strip with cortical bone on one side and many cancellous slivers are desired for each side to be fused. Half of the cancellous slivers, usually most easily obtained from the iliac crest with a gouge, are fitted against the denuded facets, the pars interarticularis, and the base of the transverse process at each level. The long strip then is firmly packed with its cancellous side down into this bed of cancellous chips. The remaining chips of cancellous bone from the ilium then are packed about the graft.

When there is no laminal defect, others such as Wiltse, Truckly, and Thompson have suggested including the lamina as well as the articular facets and transverse processes in this fusion—the posterolateral fusion.

Lateral Extrapleural and Extraperitoneal Fusion

Initially designed for treatment of tuberculous spondylitis by Alexander[17] and Capener,[18] the lateral extrapleural and extraperitoneal approach to the thoracic and lumbar spine is useful in any case in which the pathologic process is extradural and anterior to the thoracic spinal cord or cauda equina. It affords removal of lesions that cannot safely be reached by laminectomy or costotransversectomy and has a lower morbidity and complication rate than thoracotomy or laparotomy.

Lateral thoracic extrapleural fusion. The patient is placed in the prone position and a midline incision made from well above to well below the lesion, curving laterally inferiorly for about 10 cm. The back muscles are stripped from the ribs. The number of vertebral levels to be approached determines the number of ribs to be removed, but usually at least two are desirable. The rib is transected 8 cm lateral to the costotransverse joint and is removed with rongeurs (Fig. 85-7). The pleura is very carefully stripped from the endothoracic fascia with blunt finger dissection, the neurovascular bundle is located, and the intercostal nerve is separated from the vessels. The costovertebral articulation and transverse processes are removed (Fig. 85-8). The intercostal nerve is traced to its foramen and it along with the segmental artery and vein are doubly clipped and divided. The pedicle is removed with a rongeur. When the anatomy is particularly distorted, it is often advantageous to first remove the pedicle above and below the lesion. At this point, turning the operating table on a 30°–45° tilt laterally aids in viewing the spinal canal. The annulus is now incised below the level of the posterior longitudinal ligament and the entire disc and adjacent cartilaginous plates are removed with curettes. The curette stroke is always downward and laterally into the cavity. Epidural bleeding can be controlled with cottonoids. An angled dental mirror may aid in assessing the completeness of the disc excision. I prefer a Smith-Robinson type bone graft from the iliac crest that with the aid of Cloward spreaders is tapped into place with a mallet and tamper. The wound is now closed in layers. If a bronchopleural fistula has occurred, a chest tube connected to a closed drainage system is required.

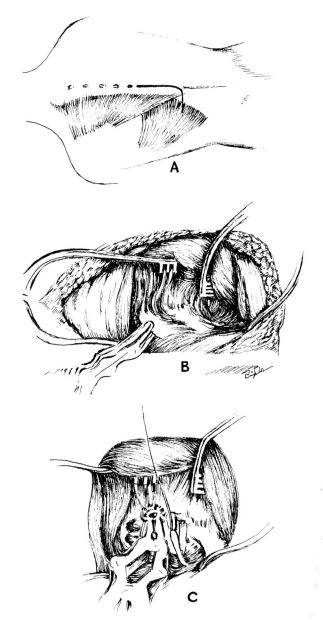

Lateral retropleural approach :
A. skin incision midline and curved laterally ;
B. muscles retracted to expose ribs ;
C. rib resected ;

Fig. 85-7.

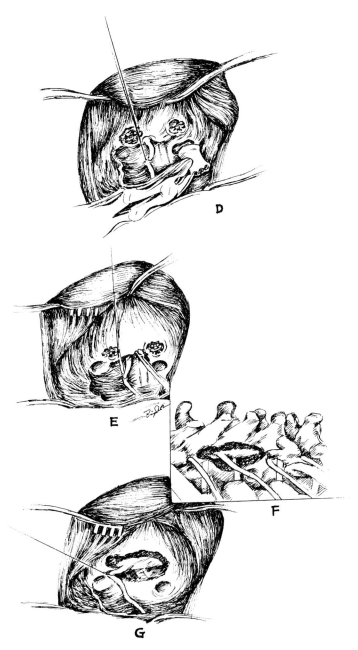

D. rib, including costovertebral articulation removed ;
E. anulus incised and disc removed ;
F, G. contiguous portions of bone removed from dorsal
      portions of vertebral bodies.

Fig. 85-8.

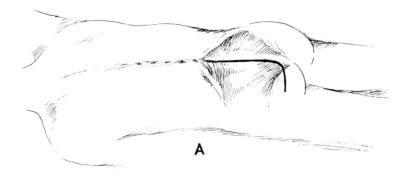

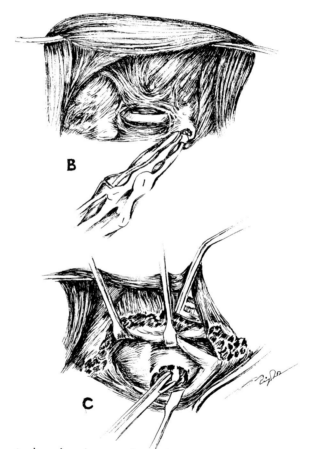

Lateral retroperitoneal approach :
A. lumbar incision is comparable to that used in thoracic area;
B. lumbar fascia is incised, transverse processes and
   intertransversarii muscles resected;
C. disc is removed;

Fig. 85-9.

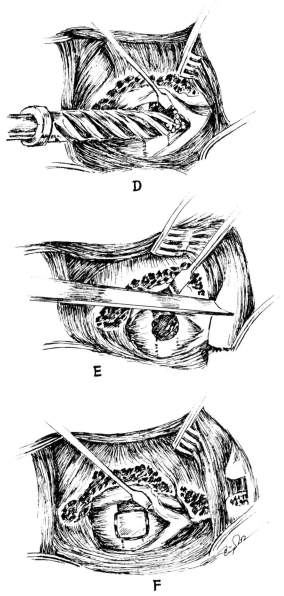

D, E, F. bone is removed from vertebral body and
fusion achieved with iliac bone graft.

Fig. 85-10.

Lateral lumbar extraperitoneal fusion.   A skin incision similar to that used for lateral thoracic extrapleural fusion is employed. The lumbodorsal fascia is incised laterally, and the latissimus and erector spinae muscles are split. At least two transverse processes are identified (an x-ray may be required), and their superior and inferior surfaces are cleared of erector spinae and quadratus lumborum muscles respectively. Then the transverse processes and associated intertransversarii muscles are removed (Fig. 85-9). The lumbar plexus now is identified and the spinal nerve, which has just exited from the level above, is noted. Complete removal of the transverse process affords exposure of the nerve at the level of the lesion. It may be necessary to remove the pedicles above and below to afford good exposure of the spinal canal. Division of connecing rami to the sympathetic chain permits sufficient mobility of the spinal nerves to allow

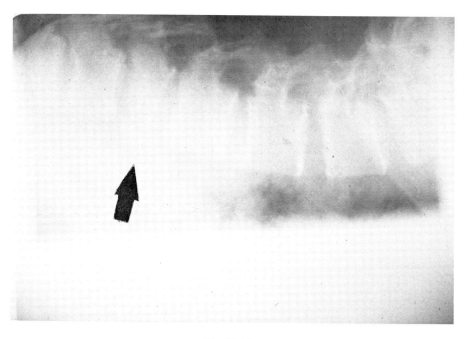

Fig. 85-11.

good exposure for removal of the disc and adjacent cartilaginous plates. The technique of disc excision and lateral interbody fusion using a Smith-Robinson bone graft is the same as that described for the thoracic spine (Fig. 85-10).

Harrington-Rod Thoracolumbar Fusion

David Yashon in Chapter 88 covers the surgical treatment of spinal trauma. I wish however, to conclude this chapter with a discussion of the Harrington distraction system. Although initially devised to treat scoliosis,[19] it has come to be widely used in the treatment of fracture of the thoracolumbar spine with and without paraplegia.

Controversy still exists regarding the treatment of unstable fractures and fracture-dislocations of the thoracic and lumbar spine. Investigators such as Frankel, Guttman, Lewis, and McKibbin support the nonoperative approach while Dickson, Harrington, Kaufer, Whitesides, Bradford, and others advocate operative management. There also is a wide divergence of opinion regarding the best operative approach. Laminectomy has recently fallen from favor because it frequently fails to relieve spinal compression and furthers instability. In the 1980 edition of *Campbell's Operative Orthopedics,* the statement is made that laminectomy "is to be condemned in these fracture-dislocations."[20]

It is my personal opinion that this is incorrect. I take issue with Guttman and Bedbrook that all neural tissue damage occurs at the time of injury.[20] Over my 15-year neurosurgical experience, I have seen incomplete compressive spinal lesions that worsen over a period of hours or several days and then rapidly start to improve with adequate relief of the block by laminectomy and, when unstable, internal fixation. When there is an incomplete lesion of the cord or cauda equina with a high-grade or complete block on myelogram, I favor relief of the block as soon as the patient is stable. I believe a needless delay in some patients will lead to vascular compression and further cord infarction. If the cord lesion is complete, then stabilization may be deferred a week or more, as the indication for stabilization is to lessen local back pain and facilitate a future wheelchair existence, not neurologic recovery.

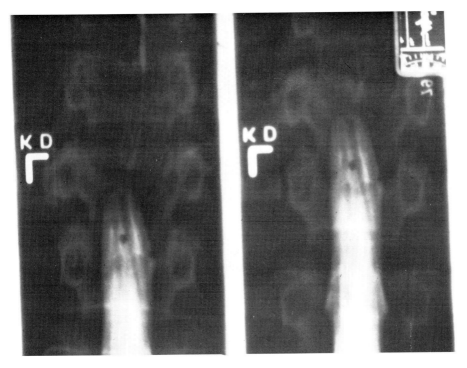

Fig. 85-12.

My own preference for relief of the block with incomplete lesions is a decompressive laminectomy—especially when there is evidence of neurologic worsening—coupled with Harrington distraction instrumentation and lateral fusion. The laminectomy should be at least a level above and below the fracture and should preserve the articular facets. I favor intraoperative x-rays to confirm the realignment with the Harrington apparatus, but also direct inspection via the laminectomy to be certain that no disc or bone fragments are left within the spinal canal. If alignment is achieved by x-ray and inspection shows no intraspinal fragments yet the dura remains tense or "apparently" bulging, then I favor opening the dura to inspect the cord. If the cord is partially pulped, I do not favor a myelotomy, but do favor a fascial-lata or sacrospinalis dural fascial graft. I believe that by combining laminectomy and Harrington distraction instrumentation and fusion that maximal cord and root decompression, anatomic alignment, and long-term stabilization are achieved. Depending on one's training, both in residency and subsequently, the above combined procedure may be carried out by a neurosurgeon or orthopedist alone or working together. Following surgery, we prefer to use a Stryker frame for 1 week. Thereafter, a body jacket is used, and the patient is ambulated. External support is continued for 5 to 6 months.

The use of this combined approach is exemplified by the case of a 26-year-old male who sustained a fracture-dislocation of L1 with a resultant incomplete conus lesion. Numbness was present in the perineal and sacral areas. The anal wink, cremasteric, and bulbocavernous reflexes were lost, but knee and ankle reflexes were preserved. The patient was incontinent of urine and stool. Figure 85-11 shows the fracture-dislocation and Figure 85-12 the high-grade but incomplete myelographic bloc. Figure 85-13 shows the Pantopaque trapped above L1. Two No. 1252 Harrington hooks were notched into the facet joints several levels about the fracture and two No. 1254 hooks several levels below the fracture. The outrigger was installed and extended to correct the dislocation and realign the spine (Fig. 85-14). With the outrigger in place, twin distraction rods were inserted until snug. X-rays then were taken to assess alignment. Some surgeons prefer to awaken the patient at this point to test neurologic function. After a final

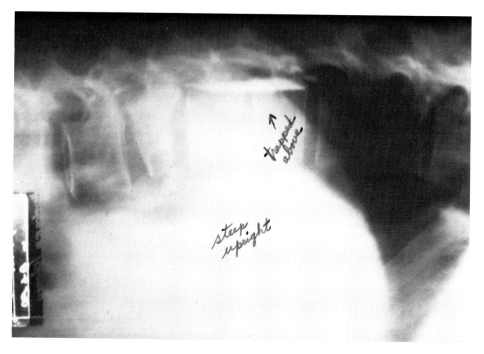

Fig. 85-13.

intraspinal inspection, a posterolateral fusion with iliac crest bone was carried out, as described earlier in this chapter, from hook to hook of the instrumentation. Figures 85-15 and 85-16 show the distraction rod and the anatomic alignment attained. Following surgery, perineal and anal sensation rapidly started to improve. Bowel, bladder, and sexual function returned within the first month.

Postoperative Care and Pseudoarthrosis

No chapter on spinal fusion would be complete without covering the postoperative care including the evaluation of the solidarity of the fusion. My comments here will apply primarily to the posterior and posterolateral fusion, as other authors have covered the anterior approach.

While there is no unanimity of opinion as to the precise day a patient should first be allowed up after surgery, most favor ambulation within a week. There is no concrete evidence that several weeks of bedrest decreases the incidence of pseudoarthrosis, but it does increase the risk of pulmonary embolism. I tend to allow age, condition of the patient, and the degree of postoperative pain to be taken into account, but I like to ambulate most patients by the third or fourth day after surgery. A rigid low-back brace or Fiberglass cast is worn for 4 to 6 months until the fusion is solid, as determined by AP and lateral forward, backward, and right and left lateral bending films. Williams low-back exercises are commenced before the brace is discarded and are recommended for the rest of the patient's life.

Pseudoarthrosis will occur in about 10 percent of lumbar one-level fusions, slightly less in cervical and thoracic fusions. The incidence increases with the number of levels fused; more than two is not recommended in the lumbar area excluding the Harrington procedure. *In this litigious era, it is especially important to frankly discuss the possibility of pseudoarthrosis preoperatively.* It is estimated that up to 50 percent of pseudoarthroses are asymptomatic.[20] In patients in whom severe pain and tenderness are sharply localized over a single level of non-union demon-

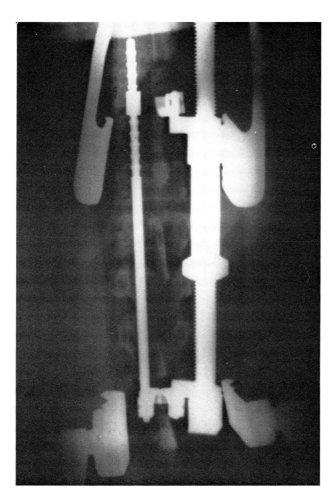

Fig. 85-14.

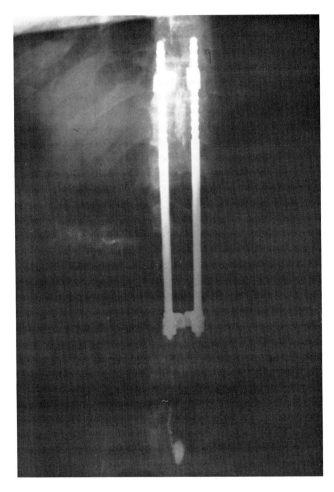

Fig. 85-15.

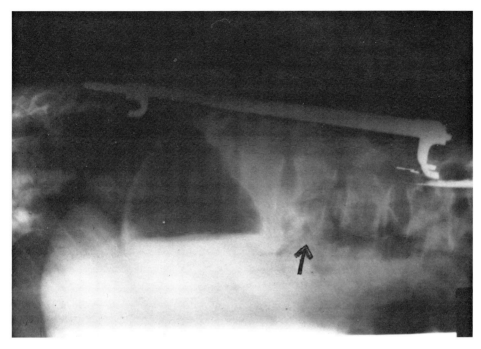

Fig. 85-16.

strated by x-ray, and who obtain significant partial relief from a brace, however, pseudoarthrosis repair should be considered. Since there are may reports of successful pseudoarthrosis repair in which pain persists, it is probably wise to insist on favorable preoperative psychometric studies; it certainly is wise to make no promises that the pain will be relieved, and to not operate on cases of pseudoarthroses in which pain is slight or absent unless unacceptable progression of deformity or disease persists.

There is no one favored technique for repair of pseudoarthrosis, as posterior, posterolateral, as well as anterior interbody fusion all can achieve the desired arthrodesis. Rather, operative judgment and technical excellence are of the utmost important.

REFERENCES

1. Bick EM: An essay on the history of spine fusion operations. *Clin Orthop 35*:9–15, 1964
2. Bick EM: *Source Book of Orthopedic Surgery*, 2nd ed. Baltimore, Williams & Wilkins, 1948
3. Goodwin GM: *Russell A. Hibbs.* New York, Columbia University Press, 1935
4. Albee FH: Transplantation of portions of the tibia into the spine for Pott's disease. *JAMA 57*:885, 1911
5. MacKenzie-Forbes A: Technique of an operation for spinal fusion as practiced in Montreal. *J Orthop Surg 2*:509, 1920
6. Kleinberg S: Operative treatment for scoliosis. *Arch Surg 5*:631, 1922
7. Ghormley RK: Low back pain. With special reference to the articular facets with presentation of an operative procedure. *JAMA 101*:1773, 1933
8. Mercer W: Spondylolisthesis. *Edinb Med J 43*:545, 1936
9. Jenkins JA: Spondylolisthesis. *Br Med J 24*:80, 1936
10. Toumey JW: Internal fixation in fusion of the lumbosacral joints. *Lahey Clin Bull 3*:188, 1943
11. King D: Internal fixation for lumbosacral fusion. *Am J Surg 66*:357, 1944
12. Jaslow IA: Intercorporal bone graft in spinal fusion after disc removal. *Surg Gynecol Obstet 82*:215, 1946
13. Cloward RB: Changes in vertebra caused by ruptured intervertebral discs. Observations on their formation and treatment. *Am J Surg 84*:151, 1952
14. Robinson RA, Smith GW: Anterolateral cervical disc removal and interbody fusion for cervical disc syndrome. *Bull Johns Hopkins Hosp 96*:223, 1955

15. Cloward RB: The anterior approach for removal of ruptured cervical discs. *J Neurosurg 15*:602, 1958
16. Cleveland M, Bosworth DM, Thompson RR: Pseudarthrosis in the lumbosacral spine. *J Bone Joint Surg 30A*:302, 1948
17. Alexander GL: Neurological complications of spinal tuberculosis. *Proc Roy Soc Med 39*:730–734, 1946
18. Capener N: The evolution of lateral rhachotomy. *J Bone Joint Surg 36*:173–179, 1954
19. Harrington PR: Treatment of scoliosis. *J Bone Joint Surg 44*:591, 1962
20. Edmonson AS, Crenshaw AH: *Campbell's Operative Orthopedics,* vol. 2. St. Louis, CV Mosby, 1980

CHAPTER 86
Posterior Lumbar Interbody Fusion

Paul M. Lin

THE CONCEPT OF INTERVERTEBRAL (INTERCORPORAL) FUSION in the cervical area has gained wide acceptance in recent years. In 1945, Cloward[1] devised the intervertebral fusion procedure, and first reported "the treatment of ruptured lumbar disc by intervertebral fusion" at the Harvey Cushing Society meeting at Hot Springs, Virginia, in November 1947. His description of the technique of posterior lumbar interbody fusion predated by 12 years his more popular cervical anterior fusion. With the exception of Cloward's own publications,[2,3] there has been astonishingly little enthusiasm for posterior lumbar interbody fusion.[4-6]

The practice of posterior lumbar interbody fusion is more popular outside the United States. Crock[7] of Australia indicates that the ideal operation for isolated "lumbar disc resorption" (localized spondylosis) is posterior lumbar interbody fusion. LeVay[8] reports that posterior lumbar interbody fusion is favored by neurosurgeons in England. In Germany, Junghanns[9] also is an advocate of Cloward's concept of the posterior lumbar interbody fusion. He feels the unstable lumbar segments not only should be fused, but also should effect an "operative unfolding" (*distraction*) of the disc space together with the fusion. "In the lumbar spine this could only be achieved posteriorly by removing disc tissue, eliminating the cartilagineous plate, unfolding (*distraction*) of the disc space and positioning of the osseous packs," Junghanns concluded (italics added). Wiltberger[10,11] also favors posterior lumbar interbody fusion. He modifies the technique by inserting dowel grafts through the facet instead of peg grafts without prior dissection or isolation of the nerve root.

In discussing posterior lumbar interbody fusion, there are two principles that should be brought into focus: (1) the concept of the lumbar intervertebral disc as part of a motion segment, and (2) tropism.

Junghanns[9] was the first to describe the lumbar intervertebral disc as only a part of the "motor segment" (or perhaps better translated as "motion segment; *bewegungssegment*) (Fig. 86-1). The "motion segment" also consists of the intervertebral disc, the intervertebral foramen, the facet, the interlaminar space, the ligamentum flavum, the spinous processes, and the adjoining ligaments. Junghanns's concept is that with a change in the disc space there also is an associated change in the entire "motion segment." When a lumbar disc degenerates or if the disc is removed surgically, the intervertebral disc space settles, and the narrowing is followed by sequential changes in the "motion segment" as a whole (Fig. 86-2). In addition to disc herniation, there would be posterior spur formation on the vertebral body, facet overriding, spur formation on the facet, or internal invagination of the ligamentum flavum. The effect of spondylosis, either degenerative or postdiscectomy, actually affects two pairs of nerve roots: the root generally im-

Department of Neurological Surgery, Temple University Health Science Center, Philadelphia, Pennsylvania

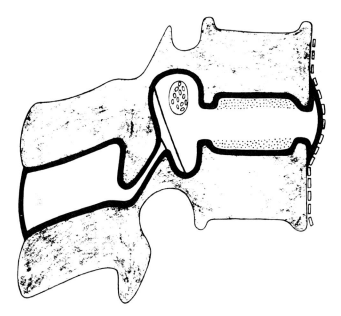

Fig. 86-1. Junghanns' concept of *bewegungssegment* or the "motor segment" or "motion segment," with the disc and the facet working as a single-motion unit. Note the ligamentum flavum covering the anterior portion of the facet.

pinged upon by the herniated disc is compressed by the lateral spinal stenosis or subarticular compression, whereas the nerve root that is above the herniated disc is impinged upon by the stenotic foramen as a result of the overriding facet impinging the nerve against the pedicle (Fig. 86-3). In various combinations this would result in neural compression at various sections of the spinal segment. Spinal stenosis, both of the intervertebral foramen and of the spinal canal, often is the result of failure of simple discectomy because attention was not given to the problem of settling at the time of surgery.

Tropism is defined as an organismatic response in a motile organism elicited by an external stimulus. It is also described as "the turning or movement of protoplasm or organistic matter." This term as applied to the facet indicates inversion or hypertrophy of the facet joint because of excessive or abnormal external stimulation, which is related to motion or static stress of the facet from an abnormal "motion segment." Hypertrophic arthrosis of the facet or inversion of the facet joint therefore is the result of abnormal external or static stress on the facet related to motion—Wolffe's Law (Fig. 86-4).

Tropism is the most frequent cause of lateral spinal stenosis. Kilbaldy-Willis et al.[12] were the first to attempt to categorize spinal stenosis into (1) general spinal stenosis, (2) lateral spinal stenosis, and (3) foraminal stenosis. Since the lumbar intervertebral foramen is not a true fora- men (at best it is a tunnel extending into the lateral spinal recess), foraminal stenosis should best be categorized with subarticular compression as part of lateral spinal stenosis.

Lateral spinal stenosis at one level would compress two pairs of intervertebral nerves: (1) a narrow lateral spinal recess with subarticular compression would compress the root that leaves the intervertebral foramen at the level below; (2) foraminal stenosis as a result of settling of the disc space, spur formation, and overriding of the facets would impinge the nerve root that leaves the intervertebral foramen at the same level of localized spinal stenosis against the pedicle (Fig. 86-5).

Computerized tomography has its limitations in diagnosing lateral spinal stenosis (subarti- cular compression and foraminal stenosis) because of the limitations of the thickness (5 mm) of each cut. Until a new generation of scanners can be developed that can reduce the thickness of

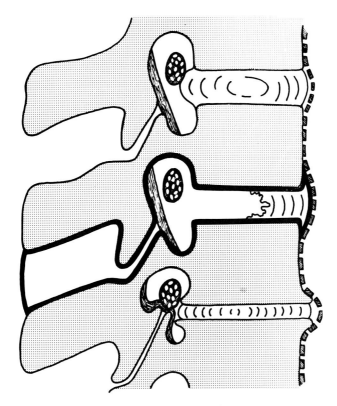

Fig. 86-2. A diagram of the sequential changes expected in a "motion segment" when disc material is extruded or removed surgically. Laterally, the ligamentum flavum lies anterior to the facet and generally is not radiologically identifiable.

each cut to 1.5 mm or that have the capability of sagittal reconstruction, the diagnosis of lateral spinal stenosis still must depend upon traditional radiologic techniques. The findings suggestive of lateral stenosis are:

1. Hypertrophic arthrosis of the facet.
2. Presence of a facet cleft on a lateral view (Fig. 86-6).
3. A long lateral defect on a myelogram (Fig. 86-7).
4. A tomogram of the intervertebral foramen. Tomograms of an intervertebral foramen are difficult to obtain because the facets often are more laterally situated. If two cuts are made, however, one visualizing the pedicle and the other the facet, the superimposed picture would give a true reading of the size of the intervertebral foramen. This overlapping technique is useful if there is only a unilateral stenosis, the diagnosis of which cannot be established by the usual lateral radiograms (especially the L5 interspace) (Fig. 86-8).
5. Hypertrophy of the pedicle and narrowing of the interpedicular space. This is seen in diffuse types of spinal stenosis and is not specific of lateral spinal stenosis.
6. An amipaque myelogram that rules out symptomatic foraminal stenosis. Amipaque myelograms sometimes can visualize the nerve roots beyond the intervertebral foramen and thus rule out any symptomatic foraminal stenosis (Fig. 86-9).

The advantages of posterior lumbar interbody fusion (PLIF) are:

1. PLIF reconstitutes the normal anatomic relationship between the motion segment and the neural structures. The narrow disc space and the "motion segment" are unfurled or restored to normal anatomic alignment.

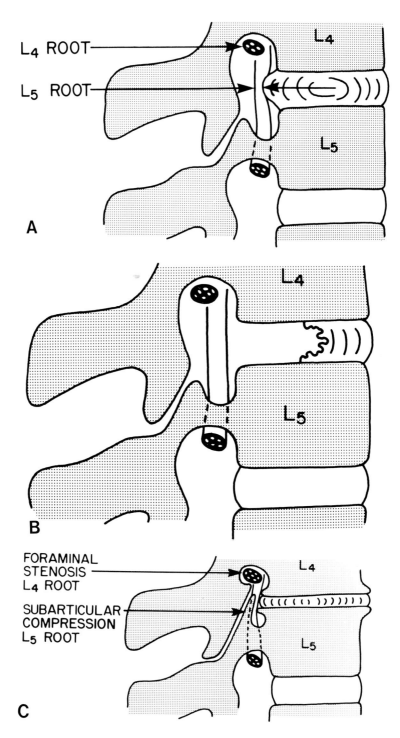

Fig. 86-3. **A.** Diagram of an L4-5 disc impinging on the L5 root. The L4 root leaving the L4-5 intervertebral foramen is rarely affected. **B.** After partial discectomy, pressure on the L5 root is released. **C.** A diagram of postdiscectomy spondylosis. The L5 root is compressed by subarticular compression and the L4 root is compressed by foraminal stenosis.

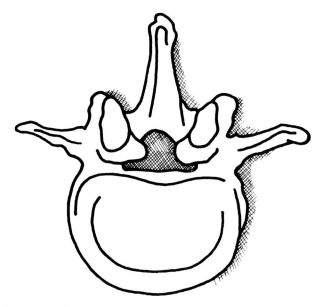

Fig. 86-4. A coronal view of tropism. The hypertrophic arthrosis and tropism of the posterior joints mainly are responsible for a localized spinal stenosis.

2. Successful PLIF would arrest the degenerative process of the fused motion segment. Because of an increased range of motion of the adjoining vertebral disc spaces, however, their degenerative processes could be enhanced by PLIF.
3. Total discectomy, which is needed for PLIF, prevents recurrent lumbar disc herniation at that level.
4. The PLIF would prevent painful nerve irritation from postoperative perineural adhesions. The lack of motion after a successful PLIF prevents mechanical pulling of the nerve root by the surrounding scar tissue.
5. Wide laminotomy in PLIF relieves all neural compression from structures other than the disc, especially in cases of lateral spinal stenosis.
6. Tropism is the result of stress and motion from an abnormal motion segment. Stabilization arrests the motion, and thus PLIF prevents recurrence of tropism or lateral spinal stenosis.

Indications

Keim[13] has listed 10 indications for fusion of the lumbar spine. Our indications parallel those of Keim.

1. An unstable joint complex associated with a long history of low back pain.
2. Spondylolisthesis with or without spondylosis.
3. Congenital anomaly, transitional transverse process, or spondylolysis without spondylolisthesis.
4. Localized lateral spinal stenosis or degenerative spondylosis at one level.
5. Facet resection from previous surgery.
6. Simple disc herniation with or without degenerative changes associated with heavy labor or sports.
7. Bilateral disc herniation or massive midline herniation.
8. Previous disc surgery at that level.
9. Reconstruction for failed back, including pseudoarthrodesis from lateral fusion.

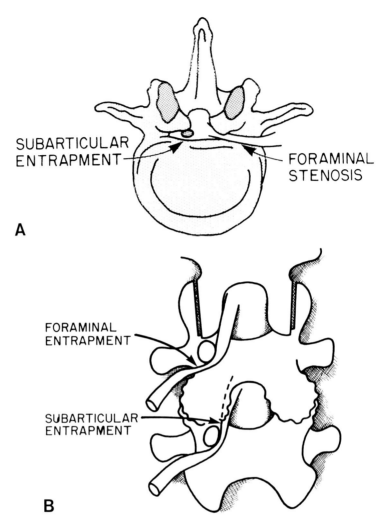

Fig. 86-5. **A.** A coronal view of lateral spinal stenosis, showing hypertrophy and tropism of the facet producing subarticular compression of the nerve leaving the level below, and foraminal compression of the nerve leaving at the same level. **B.** An anteroposterior view of lateral spinal stenosis at one level, showing compression of two pairs of intervertebral nerves—foraminal compression of the nerve leaving the same level above the disc space, and subarticular entrapment of the nerve leaving the foramen below.

10. Lateral extruded discs in obese patients; prevention of rapid postoperative settlement of the disc space.

Technique

The potential problems of Cloward's original PLIF[10] were studied and solutions were formulated (Table 86-1). A modification of Cloward's posterior lumbar interbody fusion is introduced with the following characteristics.[4-6]

1. A better technique for controlling epidural hemorrhage by emphasizing a lessening of the epidural venous pressure through proper positioning of the patient.

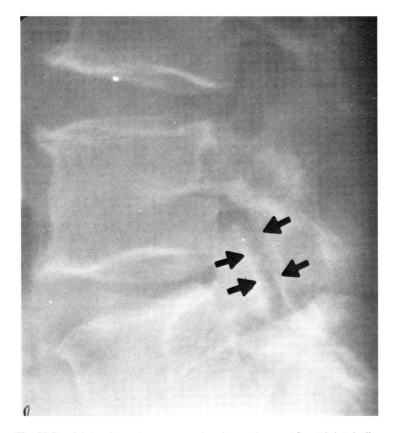

Fig. 86-6. A lateral roentgenogram showing a clear-cut facet joint, indicating that the joint is coronal in orientation—tropism.

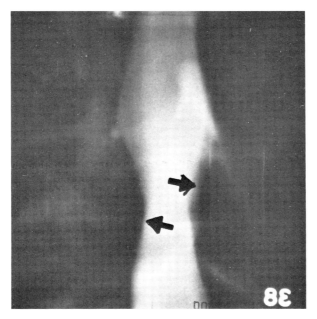

Fig. 86-7. An anteroposterior myelogram of the lumbar spine. The long lateral defects are due to dorsal and lateral compression of the whole length of the coronal-oriented facet joint.

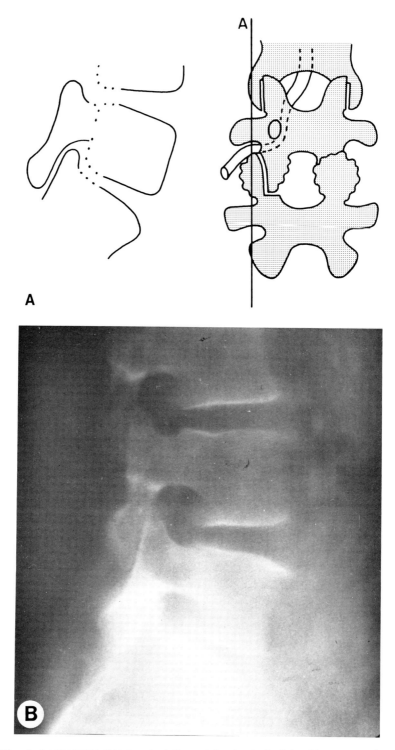

Fig. 86-8. **A.** A schematic diagram depicting a lateral cut of a lateral tomogram showing the facet. **B.** A roentgenogram of the same view in **A.** **C.** A schematic diagram of a slight medial cut, showing the posterior wall of the vertebral body and the pedicle. **D.** A roentgenogram of the same view in **C.** **E.** Superimposition of **A** and **C.** **F.** Superimposition of **B** and **D** reveals a true unilateral foraminal stenosis.

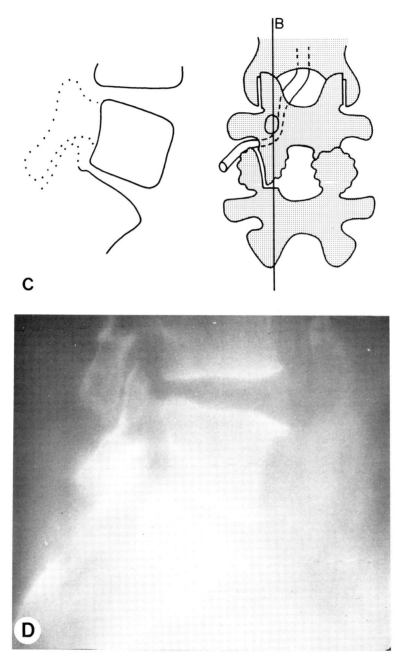

Fig. 86-8 (cont'd).

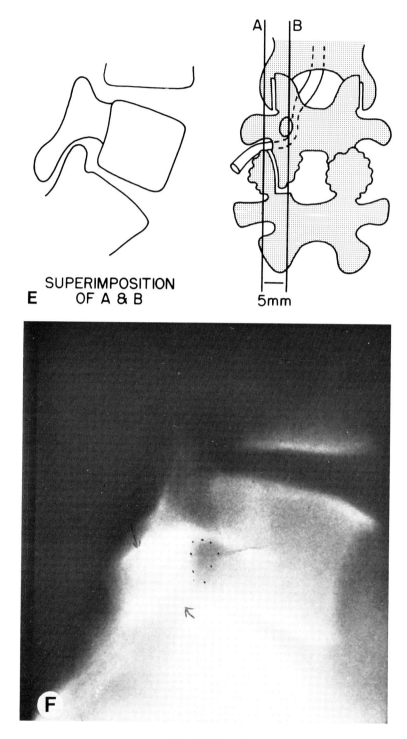

SUPERIMPOSITION
OF A & B

5mm

Fig. 86-8 (cont'd).

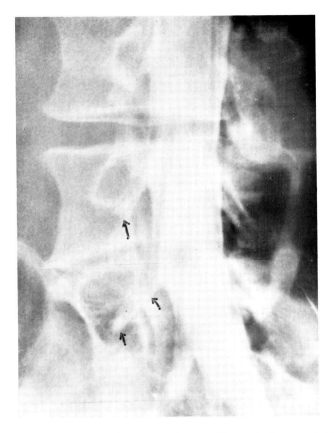

Fig. 86-9. An oblique amipaque myelogram. The root sleeve passes beyond the pedicle–facet interspace (see arrows). There is no myelographic evidence of intervertebral foraminal stenosis.

2. The use of Surgicel* in the form of tampons to control epidural bleeding, thus avoiding the excessive use of electric coagulation of the epidural venous plexus.
3. Preservation of the integrity of the facet through a more limited interlaminal approach.
4. Preservation of the cortical plate and assurance of osteosynthesis of the graft by multiple perforations of the cortical plate in accordance with the principle of Robinson as applied to anterior cervical interbody fusion.[14,15]

Illumination

Excellent illumination is critical in the success of this procedure. We routinely use a fiberoptic headlight.

Position

The patient is placed in the prone position (Fig. 86-10). Rolls used to support the patient must be firm and customized to the patient's height and weight. They must be placed laterally so that the inferior vena cava and the femoral veins are not compressed. The pressure points should be at the clavicle, ribs, and anterior iliac crest. The surgeon must place his hands between the rolls after the patient is placed on the table to be sure that the anterior abdominal wall is not tense and is suspended freely. There must not be any undue pressure on the inferior vena cava.

*Surgicel: Oxidized cellulose, Johnson & Johnson, New Brunswick, New Jersey.

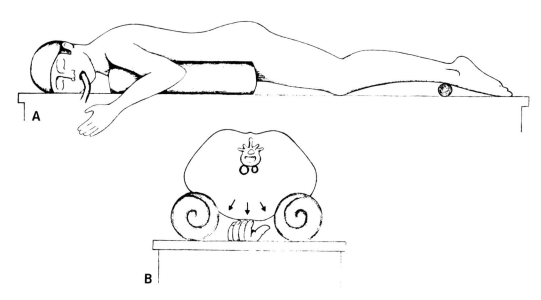

Fig. 86-10. **A.** Positioning of the patient for posterior lumbar intervertebral fusion. The rolls are firm. Flexion of the table is not needed. **B.** Testing the tension of anterior abdominal wall.

Many rolls that are commercially available have a slanting surface that will compress the inferior vena cava through lateral compression on the abdominal wall. The table is not flexed; flexing the table increases the intra-abdominal venous pressure, thus increasing epidural hemorrhage. It also could increase the incidence of thrombophlebitis from venous stagnation in the lower extremities.

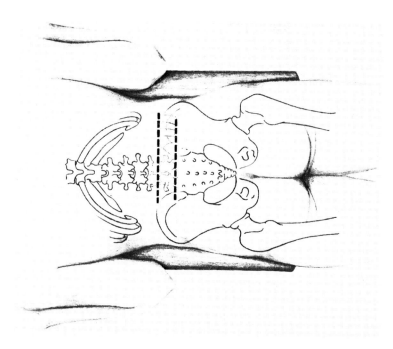

Fig. 86-11. The incision for posterior lumbar intervertebral fusion. The upper (left) dotted line is for fusion of the L4-5 discs and the lower (right) line is for fusion of the L5-S1 discs.

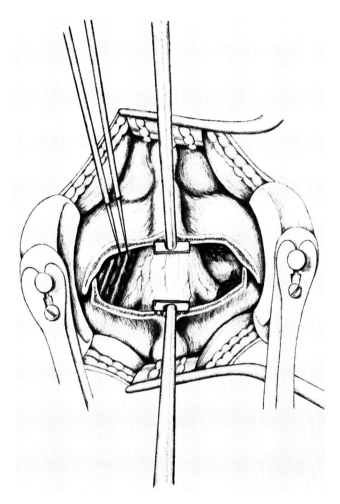

Fig. 86-12. Bilateral laminotomy with preservation of the facets. Control of epidural hemorrhage. Bipolar or insulated coagulation forceps are used on the left side. On the right side, epidural hemorrhage is controlled by packing with Surgicel tampons. The impacted Surgicel tampons also push the nerve root medially and expose the disc space without the need of a nerve root retractor.

Incision

The incision is horizontal (Fig. 86-11). Grafts can be removed from the posterior iliac crest through the same incision. Three disc levels can be explored through this horizontal approach.

Exposure

The usual bilateral laminotomy exposure is used (Fig. 86-12). The amount of bone removed is no more than that for an ordinary decompressive laminotomy for compression of the cauda equina. The facet is not totally removed as recommended by Cloward. Instead, the mesial half is chiseled away to gain exposure just lateral to the nerve root. Total removal of the facet would produce instability postoperatively, resulting in spondylolisthesis.

In cases of lateral spinal stenosis a mesial facetectomy would relieve the nerve being impinged upon by subarticular stenosis (Fig. 86-13). The distal end of a superior facet that is hyper-

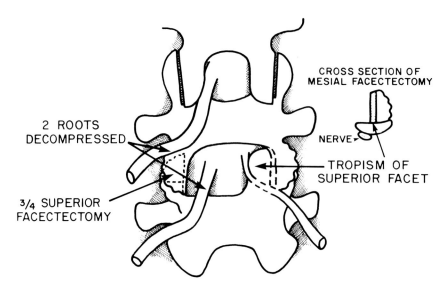

Fig. 86-13. An anteroposterior view showing that in PLIF the mesial facetectomy does decompress the subarticular nerve compression.

trophic and tropism may impinge underneath the lamina above. This must be removed to achieve decompression of the lateral gutter. The true foraminotomy for foraminal stenosis would require the amputation of the upper portion of the superior facet (Fig. 86-14). We have found that a supersonic curette aids in the removal of the hard-to-get superior tip of the superior facet, which is often laterally situated. This is in distinct contrast to the conventional foraminotomy (Fig. 86-15) where the superior laminae are unroofed over the nerve that leaves the foramen of the space below, whereas the true foraminal compression lies above the disc space (see Figs. 86-3 and 86-5).

A strong functioning posterior interspinous ligament must be preserved. This adds to the stability of the graft (Fig. 86-16).

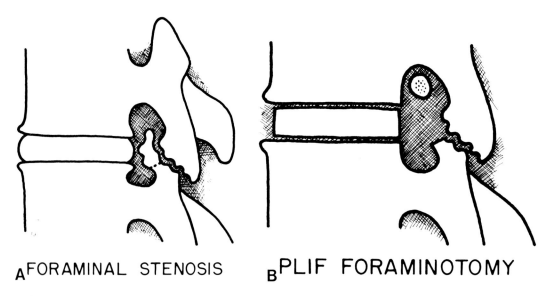

Fig. 86-14. **A.** A lateral view of an encroached intervertebral foramen. **B.** "True" foraminotomy is accomplished by partial facetectomy, especially of the superior facet.

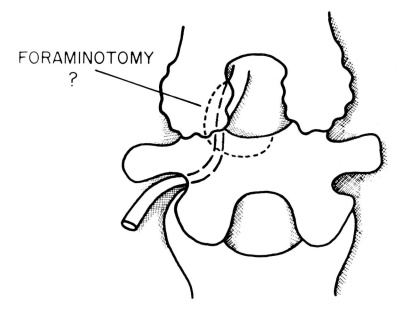

Fig. 86-15. A "conventional" foraminotomy performed by unroofing the upper laminae is *not* a foraminotomy.

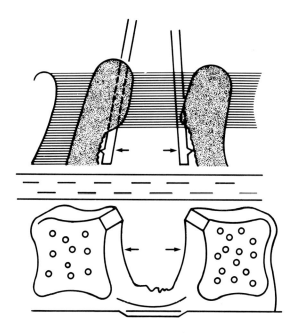

Fig. 86-16. Preservation of the posterior portion of the interspinous ligament would enhance: (1) avoidance of postoperative flexion injury, which may dislodge the grafts; and (2) the locking mechanism during the laminal distraction procedure and a more even distraction of the emptied disc space.

Table 86-1. Problems with the Original Posterior Lumbar Interbody Fusion (PLIF)
Technique of Cloward, and Their Solutions

Problem	Solution
Visibility	Fiberoptic illumination
Hemostasis	Proper positioning of patient
	Surgicel tamponade
	Bipolar coagulation
Instability—facet resection	Mesial facetectomy
Settlement and angulation— removal of cortical plates	Robinson's principle of preservation of cortical plate
Failure of osteosynthesis	Autogenous grafts
	Generous use of cancellous bone grafts mixed with cortical peg grafts
	Compression—Unipour concept
	Knight's lumbar brace—4 months

Epidural Hemostasis

The success of this operation depends upon mastering the technique of controlling epidural hemorrhage. The first prerequisite is the proper positioning of the patient so that the venous pressure within the epidural space is reduced to a minimum. Surgicel is used as a tampon to control epidural bleeding (see Fig. 86-13). The epidural veins can be cut with scissors and then pushed out of the way with a ball or tampon of Surgicel above and below the disc space. The bleeding of course could be controlled by coagulation, preferably bipolar (see Fig. 86-13). Generally the veins are longitudinal. Sectioning one or two longitudinal veins after coagulation and then by blunt dissection pushing the remaining veins out of the field with the Surgicel tampon will render the control of epidural bleeding a reasonably simple procedure. If the venous pressure within the epidural space is minimal, the bleeding can be controlled without the use of coagulation. Bleeding from the lateral gutter also can be controlled by packing a smaller piece of Surgicel into the lateral gutter. On very rare occasions there may be bleeding from a small artery that requires careful bipolar coagulation and, if necessary, the aid of a magnification device. The Surgicel tampon also would retract the dura and the nerve root medially. With the use of such tampons, the prolonged use of metallic nerve root retractors can be avoided. This is a definite advantage in minimizing injury to the nerve roots. The laminal retractor is used to distract the disc space for better exposure. When it is removed after the grafts have been inserted, compression of the grafts is enhanced. The laminal retractor should be used just before the grafts are inserted. For reasons not totally apparent, we have found that when the laminal retractor is applied and the laminae are forcibly distracted, there may be an increase in the epidural bleeding. We therefore use the laminal retractor at the completion of the total discectomy, just before the grafts are inserted. The laminal retractor may not be effective in distracting the distal disc space (Fig. 86-17). Insertion of a Cloward impactor deep to the disc space and with leverage may provide a larger entrance in the disc space to the initial central graft. The prying distraction can be repeated on the other side to facilitate the insertion of the several central grafts (Fig. 86-18).

Discectomy

The adjoining intervertebral rims first are chiseled away (Fig. 86-19). This accomplishes three objectives: (1) it enlarges the entrance to the disc space, (2) it exposes the cancellous bone posteriorly, and (3) it exposes a cleavage between the cartilaginous plate and the cortical bone.

The cortical plate is exposed after all disc material and the cartilaginous plate are energetically removed by sharp curetting and rongeuring with either upbite or downbite instrumentation. The centrum of the lower cortical plate often is slightly concave so that the cartilaginous material can be removed only by a curved upbite curette (Fig. 86-20). Total discectomy is required before the disc space is ready to receive the grafts.

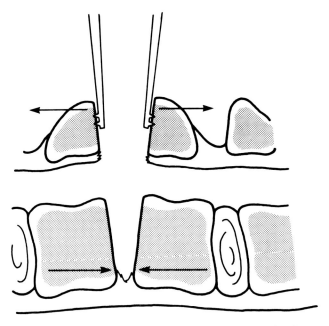

Fig. 86-17. The laminal retractor would distract the laminae, but the leverage action of the "motion segment" may actually narrow the disc space distally, making it difficult to place a rectangular peg graft.

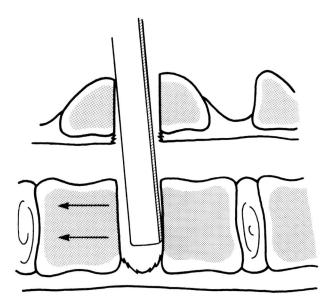

Fig. 86-18. The Cloward impactor should be inserted to the depth of the disc space and pried forcibly. This will distract the disc space evenly. A large medial graft can be inserted into the opposite side and the process reversed.

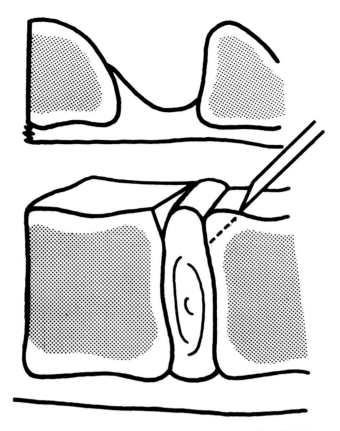

Fig. 86-19. Before attempts are made to remove the disc material radically, the intervertebral rims are first chiseled away.

Any midline bar must be removed (Fig. 86-21). This may be difficult. The annulus should be separated from the posterior longitudinal ligament with a Cloward cervical periosteal elevator and then pushed downward with a right-angle downbite curette. Often the midline bar can be removed only after it has been pushed by a medially advanced graft.

Graft Site Preparation

The cortical plate then is penetrated at many points. The use of chisel alone is not effective. To make larger and deeper penetrations into the cancellous bone, a Cloward cervical periosteal elevator is modified for use as a perforator (Fig. 86-22). This instrument is sharp pointed and has a 45° angulation. Tapping downward with this instrument should result in horizontal entrance into the cancellous bone. Radical perforation of the cortical plate would facilitate revascularization of the grafts. In effect, Robinson's cervical interbody principle is being used in the Cloward posterior lumbar interbody fusion. The preservation of the cortical plate is important in avoiding settling.

Graft Removal

A split-thickness graft then is removed from the iliac bone posteriorly. This graft is about 8 mm thick, 3 to 4.5 cm wide, and 6 to 8 cm long (Fig. 86-23). The graft is removed *en bloc* with an osteotome. Six to eight generous strips of cancellous bone also are removed to fill the available space distally and laterally in the prepared bed after total discectomy. The *en bloc* grafts then are

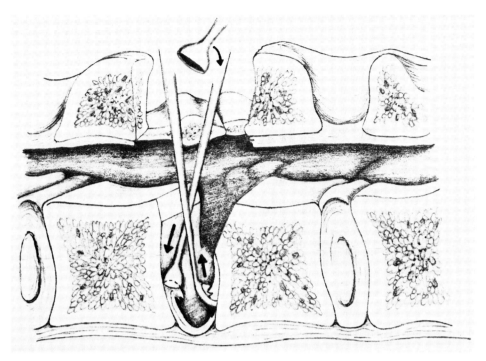

Fig. 86-20.   After the intervertebral rims are removed, the cleavage of disc attachment to the cortical plate is identified and downbite or upbite curettes are used to energetically detach the disc materials from the cortical plate. A curved upbite curette is used to remove the concave centrum of the lower cartilaginous plate. The large chunks of disc material that are detached are removed with a rongeur.

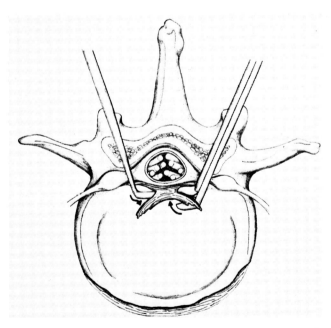

Fig. 86-21.   Removal of midline bar of the annulus fibrosus. A sharp-pointed osteophyte periosteal elevator is used to separate the disc material from the posterior limiting membrane and then is removed either with a sharp-angled upbite disc rongeur or a "pea-pod" pituitary rongeur.

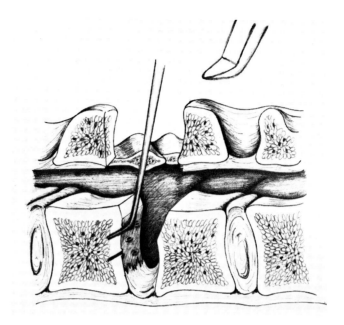

Fig. 86-22. Preparation of the graft site. The epiphyseal ring is osteotomed, the central cortical plate is preserved, and the cortical plate is perforated to enhance revascularization of grafts from the cancellous bone. The perforator (see insert) has a 45° angle and a sharpened end. A downward tap of the perforator will drive the sharp tip into the cancellous bone of the vertebral body.

cut to size depending upon the height of the disc after it is totally distracted. A power saw is used for the preparation of the grafts. Each graft is generally about 10 mm in width and about 30 mm in length. If only four grafts can be obtained, four extra half grafts can be procured by making the graft site deeper or wider.

Graft Insertion

Before the peg grafts are inserted, the depth of the disc space is filled with 1 to 2 strips of cancellous bone. The peg grafts then are inserted with the cortical bone of the graft along the longitudinal axis of the body. With the disc space fully distracted by the laminal retractor or by a deeply placed Cloward "Puka" impactor, the grafts can be pushed into the disc space with only a slight tapping. A slight swiveling movement of the blunt end of the chisel will move the graft medially to the center so that a second graft can be placed laterally (Fig. 86-24).

If the graft is firmly packed into the disc space, the Cloward "Puka" maneuver may be needed to move the first graft to the center. This maneuver entails using two blunt-end chisels and swiveling one against the other in order to propagate the graft medially. We use at least four grafts and prefer to use six grafts (Fig. 86-25). We feel that at least 50 percent of the disc space should be filled with grafts in order to avoid failure of osteosynthesis (Fig. 86-26). We also have been filling the lateral recesses laterally with strips of cancellous bone. All crevices between the peg grafts could be filled with cancellous bone (Fig. 86-27); we fully agree with Cloward's teaching to "pack them tight" (see Fig. 86-25). We firmly believe that a tightly packed disc space (a "unipour" concept), with many cancellous and peg grafts, is essential to the success of the fusion. The normal bearing of weight by the adjoining vertebral bodies results in a natural locking mechanism for the grafts.

When the intervertebral foramen is well decompressed through the mesial facetectomy and partial facetectomy of the superior facet, the nerve root that leaves the foramen of the same level

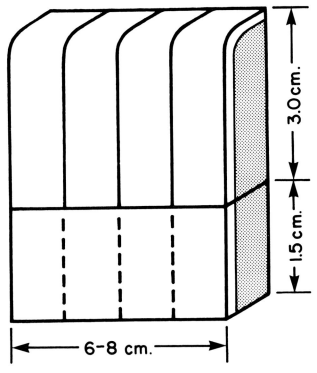

Fig. 86-23. A split-thickness en bloc graft 6–8-cm wide is removed from the posterior iliac crest. The graft is long enough to provide 4 extra half-length peg grafts.

is very close to the lateral margin of the disc space. This nerve root often can be seen after the decompression. When the lateral-most graft is packed, the graft may split and displace laterally and impinge on this nerve root (Fig. 86-28). After all grafts are inserted, care must be taken that the grafts exert no undue pressure on the nerve root that is in front and easily visible, and a search for any possible bony impingement on the lateral nerve root, which is behind and often partially hidden, should be made.

Closure

The Surgicel is removed at the end of the procedure and epidural bleeding is controlled with Gelfoam. The bleeding at the donor site can be controlled easily with Gelfoam soaked with Thrombin.* We do not use a drain. We administer cephalothin sodium (Keflin**) intraoperatively in a dose of 2 g intravenously and continue it at a rate of 2 g every 6 hours for 4 doses. We rarely use transfusions. The average blood loss is 200–400 cc.

Postoperative Care

Patients are out of bed in 2 or 3 days with a Knight lumbar spinal brace. The timing of the ambulation can be judged easily by the ease with which the patient can move himself in bed. Many patients who have had previous simple discectomies claim that the pain from the posterior lumbar interbody fusion is less than that from simple discectomy. Generally, solid fusion should occur in 4 months after surgery (Figs. 86-29, 86-30, and 86-31). Depending upon the result of the tomogram done 4 months postoperatively, we will decide when the brace should be removed. We do encourage patients to engage in physical exercise (such as brisk walking) within the confines of the Knight lumbar spinal brace during the recuperative period.

*Thrombin: topical (bovine origin), Parke-Davis, Morris Plains, New Jersey.
**Keflin: cephalothin sodium. Eli Lilly & Co., Indianapolis, Indiana.

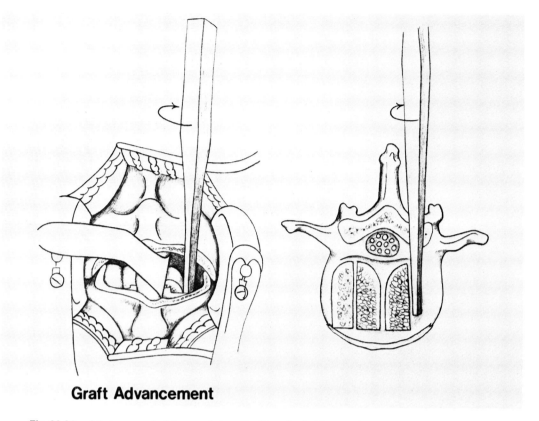

Graft Advancement

Fig. 86-24. Advancement of the medial graft with a single blunt-end chisel (Cloward's "PUKA" technique).

Complications

The first 350 cases performed by the author have shown no postoperative wound infection. There were 6 cases of postoperative thrombophlebitis, 4 during the hospital stay and 2 delayed, occurring after discharge. There were 12 cases of increased neurologic deficit manifested by a foot drop, which recovered in 6 weeks to 6 months. If a cerebrospinal (CSF) leak is encountered during surgery, the leak should be closed with sutures. If an airtight closure is not possible with sutures, the leak should be controlled by Gelfoam or a muscle graft, and the patient should be put on complete bedrest for 14 days before ambulation. In our series we have not encountered any difficulty with CSF leak.

Most patients experienced mild discomfort over the donor site. About 7 percent had transient numbness of the anterior thigh over the distribution of the anterolateral femoral cutaneous nerve, secondary to compression of the nerve by the firm rolls used to support the body.

Result

Out of a total series of 350 cases, 50 consecutive patients who were operated upon and followed for at least 24 months were invited to be studied by two Board-certified orthopedic surgeons to determine the success of fusion and the clinical improvement. Letters were sent out to the patients inviting them to return to be examined by the orthopedic surgeons. Forty-five patients responded. Of the 45 patients examined, 31 were male, 14 were female. The ages of the males varied from 20 to 60 years with an average age of 42.1 years. The ages of the females varied from 20 to 60 years with an average age of 42.8 years (Fig. 86-32A,B).

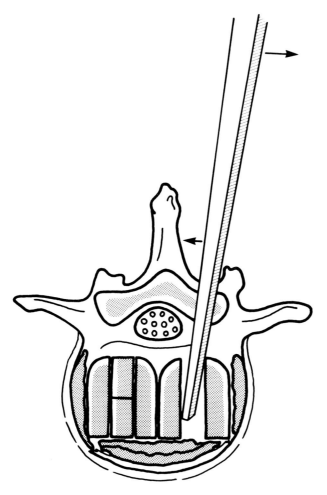

Fig. 86-25. In this diagram six peg grafts have been placed. Two are half-length peg grafts. The disc space is very tightly packed. Cancellous bone grafts are used to fill the spaces in depth and the lateral recesses of the disc space.

Of the 45 patients examined, 30 patients had surgery performed at the L4-5 level, 14 had surgery at the L5-S1 level, and 1 patient had surgery at both the L3-4 and L4-5 levels (Fig. 86-33)

The clinical results were rated:

1. Excellent—complete recovery, resumed normal activity, not on medication.
2. Good—returned to work, occasional mild analgesic, enjoys work and recreation.
3. Fair—works under duress, takes occasional medication, better than before surgery.
4. Poor—needs medication in a dependent fashion, unable to return to work, denied any improvement.

In this series, no patients claimed they were worse than before the surgery.

Thirty-seven patients had 82 percent fusion determined radiologically. This was demonstrated either by tomograms or flexion extension lateral films or both. Two had questionable fusion. Pseudoarthrodesis occurred in 6 patients or 13.3 percent (Fig. 86-34).

The clinical result was rated as excellent in 25 patients (55.5 percent), and a good result was obtained in 6 patients (13.3 percent), giving a total group composed of excellent and good results of 68.8 percent (Table 86-2). A fair result was obtained in 7 patients (15.5 percent), and a poor

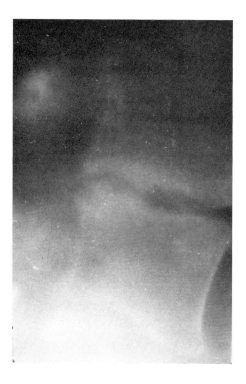

Fig. 86-26. Pseudoarthrodesis occurs when the graft occupies less than the posterior 50 percent of the disc space.

result was obtained in 7 patients (15.5 percent), thus 14 patients (31.2 percent) had a less than satisfactory result. In this group, there are 11 patients with documented secondary gain problems (compensation or litigation). Only one had an excellent result, 4 had fair results, and 6 had poor results.

If the patients who had secondary gain are eliminated, the excellent-to-good result would be elevated to 88.2 percent in contrast to 68.8 percent (Table 86-3).

In the group with excellent results, only 1 patient had questionable fusion; all of the rest had solid fusion (Fig. 86-34A). In the group with good results, 3 had fusion and 3 did not have fusion. In the 3 cases of non-union, motion was detected but the disc space was not collapsed, indi-

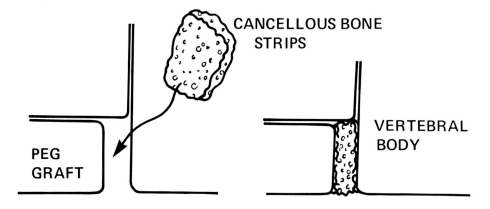

**FILL ALL CREVICES WITH CANCELLOUS BONE STRIPS
LIKE DENTAL FILLING OF CAVATIES**

Fig. 86-27. Technique for filling crevices between the peg grafts and vertebral body with cancellous bone grafts.

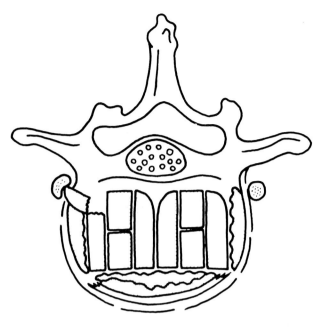

Fig. 86-28. A schematic drawing showing the danger of the lateral-most graft being broken, displaced, and impinging on the nerve behind the facet at the same level.

cating that incomplete bony union possibly may be sufficient to render a good result. Fourteen patients are in the unsatisfactory group, which includes 10 patients with secondary gain problems, and all but 1 of these patients had radiologic evidence of fusion. It appears that in the secondary gain group, the status of fusion does not correlate with the clinical result (Fig. 86-34B).

In the unsatisfactory group, however, 4 patients had no secondary gain, and 3 had evidence of motion of pseudoarthrodesis. Excluding the patients in the secondary gain category, solid bony fusion appears to be a prerequisite for an excellent result.

Our of 45 patients, 34 (75 percent) returned to work. Nine kept their previous heavy-duty jobs, and 7 had to be downgraded to lighter work even though they still performed physical manual work. If we remove secondary gain problems from this group, 33 patients (97 percent) returned to work after surgery. Sixteen patients of this group had previous disc surgery at the same level. In this category 8 had an excellent result (50 percent) and 1 had a good result (6 percent), giving a total with a satisfactory result of 56 percent. Excluding the patients with secondary gain (6) from this series, 70 percent had an excellent result and 10 percent had a good result; this gives a total of 80 percent with satisfactory result.

Table 86-2. The Clinical Results Obtained in 45 Patients with Posterior Lumbar Interbody Fusion

Result	No. of patients (%)
Excellent	25 (55.5)
Good	6 (13.3)
Total with satisfactory result	31 (68.8)
Fair	7 (15.5)
Poor	7 (15.5)
Total with unsatisfactory result	14 (31.2)

**Table 86-3. The Clinical Results Obtained in the Series Excluding Patients
with Secondary Gain Problems**

Result	No. of patients (%)
Excellent	24 (70.6)
Good	6 (17.6)
Total with a satisfactory result	30 (88.2)
Fair	3 (8.7)
Poor	1 (3.1)
Total with an unsatisfactory result	4 (11.8)
Total number of patients	35

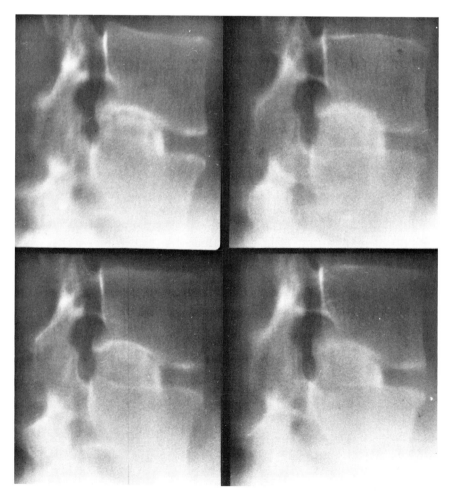

Fig. 86-29.   Four serial lateral tomograms, 4 months after surgery, show good osteosynthesis in all cuts.

Table 86-4. A Review of 120 Consecutive Lumbar Myelograms for
Mechanical Back Pain and Sciatica

Finding	Number of patients		Total (%)	Average age	
	Male	Female		Male	Female
Total	59	61	120	46.4	45.5
Lateral disc syndrome	20	10	30 (25)	34.4	38.2
Facet root syndrome of lateral spinal stenosis	28	22	50 (41.7)	40.3	48.5

Discussion

Froning[16] demonstrated the limitation of flexion extension in the majority of patients with successful discectomy. Persistent mobility, comparable with that expected in a normal individual, usually was found in patients judged to have a poor result. This corroborates the contention of the advocates of posterior interbody fusion that to achieve a better result in the surgery of prolapsed discs, there should be minimal motion of the "motion segment" after surgery.

Simeone,[4] in discussing a paper, stated: "The issue of indications for lumbar fusion remains unsettled. Classically, neurosurgeons have frequently deferred lumbar fusion procedures to their orthopedic colleagues. Independent of one's feelings about fusion . . . the surgeon who believes in lumbar fusion but who may have demurred because of technical uncertainties. The neurosurgeon is familiar with this approach, he can easily gain access to the interspace. . . . On logical grounds, one might assume that fusion by this approach is at least equal to the more formidable transabdominal anterior lumbar fusion, during which less than adequate inspection of the nerve roots is possible. Spine surgeons who believe in fusion should have this procedure in their technical repertoire."

Burton and associates,[17] in reviewing their 1000 cases of failed back, found that between 50 and 60 percent had evidence of lateral spinal stenosis at the time of their first lumbar discectomy. The clinical importance and the frequency of lateral spinal stenosis as a clinical entity with or without disc herniation has been fully appreciated only recently. Our own experience after reviewing 120 lumbar myelograms shows that 41.7 percent have facet root syndrome or lateral spinal stenosis, whereas only 25 percent have the classic lateral disc protrusion without facet abnormality (Table 86-4). We must consider posterior lumbar interbody fusion as an ideal definitive reconstructive and curative procedure for nerve compression and foraminal nerve stenosis (see Figs. 86-3, 86-4, and 86-5). When the two pairs of nerves that are compressed are effectively decompressed at the lateral recesses and at the foramen, there is a loss of stability, and unless the dysfunction of the altered dynamic motion segment is stabilized by fusion, facet hypertrophy and tropism surely recurs. The cause of tropism and hypertrophy of the posterior joints or facets is best explained by Wolffe's Law, which states that "any changes of bony architecture are the result of the external environment." Failure to eliminate the effects of lateral spinal stenosis and to prevent its recurrence is one of the most important causes of the failure to obtain relief by a simple lumbar discectomy, and repeated similar procedures lead to the so-called "failed back." We too often blame the "failed back" or the lack of motivation on the patient. We must consider that in many cases "failed back" is due to a "failed operation."

Modern improvements in operative illumination, better control of epidural hemorrhage by proper positioning of the patient, and the use of Surgicel as a tamponade in retracting epidural veins and dura definitely improve the technical feasibility of PLIF. Adherence to Cloward's teaching, i.e., packing the disc space with as many bone grafts as possible, including cancellous bone to fill all the available spaces, will ensure a higher rate of spinal fusion than shown in the earlier studies documented above.

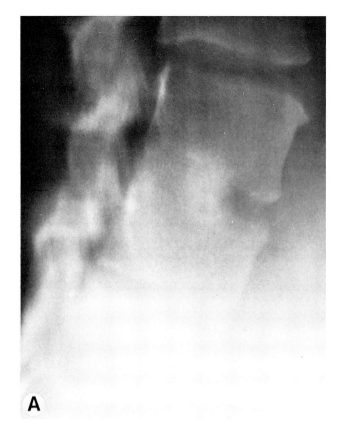

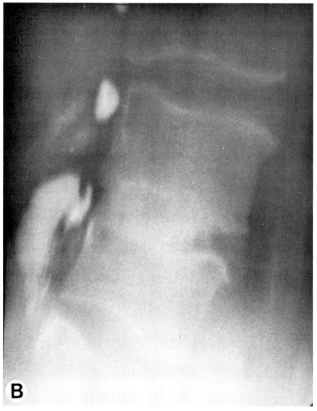

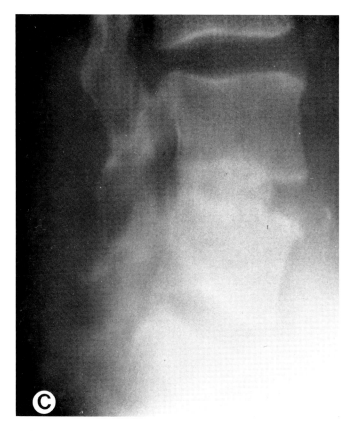

Fig. 86-30.   Tomograms taken 4 months after surgery show the beginning of good osteosynthesis.

McNab[18] in his text stated that a solitary bone graft in the disc space would be absorbed by the surrounding fibrous tissue. He advised[19] that ". . . to have a successful interbody fusion, the only substance between the vertebral bodies must be bone." The experimental work of Bunnell with anterior interbody fusion on canines also indicated that only those spaces packed tightly with graft material were likely to produce fusion.[20] His work favors cancellous bone on cortical bone as the ideal graft material in interbody fusion.

In the surgery of recurrent disc problems, it is wise not to adhere to the surgical principle that the dura and nerve root be visualized first before retracting and exposing the disc space. Where there is scar tissue, it would be wise to remove the medial half of the facet and gain entrance to the lateral gutter lateral to the nerve root. Once the disc space is entered, the scar tissue around the nerve root can be identified easily and pushed medially.

In cases of spondylolisthesis, posterior lumbar interbody fusion for slippage beyond Grade I is technically difficult but not impossible. In our series we removed only the posterior 75 to 85 percent of the disc for fear of endangering the great vessel in front of the vertebral disc. The anterior remnants of the disc material are allowed to remain attached to the anterior limiting membrane. We further believe that in posterior lumbar interbody fusion more than 50 percent of the disc space should be filled with bone grafts. Since it is difficult to reduce the slippage in spondylolisthesis even in the most ideal cases of Grade I, only about 50 percent of exposed and opposing surfaces of the intervertebral surfaces can receive bone grafts. Therefore, in cases in which there

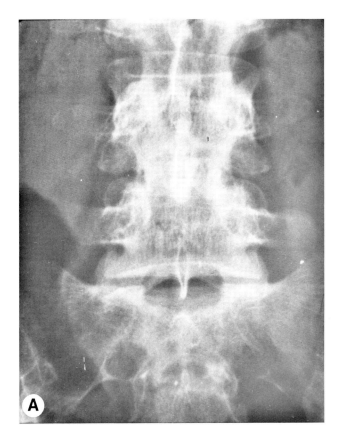

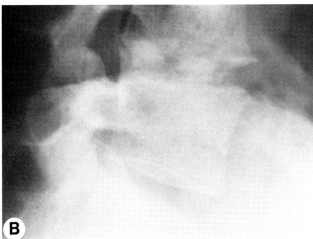

Fig. 86-31.   **A.** An anteroposterior spinal x-ray 2 years postoperatively. The films show solid bony fusion in the disc space with evidence of trabeculation. **B.** A lateral x-ray 2 years postoperatively. The x-ray shows solid bony fusion in the disc space with evidence of trabeculation.

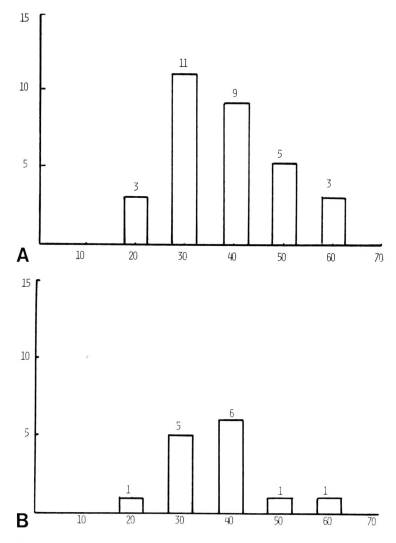

Fig. 86-32. **A.** A graph of the 2-year follow-up on 31 male patients, giving the age distribution. **B.** A graph of the 2-year follow-up of 14 female patients, giving the age distribution.

is any slippage beyond Grade I, we would recommend posterior lateral fusion alone or in combination with posterior lumbar interbody fusion.

Conclusion

Posterior lumbar interbody fusion not only has the advantage of avoiding collapse of the disc space, but also ensures stability of the "motion segment." This stability will avoid tropism of the facet, frequently a cause of recurrent lateral spinal stenosis and "failed back." It also accomplishes wide decompression of all neural components and distraction of the intervertebral disc space. The natural posterior concavity of the lumbar spine produces a firm locking mechanism for the grafts within the disc space. With a generous amount of bone grafts—both cortical peg grafts and cancellous grafts—tightly packed into the disc space, the chances for solid fusion are enhanced.

The modified technique of posterior lumbar interbody fusion with preservation of the facet and cortical plate[4] alleviates postoperative slippage and settlement. Forty-five patients who had

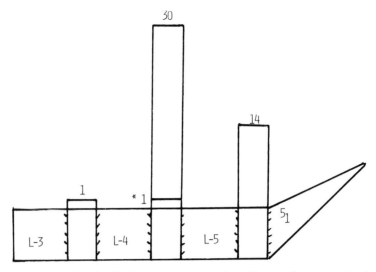

Fig. 86-33. The distribution of surgery at the different disc-space levels.
* = Two-level fusion; L3-4 and L4-5.

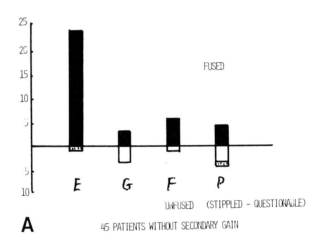

A 45 PATIENTS WITHOUT SECONDARY GAIN

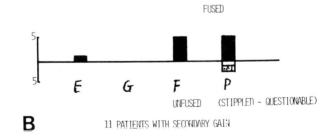

B 11 PATIENTS WITH SECONDARY GAIN

Fig. 86-34. A. The fusion rate and results in 45 patients with
secondary gain. A fusion rate of 82 percent with 2-
year follow-up correlates with the results. **B.** The
fusion rate and result in 11 patients with secondary gain problems, 2-year follow-up. E = Excellent;
G = good; F = fair; P = poor.

undergone modified posterior lumbar interbody fusion with at least 2 years of follow-up show 82 percent bony fusion as visualized by radiologic technique, with clinical results rated as satisfactory in 68.8 percent. Patients who had previous disc surgery at the same level gave a satisfactory result of 56 percent. If 11 patients who had secondary gain problems were removed from consideration, the overall satisfactory result would be 88.2 percent, and in patients who had previous disc surgery done at the same level, the satisfactory results would be increased to 70 percent.

PLIF is especially suited for treatment of lateral spinal stenosis (subarticular and foraminal compression) either with or without association of lumbar disc herniation. It provides neural decompression and establishes permanent stability of a pathologic motion segment, and so prevents recurrence of facet hypertrophy and tropism.

Experience with over 350 PLIF cases indicates that the posterior lumbar interbody fusion should be used as a reconstructive procedure for disabling lumbar disc disease. The procedure is technically feasible and should be more widely employed in patients with lateral spinal stenosis, recurrent discs, and other disabling or failing lumbar disc diseases.

REFERENCES

1. Cloward RB: New treatment of ruptured intervertebral disc. Read at the Annual Meeting of the Hawaii Territorial Medical Association, May 1945
2. Cloward RB: The treatment of ruptured lumbar intervertebral discs by vertebral body fusion. Indications, operative technique, after care. *J Neurosurg* 10:154–168, 1953
3. Cloward RB: Lesions of intervertebral discs and their treatment by intervertebral fusion method. *Clin Orthop* 27:51–77, 1963
4. Lin PM: A technical modification of Cloward's posterior lumbar interbody fusion. *J Neurosurg* 1:118–124, 1977
5. Lin PM: Posterior lumbar interbody fusion, in Schmidek HH, Sweet WH (eds): *Current Techniques in Operative Neurosurgery.* New York, Grune & Stratton, 1977, pp 357–385
6. Lin PM, Cautilli RA, Joyce MF: Posterior lumbar interbody fusion. *J Neuro Orthop Surg* 1: 1–14, 1979
7. Crock HV: Isolated lumbar disc resorption as a cause of nerve root canal stenosis. *Clin Orthop* 191:109–115, 1976
8. LeVay D: A survey of surgical management of lumbar disc prolapse in the United Kingdom and Eire. *Lancet 1*:1211–1213, 1967
9. Junghanns J, Schmorl G: *The Human Spine in Health and Disease.* 2nd ed. New York, Grune & Stratton, 1977, pp 35–37
10. Wiltberger BR: The prefit dowel intervertebral body fusion as used in lumbar disc therapy. A preliminary report. *Am J Surg 6*:723–727, 1953
11. Wiltberger BR: Intervertebral body fusion by the use of posterior bone dowel. *Clin Orthop 35*:69–79, 1964
12. Kilbaldy-Willis WH, McIvor GWD: Spinal stenosis. *Clin Orthop 115*:2–3, 1976
13. Keim HA: Indication for spinal fusion and techniques. *Clin Neurosurg 25*:266–267, 1977
14. Robinson RA: Anterior and posterior cervical spine fusion. *Clin Orthop 35*:34–62, 1964
15. Robinson RA, Smith GW: Anterolateral cervical disc removal and interbody fusion for cervical disc syndrome. *Bull Johns Hopkins Hosp 96*:223 224, 1955
16. Froning EC, Frohman B: Motion of the lumbosacral spine after laminectomy and spine fusion. Correlation of motion with the result. *J Bone Joint Surg 50*:897–918, 1968
17. Burton C, Finneson B, Kilbaldy-Willis WH: Fail back surgery. Presented at Spinal Symposium, Gainesville, Fla., April 1980.
18. McNab I: *Backache.* Baltimore, Williams & Wilkins, 1977, p 166
19. McNab I: Personal communication, December 1979
20. Bunnell WP: Anterior spinal fusion: Promising canine data. Presented at the meeting of the Eastern Orthopedic Association as an award paper for spinal research, Miami, Fla., Oct. 17–21, 1979

CHAPTER 87

Anterior Lumbar Discectomy and Interbody Fusion: Indications and Technique

J. Leonard Goldner
Kenneth E. Wood

James R. Urbaniak

IF SPINAL FUSION IS OCCASIONALLY REQUIRED for the management of patients with intervertebral disc disease, then anterior lumbar discectomy and fusion have a place in the management of patients with chronic low-back pain. We believe that regardless of the technique used, certain patients are relieved of pain if the spine is stabilized. After one operation has failed to relieve intervertebral disc symptoms, fusion of the spine should be seriously considered as a part of the second operative procedure. This is a generality and exceptions do exist, but that philosophy has been helpful in managing patients with recurrent low-back pain who are candidates for operative treatment.

Those who believe in anterior cervical discectomy and fusion should also recognize the value of the same procedure in the lower lumbar and lumbosacral segments. Removal of an intervertebral disc by the anterior approach in either the cervical or lumbar regions will decompress nerve roots without actually manipulating them. Immobilization is almost complete immediately postoperatively, and relief of nerve-root irritation is, temporarily, prompt.

The anterior procedure is not currently popular. It is reserved for *salvage* patients and is considered a last resort. Our experience is that it will resolve the problem of failed discectomy at one or two interspaces, and that it might be the procedure of choice in certain patients before posterolateral fusion, and certainly before wide extensive laminectomy is done posteriorly to relieve patients who have nerve-root irritation and who do not have free fragments compressing the roots.

Historical Review

Anterior lumbosacral fusion was first used in the mid-1930s for spondylolisthesis.[1-5] In 1948[6] the procedure was used for lumbosacral intervertebral disc disease.

Sacks,[7] in 1961, reported 150 patients treated by anterior arthrodesis. He stated that 26 percent of these patients were asymptomatic, 62 percent were improved, and 12 percent were unchanged. In 1970, the same author[4] indicated that the functional results of the anterior lumbar

Department of Orthopaedic Surgery, School of Medicine, Duke University, Durham, North Carolina

fusion series were "about the same," as those for his posterolateral fusion series. Our experience has been similar. The arthrodesis rate of posterolateral fusions at Duke University Medical Center is only slightly better than the rate of healing of anterior interbody fusion.[8-10]

In 1972, Stauffer and Coventry[11] reported on 77 patients treated by anterior lumbar fusion. They observed a single interspace fusion rate of 68 percent and reported 36 percent "good clinical results." They stated that they reserved the procedure for salvage. They do not indicate why 64 percent were considered failures.

Kotcamp[12,13] has used anterior lumbar fusion in the management of over 500 patients. He states that he frequently uses this operation as a primary method of managing discectomy, and indicates that he has observed a fusion rate of 90 percent for a single interspace.

Several years ago the results of this procedure and the fusion rate obtained by authors using calf bone[14-16] and by a technique using circular plug grafts were thought to be very high. Harmon[17] has altered his reported technique and more recently has obtained a higher fusion rate by using fibular graft and screw fixation.

Indications for Anterior Discectomy and Lumbar Fusion

The nonoperative treatment of intervertebral disc disease has a high priority in our management of patients with chronic low-back pain. We apply all currently available nonoperative techniques in an effort to "avoid the first operative procedure." If this treatment fails, then posterior nerve-root decompression and hemilaminectomy after myelography is the program selected for treating the patient with persistent radiculopathy. If this treatment fails, then reoperation and possibly posterolateral fusion are considered. The latter approach depends on whether or not the nerve roots require re-exploration and further decompression or whether the interspace, proximally or distally, requires exploration. Patients in this *first category* also have been managed by anterior discectomy and fusion. They have had one or more prior operations, but pain has not been relieved.[8-10]

A *second group* of patients may have persistent pseudoarthrosis if fusion has been attempted, or instability, incongruity, or nerve-root irritation secondary to specific pathologic conditions.

A *third group* is the fourth-decade female with a narrow lumbosacral joint, sclerosis of the interspaces, chronic severe low-back pain, and intermittent radiculopathy. The myelogram usually has been negative, but the patient does have evidence of buttock, thigh, and calf pain. Anterior discectomy and fusion usually relieve the back pain and radiculopathy without interfering with the nerve roots.

A *fourth indication* is seen in patients who have had posterior operations and developed infection. Persistent back pain and radiculopathy in these patients should be managed by anterior removal of the residual intervertebral disc material and localized arthrodesis. The interspace may or may not have been affected by the prior infection, but tissue usually is sterile after antibiotic therapy has been given.

The *fifth group* includes patients who have had posterolateral fusion and laminectomy for management of spondylolisthesis and who still have pain and pseudoarthrosis. They usually can be managed successfully by anterior discectomy and fusion. As a primary procedure for management of spondylolisthesis, however, this is not recommended.[16,18]

In the *sixth group,* patients with proven spinal stenosis and arachnoiditis have been improved by anterior discectomy and fusion, particularly if the myelogram showed anterior indentations rather than posterior compression (Fig. 87-1). A second-stage posterior laminectomy was done, with less instability resulting if vertebral bodies were fused.

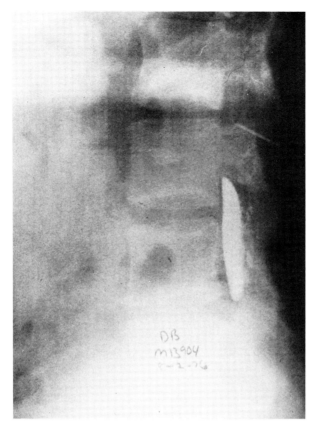

Fig. 87-1.   A lateral x-ray film of a 20-year-old man who has had three operative procedures of discectomy and hemilaminectomy for management of pain in the back and lower extremity. This myelogram shows the column of contrast blocked at the L4-5 interspace. Two years have elapsed since the original operation was done. The patient was almost completely incapacitated because of the pain in his back and lower extremity.

Diagnostic Studies

Information obtained from the patient's history, physical examination, and roentgenograms usually is essential to making the decision concerning which approach to use for spine stabilization. Other studies that can be selected, as indicated, are listed and the particular reasons for each are mentioned briefly.

1. *Laboratory studies* should include a battery of chemical analyses, including enzymes, uric acid, and blood sugar, to detect any subtle systemic disease and, particularly, to determine any elevation of liver enzymes. This study is described elsewhere. If liver enzymes are elevated, general anesthesia should be avoided until the cause of the elevation is determined. Also, studies related to rheumatoid arthritis or ankylosing spondylitis are important, as, occasionally, the patient with chronic back pain has a primary condition other than intervertebral disc disease.
2. *Roentgenograms* should be taken in multiple planes and, if the patient has been operated

upon previously, a lateral flexion and extension as well as an anterior, posterior right, and left lateral bending-stress exposure should be done. This will give information about motion at the interspaces and aid in determining whether or not pseudoarthrosis exists. Tomography also helps to determine if pseudoarthrosis is present.

3. *A differential spinal* test will aid in determining whether the patient has total relief of extremity or back pain at certain concentrations of injected anesthetic. If the patient's pain is relieved by saline, then the severity of this complaint is questioned. If pain is not relieved by a total motor and sensory block, the other considerations concerning its origin are reviewed.[18]

4. *Psychiatric consultation* is important in managing the patient who has had multiple operations and is being considered for another operation. Reactive depression, frank neuroses, or subtle psychoses may exist, and the psychiatrist can recommend appropriate medication and proper timing of an operation, if indicated, in this particular patient. The psychiatrist may be able to give advice to the family through the social worker and information to the employer that is helpful in rehabilitating the patient.

5. *Clinical psychologic* studies have proved to be valuable in assessing the patient's behavior profile, response to injury and operation, and characteristics as they appear on the scale of conversion hysteria, hypochondriasis, or depression. This information is very important in postoperative management and in deciding whether or not the operative procedure, if not clearly indicated, should be done at all.

6. *Discography* has proved to be valuable for us in reproducing pain at a space that has not been operated upon, in providing information about the amount of fluid that can be injected into an interspace, and for providing information about a normal intervertebral disc that takes a minimal amount of contrast and does not result in pain at the time of the injection. An intervertebral disc that appears abnormal but does not cause pain at the time of injection usually can be ignored. Abnormalities seen by discography are not an indication for surgery.[19] Renografin* is the contrast used for discography. If the injection is painful, it can be followed by an injection of 40 mg of Depomedrol. We believe this diminishes the irritation caused by the iodide contrast. (Fig. 87-2).

7. *Electromyography* by a trained observer, if used to sample enough muscles, will provide invaluable information about the condition of the lower extremities. There is a high correlation between positive electromyography and positive myelography and discography. If the electromyogram is positive and the myelogram is negative, that information is particularly helpful. If the electromyogram is negative and the myelogram is positive, the electrical studies should be repeated by an experienced electromyographer and special tests such as H reflex should be done.

8. *A metrizamide myelogram* is helpful in localizing root-compression lesions and in ruling out a significant posterior block or posterior compression. A large defect, noted at the time of the *initial myelogram,* usually was a contraindication to anterior discectomy (Figs. 87-1 and 87-3). Patients who have had multiple operative procedures, however, and who had perineural fibrosis or arachnoiditis demonstrated that the block was not a contraindication to anterior discectomy and fusion.

9. *Nerve-root block* has been helpful in localizing the pain and the particular nerve root that required decompression. This test is an adjunct to the differential spinal test in that it provides information about complete or partial relief of pain.

10. *Thermography* has provided some information about the inflammatory aspect of the patient's complaints. A positive thermogram suggests the process may be inflammatory rather than a primary mechanical deficiency. Occasionally this test has suggested ankylosing spondylitis and has resulted in other studies that aided proper diagnosis.

11. *Epidural venography* aids in localizing a compression lesion and may provide evidence of

*American Critical Care, McGaw Park, Illinois.

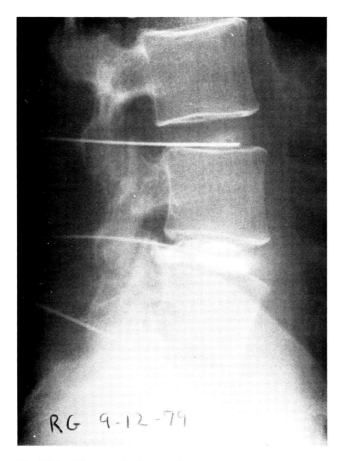

RG 9-12-79

Fig. 87-2.   Discography is an adjunct procedure that gives information about the production of pain. Renografin is injected to determine if there is a leak in the annulus and irregularity of the annulus and nucleus. An abnormal test does not require an operative procedure. A normal discogram is helpful in eliminating the diagnosis of intervertebral disc disease and directs attention to the paravertebral structures. The injection shown here between L4-5 is abnormal and shows leakage of the contrast through a defect in the posterior longitudinal ligament. The patient had pain during the injection, as the Renografin irritated sensory receptors outside of the annulus. The needle at L3-4 is not well centered and was readjusted before injection. This interspace showed a "cotton ball" appearance and was considered normal.

nerve-root involvement when the myelogram is negative. False-negative venograms may be a problem, and the data must be interpreted in conjunction with other findings (Fig. 87-4A, B).

12. *Computerized axial tomography* (CT) complements the studies already mentioned (Fig. 87-5A, B).

13. *Technetium 99 bone scan* will aid in determining the presence of nonunion, an inflammatory process, or an infection.

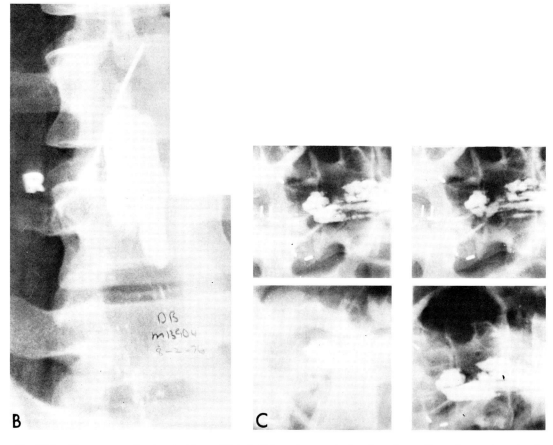

Fig. 87-3. The same patient as in Figure 87-1. **A.** This anteroposterior view shows the column of contrast blocked at the L4-L5 level. The presumptive diagnosis was arachnoiditis and perineural fibrosis. The appearance of the myelogram was the same after the second and third operations. Note that the spinous processes have been removed and that a segment of the laminal arches have been removed from the fifth lumbar vertebra and the inferior segment of the fourth lumbar vertebra. The facets are intact. **B.** A postoperative AP view of the L4-5 interspace with the bone grafts visible between the vertebral bodies and the contrast at the same level as preoperatively.

Contraindications to Anterior Lumbar Discectomy and Fusion

1. If nerve-root exploration is essential, then the posterior approach is desirable. We have not depended on nerve-root decompression from the anterior approach, although we have in the cervical spine.
2. Other contraindications are multiple interspace, advanced intervertebral disc disease (more than three interspaces), particularly in a patient over 60 years of age and in those with severe osteoporosis.

Surgical Technique

Patients usually have been operated upon under general anesthesia supplemented with muscle relaxants. The Trendelenburg position, with the head down about 10°, is desirable as it allows displacement of the abdominal contents proximally and reduces venostasis in the lower extremi-

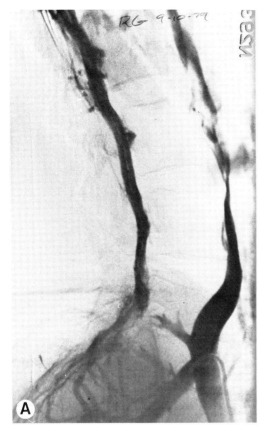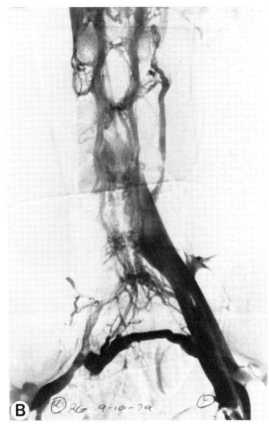

Fig. 87-4.   A. This epidural venogram subtraction film shows the pattern of the vena cava, the iliac arteries, and the anterior and posterior venous pattern over the vertebral bodies and the interspaces. This information is helpful not only in determining an extrusion from the interspace and the extent of fibrosis at the interspace but also in determining any alterations that might be present in the vena cava or the iliac vessels. **B.** Epidural venogram subtraction study shows incomplete filling of the radicular veins and the lumbar veins on the right side and cross flow of venous return from right to left through the sacral and iliac veins. This information is helpful in determining the presence of collateral circulation, the size of the venous vessels, and the areas of fibrosis.

ties. This position is arranged after induction. A thin, folded sheet is placed under the left buttock to elevate the iliac crest. The upper extremities are placed so as to avoid stretch on axillary structures and compression on ulnar nerves at the elbows.

The anesthetist then is asked to locate handles on the table that provide hyperextension of the lumbar spine. This position is not used when the incision is made, but is used while a discectomy is being done.

The abdomen and iliac crest are prepared with soap, water, and Betadine, and the skin is covered with a transparent adhesive dressing. The patient also is tilted to the left side 10° if the surgeon is standing on the left while exposure is being made, or to the right side 10° if the surgeon prefers to stand on the right while the *left* retroperitoneal exposure is performed.

The left paramedian incision is made through the skin and superficial fascia, the anterior rectus sheath is opened, and the muscle belly is retracted laterally to the lateral gutter (Fig. 87-6). If the rectus sheath is incised in the midline, the peritoneum will be entered. The retroperitoneal space is entered, initially, inferiorly at the linea semilunaris, and the peritoneum is carefully and slowly separated by blunt dissection from the undersurface of the rectus sheath. The proximal incision into the posterior sheath should not be made until the peritoneum is separated from the fascia. Small peritoneal tears may occur during this step in the procedure, and they should be

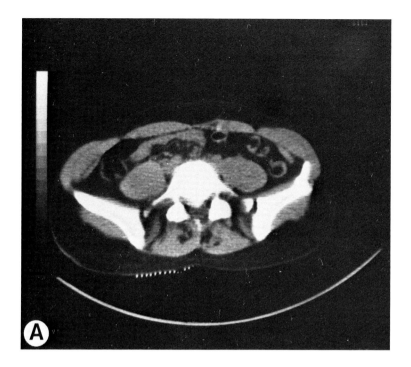

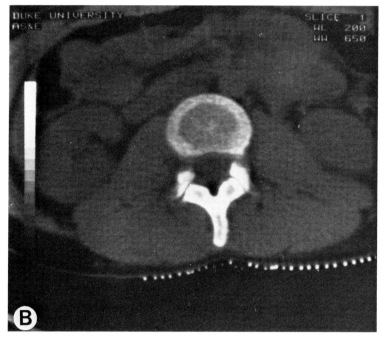

Fig. 87-5. A. Computerized axial tomography shows the absence of the
spinous process and part of the laminal arch and impingement
in the region of the lateral recess. The bulging in the posterior
aspect of the vertebral body is significant only after sections
above and below this location are reviewed. **B.** This CT exposure
through the L3 spinous process and vertebral body shows slight
irregularity of the facets but no impingement from the vertebral
body. This method of diagnostic study is important in determining "napkin-ring" constriction proximal to the site of a prior posterior fusion or spontaneous spinal stenosis.

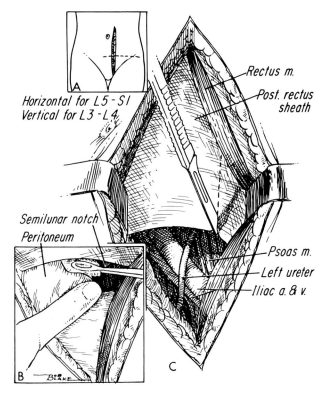

Fig. 87-6.   A periumbilical incision has been made, the anterior sheath of the rectus has been incised, and the rectus muscle has been retracted laterally. The posterior rectus sheath is identified anteriorly and far laterally. The semilunar notch is used as a guide for reflecting the peritoneum from the undersurface of the rectus sheath. The peritoneum and abdominal contents are swept medially. The posterior rectus sheath is incised laterally and proximally and these same flaps are sutured with nonabsorbable suture at the time of closure.

repaired with chromic catgut. The rectus sheath is incised from the semilunar notch inferiorly to its superior border proximally. The psoas muscle is identified, and the iliac artery and vein then are palpated or visualized on the left side. The left ureter is located, after which the lumbosacral interspace is palpated. This space is identified between the right and left iliac arteries and veins (Fig. 87-7). The sacral promontory is identified by palpation without disturbing the sympathetic nerves crossing over the sacral promontory or the major sympathetic nerves on either side of the lumbar vertebrae. The soft tissue over the interspace of the vertebrae and lower half of the fifth lumbar vertebral body is dissected off with a small dissector, and the venous tributaries from the iliac vein and vena cava are clamped with silver clips. The lumbosacral interspace is exposed by retracting the left iliac artery and vein to the left side and the right iliac artery and vein to the right side with blunt vein retractors (Fig. 87-8). Spike retractors, driven into the body of the fifth lumbar vertebra, are helpful in maintaining the exposure (Fig. 87-9A). The vessels are protected from the spike by a small abdominal pack, and the peripheral pulse is palpated distal to the spike, indicating that excessive tension is not placed on the artery or vein. No dissection is done on the first sacral segment. Bleeding and the decussating fibers of the sympathetic chain, which partially control ejaculation, are avoided. Venous bleeding is avoided by frequent use of vascular clips, both large and small, by preclamping of venous tributaries, and by slow and deliberate mobiliza-

1382   GOLDNER, WOOD, AND URBANIAK

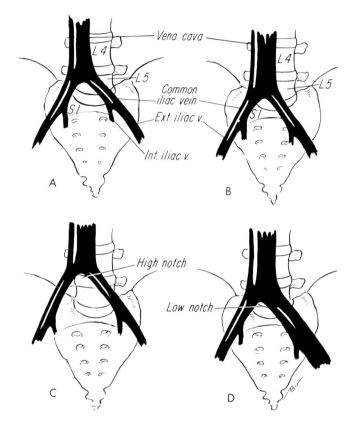

Fig. 87-7. Several patterns of bifurcation of the vena cava into the iliac veins exist. The bifurcation may be opposite the middle of the fifth lumbar vertebra, at the level of the last intervertebral disc space, or even as high as the middle of the fourth lumbar vertebral body. The decision to reflect the artery, vein, and ureter to the right, in order to expose L4-5, depends on the height of the notch. Over 90 percent of the time, this reflection is necessary and makes the exposure easier. In each instance, isolation of the L5-S1 interspace has been possible just below the bifurcation.

tion of the vena cava. This structure may be adherent and may require partial clipping or suturing to prevent tearing. Angulated vascular clamps in addition to the vascular clips should be readily available. Also, synthetic clotting material should be readily available to stop bleeding from an irregular surface. A fiberoptic headlight provides visibility.

In exposing the fourth lumbar interspace, the left iliac artery and vein and the ureter are displaced to the right side of the spine and are held in place by spike retractors. During exposure of this interspace there is even more likelihood of obliterating the left iliac artery by applying excessive tension on the retractor.

The anterior longitudinal ligament at the L5-S1 interspace is elevated from the annulus as a flap, with the base attached at the left (Figs. 87-8 and 87-10). This flap, when tagged with sutures, affords additional retraction and protection for the vessels. Hyperextension of the operating table brings the spine closer to the surface of the wound and affords better exposure of the interspace (Fig. 87-11). The intervertebral disc and the annulus are separated from the cartilaginous plates of the vertebra with a knife or a thin osteotome. Once detached from the vertebral body above and below, the disc complex can be removed easily with a large pituitary rongeur and large curettes (Fig. 87-9B). The space is cleaned out thoroughly, back to the posterior longitudinal ligament, before any bone is removed. In this way, bleeding is minimal and dissection

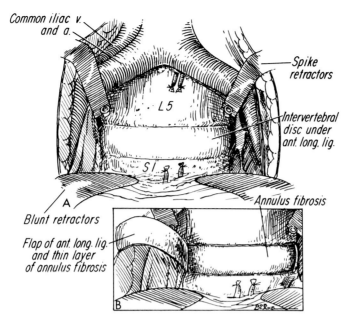

Fig. 87-8. The notch of the vena cava, where it divides into the iliac veins, may be high or low. In this instance the midportion of the fifth lumbar vertebra is clearly visible, the intervertebral disc is exposed widely to the right and left, and no dissection is carried out over the sacral prominence other than to interrupt the veins and arteries with silver clips. Spikes are not inserted into the sacrum, since this may result in additional dissection and cause trauma to the decussating nerve fibers over the first sacral segment. These fibers should be avoided. A long flap of anterior longitudinal ligament, to which is attached a thin layer of the annulus fibrosis, is isolated and reflected either right or left, depending upon which interspace is involved. This flap will protect the artery and vein at the fourth interspace.

can be done under direct vision. The lateral recesses are cleaned thoroughly. Cartilage surfaces are removed from the vertebral bodies with an osteotome until bleeding bone is encountered. Vigorous bleeding may occur from the posterior aspect of the vertebral bodies and can be controlled with small amounts of bone wax or cautery. The undersurface of the L5 vertebra is concave and requires special attention in removing soft tissue.

After the soft tissue and cartilage have been removed from the interspace, the dimensions of the interspace are measured with a caliper and ruler. The grafts then are cut individually from the left ilium, which is prepared by subperiosteal dissection so that full-thickness grafts, with inner and outer cortex of the ilium, can be obtained.[11] The graft is cut slightly larger than the height of the interspace so that firm impaction can be obtained (Fig. 87-12A and B). The lateral recesses of the intervertebral space are packed first with short vertical struts, with the cortices at right angles to the vertebral bodies. The central graft is usually 3.5 cm deep and the width varies from 0.8 to 1.0 cm. After the lateral grafts are placed, the center graft is packed into place so that the anterior edge is countersunk about 2 mm. The second center graft then is inserted and compressed, both to the right and to the left sides. A wedging technique is used by inserting two osteotomes between the center grafts and spreading the osteotomes to the right and to the left, thereby compressing the grafts and allowing space for an additional piece of bone (Fig. 87-11C). Small segments of cortical and cancellous bone can be packed between the grafts. The grafts

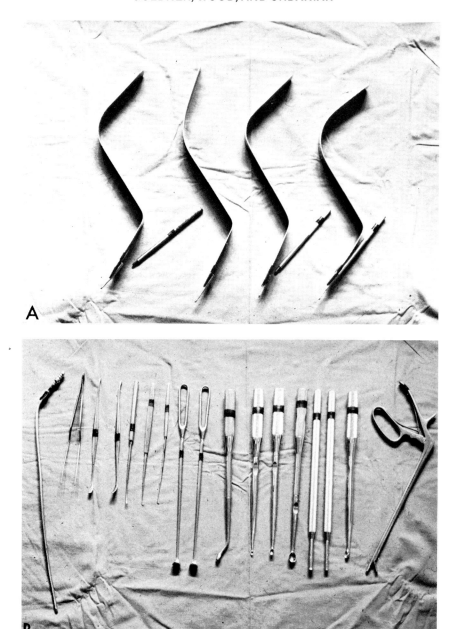

Fig. 87-9. **A.** The spiked retractors are very helpful in doing the procedure. The extension screws on and off and is used to impact the spike into the vertebral body. Two retractors usually are used with one being placed on the right and one on the left in order to retract the artery and vein. The spike should be covered with a sponge pack on one side so that pressure from the metal does not irritate the vessels. When the spikes are removed, a small amount of bone wax is used to fill the bone hole in order to diminish bleeding. **B.** Special instruments used in doing anterior lumbar discectomy and fusion. The large pituitary ronguer was made by an instrument company at our request. The large curettes and long-handled impactors are helpful in cleaning out the interspace and in placing the bone grafts. The long-handled vein retractors are helpful in displacing the iliac vein and the vena cava, while silver clips are used to clamp the small tributaries.

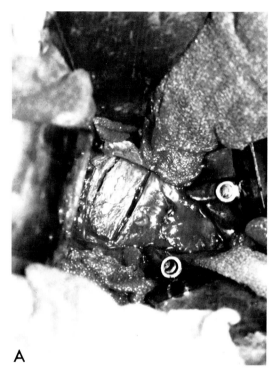

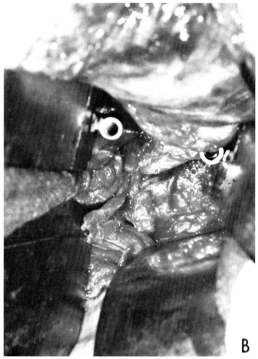

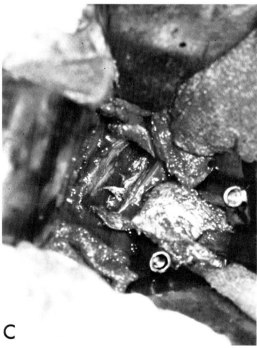

Fig. 87-10. **A.** The anterior ligament has been removed and the annulus incised. The soft tissue remaining in the interspace is made up of residual fragments of annulus, fibrous tissue, cartilaginous fragments, and minimal nucleus. All of this material is removed completely until the cartilage plates are clearly visible. **B.** The 2.0-cm spikes of the metallic retractor are driven into the L5 vertebral body. Cuts have been made into the anterior longitudinal ligament superiorly and inferiorly. A flap of anterior longitudinal ligament has been elevated and retracted to the patient's right. Packs are used to protect the vessels, the ureter, the sympathetic chain, and the presacral decussation. **C.** The anterior longitudinal ligament flap has been elevated, the anterior, medial, and lateral segments of the annulus have been removed, and the soft tissues remaining superiorly, interiorly, and posteriorly must be removed so that good bone contact can be obtained between the autogenous bone graft and the vertebral bodies.

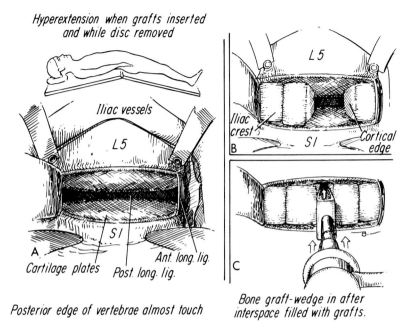

*Hyperextension when grafts inserted
and while disc removed*

Posterior edge of vertebrae almost touch

*Bone graft-wedge in after
interspace filled with grafts.*

Fig. 87-11. The intervertebral disc, which is relatively avascular, has been removed without breaking through the cartilage plates. After the annulus and nucleus have been excised, the cartilage plates are partially removed, perforated, and roughened, so that bone surfaces that bleed exist. Lateral bone grafts are packed so that the right and left edges of the interspace are filled with a graft. Additional bone grafts then are placed in the center of the interspace and the last bone graft is wedged in between the seemingly tight impacted grafts.

should not be countersunk excessively as they may extend posteriorly through holes in the posterior longitudinal ligament and irritate the nerve roots.

The spine then is straightened by correcting the hyperextended position of the table. This holds the grafts in place by wedging the vertebral bodies.

The L4-5 interspace is exposed by retracting the left iliac artery, vein, and ureter toward the right side and replacing the spike retractors in the L5 vertebral body. The spine then is hyperextended and the L4-5 interspace is cleaned out and prepared for insertion of the iliac bone graft (Fig. 87-13). If the L3-4 interspace is to be done, the dissection is completed proximally and the lumbar artery and vein ligated.

After the bone grafts are in place, a small piece of Surgicel is placed over the grafts, and the anterior longitudinal flaps are replaced with a single nonabsorbable suture. All deep fascia layers are closed with nonabsorbable sutures and subcutaneous tissues are closed with absorbable sutures. Four tension sutures of nylon are placed through the skin, subcutaneous tissue, and fascia and the dressing is sutured in place in order to absorb hematoma. This is removed after 5 days.

The average blood loss for a one-interspace operation is 500 ml and 1200 ml for a two-interspace operation. Replacement is done during the operative procedure with whole blood or packed cells; selection depends upon the volume of blood and the rapidity of loss. Packed cells may be given postoperatively if necessary.

Postoperative Management

Nasogastric intubation is not always necessary but is used in some patients for maximum abdominal comfort, even though the tube itself may be uncomfortable. A low negative pressure is connected to the nasogastric tube until active peristalsis occurs, which is usually within 36 to

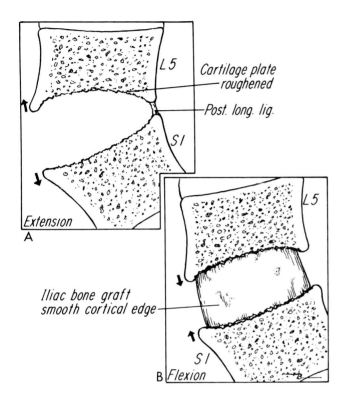

L5

Cartilage plate
roughened

Post. long. lig.

S1

Extension

A

Iliac bone graft
smooth cortical edge

L5

S1

B *Flexion*

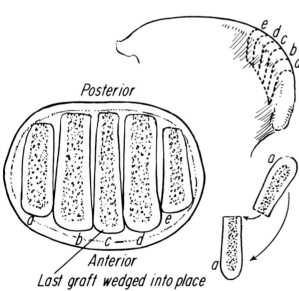

Posterior

Anterior
Last graft wedged into place

Fig. 87-12. A lateral view of the vertebral bodies in the hyperextended position showing the posterior longitudinal ligament intact, the roughened edges of the cartilage plates, and perforations into the subchondral bone. After the bone graft is inserted and the convex edge is placed into the inferior surface of the upper vertebra, the trunk is flexed for impaction and compression. The graft is countersunk, with the anterior edge resting just below the edge of the vertebral bodies. The muscle origins attached to the anterior iliac spine are left in place and the anterior-superior iliac spine is not removed. The full-thickness grafts then are rotated before insertion, so that the cortical edges provide vertical support for the vertebral bodies. The bone grafts are contoured so that there is a convex edge superiorly and a straight edge inferiorly. The iliac crest eventually rests in the outer two-thirds of the interspace, and the narrower portion of the graft is deep. Wide exposure of the interspace is needed in order to place bone at the periphery of the interspace. The width of the iliac crest and the size of the lumbar interspace determine the number of bone grafts that can be pressed into the interspace.

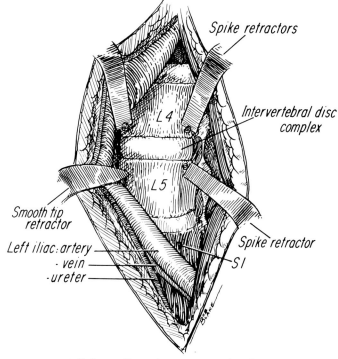

Retroperitoneal exposure of spine

Fig. 87-13. Retroperitoneal exposure of L4, L5, and S1 through a retroperitoneal incision. The iliac artery, vein, and ureter have been displaced medially, the left sympathetic chain is recognized and
avoided, and the spike retractors are used to provide exposure
of the intervertebral disc complex. Compression of the artery
and vein by the retractors must be avoided and the pulsation of
the vessels should be felt from time to time. If L3 is to be exposed, the lumbar artery and vein must be ligated and the vessels dissected to the level of the upper edge of the third lumbar
vertebra.

48 hours. The patient's head and chest are elevated slightly; also, *the lower extremities should be
higher than heart level.* Elastic stockings are used immediately postoperatively, but no elastic
wrappings are used during the operation. The patient is encouraged to initiate active motion of
the feet immediately upon awakening. The patient should be encouraged to turn frequently,
to place a pillow on the abdominal wall in order to decrease pain of coughing, and to
breathe deeply several times each hour. A trapeze is placed on the bed and the patient encouraged to use it.

Anticoagulation has been used in all patients who have anterior lumbar fusion. Our current
anticoagulation routine is therapeutic low-dose heparin; 5000 units are given subcutaneously on
call, and 3000 subcutaneously postoperatively, with the first dose beginning about 6 hours after
the operation has been completed. The heparin is monitored daily by activated partial thromboplastin time. High therapeutic levels are not necessary. The level should be prolonged only
slightly more than normal. Heparin is continued about 5 days, the platelet count is observed
every third day, and the patient is started on Coumadin on the fourth postoperative day. Heparin
is continued until the ratio of Coumadin is 1.5:1. Coumadin is monitored for a total of 3 weeks.
Prothrombin time is maintained at 1.5 times normal level. The patient may leave the hospital 10
to 14 days after the procedure, and the family physician is asked to monitor the anticoagulant.
Certain medications alter the prothrombin time and the physician should be familiar with these.

Straight-leg raising is started on the third postoperative day and continued for several months. By the fifth postoperative day, the patient is allowed to sit and to walk. A low-back corset has been used to support abdominal muscles and to encourage deep breathing and coughing. The iliac donor site usually is more painful than the abdomen or back.

The pain relief associated with radiculopathy has been consistently noted on the day after surgery. Because of early relief of pain, many patients tend to overexert physically, and they must be warned that total pain relief will not persist and may not be present for several months. Recurrent episodes of discomfort are to be expected.

Patients are asked to avoid driving an automobile for 6 to 8 weeks. Walking should be increased in a graduated way and the patient should attempt to go 2 to 3 miles daily after 4 to 6 weeks have passed. Isometric, abdominal, and gluteal exercises are encouraged. The patient is maintained on a high-protein, low-fat diet with adequate daily vitamin intake and modest doses of anti-inflammatory medication.

Anteroposterior and lateral roentgenograms of the lumbosacral spine are taken just before the patient leaves the hospital. These provide a base line for judging the appearance of the graft, psoas shadows, bone density, and the height of the interspace. Three months after surgery, lateral flexion and extension roentgenograms are taken with the patient in the standing position. Radiographic studies are repeated again at 6 to 12 months. A solid fusion cannot be confirmed until at least a year after the operation, and even at that time trabeculations across both sides of the interspace are not always present. Delayed union can be established at 12 months after surgery, and nonunion can be established at 18 to 24 months if the condition is relatively static.

Complications and Sequelae

Immediate complications have occurred infrequently. These diminished as experience with the procedure increased. Complications have included thromboembolism and pseudoarthrosis.

Thromboembolism

This has been avoided by the use of anticoagulation therapy in all of the patients done during the past 6 years. Low-molecular weight or regular dextran was used for 3 or 4 years, with a diminished incidence of venous thrombosis. About 1970, therapeutic low-dose heparin was introduced. After 7 to 10 days of receiving heparin, the patient was given Coumadin and maintained on a limited anticoagulation regimen for a total of 4 weeks. Coumadin alone, or dextran and aspirin, or aspirin alone also are used by certain members of the staff. A recent review of all patients who had major orthopedic operations and received anticoagulation showed that therapeutic low-dose heparin had a predictable protective effect against thromboembolism. Other preventative measures, such as elevation of the extremities during and after the procedure, adequate hydration, and early ambulation (on the third or fourth day), are important measures in diminishing the incidence of thromboembolism. The high-risk patient is defined as one who is known to have had thromboembolic disease or who has a known collagen disease or a family history of hypercholesterolemia. Obesity also is a factor associated with an increased incidence of thromboembolic disease.

Pseudoarthrosis

As the number of spaces operated upon increases in a particular patient, the pseudoarthrosis rate also increases. Studies of successful fusion in the first 100 cases operated upon in our series are listed in Table 87-1. Patients with successful fusion cannot be determined for at least 1 year after the operative procedure has been completed, and, preferably, follow-up should be at least 2 years; nonunion not evident at 1 year may be evident at 2 years. Likewise, what appeared to be an early pseudoarthrosis may progress to a stable spine at about 1 year.

Table 87-1. Anterior Discectomy and Fusion: Incidence of Successful Fusion

	Patients	Successful fusion	% Fusion
Single-space	46	42	91
Two-space	46	33	72
Three-space	8	5	62
Total	100	80	

The arthrodesis rate has been reviewed for the second 100 cases, and patients who have had one interspace arthrodesed showed a rate of fusion of about 90 percent; those who had two spaces arthrodesed had a fusion rate of about 80 percent. Individual surgeons, however, demonstrated smaller series in the group with a higher fusion rate, indicating that there is a direct relationship between the technique used, the placement of the bone grafts, the stability of the interspace after the operative procedure has been completed, and the patient's activities during the next several months.

Our analysis of the last 200 patients shows a definite correlation between successful spine arthrodesis, subsequent relief of symptoms, and diminution of pathologic physical findings. A few patients who were relieved of radiculopathy did not have a solid fusion. Their back pain usually persisted. Other patients obtained a solid fusion and were not relieved of all their complaints. Factors known to be related to the persistence of pain, such as perineural fibrosis, intraneural fibrosis, and involvement of areas outside the spine as well as the interspaces proximally, must be considered in the total management of these patients.

When arthrodesis failed in patients who had undergone a two-space fusion, the pseudoarthrosis was usually in the upper interspace. Stress, torque, and abnormal motions persist at that space, whereas the L5-S1 interspace is compressed more readily. Almost all patients who developed anterior pseudoarthrosis were managed subsequently by posterior lateral fusion. A combination of prior anterior and additional posterior fusion provided a high degree of success in obtaining fusion in these patients (98%). A prior ununited anterior fusion always showed evidence of union, with trabeculations crossing the vertebral bodies within a year after the posterior lateral fusion was done. Anterior fusion enhanced a failed posterior fusion as well. Reoperation anteriorly was done only if there was a contraindication to posterior exposure, such as prior infection or small transverse processes.

We advise patients who are to have an anterior discectomy and fusion to expect about a 20 percent chance of having to undergo an additional operative procedure in order to obtain a solid fusion. Considering the fact that many of these individuals have anywhere from two to five prior operations, we feel that this is an acceptable method of management.

If prior discectomy without fusion has resulted in persistent signs and symptoms that interfere with the patient's daily activities, then anterior discectomy and fusion are performed. If pain relief has not been acceptable and if evidence of progressive arthrodesis has not occurred within 6 to 12 months, the additional procedure of supplementary posterior lateral fusion or decompression and fusion are included.

Discussion of Other Complications and Sequelae

Donor Site Disturbance

This can be avoided if the anterior superior spine is not removed when the bone graft is taken. The lateral femoral cutaneous nerve should not be subjected to traction or laceration, as this is the most common cause of postoperative discomfort. Pain at the site of the bone graft after operation usually is more noticeable than abdominal pain. Gluteal and abdominal muscles should be removed with a small flake of bone attached to them. An osteotome is used to do this. This allows firm closure of periosteum with a bone attachment. There usually is quicker recovery of muscle tone and less pain if this is done. Suction draining is always used. Bone wax is used to cover the bleeding surfaces. "Hip limp" may persist for 3 months, but there have been no permanent problems from the bone graft site after 6 months. Even after the entire iliac crest is used for full-thickness bone for three interspaces, the reconstitution of stability of the origin of the gluteus muscles and the external oblique muscles has been adequate and allowed unimpeded gait and resumption of ordinary activity.

Thromboembolism

This has been avoided by administering anticoagulants as mentioned; elevating the foot of the operating table during the procedure; maintaining the lower extremities higher than the heart level postoperatively; and ensuring that the patient is active in bed postoperatively, using foot exercises and an overhead trapeze, coughing frequently, using blow bottles, and maintaining adequate hydration. Antithromboembolic stockings are used and these must contour above the knee, or below knee stockings are selected. Aspirin is used for several weeks after the primary anticoagulant is stopped.

Urinary Tract Disturbance

Indwelling catheters are avoided. Preoperative assessment for bacterial infection is done and the patient is not operated upon if there is evidence of a symptomatic bacterial infection. These infections are treated initially. Postoperatively, Urecholine, manual compression, and other methods are used to maintain adequate bladder tone. One patient in 200 received a small puncture wound of the left ureter. This was demonstrable postoperatively by retroperitoneal urinoma. This was treated by an indwelling catheter and healed.

Impotence (Retrograde Ejaculation)

In none of the 200 patients, both males and females, and in no instance in the management of a male was impotence related to neurogenic involvement recognized. Those patients who had difficulty with erection several weeks or months postoperatively had the same problem preoperatively. Three of the 200 patients demonstrated retrograde ejaculation. They were included in the first 30 patients done, and more extensive dissection over the first sacral segment anteriorly had been performed. The decussating fibers of the upper sacral plexus may have been involved in this dissection. No dissection is carried below the anterior edge of the L5-S1 interspace. Hand-held, blunt-nosed retractors are used over the superior body of S1. No cauterization is done over the superior sacral segment and none over the body of L5. Soft tissues are swept aside with blunt dissectors and silver clips are used to manage the venous collaterals. We are confident that if this technique is followed, the procedure can be done in male patients of any age without affecting sexual function.

Fear of sexual dysfunction associated with anterior lumbar fusion has been emphasized in the literature. That possibility, of course, does exist because of the anatomic location of the operative procedure. Our experience has shown, however, that this is not an expected or necessary complication of this operative procedure.

Infection

Bacterial infection occurred in 2 patients of the initial 100; both of these infections were accounted for by gram-negative involvement from the urinary tract. Infection was controlled by draining the hematoma and by antibiotics. The fusion rate was not affected. No infections have occurred in the last 100 cases, and the senior author has performed approximately 200 anterior discectomies and fusions during the past 15 years with no deep infections. Ultraviolet light was used during the procedure on each of these patients and one-half of the patients received prophylactic antibiotics.

Postoperative Hematoma

Persistent bleeding from an epigastric vessel resulted in a large progressive retroperitoneal hematoma in 1 patient, which was managed by evacuation and by ligating the vessel on the sixth postoperative day. The patient's progress was satisfactory subsequent to that. If the hematocrit drops and if the patient shows evidence of enlarged abdominal girth, re-exploration is essential in order to locate the bleeding point. This usually will be either on a branch of the iliac artery, a branch of the vena cava, or an abdominal vessel. Re-exploration was required in 2 of 200 patients.

Prolonged Abdominal Ileus

Prolonged abdominal ileus is prevented by inserting a nasogastric tube if the patient does not show rapid recovery of bowel sounds after the operative procedure. We do not use the nasogastric tube routinely, although there is much less likelihood of ileus if this is done. The patient is encouraged to assume a side-lying position and to avoid intake by mouth until bowel sounds occur and flatus is passed. A rectal tube is helpful.

Intraoperative Hemorrhage

Excessive blood loss during the operative procedure has rarely occurred. The surgeon must be prepared, however, to manage a tear in the thin or adherent vena cava, bleeding from a retracted lumbar vein, bleeding from sacral veins that might be punctured from insertion of the spiked retractors into the sacrum (this procedure is not recommended), and arterial bleeding from branches of the iliac artery that might be torn during retraction. Patients who have had prior interspace infection or multiple posterior discectomies show significant reaction around the vena cava and the iliac vessels anteriorly. The surgeon should have available small and large hemoclips, blood vessel sutures, right-angle hemostats, and bipolar cautery. Avitine,[*] Gelfoam,[**] and thrombin, and direct compression all aid in stopping venous bleeding. Blood replacement has averaged 3 units per patient but larger quantities must be available if an emergency occurs.

Problem-Oriented Patients

Case 1. A 22-year-old nurse gave a history of having had acute back and lower extremity pain, initially treated by bedrest and anti-inflammatory agents. Recurrent radiculopathy was followed by a myelogram by her attending neurosurgeon, who subsequently performed a hemilaminectomy and removed a soft, bulging intervertebral disc. The patient's symptoms improved during the subsequent 4 months, but back pain and buttock aching persisted. Serial x-ray studies showed rapid narrowing of the interspace. Her pain worsened, straight-leg raising tests became strongly positive, and a second myelogram was done. A decompressive laminectomy was performed as the second operation, and spinal fusion was not done at that time. Improvement was slight. Several months elapsed, and she was unable to work at her nursing job. She continued to have evidence of nerve-root irritation and facet joint and interbody pain. One and one-half years after her initial onset of pain and radiculopathy she was still disabled.

Diagnostic studies included electromyography, which showed abnormal polyphasic action potentials in the S1 root distribution. The differential spinal test gave a physiologic response and the clinical psychologic studies showed the patient was not an hysterical type, nor was she somatizing. A discogram was done at the L4-5 level while the patient was awake. There was no pain associated with injection of the contrast and only 0.8 ml could be injected. The retroperitoneal approach was selected for the anterior discectomy and fusion. Only the L5-S1 interspace was included because of the

*American Critical Care, McGaw Park, Michigan.

**Upjohn, Kalamazoo, Michigan.

normal discogram. Postoperatively, the straight-leg raising tests were possible to 70° as compared with 30° preoperatively. Her relief of extremity pain was almost immediate. The nerve root that is fibrotic or compressed in a small canal can be decompressed by immobilizing the interspace and distracting it minimally with the bone graft. By 3 months her back pain had been eliminated, and by 6 months she was doing limited nursing. Within 1 year there were trabeculations across the interspace, and she was fully active in her occupational and social life.

There are many advantages to directly decompressing a nerve root. Spinal fusion will not cure a nerve root with intraneural fibrosis, but perineural fibrosis may be helped by immobilization. At least the constant trauma of incongruity and instability are removed and the root is protected somewhat.

If anterior discectomy and fusion and posterior discectomy and interbody fusion are compared, greater ease in cleaning out the intervertebral space, placing the bone grafts under compression, and placing the grafts in such a way that they follow the contour of the vertebral bodies will be noted if performed through an anterior approach. If the nerve roots do not require retraction, there is much less chance of involving the dura or the roots during the operative procedure. Anterior stabilization provides a safe way of obtaining stability of the spine and of cleaning out the interspace before posterior decompression if prior posterior operations have been completed.

If there continues to be evidence of anterior-posterior narrowing of the spinal canal or nerve root compression, appropriate decompression is performed posteriorly at a time when the vertebral bodies are relatively stable as a result of the anterior discectomy and fusion. Enhanced computerized tomography with metrizamide is helpful in determining the need for posterior decompression.

Case 2. A 19-year-old male developed acute back pain with radiculopathy and had the physical findings and myelographic defect compatible with a ruptured disc at the L4-5 interspace. A hemilaminectomy was done by the attending neurosurgeon, and a soft, bulging disc was removed. Temporary improvement occurred, but with increased physical activity, pain recurred in approximately 6 months. A second myelogram was done followed by a second decompression, and neurolysis was performed. Temporary improvement occurred while the patient was at bedrest, but within 4 months severe back pain and lower-extremity radiculopathy were present. The x-ray films showed gradual narrowing of the L4-5 interspace and the myelogram showed a partial block and a defect at L4-5 (Figs. 87-1A, B, and C). The patient had a physiologic response to the differential spinal test, the electromyogram was positive, involving the L5 root on the left, and a discogram at L3-4 was normal, but resulted in pain at both L4-5 and L5-S1. An anterior discectomy and fusion through a retroperitoneal approach were done at L4-5 and L5-S1. Full-thickness iliac bone grafts were used and both spaces were adequately immobilized by the procedure. Immediately postoperatively, straight-leg raising was possible to 70° on the left and was painful on the right at about 60°, which had not been the case preoperatively. After 6 months, straight-leg raising was possible on both sides to 70° and back pain was eliminated about 80 percent. The x-ray study shows fusion is progressing satisfactorily.

The diagnosis was arachnoiditis and perineural fibrosis, and incongruity and instability secondary to removal of the intervertebral disc in the young male.

Spinal fusion is recommended in young people, particularly if the first operation for bulging or soft intervertebral disc fails and definitely if a second procedure fails. Discography is helpful, if performed properly and interpreted correctly. An abnormal discogram means that a pathologic lesion exists, but this does not mean that an operative procedure is necessarily indicated. If the clinical findings are abnormal, however, and if the electromyogram coincides, then operative treatment may be indicated. Furthermore, a normal discogram is much more helpful in many instances than an abnormal one (see Fig. 87-2).

Case 3. A 28-year-old female pharmacist with an intervertebral disc syndrome at L4-5 had a 4-year history of back pain with radiculopathy. A bulging disc had been removed initially with temporary relief. Six months later the persistent pain resulted in re-exploration of the lower two interspaces posteriorly. Minimal improvement occurred temporarily and worsened as time passed. Serial x-ray studies showed moderately rapid narrowing of both lower interspaces. Because of her slow response, the question of emotional problems and the influence of possible litigation had been introduced by the attending neurosurgeon.

Our studies included an electromyogram, which was positive for S1 nerve-root irritation. The differential spinal test was physiologic, a selective nerve block gave temporary relief of pain in one extremity, and the discogram was normal at the L3-4 space. We do not usually include spaces operated upon previously in the discogram procedure, although this is done occasionally to determine if pain can be reproduced. A selective nerve block will provide the same information by encouraging the patient to undergo physical activity in order to aggravate the pain and then attempt to relieve it with the nerve block.

A two-space anterior lumbar discectomy and fusion was done. Radiculopathy was diminished, back pain improved gradually, and by 1 year after the procedure, the L5-S1 interspace was solid but a fibrous union was present at L4-5 space. The patient had buttock and thigh pain on the left side after standing and walking for moderately long distances. This root was decompressed by hemilaminectomy and neurolysis with unroofing of the foramen. A posterior lateral fusion was then done from L4 to L5 using iliac bone. The patient's radiculopathy was improved within 2 months and the back pain improved during the next 6 months. Both interspaces were solid at 1 year, and the patient was back at work.

Case 4. A 21-year-old doctor's daughter with back pain and radiculopathy was treated by excision of a bulging intervertebral disc at L5-S1. Pain and limitation of motion persisted and several months later the myelogram showed a bulging intervertebral disc at L4-5. This was excised with temporary relief, but back and buttock pain persisted. A third exploratory operation was done at the lower two spaces, four nerve roots were decompressed, and hemilaminectomies were done bilateral. Subsequent to this procedure, the patient was unable to sit more than 30 minutes without developing severe pain, she walked with the trunk flexed about 30°, and she was comfortable only when lying flat on her back with the hips and knees flexed.

We performed a discogram at the L3-4 level, which was normal. An electromyogram was positive with abnormal action potentials at the L4-5 and L5-S1 roots. X-rays showed the interspaces to be narrowed about 70 percent of normal, and flexion-extension stress x-ray studies showed distinct motion at the interspaces. A two-space anterior discectomy and fusion through a retroperitoneal approach, using iliac bone graft, was done. Recovery was moderately slow, and pain, although improved, persisted for 4 additional months. The patient could sit for longer periods of time, however, could stand erect, and by 4 months after surgery was able to drive her car. X-ray studies showed evidence of a solid fusion by 1 year; the radiculopathy had been eliminated and she returned to school.

Case 5. A 35-year-old female physician had been partially incapacitated because of chronic low back and lower extremity pain for over 5 years. She had been managed by laminectomy, attempted stabilization by posterior lateral fusion with a total of four previous operations. She was using two canes, was required to spend half the day in bed, and was carrying out limited general practice. The physical findings showed positive stretch tests, pain on manipulation of the spine, and weakness of dorsiflexion of the foot.

She was taking Urecholine, 25 mg three times a day, for management of her atonic bladder. Cystometrograms showed minimal neurogenic involvement.

A differential spinal test was physiologic, the discogram was negative at L3-4, and the electromyogram was strongly positive, involving the L4-5 and L5-S1 nerve roots bilaterally. There was no evidence of spinal infection. The sedimentation rate was normal, and a thermogram showed no excessive increase in heat.

A psychiatric assessment and clinical psychologic testing showed that the patient did need treatment for reactive depression and anxiety.

Stress x-rays in the right and left lateral position and forward flexion and extension showed definite motion at both spaces with evidence of pseudoarthrosis and incongruity.

Anterior discectomy and fusion were done through a retroperitoneal approach including the L4-5 and L5-S1 interspaces. A minimal amount of material was found at L5-S1, but a considerable amount of annulus and fibrous tissue was removed from the L4-5 interspace. Full-thickness iliac bone grafts were used to stabilize the two lower intervertebral spaces.

Postoperatively, the straight-leg raising improved, over a period of 2 weeks, to about 60°. Bladder function improved to where Urecholine was reduced to 10 mg/day. During the next 3 months, the patient's progress was one of slow but steady improvement, with diminution of pain, increased strength, and increased activity. By 6 months after the operation, she was ready to return to work for half a day. Foot dorsiflexion had improved and bladder control was almost normal. One and one-half years postoperatively this patient was working full time and was relatively free of back and lower extremity pain.

Results

One hundred patients were followed for a minimum of 8 years and a maximum of 15 years after anterior discectomy and fusion as part of their total management. The results were based on the patients' subjective descriptions, the physician's objective findings, and the patients' activity pattern at least 4 years after treatment was completed. The results of this study were based on an assessment of the degree of relief of back or lower extremity pain and rated as excellent, good, fair, slight, or none, or worse (Fig. 87-14).

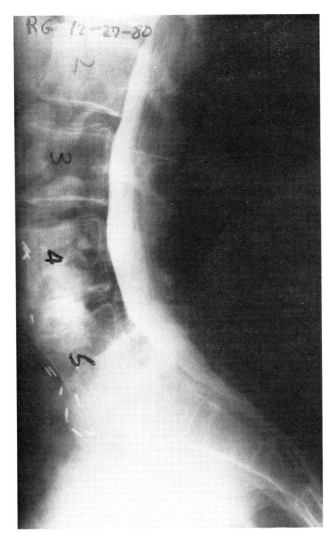

Fig. 87-14. A postoperative anterior discectomy and fusion at L4-5, L5-S1, approximately 8 months after surgery. The hemoclips controlled bleeding from branches of the iliac vessels and the vena cava and small arterioles. The bone graft between L4-5 is definitely fused to L5 and shows early fusion to L4. The interspace has been widened moderately, both anteriorly and posteriorly. The bone graft between L5 and S1 has healed and trabeculae are forming across this interspace. A myelogram was performed because the patient had recurrent lower extremity pain indicative of persistent posterior fibrosis around one root. His back pain had been relieved, and the pain in his opposite extremity had been eliminated. Posterior nerve-root decompression and wide foraminotomy and partial facetectomy diminished the extremity pain. A fusion of the posterior lateral transverse process was performed at the same time and the spine was solid within 1 year after the anterior and posterior procedures. The patient's pain has been eliminated significantly, and he has now returned to work as a truck driver.

Table 87-2. Overall Results of Anterior Lumbar Fusion 100 Patients

	Complete relief	Moderate relief	Slight relief	No change	Worse
Lower back pain	47	31	15	7	0
Lower extremity pain	58	27	12	3	0

Table 87-2 can be interpreted as showing that 78 percent of the patients had moderate or complete relief of low-back pain, and 85 percent had complete or moderate relief of lower extremity pain. No patients were worse after treatment. Eighty-five percent of the patients who had one or two interspaces fused were shown to have had complete or moderate relief. Eighteen of the 100 patients continued to have pain and accepted additional back operations after the anterior discectomy and fusion. Fifteen of these had posterior lateral fusions and some had nerve-root decompressions. Nine of these patients were improved significantly by the additional surgery. None of these patients were worse; 3 were subjectively the same, but were objectively improved significantly.

Accessory characteristics, such as personality and occupation, of 200 patients were reviewed in 1975. Patients who were considered to have good results were analyzed from an occupational as well as an emotional standpoint. About one-half of those with good results were sponsored by workers' compensation. About one-half had abnormal clinical psychologic findings, even though the result was satisfactory, and about two-thirds of the total patients had a "normal" emotional profile. Those patients with abnormal clinical psychologic results required a longer time to reach maximum improvement than did those individuals without personality conflicts and significant secondary gain or other reasons why they did not return to their usual work.

Conclusions

1. No single method of treatment is sufficient to treat all patients with low-back pain and radiculopathy successfully.
2. There is a direct relationship between patients who obtain a solid fusion and those who show improvement or relief of pain. Patients with persistent pseudoarthrosis have a greater chance of having persistent pain.
3. Detailed preliminary assessment is necessary, using several diagnostic studies as aids in determining the proper method of management and prognosis.
4. Anterior discectomy and arthrodesis with autogenous bone is a safe procedure that allows the diminution of radiculopathy and back pain by removing fragments from the interspace and stabilizing the vertebral bodies.
5. The pseudoarthrosis rate associated with anterior lumbar fusion has been diminished by meticulous removal of the intervertebral soft tissue, by shaping the bone graft, and by the addition of a maximum amount of autogenous bone wedged into the interspace under compression.
6. Bone union as determined by roentgenography may not be accurate with plain films or stress x-rays until at least 1 year after the interbody fusion.
7. Spondylolisthesis, in our experience, should be managed by nerve root decompression and posterior lateral fusion at a single interspace if mild grade 1 or 2 and two spaces if severe grade 3 or 4. If pseudoarthrosis develops, anterior interbody spinal fusion of the involved interspace can be done provided that the degree of displacement is not excessive. If the spondylolisthesis is graded 3 or 4, the plan is to arthrodese L4 to L5 and remove the disc and insert the iliac bone grafts at that level only. If L4 fuses to L5, the severe forward displacement and movement of L5 on S1 will be diminished. This additional single anterior

vertebral body fusion of the superior aspect of the involved vertebra proximal to the defects of the neural arch usually stabilizes the severely displaced spine and avoids extensive dissection about the venous and arterial channels as well as the sympathetic nerve fibers in the region of excessive forward displacement of L5 on S1.

8. Anterior discectomy and fusion have been helpful in diminishing pain and radiculopathy associated with perineural fibrosis and arachnoiditis.

9. Anterior interbody fusion is helpful in treating spinal stenosis and nerve-root stenosis. A stable spine anteriorly allows wide decompression posteriorly without causing incongruity and instability. We have observed several patients who had direct midline posterior fusions who subsequently developed napkin-ring constriction at the upper end of the fusion, encroachment of the fusion on the superior facets, and stenosis of the meninges associated with overgrowth of bone from the laminal arches and facets. A posterior decompression may be performed initially if stenosis is obvious on the CT scan. The surgeon may consider anterior discectomy and fusion if instability is an evident problem after decompression or if it becomes a problem eventually.

10. Sexual dysfunction associated with anterior discectomy and fusion has not been a problem for these patients.

11. A meticulous surgical technique is essential in order to obtain a high rate of fusion of the vertebral bodies.

REFERENCES

1. Burns BH: An operation for spondylolisthesis. *Lancet 224*:1233, 1933
2. Capener N: Spondylolisthesis. *Br J Surg 24*:80–85, 1936
3. Hartman JT, Kendrick JI, Lorman P: Discography as an aid in evaluation for lumbar and lumbosacral fusion, *Clin Ortho Related Res 81*:77–81, 1971
4. Sacks S: Anterior spinal surgery and ballarat. *J Bone Joint Surg 52-B*:392–393, 1970
5. Speed K: Spondylolisthesis. Treatment by anterior bone graft. *Arch Surg 37*:175, 1938
6. McCollum DE, Stephen CR: The use of graduated spinal anesthesia in the differential diagnosis of back and lower extremities. *So Med J 57*:410–416, 1964
7. Sacks S: Intervertebral disc excision and lumbar spine fusion by transperitoneal approach. *J Bone Joint Surg 43-B*:401, 1961
8. Goldner JL, McCollum DE, Urbaniak JR: Anterior disc excision and interbody spine fusion for chronic low back pain. American Academy of Orthopaedic Surgeons, Proceedings–Symposium on the Spine. St. Louis, CV Mosby, 1969
9. Goldner JL, McCollum DE, Urbaniak JR: Anterior intervertebral discectomy and arthrodesis for treatment of low back pain with or without radiculopathy, in Ojemann RJ (ed): *Clinical Neurosurgery*, vol. 15. The Congress of Neurological Surgeons, 1968, pp 352–383
10. Goldner JL, Urbaniak JR, McCollum DE: Anterior disc excision and interbody spinal fusion for chronic low back pain. *Orthop Clin North Am 2*:543–567, 1971
11. Stauffer RN, Coventry MB: Anterior interbody spine fusion. *J Bone Joint Surg 54A*:756–768, 1972
12. Kotcamp WW: Indications for anterior spine fusion. *Clin Ortho Related Res 70*:235, 1970
13. Hodgson AR, Stock FA: Anterior spine fusion for treatment of tuberculosis of the spine. *J Bone Joint Surg 42A*:295, 1960
14. Harmon P: Anterior extraperitoneal disc excision and vertebral body fusion. *Clin Orthop 18*:169, 1961
15. Harmon P: Anterior disc excision and fusion of the lumbar vertebral bodies. *J Int Col Surg 40*:572, 1963
16. Shanewise RP: Anterior intervertebral lumbar spine fusion. *West J Surg 71*:212, 1963
17. Harmon P: Personal communication, 1975
18. Freebody D: Motion picture shown at the Vancouver Meeting of the American Orthopaedic Association, 1965
19. Collis JS Jr: *Lumbar Discography*. Springfield, Ill., Charles C Thomas, 1963

CHAPTER 88
Surgical Management of Trauma to the Spine

David Yashon

FRACTURE-DISLOCATION OF THE VERTEBRAL COLUMN with or without involvement of the spinal cord or nerve roots continues to present a series of difficult therapeutic problems. Various modes of treatment, including skeletal traction, Halo jacket, neck brace, open fixation, posterior fusion, anterior fusion, or decompressive laminectomy followed by fusion and stabilization, entail immobilizing and hospitalizing the patient for long periods of time. The value of any one form of treatment has been difficult to assess in terms of neurologic recovery, and, indeed, the indications for surgery as well as the virtues of particular operations are controversial. The indications for surgery are not absolute, and this will be discussed when possible. This chapter concerns itself with surgical indications and the types of surgical treatment currently available for injuries to the vertebral column, beginning with the methods of skeletal traction and the anesthetic considerations in the patient with a spinal injury.

Skeletal Traction

The use of skull tongs to reduce fracture-dislocation and to maintain alignment of fractures of the cervical spine is now universal[1] and offers an important means of protecting and internally decompressing the cervical spinal cord and nerve roots following cervical spinal injury. Traction for injuries of the thoracic and lumbar spine is not feasible because of the enormous forces required for distraction and realignment.

The most widely used device for applying skeletal traction was described by Crutchfield in 1933.[2] These tongs were modified in 1938 by Barton,[3] and in 1948 by Vinke.[4] Vinke described a set of tongs based on Barton's modification that had interlocking devices between the inner and outer tables of bone to prevent their inadvertent release. Gardner-Wells tongs (Fig. 88-1) represent a major advance in the design of these devices and are now the preferred tongs in most spinal cord injury units.

Tongs should be placed as soon as possible after the injury, since realignment affects internal decompression of the spinal contents. Tongs should not be placed near a skull fracture. Delay in treatment following an injury poses a philosophical question much akin to that concerning laminectomy, i.e., whether or when tongs should be placed and reduction carried out. We generally place tongs even after 1 week has elapsed, since adequately aligned healing bone diminishes the chance of further neurologic damage, even damage confined to a single nerve root. Also, ad-

Division of Neurological Surgery, Ohio State University, Columbus, Ohio

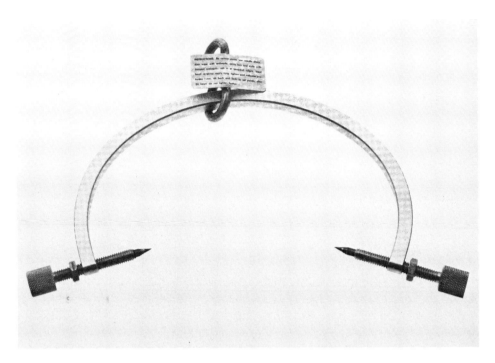

Fig. 88-1. The Gardner-Wells traction tongs. (Courtesy of Codman and Shurtleff, Inc.)

equate bone healing lessens the possibility of later pain. The second indication for placement of tongs is to achieve immobilization.

The length of time that tongs should be left in place varies. We have left tongs in place for 12 weeks without ill effect. The tong sites are treated with antibiotic ointment and kept clean with soap and water. With the exception of Gardner-Wells tongs, tongs must be gently tightened frequently, and even Gardner-Wells tongs may need occasional tightening. Skull x-rays can be valuable in detecting complications, and the position may be changed if skull penetration or osteomyelitis becomes a problem. At the present time in our hospital, tongs are left in place up to 8 weeks, depending upon the fracture, but usually halo traction is substituted much earlier. Tongs are used during cervical surgery (both fusion and laminectomy) for maintenance of alignment and are left in place until fusion occurs spontaneously or is surgically induced.

In deciding the amount of weight that is to be applied to the tongs, it should be remembered that skeletal traction is employed for both alignment and reduction. To maintain alignment, 5 to 25 pounds of weight represents the usual range needed. In the four decades since Crutchfield[2] reported tong traction to reduce a fracture-dislocation of the upper cervical spine, the amount of weight acceptably applied to achieve traction reduction has remained in doubt. Although weights of more than 35 pounds applied over hours or days have been used to reduce cervical fracture-dislocations complicated by locked facets,[5-7] Bailey,[8,9] Bovill et al.,[5] and Hollin and Gross[10] have suggested that weights greater than 50 pounds are dangerous and that operative reduction is indicated when such weights fail to produce satisfactory vertebral alignment in 24 to 48 hours. Crutchfield[11,12] cautioned against using heavy weights to achieve more rapid reduction, believing that force sufficient to speed reduction would further injure supporting tissues and endanger the spinal cord. Instead, he advocated a minimal corrective pull of up to 18 pounds followed by gradual completion of reduction with no more than double this weight.

There is at least a theoretical argument in favor of more rapid reduction, and this is our preference.[13,14] Cervical fracture-dislocations often represent emergencies in which the extent and duration of neurologic dysfunction may depend upon the time interval between the injury and decompression of the spinal cord.[15,16] A minimum of 60 to 90 minutes commonly elapses before a patient with a cervical fracture-dislocation is brought to the emergency room and placed in skull traction, and most often there are delays of upward of 6 hours. In many cases, little information is available concerning improvement or deterioration in the patient's neurologic status during this delay. Also, at least theoretically, prompt closed internal reduction provides relief of direct bony pressure on the spinal cord, thus diminishing damage.

In the presence of severe cord injury and radiographic evidence of a cervical fracture-dislocation with or without locked facets, application of a minimal corrective pull to protect neural structures from further injury may represent less than optimal acute treatment. When no neurologic functional loss is apparent, haste is not necessary. On our service, we reduce the dislocation as completely as possible, no longer than 2 hours after traction is applied.[14,15] The goal is to decompress the spinal cord quickly by restoring the anteroposterior diameter of the cervical spinal canal and achieving satisfactory positioning of bone fragments. Sector computed tomographic (CT) scanning of the vertebral column has been becoming a useful tool in assessing impingement on the spinal canal.

The technique consists of intravenous administration of muscle relaxants to reduce paraspinous muscle spasm, elevation of the head of the frame to exert countertraction, and the initial application of 20 to 30 pounds to appropriate tongs inserted in a coronal plane determined by the cervical transverse processes and the external auditory meati. Traction force thus is exerted along the longitudinal axis of the vertebral bodies with the neck in a neutral position. Five to ten pounds are added every 10 minutes, and brief appropriate neurologic examinations and lateral cervical spine films are repeated after the addition of each increment of weight. Occasionally, manual traction on the occiput and jaws also is required. Once reduction is achieved, traction is maintained with minimum weight (10 to 30 pounds). During reduction, attention must be paid to the patient's reports of additional neurologic symptoms, such as parasthesiae, pain, and neurologic loss. In patients without neurologic deficit the same technique and precautions may be employed without the same degree of urgency.

On our service over the past years the greatest amount of weight that has been used successfully to treat a patient in this manner in the first hour was 75 pounds. Operative reduction and decompression are indicated in patients with severe neurologic signs when the anteroposterior diameter of the cervical spinal canal cannot be restored to within approximately 3 mm of normal with 60 to 70 pounds of traction applied over 1 to 2 hours. The inability to establish appropriate alignment by traction usually signifies locked or jumped facets that probably should be treated by an open surgical maneuver. This remains a controversial issue, however, and acceptance of imperfect alignment occasionally is necessary for practical reasons.

The sharp points of the Gardner-Wells tongs should be used with caution in pediatric patients. We use Crutchfield tongs at our center and reduce the weight accordingly for pediatric patients.

Anesthesia

The risk of further damage as a result of movement of the head, neck, or vertebral column is a prime concern after cervical, thoracic, and lumbar injuries. Because damage may occur during transport, the induction of anesthesia, intubation, or positioning before surgery, both the anesthesiologist and the surgeon must be extremely careful to avoid moving the patient excessively. In cervical spine injuries, such movement can be minimized by skeletal traction during induction of anesthesia, intubation, throughout the operative procedure, and during the postoperative course.

In patients undergoing emergency surgery for cervical or thoracic spinal cord injury, a full stomach is a particular hazard during the induction of anesthesia. Regurgitation of the stomach contents is more probable than vomiting, because of paralysis of the abdominal muscles. Head-down tilt, airway obstruction, intermittent positive pressure breathing before intubation, and the use of depolarizing muscle relaxants are factors that predispose the patient to regurgitation. Emptying of the stomach contents by nasograstic tube before induction of anesthesia not only does not guarantee an empty stomach, but may, in fact, facilitate regurgitation if the nasogastric tube is left in place during induction. The likelihood of regurgitation is decreased if the head is kept elevated and the legs are tilted down; however, this position may initiate or aggravate hypotension and may add to the technical difficulty of intubation.

A specific consideration in the selection of the anesthetic technique to be used in the patient with a major spinal cord injury is the syndrome of massive hyperkalemia and cardiac arrest following relaxation of muscles with succinylcholine. The increase in serum potassium is thought to occur because the denervated muscle cell membrane is altered. This phenomenon begins about 6 days after injury and may continue for several months. As a result, depolarization with succinylcholine during anesthetic induction can precipitate the massive release of potassium and its attendant complications.

Other particular concerns in patients with injured spines are problems resulting from renal disease, decubitus ulcers, metabolic disorders, decreased serum proteins, altered liver function, autonomic hyperreflexia, and the inability of the vasomotor system to respond normally to blood loss.

Endotracheal intubation in the awake patient is advocated widely because it protects against possible failure to intubate the trachea, with loss of patent airways, and somewhat decreases the risk of inhalation of vomitus. Attempts to visualize the larynx and intubate the trachea by direct oropharyngeal laryngoscopy in a patient with severe cervical muscle spasm may be difficult and traumatic, however. As an alternative, blind nasotracheal intubation in the awake patient is the procedure we prefer under these circumstances.

Blind nasal intubation does not require a deep level of anesthesia and obviates the need for muscle relaxants and traumatic endoscopy. Lubrication of the tube with a nonanesthetic bland jelly and prespraying the nose with a 5% cocaine solution to shrink nasal mucosa will lessen the likelihood of epistaxis. A tube about 1 to 2 mm smaller than an oral tube, with its bevel directed toward the nasal septum, is introduced most easily. The tube is easier to fix in place than an oral tube and is well tolerated by the conscious patient after surgery. Suctioning the trachea is more difficult through a nasotracheal tube. Risk of damage to the mucous membrane of the nose and nasal pharynx is high, but this is balanced against the greater importance of nontraumatic intubation.

Intubation in the awake patient may be carried out by nasal passage of the endotracheal tube. Blind oral or nasal intubation while the patient is awake helps to prevent additional injury, since the patient can report untoward neurologic symptoms. The patient can be serially examined neurologically during and after intubation. Tracheostomy can be performed in those patients in whom intubation cannot be achieved. The necessity of this procedure, however, has become distinctly unusual for anesthesia.

A patient positioned on the Stryker frame may be anesthetized, intubated, and operated upon in either the prone or supine position with the neck maintained in a neutral position. By contrast, use of the circelectric bed specifically is discouraged because of the dangers of hypotension and loading forces exerted on the fracture with the head elevated, which may result in further damage. Problems associated with the prone position include prolonged pressure on the patient's eyes. Such pressure is particularly likely to occur under anesthesia and may exceed the normal retinal artery pressure and result in thrombosis and permanent blindness. Severe uneven and prolonged pressure has resulted in necrosis about the zygomatic arch, the supraorbital ridges, the mandible, the feet, the breasts, and the genitalia.

Surgical Technique

As a result of an injury to the spine, the bony structures, ligaments, and muscles may be stretched, crushed, fractured, or dislocated, and the spinal cord and nerve roots may be crushed, contused, compressed, or severed. Fracture-dislocation of the cervical spine is not always accompanied by a neurologic deficit; however, when it is present the disruption of the spinal cord may be irremediable. On the other hand, secondary effects such as circulatory impairment, vasomotor disturbances, venous stasis, secondary hemorrhage, thrombosis, and edema may convert a partial cord injury to a complete one, and these reversible events may occur after the initial injury. This may be produced by destruction of the intervertebral disc and herniation of the nucleus pulposus, which causes injury to the spinal cord and nerve roots. Rupture of a disc may not cause a subarachnoid block to myelography or spinal puncture, but may cause very severe neural damage, possibly because of compression of the anterior spinal artery.

The goal of surgical treatment, including skeletal traction, laminectomy, or fusion, is manifold. In the acute stage it is to furnish the spinal cord and nerve roots with the best possible conditions for improvement and recovery. There are legitimate differences of opinion among neurosurgeons concerning the optimal approach to any particular problem of spine or spinal cord injury; however, the sparing of even a single nerve root is often crucial to the quadriplegic because it may provide some hand function and may make the difference between total dependence and some ability to care for himself. Judicious surgical treatment may prevent future pain resulting from spinal instability and compression of nerve roots that can seriously hinder the patient's rehabilitation either acutely or in months after injury.

Timing of surgical intervention for acute spinal injury remains controversial, although early realignment or decompression or both is my own preference.

It should be stressed that no absolute criteria exist for either operative or nonoperative treatment in the closed, acute spinal cord injury. Various degrees of functional improvement have been reported in patients treated either operatively or nonoperatively. Both points of view have strong advocates, although no statistically significant study has been carried out or is likely to be carried out soon.

Anterior Fusion

Anterior fusion operations have been devised to allow anterior stabilization of the injured spine in any of its regions from the base of the skull to the sacrum.

Upper cervical spine anterior fusion. Several authors have described anterior approaches to the C1-C2-C3 region either through the oropharynx[17] or by an extrapharyngeal approach.[18] Murray and Seymour[18] described an anterior extrapharyngeal suprahyoid approach to the first, second, and third cervical vertebrae. Grote et al.[17] described removal of the odontoid process (dens epistropheus) by a transpharyngeal approach. Indications for removal of the dens are very uncommon and include situations in which a persistently dislocated dens continues to impinge on the spinal cord anteriorly following posterior cervical fusion. Stabilization of the upper cervical spine by the transoral transpharyngeal route also has been described by Bonney,[19] Fang and Ong,[20,21] Grote et al.,[17] as well as Estridge and Smith.[22]

In performing a transoral fusion, the palate is elevated, the mouth held open with a McIvor gag, and a 3–4-cm vertical incision is made into the pharynx overlying the involved segment of the spine. Using periosteal elevators, fibrous tissue and soft tissue are removed to expose the fracture site. The bone in the area then is removed under magnification with a high-speed burr, and a bone dowel is positioned for insertion into the defect using the technique of Estridge and Smith.[22] The dowel graft of bone is inserted as manual traction is applied to the head. When the traction is released, the graft is locked in position. Bonney[19] recommended preoperative tracheostomy. Stabilization is secured by inserting two struts of cortical bone into the body of the axis. These are notched into the anterior arch of the atlas with the space between them packed with cancellous bone. Alternatively, Bonney stated that stability could be assured by packing with cancellous chips after partial decortication of the upper vertebra. He then used halo traction. Fang and Ong[21] describe various approaches to the upper cervical spine. The transpharyngeal, transoral route was advocated, and they placed bone from an iliac crest into the lateral masses

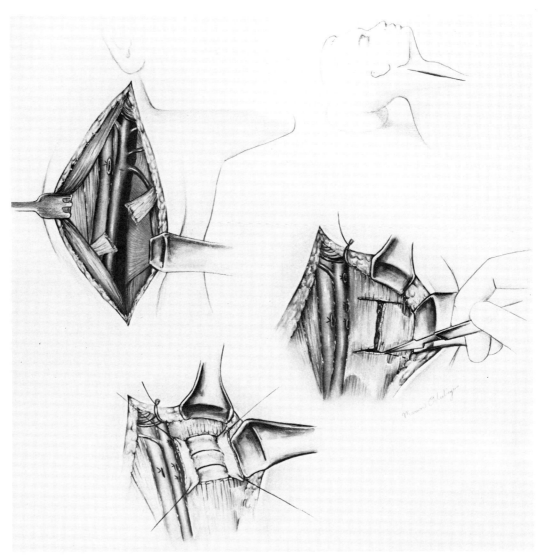

Fig. 88-2. The anterolateral approach to the upper cervical spine (after De Andrade and MacNab).[30] (Reprinted from Yashon D: *Spinal Injury.* New York, Appleton-Century-Crofts, 1978. With permission.)

between the atlas and axis to achieve fusion following removal of the anterior arch of the atlas and odontoid process in certain cases.

The anterior extrapharyngeal suprahyoid approach is described by Murray and Seymour[18] as well as Fang, Ong, and Hodgson[20] (Fig. 88-2). A collar incision is made along the uppermost crease of the neck at the level between the hyoid bone and the thyroid cartilage, extending as far as the carotid sheaths. The sternohyoid and the sternothyroid muscles are divided, and the thyrohyoid membrane is exposed and detached as close to the hyoid bone as possible to avoid damage to the internal laryngeal nerve and superior laryngeal vessels. The hypopharynx is entered by cutting into the exposed mucous membrane from the side to avoid damaging the epiglottis. Traction on the hyoid bone and epiglottis exposes the posterior pharyngeal wall, and a midline vertical incision is made to bone; the bodies of the second and third or fourth vertebrae can be exposed sufficiently to remove diseased or abnormal bone or to achieve fusion, although it may be necessary to dislocate the jaw to attain adequate exposure. Fusion is achieved by inserting strut grafts of autogenous bone into a prepared graft with slots made in the opposing vertebral bodies. The insertion of the grafts is made easier by extending the cervical spine during the operative procedure and then permitting resumption of the original somewhat flexed or neutral position. The need for tracheostomy may be avoided by this approach.

Middle and lower cervical anterior fusion.　　The introduction of the anterior approach to the management of fractures and dislocations of the cervical, thoracic, and lumbar spine has added a new dimension to the treatment of spinal injury. The work of Smith and Robinson[23] and Bailey and Badgley[24] first drew attention to the feasibility of the anterior approach in cervical fracture dislocations. Cloward[25-27] popularized the concept and introduced a set of instruments that has made this operation considerably simpler. That technique generally is satisfactory.

In bursting fractures of an anterior cervical body, at least two levels of fusion followed by

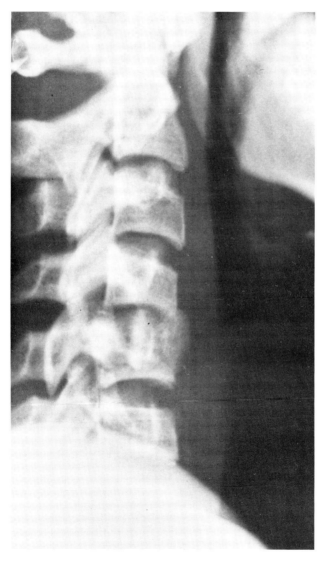

Fig. 88-3.　A recent cervical interbody fusion at C4-5. Fusion is adequate but has less purchase than would be ideal. (Reprinted from Yashon D: *Spinal Injury.* New York, Appleton-Century-Crofts, 1978. With permission.)

prolonged immobilization may be required for adequate healing without subsequent angulation. Anterior cervical fusion between C3 and C7 may be performed through a transverse or longitudinal skin incision. The recommended transverse skin incision is sufficient for exposing three consecutive vertebral bodies and two consecutive intervertebral discs. A longitudinal skin incision should be used in the unusual circumstance that a longer segment of the cervical spine is to be exposed. The landmark for placing either incision is the palpable anterior border of the sternomastoid muscle. A transverse skin incision should be centered over the anterior border of the sternomastoid muscle overlying the segment of the spine to be exposed. Generally the fifth, sixth, and seventh cervical segments should be approached through a transverse skin incision laced two to three finger breadths superior to the clavicle, and the third, fourth, and fifth cervical segments through a transverse incision placed three to four finger breadths superior to the clavicle.

A longitudinal incision should be made in the skin overlying the anterior border of the sternomastoid muscle and may be extended from the tip of the mastoid process to the suprasternal notch. The platysma muscle is grasped between forceps and sharply incised at the lateral limb of the transverse incision or at the caudal limb of the longitudinal incision, bluntly separated from the underlying structures by passing a blunt, curved hemostat or Metzenbaum scissors deep to the muscle, and sharply incised in line with the skin incision. If the platysma muscle is bluntly separated from the deeper structures before it is incised, inadvertent incision of the underlying sternomastoid muscle will be avoided. The anterior border of the sternomastoid muscle must be clearly identified and mobilized throughout the boundaries of the incision. The middle layer of cervical fascia is demonstrated as the sternomastoid muscle is retracted laterally. The omohyoid muscle may be seen crossing the field in the midportion of the neck at this level and may be mobilized and retracted inferiorly or superiorly, or transected to secure adequate exposure. The carotid artery then is palpated. After accurately identifying the artery, the middle layer of cervical fascia is sharply incised just medial to and parallel with the carotid sheath. As the

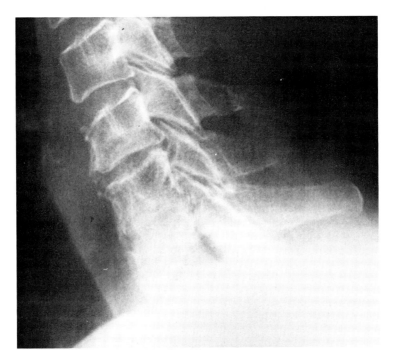

Fig. 88-4. An interbody fusion. 3 months after it was done. (Reprinted from Yashon D: *Spinal Injury*. New York, Appleton-Century-Crofts, 1978. With permission.)

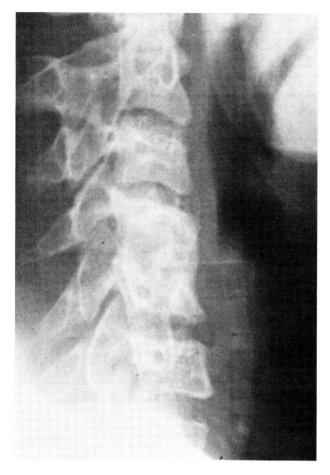

Fig. 88-5. An ancient interbody fusion at C4-5. (Reprinted from Yashon D: *Spinal Injury.* New York, Appleton-Century-Crofts, 1978. With permission.)

sternomastoid muscle and the carotid sheath are retracted laterally, the anterior surface of the cervical spine may be palpated.

The esophagus lies just posterior to the trachea, or more superiorly, posterior to the larynx. After having retracted the esophagus, trachea, and thyroid gland medially, the prevertebral fasciae are incised longitudinally in the midline of the neck and retracted to either side by periosteal elevation. It is important that the palpable anterior tubercles of the transverse processes not be mistaken for the vertebral bodies, or an incision, which should be made through the prevertebral fasciae in the midline, will be made through the longus colli muscle with resulting damage to the cervical sympathetic chain or to the vertebral artery, which lies deep to the longus colli muscle. The longus colli muscle may be sharply elevated from the intervertebral discs and the vertebral bodies in order to allow more complete exposure of the entire segment of the vertebral bodies and the intervertebral discs.

The resulting exposure is sufficient for anterior cervical discectomy and fusion, and anterior decompression of the cervical portion of the spinal cord following comminuted fractures of the vertebral bodies.

Identification of the space usually is done by x-ray after a needle is inserted into the disc space or by palpation of bony displacement. The dislocation can also be palpated for identification. At this point the graft can be prepared. The hip has been previously elevated on a sand bag. An incision 8 cm long is made parallel to and 2–4 cm below the crest of the ilium. Following skin retraction, the aponeurosis and muscles are cut perpendicular to the iliac crest. Dissection of the muscles from the external side of the crest to allow placement of the Cloward dowel cutter for removal of one or two grafts is sufficient. The dowel cutter is impinged against the bone and always is placed perpendicular to its surface. To ensure this, a cerebellar extension with the Hudson brace is useful. The dowel must be cylindrical in shape with the end surfaces at right angles, otherwise a poorly fitting dowel that is cut at an odd angle may result. This may cause poor fusion and vertebral collapse (Fig. 88-3). We have not advised the use of Kiel bone in fracture-dislocations.

Returning to the neck, the selected space then is drilled with Cloward instruments with due consideration for the angle of the intervertebral space. The drilling should be in the plane of the space between the bodies to avoid undesirable angulation and excessive bleeding from venous channels in bone. The offset position of the dowels when two or more spaces are used also is important, as is leaving sufficient bone tissue between the drilling spaces. Initial drilling is carried to a depth of 20 mm in adults. Further drilling is done cautiously in 2-mm steps. The posterior longitudinal ligament may be removed with angular cervical punches. The remaining pieces of disc may be removed with small curettes or rongeurs.

The bone dowel is inserted with either traction or the vertebral spreader. It is desirable that the anterior cortical surface of the dowel be inserted to a depth of at least 1–2 mm below the surface of the vertebral bodies. The strength of the fusion rests mostly on the cortical segment and

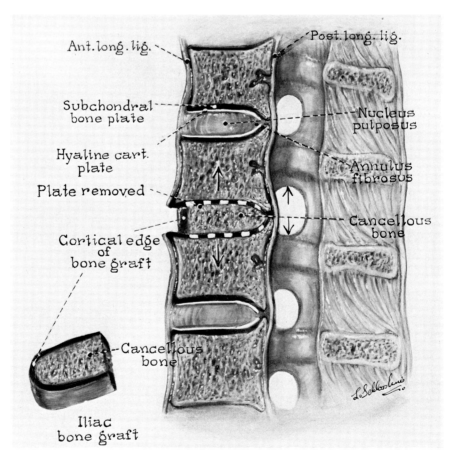

Fig. 88-6. A Smith-Robinson cervical graft. (Reprinted from Robinson RA, Walker AE, Ferlic DC, et al: The results of anterior interbody fusion of the cervical spine. *J Bone Joint Surg 44A*:1569–1587, 1962. With permission.)

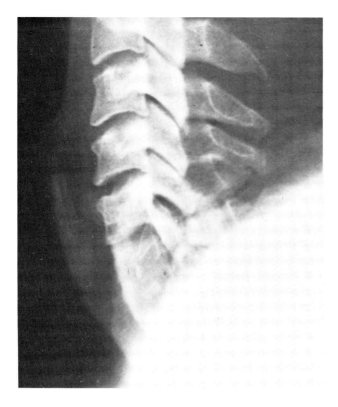

Fig. 88-7. Replacement of a vertebral body after a burst fracture. (Reprinted from Yashon D: *Spinal Injury.* New York, Appleton-Century-Crofts, 1978. With permission.)

not on the cancellous portion of the dowel (Figs. 88-4 and 88-5). Additional fixation for increased stability can be obtained by the use of an H or HH AS IF plate. Closure of the incision is accomplished by approximation of the platysma muscle and skin edges.

The Smith-Robinson type of graft, which is not prefitted as in the Cloward technique, does not seem as efficacious in cervical spine injury. In this technique the iliac bone is fashioned into a plate that is placed between the vertebral bodies after traction, or a vertebral body spreader is used to distract the vertebral bodies (Fig. 88-6). Robinson emphasizes perforation of the subchondral bony end plates for vascular access to the graft.

A vertebral body that has been crushed may be excised and replaced with a bone graft (Fig. 88-7). Complete excision of one or more vertebral bodies may be required when a fracture is extensive. A tibial, iliac, or fibular bone graft then can be used to maintain alignment and stability. With exposure of the involved vertebral body by the anterior approach, the involved vertebra is resected with rongeurs and curettes. Care must be exercised to prevent further injury to the spinal cord. Often the posterior longitudinal ligament is torn or frayed. After several days, the natural line of demarcation between the posterior longitudinal ligament and the vertebral body is lost. The vertebra may be vascular, and hemorrhage may be encountered. The upper and lower intact vertebral bodies should be notched so that the graft can be fitted into a trough and lodged tightly. The cervical spine may be extended for insertion of the graft. Cancellous bone chips then can be laid over the graft before replacement of the longitudinal vertebral muscles. The anterior longitudinal ligaments then may be approximated.

Certain pitfalls must be avoided in surgery of the anterior cervical spine. These include paralysis of the recurrent laryngeal nerve, collapse of vertebrae, nonfusion, and infection. Al-

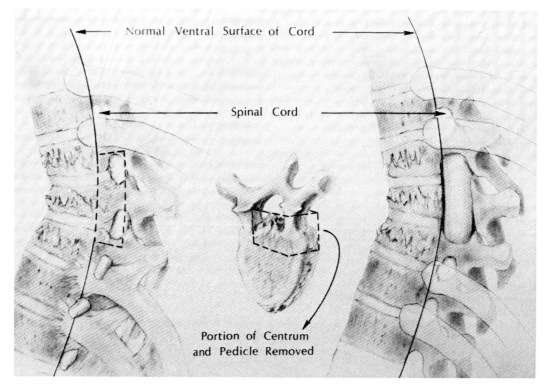

Fig. 88-8. (Left) The heads of the fifth and sixth ribs have been removed to expose the foramina between T5-7. Compression of the ventral spinal cord is in the area outlined by the broken rectangle. The osteotomy begins with resection of the pedicle of T6 (center). The extent of the completed bone resection in the coronal plane is outlined by the broken line. (Right) The completed resection in the longitudinal plane. The facets remain intact. (Reprinted from Paul RL, Michael RL Dunn JE, et al: Anterior transthoracic surgical decompression of acute spinal cord injuries. *J Neurosurg* 43:299–307, 1975. With permission.)

though complications are uncommon, some have occurred and spinal paralysis following such complications has been reported.

Transthoracic surgical decompression of acute spinal cord injuries can be accomplished. The thoracic cord is decompressed by removal of the pedicle (Figs. 88-8 and 88-9). The vertebral column is stabilized by fixing a bone graft in place with screws. In the lumbar region, anterior transperitoneal fusion also has been advocated. This operation is uncommonly used for lumbar stabilization following fracture-dislocation.

Acrylic plastics have been used for stabilization of the spine. Kelly et al.[28] as well as Stowsand and Muhtaroglu[29] used acrylic fixation in atlantoaxial dislocation for posterior stabilization. It is our view that in fracture-dislocation use of autologous bone is preferred since it appears to be more stable in the long run and possibly has a lower incidence of infection.

Anterolateral Approach to the Upper Cervical Spine

DeAndrade and MacNab[30] described an approach to the basiocciput and anterior upper cervical spine. Figure 88-2 shows this lateral approach and the anatomic structures involved. Access to the basiocciput anteriorly is limited by the mandible and subglottic structures superficially and by the internal carotid artery, cranial nerves, and pharynx deeper. Access to this area is limited, and the potential hazards are many. Such an approach generally is not useful in spinal injury, but possibly could be employed for fusion using autologous bone. A trough is fashioned and bone is laid into the trough. Some surgeons advocate preliminary tracheostomy, but this is not necessary in all cases. The patient should be immobilized for about a month; some of this

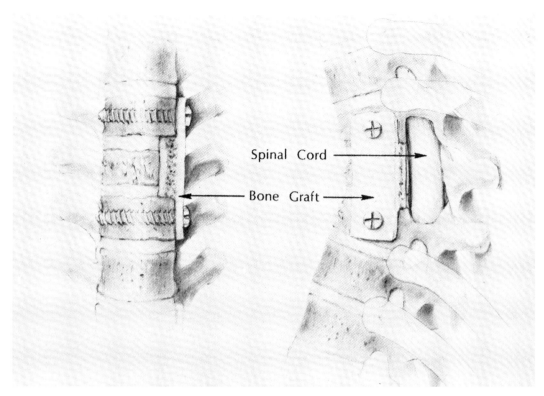

Fig. 88-9. Lateral fusion after the decompression illustrated in Figure 88-8. The template of bone is shown in both arteroposterior and lateral views. The screws should pass from cortex to cortex of the vertebral body. (Right) The relationship of the graft to the decompression. (Reprinted from Paul RL, Michael RL, Dunn JE, et al: Anterior transthoracic surgical decompression of acute spinal cord injuries. *J Neurosurg 43*:299–307, 1975. With permission.)

time should be spent in skeletal traction. External stabilization is maintained by bracing until fusion is established radiographically in 4 to 6 months. Halo traction may replace a long period of recumbency. This approach can be used for fusing the occiput to C1 and C2, but inclusion of the occiput is not necessary in most cases.

Posterior Spinal Fusion

Posterior spinal fusion is a widely accepted technique in the cervical, thoracic, and lumbar spine (Figs. 88-10 through 88-20). Indications for this procedure frequently overlap those for anterior fusion, particularly in the cervical spine. We prefer posterior cervical fusion only in burst fractures of the vertebral bodies when multiple levels are involved and in atlantoaxial dislocations. Thus, in the cervical spine it is not used as frequently as anterior fusion. Posterior fusion is most frequently employed in the thoracic and lumbar spine.

Several different operations have been advocated for the treatment of atlantoaxial fracture-dislocations. Posterior fusion of the C1 and C2 vertebrae seems to be the procedure most often chosen (Figs. 88-10, 88-11, and 88-12). Mixter and Osgood[31] originated the concept of posterior fixation of C1 and C2. They described a technique that makes use of a strong silk thread wound around the posterior arch of the atlas and tied to the spinous process of the axis. Cone and Turner[32] were pioneers in the use of wires and bone grafts for C1 and C2 fusions. Gallie[33] fused the adjacent articular facets while also wiring C1 to C2. Although they reported good results with early fusion for the treatment of atlantoaxial fracture-dislocations, neither Gallie[33] nor Cone and Turner[32] published sufficient details for comparison with other methods of treatment.

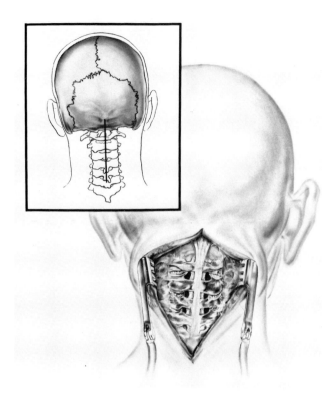

Fig. 88-10. The incision and exposure for a C1-C2 fusion. (Reprinted from Yashon D: *Spinal Injury.* New York, Appleton-Century-Crofts, 1978. With permission.)

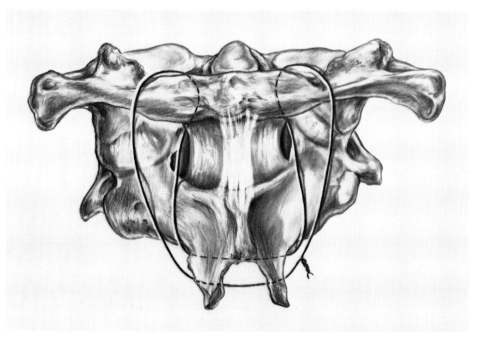

Fig. 88-11. The wiring configuration for a C1-C2 fusion. (Reprinted from Yashon D: *Spinal Injury.* New York, Appleton-Century-Crofts, 1978. With permission.)

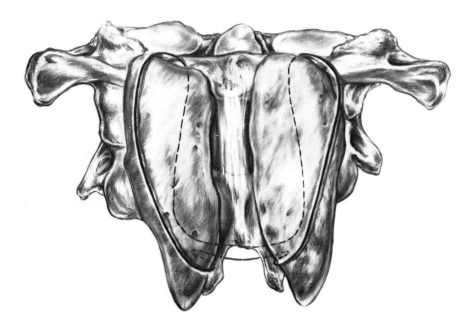

Fig. 88-12. The bone wired into place—C1-C2 fusion. (Reprinted from Yashon D: *Spinal Injury.* New York, Appleton-Century-Crofts, 1978. With permission.)

Alexander et al.[34] claimed that fusion of only C1 and C2 gave unsatisfactory results. Fusion from C1 to C3 was advocated.

The general principles of posterior cervical fusion are virtually identical, whether the upper, middle, or lower cervical spine is to be fused. Once the normal relationships between the vertebrae are established, and following exposure of the spinous processes and lamina from behind, wires are passed under the affected laminae bilaterally (Figs. 88-13 through 88-20). An alternative approach is to pass wires around only the normal vertebral laminae above and below the fracture site. Passage of the wire is facilitated by removal of small portions of the laminae with a Kerrison punch using No. 20 or 22 wire (Fig. 88-14). The dura is separated from the lamina with a small periosteal elevator (Fig. 88-15). The cortical bone of the lamina and spinous process is denuded of periosteum and a high-speed drill is used to roughen the bone. Autogenous bone struts, usually obtained from the iliac crest (Fig. 88-20) then are wired into place. As an alternative, wires may be passed through bone beneath the spinous processes. A towel clip can provide the passage hole, and the bone struts are wired (Fig. 88-15). The periosteum should be denuded from the graft. Small bone chips are packed in the crevices. Fusion of the occiput to the atlantal arch and axis has been advocated but is not used by most surgeons at present because dislocation between the occiput and the atlas is rare. Including the occiput in the fusion for a C1-C2 dislocation does not add to stability, but C3 may be added.

Lewis and McKibben[35] described treatment of unstable fracture-dislocations of the thoracolumbar spine accompanied by paraplegia. They concluded that to preserve long-term spinal function, open reduction and internal fixation are indicated in displaced fractures. Although no differences in the degree of neurologic recovery could be detected between the surgically and nonsurgically treated groups, the surgically treated patients had significantly less residual spinal deformity and significantly less serious pain. In fact, they stated that no serious pain developed in any of their surgically treated patients.

Schmidek et al.[36] employ a one-stage anterolateral decompression of the thoracolumbar

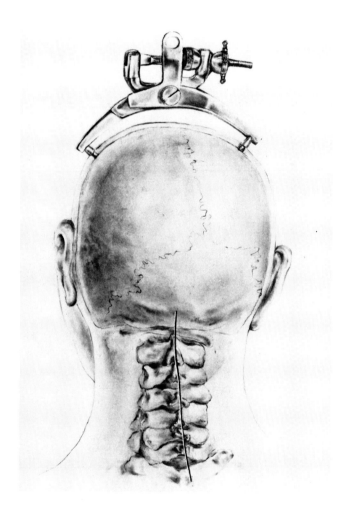

Fig. 88-13. The incision for posterior cervical fusion. (Reprinted from Yashon D: *Spinal Injury.* New York, Appleton-Century-Crofts, 1978. With permission.)

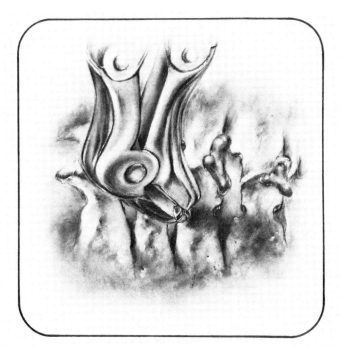

Fig. 88-14. Removal of part of the lamina for passage of the wire. (Reprinted from Yashon D: *Spinal Injury.* New York, Appleton-Century-Crofts, 1978. With permission.)

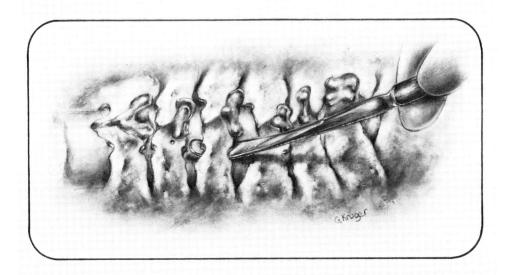

Fig. 88-15. A periosteal elevator is placed under the lamina in preparation for passing the wire. (Reprinted from Yashon D: *Spinal Injury.* New York, Appleton-Century-Crofts, 1978. With permission.)

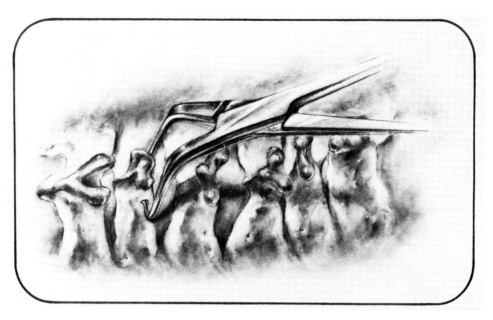

Fig. 88-16. A towel clip is used for a wire hole at the base of the spinous process. (Reprinted from Yashon D: *Spinal Injury.* New York, Appleton-Century-Crofts, 1978. With permission.)

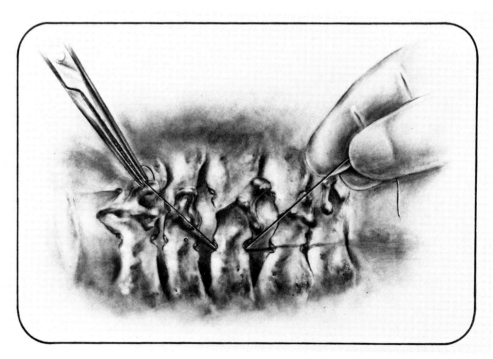

Fig. 88-17. The wires are passed for posterior fusion. (Reprinted from Yashon D: *Spinal Injury.* New York, Appleton-Century-Crofts, 1978. With permission.)

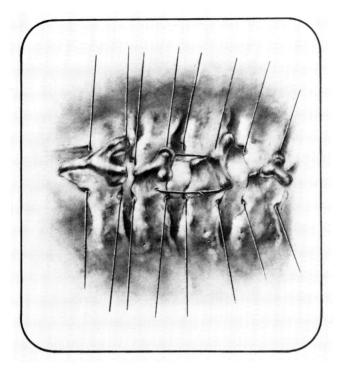

Fig. 88-18. The wires are passed under the laminae and at the base of the spinous processes. Generally the wires need not be passed around each lamina. (Reprinted from Yashon D: *Spinal Injury.* New York, Appleton-Century-Crofts, 1978. With permission.)

spine with Harrington rod alignment and posterior fusion with bone grafting. As adjuncts, they use somatosensory-evoked responses both preoperatively and postoperatively and intraoperative myelography to confirm the adequacy of decompression.

Laminectomy

For many years laminectomy has been carried out to relieve compression on the injured spinal cord. A block to lumbar puncture demonstrated by myelography has been suggested as a prerequisite. We do not subscribe to this, since an opening only the size of the spinal needle need be present for normal cerebrospinal fluid (CSF) dynamics, and have carried out decompressive laminectomy without prior myelography in the presence of severe neurologic deficit and spinal dislocation. Vertebral CT scan has been helpful in delineating candidates for laminectomy.

Whether the dura should be opened at the time of laminectomy is a matter of individual preference. If the dura is not opened, a significant intradural hematomata may be overlooked; however, if the dura is opened, closing it frequently is difficult, so that it either must be left open or a dural substitute must be used for closure. The herniation of a swollen and acutely injured spinal cord may result in neurologic worsening in the patient with a partial lesion or the development of a cerebrospinal fluid leak if the dura is not closed. After laminectomy, posterior fusion is possible and frequently is carried out. The fusion need be only lateral, involving facets and transverse processes.

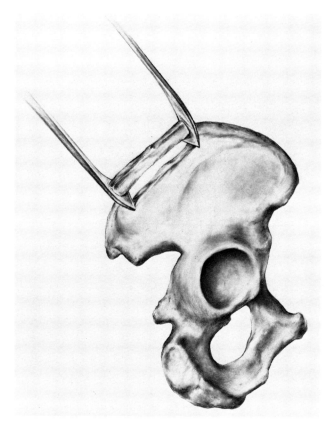

Fig. 88-19. The technique for removing bone from the iliac
crest. (Reprinted from Yashon D: *Spinal Injury.*
New York, Appleton-Century-Crofts, 1978. With
permission.)

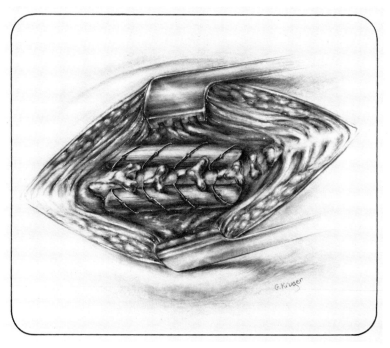

Fig. 88-20. The bone is wired into place—fusion is completed. (Reprinted
from Yashon D: *Spinal Injury.* New York, Appleton-Century-
Crofts, 1978. With permission.)

Posterior Lateral Facet Fusion

The technique for posterior lateral facet fusion has been described by Robinson and Southwick.[37] The facet surfaces are fused from one level above the area of laminectomy to one level below, using corticocancellous bone wired to the facets at each level. A small drill hole is made with a 7/64-inch drill in the inferior articulating facet with a periosteal elevator wedged between the inferior and superior articulating facets. The wire then is brought out above the superior articulating facet, and the longitudinal graft from the iliac crest is wired into place at several levels. This technique may be used when a laminectomy has been performed. The procedure is carried out bilaterally. The facet fusion extends over four levels. A posterior intraspinal fusion is carried out below the fused facets to the second thoracic spinous process. This prevents subsequent development of kyphosis below the fused facets. Support in the form of tong traction or halo traction should be maintained for a considerable period of time.

Thoracoabdominal Approach to the Lower Thoracic and Upper Lumbar Spine

It is occasionally necessary to expose the lower thoracic and upper lumbar spine in continuity (see Figs. 88-8, and 88-9). This presents a problem in exposure because of the diaphragm. A lower thoracotomy incision is made at the level of the seventh to the eleventh rib depending upon the desired level of the section. The incision extends from the plane of the scapula to the anterior margin of the rib cage. The latissimus dorsi muscle is transected across its fibers and the serratus anterior is divided and spread over the intended rib level. Intercostal muscles are divided and the thoracic cavity is opened, using a self-retaining retractor. The lung is deflated and retracted anteriorly and superiorly. A circumferential incision is made in the muscular portion of the diaphragm adjacent to the costal margin. This should be extended posteriorly to the area of the

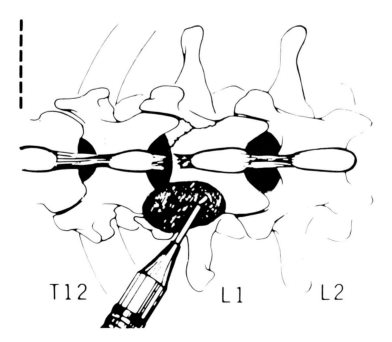

Fig. 88-21. Initiation of lateral decompression in a one-stage decompression-stabilization for a thoracolumbar fracture. Dorsoventral view. Note the use of the air drill for removal of the lateral lamina, facet, and pedicle. (Reprinted from Erickson DL, Leider LL Jr, Brown WE: One stage decompression-stabilization for thoracolumbar fractures. *Spine* 2:53–56, 1977. With permission.)

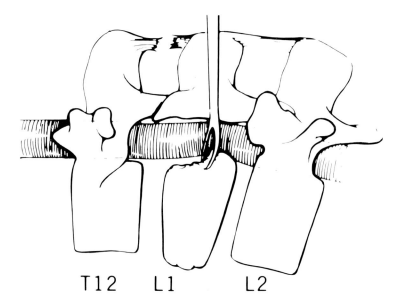

T12   L1   L2

Fig. 88-22. Removal of the retropulsed portion of a comminuted vertebral body in a one-stage decompression-stabilization for a thoracolumbar fracture. Lateral view. (Reprinted from Erickson DL, Leider LL Jr, Brown WE: One stage decompression-stabilization for thoracolumbar fractures. *Spine 2*:53–56, 1977. With permission.)

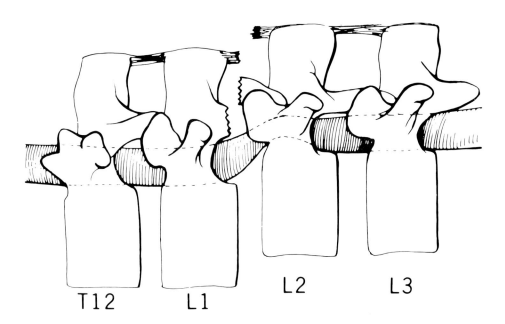

T12   L1   L2   L3

Fig. 88-23. Thoracolumbar dislocation before realignment, relocation, or removal of the retropulsed portion of a vertebral body. Lateral view. (Reprinted from Erickson DL, Leider LL Jr, Brown WE: One stage decompression-stabilization for thoracolumbar fractures. *Spine 2*:53–56, 1977. With permission.)

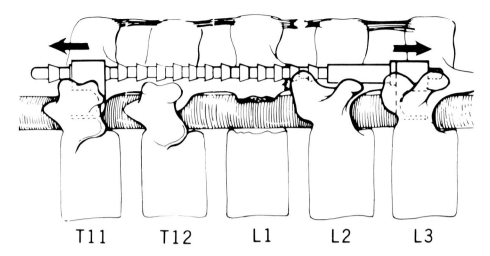

Fig. 88-24. Restoration of alignment after placement of a Harrington rod. Lateral view. In addition, intervening zygaphophyseal joint fusion and the addition of autologous bone can enhance fusion. (Reprinted from Erickson DL, Leider LL Jr, Brown WE: One stage decompression-stabilization for thoracolumbar fractures. *Spine* 2:53–56, 1977. With permission.)

lateral arcuate ligament. The incision then is extended through the peritoneal reflexion of the diaphragm, and the spleen and the contents of the left upper quadrant of the abdomen are exposed. The retroperitoneal space is opened by blunt dissection. Abdominal organs are gently retracted medially with a Deaver retractor. The vertebral bodies and aorta then are exposed. The aorta is mobilized by a combination of sharp and blunt dissection, and segmental vessels are ligated and divided to permit visualization of the involved vertebral bodies. Grafting and even resection of a vertebral body can be carried out. Fusion and inlayed bone grafting in a trough can be accomplished through this exposure. The anterior longitudinal ligament may be closed over the vertebral bodies. Various anatomic structures are reapproximated, and chest tubes attached to water-seal suction should be employed. Erickson et al.[38] advocated internal decompression stabilization for fracture-dislocation (Figs. 88-21 through 88-24).

Anterior Lateral Approach to the Lumbar Vertebral Bodies

An anterior lateral approach to the lumbar vertebral bodies through a long, oblique flank incision can provide direct access to all lumbar vertebral bodies. In the case of spinal injury, grafting can be carried out for anterior interbody fusion, but abdominal viscera and major vessels must be carefully retracted. In addition, the hypogastric nerve plexus should be protected to avoid postoperative complications of impotence and sterility in males. The anterior lateral approach to the lumbar vertebrae is similar to that used for lumbar sympathectomy.

Myelotomy

A myelotomy is an opening into the posterior substance of the spinal cord at the posterior longitudinal fissure following laminectomy and opening of the dura. Allen[39] performed experimental myelotomies on a series of dogs and then on 3 patients in the early 1900s. Slight improvement in neurologic functions below the level of injury was noted postoperatively in all 3 patients. Freeman and Wright[40] described functional recovery in dogs in whom paraplegia would otherwise have been permanent. They implied that the rapid internal decompression of traumatized necrotic tissue was responsible for the improvement in function. Benes[41] discussed his experience in 20 patients undergoing myelotomy, and seemed convinced that no further damage, beyond that incurred at injury, was done to the spinal cord by the procedure. Wagner and Rawe[42] performed an anterior cervical myelotomy, using the operating microscope and bipolar coagulation. They emphasized the ease with which hemorrhagic gray matter could be separated from normal gray matter and surrounding white matter. The issue of performing myelotomies in these patients is still open, but most neurosurgeons currently do not perform this adjunctive procedure.

REFERENCES

1. Yashon D: *Spinal Injury*. New York, Appleton-Century-Crofts, 1978
2. Crutchfield WG: Skeletal traction for dislocation of cervical spine. Report of a case. *Southern Surg* 2:156–159, 1933
3. Barton LG: The reduction of fracture dislocations of the cervical vertebrae by skeletal traction. *Surg Gynecol Obstet* 67:94–96, 1938
4. Vinke TH: A skull-traction apparatus. *J Bone Joint Surg* 30A:522–524, 1948
5. Bovill EG, Eberle CF, et al: Dislocation of the cervical spine without spinal cord injury. *JAMA* 218:1288–1290, 1971
6. Dowman C: Reduction of cervical fracture dislocation with locked facets. *JAMA* 219:1212, 1972
7. Rogers WA: Fractures and dislocations of the cervical spine. *J Bone Joint Surg* 39A:341–376, 1957
8. Bailey RW: Fractures and dislocations of the cervical spine. Orthopedic and neurosurgical aspects. *Postgrad Med* 15:588–599, 1964
9. Bailey RW: Fractures and dislocations of the cervical spine. *Surg Clin North Am* 41:1357–1366, 1961
10. Hollin SA, Gross SW: Management of cervical spine dislocations with locked facets. *Surg Gynecol Obstet* 124:521–524, 1967
11. Crutchfield WG: Further observations on the treatment of fracture dislocations of the cervical spine with skeletal traction. *Surg Gynecol Obstet* 63:513–517, 1936
12. Crutchfield WG: Skeletal traction in treatment of injuries to the cervical spine. *JAMA* 155:29–32, 1954
13. Yashon D, White RJ: Injuries of the vertebral column and spinal cord, in Feiring EG (ed): *Brock's Injuries of the Brain and Spinal Cord and Their Coverings.* New York, Springer, 1974, pp 688–743
14. Yashon D, Tyson G, Vise WM: Rapid closed reduction of cervical fracture dislocations. *Surg Neurol* 4:513–514, 1975
15. Ellis VH: Injuries of the cervical vertebrae. *Proc R Soc Med* (Secton of Orthopaedics) 40:19, 1946
16. Evans DK: Reduction of cervical dislocations. *J Bone Joint Surg* 43B:552–555, 1961
17. Grote W, Romer F, Bettag W: Der ventrale zugang zum dens epistropheus. *Langenbecks Arch Chir* 331:15–22, 1972
18. Murray JWG, Seymour RJ: An anterior, extrapharyngeal suprahyoid approach to the first, second and third cervical vertebrae. *Acta Orthop Scand* 45:43–49, 1974
19. Bonney G: Stabilization of the upper cervical spine by the transpharyngeal route. *Proc R Soc Med* 63:40–41, 1970
20. Fang HSY, Ong GB: Anterior spinal fusion. The operative approaches. *Clin Orthop* 35:16–33, 1964
21. Fang HSY, Ong GB: Direct anterior approach to the upper cervical spine. *J Bone Joint Surg* 44A:1588–1604, 1962
22. Estridge MN, Smith RA: Transoral fusion of odontoid fracture. Case report. *J Neurosurg* 27:462–465, 1967
23. Smith GW, Robinson RA: The treatment of certain cervical-spine disorders by anterior removal of the intervertebral disc and interbody fusion. *J Bone Joint Surg* 40A:607–624, 1958
24. Bailey RW, Badgley CE: Stabilization of the cervical spine by anterior fusion. *J Bone Joint Surg* 42A:565–594, 1960
25. Cloward RB: The anterior approach for removal of ruptured cervical discs. *J Neurosurg* 15:602, 1958
26. Cloward RB: Treatment of acute fractures of the cervical spine. *J Neurosurg* 18:201–209, 1961
27. Cloward RB: Lesions of the intervertebral discs and their treatment by interbody fusion methods. The painful disc. *Clin Orthop* 27:51–77, 1963
28. Kelly DT Jr, Alexander E Jr, Davis CH Jr, et al: Acrylic fixation of atlanto-axial dislocations. Technical note. *J Neurosurg* 36:366–371, 1972
29. Stowsand D, Muhtaroglu U: Dorsale stabilisierug bei luxations-frakturen des 1. and 2. halswirbels mit palacos und drahtumschlingung. *Neurochirurgia (Stuttgart)* 18:120–126, 1975
30. De Andrade JR, MacNab I: Anterior occipito-cervical fusion using an extra-pharyngeal exposure. *J Bone Joint Surg* 51:1621–1626, 1969
31. Mixter WT, Osgood RB: Traumatic lesions of the atlas and axis. *Am J Orthopaed Surg* 7:348–370, 1910

32. Cone W, Turner WG: The treatment of fracture-dislocations of the cervical vertebrae by skeletal traction and fusion. *J Bone Joint Surg 19*:584–602, 1937

33. Gallie WE: Fractures and dislocations of the cervical spine. *Am J Surg 46*:495–499, 1939

34. Alexander E Jr, Davis CH Jr, Forsyth HF: Reduction and fusion of fracture dislocation of the cervical spine. *J Neurosurg 27*:588–591, 1967

35. Lewis J, McKibben B: The treatment of fracture dislocation of the thoracolumbar spine. *J Bone Joint Surg 56B*:391, 1974

36. Schmidek HH, Gomes FB, Seligson D, et al: Management of acute unstable thoracolumbar (T11-L1) fractures with and without neurological deficit. *Neurosurgery 7*:30–35, 1980

37. Robinson RA, Southwick WO: Surgical approaches to the cervical spine. Instructional course lecture. The American Academy of Orthopaedic Surgeons, publ. XVII, St Louis, CV Mosby, 1960, pp 299–330

38. Erickson DL, Leider LL Jr, Brown WE: One-stage decompression-stabilization for thoracolumbar fractures. *Spine 2*:53–56, 1977

39. Allen A: Remarks on the histopathological changes in the spinal cord due to impact: An experimental study. *J Nerv Ment Dis 41*:141–147, 1914

40. Freeman L, Wright T: Experimental observations of concussion and contusion of the spinal cord. *Ann Surg 137*:433–443, 1953

41. Benes V: *Spinal Cord Injury*. London, Balliere, Tindall, and Cassell, 1968, p 202

42. Wagner FC, Rawe SE: Microsurgical anterior cervical myelotomy. *Surg Neurol 5*:229–231, 1976

CHAPTER 89
Metastatic Tumors of the Spine

Eugene A. Quindlen

INCREASINGLY, NEUROSURGEONS ARE ASKED TO EVALUATE and treat patients with metastatic tumors of the central nervous system. As the average age of the population increases and the prevalence of cancer increases, this trend is likely to continue. The increased use of chemotherapy and other adjuvant therapy for cancer also may increase the numbers of patients who survive to develop metastatic cancer to the spine. Approximately 5 percent of all cancer patients will develop metastatic tumors to the spine.[1] Since most of these patients present with an evolving paraparesis or other neurologic syndrome, there is often great anxiety surrounding their care and treatment. The neurosurgeon should know not only what surgical treatment can offer, but also what medical treatment can offer these patients.

Radiation Therapy versus Surgery

Several retrospective studies of patients with spinal metastases[1] and a recent small prospective study[2] have indicated that radiation therapy alone achieves results equal to or superior to either surgery alone or surgery and radiation therapy. These studies, however, combine patients with many different types of tumors and different types of clinical presentation, which makes it difficult to draw clear indications for the type of treatment to be instituted. At the same time it is also clear that the clinical result depends most on the type of tumor and the neurologic condition of the patient before treatment, regardless of the mode of therapy.

Radiation therapy is clearly the treatment of choice for all tumors that are highly sensitive to radiation, such as lymphoma, Ewing's sarcoma, myeloma, and neuroblastoma, even in the presence of spinal block or paraplegia. The treatment should be instituted immediately on an emergency basis. Most other cancers are radiation sensitive to some degree and should be treated with radiation therapy as long as there appears to be any beneficial effect.

Despite the apparent usefulness of radiation therapy, the following is a list of the many clinical situations in which surgery should be considered as the optimal therapy:

1. To achieve a histologic diagnosis in a patient without a known primary tumor.
2. To decompress a known radioresistant tumor.
3. To decompress the spinal cord of the patient who is deteriorating neurologically during radiation therapy.
4. To decompress the spinal cord compressed by bony encroachment of the canal caused by vertebral body collapse or displacement.
5. To decompress the spinal cord with recurrent tumor in an area with previous maximal irradiation.

Surgical Neurology Branch, National Institute of Neurological and Communicative Disorders and Stroke, National Institutes of Health, Bethesda, Maryland, and Division of Neurosurgery, George Washington University Hospital, Washington, D.C.

If the neurologic condition permits, a metastatic work-up can be instituted in the patient who presents with a spinal metastasis and unknown primary tumor. The surgeon should determine if the patient has previously received radiation therapy for the primary tumor or other metastatic lesion; if this radiation was not effective in reducing tumor growth, surgery should be performed to decompress a spinal metastasis. Certain tumors are known for their relative radioresistance, such as prostatic carcinoma and renal cell carcinoma. Occasionally these tumors do respond to radiation, however, and this may be tried if the patient's neurologic condition permits. Otherwise, surgical decompression of epidural tumors is warranted if the patient has severe pain or is rapidly developing paraparesis.

It is felt that in some cases of epidural tumor, the tumor swells and increases its bulk during radiation therapy. This would explain why some patients begin to deteriorate rapidly after radiation therapy has been instituted. Surgical decompression may be of benefit in that situation. Although the neurologic decline of most patients is directly related to the presence of an epidural tumor, the surgeon should be alert to the possibility that a few patients have their spinal cords compromised by a collapsed vertebral body that has been displaced posteriorly into the spinal canal. This mechanical compromise of the canal will obviously not be relieved by radiation, and surgical decompression should be performed.

Clinical Presentation

The clinical presentation of a patient with a spinal tumor metastasis is fairly typical and was well characterized by Wright.[3] The patient first experiences vague back pain or local root pain. This symptom may precede the onset of neurologic deficit by weeks to months and is such a constant finding that cancer patients with this first symptom should be regarded as having a spinal metastasis until it is proven otherwise. Since the results of treatment so heavily depend on the early recognition and treatment of the spinal metastasis, this symptom must be recognized as important by any physician caring for cancer patients.

Motor weakness is the next stage in the illness. It is often subtle and not recognized initially in a patient who is already ill and weak. The patient may notice increased difficulty in getting out of a chair or climbing stairs, or may experience unsteadiness while walking. The patient who goes to bed because of back pain may feel that he is weaker because of the bedrest.

Although the initial motor loss may be subtle and gradual, the next stage of the illness tends to evolve over a matter of a few days. The patient notices daily decreases in the strength in the lower extremities, and about the time the patient can no longer walk, he begins to develop numbness in the distal extremities. Bladder or bowel incontinence rapidly follows, which heralds complete physiologic transection of the spinal cord.

When the surgeon sees the patient for the first time, it is important to do a careful neurologic examination so that the surgeon can arrive at some impression of the stage the patient's illness has progressed to and what level of the spinal column is affected. In a patient with a single metastasis, local percussion tenderness may locate the affected level of the spine. In testing muscle power, one finds that the hip flexors usually are the most prominently affected group. Careful examination of the skin with a pin may demonstrate a sensory level or a dermatomal sensory loss. The abdomen should be examined for a distended bladder and the anal sphincter checked for tone.

In general, a few tests that are repeated often will give the surgeon a clear idea of the progress of the patient's illness. The majority of patients present with myelopathic signs referable to the lower extremities in both cervical and thoracic tumors. Cauda equina compression may be similar in presentation to an early cord compression, and because the latter can progress much more rapidly and with more irreversible potential, early radiologic evaluation should be instituted regardless of the clinical diagnosis. Roughly two-thirds of the patients will have metastatic tumors in the thoracic region, while the remainder are divided between the cervical and lumbar areas.

Radiologic Investigations

Radiologic procedures that are performed properly are crucial in understanding the location and extent of the patient's disease as well as the best approach to treatment. Early in the course of spinal metastasis, radionucleide scanning of the spinal column may be the most sensitive technique available to detect the presence of tumor. If the tumor is confined to the epidural space, however, and has not involved the bony vertebra, bone scan and plain radiograms of the spine may be negative. Consequently, even in patients who present only with back pain or root pain, myelography should be the next step. Bone scans and radiographs of the spine, however, should not be omitted since these studies may alert the surgeon and radiotherapist to other areas of the spine that may require treatment and that may not be seen in myelography.

The plain radiographs of the spine may disclose vertebral collapse or, characteristically, the destruction of a pedicle (Fig. 89-1). In the case of palpable tumors of the paravertebral soft tissues, the plain x-ray can nicely demonstrate the extent of local invasion of the bony spinous process (Fig. 89-2). If the plain x-rays show vertebral collapse or instability, polytomography should be performed to assess the diameter of the spinal canal and the extent of bony destruction.

The recent introduction of "fourth-generation" computed tomographic (CT) scanners with bone-review options has allowed the physician to scrutinize the spine and its associated soft tissue structures on the same scan. In this mode the section is scanned with the normal window width up to 300 and the high-density window up to 4000; both can be presented on the same scan

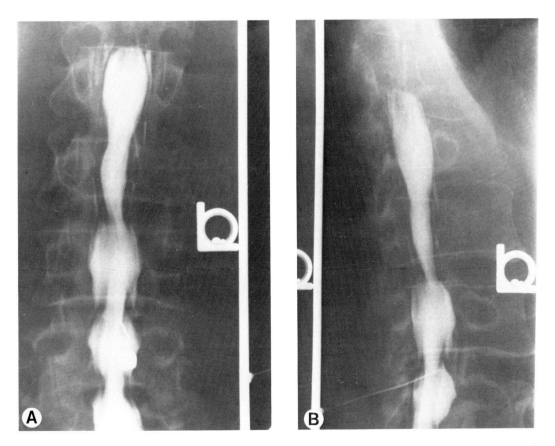

Fig. 89-1. Anteroposterior (**A**) and oblique (**B**) lumbar Pantopaque myelograms in a patient with root pain and metastatic breast cancer. Note the hour-glass configuration of the thecal sac caused by lumbar spondylosis. The absent pedicle and the compression of L3, however, are the clues of metastatic involvement of the spine.

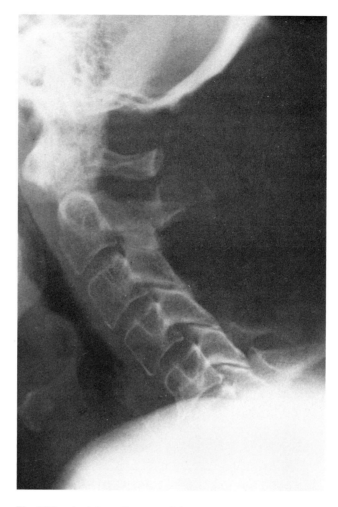

Fig. 89-2.   A plain radiogram of the lateral cervical spine of a patient with a locally invasive sarcoma of the neck, showing extensive destruction of the spinous processes and lamina.

This allows detailed examination of the bone structure and the soft tissue, as demonstrated in Figure 89-3.

Myelography is the most important investigation to pursue in patients with spinal metastasis, as it is in patients with primary intraspinal tumors. It should be considered even in patients with back pain or root pain only since it may disclose disease much more extensive than suspected by clinical examination or routine radionucleide scanning (Fig. 89-4).

The most widely used form of myelography is Pantopaque fluorography. When a spinal block is suspected, as in a patient with a progressing myelopathy, 2–3 cc of Pantopaque are instilled into the subarachnoid space via a lumbar needle (Fig. 89-5). If no block is found, more Pantopaque can be instilled to obtain adequate visualization of the thecal sac. In a patient who has a complete block to the dye column, or is suspected of having a lumbar epidural tumor, a C1-C2 lateral cervical puncture of the subarachnoid space is used to introduce the contrast agent. Instilling the dye in both the cervical and lumbar segments in a case of complete block will nicely define the upper and lower extent of the tumor.

At the time of myelography it is convenient to mark the level of the block on the patient's skin by making a scratch with a sterile needle under fluoroscopic control. Alternatively, a radi-

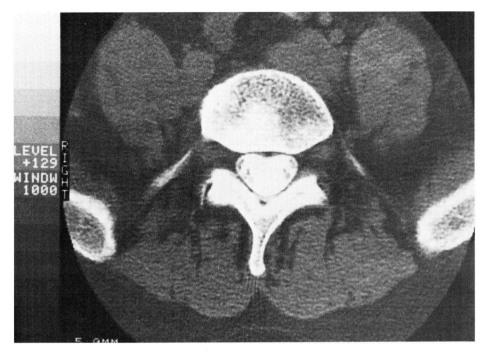

Fig. 89-3. A CT scan of a patient with a painful neuropathy caused by prostate carcinoma involving the pelvic nerves. The scan was performed during metrizamide myelography at the level of L5 on a General Electric 880 scanner with a bone-review option. Note the fine detail of the bony structures and soft tissue on the same scan. Review of this scan and the other slices indicated that the patient's disease had not spread into the canal or spine.

opaque marker such as a paper clip can be taped to the skin at the site of the block. This maneuver will greatly aid in planning the incision for subsequent surgery.

Another form of myelography is now being used with increasing frequency with the advent of CT scanning and water-soluble contrast agents. Metrizamide myelography combined with CT scanning can quickly and easily locate the site of an epidural tumor with minimal discomfort to the patient.

This procedure requires much less contrast agent than standard metrizamide myelography. The usual procedure consists of the introduction of 4–5 cc of metrizamide at a concentration of 170–200 mg/ml of iodine. After allowing 30 to 60 minutes for diffusion of the agent in the subarachnoid space, the patient is scanned at consecutive levels above and below the site of the suspected tumor (Fig. 89-6). This type of myelography is extremely useful in demonstrating ventral and ventrolateral lesions in the canal that at times may be difficult to see by standard myelography (Fig. 89-7). Newer CT machines can produce a scout film of the area examined with a slice location marker on the plain x-ray.

Preoperative Evaluation and Preparation

In addition to a thorough physical examination, adequate laboratory investigations should be performed, including chest x-ray, electrocardiogram, complete blood count, platelet count, prothrombin time, partial thromboplastin time, liver function tests, urea nitrogen, creatine level, and urinalysis. Specific tests that may aid in the diagnosis of a particular tumor, such as acid phosphatase in prostate carcinoma, also should be performed. The clotting function test and platelet count are important if one is contemplating surgery; any deficiencies should be cor-

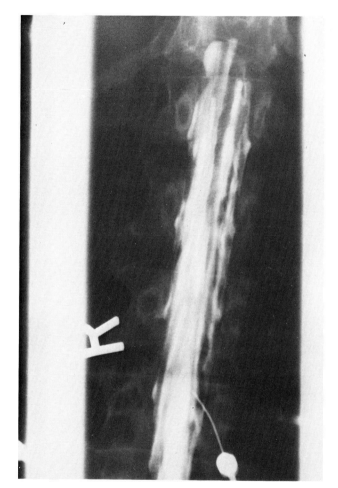

Fig. 89-4. A Pantopaque myelogram of a patient with metastatic adenocarcinoma of the colon. The patient presented with back and root pain. Plain x-rays and bone scan were normal. The myelogram shows the thickened irregular roots characteristic of carcinomatous radiculopathy of the cauda equina.

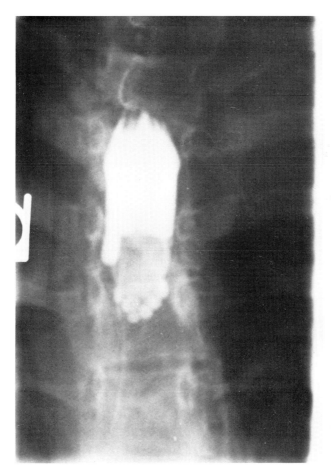

Fig. 89-5. A Pantopaque myelogram of a patient with Ewing's sarcoma presenting with back pain and mild para paresis. Three cubic centimeters of Pantopaque were instilled via a lumbar needle. Note the characteristic "paintbrush" appearance of the dye block caused by the epidural tumor.

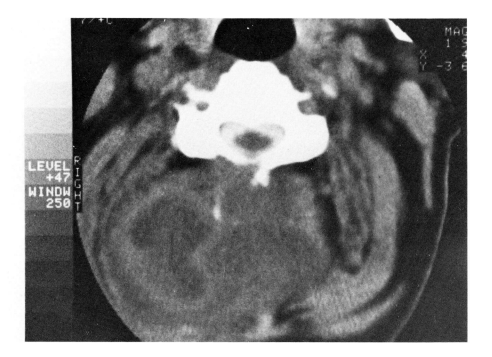

Fig. 89-6. Metrizamide myelogram of the patient in Figure 89-2. The scan demonstrates the extensive tumor of the soft tissue of the neck with involvement of the posterior arch of the spine, but no distortion of the subarachnoid dye column. At operative resection, the tumor extended down to but did not invade the dura.

rected before the operation. In addition, four units of packed red cells or whole blood should be cross-matched for the preoperative patient, and the possibility of more blood for transfusion should be available since some epidural tumors can occasionally be quite vascular and produce bleeding that is difficult to control.

If the patient does not have a rapidly progressing myelopathy and the diagnosis is unknown, then a thorough metastatic work-up can be initiated. This might include a metastatic bone series, lung tomography, and contrast studies of the gastrointestinal and urinary tracts. A bone marrow test may show lymphoma or other metastatic tumor.

If the patient's myelopathy is progressing rapidly and surgery rather than radiation therapy is decided upon as discussed above, then one should proceed with the operation after the basic laboratory studies listed above have been performed.

As soon as the diagnosis of a progressive myelopathy is made, the administration of high-dose steroids such as dexamethasone (4 mg PO/IM/IV every 6 hours) has been found to temporarily improve or reduce a progressing neurologic deficit. Most surgeons today are convinced that steroids can reduce spinal cord edema resulting from compression to such an extent that steroids are continued through the operative and postoperative periods. It should be emphasized, however, that improvement in the patient's condition may be minimal or very brief and that steroids are no substitute for a timely decompressive operation.

Decompressive Laminectomy

A decompressive laminectomy is the most common procedure required for alleviating spinal cord compression from a posteriorly situated epidural tumor. If the myelogram shows the tumor mass to be predominantly posterior or posterolateral with little or no ventral body encroachment on the canal, then this is the procedure of choice.

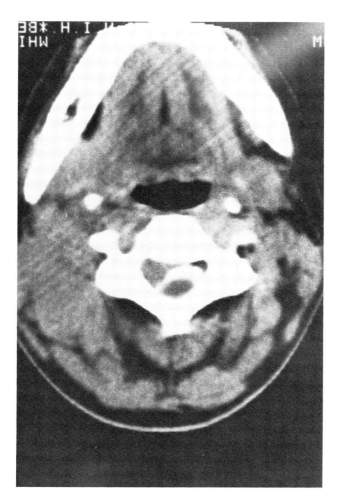

Fig. 89-7. A metrizamide myelogram with CT scan imaging of a patient with a metastatic hemangiopericytoma involving the cervical spine. The patient presented with neck pain. The ventrolateral tumor mass is easily seen on this scan.

After the patient has been intubated and general anesthesia has been instituted, the patient is carefully rolled into the prone position on the operating table. The body is supported by pillows or blanket rolls extending along the anterolateral chest wall to the anterior iliac crests (Fig. 89-8). Alternatively, a padded laminectomy frame may be used. The supports used should be high enough so that the abdomen will not be compressed, thus preventing high pressure and distention in the epidural and paravertebral veins. The operating table is flexed slightly to allow expansion of the interlaminar spaces. The arms can be brought forward and above the head and should be properly padded and supported on arm boards. The surgeon should keep in mind that the emaciated cancer patient is much more susceptible to compression neuropathy than a normal individual, and great care is needed in positioning the patient.

In the case of cervical epidural tumors, the three-point Mayfield or Gardner type of head prongs is a sure way to fix the head and give controlled neck flexion and stability for the operation. If preoperative x-rays and tomography indicate an unstable spine because the tumor has invaded the cervical vertebral bodies, then preoperative stabilization should be instituted before general endotracheal anesthesia. This can be accomplished by placing the patient in a Halo jacket and adjusting the support rods until satisfactory reduction and alignment of the spine is achieved. The patient then is anesthetized and operated upon while in the Halo jacket.

Another technique is to place the patient in cervical traction with skull tongs and to operate using a horseshoe headrest. A pulley placed superior to the headrest is used to give continuous traction. The patient then is nursed postoperatively in cervical traction. Of the two techniques, this author feels the Halo jacket gives the most secure reduction and fixation and allows more rapid postoperative mobilization of the patient.

After the patient has been positioned properly, a wide area of the trunk or neck is shaved and prepared. The skin is marked with a marking pen or gentian violet for a sagittal midline incision that is bisected by the previously marked level of tumor determined at myelography. The drapes should be placed so that the incision can be extended superiorly or inferiorly if necessary.

The skin is incised with a blade down through the dermis. The electrocautery then is used to divide the subcutaneous tissue. Small bleeding points can be coagulated using the electrocautery and insulated forceps. The spinous processes are palpated and the paraspinal muscle fascia divided in the midline with the electrocautery. The attachments of the paraspinal muscles to the spinous processes are divided with the electrocautery and the processes palpated to determine if they are loose or destroyed by tumor. Infiltration and softening of the spinous processes and lamina by tumor should be suspected in every case, and as a result the paraspinal muscles are

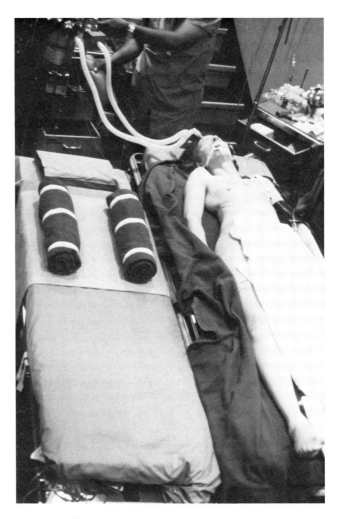

Fig. 89-8. The patient is anesthetized on the mobile stretcher and will be turned prone and lifted onto the blanket rolls on the operating room table.

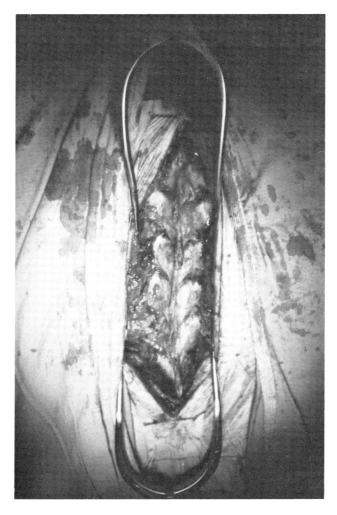

Fig. 89-9.   A decompressive thoracic laminectomy. The dissection of the paraspinal muscles from the spinous
processes and lamina has been carried out. Self-
retaining retractors have been inserted and hemostasis has been achieved.

best removed from these structures by sharp dissection. Then gentle blunt dissection of the
paraspinal muscles laterally can be achieved. Self-retaining retractors are used to hold the muscles and wound open (Fig. 89-9). Attempted movement of the processes may confirm instability
or softening of the vertebra, usually at the level of the spinal block. In any case, the spinous
processes are removed using bone cutters (Fig. 89-10). The remnants of the processes and the
lamina are then thinned and nibbled away with bone rongeurs (Fig. 89-11).

The actual laminectomy is begun at a location away from the suspected site of the epidural
tumor so that normal tissue and structure can be recognized. Ideally this should be at a site
above the level of the block, since sudden decompression of the canal below may cause the tumor to shift caudally and further impact against the cord. In the lumbar region this mechanism
may not be as important as in areas over the spinal cord proper.

The removal of the lamina is accomplished with a Kerrison punch inserted beneath the
bony inferior edge of the lamina and above the ligamentum flavum (Fig. 89-12). Once one
lamina is removed, the ligamentum flavum can be removed along with the bone with the Kerrison punch. The punches used should be sharp and the bone removed by a biting action rather

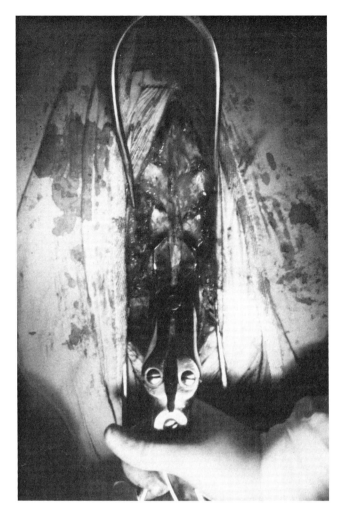

Fig. 89-10. Decompressive thoracic laminectomy. The laminectomy is begun with the sharp removal of the
spinous processes with bone cutters and without
twisting or tearing.

than a twisting or tearing action, which could turn a fragment of bone into the spinal cord. The
bone may be soft and infiltrated with tumor, and it is a good practice to send all of the bone removed to the pathology laboratory for examination. Occasionally this can aid the pathologist in
making a diagnosis.

When the epidural tumor is encountered, normal epidural fat will disappear or will be infiltrated with tumor. The laminectomy is continued right over the surface of the tumor and beyond
until normal epidural fat is encountered again. This usually can be accomplished without taking
a bite of the tumor, which will result in bleeding. If bleeding is encountered, the bipolar coagulating forceps can be used to gently coagulate the surface of the tumor or surrounding veins. At
times, even though the laminectomy is carried out two levels above and below the level of the
block, the epidural tumor is found to extend much further in the epidural space than the laminectomy has exposed. If one is sure that the level of the block has been uncovered, then this continuation of tumor, which is usually diminutive, is left alone. If, however, the tumor still
occupies a considerable portion of the canal, extension of the laminectomy should be done until
the tumor bulk becomes insignificant. Bleeding from the bone edges is controlled with bone wax.

The tumor generally receives its blood supply from the epidural arteries and veins situated

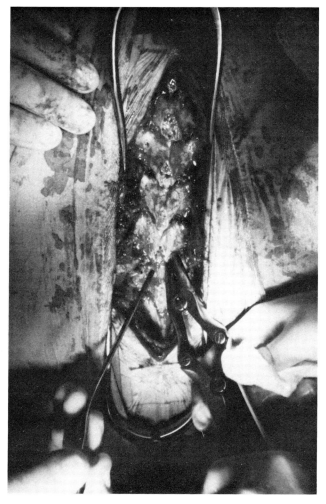

Fig. 89-11. Decompressive thoracic laminectomy. Bone rongeurs are used to nibble away the remaining
stumps of the spinous processes and to thin the
lamina so that minimal force will be exerted with
the Kerrison punches.

laterally in the canal. After identifying normal dura, the epidural tumor is grasped laterally with
the bipolar forceps and coagulated. If this maneuver is repeated on each side for a distance of 1
cm, the coagulated tumor can be cut and the process repeated. In this way the tumor can be rolled
up like a rug with minimal bleeding and without tearing the epidural veins (Fig. 89-13).

Some tumors have minimal blood supply and can be elevated right off the dura with a No. 3
Penfield dissector and coagulation of a few feeding vessels. Others are tenaciously bound to the
dura and cannot be removed by blunt dissection. These tumors often bleed extensively when removal with sharp dissection is attempted. In such a case it is best to remove enough tumor for
pathological examination and to leave the decompressed tumor attached to the dura. Although
any metastatic tumor can be hemorrhagic, melanoma, hypernephroma, and some breast tumors
can bleed profusely. This often occurs when the lamina are removed from the tumor. Control of
the bleeding may not be possible with the bipolar cautery, in which case oxidized cellulose or gelatin sponge and gentle pressure with a cotton patty will often control the bleeding. After the tumor is removed or at least decompressed, the normal respiratory pulsations of the dural sac will
often, but not always, return.

A frozen section of the tumor tissue performed at the time of surgery is useful in helping the

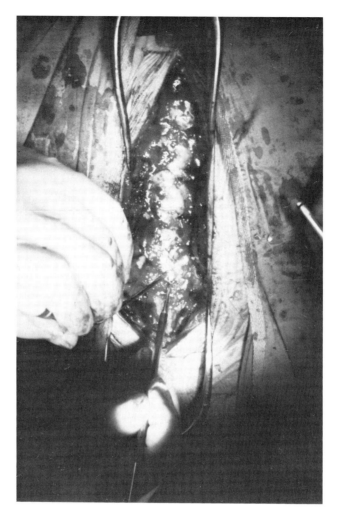

Fig. 89-12. Decompressive thoracic laminectomy. The lamina have been thinned and waxed with bone wax. The dental instrument is used to create a plane beneath the edge of the lamina that will accept the foot-plate of the Kerrison punch visible on the right.

surgeon conduct the operation. If the pathologist reports that the tumor is a lymphoma or some other radiation-sensitive tumor, the surgeon can be less aggressive in removing all the tumor that can be seen, knowing that radiation will be effective in controlling any residual tumor.

After the removal of the tumor is completed, hemostasis is achieved by waxing all bone edges and coagulating any epidural veins with the bipolar cautery. Any bleeding points not discrete enough to be coagulated can be controlled with cellulose or gelatin sponge. Despite extensive hemostatic maneuvers, there still may be a slow ooze of blood from the epidural space, in which case the surgeon should consider placing a drain tube in the epidural space and bringing it out to drain through a separate site (Fig. 89-14). Drains connected to a closed container system that allows gentle suction on the draining tube are particularly valuable for this purpose. The drain is rarely required for more than 12 to 24 hours after the operation.

The paraspinal muscles and fascia are reapproximated in the midline over the drain tube with interrupted 0 silk or synthetic absorbable sutures. The subcutaneous tissue is closed with in-

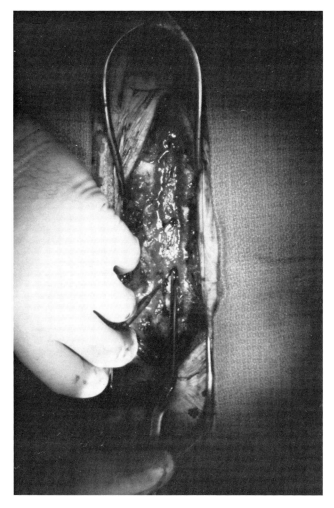

Fig. 89-13. Decompressive thoracic laminectomy. The laminectomy has been completed. A plane between
the normal dura and the epidural tissue is developed at the lower edge of the wound. The bipolar
forceps then are used to coagulate the lateral epidural veins and tumor tissue as the mass is gently
elevated from the dura.

terrupted 3-0 silk or synthetic absorbable sutures. The skin is best closed with interrupted 3-0 nylon sutures. Because of its nonreactive quality, this suture material may be left in the skin for up
to 14 days with minimal skin reaction. Some surgeons prefer wire sutures for this purpose. A
sterile gauze dressing taped in place completes the operation.

Generally most patients with epidural metastatic tumors have adequate stability of the
spine. Since most of the epidural metastases occur in the thoracic region, the surgeon can rely on
the ribs and chest wall to stabilize this area, provided extensive destruction of the vertebrae has
not taken place. The patient can be simply nursed flat on the bed with appropriate "log-rolling"
maneuvers. Often, after postoperative radiation therapy, x-rays will show healing of the affected
vertebrae. In the case of extensive destruction of the thoracic and lumbar vertebrae with gross
kyphosis, however, the insertion of Harrington rods at the time of decompression should be
considered and an orthopedic colleague consulted. The cervical spine is best stabilized with a
Halo jacket as described earlier.

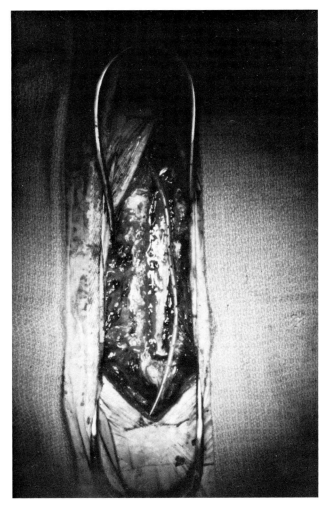

Fig. 89-14. Decompressive thoracic laminectomy. The tumor mass has been successfully removed from the dura and a perforated drain tube has been inserted into the epidural space and is brought out through a separate stab wound before the wound is closed.

In the uncommon situation in which only one vertebra is completely destroyed and presents with angulation, one can perform intraoperative methyl-methacrylate fusion using a technique similar to that described for vertebral fractures of the spine.[4] In order to apply this technique, firm and sound spinous processes and lamina should be present above and below the two or three segments that have been decompressed. Instead of making logs of plastic as originally described, this surgeon prefers to pass heavy stainless wires through and around the spinous processes above and below the decompression site. Then the methyl-methacrylate plastic is molded on top of and around the wires to form a single large strut of posteriorly situated plastic. The underlying dura is protected with several sheets of gelatin sponge, which can be removed after the plastic hardens. It is important to use the skeletal type of methyl-methacrylate that is designed for orthopedic uses. This plastic sets more slowly than the material used by neurosurgeons for cranioplasty, which allows the plastic to be modeled while it is in its puttylike state. In addition, it is radiopaque and can be visualized by standard x-ray for continuity and position.

Anterior Decompression of the Spinal Canal

All of the techniques developed for the anterior decompression of the spinal canal in cases of disc herniation and vertebral fracture can be used with modification to remove ventrally placed tumor masses.

Usually the mass consists of a vertebral body that has been replaced by tumor and has impinged on the cord, which results in a myelopathy. The posterior elements—lamina, spinous processes, and facets—may also be invaded by tumor. This fact usually requires that intraoperative stabilization or fusion be performed. Anterior decompression is required in only a minority of patients presenting with metastatic spinal disease, but it is important to recognize those that require it since posterior laminectomy may not achieve a satisfactory result. The description of the general operative technique for approaching the anterior spine is already adequately outlined in the literature and in the chapters dealing with disc disease. It would therefore be best to comment on those modifications and salient features that pertain to metastatic involvement of the spine.

The general operative approach of Cloward can be used to perform a vertebral corpectomy in the cervical region.[5] Instead of using the Cloward drill, however, the softened vertebral body is best removed piecemeal with sharp bone curettes and a high-speed drill with dental burrs. This prevents the displacement of infiltrated and loosened bone fragments into the canal, which can be a problem with the Cloward drill. The disc material is likewise removed with a bone curette until normal vertebral bodies are encountered above and below the lesion. If fragments of the diseased vertebral body remain attached to the underlying dura but are decompressed, they are best left in place. Rarely, more than one vertebral body must be removed. After the decompression has been achieved, a bone graft or plastic vertebral body replacement may or may not be necessary. When a single diseased vertebral body is removed along with the adjacent discs and cartilaginous plates, no fusion is necessary. In fact, the diseased vertebral body usually has already collapsed in height and the small defect left after its removal is easily bridged by the settling of the spine. The patient's neck of course should be immobilized with a Halo jacket, or, if there is no involvement of the posterior elements, a rigid cervical collar.

When two or more vertebral bodies are removed, the resulting defect must be bridged with a bone graft or a methyl-methacrylate strut. The fibula provides a bone graft that is easy to obtain and has the ideal dimensions. The remaining normal superior and inferior vertebral bodies should be hollowed slightly with a drill to accept and secure the correct length of fibula. If a plastic graft is used, short K-wires or screws are driven into the vertebral bodies at either end of the defect.[6] The underlying dura is protected with 2 to 3 layers of gelatin sponge, and the plastic is molded into place when it has a puttylike consistency. In order to dissipate the heat of polymerization, the plastic is irrigated continuously with water while it is curing. After the plastic has set, excess gelatin sponge is removed from beneath the graft. Immobilization of the neck with a rigid collar is maintained for 6 weeks.

The techniques of vertebral body removal in the thoracic region are similar to those described above for the cervical region. There are two major approaches to the thoracic vertebral bodies. One approach is by a thoracotomy at the level of interest, which gives a view of the vertebral bodies that is almost directly anterior. This technique gives the best exposure and is technically quite simple.[7,8] Likewise, a bone graft or plastic graft is used. Recently, the use of stainless steel mesh for reinforcing a thoracic plastic graft has been reported.[9] This technique does expose the patient to the possible pulmonary complications of a thoracotomy. The other approach is a costotransversectomy, which does not require entering the pleural space but gives a more limited and strictly lateral approach to the vertebral bodies. This operative approach has been used for many years, first to treat Potts' disease of the spine and presently for thoracic disc herniations. The actual technique is described in detail elsewhere.[10]

Several points about this technique are worth mentioning, however. The exposure is quite limited and generally affords access to only one vertebral body. The surgeon must therefore be sure to operate at the correct level and use intraoperative x-rays if necessary. Although the thoracic cavity is not intentionally opened, the parietal pleura may be violated with a resulting pneumothorax. This may not be noticed at the time of the operation, making an immediate postoperative chest x-ray mandatory. The surgeon should be prepared to insert a chest tube if necessary. Finally, the operation is easiest in patients with a slender build who already have a dorsal kyphosis caused by vertebral collapse and angulation.

Postoperative Care

Following decompressive laminectomy, patients are nursed flat in bed using log-rolling techniques for the first 3 or 4 days. After this they are mobilized into a chair or are assisted in walking if their condition permits. The same regimen is followed for patients who have had an anteriorly placed bone graft or plastic fusion. Prolonged unnecessary bedrest will invite complications such as pulmonary embolism or pneumonia. Periodic postoperative x-rays of the spine should be performed, however, to detect any early subluxation or graft displacement. The dressing is checked daily for any evidence of cerebrospinal fluid (CSF) leakage. If it is found, the wound is immediately oversewn with a running suture of 4-0 or 3-0 nylon.

Preoperative antibiotics are used only in those patients who have a current bacterial infection and require emergency decompressive surgery. Cancer patients are known to be more susceptible to sepsis, however, so that postoperative atelectasis, pneumonia, or urinary tract infection should be diagnosed and treated promptly. Steroids are given to those patients who had a progressing myelopathy preoperatively and are continued for 7 to 10 days or until the neurologic condition stabilizes.

Results and Complications

In general, the neurologic condition of the patient at the time of surgery can be the expected postoperative condition. A survey of several different operative series showed an overall improvement of only 30 percent.[1] In most cases operative intervention prevented the patient from worsening. This same survey found an average mortality rate of 9 percent, with 12 percent of the patients becoming neurologically worse. Postoperative complications such as wound infection, CSF fistula, epidural hematoma, and spine subluxation occurred in 11 percent of the cases. Complications such as wound infection or hematoma should be treated promptly by a second operation and suitable debridement or closure of the wound. If postoperative x-rays show gross displacement of a bone or plastic graft, surgery may be required when the patient's neurologic condition is threatened.

REFERENCES

1. Black P: Spinal metastasis: current status and recommended guidelines for management. *Neurosurgery* 5:726–746, 1979
2. Young RF, Post EM, King GA: Treatment of spinal epidural metastases. *J Neurosurg* 53:741–748, 1980
3. Wright RL: Malignant tumors in the spinal extradural space: Results of surgical treatment. *Ann Surg* 157:227–231, 1961
4. Kelly DL, Alexander E, Davis CH, et al: Acrylic fixation of atlanto-axial dislocation. *J Neurosurg* 36:366–371, 1972
5. Cloward RB: The anterior approach for removal of ruptured cervical discs. *J Neurosurg* 15:602–617, 1958
6. Cross GO, White HL, White LP: Acrylic prosthesis of the fifth cervical vertebra in multiple myeloma. *J Neurosurg* 35:112–114, 1971

7. Perot P, Munro DD: Transthoracic removal of midline disc protrusions causing spinal cord compression. *J Neurosurg* 31:452–458, 1969
8. Paul RL, Michael RH, Dunn JE, et al: Anterior transthoracic surgical decompression of acute spinal cord injuries. *J Neurosurg* 43:299–305, 1975
9. Galicich, JH: Management of metastatic tumors to the nervous system at the Sloan-Kettering Institute. Presented at the Central Neurosurgical Society Meeting, Chicago, 1980
10. Hulme A: The surgical approach to thoracic intervertebral disc protrusions. *J Neurol Neurosurg Psychiatry 23*:133–137, 1960

CHAPTER 90
Surgical Management of Spinal Cord Tumors and Arteriovenous Malformations

Kalmon D. Post   Bennett M. Stein

Intramedullary Spinal Cord Tumors

ALTHOUGH VON EISELSBERG TOTALLY EXCISED A NEUROFIBROSARCOMA from the spinal cord in 1907 and Cushing operated on an 8-year-old child and completely removed an intramedullary ependymoma extending from C1 to T2 in 1924,[1] the first well-documented surgical effort to remove an intramedullary tumor was reported by Elsberg[2] in 1925. Of the 13 tumors he reported on, 3 were totally removed and the remainder were partially removed. He stressed that because some of these tumors were infiltrating, they defied removal; nevertheless, he emphasized that the surgeon must search out those tumors with well-defined cleavage planes that permit total removal of the neoplasm. Considering his lack of magnification techniques and previous surgical experience with such tumors, these results were remarkable. When a definitive plane between the tumor and the spinal cord was not visible, Elsberg proposed a second operation when the tumor might present through the myelotomy, making total removal possible. Later, Matson[3] also advocated this technique. With the exception of these reports, little experience with two-stage removal has been published. Following Elsberg's early reports, others[1,3-8] have described successful removals of intramedullary tumors. Successful surgical removal of these tumors was mounted on a firm foundation when Greenwood presented his experience with 10 intramedullary tumors, primarily ependymomas, which he totally removed with no mortalities.[5] These results, with useful survival, justified his enthusiasm for an aggressive surgical approach to these lesions. He also emphasized the use of magnification techniques and microsurgical instrumentation.

Guidetti[6] published his experience with a large group of intramedullary tumors and noted the difficulty in totally removing astrocytomas. In the presence of intramedullary ependymomas and other tumors, however, he felt that every effort should be made to achieve total removal, although only a line of cleavage between the normal spinal cord and the tumor would make this possible. Once a cleavage was established, gentle dissection separated the tumor from the normal spinal cord on each side; then the tumor could be lifted carefully by one end or the other and slowly removed from its bed. Blood vessels were severed close to the tumor by bipolar cautery with irrigation. Guidetti achieved an overall total removal of 24 of 71 tumors, representing a wide variety of histologic types, with a 10 percent operative mortality.

Department of Neurosurgery, College of Physicians and Surgeons, Columbia University, New York, New York

Table 90-1. Intramedullary Spinal Cord Tumors

No.	Age	Location	History	Removal	Result	Follow-up	
1	26	C	Ependymoma	T	I	3	mos.
2	24	Conus	Ependymoma	T	I	1½	yrs.
3	49	C	Ependymoma	T	I	5	yrs.
4	28	C-D	Ependymoma	T	S	4½	yrs.
5	38	C	Ependymoma	T	S	4½	yrs.
6	45	Conus	Ependymoma	T	S	2	yrs.
7	35	Conus	Ependymoma	T	S	2	yrs.
8	20	Conus	Ependymoma	T	S	2	yrs.
9	35	C	Ependymoma	T	I	1½	yrs.
10	12	C	Astrocytoma	P	S	6	mos.
11	60	C-D	Astrocytoma	90%	S	6	yrs.
12	13	D-L	Astrocytoma	T	S	4	yrs.
13	3	C-D	Astrocytoma	95%	I	4	yrs.
14	48	C	Astrocytoma	T	I	4½	yrs.
15	38	C	Astrocytoma	T	I	5	yrs.
16	7	C	Astrocytoma	T	I	1½	yrs.
17	5	C-D-L-S	Astrocytoma	50%	S	1	yr.
18	14	C	Malignant glioma	P	W	1	yr. (died)
19	20	C	Malignant glioma	P	W	6	mos. (died)
20	13	D	Teratoma	T	I	4½	yrs.
21	12	Conus	Dermoid	T	I	11	yrs.
22	4 mos.	Conus	Epidermoid	T	I	11	yrs.
23	28	D-L	Mixed	P	W	2	yrs.
24	52	D	Metastatic	P	S	1	mo. (died)
25	57	C	Hemangioblastoma	T	I	2	mos.

C = cervical; D = dorsal; L = lumbar; T = total; P = partial; I = improved; S = same; W = worse.

In the famous case of Horrax and Henderson,[7] an intramedullary ependymoma extending the entire length of the spinal cord was totally enucleated during a series of operations, resulting in recovery and long-term survival.

Our series comprises 25 cases of intramedullary tumor, with 17 total removals (Table 90-1). A range of histology is represented, with astrocytoma and ependymoma the most common tumors and teratomatous types less frequent. No lipomas are included in this group.

Some patients had undergone previous treatment, including decompressive laminectomy, tapping of cysts associated with the tumors, and radiotherapy. The effects of treatment other than total removal are difficult to evaluate. It is clear, however, that the degree of neurologic deficit caused by the disease process before surgery often determined the postoperative result.

Clinical Presentation

Although intramedullary tumors occur most commonly in adults,[2,4-6] a significant incidence has been reported in children.[3,9] The symptomatology in both age groups is similar. It is quite amazing at times to see an extensive tumor filling the majority of the intramedullary space yet causing few symptoms. Often, however, an end point is reached when compensatory ability fails, and marked neurologic deterioration occurs rapidly. Persistent pain involving the dorsal root dermatomes in the area of tumor involvement is often the signature of an intramedullary neoplasm. Dysfunction of the posterior column may occur in a progressive fashion, with sensory dysesthesias in the arms, torso, and legs, depending upon the site of the intraspinal neoplasm. Sacral sparing may or may not be present and is not an invariable finding with intramedullary neoplasms. Lower motor neuron symptomatology and signs usually occur at the level of the tumor. Well-defined central cord syndromes, as seen in syringomyelia, with disassociated sensory loss and the classic signs of anterior horn cell involvement may be lacking. Children often present with a scoliosis. The symptomatology generally is progressive with few

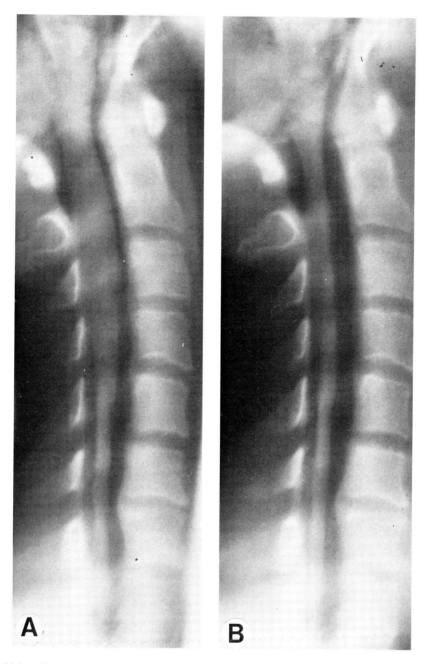

Fig. 90-1. Air myelogram demonstrating the "collapsing cord" sign of syringomyelia. **A.** Head-up position with cervical cord enlarged. **B.** Head-down position with cervical cord narrow.

remissions or exacerbations. Symptoms are usually bilateral, but in rare instances neurologic abnormalities are confined to one extremity. The duration of symptoms generally is measured in years, although some neoplasms may present with histories of 6 months or less.

Diagnostic Evaluation

The radiologic demonstration of intramedullary tumors depends upon myelography with either amipaque-lyophilized metrizamide,* or Pantopaque-Iophendylate.** A fusiform dilata-

*Winthrop Laboratories, Division of Sterling Drug, Inc., New York, New York.
**Lafayette Pharmacological, Inc., Lafayette, Indiana.

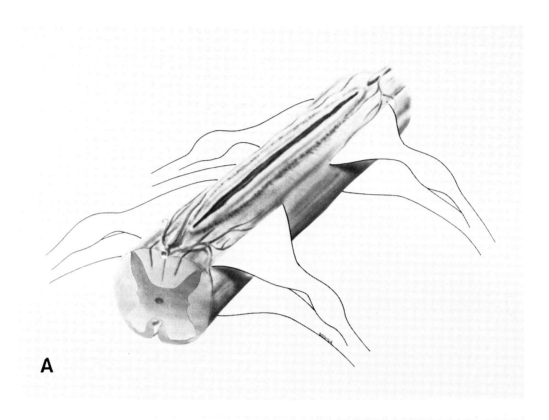

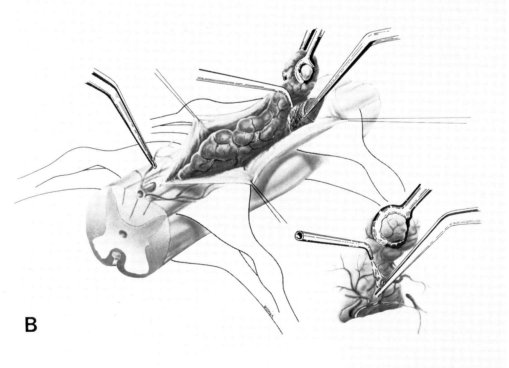

Fig. 90-2.   **A.** Drawing of a myelotomy over an intramedullary tumor. **B.** Drawing showing removal of an intramedullary tumor. **C.** Drawing of the open cord after the removal of
an intramedullary tumor.

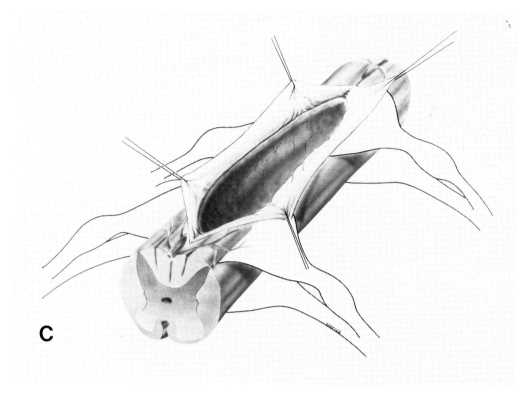

C

Fig. 90-2 (cont'd.)

tion of the cord in the region of the tumor usually is seen, while a complete block is not generally present (Fig. 90-3A and 90-4A). If a block is present, dye should also be instilled from the opposite end of the spinal canal to define the complete extent of the tumor. Since the introduction of water-soluble contrast agents, radiologic definition has been significantly improved. Dilated venous channels at the caudal aspect of small intramedullary tumors may suggest the differential diagnosis of a vascular malformation. This differential is rarely a problem, and spinal angiography has not been of diagnostic value except for the identification of an intramedullary hemangioblastoma. The differential diagnosis between syringomyelia and intramedullary tumor sometimes presents a perplexing problem and air myelography has been useful in distinguishing these two conditions. In the case of syringomyelia, a "collapsing cord" sign may be demonstrated, whereas in intramedullary neoplasms the cord width will remain uniform regardless of the patient's position (Fig. 90-1).

Routine computed tomographic (CT) scanning of the spinal canal has not been of practical use in the diagnosis of these neoplasms. We have retrospectively scanned a number of patients with large tumors, failing to visualize the tumors. CT scanning of the spinal canal with water-soluble contrast agents promises to assist in the definitive diagnosis of syringomyelia. CT scanning has shown metrizamide leaking into the fluid within a syrinx.[10]

Percutaneous cord puncture and myelocystography have been reported,[11] and were performed once in our series. Our patient had a percutaneous puncture to distinguish a cord tumor from a syrinx rather than for relief of symptoms.

Surgical Pathology

Intramedullary spinal cord tumors account for one-third of primary intraspinal neoplasms.[2,6,8,12] Astrocytomas and ependymomas comprise the largest group of intramedullary tu-

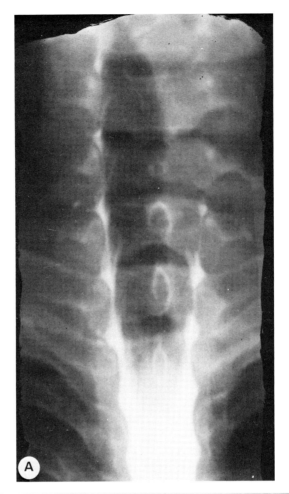

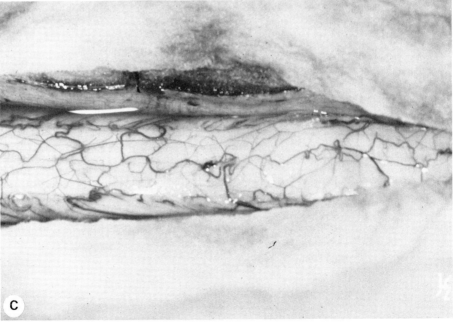

Fig. 90-3. **A.** AP view of cervical myelogram showing widened spinal cord (Case 1). **B.** Lateral view of cervical myelogram showing widened spinal cord (Case 1). **C.** Operative

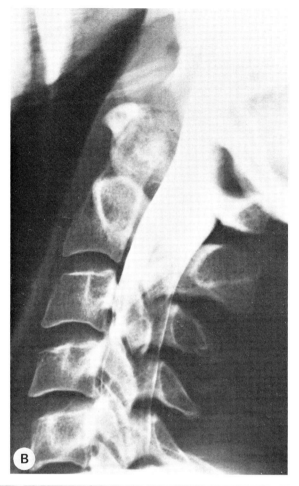

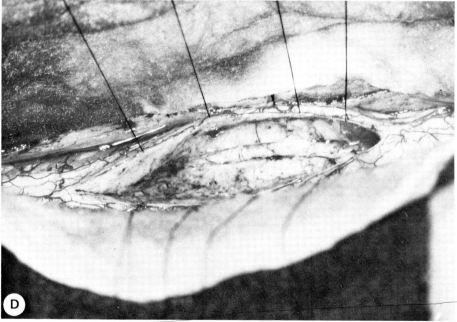

view of exposed spinal cord C2-T2. Note widened full appearance (Case 1). **D.** Operative view of spinal cord after cystic ependymoma was removed (Case 1).

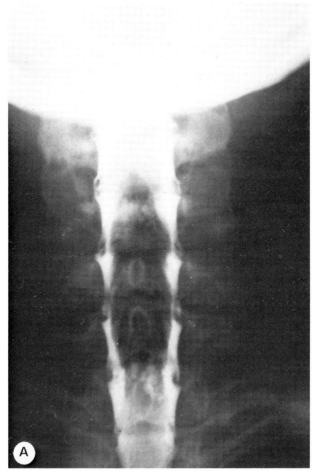

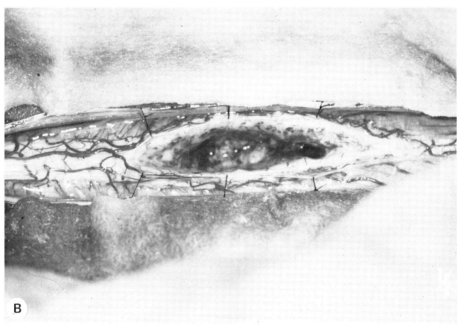

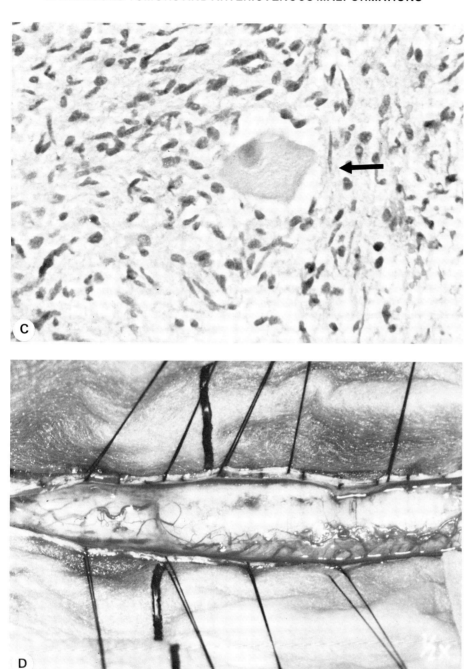

Fig. 90-4. **A.** AP view of cervical myelogram showing widened spinal cord (Case 2). **B.** Operative view of exposed spinal cord during first operation (Case 2). **C.** Microscopic picture of tissue removed during first operation (Case 2). Pathology was mixed ependymoma-astrocytoma grade II. Note invasion with the tumor surrounding a neuron. **D.** Operative view of exposed spinal cord during second operation (Case 2). Note extreme fullness of the spinal cord. **E.** Microscopic picture of tissue removed during second operation (Case 2). Pathology was glioblastoma. Note giant cell. **F.** Pathologic specimen, postmortem (Case 2). Note metastatic nodules along the floor of the fourth ventricle.

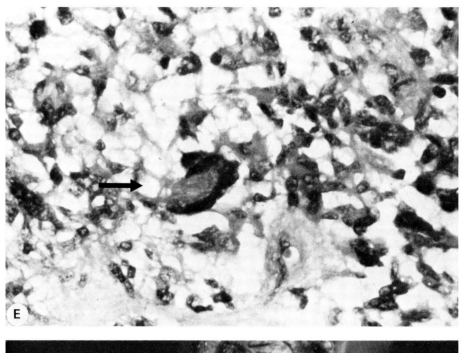

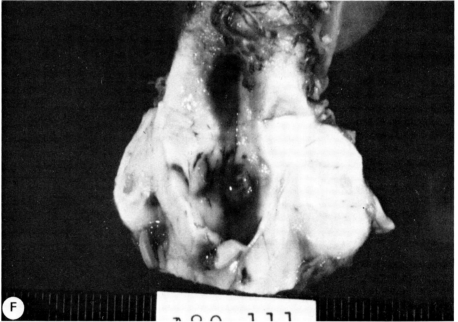

mors and occur with about equal frequency. They are generally low grade and extend over many segments of the spinal cord. Astrocytomas most commonly appear in the cervical and thoracic regions of the spinal cord, whereas the ependymomas have a higher incidence in the caudal regions because of their prevalence in the conus medullaris and filum terminale.

Tumors that occur less frequently include dermoids, epidermoids, teratomas, oligodendrogliomas, hemangioblastomas, and either primary or metastatic malignant tumors. Lipomas, common in children, have different growth patterns and therapeutic implications and will not be discussed further.

Intramedullary ependymomas often have a distinct plane between the neoplasm and spinal cord tissue. These tumors generally are soft, solid, and have a pseudocapsule. They are not highly vascular and may have necrotic areas. Astrocytomas usually are infiltrative with an ill-defined margin between the neoplasm and the normal spinal cord tissue. Where a well-defined margin between the neoplasm and the normal spinal cord exists, a pseudocapsule is found. This variety is similar to the cerebellar astrocytoma, which has a uniformly soft consistency and minimal vascularity sometimes associated with cysts containing yellow fluid high in protein.

At times, astrocytomas may appear to have a plane between the tumor and the normal cord tissue, yet pathologically they demonstrate infiltration (Fig. 90-4C). The pathologic grade may also vary in different parts of the tumor, just as it does within brain tumors. Astrocytomas and ependymomas produce a fusiform enlargement of the spinal cord, often without any indication of their presence on the surface of the cord other than an occasional dilated vein at the caudal end of the tumor. In some cases the dorsal surface of the cord will be so thin that it will be transparent. Glioblastomas produce a discoloration of the cord and are associated with a plethora of enlarged arterialized veins and obvious feeding arteries. Ependymomas of the conus or filum terminale region often grow in an exophytic fashion from the intramedullary locus into the cauda equina, displacing and sometimes adhering to the nerve roots. Because of the expanding nature of these neoplasms, structural changes in the osseous spinal canal may be produced.

Teratomas and dermoid tumors have varying amounts of grumous material in their central portions, are frequently variegated, and have a capsule that is adherent to the surrounding spinal cord tissue; often there is a pedicle of fibrous tract involving the dura and overlying bone and soft tissues. Radiographic defects may be present in the overlying bone if a fibrous tract is present.

Intramedullary tumors receive their blood supply from perforating branches of the anterior spinal artery that enter the ventral aspect of the tumor. These vessels are small and are not associated with a high degree of vascularity within the tumor. Small vessels also enter the tumor from the dorsal and lateral positions of the spinal cord. The tumors tend to be eccentric and located in the more dorsal portion of the spinal cord. Invariably there is a thin layer of compressed spinal cord tissue overlying the dorsal surface of these tumors, and they rarely present directly on the surface of the cord.

Surgical Technique

Turnbull[1] stated: "A surgeon exploring a spinal cord for a suspected intramedullary tumor must be prepared to face a formidable problem and also have the courage of conviction to make every attempt to remove the tumor. Anything less than this, with a cursory inspection of the spinal cord or aspiration thereof, can only create problems of a more complex nature for the subsequent surgical effort to remove such tumors."

The prone position is generally used now for all intramedullary cord tumors, although early in our experience the sitting position was used for some cervical cord cases. The prone position is preferred now because it decreases the potential for vasomotor collapse, which can be significant when the autonomic pathways are compromised by the tumor or surgery; it also allows the assistant to take a more active role in the operation, providing traction, irrigation, or assistance with the dissection.

The full extent of the tumor must be known before the surgery. This usually is demonstrated on a myelogram, often taken from above as well as from below. In the case of a suspected hemangioblastoma, the vasculature should be demonstrated by arteriography to aid in the surgical removal. A wide laminectomy then is performed over the entire extent of the tumor, extending to a level above and below. The dura must be opened carefully since the pia-arachnoid of the enlarged spinal cord often adheres to the underside of the dura. It is important to prevent any injury to the cord vasculature since hemorrhage during this phase of the operation will obscure all landmarks and significantly compromise the surgical effort. In the event of previous surgery, particularly if the dura has been left open, this early dissection is tedious, but care must be taken to re-establish all anatomic landmarks. In those cases, both with and without previous surgery, the initial appearance of the cords generally was similar; the cords appeared widened, often without evidence of tumor on the surface. The widening of the spinal cord and the presence of dilated veins at the caudal end of the tumor site were indications of the underlying pathology. When observing a widened spinal cord, the surgeon must not be misled in those rare instances of anterior extramedullary lesion, in which the cord is splayed out over the lesion.[13]

The dorsal surface of the cord at the area of greatest enlargement then is inspected for the site of the myelotomy. Generally, myelotomies are performed in the midline with a preference for the thinnest and most avascular areas; at times, however, it is more expeditious to use a paramedian approach (Fig. 90-2A).

Some of the vasculature will be sacrificed during this myelotomy. An initial incision of approximately 1–2 cm is performed over the greatest enlargement of the spinal cord to evaluate the plane between the tumor and the spinal cord tissue. In some instances the presence of a cyst associated with the tumor may be easily noted; if so, additional room may be gained by aspirating some of the cystic contents through a small-bore needle. To facilitate dissection, however, these cysts should not be completely evacuated. Once it is determined that the neoplasm is cystic or has well-defined planes, the myelotomy is lengthened over the extent of the tumor. With teratomas, a stalk between the cord and the dura should be removed as an integral part of the lesion. With ependymomas extending from the conus, the extra-axial portion in the cauda equina may be removed first, providing adequate decompression and visualization of the residual tumor involving the intramedullary portion of the conus. The draining veins of intramedullary hemangioblastomas must be left to the latter part of the surgical resection.

Following the myelotomy, 6-0 or 7-0 traction sutures are placed through the pial margins on either side to expose the interior of the spinal cord (Fig. 90-2B). Generally, the tumor is visible a few millimeters under the dorsal surface of the spinal cord. There is often a soft gliotic interface between the tumor and the spinal cord proper. With the operating microscope and microsurgical techniques, using bipolar cautery, small suction tubes, and various dissectors, a plane is developed around the margin of the tumor, taking care to retract primarily on the tumor and not on the spinal cord. The surgeon works to one or the other end of the tumor. At the pole where the tumor is the narrowest, it may be possible to grasp the end and gently extract it from the interior of the cord. All the fine vascular adhesions to the spinal cord, especially on the ventral aspect of the tumor, should be cauterized with bipolar cautery and sharply divided. No blunt dissection should be carried out in areas where vascular channels connect the tumor to the spinal cord. Most tumors are amazingly avascular and present no threat of hemorrhage or the loss of control of large blood vessels. It is important to keep the operative field meticulously dry so that the plane between the tumor and the spinal cord may be readily identified (Fig. 90-2B). If the tumor is too large to remove in toto or necessitates too much retraction on the spinal cord, its interior may be decompressed. Cystic collections at the margins of the tumor, as in the case of astrocytomas, facilitate the tumor resection. We make no attempt, however, to remove the wall of the cyst, which is thin and nonneoplastic. If there is any doubt about the totality of removal, small biopsies may be obtained from the margin of the resection and evaluated by frozen section during surgery. In most instances, the margins are well defined and there is no question about the removal of the tumor (Fig. 90-2C).

In cases in which the tumor has been treated with radiation previously, we have noted intense intramedullary gliosis by biopsy, distinctly separate from the margin of the tumor, usually at the caudal or rostral interface. It is assumed that this is an adverse effect of preoperative radiation. Previous surgery with aspiration of a cyst but without definitive removal of the intramedullary tumor has provided transient benefits and reaccumulation of the cyst fluid.

In teratomas, the border of the tumor, although well defined, may be densely adherent to the surrounding spinal cord. Every attempt should be made to remove this capsule, which is a potential source of regrowth. There may be extensive involvement of central areas of the spinal cord and the tumors may extend from the posterior to the anterior surface. Teratomatous tumors also may have a dumbbell configuration within the substance of the spinal cord, and the surgeon must be wary not to miss satellite portions of the primary tumor.

When the margins of the cord are allowed to fall back into position, the remarkable decompressive effect of tumor removal is quite apparent. The dorsal columns are often thin to the point of being transparent. If there has been minimal retraction on the cord, these fiber tracts function in a satisfactory way and will show progressive functional recovery. Rarely has the function of the spinal cord been made permanently worse by this dissection. Thus far we have not routinely used evoked-potential monitoring during surgery, but this may hold promise for the future.[14] Gentleness of dissection may be gauged by the vascular pattern on the dorsal surface of the cord at the completion of tumor resection. Distended veins that were present before removal, usually at the caudal end of the tumor on the surface of the spinal cord, will not be less prominent. No attempt has been made to sew the pial surfaces of the spinal cord together. The dura is closed in a watertight fashion; it is rarely necessary to use a fascial graft other than in those cases in which the dura was left open after previous surgery. If total removal of an intramedullary tumor is not feasible, the dura should be reconstructed, preferably with a fascial graft, so that subsequent surgical endeavors may be facilitated.

The single most important factor determining the ease of the operation is the presence and nature of previous operations. In patients who have had previous surgery and in whom the dura mater was left open, the initial exposure of the tumor and the dissection of adjacent tissues from the spinal cord has prolonged the operating and made exposure more difficult. In those cases in which radiation was administered previously, gliotic areas in the dorsocentral portion of the spinal cord have been verified by biopsy. There have been no histologic changes in the tumor that were attributed to radiation. Similarly, none of the tumors that were previously irradiated showed malignant changes. Problems with wound healing also were encountered frequently in those cases in which radiotherapy was used previously.

Postoperative Treatment

Steroids are routinely used pre- and postoperatively in high doses (Dexamethasone 10-20 mg IV q4h) with a slow taper dependent upon the neurologic condition. Prophylactic antibiotics are used intraoperatively and for 48 hours postoperatively. If the surgery involved extensive areas of the cervical region, the endotracheal tube is left in place for at least 24 hours, regardless of the patient's condition at the termination of surgery.

Radiation therapy is considered postoperatively for children with astrocytomas, but we generally wait with adults and consider re-operation if recurrence should occur.

Careful orthopedic follow-up and possible bracing are necessary for the pediatric patients.

Results

Removal of large intramedullary tumors can be performed with a fair degree of safety (Table 90-2) and can offer significant neurologic improvement in many situations. Generally, those patients with only mild to moderate neurologic deficit before surgery did extremely well, regardless of the size of the tumor (Table 90-1). The total removal of these tumors offers a much im-

Table 90-2. Intramedullary Spinal Cord Tumors

Author	Cases	Total Removal	Mortality
Elsberg[2] 1925	13	3	15%
Greenwood[5] 1963	10	10	0%
Guidetti[6] 1967	71	24	10%
Stein 1980	25	17	0%

proved outlook for patients who have not responded to previous decompressive laminectomy and radiotherapy. Our follow-up in the astrocytoma and ependymoma group has been too short to draw definite conclusions regarding a recurrence rate, although several patients are now 5 years or more postoperative without evidence of recurrence. Experience would indicate that the recurrence rate should be low following total removal.[2,5,7,8,15,16]

Case 1. A 35-year-old woman was asymptomatic until 6 months before admission when she developed sharp pains radiating around the right breast, as well as progressive numbness in a suspended pattern over the right side from the nipple line to the umbilicus level. Subsequently, she developed numbness in the right V2 distribution as well as around the shoulders. Minimal weakness was present in the upper arms.

Examination showed hypalgesia in the right V1 and V2 distribution. Strength was uniformly good except for minimal weakness of the left biceps muscles. Sensory examination showed a marked suspended sensory level loss from T1 to T8 with a lesser loss extending up to C2. Posterior column function was good. Reflexes were decreased in the left biceps, while slightly increased in the lower extremities. Babinski signs were absent.

Myelography was performed, which demonstrated a widened cord extending from T2 to C2 (Fig. 90-3A). Subsequently, a laminectomy from C2 through T2 was performed with myelotomy and total removal of a cystic ependymoma (Fig. 90-3B and C). Follow-up examination at 1½ years postoperatively showed the patient to be functioning extremely well at home. She noted some numbness under the right breast and tingling in her left fingers. Examination showed full muscle power with a decreased left biceps and triceps reflex. Joint position sense and vibratory sensation were decreased in the lower extremities but normal in the uppers.

Until recently we had not seen a recurrence in our series of low-grade astrocytomas and ependymomas. The following case, however, shows the potential for recurrence in some of the more aggressive tumors.

Case 2. A 20-year-old right-handed female college student presented with sudden onset of right hand weakness 1½ years before admission. The weakness lasted 30 minutes and was not associated with sensory phenomenon. Two similar episodes occurred 6 months and 3 months before admission. Two months before admission, progressive weakness of the right upper extremity developed with hand function far worse than arm strength. Sensory complaints were absent.

On examination, marked weakness and atrophy were noted in the right hand with moderate weakness in the forearm and upper arm. The left upper extremity and lower extremities were normal. Sensory loss to pin was noted only in the left lower extremity. Reflexes were normal without Babinksi's signs.

Pantopaque and gas myelography demonstrated a widening of the spinal cord between C5 and C7 without collapse during position change (Fig. 90-4).

A cervical laminectomy was performed and a well-demarcated tumor was excised (Fig. 90-4B). The tumor was a mixed astro-ependymoma, grades II–III with tumor surrounding anterior horn cells (Fig. 90-4C). It was thought that a total removal had been achieved. Postoperatively, strength was little changed, but sensory examination showed a moderate decrease in proprioception and vibratory sense of the right and mild hypalgesia to T1 bilaterally.

Intense physical therapy was given with marked improvement, so that she was able to return to work and function completely independently. Two and one-half months later, however, she returned with pain in her scapular regions and further hand weakness bilaterally. Sensory examination was slightly improved. Steroids were reinstituted.

Four months following surgery she had marked increase in neck pain and sudden quadraplegia. With the anticipation of finding either a cyst or a hemorrhage, re-operation was carried out; a highly malignant glioma, which was nonresectable, was encountered (Fig. 90-4D). Pathologically, the lesion was markedly different with multiple mitoses. Biopsy and duroplasty were performed (Fig. 90-4E). Postoperatively, she showed steady decline with intractable nausea until her eventual death 2 months later. Before her death cerebrospinal fluid cytology was positive and radiation therapy was given without palliation. Postmortem study showed an extensive tumor with seeding in the spinal and craniosubarachnoid spaces (Fig. 90-4F).

Radicular pain in the distribution of the nerve roots associated with the tumor has been a distressing postoperative problem. This pain has a burning quality, severely disturbing to the patient and extremely difficult to control. Derangement of the physiologic pathways for pain at the dorsal route entry zone has been postulated as the cause. Unfortunately, we have not had satisfactory results in the treatment of these postoperative dysesthetic or pain syndromes.

Our experience[4,17] and that of others[5,6] indicate that a decompressive laminectomy, whether or not a tumor cyst has been evacuated, with or without radiotherapy, has had little beneficial effect on the course of most intramedullary spinal cord tumors. Some reviews[6,8,12,18] of the effects of radiation on these tumors are clouded by incomplete knowledge of the pathology, the natural course of these tumors, and the number of associated variables, including decompression and partial surgical removals. Publications by Guidetti,[6] Woltman et al.,[12] and Woods and Pimenta[8] suggest that even with partial removal, long-term survival with static neurologic deficit may be expected. Radiation has apparently yielded beneficial effects,[18] but this report has a high percentage of histologically unverified tumors.

One report by Schwade et al.[19] retrospectively reviewed 34 patients, 25 of whom had confirmed histology. They recommended conservative surgery to remove as much tumor as safely possible. Postoperative radiation therapy was given to 4500–5000 rads in 5 to 6 weeks, through portals that cover the tumor generously. Twelve of 12 patients with ependymomas were alive without recurrence with a minimum follow-up of 3 years. Five of 6 patients with low-grade astrocytomas survived longer than 3 years. Although encouraging, longer follow-up may be needed to evaluate this fully. In most reports there has been little objective follow-up of reduction in tumor size following radiation therapy. A significant number of reports indicate that surgical removal is the treatment of choice.[3–6,8,9] Improvement in the patient's condition or at least an arrest of the neurologic deterioration may be anticipated in most cases following surgery. Postoperative result is determined by the degree of preoperative neurologic involvement. Many surgeons have reported difficulty in totally removing astrocytomas. In our series we were able to totally remove 4 of 8 astrocytomas with no more significant problems than those encountered in the removal of ependymomas. In 2 other cases, near-total removals were performed with a definitive plane observed around most of the tumor.

Through the use of microsurgical techniques and strict attention to postoperative pulmonary function, negligible mortality and morbidity rates can be expected, even with removal of extensive tumors in the cervical region. Similar experiences have been reported by Greenwood.[5] Guidetti[6] supports radical removal of these tumors, except where ill-defined planes do not permit this to be accomplished. In such cases he feels that subtotal resection produces no better result than biopsy. In those cases of astrocytoma in which only a biopsy was performed and presumably postoperative radiation given, the average survival rate was 5 years. Guidetti suggests that when attempts with microsurgical techniques are made, a significant number of the astrocytomas may be totally removed.

We have not used postoperative radiation for intramedullary tumors that have been totally removed and do not advocate postoperative radiation for benign intramedullary tumors that have been incompletely removed, except occasionally in children. The patient's course should be monitored closely, facilitated by the use of water-soluble contrast agents and CT scanning. A second surgical attempt should be made to remove the tumor at the time of recurrence. Following this, radiation may be considered. Experience with a significant number of cases demonstrates that recurrence should not be a problem. Greenwood's series[5] was comprised almost exclusively of ependymomas, and his long-term survivals, as well as those of Guidetti[6] and others,[7,8,12] have been gratifying.

Spinal Cord Arteriovenous Malformations (AVMs)

AVMs of the spinal cord are relatively rare, being only one-tenth as common as cerebral AVMs and one-tenth as common as primary spinal neoplasms. They appear more commonly in males (4:1) and generally occur in an older age group than those of the brain. Eighty percent occur in the thoracolumbar spinal cord, although they may involve the entire cord from cervical to sacral levels.[20,21]

Anatomy

There are two arterial systems of the spinal cord: an anterior one and a posterior one. These are supplied by the anterior and posterior radiculomedullary arteries, respectively. The anterior spinal artery usually is a well-defined single artery running in the anterior-median fissure and supplying approximately the anterior two-thirds of the spinal cord.[22] The posterior arteries while paired on either side of the midline are variable and often are represented by numerous interlacing smaller arteries. They supply the posterior one-third of the cord.[22] The largest and most important radicular artery supplying the cord is the artery of Adamkiewiez (great anterior medullary artery), which arises most frequently in the left side between T8 and L4.[23] After entering the spinal canal, it ascends and makes a hairpin turn with its largest branch directed caudally and a smaller branch cephalad. It anastomoses caudally with the artery accompanying the first sacral root. The posterior arteries have rich anastomoses with the anterior ones around the circumference of the cord.[22,24,25]

The artery of Adamkiewiez often contributes to spinal AVMs, as it supplies the most commonly involved area of the spinal cord. The intercostal arteries, the dorsal segmental arteries, and the lumbosacral radicular arteries also may contribute blood supply to the AVM. In the cervical region, the vertebral arteries and the costocervical or thyrocervical trunks of the subclavian artery may also supply the AVM. The majority of these AVMs are supplied by the dorsal radicular arteries, as the AVMs tend to be dorsal. In some instances, however, the anterior spinal artery sends perforating branches to supply portions of the AVM in the central or dorsal portion of the cord. The feeding arteries often are limited to a few radicular arteries, but on occasion there may be multiple small twigs at numerous levels shunting into an extensive venous draining system. These lesions primarily involve the pial surface of the cord rather than the parenchyma, but at times a portion of the malformation or a venous aneurysm may extend into the center of the spinal cord. Because of the dorsal pial position, their surgical removal is often feasible.

In the past, such terms as "cavernous" and "racemous" angiomas, both arterial and venous, were often used descriptively[26,27]; with the advent of spinal angiography, however, and the operating microscopic exposure, a more practical scheme has been developed.[28-30]

The majority of these lesions represent arteriovenous communications of varying extent and degree. The communication between arteries and veins develops primarily between the dorsal radicular arteries and the dorsolateral veins of the spinal cord. The classification of Ommaya is useful in the surgical evaluation of these lesions.[29] His type 1, the most common, represents an extensive single-coiled vessel with one or two arterial feeders entering at various levels. The flow is slow and the blood supply appears distinct from that of the cord. Type 2 is a more discrete glomus type of lesion, again an arteriovenous communication, in which a small discrete coil of arteries connects to the venous system. The flow is slow. Type 3, the so-called juvenile type, most commonly seen in children, is a more diffuse, comprehensive arteriovenous lesion of the cord, which often encircles it in a cuirass configuration (Fig. 90-5). Flow is rapid and the blood supply of the AVM and the cord may be closely related. Doppman[31] emphasizes the "nidus" concept in regard to some of these lesions. In these cases, angiography will demonstrate discrete arteriovenous communications with limited involvement of the rostrocaudal extent of the spinal cord. A detailed picture of the vascular anatomy is therefore essential when one is considering the extent of laminectomy and whether or not a lesion can be totally removed. Ventral lesions are most difficult to treat surgically.

The lesions that do not have arteriovenous communications and that represent pure venous

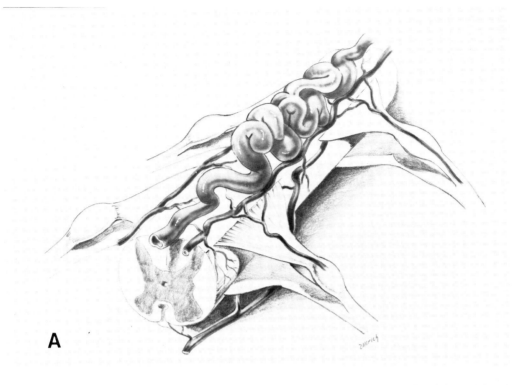

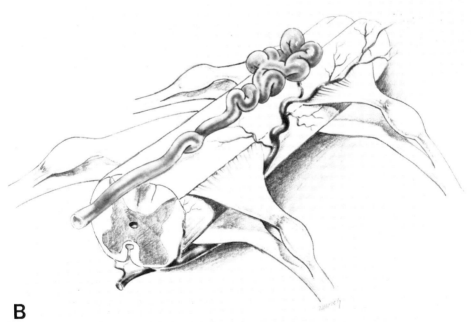

Fig. 90-5.   AVMs of the spinal cord. **A.** Abnormal arterialized tortuous veins cover the dorsal aspect of the cord (lighter and larger vessels). These are fed by numerous arterial branches at multiple levels (smaller and darker vessels). **B.** A nidus with a feeding artery (dark vessel) and a localized tangle of abnormal draining veins (lighter and larger vessels). **C.** This AVM lies both within and on the surface of the spinal cord. It consists of large cavernous channels and multiple arteriovenous shunts. (Reproduced with permission of Baker HL Jr, Love JG, Layton DD Jr: Angiographic and surgical aspects of spinal cord vascular anomalies. *Radiology 88*:1078–1085, 1967.)

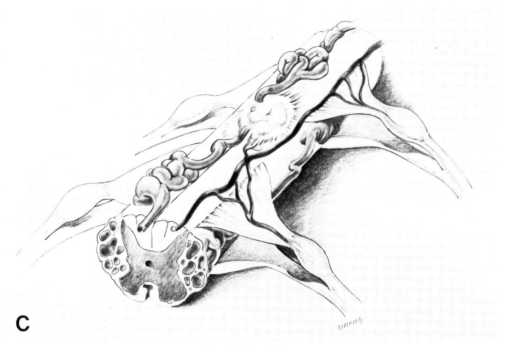

C

Fig. 90-5 (cont'd.)

or arterial abnormalities are exceedingly rare and have not been demonstrated by arteriography. The concept that such lesions exist is primarily based on data from autopsy specimens. Whether this concept has any validity in the present-day evaluation of these lesions is open to question.

Clinical Presentation and Natural History

Spinal AVMs tend to occur in males (2–4:1, male: female) in the 30 to 70-year age group, primarily at the thoracolumbar levels.[20] Frequently, AVM is not suspected and a diagnosis of tumor or disc disease is made. In the planning of therapy, which may involve procedures of considerable risk, the natural history of these lesions must be considered. Aminoff and Logue,[32,33] in an extensive review of 60 cases, reported that the vast majority had an insidious onset with progressive deterioration, while 50 percent of the patients were severely disabled within 3 years of the onset of the disorder. Only 20 percent of the cases had an acute onset, and subsequently many of these had progression of symptoms. Subarachnoid hemorrhage occurred at one time or another in 10 percent of the cases, but was a presenting symptom in only 5 percent. Herdt et al.[34] found that only 6 percent of the patients had definite proof of subarachnoid hemorrhage. Tobin and Layton,[20] reviewing the Mayo Clinic experience with 71 patients, found a slowly progressive course in 73 percent and an abrupt onset with subarachnoid hemorrhage in 10 percent. The symptom complex of leg weakness, sensory loss, pain, and early sphincteric involvement was the most common presentation. The prognosis once the lesion becomes symptomatic generally is poor and is represented by a progressive and disabling disease. In a small number of cases the threat of instantaneous neurologic disaster is present. In such instances the onset may be devastating with all of the manifestations that go with a ruptured intracranial aneurysm. The following history of a 36-year-old female typifies the sudden but unusual nature of the symptoms related to these malformations.

Case 3. The patient had a vague past history of low back and right leg pain with dysuria. No cause for these symptoms had been elicited. On June 7, 1975, while parking her car, she had the sudden onset of severe occipital pain—"as though someone had stuck me from behind." She became confused and semi-comatose. Evaluation at that time showed massive subhyaloid hemorrhages in both eyes and a confused disoriented patient with severe meningismus. Sensory examination suggested a T3 level to pain sense. A myelogram in the face of grossly bloody spinal fluid suggested a block at the upper thoracic level. Laminectomy at that level showed only subdural and subarachnoid blood.

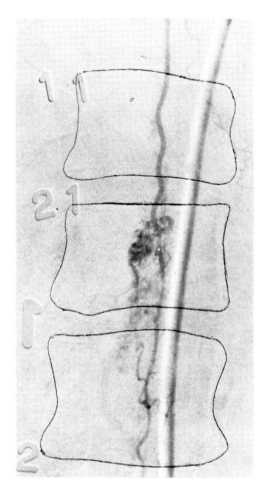

Fig. 90-6. Anteroposterior spinal cord arteriograms with subtraction technique. The nidus of the AVM is seen at the small arrows. The feeding artery is present at the open arrow (Case 3). (Reproduced with permission of Kasdon DL, Wolpert SM, Stein BM: Surgical and angiographic localization of spinal arteriovenous malformations. *Surg Neurol* 5:279–283, 1976.)

She was admitted to the New England Medical Center on June 13, 1975, and because the history seemed so typical of the rupture of a cerebral aneurysm and because of the lack of focal neurologic findings at this point, four-vessel arteri-columbar spinal cord (Fig. 90-6). On July 23, 1975, the lesion was totally resected. The patient made a good neurologic recovery except for slow resolution of blindness in the right eye secondary to the subhyaloid hemorrhage. She has subsequently returned to full employment.

The catastrophic onset of symptoms related to this malformation was quite typical of those of a ruptured cerebral aneurysm. The myelogram done in the face of significant subarachnoid hemorrhage was misleading. It was only after an exhaustive evaluation of the cerebral vascular system had proved negative that spinal angiography uncovered the true nature of this woman's problem.

Subarachnoid hemorrhage with the sudden onset of neurologic symptomatology is unusual, however, except in patients under 30 years of age.[35] An insidious progressive course is most common; it is accentuated by pain of radicular origin, depending upon the location of the lesion. The location of the pain, however, is often not a reliable indication of the levels of involvement.[20] Progressive upper or lower motor neuron involvement is the rule, with spasticity or absent reflexes, depending upon location. Involvement of the dorsal columns with paresthesias, loss of position, and other sensory modalities is also part of the progressive picture.

These lesions appear to produce symptoms because of ischemic changes in the spinal cord secondary to a vascular steal and the mass effect of the lesion.[30,36] On occasion, the arterialized veins that compose these malformations are layered four to five deep on the surface of the spinal cord (Fig. 90-7). When the lesions are removed, grooves from the dilated vascular channels can be noted on the surface of the spinal cord.

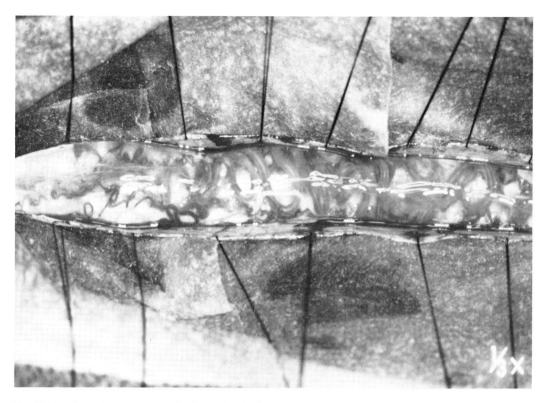

Fig. 90-7. Operative exposure of a large AVM of the spinal cord composed principally of tortuous, distended, arterialized veins.

Diagnosis

On examination, two signs are helpful if present. A bruit over the spine is virtually diagnostic[37] and the presence of a cutaneous angioma helps diagnostically and also in localizing the level of the lesion.[38] Plain x-rays of the spine generally are noncontributory, while tomography may show occasional changes (Fig. 90-8). Cerebrospinal fluid evaluation shows some abnormality in 75 percent with protein elevation and pleocytosis being most common.[20,39]

Myelography is often diagnostic of the lesion but does not define its nuances. In one series,[32,33] 90 percent of the myelograms that were done in the supine position with a generous amount of dye were abnormal. From 12 to 30 cc of Pantopaque should be used; if a block is present, a dehydrating agent may be given to relieve it. Because of the dorsal location of most lesions, supine myelography is more definitive. The presence of a septum posticum connecting the dorsal aspect of the cord to the dura may result in confusing defects, however, mimicking a small AVM. False positives include spinal cord tumors with seeding throughout the spinal axis or metastases from malignant tumors elsewhere, as well as redundant nerve roots (Fig. 90-9), and arachnoiditis.

The introduction of a less dense contrast medium, such as the water-soluble compounds, may increase the accuracy of diagnosis and better define these lesions.

For one to thoroughly evaluate these lesions, spinal angiography with selective injection of the relevant arteries and a serial study with subtraction technique are important. In the cervical region, selective injection of the subclavian branches, including the vertebral, thyrocervical, and costocervical trunks, should be done. Spinal angiography must be comprehensive. If there is no myelographic clue to the location of the AVM, the procedure is extremely laborious and tedious.

Unfortunately, a lesion must represent a significant arteriovenous shunt or arteriography may be unsuccessful in the demonstration of all of the ramifications of the lesion. Opacification

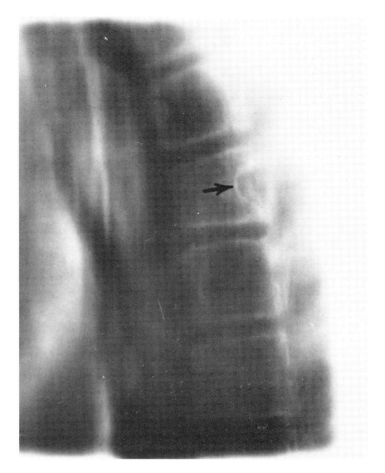

Fig. 90-8. Lateral tomogram of midthoracic spine demonstrating erosion (arrow) of the posterior vertebral body caused by an arteriovenous malformation (Case 4). (Reproduced with permission of Post KD, Levitsky S, Doppman JL, et al: Transthoracic ligation of intercostal arteries of arteriovenous malformations of the spinal cord. *Ann Surg 173*:152–156, 1971.)

of the posterior spinal arteries is rare, while the thoracic anterior spinal artery is small and often hard to visualize under normal circumstances.

A flush of the aorta may show a flash filling of the lesion but is contraindicated because of spinal cord toxicity. Selective arteriography must be done at individual levels to demonstrate these malformations properly. In some instances, arteriography may fail to define the arterial contribution to an extensive malformation of dilated arterialized veins extending over multiple segments of the spinal cord. In other instances, where a nidus exists, it may be difficult to tell from angiography whether the lesion is intra- or extramedullary in location.[40]

The variability of the position of the spinal cord in the anterior-posterior plane within the spinal canal plays a major role in the difficulty of precise localization. Displacement of the spinal cord by thrombosed portions of malformations, which are not visualized with contrast material, is an additional source of error in localization by spinal angiography. CT scanning of the spine with intravenous contrast enhancement may hold some promise for screening and follow-up of patients with spinal AVMs. The axial-transverse view of the lesion may permit a better appraisal of the anatomic relationships of the extrathecal extension of the malformation.[41] Because the prognosis is poor for patients with spinal arteriovenous malformations that are untreated or

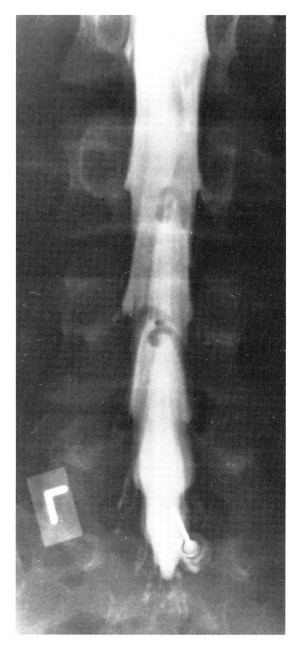

Fig. 90-9. Lumbar thoracic myelogram demonstrating tortuous shadows suggestive of abnormal vascular channels but representing redundant nerve roots (arrows). (Reproduced with permission of Stein BM: Arteriovenous malformations of the brain and spinal cord, in *Practice of Surgery,* Hagerstown, Md., Harper & Row, 1979.)

simply decompressed, we feel that surgical exploration to assess resectability is important. This should be carried out in spite of an angiographic appearance suggesting a largely intramedullary localization of the malformation.

Treatment

The only completely satisfactory treatment for spinal AVMs is total obliteration or excision. Thus far, the usefulness of embolization has been limited.

Embolization.   Various techniques have been used, including silicone emboli that are placed via catheter into the feeding arteries.[42,43] This technique is limited because of the small size of the feeding arteries and the fact that these arteries, which are proximal to the lesion, may be significant contributors to the normal spinal cord circulation. Furthermore, in lesions with comparatively low blood flow there is an additional hazard of inadvertent embolization of normal vessels. Of more promise is the technique in which polymerizing agents or "glues" are placed directly into the malformation.[44] Where the arterial supply enters a nidus, this may be done with fine, flow-directed catheters and specialized materials. Because of the limited arterial supply to these lesions, such a technique affords the hope that the lesion may be totally obliterated.

Surgical excision. The cornerstone of treatment for spinal AVMs is microsurgical obliteration.[28-30,35,40,45] The lesions lend themselves to surgery since the vast majority lie on the dorsal surface of the spinal cord and are thereby accessible (Figs. 90-7 and 90-13). They also represent low flow and low pressure systems in which there is a limited arterial contribution with a significant venous component that is readily visualized on the surface of the spinal cord. Uncommonly, the lesion invades portions of the spinal cord. Even in such instances the AVM occasionally may be removed microsurgically with satisfactory results.

Doppman[31] has emphasized that only the nidus of the AVM, as demonstrated by arteriography, must be excised. The venous channels need not be removed. Since angiography may not demonstrate all the feeding arteries, however, excision of the "apparent nidus" alone may not be sufficient and the veins may remain arterialized. In this situation, the abnormal venous channels should also be excised to the point where the shunting is eliminated. This may require a very extensive laminectomy and possibly staging. Selective ligation of feeding arteries without removal of the AVM has been recommended.[29,46,47] This presumes a small, completely defined number of feeding arteries demonstrated by arteriography. This is too often not the case, however, and all feeders are not seen on arteriography. Although not optimal, the results of this treatment have been good, with stabilization of the disease process and occasional improvement. There is rarely an immediate collapse or marked change in the arterialization of the veins of the malformation.

Case 4. A 12-year-old girl was in excellent health until she had a sharp pain in the left side of her chest. This persisted intermittently and 11 days later numbness and weakness in her legs appeared. Within 3 days this progressed to complete paraplegia, paresthesia, and areflexia in the lower extremities with analgesia in the left T7 dermatome. Urinary function remained normal until 1 week later when incontinence appeared. She was admitted to a hospital, where erosion of the dorsal aspect of one thoracic vertebra was found on spinal tomography (Fig. 90-8) and a myelogram demonstrated a serpiginous filling defect in the spinal canal, extending from T3 to T9. A transfemoral midthoracic arteriogram showed a large, rapidly filling intra- and extrathecal arteriovenous malformation extending from T3 to T10 and appearing to extend into the spinal canal and the pleural gutters bilaterally (Fig. 90-10).

Neurologic examination showed normal cranial nerve and upper extremity function. There was no voluntary or involuntary motor activity below the hips; muscle tone was diminished and reflexes were absent. Sensory examination revealed complete loss of fine touch, pin prick, and position sense below L3, and diminished sensation from T7 to L3 bilaterally. Perception of deep pain was present in the right Achilles tendon. No bruit was audible, but there was a hyperpigmented area that darkened with a Valsalva maneuver over the entire thoracodorsal spine. A transfemoral selective arteriogram demonstrated large feeding vessels at T5 and T6 on the right and left. Smaller feeders were seen to arise at T7 and T9.

The lesion was approached via a left thoracotomy with rib resection immediately following arteriography. Several enlarged anomalous and intercostal arteries were found (Fig. 90-11). Two short dilated vessels directed posteriorly were divided as they disappeared into the paravertebral musculature. A total of 10 arteries were ligated and divided between T4 and T10 and stainless steel clips were placed on the distal ends to mark the sites of division.

The postoperative course was marked by steady neurologic improvement. There were no pulmonary complications related to the thoracotomy. Within 24 hours the patient was moving her left leg and within 48 hours this motor recovery extended to her right leg and foot. After 10 days she was able to stand in parallel bars, and in 2 weeks following the operation she was walking with crutches.

The patient was re-evaluated 7 months after surgery and was neurologically intact except for mild hyperreflexia in the left leg. An arteriogram showed only a faint blush at T5 from a medium-sized artery originating at the left subclavian artery. No collateral filling had occurred in the previously ligated vessels.

In preparation for surgery, the patients are positioned so as to prevent any abdominal compression, which would adversely affect the surgery by distending the venous channels. The laminectomy should encompass the extent of the malformation as visualized at spinal arteriography

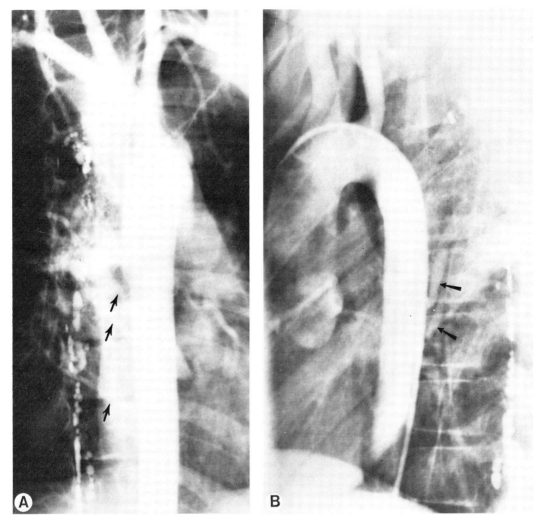

Fig. 90-10. **A.** Preoperative aortogram revealing abnormal vessels adjacent to and overlying the midthoracic spinal cord. Note the enlarged intercostal arteries (arrow) supplying the malformation (Case 4). **B.** Lateral aortogram, early phase, showing enlarged intercostal arteries (arrows) (Case 4). (Reproduced with permission of Post KD, Levitsky S, Doppman JL, et al: Transthoracic ligation of intercostal arteries for arteriovenous malformations of the spinal cord. *Ann Surg* *173*:152–156, 1971.)

or at myelography. It is possible but awkward to extend the laminectomy should there be evidence of residual arterialized veins beyond the area of resection. At this point the operating microscope is brought into use. With a binocular observer tube it is possible for the surgeon and the assistant to stand face to face across the operating table, thereby allowing the assistant to be of most help. The dura should be opened with caution, since adhesions may be present between the malformation and the dura. The benefit of a wide laminectomy will be appreciated as the dura is held open by traction sutures. In cases in which subarachnoid hemorrhage has occurred, it may take many weeks for the fibrin and other blood products from the subarachnoid spaces to clear. The presence of the fibrin and other blood products obscures important landmarks and makes the dissection more difficult. It is critical to keep the operative field dry, as any blood staining of the pia-arachnoidal spaces will obscure the plane of dissection and make meticulous removal of the lesion next to impossible. A bipolar cautery with irrigation is used throughout. Major feeding arteries as defined by arteriography then are sought along the lateral margins of the cord and

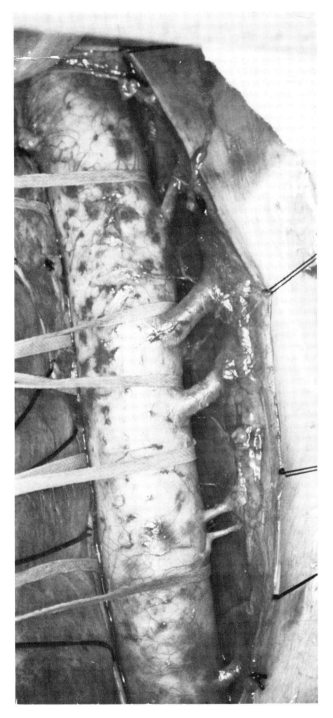

Fig. 90-11. View of the aorta and intercostal and anomalous arteries as viewed through a left thoracotomy with a sixth rib resection (Case 4). (Reproduced with permission of Post KD, Levitsky S, Doppman JL, et al: Transthoracic ligation of intercostal arteries for arteriovenous malformations of the spinal cord. *Ann Surg 173*:152–156, 1971.)

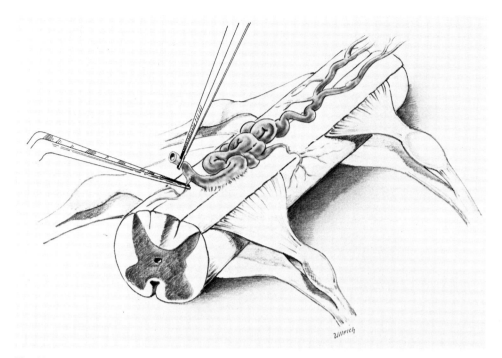

Fig. 90-12. Drawing of the surgical resection of an AVM showing meticulous cautery of the feeding arteries and gradual peeling away of the abnormal venous channels from the surface of the spinal cord. (Reproduced with permission of Stein BM: Arteriovenous malformations of the brain and spinal cord, in *Practice of Surgery,* Hagerstown, Md., Harper & Row, 1979.)

malformation. They are identified by their size, color, and location. The arteries then are coagulated, clipped, and divided. Beginning at one end of the lesion or at the margin of an obvious nidus, the surgeon cauterizes and divides the smaller feeding vessels while the lesion is gradually peeled away from the dorsal surface of the spinal cord (Figs. 90-12 and 90-13). Numerous small vascular or arachnoidal adhesions may exist between the malformation and the spinal cord (Fig. 90-13E). The removal of a significant shunt improves the circulation, however, through the remaining normal medullary arteries and veins. In some instances numerous small arterial feeders accompany the dorsal roots to supply distended and tortuous veins that extend over numerous segments. Because of their tortuosity, these veins may engulf the nerve roots or extend along the lateral margins of the spinal cord. Extensions of the malformation, such as venous aneurysms, may be encountered within the spinal cord. Rarely, a significant but discrete portion of the malformation receives its blood supply from perforating branches of the anterior spinal artery and lies within the cord. With meticulous microdissection, these components may be removed without permanently damaging the spinal cord.

Although not always predictable from the preoperative angiogram, a large portion of the malformation may lie within the spinal cord. In such cases it may be impossible to remove the lesion without incurring major neurologic deficit.

Ommaya et al.[29] have recommended ligation of major feeding arteries in those patients in whom total resection is not feasible. Their follow-up evaluations would indicate a beneficial effect from this operative procedure. Such procedures do not, however, extend to the indiscriminate ligation of the artery of Adamkiewicz, which is a vital source of blood for the normal spinal cord.

We believe that most spinal AVMs should be explored regardless of the angiograms, for although the x-ray studies yield important information, they may be misleading as to operability. Only by direct inspection can operability be truly assessed.

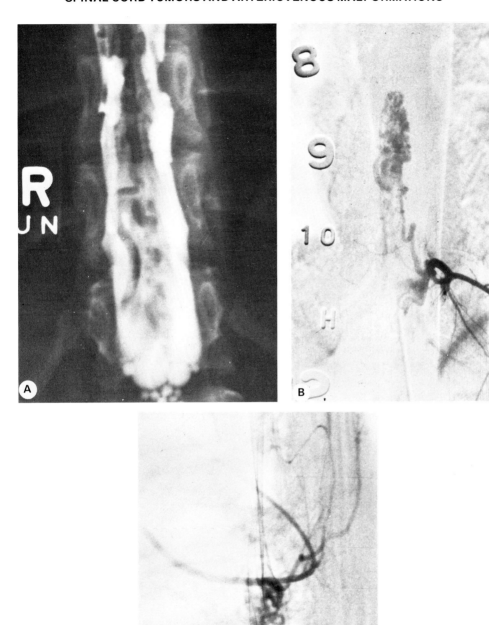

Fig. 90-13. **A.** AP view of low thoracic myelogram demonstrating serpiginous filling defect suggestive of an AVM (Case 5). **B.** AP view of selective spinal arteriogram demonstrating spinal AVM opposite T8-T10 (Case 5). **C.** Later view of selective spinal arteriogram demonstrating spinal AVM with components appearing dorsal, ventral, and possibly within the spinal cord (Case 5). **D.** Operative exposure of spinal cord from T7-T11 with extensive AVM. (Case 5). **E.** Operative view after dorsal and lateral portions of the AVM were removed (Case 5).

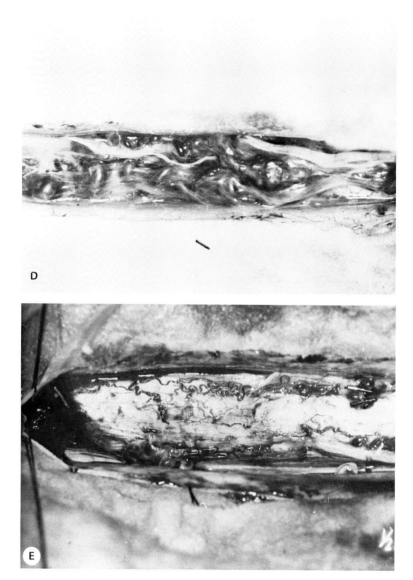

Fig. 90-13 (cont'd.)

Lesser surgical procedures such as decompressive laminectomy with or without opening the dura appear to have little or no merit in the treatment of these malformations. In fact, such operative "explorations" may be detrimental in that they make future definitive surgery more difficult. If the lesion is found to be inoperable and all that can be offered is decompression with opening of the dura, then the dura should be closed with a patch graft of fascia to prevent adhesions to the surface of the spinal cord. If there is a possibility that surgery will be performed in the future, it is mandatory to close the dura, since the adhesions that will otherwise form will preclude subsequent, definitive surgical ventures.

Case 5. An 18-year-old female was initially seen for a 4-month history of a burning sensation in her right leg of insidious onset. Over the next few months this "hot, pokerlike" sensation involved her thorax and abdomen. Past history was benign except for being told of a "crooked leg" at age 7.

Examination showed a mild decrease of deep tendon reflexes on the right side with a dysesthesia and loss of sensation involving the entire right leg except the L2 dermatome. Motor function was slightly decreased on abduction and adduction of the right thigh and extension of the right foot.

A myelogram (Fig. 90-13A) demonstrated a serpiginous defect in the lower thoracic region and conus region consistent with an AVM. CT scan with contrast showed no abnormalities.

Spinal arteriography demonstrated an AVM opposite T8-T10. Feeding arteries were seen from the right and left T8 level, as well as from the left T10 level. The artery of Adamkiewicz filled bilaterally from T8. The AVM appeared both anterior to, posterior to, and possibly within the cord (Fig. 90-13B and C).

On August 21, 1978, the patient underwent laminectomy of T7-T11 and subtotal removal of the AVM. Portions of the malformation were anterior and intramedullary and these remained. All known feeding arteries were divided. The entire dorsal and lateral portions of the AVM were excised (Fig. 90-13D and E). The intramedullary portion of the AVM that remained appeared to collapse.

Postoperatively, she showed hypesthesia on the left below L1 and a band of hypalgesia from L1 through L3. Posterior column function was completely normal. Minimal left hamstring weakness was noted, but gait was normal.

Follow-up examination at 2 years showed the same sensory findings and minor complaints of anterior thigh dysesthesias.

Results

In those patients in whom surgical obliteration or resection of the lesion has been accomplished, good results in terms of an improved or arrested neurologic status are seen in approximately 80 to 90 percent of the patients.[29,30,32,33,35] Unfortunately, the results are often predicated on the preoperative condition of the patient, so that those with neurologic devastation or severe advanced disease are less apt to make gratifying recoveries following successful resection of the lesion. On the other hand, individuals who have mild or modest neurologic deficits before surgery will receive the most benefit and often return to normal or near normal status. Resection of these malformations precludes the possibility of devastating neurologic deficit from subsequent hemorrhage.

Luessenhop and Dela Cruz[28] report, in a broad review of the literature, that decompressive procedures resulted in improvement in 19 percent and deterioration in 81 percent, while ligation of some feeders resulted in improvement in 34 percent and worsening in 66 percent. When these figures are compared with those of surgical resection, it is clear that the latter procedure, if feasible, is preferable. Radiation plays no role in the therapy of these lesions and may be deleterious, producing scar tissue that would make subsequent definitive operative procedures on these lesions difficult or impossible.

A postoperative arteriogram may or may not be done to define the completeness of resection. We do not feel postoperative angiography is as important in these cases as in the treatment of cerebral AVMs, since one is better able to gauge the effectiveness of resection while at the same time realizing the limitations of spinal arteriography in fully defining these lesions.

In addition to the AVMs that directly involve the spinal cord, there are similar situations existing in the meninges or parameningeal areas. These are often represented by enormous arteriovenous communications involving the intercostal or cervical arteries and involving not only the dura and sometimes the spinal cord but also often extensively the muscles and surrounding soft tissues. These are associated with bruits and may not manifest themselves with the spinal cord syndrome so familar to true AVMs of the spinal cord. Unfortunately, these lesions, being extensive with large shunts between arteries and veins, are difficult to treat by embolization, surgery, or both. In many instances, emboli will transverse the fistula and enter into the systemic venous circulation. Because of the extensive nature of these lesions, it is often impossible to remove the entire lesion, even with thoracotomy and massive resection. They are similar to cirsoid aneurysms of the scalp and some of the soft-tissue AVMs that involve the face and tissues at the base of the skull.

REFERENCES

1. Turnbull F: Intramedullary tumors of the spinal cord, in *Clinical Neurosurgery,* vol. 8. Baltimore, Williams & Wilkins, 1962, pp 237–247
2. Elsberg CA: *Tumors of the Spinal Cord.* New York, Paul B. Hoeber, 1925, pp 206–239

3. Matson DD: *Neurosurgery of Infancy and Childhood.* Springfield, Ill, Charles C Thomas, 1969, pp 647–688

4. Garrido E, Stein BM: Microsurgical removal of intramedullary spinal cord tumors. *Surg Neurol* 7:215–229, 1977

5. Greenwood J Jr: Surgical removal of intramedullary tumors. *J Neurosurg* 26:276–282, 1967

6. Guidetti B: Intramedullary tumors of the spinal cord. *Acta Neurochir (Wien)* 17:7–23, 1967

7. Horrax G, Henderson, DG: Encapsulated intramedullary tumor involving whole spinal cord from medulla to conus: complete enucleation with recovery. *Surg Gynecol Obstet* 68:814–819, 1939

8. Woods WW, Pimenta AM: Intramedullary lesions of the spinal cord: a study of 68 consecutive cases. *Arch Neurol Psychiatry* 52:383–399, 1944

9. Rand RW, Rand CW: *Intraspinal Tumors of Childhood.* Springfield, Ill, Charles C Thomas, 1960

10. Vigneud J, Aubin MD, Jardin C: CT in 40 cases of syringomyelia (abstract). *AJNR* 1:112, 1980

11. Quencer RM, Tenner MS, Rothman LM: Percutaneous spinal cord puncture and myelocystography. *Radiology* 118:637–644, 1976

12. Woltman HW, Kernohan JW, Adson AW, et al: Intramedullary tumors of spinal cord and gliomas of intradural portion of filum terminale: fate of these patients who have these tumors. *Arch Neurol Psychiatry* 65:378–395, 1951

13. Stein BM: Case records of the Massachusetts General Hospital—case 26. *N Engl J Med* 293:33–38, 1975

14. Brown RH, Nash CL Jr: Current status of spinal cord monitoring. *Spine* 4:466–470, 1979

15. Greenwood J Jr: Intramedullary tumors of the spinal cord. A follow-up study after total surgical removal. *J Neurosurg* 20:665–668, 1963

16. Love JG, River MH: Thirty-one year cure following removal of intramedullary glioma of cervical portion of spinal cord. Report of case. *J Neurosurg* 19:906–908, 1962

17. Stein BM: Surgery of intramedullary spinal cord tumors, in *Clinical Neurosurgery,* vol. 26. Baltimore, Williams & Wilkins, 1979, pp 529–542

18. Wood EH, Berne AS, Taveras JM: The value of radiation therapy in the management of intrinsic tumors of the spinal cord. *Radiology* 63:11–24, 1954

19. Schwade JG, Wara WM, Sheline GE, et al: Management of primary spinal cord tumors. *Int J Radiat Oncol Biol Phys* 4: 389–393, 1978

20. Tobin WD, Layton DD: The diagnosis and natural history of spinal cord arteriovenous malformations. *Mayo Clin Proc* 51:637–646, 1976

21. Krayenbuhl H, Yasargil MG: Die Varicosis spinalis und ihre Behandlung. *Schweiz Arch Neurol Psychiatr* 92:74–92, 1963

22. Doppman JL, DiChiro G, Ommaya AK: *Selective Arteriography of the Spinal Cord.* St. Louis, Warren Green, 1969

23. DiChiro G, Doppman J, Ommaya AK: Selective arteriography of arteriovenous aneurysms of spinal cord. *Radiology* 88:1065–1077, 1967

24. Djindjian R, Faure C, Houdart R, et al: Exploration angiographique des malformations vasculaires de la moelle epiniere. *Acta Radiol (Diagn) (Stockhl)* 5:145–162, 1966

25. Djindjian R: Arteriography of the spinal cord. *Am J Roentgenol Radium Ther Nucl Med* 107:461–478, 1969

26. Bergstrand A, Hook O, Lidvall H: Vascular malformations of the spinal cord. *Acta Neurol Scand* 40:169–183, 1964

27. Wyburn-Masson R: *The Vascular Abnormalities and Tumors of the Spinal Cord and Its Membranes.* London, Krimptom, 1943

28. Luessenhop AJ, Dela Cruz T: Surgical excision of spinal intradural vascular malformations. *J Neurosurg* 30:552–559, 1969

29. Ommaya AK, DiChiro G, Doppman, JL: Ligation of arterial supply in the treatment of spinal cord arteriovenous malformations. *J Neurosurg* 30:679–692, 1969

30. Krayenbuhl H, Yasargil MG, McClintock HG: Treatment of spinal cord vascular malformations by surgical excision. *J Neurosurg* 30:427–435, 1969

31. Doppman JL: The nidus concept for spinal cord arteriovenous malformations. A surgical recommendation based on angiographic observations. *Br J Radiol* 44:758–763, 1971

32. Aminoff MJ, Logue V: Clinical features of spinal vascular malformations. *Brain* 97:197–210, 1974

33. Aminoff MJ, Logue V: The prognosis of patients with spinal vascular malformations. *Brain* 97:211–218, 1974

34. Herdt JR, DiChiro G, Doppman JL: Combined arterial and arteriovenous aneurysms of the spinal cord. *Radiology* 99:589–593, 1971

35. Houdart R, Djindjian R, Hurth M: Vascular malformations of the spinal cord; the anatomic and therapeutic significance of arteriography. *J Neurosurg* 24:583–594, 1966

36. Kaufman HH, Ommaya AK, DiChiro G, et al: Compression vs. "steal." The pathogenesis of symptoms in arteriovenous malformations of the spinal cord. *Arch Neurol* 23:173–178, 1970

37. Matthews WB: The spinal bruit. *Lancet 2*:1117–1118, 1959
38. Doppman JL, Wirth FP Jr, DiChiro G, et al: Value of cutaneous angiomas in the arteriographic localization of spinal cord arteriovenous malformations. *N Engl J Med 281*:1440–1444, 1969
39. Yasargil MG: Diagnosis and treatment of spinal cord arteriovenous malformations. *Prog Neurol Surg 4*:355–428, 1971
40. Kasdon DL, Wolpert SM, Stein BM: Surgical and angiographic localization of spinal arteriovenous malformations. *Surg Neurol 5*:279–283, 1976
41. DiChiro G, Doppman JL, Wener L: Computed tomography of spinal arteriovenous malformations. *Radiology 123*:351–354, 1977
42. Doppman JL, DiChiro G, Ommaya AK: Percutaneous embolization of spinal cord arteriovenous malformations. *J Neurosurg 34*:48–55, 1971
43. Hilal SK, Sane P, Michelson WJ, et al: The embolization of vascular malformations of the spinal cord with low-viscosity silicone rubber. *Neuroradiology 16*:430–433, 1978
44. Kerber C: Intracranial cyanoacrylate: a new catheter therapy for arteriovenous malformations. *Invest Radiol 10*:536, 1975
45. Kunc Z, Bret J: Diagnosis and treatment of vascular malformations of the spinal cord. *J Neurosurg 30*:436–445, 1969
46. Bailey WL, Sperl MP: Angiomas of the cervical spinal cord. *J Neurosurg 30*:560–568, 1969
47. Baker HL Jr, Love JG, Layton DD Jr: Angiographic and surgical aspects of spinal cord vascular anomalies. *Radiology 88*:1078–1085, 1967
48. Stein BM: Anteriovenous malformations of the brain and spinal cord, in *Practice of Surgery,* Hagerstown, Md., Harper & Row, 1979
49. Post KD, Levitsky S, Doppman JL, et al: Transthoracic ligation of intercostal arteries for arteriovenous malformations of the spinal cord. *Ann Surg 173*:152–156, 1971

CHAPTER 91

Surgical Treatment of Rheumatoid Arthritis, Ankylosing Spondylitis, and Paget's Disease with Neurologic Deficit

Ghaus M. Malik

Rheumatoid Arthritis

RHEUMATOID ARTHRITIS OF THE SPINE involves the cervical region more often than any other. Chronic inflammation may lead to erosion of the bone and ligaments with subsequent loss of stability. Involvement of the cervical spine may cause sudden death or symptoms of vertebrobasilar ischemia, tetraparesis, and neck pain.

Both juvenile and adult rheumatoid arthritis carry a high incidence of involvement of the cervical spine. Isdale and Conlon, in a long-term follow-up of rheumatoid patients, reported that 80 percent showed radiologic changes in the cervical spine and 50 percent showed atlanto-axial subluxation.[1]

Rheumatoid arthritis most often affects the upper levels of the cervical spine and produces different clinical features at different ages. In children, the apophyseal joints often fuse and growth is deficient, while subluxation is the predominant feature in adults. In addition to the bony and ligamentous involvement, the presence of rheumatoid nodules, which can lead to destruction and collapse of the vertebral bodies as well as marked thickening and fibrosis of the dura mater, have been reported. The involvement of the spine may be evident in different forms (Table 91-1).

Anterior Atlanto-Axial Subluxation

The single most common spinal condition associated with rheumatoid arthritis is the anterior atlanto-axial subluxation, which is felt to be caused by destruction or laxity of the transverse ligament or from erosion or fracture of the odontoid process. Davis and Markley have been credited with the first documented case of atlanto-axial subluxation in rheumatoid arthritis causing neurologic deficits.[2]

Atlanto-axial subluxation is considered to be present if the distance between the posterior

Department of Neurological Surgery, Henry Ford Hospital, Detroit, Michigan

Table 91-1. Forms of Involvement of the Spine in Cases of Rheumatoid Arthritis

Cervical Spine
  Craniovertebral region
    1. Anterior atlanto-axial subluxation
    2. Vertical atlanto-axial subluxation
    3. Posterior atlanto-axial subluxation
    4. Transverse or rotatory subluxation
  Subaxial region
    1. Subluxation—single or multiple levels
    2. Vertebral endplate erosion and disc involvement
      (simulating infection)
    3. Apophyseal joint involvement with erosion or ankylosis
    4. Intervertebral disc herniation
  Miscellaneous
    1. Pachymeningitis
    2. Rheumatoid granulation tissue
Thoracic and Lumbar Spine
    1. Osteoporosis with compression fractures
    2. Subluxation in lumbar region
    3. Rheumatoid nodules
    4. Vertebral endplate erosion

aspect of the anterior arch of atlas and the anterior aspect of the odontoid is more than 2.5 mm in adults and 4.5 mm in children (measured in flexion). Nakano has reported a 30 to 40 percent incidence of cervical subluxation in patients admitted to the hospital with rheumatoid arthritis.[3] Often these radiologic findings are not associated with neurologic symptoms.

Determination of the exact incidence of neurologic manifestations in atlanto-axial subluxation is difficult, owing to a number of variable factors. Because of the disabling deformities and involvement of major joints causing difficulty in ambulation, some of the symptoms may be disregarded. Sensory symptoms, at times, are considered to be caused by peripheral neuropathy, which also is associated with rheumatoid arthritis. The neurologic examination is frequently difficult to perform adequately. Conlon et al. found 84 subluxations without any neurologic manifestations in the follow-up of 333 cases of rheumatoid arthritis for 6 years.[4] On the other hand, Stevens et al. had 24 cases with neurologic changes out of 36 patients with subluxations in their study of 100 cases.[5]

Clinical Presentation

Rheumatoid subluxation may present as a neurologic syndrome requiring urgent treatment, or even as a cause of sudden death. In addition to direct compression, neurologic symptoms may result from occlusion of the vertebral arteries or intrinsic vascular disease in the spinal cord or the brainstem. Rheumatoid inflammatory tissue also may act as a compressive lesion in the spinal canal. Several factors may be involved in a single patient.

Neck pain is the most frequent symptom. The pain is usually in the upper cervical or suboccipital area with variable radiation to the mastoid, occipital, temporal, or frontal regions. Sometimes this specific information may have to be sought by the examining physician. Paresthesias can be caused by head or neck movement, and Lhermitte's sign produced by sudden flexion of the neck may be elicited. Rarely, complaints of vertebrobasilar ischemia (transient visual disturbances, diplopia, vertigo, and sensory or motor phenomena) may be present. Smith et al. reported that in their follow-up of 130 patients with subluxation for an average period of 7 to 8 years, 6 patients developed symptoms consistent with involvement of the vertebral artery.[6]

Compression or ischemia of the spinal cord may produce spastic quadriparesis. As stated earlier, in the majority of the cases, subtle deficits are confused with disability caused by general debilitation and joint involvement. Hyperreflexia and Babinski's sign are probably the most reliable indicators of the involvement of the spinal cord. Paresthesias of the hands and feet are quite common. A significant number of patients have involvement of the first division of the trigeminal nerve as well as sensory disturbance in the distribution of C2.

Diagnostic Studies

Lateral x-rays of the cervical spine made in neutral, flexion, and extension positions are necessary. In addition to confirming the diagnosis, they serve to demonstrate whether or not subluxation is spontaneously reducible. Lateral tomograms of the craniovertebral junction may be needed if visualization of the odontoid process and other structures is not adequate on regular films. It is also important to know the status of the lower cervical spine. Visualization generally is difficult because of shoulder deformities and, again, tomography may be necessary. If neurologic examination points to a lower cervical lesion because of root symptoms or sensory level, this evaluation is even more important. Myelography is indicated whenever involvement of the lower spine is suspected or if the spine films do not show sufficient changes to account for the patient's symptoms. In the latter instance, compression might be due to granulation tissue or pachymeningitis. This was exemplified by a recent patient of ours who had advanced rheumatoid arthritis and presented with myelopathy. There was a 6-mm anterior atlanto-axial subluxation on flexion, but he complained of Lhermitte's-type phenomena with extension of the neck, in contrast to flexion. Myelography showed an almost complete block opposite the C3-4 disc space from hypertrophic changes.

In patients presenting with symptoms of vertebrobasilar ischemia, vertebral angiography is indicated. For more detailed radiologic aspects, the reader is referred to the monograph by Yves Dirheimer.[7]

Treatment

Unless the patient's condition poses definite contraindications to treatment, we feel that patients presenting with neurologic involvement need stabilization of the subluxation. Different types of operative procedures have been described for atlanto-axial subluxation. Most of these utilize a posterior approach. These methods range from a simple internal wire fixation to bony or acrylic fusion. Newman has described an occipitocervical fusion,[8] as has Hamblen,[9] but with different techniques. Others advocate only fusion of C1-C2, since there is less limitation of neck motion and a decreased incidence of nonunion. Alexander and his group have reported that acrylic provides adequate support, and the need for a bone graft is eliminated.[10] With this technique, however, there is long-term reliance on wire, since eventual bony fusion may not occur. Even if minimal displacement persists following the fusion, the stability provided by the fusion prevents further neurologic deterioration by avoiding constant slipping and spinal cord trauma during flexion and extension of the spine.

Ideally, considering the debilitation and disability of these patients, the procedure of choice would be one that provides immediate and long-term stabilization and early ambulation without the necessity of being in heavy orthotic devices. We currently use a modified Gallies fusion, utilizing a bicortical iliac bone H-graft so that two cortical surfaces provide greater immediate strength, and the bony fusion gives long-term stability.[11] The technique of this procedure is described in some detail.

C1-C2 Fusion for Atlanto-Axial Subluxation

Preparation. The patient is placed in Gardner-Wells tong traction, particularly if the patient has a significant or progressive deficit. Coagulation studies are done, and the patient receives additional steroids, since the majority of these patients have been on long-term steroid therapy. We prefer to use cortisone acetate, 100 mg the night before surgery, and another 100 mg with preoperative medication on the morning of the operation.

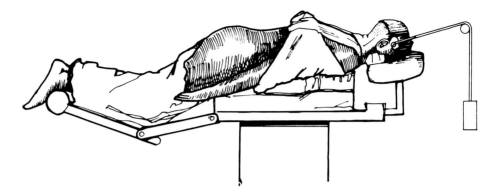

Fig. 91-1. Positioning of the patient.

Anesthesia.   Since the majority of these patients have joint deformities as well as a limited range of neck motion with subluxation causing neurologic deficit, great care is taken in the induction of anesthesia. We prefer to intubate the patient while he is awake, without undue flexion or extension of the neck while the patient is still in traction. The throat is sprayed with Cetacine.[*] If the patient is apprehensive, slight sedation with a small dose of Valium is used. We have found that blind nasotracheal intubation while the patient is breathing is well tolerated; however, endotracheal intubation could be done using a fiberoptic laryngoscope.

Positioning.   The patient then is turned over to the operating table in the prone position, supported on rolls, while skeletal traction is maintained over an anesthesia screen (Fig. 91-1). The head is supported on a horseshoe headrest and held in extension. The pressure points are

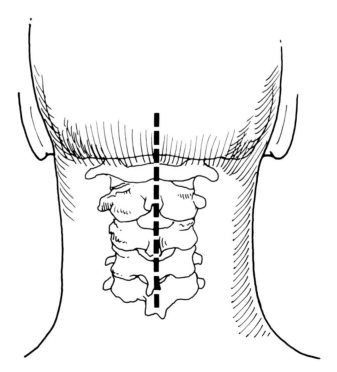

Fig. 91-2. The line of the incision.

*Cetylite Industries, Inc., Pennsauken, New Jersey.

padded. The table is flexed to avoid hyperextension of the lumbar spine, and a pillow or rolled blanket is used to avoid pressure on the feet. The draw sheet is brought together in such a way that the arms are supported while the upper part of the chest and right flank and buttock areas are left exposed. The right iliac crest is used for the graft, unless other factors dictate differently. A lateral film of the cervical spine is obtained in this position to assess the reduction of the sub-luxation.

Operation.   A midline skin incision is made from the inion to the midcervical region following appropriate preparation and draping (Fig. 91-2). The dissection is continued strictly in the midline. The muscles are dissected off the occipital bone and the laminae of C1, C2, and C3. Particular attention is given to the posterior arch of the atlas where, after the muscles in the midline are sharply divided, a periosteal elevator is used gently to dissect the muscles laterally, without disturbing the vertebral arteries or venous plexuses. The exposure is maintained with self-retaining retractors (Fig. 91-3). A transverse incision is made over the dorsal aspect of the

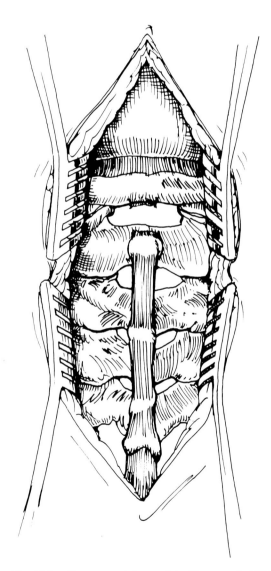

Fig. 91-3.   Exposure of the occipital bone and upper cervical laminae.

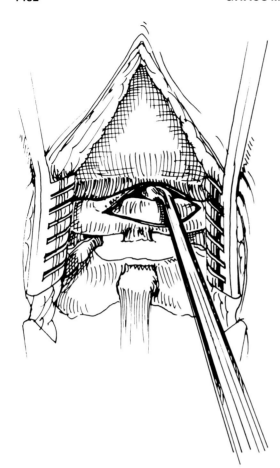

Fig. 91-4. The periosteum is stripped off the posterior arch of C1 with a small angled curette.

posterior arch of the atlas with a No. 15 blade, and the periosteum is dissected off the arch, both on the dorsal and ventral surfaces, using a small, angled curette (Fig. 91-4). The bony surfaces are roughened with a bone rasp. A notch, about 5 mm in depth, is made at the superior aspect of the base of the C2 spinous process with a narrow-beaked rongeur, and a hole is made through the spinous process with a sharp right-angled awl. Once the arch has been freed, a loop of No. 20 monofilament wire is passed underneath C1 from below, while the arch is gently retracted backward with the curette (Fig. 91-5). As the loop becomes slightly visible, it is pulled up with a nerve hook (Fig. 91-6). At the same time, a bicortical iliac bone graft is removed (Fig. 91-7). This requires stripping of abdominal, iliacus, and gluteal muscles from their attachments to the upper, inner, and outer surfaces of the ilium. Four notches are cut on the graft, allowing a close fit between the graft and the posterior elements of C1 and C2. The wire is looped around the graft. A second wire is placed through the hole made in the spinous process, and its ends are twisted together (Fig. 91-8). The wire loops are tightened around the graft, pulled downward under tension, and tightly twisted to the wire already fixed to the spinous process of C2 (Fig. 91-9). Cancellous bone chips then are packed into the crevices underneath the iliac graft. Both incisions are closed carefully in layers.

Postoperative care. The patient is left in traction for 24 to 48 hours, after which time ambulation is encouraged with a light collar. Radiograms of the cervical spine are obtained for 2 to 4 months postoperatively to ensure that adequate reduction and fusion have taken place (Fig. 91-10).

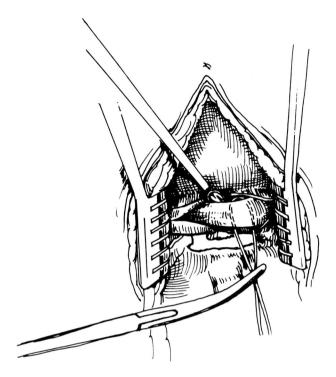

Fig. 91-5. A wire loop is passed underneath the posterior arch of C1 while the arch is gently pulled back with the curette.

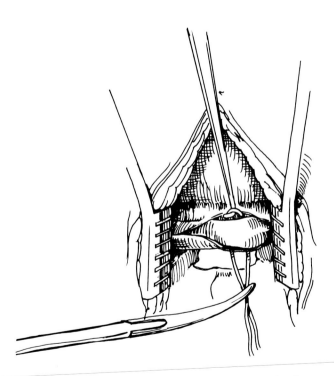

Fig. 91-6. The wire loop is pulled with a nerve hook.

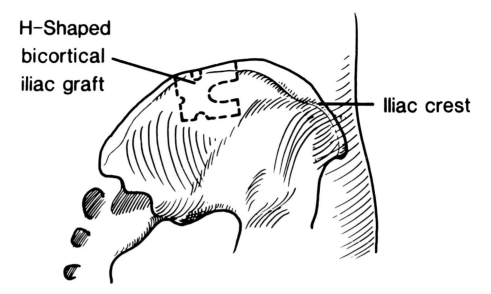

Fig. 91-7. Diagram outlining the donor site for the bicortical iliac bone graft. (Reproduced from Wu KK, Malik GM, Guise ER: *Orthopaedics,* 1982. With permission.)

Vertical Atlanto-Axial Subluxation

Greater attention has been given to vertical atlanto-axial subluxation in recent years.[12-14] It has been known by different names such as vertical atlanto-axial dislocation, basilar invagination, upward atlanto-axial dislocation, or upward odontoid dislocation. Vertical subluxation results from: (1) destruction of the ligaments, and (2) erosive changes with bone resorption in the basilar aspect of the skull, the occipital condyles, and the lateral masses of the atlas. The odon-

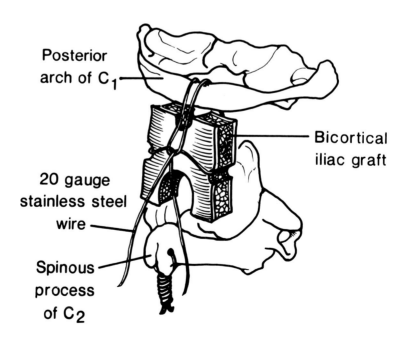

Fig. 91-8. An exploded view of C1 and C2 showing the technique for looping the wire and placing the graft. (Reproduced from Wu KK, Malik GM, Guise ER: *Orthopaedics,* 1982. With permission.)

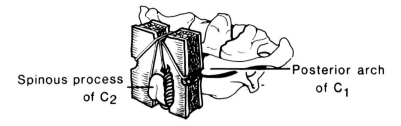

Spinous process of C$_2$

Posterior arch of C$_1$

Fig. 91-9. Diagram of the bicortical iliac "H" strut graft in place after it has been intimately wired to the posterior arch of the atlas and the spinous process of the axis. (Reproduced from Wu KK, Malik GM, Guise ER: *Orthopaedics,* 1982. With permission.)

toid process projects up into the foramen magnum and generally is associated with some degree of atlanto-axial subluxation, so the odontoid process also is placed posteriorly in the canal. This causes direct compression of the medulla, along with potential ischemia from compression of the vertebral arteries, the anterior spinal arteries, or small perforating vessels of the brainstem and spinal cord.

Several fatal cases, with death caused by sudden-onset medullary ischemia, have been reported.[15,16] In a survey of 476 patients with rheumatoid arthritis admitted to the hospital, Henderson found that 13 cases (3.7 percent) had vertical atlanto-axial subluxation.[12] This form of subluxation was considered to be present if the tip of the odontoid process lay more than 4.5 mm above McGregor's line. Five of these patients had definite involvement of the brainstem, cervical cord, or upper cervical nerve roots, and two others had pyramidal signs without subaxial subluxation.

The development of brainstem symptoms, especially dysphagia, hoarseness, periods of unconsciousness, and respiratory difficulty, is an ominous sign and requires urgent treatment. The patient should be placed in skeletal traction. Some improvement or stabilization of the neurologic deficit may be obtained with occipito-axial fusion, with or without removal of the posterior arch of the atlas. When medullary involvement is noted, however, the transoral approach with

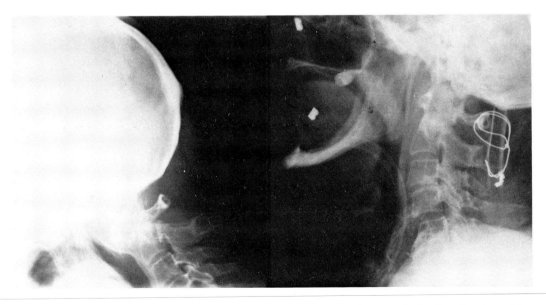

Fig. 91-10. Pre- and postoperative radiograms: (left) a flexion view of the cervical spine showing subluxation; and (right) a lateral film demonstrating reduction of subluxation and position of the graft.

removal of the odontoid and overlying synovial tissue is recommended.[17,18] This provides the best opportunity to decompress the brainstem. The patient obviously requires a tracheostomy, and transoral decompression has to be followed with occipital-cervical fusion.

In rare cases of atlanto-axial subluxation, as in the one described by Kao et al., reduction is not possible because of the presence of rheumatoid granulation tissue between the anterior arch of the atlas and the odontoid process.[19] Under these circumstances, the transoral approach provides a means of removal of granulation tissue and reduction of the subluxation. This can be followed later with occipitocervical fusion. The alternative method would be resection of the posterior arch of the atlas before fusion of the occiput to C2-3.[20]

Subaxial Subluxation

Spontaneous rheumatoid subluxation below the axis also occurs with some frequency and may cause severe cord damage.[21] Multiple levels may be involved; however, the C4-5 level is most commonly affected. Cervical myelopathy may be caused by intervertebral disc extrusion or rheumatoid granulation tissue in addition to, or at a level different from, that of the subluxation. As pointed out earlier, it also may be associated with atlanto-axial involvement. The difficulty of evaluating lower cervical segments cannot be overemphasized and, therefore, tomography may be necessary. Myelography is considered advisable before surgical treatment unless the clinical level of the involvement of the spinal cord exactly matches the level of subluxation.

Tong traction, followed by anterior cervical fusion by the Cloward method, is the treatment of choice for single-level subluxation.[22] Spinal cord compression from granulation tissue or intervertebral disc herniation also may be treated adequately by this approach. The only problem, encountered occasionally, is the poor quality of graft obtained from the ilium because of severe osteoporosis. One might therefore have to use a strut graft rather than a Cloward plug. A fibular graft could certainly be used, particularly if more than one level is to be treated.

In some patients, however, the only reasonable way to decompress the spinal cord is by cervical laminectomy. If subluxation is already present at this level, this can be treated by anterior fusion. In other cases, one should follow the patient very closely for possible future subluxation. Similarly, if the myelogram reveals compression because of pachymeningitis,[23] decompressive laminectomy and placement of a fascial graft in the dura are necessary.

Obviously, all of these procedures are helpful only if the patient has some neurologic function remaining. Major surgical procedures are fruitless and probably unjustified in a patient who is quadriplegic or on a respirator. It therefore cannot be stressed enough that, despite some reports indicating lack of major neurologic deterioration on long-term follow-up, a thorough initial neurologic evaluation and close follow-up are necessary. If a potentially hazardous situation exists, treatment is necessary before irreversible cord damage occurs.

Thoracic and Lumbar Spine Involvement

The neurologic complications from involvement of the thoracic and lumbar spine are rather uncommon.[24] Rheumatoid nodules have been reported to cause nerve root compression.[25] Subluxations are seen in rheumatoid patients, but generally it is difficult to differentiate this from the degenerative disc disease. If the symptoms are referable to the thoracic or lumbar region, myelography is necessary. Occasionally the vertebral end-plate may be destroyed and this may simulate osteomyelitis or discitis. The treatment depends on pathology.

Obviously a patient suffering from rheumatoid arthritis is not immune to other intraspinal lesion-causing myelopathy or radiculopathy that may require appropriate investigations and treatment.

Ankylosing Spondylitis

Ankylosing spondylitis is a chronic inflammatory disease that most frequently affects the sacroiliac joints of young men and synovial joints of the whole spine. Bony fusion of these joints and ossification along the longitudinal ligaments lead to total immobility of the vertebrae. The condition has been known by different names, such as rheumatoid spondylitis, rheumatoid arthritis of the spine, Marie-Strumpell disease, Bechterew's disease, and pelvospondylitis ossificans.

Early symptoms include low back pain or lumbar stiffness or both, which is usually increased in the morning or after periods of inactivity. In 65 to 70 percent of the patients, the initial symptom is intermittent or persistent low back pain. In rare instances the back pain may be hyperacute and resemble an acute herniated lumbar disc. The possibility of early ankylosing spondylitis must therefore be kept in mind while evaluating patients with low back pain and suspected disc disease. Particular attention should be given to sacroiliac joints in patients who do not have neurologic changes of nerve root involvement. The erythrocyte sedimentation rate is elevated in 80 to 90 percent of the patients with obvious active disease, and HLA B-27 antigen is present in 90 to 95 percent of the patients.[26]

The most common neurologic complications in patients with ankylosing spondylitis are caused by: (1) fracture-dislocation of the spine; (2) atlanto-axial subluxations; (3) intraspinal ossifications or pachymeningitis; and (4) cauda equina syndrome.

Fracture-Dislocation of the Spine

A rigid spine and fragile osteoporotic vertebrae in ankylosing spondylitis make the patient especially susceptible to spinal fracture-dislocation. Unlike an ordinary spinal fracture, the ankylosed spine breaks like a long bone. The fracture line tends to be transverse and may extend to involve more posterior structures. Bergmann stated that the fractures occurred through what had formerly been an interspace.[27] Others have reported cases, however, in which fracture was primarily through the vertebral body.[28] Hyperextension injuries are more likely to cause a fracture. The spine may be locked in hyperextension, either because of locking of the facets or locking of the neural arches. The more advanced the process of ankylosing spondylitis, the less trauma appears necessary to break the brittle bone and calcified ligaments. At times there may be no definite history of trauma. Woodruff and Dewing reported a case in which the momentary unsupported weight of the head while the patient was being turned on a Stryker frame was enough to result in a fracture of C5-6.[29] The cervical spine is the most commonly involved, although fractures of the thoracic and lumbar spine have been observed. In the cervical region, C5-6 and C6-7 levels are the most frequently affected.

Patients may only complain of pain, but the most dramatic symptom is quadriplegia. Fracture or fracture-dislocation of the vertebral column should be suspected in any patient with severe ankylosing spondylitis who has had trauma, especially if there are complaints of neck or back pain. Such a patient should be handled as if he had an unstable fracture until thorough clinical and radiologic assessment have ruled out the presence of such a lesion.

Just as in the case of rheumatoid arthritis, certain areas of the spine, particularly the lower cervical and upper thoracic portions, may be difficult to visualize because of the deformities produced by the disease. Tomograms should be obtained if complete visualization is not possible by other means.

A complete transverse fracture converts the spine into two rigid segments. The calcified longitudinal ligaments also may be fractured and are no longer available to assist in maintaining the alignments of the two segments, which move as independent units. Once the diagnosis has been established, every effort should therefore be made to prevent or minimize spinal cord injury.

If there is no neurologic deficit and the subluxation is slight, an efficient immbolization with a

Halo or Minerva jacket would be sufficient. The majority of fractures heal within 8 to 10 weeks, although evident nonunion has been reported as late as 6 months.[30] When there is appreciable displacement or instability, however, skeletal traction is needed as initial treatment. The traction should be applied in a neutral position along the long axis of the cervical spine. This axis also might be distorted because of flexion deformity of the cervical spine in advanced ankylosing spondylitis. Any hyperextension may cause further compromise of the spinal canal and potential neurologic deterioration. If reduction is achieved, the spine may be stabilized by an anterior approach or simply treated with immobilization.

When reduction is not possible with traction or there is progressive neurologic deficit, immediate operative intervention is necessary. The fracture-dislocation may be associated with epidural hematoma. Open reduction and decompressive laminectomy, followed by a stabilizing procedure, using internal fixation and bone graft at the same time, are essential.[31] The patient then needs to be immobilized in a brace for 2 to 3 months.

If operative intervention becomes necessary, several factors have to be taken into consideration. Endotracheal intubation might risk further neurologic damage because of hyperextension of the neck. Nasotracheal intubation or elective tracheostomy, with the patient awake, may therefore be necessary.

Several cardiovascular abnormalities are associated with ankylosing spondylitis, including aortic insufficiency, persistent conduction disturbances, cardiomegaly, pericarditis, and angina.[32] Complete atrial-ventricular blocks, causing Stokes-Adams attacks, have been reported. Similarly, diffuse rib cage involvement by the ankylosing process leads to the restriction of chest expansion. A peculiar apical or upper lobe fibrosis with occasional cavitation also has been noted. These factors have to be assessed along with the commonly associated problem of severe kyphoscoliosis. These patients generally have been on long-term steroid therapy and require additional steroids at the time of surgery.

The prognosis, in general, is much less favorable in fracture-dislocation of the ankylosed cervical spine than in a similar injury of the normal spine. Hollin et al. reported a 45 percent mortality in their review of 38 cases.[33]

Atlanto-Axial Subluxations

All types of atlanto-axial subluxations, as described in the section on rheumatoid arthritis, also are seen in ankylosing spondylitis. The frequency, however, is much less and generally is in the range of 2 to 8 percent. When symptomatic, similar treatment is indicated. The problems of a rigid, brittle lower cervical spine and associated cardiovascular and respiratory difficulties need to be taken into consideration when surgical intervention is necessary.

Intraspinal Ossification or Pachymeningitis

Intraspinal ossification of the posterior longitudinal ligament, as well as the dura, has been reported as a cause of myelopathy in ankylosing spondylitis. Evidently it is more commonly seen in Japanese, and Briedal called this syndrome "the Japanese Disease."[34] Dirheimer, however, reported 2 cases of meningeal ossification evident on radiologic studies.[7] Any patient with ankylosing spondylitis presenting with myelopathy not explained by radiographic changes needs myelography. If a compressive lesion is found, surgical decompression is indicated. If the thickening or ossification of the dura is the source of compression, placement of a fascial graft in the dura is needed.

Cauda Equina Syndrome

There are several case reports in the literature of slowly progressive cauda equina syndrome in patients with long-standing ankylosing spondylitis.[35-37] There is loss of function of the lower spinal roots, both motor and sensory. Generally the presenting symptom is disturbance of sphincter control. Changes in ankle reflexes and cutaneous sensation, particularly in the sacral dermatomes, are evident. There is variable involvement of the lower nerve roots. Surprisingly, no compressive lesion has been found on myelography in these patients. The spinal canal is said to be quite wide. In some cases, however, posterior diverticula have been noted.[38] In one postmortem evaluation reported by Matthew, the posterior aspect of the lower spinal canal was found to be eroded by numerous large arachnoid cysts, and arachnoid adhesions were present above the level of the diverticula.[39] There also were some degenerative changes in the nerve roots of the cauda equina. No definite cause has been determined; however, Matthew suggested the possibility of arachnoiditis occurring at an earlier stage of the disease and possibly being responsible for this syndrome later on. Nothing surgical can be done about it; however, the patient certainly needs investigations, including myelography.

Paget's Disease

There is some involvement of the spine in almost all patients with Paget's disease. The risk of neurologic involvement is inversely related to the frequency with which the vertebrae are involved, being greatest in the cervical spine where Paget's disease is least common, and least in the lumbar spine where the disease is most common. The thoracic spine is intermediate in both respects.[40] Although the neurologic complications are relatively uncommon considering the frequency of the disease, they may be treatable and should therefore be recognized. There is a broad spectrum of neurologic sequelae,[41] but only the ones associated with spinal involvement will be discussed here.

Several mechanisms are involved in the etiology of neurologic changes,[41] including:

1. Pressure exerted by pathologic bone on neural structures.
2. Changes in the ability of the bone to bear weight.
3. Malignant change of the involved bone.
4. Compromise of the vascular supply of neural structures.

Spinal cord compression is a well-known complication of Paget's disease of the vertebral column, and was first described by Wyllie in 1923.[42] Sadar et al., in 1972, presented a review of 86 cases, already reported, and 4 of their own with neurologic dysfunction attributable only to Paget's disease of the vertebral column.[43] Eighty-nine percent of the patients were men and 11 percent women. Progressive paraparesis or quadriparesis was the presenting feature in most patients. Pain was the only symptom in 5 patients; however, it is a complaint frequently associated with Paget's disease and is secondary to either local bony changes, radicular compression, or flexor spasm at a later stage.

The bony changes in Paget's disease of the spine result from relative effects of the destructive and reparative processes.[41] There is thickening of the pedicles and laminae, and the destructive process causes softening of the bone resulting in the compression of the vertebral bodies. At the same time, reparative changes occur, mainly along the periphery, increasing the width of the vertebral body, which is already increased because of the decreased height secondary to compression. These changes, thus combined, cause narrowing of the spinal canal and the intervertebral foramina, resulting in the compression of the neural elements, i.e., the spinal cord and the nerve roots.

The upper thoracic spinal cord is most vulnerable to the effects of Paget's disease. Normally the vertebral canal is narrowest in this area and the vascular compromise also is more likely to occur, since this is considered to be the watershed area. Neurologic involvement may follow either diffuse changes affecting a considerable length of the vertebral canal, or a monostotic lesion. The radiologic demonstration of a paraspinal mass with neural arch involvement is undoubtedly the most vital clue to the diagnosis.

The patient usually presents with symptoms of progressive spinal cord involvement. The course is slow with symptoms usually being present for more than a year and rarely less than 6 months. Sensory and motor symptoms generally start simultaneously. As noted earlier, the upper thoracic spinal cord is most commonly affected and, therefore, the patient generally first notices numbness and weakness in the legs. With further progression, spasticity and other upper motor neuron signs appear, and the patient may develop sphincter disturbances. A typical history, however, does not always signify a compressive etiology as explaining the spinal cord dysfunction.[43] Petit-Dutailis et al.[44] described a patient with Paget's disease and progressive paraparesis who had a negative myelogram, but the cerebrospinal fluid protein was high. Two years later, however, a repeat myelogram showed evidence of spinal cord compression, and decompression resulted in improvement. Similar cases in patients who have had neurologic deficit but no myelographic block have been reported since then. Under these circumstances, vascular insufficiency of the neural elements would have to be considered as the most likely etiologic factor.

Involvement of the atlas and axis with spinal cord compression and subsequent quadriplegia has been reported.[45-47] The involvement of the craniospinal junction results in basilar impression, as described by Wycis.[48] This can be associated with occipital neuralgia, lower cranial nerve signs, medullary compression, cerebellar compression, syringomyelia with ventricular obstruction, hydrocephalus, and vertebrobasilar insufficiency.

Symptoms of compression of the cauda equina result from involvement of the lumbar spine, characteristically of a single vertebra. Paget's disease can be a cause of sciatica through encroachment of the vertebral foramen, through the well-known pelvic outlet (pyriformis) syndrome, or through a lower nerve entrapment between the enlarged ischium and the lesser trochanter.[49]

Malignant degeneration, resulting in osteogenic sarcoma, has been reported.[50] The incidence of malignant change in the spine is extremely infrequent in comparison to the humerus and skull. Sadar et al. found only 7 documented cases.[43] In contrast to slowly progressive neurologic deficit with Paget's disease of the spine, the patient with osteogenic sarcoma has a rapidly deteriorating course over a period of a few weeks. Pain is a prominent symptom, and generally when the patient is first seen, pulmonary metastases are already evident. Operative decompression, in 4 of the 7 patients reported, resulted in minimal and temporal improvement with the longest survival being 5.5 months.

Treatment

At the present time, myelography is the only definitive way to determine the extent to which the subarachnoid space is compromised. Myelography, through lumbar puncture, might be difficult if there is involvement of the lumbar spine. In these cases, a lateral C1-2 puncture could be used safely to introduce contrast material.

Computed tomographic scanning of the spine is certainly helpful in delineating the extent of bony involvement. Regional angiography is recommended to assess the vascularity of an area before surgery, particularly in the presence of very active or neoplastic disease. It then may be appropriate to consider occlusion of the major arterial feeders to the involved bone before decompression or excision of tumor.

Several medications are being used in the treatment of Paget's disease of the bone. Calcitonin has proven effective in the relief of pain. The medication, however, has to be given over a long period of time. In a case reported by Melick et al.,[51] it appeared to relieve neurologic dysfunction resulting from spinal compression. This patient showed slow improvement over a period of 8 months. Coincident with therapy, urinary hydroxyproline and serum alkaline phosphatase levels fell. The mechanism of the improvement is unclear, but may be secondary to a reduction in the volume and vascularity of the bone. Improvement in cranial nerve palsies, ataxia, and myelopathy with spastic paralysis and paraplegia all have been noted during Calcitonin therapy, but it must be remembered that only a small number of patients have been documented.[52]

Similarly, other agents such as Mithramycin, EHDP, and diphosphonates are being used in the treatment of Paget's disease and have shown some effectiveness in pain control. Ryan reports having seen considerable return of function in patients with neurologic involvement using Mithramycin.[53] Evidently Mithramycin provides a very rapid reduction in disease activity, but there is associated higher toxicity.

The medical therapy should be considered in the patient experiencing bone pain without neurologic deficit. Similarly, in the case of a very slow, progressive lesion, drug therapy would be attractive since one is able to monitor the changes on close follow-up. In a patient with very active disease but relatively slow progression, Calcitonin or Mithramycin could be used in an effort to reduce the activity before surgical intervention.

When the progression of neurologic deficit is more rapid, or other factors dictate early decompression of neural elements in the hope of preserving neurologic function, surgical decompression has to be carried out. The value of surgery in the presence of myelographically documented compression has been repeatedly proven. Sadar et al. reported 55 cases out of 65 treated with decompressive laminectomy showing variable but definite improvement.[43]

The general principles of decompressive laminectomy are the same as they would be for any other similar compressive lesion, such as a metastatic epidural tumor. A few points, however, should be stressed. The bone involved by Paget's disease is extremely vascular and soft. Similarly, the attachments between the paraspinal muscles and laminae are very vascular. The most prominent feature of surgical decompression is difficulty with the hemostasis. The bone bleeds very easily and profusely, making the operation very difficult. Extra attention is therefore necessary in stripping the paraspinal muscles, and judicious use of bone wax helps in reducing blood loss. Excessive blood loss has to be anticipated and appropriate arrangements have to be made for type and cross-match of adequate quantities of blood. It generally is not necessary to open the dura, but one has to make sure that adequate bony decompression has been carried out on both sides of the block.

Following an initial response to decompression, recurrent neural compression may occur in the course of the disease, secondary to new bone formation, fracture-dislocation, or malignant degeneration. This occurred in 6 out of 65 patients undergoing decompressive laminectomy in the review by Sadar; one patient, however, did not show any improvement following repeat laminectomy. Plaut also added a representative case in which the patient responded favorably to a second laminectomy.[54]

REFERENCES

1. Isdale IC, Conlon PW: Atlanto-axial subluxation. *Ann Rheum Dis 30*:387–389, 1971
2. Davis FW, Markley ME: Rheumatoid arthritis with death from medullary compression. *Ann Intern Med 35*:451–454, 1951
3. Nakano KK: Neurological complications of rheumatoid arthritis. *Orthop Clin North Am 6*:861–880, 1975
4. Conlon PW, Isdale IC, Rose BS: Rheumatoid arthritis of the cervical spine—an analysis of 333 cases. *Ann Rheum Dis 25*:120–126, 1966
5. Stevens JC, Cartlidge NEF, Saunders M, et al.: Atlanto-axial subluxation and cervical myelopathy in rheumatoid arthritis. *Q J Med 40*:394–408, 1971
6. Smith PH, Benn RT, Sharp J: Natural history of rheumatoid cervical luxations. *Ann Rheum Dis 31*:431–439, 1972
7. Dirheimer Y: *The Cranio-Vertebral Region in Chronic Inflammatory Disease.* Berlin, Springer-Verlag, 1977
8. Newman P, Sweetnam R: Occipito-cervical fusion—an operative technique and its indications. *J Bone Joint Surg 51B*:423–431, 1969
9. Hamblen DL: Occipito-cervical fusion: Indications, technique and results. *J Bone Joint Surg 49B*:33–45, 1967
10. Kelly DL, Alexander E, Davis C, et al.: Acrylic fixation of atlanto-axial dislocation: Technical note. *J Neurosurg 36*:366–371, 1972

11. Wu KK, Malik GM, Guise ER: Atlanto-axial arthrodesis: A clinical analysis of twenty-two consecutive cases performed at Henry Ford Hospital. *Orthopedics* 5:865–871, 1982

12. Henderson, DRF: Vertical atlanto-axial subluxation in rheumatoid arthritis. *Rheumatol Rehabil* 14:31–38, 1975

13. Rana NA, Hancock DO, Taylor AR, et al: Upward translocation of the dens in rheumatoid arthritis. *J Bone Joint Surg* 55B:471–477, 1973

14. Swinson DR, Hamilton EBD, Matthews JA, et al: Vertical subluxations of the axis in rheumatoid arthritis. *Ann Rheum Dis* 31:359–363, 1972

15. Martel W, Abell M: Fatal atlanto-axial luxation in rheumatoid arthritis. *Arthritis Rheum* 6:224–231, 1963

16. Web FWS, Hickman JA, Drew D: Death from vertebral artery thrombosis in rheumatoid arthritis. *Br Med J* 2:537–538, 1968

17. Brattström H, Elner A, Granholm L: Transoral surgery for myelopathy caused by rheumatoid arthritis of cervical spine. *Ann Rheum Dis* 32:578–581, 1973

18. Smith HP, Challa VR, Alexander E: Odontoid compression of the brain stem in a patient with rheumatoid arthritis. *J Neurosurg* 53:841–845, 1980

19. Kao CC, Messert B, Winkler SS, et al: Rheumatoid C1-C2 dislocation—pathogenesis and treatment reconsidered. *J Neurol Neurosurg Psychiatry* 37:1069–1073, 1974

20. Thomas WH: Surgical management of rheumatoid servical spine. *Orthop Clin North Am* 6:793–800, 1975

21. Hopkins JS: Lower cervical rheumatoid subluxation with tetraplegia. *J Bone Joint Surg* 49B:46–51, 1967

22. Lidgren L, Ljunggren B, Ratcheson RA: Reposition, anterior exposure and fusion in the treatment of myelopathy caused by rheumatoid arthritis of the cervical spine. *Scand J Rheumatol* 3:195–198, 1974

23. Gutmann L, Hable K: Rheumatoid pachymeningitis. *Neurology* 13:901–905, 1963

24. Lawrence JS, Sharp J, Ball J, et al: Rheumatoid arthritis of the lumbar spine. *Ann Rheum Dis* 23:205–217, 1964

25. Friedman H: Intraspinal rheumatoid nodule causing nerve root compression. *J Neurosurg* 32:689–691, 1970

26. Neustadt DH: Ankylosing spondylitis. *Postgrad Med* 61:124–135, 1977

27. Bergman EW: Fractures of ankylosed spine. *J Bone Joint Surg* 31A:669, 1949

28. Rand RW, Stern WE: Cervical fractures of anklosed rheumatoid spine. *Neurochir* (Stuttgart) 4:137, 1961

29. Woodruff FP, Dewing SB: Fracture of the cervical spine in patients with ankylosing spondylitis. *Radiology* 80:17–21, 1963

30. Lemmen LJ, Laing PG: Fracture of the cervical spine in patients with rheumatoid arthritis. *J Neurosurg* 16:542–550, 1959

31. Grisolia A, Bell RL, Peltier LF: Fractures and dislocations of the spine complicating ankylosing spondylitis. *J Bone Joint Surg* 49A:339–344, 1967

32. Calabro JJ: Medical and surgical management of ankylosing spondylitis. *Clin Orthop* 60:125–148, 1968

33. Hollin SA, Gross SW, Levin P: Fracture of the cervical spine in patients with rheumatoid spondylitis. *Am Surg* 31:532–536, 1965

34. Briedal P: Ossification of the posterior longitudinal ligament in the cervical spine. "The Japanese Disease" in patients of British descent. *Australas Radiol* 13:311–313, 1969

35. Bowie EA, Glasgow GL: Cauda equina lesions associated with ankylosing spondylitis. *Br Med J* 2:24–27, 1961

36. Lee MLH, Waters DJ: Neurological complications of ankylosing spondylitis. *Br Med J* 1:798, 1962

37. Russell ML, Gordon DA, Ogryzlo MA, et al: The cauda equina syndrome of ankylosing spondylitis. *Ann Intern Med* 78:551–554, 1973

38. Rosenkranz W: Ankylosing spondylitis—cauda equina syndrome with multiple spinal arachnoid cysts. *J Neurosurg* 34:241–243, 1971

39. Matthews WB: The neurologic complications of ankylosing spondylitis. *J Neurol Sci* 6:561–573, 1968

40. Parfitt AM, Duncan H: Metabolic bone disease affecting the spine, in Rothman RH and Simeone FA (eds): *The Spine.* Philadelphia, W.B. Saunders, 1978, pp 696–702

41. Schmidek HH: Neurologic and neurosurgical sequalae of Paget's disease of bone. *Clin Orthop* 127:70–77, 1977

42. Wyllie WG: The occurrence in osteitis deformans of lesions of the central nervous system with a report of four cases. *Brain* 46:336–351, 1923

43. Sadar ES, Walton RJ, Gredssman HH: Neurologic dysfunction in Paget's disease of the vertebral column. *J Neurosurg* 37:661–665, 1972

44. Petit-Dutailis D, Marchand J, Garcia Calderon J: Un cas de compression médullaire par maladie osseuse de Paget grandement amelioré par la laminectome. *Rev Neurol* 66:71–78, 1936

45. Whalley N: Paget's disease of atlas and axis. *J Neurol Neurosurg Psychiatry* 9:84–86, 1946

46. Ramamurthi B, Visvanathan GS: Paget's disease of the axis causing paraplegia. *J Neurosurg* *14*:580–583, 1957

47. Feldman F, Seaman WB: The neurological complications of Paget's disease in the cervical spine. *AJR* *105*:375–382, 1969

48. Wycis HT: Basilar impression (platybasia), a case secondary to advanced Paget's disease with severe neurologic manifestations; successful surgical results. *J Neurosurg 1*:299–305, 1944

49. Christman OD, Snook GA, Walker HR: Paget's disease a differential diagnosis in sciatica. *Clin Orthop* *37*:154–159, 1964

50. Finneson BE, Goluboff B, Shenkin HA: Sarcomatous degeneration of osteitis deformans causing compression of cauda equina. *Neurology (Minneap) 8*:82–84, 1958

51. Melick RA, Ebeling P, Hjorth RJ: Improvement in paraplegia in vertebral Paget's disease treated with Calcitonin. *Br Med J 1*:627–628, 1976

52. MacIntyre I, Evans IMA, Hobitz HHG, et al: Chemistry, physiology and therapeutic applications of Calcitonin. *Arthritis Rheum 23*:1139–1147, 1980

53. Ryan WG, Schwartz TB: Mithramycin treatment of Paget's disease of bone. *Arthritis Rheum 23*:1155–1161, 1980

54. Plaut M: Paget's disease of the vertebrae. *J Neurosurg 40*:791, 1974

CHAPTER 92
Surgery of the Peripheral Nerves and Brachial Plexus

Robert D. Leffert

"I would like to see the day when somebody would be appointed surgeon somewhere who has no hands, for the operative part is the least part of the work."   Harvey Cushing
November, 1911[1]

ACCOMPLISHMENTS IN PERIPHERAL NERVE SURGERY in the 70 years since this was written are undeniable proof that it cannot be accepted verbatim. It is, however, immediately apparent to anyone with more that trivial clinical experience that re-establishment of axonal continuity with the end organ, although of major importance to functional recovery, cannot guarantee it. Restoration of function of the paralytic or sense-deficient part depends on a variety of operative and nonoperative techniques involving such nonneural tissue as skin, muscle, bone, and joint. To achieve optimal functional results from the nerve operation, a surgeon must be familiar with these techniques as well as their indications and timing so that alternatives can be evaluated and proper decisions made. Above all, these must be relevant to the patient and his particular needs.

The focus of this work is on current operative neurosurgical techniques, so these will be described in detail and context. Since a thorough and all-inclusive discourse on the subject is impossible in the space available, the reader is referred to an extensive array of pertinent literature, including several major texts and monographs devoted to the subject.[2-5] The advances since Cushing's day have come largely from the carefully documented clinical experience of two world wars[3,6] (and several lesser ones) as well as laboratory research. Technologic improvements in optics and suture material have made microsurgery possible. Without it, the current state of the art would be severely lacking.[7,8]

Many of the peripheral nerve techniques are identically applicable to the brachial plexus, but the specialized nature of this area makes certain individual considerations of diagnosis and treatment necessary. These will be described later.

Before proceeding further, a brief comment should be made on some anatomic, physiologic, and pathologic features of the peripheral nervous system that define it from the central nervous system. The unique potential, under optimal circumstances, for regeneration in the periphery makes successful surgical manipulation possible. This phenomenon, however, primarily depends upon survival of the cell body, without which new axoplasm cannot be synthesized. Then if the supporting stroma of the injured nerve is in continuity, or if alignment of the severed distal segment can be restored and scar does not unduly obstruct the juncture, regeneration can

Department of Orthopaedic Surgery and the Department of Rehabilitation Medicine, Massachusetts General Hospital and the Harvard Medical School, Boston, Massachusetts

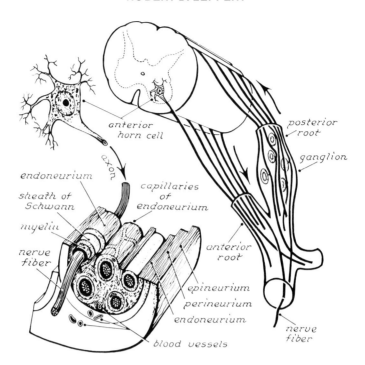

Fig. 92-1. The structure of a typical myelinated peripheral nerve. (Reproduced from Bateman JE: *Trauma to Nerves in Limbs.* Philadelphia, W.B. Saunders, 1962, p 20, with the permission of the author and publisher.)

take place. The metabolic background within which this occurs is complex and only partly understood.[9] In addition to the interdependence of the cell body and axon, the complex structure of the peripheral nerve itself contributes to the difficulty of repair. Although the axon is the conducting medium for the nerve impulse, the supporting fibrous elements and myelin sheathing are of great importance, both under normal and pathologic conditions (Fig. 92-1).

Unfortunately, the simplistic comparison of the peripheral nerve with a telephone cable has

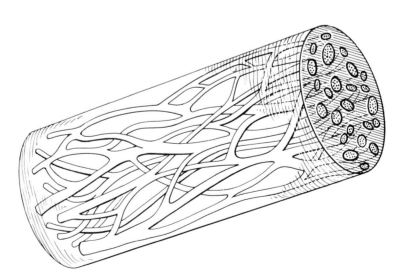

Fig. 92-2. The intraneural topography of a peripheral nerve, adapted from Sunderland.

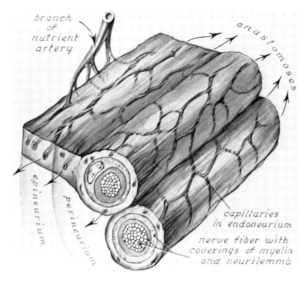

Fig. 92-3. The blood supply of a peripheral nerve. (Reproduced from Bateman JE: *Trauma to Nerves in Limbs*. Philadelphia, W.B. Saunders, 1962, p 29, with the permission of the author and publisher.)

led to many illogical and unsuccessful attempts at surgical repair of damaged nerves. The monumental work of Sunderland[5] in demonstrating the intraneural topography of major peripheral nerves has provided an anatomic substrate within which the surgeon may work (Fig. 92-2).

The constantly changing pattern of groups of fibers within a nerve, as it traverses the limb, helps to explain why long gaps caused by injury, even if they can be overcome, often lead to poor operative results. Since the pattern does not remain constant for more than 1.5 cm, this imposes a limit on just how many potential axon-bearing sheaths may be reunited following a lengthy resection.

Furthermore, even though peripheral nerves are abundantly supplied with blood vessels at all structural levels (Fig. 92-3) and these are arranged both segmentally and longitudinally, it cannot be assumed that extensive mobilization will not have an adverse effect on their nutrition, or that destruction or ligation of adjacent vessels will not prejudice the ultimate result.

There are two specific situations wherein the presence of an intraneural artery may prove troublesome. Both the sciatic nerve and the median nerve have well-developed and relatively constant arteries. In the sciatic, a laceration of the intraneural artery that leaves the bulk of the nerve intact can cause catastrophic pressure necrosis of the surrounding fascicles, if it is not relieved promptly. A suture of the median nerve under tourniquet ischemia may rupture once arterial flow is re-established, if the artery is not microcoagulated and the epineural closure is tight.

Mechanism of Injury

The peripheral nerves may be injured by a variety of types of trauma, which can act singly or in combination (Table 92-1).

Table 92-1. Mechanism of Injury

Compression	Ischemia
Traction	Chemical injury
Laceration	Thermal or cold injury

Table 92-2. Three Types of Nerve Injury

	Neurapraxia	Axonotmesis	Neurotmesis
Common causes	Compression Traction Freezing Ischemia Missiles	Compression Traction Missiles Ischemia Freezing Friction	Lacerations Missiles Traction Injections Ischemia
Pathology (may involve all or part of anatomical nerve circumference)	Local Demyelination, *no* axonal interruption	Axonal interruption, supporting stroma (Schwann sheaths intact)	Axonal and sheath interruption
Clinical findings	Complete motor paralysis, incomplete or lesser sensory loss	Complete motor and sensory loss	Complete motor and sensory loss
EMG	Rare fibrillations, no voluntary action potentials	Fibrillations > 3 wk. No voluntary action potentials	Fibrillations > 3 wk. No voluntary action potentials
Operative findings	Continuity preserved	Continuity preserved. Occasional neuro- matous swelling	Anatomic gap surgically repaired, then 1 mm/day with delays
Spontaneous recovery and timing	Usually by 4-6 wk, in no regular order of innervation	1 mm/day in order of innervation	None unless surgically repaired, then 1 mm/day with delays
Quality of recovery	Normal	Usually normal	Never completely normal even after surgical repair

Adapted from Seddon.[10]

These may not only involve different components of the nerve, but different lengths as well. For example, knife wounds are characteristically discrete and involve small segments, while traction injuries usually involve longer lengths and are harder to delineate.

In addition, the injury may be immediate, such as a gunshot wound, or delayed, as in the traction-friction neuritis presenting as a tardy ulnar palsy years after an elbow fracture. Therefore, an almost infinite variety of clinical presentations of nerve injury is possible, leaving the surgeon with a very difficult-to-definite state of pathology on which to attempt to define rational management. Fortunately, however, traumatized nerves react in a reasonably predictable fashion. Although a number of classifications and descriptions of the type of nerve injury have been advanced, that of Seddon,[10] who defined three basic varieties of nerve injury, has, in my opinion, proved most workable (Table 92-2).

Degeneration and Regeneration

A brief discussion of the sequence of events involved in the process of degeneration of a transected nerve and regeneration following repair will serve as a physiologic background against which to interpret the technical procedures available.

Within 4 days after the nerve is severed, all conductivity in the distal segment is lost. Axons and myelin sheaths disintegrate and are ingested by macrophages and Schwann cells. This active process is called *Wallerian degeneration*. A proliferation of Schwann cells and endoneurial fibrocytes causes the cut end of the distal stump to swell, with the result that it is initially enlarged. With time, the cellular population diminishes, endoneurial tubes shrink, and collagen is laid down around them so that the whole distal part of the nerve shrinks. The proximal segment undergoes similar changes in its distal stump, over a very short segment, without shrinkage, but significant effects of the injury also are recorded in the parent cell body. Depending upon the severity and proximity of the injury, the neuron may undergo complete destruction, or more usually, begin manufacturing increased amounts of RNA in preparation for regeneration. The axoplasm streams out of the tangle of Schwann cells and collagen to form a randomly arranged and bulbous neuroma. If, however, with a primary suture, the supporting elements of the nerve have been accurately aligned and opposed, vigorous proliferation of Schwann cells and fibroblasts of the distal segment causes them to reach proximally, in an orderly fashion, and align themselves longitudinally. With correct orientation, then, more of the axons may find their way into the proper distal endothelial tubes. Suture within 3 months of injury is called *early secondary suture*. The cellular hyperplasia is then at its highest level and the epineurium is thickened, so that if epineurial sutures are used, they will hold solidly. The extent of scarring is delineated more easily than immediately post injury, but greater resection usually is necessary. Beyond 3 months, suture will be *late secondary*, and although Schwann tubes may remain open for longer than 6 months, there is proportional diminution in their available number and size, with decreased quality of the end result.

Diagnosis of Peripheral Nerve Injury

"When in doubt, do a history and physical. . . ."   Anon.

Although this maxim would seem both inappropriate and unnecessary, many nerve injuries escape initial detection in a massively traumatized patient or a situation wherein a surgeon caring for an injured extremity is introduced to a patient already under anesthesia. The implications of first noting the nerve deficit after treatment are obviously unfortunate. Careful notation of when the neurologic loss occurred is mandatory, both in fresh cases and those seen after a delay. Since many patients are seen late, it is necessary to establish whether motor and sensory loss have changed in the interval. The presence of associated injuries in the limb and their sequelae must be considered, since they can affect what is done to a significant degree. Information about the patient's occupation and previous function, as well as the circumstances and mechanism of injury, are pertinent parts of the record, as is the presence or absence of pain.

Physical examination, in addition to discrete neurologic examination, must include an accurate assessment of the position of wounds, character of scarring, and tissue quality, as well as the range of motion of joints, the presence of contractures, and vascular status.

For peripheral nerve injuries involving the limbs, it is necessary to determine that there are no nerve lesions proximal to the obvious one under consideration.

The assessment of motor power depends on the ability of the examiner to perform manual muscle tests accurately and with full knowledge of so-called trick and supplementary motions. Although the virtual disappearance of paralytic poliomyelitis has made this technique harder to master, several available manuals are quite helpful.[11] Records should be detailed, accurate, and standardized. An acceptable scale is that of the British Medical Research Council.[3]

Sensory testing in the presence of nerve injury should include determination of light touch, using a fine brush or wisp of cotton, and a pin for pain sensibility. Where applicable, in the fingertips, two-point discrimination should be tested with a blunt caliper or two paperclips held in such a way that the distance between their ends is constant. This last examination is an indication of stereognosis, a higher type of sensory function, without which the hand may have protective sensibility but still be *blind*, especially for activities where eye-hand coordination cannot compensate for deficient feedback. The *coin test* provides additional data on function of the hand. This and other functional evaluations may be far more informative than the standardized neurologic testing of individual modalities.

The value of Tinel's sign, eliciting paresthesias in the distribution of an injured peripheral nerve by percussion over its course, has been much debated and misunderstood.[13,14] If one taps over the point of injury, assuming the nerve is not deeply buried, a tingling sensation will be felt distally. Since it is a central phenomenon, this would happen even if the limb were amputated at that level. If some time has elapsed during which regeneration could have taken place, however, and tapping over the nerve distal to the injury produces tingling, then one can assume that at least some axons have reached this point. If, with further passage of time, the sign becomes less positive at the point of injury and more distal, this indicates that further downgrowth of axons has occurred. A persistently positive response at the site of injury and nothing distally bodes ill for recovery, but since only part of the total area of a nerve may have been injured and has been providing this response, an advancing Tinel's sign cannot be taken as assurance that functional recovery will ensue. Furthermore, since smaller and immature axons are responsible for the response, there is no way of determining that more and larger-diameter axons eventually will follow.

Objective electrodiagnostic testing in the form of electromyography and nerve conduction velocity determination has emerged from studies of nerve in the neurophysiologic laboratory to provide a most useful adjunct to the management of nerve injuries.[15] Although an inexperienced or ill-advised electromyographer may serve only to obfuscate, when viewed within the perspective of the clinical situation, the test is often of critical value.

By means of small percutaneous needle electrodes, fibrillation potentials may be detected at rest in partially or completely denervated muscle after about 3 weeks, when Wallerian degeneration has taken place. Since they are entirely outside of the patient's control, they have total objectivity, dependent, of course, on the ability of the observer to correctly interpret them. The pattern, on attempted voluntary contraction, may indicate partial denervation, or sequential observations may document recovery before it can be detected clinically.

Nerve conduction velocity determination,[16] an offshoot of electromyography, may be used to localize the site of a lesion of a peripheral nerve, and is particularly useful in compression lesions. Both motor and sensory components may be measured. Measurement of *evoked potentials* in the evaluation of neuromas-in-continuity at surgery has greatly expanded the use of this modality.[17]

Although of historic interest, the use of chronaxie and strength-duration curves has declined with the refinement of the preceding modalities.

Since the autonomic fibers supplying the skin have the same distribution as sensory fibers, observation of sudomotor function can be a useful adjunct to evaluation. A magnifying glass for visualization, a micro-ohmeter to measure electrical skin resistance, or Moberg's ninhydrin test all essentially provide the same information.

General Operative Indications

It is most important to know when not to attempt to repair an injured peripheral nerve. Although few dicta can realistically be accepted as absolute, the following can be useful in formulating operative indications in particular cases.

When the muscles to be reinnervated are severely atrophic, fibrotic, or so distant that years would be required for recovery; if sensation is present or of much lesser importance; or if the motor lesion is partial, then restoration of deficient motor function by appropriate tendon transfers rather than by nerve repair should be done. This is particularly applicable to intrinsic muscles in the hand but is applicable in other areas as well. Lesions that have a generally poor prognosis, such as severe traction injury of the peroneal nerve accompanying rupture of the lateral knee ligaments in adults, often are better not explored secondarily to "see what happens," although individual cases may be benefited. The use of tendon transfers or light plastic braces or both may prove more satisfactory. An elderly patient with a high radial nerve lesion caused by laceration usually will derive considerably more functional benefit immediately and in the long term from tendon transfer to restore wrist and finger extension than from attempts to suture or graft the nerve. A patient seen years after a median nerve injury may not regain motor function after surgery, but since median nerve sensibility is so important, an attempt to restore it even partially is reasonable as long as 5 years later. If the ulnar nerve is intact, thought should be given to neurovascular island pedicle transfer to restore sensibility to the thumb if nerve repair cannot be done or if repair fails.[13] Long-term follow-up of these patients, however, often reveals that although sensation is restored to the thumb, the patient still will refer it to the donor finger and not make the transfer. Recent developments in free tissue transfer have enlarged the possibilities for sensory reconstruction considerably. Isolated complete lesions of the posterior tibial nerve low in the adult leg may, if repaired, regenerate imperfectly and result in disabling dysesthesia of the skin of the plantar surface of the foot. This lesion must be carefully considered preoperatively, since if the adjacent cutaneous nerves are intact, the sole rarely will be completely anesthetic.

Finally, local conditions in the limbs, such as poor soft tissue cover for the proposed repair, which will predispose to scarring, must be corrected preoperatively. If posturing of joints will be necessary to accomplish mobilization and coaptation of a nerve, then they must be mobile to allow for this maneuver.

Gunshot wounds constitute a dilemma in that often the nerve deficit is caused by a *near-miss* and the shock wave that momentarily deforms the nerve. Unless there is concomitant bone or vascular injury that requires immediate attention, or the track of the bullet, as measured by entrance and exit wounds, could not possibly have missed cutting the nerve, there is little to be gained from immediate exploration, and one should wait out the period of neurapraxia—usually 6 weeks.

Because of the likelihood of neurotmesis when a sharp object, such as a knife or glass, has caused a significant nerve injury, all such wounds should be explored, although a small percentage of them will recover spontaneously. The timing of the procedure, however, continues to be a controversial issue between those who favor immediate primary repair, and those who will electively postpone definitive surgery. Although numerous clinical theories endorsing each approach exist,[4,5,19] they generally suffer from a lack of precise statistical comparability to account for all pertinent factors. Rather than endorse one method or the other as in "voting the straight ticket," the surgeon should be aware of the advantages and disadvantages to be weighed in his particular case. In order to allow for primary repair, a nerve wound should be a clean laceration, without significant additional tissue damage or contamination in a patient whose general condition will not be endangered by what could be a lengthy operative procedure. An experienced surgeon and operating team should be available and the wound should not be over 24 hours old. The patient should have been on antibiotics during the interval. Children are good candidates for primary repair, since their prognosis for nerve repair is superior. Digital nerves and clean cuts of median and ulnar nerves at the wrist should be repaired primarily, since in the latter case the fascicles are readily identifiable. Because of the high percentage of nonfascicular tissue in the nerves at this level and the pure composition of the bundles themselves, the penalty for malrotation is severe in terms of axons that go astray.

The negative side of primary repair, in addition to the possibly increased risk of infection because of additional surgical manipulation and the time required to accomplish it, is the very real difficulty of being able to accurately assess the condition of the nerve ends in a fresh wound. Obviously, repair of compromised tissue that commits the patient to a long wait, only to realize an unsatisfactory result, is to be avoided. If there is significant doubt, one should wait and do a secondary repair when the wound has healed per primum and delineation is easier; however, this usually requires greater resection of the nerve ends. The issue has become less of a problem since the operating microscope has been available; at high magnification, a more informed picture of the condition of the fascicles is possible.

Despite what could be intuitively concluded about the treatment of nerves in limbs re-planted following traumatic amputation, it is now generally believed by those with the greatest experience in this area, including the Chinese, that primary repair of these nerves is preferable. Documentation of these results will take years to accumulate, however.

The management of nerve injuries accompanying fractures and dislocations should be divided into: (1) closed injuries, where a skeletal injury may be assumed to have caused the nerve injury; and (2) open injuries, where the fracture usually is incidental to the wounding agent that also injures the nerve. In the latter case, indications are those of the isolated nerve injury. Closed fractures and dislocations rarely cause neurotmesis, and in most cases expectant treatment eventuates in recovery. The best example of this is a closed transverse fracture of the midshaft of the humerus with a radial palsy. The anatomic position of the nerve relative to the fracture makes it unlikely that the nerve is caught in fracture fragments. Therefore, knowing the level of fracture and nerve injury and the distance to the first motor branch, the brachioradialis, calculation at the rate of 1 inch per month should set an outer limit of time allowed for spontaneous recovery. If this interval is exceeded, and neither electromyographic nor clinical evidence of recovery is present, then the nerve should be explored. It is important to recognize that the radial palsy accompanying long oblique fractures of the humerus at the junction of the upper two-thirds and lower one-third is likely to result from the anatomic propensity of the nerve at this level to be entrapped in the fracture. These should be explored primarily and the nerve decompressed while the fracture is fixed internally.[20]

In general, sciatic nerve injury accompanying hip dislocations recovers spontaneously, while those injuries with acetabular fractures more often require operative release. A palsy that arises after manipulation of a fracture or dislocation, when no such lesion pre-existed, in my opinion, usually should be explored.

Anesthesia

The prolonged and meticulous nature of peripheral nerve surgery makes general anesthesia preferable in most cases. Since nerve grafts may have to be obtained from the lower extremities in procedures on the upper extremity, this would necessitate a general anesthetic. Since the continued use of muscle relaxants may interfere with intraoperative diagnostic nerve stimulation, this phase of the procedure must be discussed with the anesthetist in advance. Undoubtedly, there are many operations of lesser magnitude, such as carpal tunnel release or other decompressions, or even sutures, that can be performed in satisfactory fashion under regional anesthesia. Some patients, however, dislike experiencing additional numbness, even temporarily, in a limb that is already neurologically abnormal. Intravenous regional anesthesic, however, precludes letting down of the tourniquet, so that hemostasis may be assured before completing a neurorrhaphy.

Aids to Surgery

Time is well spent in planning the sequence of maneuvers in an operation on a peripheral nerve, especially if it is done along with tendon, bone, or vascular repair. This precaution usually will avoid embarrassing compromise during or after the procedure. Assuming it will not impose additional hazards to the patient under anesthesia, the position chosen should be selected for ease of surgical approach. The surgeon and operating team are comfortably seated at an absolutely steady table that will permit the surgeon to support his forearms to avoid fatigue. A number of *hand tables* have been designed and are available, but they need not be elaborate as long as they fulfill the above criteria. In addition, as a result of the technologic explosion accompanying microsurgery, a number of complicated, motorized surgeon's chairs have been suggested. We continue to use conventional operating room stools.

Preparation and draping should be done to allow for extensile exposure, and, if necessary, posturing of the limbs. Potential graft sites are covered with sterile drapes before the procedure begins so that if the sites are needed, breaks in technique will not be likely. If sural nerve grafts are to be used, the lower extremity should be prepared to the tips of the toes, and the limb left mobile and draped free to avoid the aggravation of having to "stand on one's head" to harvest the grafts.

Although tourniquet ischemia and a bloodless field are not absolutely essential to peripheral nerve surgery, they can markedly facilitate exposure and identification of vital structures, especially in a scarred or previously explored area. Unless there is an anatomic or physiologic contraindication to the tourniquet, I use it routinely for at least the preliminary exposure and preparation of the nerve. Obviously it is contraindicated in the presence of significant vascular disease. In some situations in which the configuration of the part or position of the wound prevents the use of a standard pneumatic tourniquet, a pediatric-sized cuff may be used with benefit. A gas-sterilized or disposable pneumatic cuff also is a possibility, but the Esmarch or Martin bandage should be restricted to preliminary exsanguination rather than used as the definitive tourniquet in an awkward situation. If it is used, there is no way of quantitating the amount of compression produced by multiple turns of the rubber bandage at the root of the limb. The risk of tourniquet palsy with this method is significant, but it may be considered acceptable under some circumstances.

Even with commercially available pneumatic tourniquets, the continued accuracy of a pressure gauge cannot be ensured, so periodic and frequent calibration against a mercury manometer standard is a good safety measure. Recommended inflation pressures for the adult upper extremity range from 250 to 375 mm Hg, and for the lower extremity, 350 to 550 mm Hg. These should be adjusted according to measured systolic blood pressure and the size of the patient's limb. There is no universally accepted time limit for tourniquet ischemia. My own practice is not to exceed 2.5 hours in the upper extremity. By the end of this period, that part of the procedure requiring the tourniquet usually has been accomplished. A double tourniquet cuff may be used in situations in which prolonged ischemia is required, since alternating the portion of the cuff that is inflated will diminish the total time that any particular segment of nerve is subjected to significant compression. It should be remembered that if electrical stimulation of the nerve is to be part of the procedure, it will have to be accomplished before 20 to 30 minutes of ischemia have passed, since nerve transmission normally ceases under these circumstances.

Use of the nerve stimulator to assess the condition of a neuroma-in-continuity is an extremely valuable technique. Even though voluntary contraction of a paralyzed muscle may not be possible, direct nerve stimulation at open operation may identify axonal continuity and prevent unnecessary resection of damaged but recovering nerves. Neurolysis in the midst of dense scar may be impossible without a stimulator. Kline and Nulsen[17] have described in detail the technique of evoked potentials in the evaluation of lesions in continuity. It is extremely useful, but requires sophisticated electromyographic equipment at the operating table.

The proliferation of specialized instruments for microsurgery has created a bewildering array of available equipment that can be used for nerve suture. In addition to the usual forceps, needle holders, and scissors, which are part of the armamentarium of any neurosurgical cabinet, many new instruments have evolved from microvascular surgery. These are well suited to peripheral nerve repair, and each surgeon tends (often quite arbitrarily) to prefer one instrument type or another. In general, needle holders that do not lock are advantageous, since they do not jar when opened and closed under high magnification. Forceps, too, are almost infinite in their variety and advocates, but we tend to use the simple *watchmaker's* or *jeweler's* forceps without teeth. They are minimally traumatic to delicate tissues, but, as with all such instruments, their tips must be protected against damage, especially during sterilization and storage, when it is wise to keep them and all microinstruments in cases specially designed for the purpose.

If a neuroma that occupies the entire circumference of a nerve is to be resected or if epineurial suture or a cable graft is to be performed, then it will be desirable to cut all fascicles at the same level and at right angles to the length of the nerve. Since normal peripheral nerve fascicles have the consistency and rigidity of wet spaghetti, it is often difficult to achieve the desired neat, sharp cut by simply drawing a scalpel blade across the nerve. The nerve tends to deform as it is cut, with the result that the epineurium may shred, or fascicles may be cut on the bias or at different levels. To obviate this problem, a number of ingenious neurotomes and miniature miter boxes have been designed.[21] They may be helpful in achieving the desired result. In the hands of a very experienced surgeon, a very sharp manual dermatome blade or a fresh razor blade can be used, while steadying the nerve against a wooden tongue depressor. The indelicate practice of pinning the nerve to the tongue depressor proximal to the line of section to steady it so it can be tensioned is to be avoided. A diamond knife for microsurgical repair of nerves has been adapted from one introduced into microsurgery by Microsurgical Instrument Research Association.[22] This is said to be valuable in interfascicular dissection of neuromas. A simple, practical, and economic way of aiding the right-angle section of nerves before repair has been proposed by Clark.[23] He encloses the nerve within a paper sheath and grasps the free leaves of paper with a right-angle clamp before sectioning through it. This allows the axons to be held in a cyclindric form without being crushed or rolled under the pressure of a razor blade.

Suture material has been the subject of much discussion. There are many advantages and disadvantages of various materials demonstrated in animal experiments. Although there have been great technical advances in the uniformity, tensile strength, and reactivity of suture material, there is still no ideal material. The search goes on. At the present time, 8-0 and 10-0 monofilament nylon swaged on needles are the sutures of choice for most peripheral nerve repairs. The use of plasma clot as a means of joining nerves has been shown to be effective by Tarlov and others;[24,25] however, there has been little recent enthusiasm for the method.

There is now no serious doubt that magnification must be employed in the surgery of peripheral nerves. What remains to be seen is just how much magnification is necessary, assuming a constant degree of surgical ability and visual acuity. From a purely practical point of view, most surgeons (and nurses) can barely see 10-0 suture without magnification. This should not lead to an immediate mandate that all sutures be done with $25,000 microscopes at 40X magnification, however. The simpler devices available to achieve magnification range from loupes to operating telescopes on eyeglass frames. The former are inexpensive but rarely give more than 2X, and the operating telescopes come in various strengths up to 6X. The depth of field with these is very shallow and they do not have a focused light source. A practical compromise are the eyeglass telescopes with 3.5X magnification, which can be used for preliminary dissection.

The market in operating microscopes can readily be compared, somewhat facetiously, to the used-car market, with a bewildering array of basic models and numerous options and accessories, including power controls. Interestingly enough, the prices tend to parallel and even exceed automobile prices. Very simply, there are less expensive models that clamp on to the operating table and more elaborate ones with fiberoptic light sources and multiple heads as well as provisions for photography and TV.

The addition of a counterbalanced portable floor mount conveys stability, which at extremely high magnifications may be further enhanced by permanent floor or ceiling mounts.

The optical characteristics of the system and, therefore, the degree of magnification and clarity depend on the combination of ocular and objectives. For most types of microsurgery, a 200- to 300-mm focal-length objective will be suitable. The focal length of the objective will determine the working distance, which can be varied according to the topography and location of the operative field. Eyepieces ranging from 10X to 20X are available.

Most microscopes have a magnification-changer setting that can be applied to a particular combination of ocular and objective to achieve a desired result. The actual degree of magnification cannot, as one would assume, be read directly from the changer setting on the microscope, but will be found by consulting the chart that comes with each instrument. Although the degree of available magnification may, in some systems, vary from 1.5 to 40X, the degree of magnification actually employed at any time will vary according to the specific part of the procedure being done and the preferences of the surgeon. Some surgeons find that for peripheral nerve repair, the six-fold magnification provided by the operating telescopes is sufficient, while others prefer the microscope. Ease of modifying the field and magnification is greatly enhanced by motorized zoom, positioning, and focusing with foot controls. Obviously this adds to the cost. Finally, the sterile draping of the microscope and stand may prove to be a logistic annoyance. To obviate this, commercial plastic microscope drapes are available, and some microscopes are designed with autoclavable handles and do not require sterile draping.

Technique

The operative approaches to major peripheral nerves in the limbs have been well illustrated in standard references.[2,4,26] Time and space do not permit their recapitulation here. The peripheral nerve surgeon must be prepared to expose a nerve throughout its length, with due regard for avoiding vital structures and producing hypertrophic scars and contractures, but without apology for the length of the incision, if anatomic considerations so dictate. In the presence of scarring and neuroma formation, the dissection should begin in normal tissue, both proximally and distally if possible, so that all important structures can be identified and preserved. Dissection then is carried centripetally to expose the area of nerve damage.

If one is dealing with a compression lesion, or by reason of the pathogenesis, an incomplete clinical deficit, then simple decompression is indicated, and the prognosis for recovery should be favorable. A common example of this is the carpal tunnel release. Even here, however, if the nerve shows evidence of epineurial thickening, or the surface vascular pattern remains interrupted after the transverse carpal ligament has been divided, then careful circumferential removal of the epineurium under magnification is indicated. I do not use saline injection under the epineurium as a test of the adequacy of decompression, or a substitute for manual neurolysis, since without relieving the constriction of tight epineurium, little would appear to be gained. Whether one should perform an additional interneural lysis under magnification[27] is debated, since cross connections between fascicles, or the bundles themselves, could conceivably be injured during the dissection.

Neurolysis—the act of mechanically freeing a nerve from scar—would appear to be a logical and reasonable operation. Yet there are fewer procedures more often done for poorer indications than this one, and quite commonly, either nothing positive is accomplished, or the recovery that is observed postoperatively would have occurred spontaneously had the surgeon waited a while longer.[28]

The least controversial and best indication for neurolysis is documented compression, and if it can be relieved without likelihood of supervening scarring, then the chances of recovery are significantly enhanced. If, however, nothing more is done than to simply incise the scar and observe the nerve, the procedure will produce at best a temporary improvement. If the basic anatomic surroundings of the nerve or its blood supply can be favorably influenced, however, there may be substantial benefit. A transposition of a nerve into a favorable bed would be a positive example, as for traction-friction neuropathy of the ulnar nerve at the elbow, while exploration of nerves scarred by radiation fibrosis would be unfavorable. In addition, there is always the risk of intraoperative mechanical injury to the nerve itself or of stripping it of its remaining blood supply. Neurolysis in situations where recovery has been documented as having ceased or actually regressed is legitimate. The treatment of various types of injection injury to nerves remains controversial and specific to the nature of the noxious agent and time elapsed since injury. Penicillin is particularly neurotoxic, and injection injuries caused by penicillin should be subjected to neurolysis if they are seen within the first day or so. The indication for neurolysis for infections is extremely narrow since peripheral nerves are ordinarily remarkably resistant to infection, with the leprosy bacillus being a significant and invasive exception. The two final conditions often cited as reasons for doing a neurolysis—pain and poor result from suture—are, in my opinion, rarely proper indications, although the occasional case for the former situation may occur.

If the lesion is of long duration, the neurologic deficit is complete, and a neuroma in continuity is encountered at surgery, it still may be possible that the lesion is an axonotmesis rather than a neurotmesis. Obviously, to experience recovery without having to do a formal resection and neurorrhaphy or graft would eventuate in a better result, but the proper identification of the nature of the lesion may be difficult. The appearance of the neuroma may be deceptive, although the extremely attenuated or very large and firm ones usually are not functional and require resection. The intraoperative use of a nerve stimulator may provide valuable information, and the measuring of nerve action potentials directly from the nerve, as described by Kline and Nulsen[17] is a refinement that can be of benefit, although it requires specialized equipment and expertise.

Closed injuries to peripheral nerves resulting from fractures and dislocations must be evaluated in light of the magnitude and nature of the trauma that produced them as well as the pathomechanics of the lesion and its specific location. This has already been commented upon.

The management of documented complete transections of peripheral nerves is the most difficult and controversial aspect of the subject under discussion. Simply stated, the object of the procedure is to re-establish axonal continuity with the periphery in such a fashion that maximal neurologic function is restored. An ecumenical and complete historical review might prove interesting (or tedious), but a series of straw men erected only to be knocked down is of little comfort to the surgeon faced with the immediate problem of managing a neurotmesis. The question of primary or secondary nerve repair already has been discussed. Having made either choice, the remaining decisions concern how to get the correct fascicles together when that part determined to be damaged has been resected. Inspection of the cut end of the nerve under magnification is an indicator of adequate resection but does not assure the absence of fibrosis or other impediments to regeneration. The variable gap that results may call for more than a single solution, and one ought to be prepared to consider alternatives. There is general agreement that excessive tension on the suture line is the most deleterious factor mitigating against success in nerve repair, assuming fascicular orientation is correct. In order to avoid tension at the suture line, mobilization of the nerve from its bed (and segmental blood supply) may be carried out. The question remains just how far this can be done before it becomes self-defeating.

The first half of this century saw the establishment of empirically determined *critical resection lengths*[4] for each nerve, limits within which one could expect regeneration following neurorrhaphy. Of course, the absolute lengths of nerve were really very rough guides, not referable to the height and length of the extremity of the patient under consideration, and based on rather indefinite criteria for success of the procedure. They are, therefore, of very limited value. Assuming the nerve was sufficiently mobilized proximally and distally, then, in order to coapt the ends, the adjacent joints would have to be postured accordingly and held with a splint or cast for 3 weeks until healing at the suture line was sufficient to allow gradual stretching. Although it may be possible by total mobilization, transposition, and acute posturing of all joints to actually get the nerve ends together, such maneuvers usually end in failure because when the extreme position is reduced, the result is either a rupture, or more likely, a severe traction lesion of the nerve that precludes recovery. In general, for repairs of the median or ulnar nerves, if the elbow must be flexed more than 90° or the wrist 40° to achieve coaptation, then excessive tension will be present when full range is resumed, and the prognosis is poor. At the knee, 90° of flexion, with the hip in neutral, should not be exceeded.

Epineurial suture, in which sutures are placed only in the outer layer of the epineurium without surgical manipulation of the fascicles themselves, has been the accepted and most widely employed method of joining severed nerves until the recent emergence of microsurgical techniques. As surgeons realized that they not only could clearly visualize individual fascicles within a nerve, but actually could place sutures in them, enthusiasm grew for repairing progressively smaller subunits of peripheral nerves until virtually no fascicle was immune to the needle and thread of the aggressive repairer of nerves. The controversy over this subject is still raging, but I believe that Sir Sidney Sunderland's observations[5,29] as well as recent experimental work[30,31] have helped considerably in providing perspective in a field where the "triumph of technology over reason" is a constant threat. In general, I believe that with the exceptions to be described, if suture is possible (rather than a graft), then it should be epineurial rather than fascicular, since the evidence is not convincing that the additional time, obligatory intraoperative trauma, and additional suture material that undoubtedly causes scarring will eventuate in a superior result. The exception to this dictum is in situations where the ratio of intraneural epineurium to fascicles is high or the fascicles are quite discrete and identifiable as specific branches. In these situations, which pertain at the elbow and wrist, groups of like fascicles may be sutured in order to avoid having their axons misdirected into intraneural epineurium or foreign endoneural tubes. It should be stated, however, that the sutures actually are placed in the condensed internal epineurium that surrounds the groups of fascicles and the external epineurium actually is removed over the repair, as suggested by Millesi et al.[32]

In all nerve repair, the handling of the nerve must be minimized, and then handled only gently, with microinstruments, rubber drain retractors, or fingers. Hemostasis is essential, so the tourniquet should be down and all bleeding points stopped before suture is performed. A suitable background that will allow visualization of the fascicles and fine sutures may be provided by a piece of sterilized, light-colored plastic, such as that used for household garbage bags.[33] Correct fascicular orientation may be aided by matching the alignment of surface blood vessels, if these are visible. Sometimes the nerve will simply lie in correct rotatory position, but it may not, especially if it has been malrotated by a previous attempt at repair. Inspection under magnification of the fascicular pattern at the resection surfaces is the best guide to alignment, and although exact correspondence usually is not found, major groups of bundles can be identified and approximated. Once this has been established, the epineurial repair is commenced by means of two traction sutures introduced at the edges 180° apart and left long so that they may be held by micro bulldog clamps. This maneuver will permit turning the nerve so that simple interrupted sutures may be used to close the circumference of the epineurium without deforming the fascicles. Only as many sutures as are required to achieve this are used, according to the size of the nerve. It should be remembered that the suture material is a foreign body that may, with remodeling, actually become incorporated within the substance of the nerve. Usually no more than six to eight sutures, and preferably fewer, are needed. Despite claims that wrapping the suture line with foreign material will diminish fibrosis and improve results, there is no conclusive proof that this is so, but the list of materials so employed is long and varied. A number of these actually have proved to be deleterious on long-term evaluation. To date, there is no ideal substance for this purpose, and their use is not recommended.

For lesions that result in gaps that cannot be overcome, as described with posturing the joints or anatomic maneuvers such as anterior transposition of the ulnar nerve, grafting provides a useful alternative. After years of uncertainty, it is quite clear now that fresh autogenous grafts are the donor material of choice. Usually cutaneous nerves are preferred because they can be sacrificed with less significant residual deficit, and their smaller diameter makes central necrosis during revascularization less likely. The sural nerve has become the most popular donor, and in an average adult as much as 35 cm may be obtained by multiple transverse incisions in the calf and mobilization in the intervals. A long incision from the popliteal space to the lateral ankle is easier technically and even may be necessary, but it is less desirable in its ultimate appearance. Cutaneous nerves in the upper extremity may be used, but it would be imprudent to sacrifice one that is providing sensation to an area adjacent to that already denervated. If a mixed nerve has been severed and is not to be reconstituted, it may serve as donor, but this situation is becoming progressively less common, and the risk of central necrosis of the thicker graft is a disadvantage in their use.

The grafts may be employed in several ways. They may be placed side by side in the manner of the cable and sutured to the epineurium of the host proximally and distally, usually with one

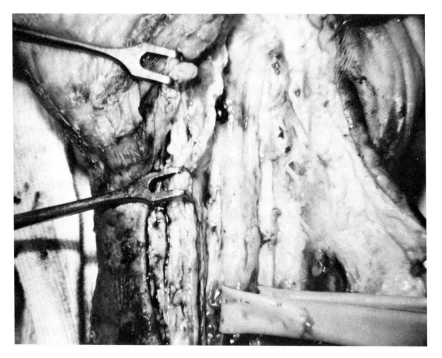

Fig. 92-4. The volar aspect of the distal forearm 5 months following a close-range shotgun wound. The median nerve is embedded in the scar in the carpal tunnel.

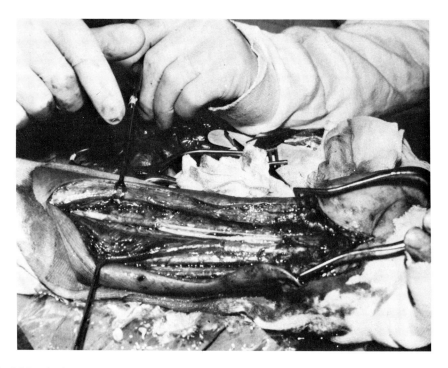

Fig. 92-5. A 10-cm segment of the scarred median nerve has been replaced by four cables of sural-nerve graft.

suture per strand. It then is possible to cover the cross-sectional area of the nerve and preserve longitudinal orientation. Presumably the fascicles will find their way to the corresponding radial segment of the distal end of the nerve (Figs. 92-4, 92-5, and 92-6). This type of repair by graft is only indicated in situations where the fascicular pattern is not readily apparent or clearly defined, and the gaps are long, as in the illustration. When groups of fascicles are recognized, it is preferable to excise host epineurium and suture the grafts between corresponding groups in order to preserve orientation and apposition that might otherwise be lost. For partial lesions, or lateral neuromas, an inlay graft of this type rather than a *loop suture* may provide good results, despite the theoretical objections to two suture lines as opposed to one.

The foregoing discussion describes the general concept of nerve grafting as a salvage procedure, and although some workers devoted to meticulous technique were able to document results that were satisfactory,[34] the overall impression was not particularly favorable. The presentation of the concept of grafting a priori, by Millesi and his colleagues,[31,32] is a radical departure from past practice. It evolved from realization of the deleterious effects of tension at the suture line as well as their laboratory studies showing that the epineurium contributed significantly to the fibrosis that impeded regeneration past the suture. This, then, while a technique for secondary nerve repair, is an alternative to attempting mobilization, and if it is not feasible, grafting should be used. The criteria for the median and ulnar nerves of Millesi et al. are as follows.

All cases are grafted except:

1. If the gap in the nerve is 2 cm or less and the nerve ends can be approximated without tension when the joints of the extremity are in full extension.
2. For the ulnar nerve at the elbow, gaps of up to 4 cm that can be closed without tension by anterior transposition.
3. A nerve gap accompanying nonunion of a fracture that requires surgery may be closed and sutured following shortening of the bone.[32]

The important differences between this technique and that of the cable graft should be noted. Millesi advocates interfascicular grafting rather than epineurial bridging. Under magnification, the neuroma is approached from both ends, but rather than preserving the epineurium and transecting all fascicles at the same level, he dissects and transects each major fascicle and group of minor ones at the point of injury and then maps them before proceeding to the distal stump, where the same process is repeated. The epineurium is resected from both ends, and then corresponding fascicles or groups are united by interposed grafts, usually of sural nerve, with the epineurium of each graft fixed by one fine suture to the internal epineurium surrounding the host fascicles. The suture lines are, therefore, staggered as the pathology dictates. The limb is immobilized for 10 days, following which active exercises can begin. The results of this technique have been described by Millesi to be at least as good as those achieved after epineurial suture under ideal conditions and better than those after neurorrhaphy under tension.[35]

One hopes that the long-term evaluation of a strictly controlled and comparable clinical series of peripheral nerve injuries managed by these alternate methods will eventually clarify these issues.

A number of unusual methods of handling special situations in peripheral nerve surgery have been developed. Both nerve transfer and pedicle grafts[36] have proved useful in some cases. For details the reader may consult several excellent references.[4,5]

Postoperative Management

If a suture repair has been done that involves posturing of joints, immobilization normally is maintained for 3 weeks before the limb is begun on range-of-motion exercises. During this time, adjacent joints must be kept mobile, and contractures must be prevented by splinting and

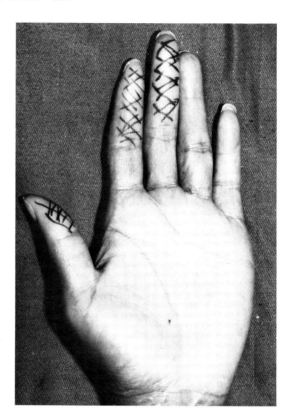

Fig. 92-6. Clinical appearance of the hand 10 months after grafting. The thenar muscle bulk had been regained and protective sensibility had returned proximal to the cross-hatched area. The patient lost to follow-up thereafter.

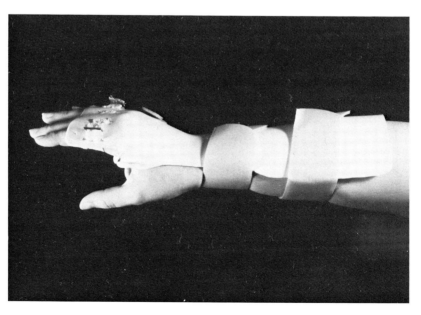

Fig. 92-7. A low-profile radial palsy splint made by occupational therapists at the Massachusetts General Hospital.

passive exercise (Fig. 92-7). It is indeed unfortunate to regain motor power after many months of waiting for nerve regeneration only to find that it is functionally useless because the joints are stiff. Not all patients require formal physical or occupational therapy, and these treatments must be individualized. The efficacy of electrical stimulation during the period of regeneration has not been clearly established. Many of the studies that have been done have been on animal models[37] and some have been poorly controlled. I do not believe that sufficient evidence, based on experience with humans, exists either to have my patients come to the hospital for daily stimulation or to urge them to buy home stimulators.

Factors Influencing Results of Nerve Repair

A number of technical factors that influence the result of nerve repair have been mentioned. In addition, there is little question that the experience and technical skill of the surgeon are of tremendous import.

Other factors independent of the surgeon or control, however, are significant determinants of the result:

1. *Age.* The power of regeneration and adaptability of children gives them considerably better results than those obtained in comparable situations in adults.
2. *Mechanism of injury.* In general, those wounds caused by greater trauma tend to exert a more deleterious effect on the nervous system than those of lesser magnitude, i.e., blast wounds tend to do worse than clean knife wounds.
3. *Length of resection.* In general, lesions involving greater length require more elaborate maneuvers for repair, have greater dissimilarity of the fascicular pattern, and tend not to do as well.
4. *Duration between injury and repair.* Ordinarily, after 3 months, the greater the delay in repair, the poorer the result.
5. *Location of the lesion.* The closer to the spinal cord, or the more proximal the lesion, the poorer the prognosis. This may result from retrograde neurologic change, exhaustion of axoplasm production, atrophy of the end organ with time, or a combination of all of these factors.

In the final analysis, there are many unsolved problems in surgery of peripheral nerves. Most of our efforts have been of a mechanical nature, but the greatest single impediment to success is the production of scar. It may well be that we really are very primitive in our thinking about this type of surgery, and that the ultimate solution is a biochemical or neurophysiologic one that will correctly direct the down-growing axon, preserve the waiting end-organ, and above all, prevent the formation of scar. Some interesting work is already going on in this area.[38,39]

Surgery of the Brachial Plexus

Many of the diagnostic and therapeutic techniques already discussed in detail are directly applicable to surgery of the brachial plexus. Sufficiently specialized differences exist, however, to merit separate consideration.

The anatomic complexity of the brachial plexus makes both diagnosis and treatment considerably more difficult than the problem posed by single or even multiple peripheral nerve injuries. If compression lesions are excluded, most of the remaining trauma can be considered under the general headings of *closed* and *open* injury. The latter will be considered first.

Open Wounds of the Brachial Plexus

Open wounds of the brachial plexus often are accompanied by serious vascular or pulmonary complications that may obscure recognition of the nerve injury or even kill the patient.[40] Surgical maneuvers to treat these problems obviously must take precedence over treatment of the nerve lesion. But what are the indications for surgical exploration of open wounds of the plexus? The answer depends, in addition to the above considerations, on several factors. The first of these is the nature of the wound. A knife or glass cut is unlikely to be anything less than a neurotmesis, so that awaiting recovery calculated at the rate of 1 inch a month is pointless. If the upper or intermediate trunk or their distal outflow is injured, it is worth exploring the lesion, since a discrete injured area may be amenable to suture or graft. The muscles innervated are mainly proximal, often large, and not of great functional complexity (but not invariably). Careful neurorrhaphy, therefore, has at least a chance of improving function. For the lower trunk and its terminal branches, the prognosis for recovery is so poor that in my opinion it is not worthwhile.

Gunshot wounds, however, constitute a completely different situation, and they are much harder to assess. The passage of a bullet through the tissues causes momentary deformation that spreads like a wave through the surrounding area. Hence, the spectrum of injury may be quite broad in an individual case, and there is no way of knowing immediately which parts actually are transected and which are going to recover. The carefully documented work of Donal Brooks[41] in World War II demonstrated how difficult it is to assess open wounds of the brachial plexus at surgery. He explored 54 cases, thought 16 to be amenable to surgical repair, and achieved a functional result in only 1, a lesion of an upper trunk.

The indication for exploration of the gunshot wound, therefore, is far less urgent than that of the sharp transection, although the operating microscope has brightened the outlook for treatment of open wounds.

Closed Wounds of the Brachial Plexus

These can be divided into supraclavicular and infraclavicular injuries, and since they have significantly different prognoses, they will be considered separately. Infraclavicular injuries of the brachial plexus result from skeletal injuries in the region of the shoulder girdle.[42] Often accompanying shoulder dislocations or fractures, they are of lesser severity than the supraclavicular variety because the bony lesions are the cause of the nerve injury by direct compression or traction, and root avulsion or infraganglionic neurotmesis usually do not occur. The prognosis for recovery, even of hand function, is generally good, and their treatment differs considerably from the larger group of supraclavicular injuries. Criteria for their identification and management have been advanced by Leffert and Seddon.[42] Rarely, because of sharp bone fragments, neurotmesis of the infraclavicular plexus may occur and require surgical repair. Plain radiograms may provide important evidence in these cases.

The supraclavicular injuries usually are caused by high-velocity vehicular accidents, and most often by falls from motorcycles. The patient often falls so that the shoulder and neck are forced apart, and great force is brought to bear in producing a traction lesion of the plexus. The damage may vary from frank avulsion of cervical roots from the spinal cord (a supraganglionic lesion) to lesser or greater degrees of damage to the trunks or divisions (infraganglionic), which can range from neurapraxia to neurotmesis. Differential involvement of motor and sensory components also is possible, so that an almost infinite spectrum of pathology can be observed. Detailed and accurate anatomic knowledge is essential for diagnosis. In addition to the usual techniques of clinical and electrodiagnostic evaluation, several indirect methods of study are useful in arriving at an accurate picture of the damage before surgery is considered.[43,44]

The presence of a Horner's syndrome usually indicates a supraganglionic avulsion of T1. Paralysis of the rhomboids, diaphragm, or serratus anterior are found in patients with supraganglionic lesions of C5, C6, and C7, since the nerves to these muscles usually are given off immediately after exit from the foramina.

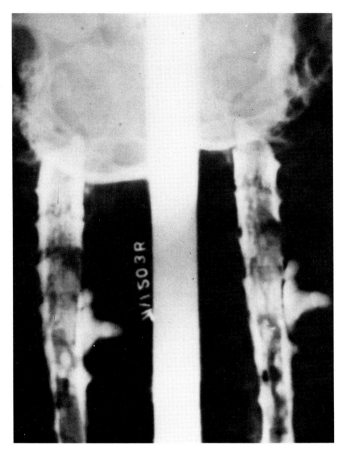

Fig. 92-8. Traumatic pseudomeningoceles seen on the cervical myelogram of a patient who has sustained avulsion of three roots in a
traction injury.

Plain films of the cervical spine and shoulder girdle can provide clues to the fate of the un-
seen plexus. If transverse processes are avulsed, this is a generally reliable indication that the
nerve root at that level has suffered a like fate. If the clavicle is fractured, it almost always accompanies a supraclavicular rather than an infraclavicular injury because of the greater excursion that it allows between the head and the shoulder, and prognosis is correspondingly worse.

Cervical myelography can demonstrate root avulsion by the presence of traumatic pseudomeningoceles.[45] It should be performed no sooner than 1 month following injury to allow the
meninges to retract at the site of avulsion and form pockets that will allow the dye to pool and be
seen on x-ray (Fig. 92-8). It should be noted that because of variations in the root innervation,
the observed pseudomeningoceles may not correspond exactly to the level of presumed injury arrived at by clinical neurologic deduction. Usually, the variation is not greater than a single segment, however. Furthermore, both false positive and false negative deductions do
occur[46,47]—especially if the only criterion is the presence or absence of a pseudomeningocele.
The use of water-soluble contrast material and improved imaging with polytomography may
make it possible to better delineate the presence or absence of the rootlets at cord level and improve the reliability of the test.

The use of the axon reflex by studying the response to intradermal histamine can provide an
additional indicator of the level of the lesion.[48] Yeoman's excellent article evaluating these methods can be consulted for details.[49] The improvement of other means of evaluation and the relatively lower yield of this test, however, have discouraged me from its routine use.

Because the erector spinae musculature posterior to the cervical spine is innervated segmentally in its deepest layers by the posterior primary rami of the same spinal nerves that provide the

anterior primary rami forming the brachial plexus, electromyographic examination of these muscles, as described by Bufalini and Pescatori,[50] may provide yet another means of determining whether a particular root is likely to have been avulsed as a supraganglionic lesion. Nerve conduction velocity determinations and evoked potentials may contribute similar information.

All of these methods of evaluation, used in conjunction with the clinical and electromyographic studies, usually make cervical laminectomy unnecessary in determining the presence of root avulsion, which, with the present state of the technology, is not amenable to surgical repair. pair.

The patient with a flail-anesthetic arm was, until recently, felt not to be a candidate for any attempt at surgical reconstruction of the plexus, especially if there were two or more traumatic pseudomeningoceles seen on myelography. Seddon, who had probably the greatest accumulated experience in the evaluation and management of traction injuries, taught that exploration in such cases was only for the purpose of clearly establishing a prognosis, since in the presence of a combination of multiple root avulsions and distal rupture within the plexus, one then could proceed with amputation of the arm and the fitting of a prosthesis.[51] In this way the patient with a flail-anesthetic arm could preserve some semblance of bimanuality. The pioneering work of Millesi et al.[52,53] and Narakas[54,55] as well as Lusskin et al.,[56] Alnot,[57,58] and Allieu[59] in the mid-1960s and 1970s has shown that it is possible to restore the function mediated by parts of the plexus damaged by traction if they are ruptured in the infraganglionic portion. Although the results differ between different centers, it generally is agreed that for the patient with a total plexus lesion, the strong recommendation should be for surgical exploration if any portion is felt to be ruptured distally and therefore is potentially reparable. As a practical matter, this usually is confined to the upper three roots and their outflow. The prognosis for recovery of voluntary elbow flexion has been the best of all the functions sought, but some success has been achieved in restoration of shoulder control, wrist extension, and to a lesser degree in finger flexion. For details of the results of individual workers, the reader is directed to their publications.[52-59] In general, such explorations should, after appropriate work-up, be done as early as 2 to 3 months following injury, and are not worthwhile after 18 months. In patients in whom the entire plexus has been irrevocably damaged at the level of the spinal cord, it still may be possible to provide some function by neuroticization from innervation either above or below the level of the plexus. The spinal accessory nerve had been used in part,[59] as have the intercostal nerves.[60] The general level of reliability of these procedures would, in my opinion, reserve them for very special and infrequent situations.

Exploration of the plexus requires extensive exposure, long operating time, and a surgical team thoroughly familiar with the regional anatomy and the specialized techniques specific to this type of surgery. In addition to the sterile field encompassing the neck, hemithorax, and arm, both legs must be sterilely prepared should the harvesting of the sural nerves be required. The incision begins in the supraclavicular fossa at the midpoint of the posterior border of the sternomastoid and drops vertically to 1 inch below the midpoint of the clavicle. It then proceeds laterally beneath the clavicle and then into the deltopectoral groove, from which it can be extended into the arm. The platysma muscle is carefully divided and retained for layered closure, and usually the external jugular vein must be ligated and removed. The transverse cervical and suprascapular vessels as well as the omohyoid muscle are oriented transversely to the plexus and all must be divided. Even though the clavicle would seem to be an impossible barrier without dividing it for exposure, all efforts should be made to avoid osteotomy, since there is a risk of nonunion or osteomyelitis, both of which are preventable and very nasty complications. Meticulous dissection through dense scar may be required to delineate the nerves and to decide which are potentially reparable. High magnification and electrical stimulation may be of great assistance at this stage, as may be the ability to record evoked potentials as reported by Landi et al.[61] If grafting can be accomplished, it is more likely to succeed the further it is done from the intervertebral foramen, but cables may be directed from the proximal intact portions of the plexus distally as shown in Figure 92-9. The goals of such surgery often are limited, but they may be

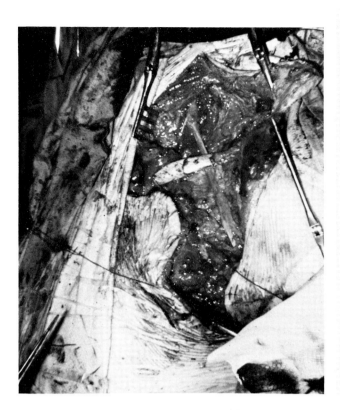

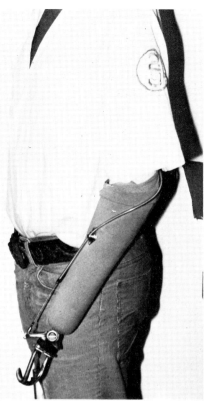

Fig. 92-9. (upper left) A 16-cm sural-nerve graft of four cables from the upper trunk to the lateral cord in a patient whose C7, C8, and T1 have been avulsed. (Right) Eighteen months following nerve grafting with shoulder fusion, forearm amputation, and prosthetic fitting. The active elbow flexion is of significant benefit to the patient's ability to use the prosthesis.

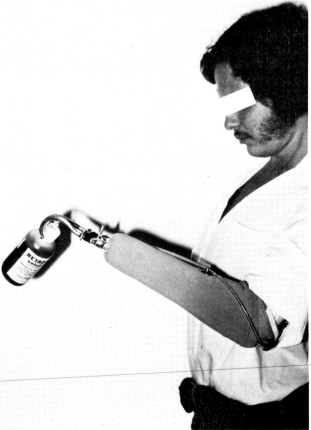

extremely gratifying, even if combined with other conventional methods of management. For the patients who would otherwise have nothing, a little gained is a lot. The alternative of primary amputation or surgical reconstruction of the flail-anesthetic limb, as advocated by Hendry,[62] has, in my opinion, considerably less to offer.

As greater experience is gained with direct surgical attack on the plexus, more patients who formerly either would have had amputations[51] or no treatment are being considered for neurologic reconstruction or neurolysis. Neurolysis is particularly indicated in patients with documented infraganglionic lesions whose recovery does not proceed as expected, or who actually experience a plateau or reversal of this process.[56]

It is obvious, then, that the management of patients with brachial plexus injuries has undergone important and continuing changes within the past few years in response to improvements in technology. The surgeon who must advise and treat a patient with a brachial plexus injury must have a well-ordered concept of not only what is available in neurosurgical treatment, but what peripheral reconstruction can offer as well. To attempt to graft the lower trunk of the plexus when chances for restoring the intrinsics by this means are virtually nil, especially when tendon transfer in the hand usually is successful, is to ignore the goal of a functional outcome. The burden imposed on the surgeon is, therefore, one that crosses specialty borders, and must be dealt with. In patients with lesser degrees and distribution of neurologic loss, successful rehabilitation of the upper limb depends on whether a useful hand potentially or actually is present. Many of the peripheral reconstructive procedures may be adapted from their use in poliomyelitis, with the important difference that, in the latter disease, sensation is preserved. The same procedure may be employed in patients with peripheral nerve injuries, where deficits usually are less extensive than in the brachial plexus population. A detailed discussion of these operations is beyond the scope of this chapter.

The problem of pain in patients with brachial plexus injuries is both major and unsolved. Many patients have severe pain, which can be unresponsive even to narcotics. Fortunately, it tends to abate with time, but for some it is intractable. Neurolysis usually is not effective treatment, and although some successes for the various operative maneuvers have been recorded, the overall record is a dismal one.[63] Amputating the arm does not help to cure the pain and actually may be contraindicated when pain is significant.[64,51]

REFERENCES

1. Strauss MB: *Familiar Medical Questions.* Boston, Little, Brown, 1968
2. Bateman JE: *Trauma to Nerves in Limbs.* Philadelphia, W.B. Saunders, 1962
3. Seddon HJ: *Peripheral Nerve Injuries.* London, Her Majesty's Stationery Office, 1961
4. Seddon HF: *Surgical Disorders of the Peripheral Nerves,* 2nd ed. Edinburgh, Churchill Livingstone, 1975
5. Sunderland S: *Nerves and Nerve Injuries,* 2nd ed. Edinburgh, Churchill Livingstone, 1978
6. Spurling RG, Woodhall B: *Surgery in World War II, Neurosurgery,* vol. 2. Washington, D.C. Office of the Surgeon General, Department of the Army, 1959
7. Smith JW: Microsurgery of peripheral nerves. *Plast Reconstr Surg 33*:317, 1964
8. Khodadad G: Microsurgical repair of peripheral nerves. *Surg Clin North Am 52*:1157, 1972
9. Ducker TB, Kempe LG, Hayes CJ: The metabolic background for peripheral nerve surgery. *J Neurosurg 30*:270, 1969
10. Seddon HJ: Three types of nerve injury. *Brain 66*:237, 1947
11. Kendall HO, Kendall FP, Wadsworth GE: *Muscles, Testing, and Function,* 2nd ed. Baltimore, Williams & Wilkins, 1975
12. Moberg E: Methods for examining sensibility of the hand, in Flynn (ed): *Hand Surgery.* Baltimore, Williams & Wilkins, 1975
13. Tinel J: Le signe du fourmillement dans les lesions des nerfe peripheriques. *Presse Med 47*:388, 1955
14. Henderson WR: Clinical assessment of peripheral nerve injuries. Tinel's test. *Lancet 2*:801, 1948
15. Licht S (ed): *Electrodiagnosis and Electromyography.* New Haven, E. Licht, 1971
16. Leffert RD, Frankel VH: The value of determination of conduction velocity of peripheral nerves in orthopaedic surgery. *Bull Hosp Joint Dis 25*:32, 1963

17. Kline DG, Nulson FE: The neuroma incontinuity, in symposium on operative nerve injuries and their repair. *Surg Clin North Am* 52:5, 1972
18. Littler JW: The neurovascular pedicle transfer of tissue in reconstructive surgery of the hand. *J Bone Joint Surg* 38:917, 1956
19. Michon J, Moberg E: *Traumatic Nerve Lesions of the Upper Limb.* Edinburgh, Churchill Livingstone, 1975
20. Holstein A, Lewis GB: Fractures of the humerus with radial nerve paralysis. *J Bone Joint Surg* 45A:1382, 1963
21. Gabrielsson GH, Stenstrum SJ: Contribution to peripheral nerve suture technique. *Plast Reconstr Surg* 38:68–71, 1966
22. Terzis J, Faibisoff B, Williams HB: A diamond knife for microsurgical repair of peripheral nerves. *Plast Reconstr Surg* 54:102–103, 1974
23. Clark GL: Method of preparation of nerve ends for suturing. *Plast Reconstr Surg* 34:233–235, 1964
24. Young JZ, Medawor PB: *Fibrin Suture of Peripheral Nerves and Nerve Roots.* Springfield, Ill., Charles C Thomas, 1950
25. Tarlov IM: *Plasma Clot Suture of Peripheral Nerves and Nerve Roots.* Springfield, Ill., Charles C Thomas, 1950
26. Henry AK: *Extensile Exposure,* 2nd ed. Baltimore, Williams & Wilkins, 1957
27. Curtis RM, Eversmann WW: Internal neurolysis as an adjunct to the treatment of the carpal tunnel syndrome. *J Bone Joint Surg* 56A:733, 1973
28. Omer GE: Injuries to nerves of the upper extremity. *J Bone Joint Surg* 56A:1615, 1974
29. Sunderland S: The pros and cons of fascicular nerve repair. *J Hand Surg* 4:201, 1979
30. Bora FW, Pleasure DE, Didizian NA: A study of nerve regeneration and neuroma formation after nerve suture by various techniques. *J Hand Surg* 1:138, 1976
31. Caband HE, Rodkey WG, McCarroll HR, et al: Epidural and perineurial fascicular nerve repairs: A critical comparison. *J Hand Surg* 1:131, 1976
32. Millesi H, Meiss G, Berger A: The interfascicular nerve grafting of the median and ulnar nerves. *J Bone Joint Surg* 54A:727, 1972
33. Terzis J, Faibisoff B, Williams HB: Use of polyethylene bag background in microsurgical repair of peripheral nerves. *Plast Reconstr Surg* 53:596–597, 1974
34. Seddon HJ: Nerve grafting. *J Bone Joint Surg* 45B:447, 1963
35. Millesi H, Meissi G, Berger A: Further experience with interfascicular grafting of the median, ulnar, and radial nerves. *J Bone Joint Surg* 58A:209, 1976
36. Strange FGStC: An operation for nerve pedicle grafting, preliminary communication. *Br J Surg* 34:423, 1947
37. Gutmann E, Guttmann L: Effect of galvanic exercise on denervated reinnervated muscles in rabbit. *J Neurol Neurosurg Psychiatry* 7:7, 1944
38. Bora FW, Lane JM, Prockop DJ: Inhibitors of collagen biosynthesis as a means of controlling scar formation in tendon injury. *J Bone Joint Surg* 54A:1501, 1972
39. Pleasure D, Bora FW, Lane J, et al.: Regeneration after transection: effect of inhibition of collagen synthesis. *Exp Neurol* 45:72–78, 1974
40. Nelson KG, Jolly PC, Thomas PA: Brachial plexus injuries associated with missile wounds of the chest. *J Trauma* 8:268, 1968
41. Brooks DM: Open wounds of the brachial plexus. *J Bone Joint Surg* 31B:17, 1949
42. Leffert RD, Seddon HJ: Infraclavicular brachial plexus injuries. *J Bone Joint Surg* 47B:9, 1965
43. Leffert RD: Brachial plexus injuries. *N Engl J Med* 291:1059–1067, 1974
44. Leffert RD: Lesions of the brachial plexus, including thoracic outlet syndrome. Instructional course lectures, vol. 31, American Academy of Orthopedic Surgeons. St. Louis, CV Mosby, 1977
45. Murphy F, Hartung W, Kirklin JW: Myelographic demonstration of avulsing injury of the brachial plexus. *AJR* 58:102, 1947
46. Heon M: Myelogram: a questionable aid in diagnosis and prognosis in avulsion of brachial plexus components by traction injuries. *Conn Med* 29:260, 1965
47. Jelasic F, Piepgres U: Functional restitution after cervical avulsion injury with "typical myelographic findings." *Eur Neurol* 11:158, 1974
48. Bonney G: The value of axon responses in determining the site of the lesion in traction injuries of the brachial plexus. *Brain* 77:588, 1954
49. Yeoman PM: Cervical myelography in traction injuries of the brachial plexus. *J Bone Joint Surg* 50B:2, 1968
50. Bufalini C, Pescatori G: Posterior cervical electromyography in the diagnosis and prognosis of brachial plexus injuries. *J Bone Joint Surg* 51B:627, 1969
51. Yeoman PM, Seddon HJ: Brachial plexus injuries: treatment of the flail arm. *J Bone Joint Surg* 43B:3, 1961

52. Millesi H, Meissl G, Katzer H: Therapy of brachial plexus injuries: proposal for an integrated therapy (German). *Bruns Beitr Klin Chir 220*:429–446, 1973
53. Millesi H: Surgical management of brachial plexus injuries. *J Hand Surg 2*:367, 1977
54. Narakas A: Plexo braquial terapeutica quirigica directa. *Rev Orthop Traumatol 16*:855, 1972
55. Narakas A: Surgical treatment of traction injuries of the brachial plexus. *Clin Orthop 133*:71, 1978
56. Lusskin R, Campbell JB, Thompson WAL: Post-traumatic lesions of the brachial plexus: treatment by transclavicular exploration and neurolysis or autograft reconstruction. *J Bone Joint Surg 55*:1159–1173, 1973
57. Alnot JY: Technique chirgicale dans les paralysies du plexus brachial. *Rev Chir Orthop 63*:75, 1977
58. Alnot JY, Augereau B, Frot B: Traitement direct des lesions nerveuses dans les paralysies traumatiques par elongation du plexus brachial chez l'adulte. *Chirurgie 103*:935, 1977
59. Allieu Y: Exploration et traitement direct des lesions nerveuses dans les paralysies traumatiques par elongation du plexus brachial chez l'adults. *Rev Chir Orthop 63*:107, 1977
60. Tsuyama N, Hara T: Intercostal nerve crossing in the treatment of brachial plexus injury of root avulsion type. Proceedings of the 12th Congress of the International Society of Orthopaedic Surgery and Traumatology Tel Aviv 1972. Amsterdam, Excerpta Medica, 1972, p 351
61. Landi A, Copeland SA, Wynn Parry CB, et al.: The role of somatosensory evoked potentials and nerve conduction studies in the surgical management of brachial plexus injuries. *J Bone Joint Surg 62B*:492–496, 1980
62. Hendry AM: The treatment of residual paralysis of brachial plexus injuries. *J Bone Joint Surg 31*:42–49, 1949
63. Taylor PE: Traumatic intradural avulsion of the nerve roots of the brachial plexus. *Brain 85*:579–602, 1962
64. Fletcher I: Traction injuries of the brachial plexus. *Hand 1*:129, 1969

CHAPTER 93

Surgical Management of Peripheral Entrapment Neuropathy

Henry A. Young

EXPERIMENTAL AND CLINICAL OBSERVATIONS on the etiology and pathogenesis of peripheral entrapment neuropathy suggest that the two predominant causative agents are ischemia and compression. The precise role of each factor is not established, although the more recent studies emphasize the importance of direct mechanical compression of the nerve.

Local compression results in damage to peripheral nerves. Severe compression may crush fibers and lead to Wallerian degeneration with a loss of distal excitability that requires months to resolve. Very mild compression produces physiologic block, which is reversed as soon as the pressure is released. Based on studies with pneumatic cuffs or clamps in humans, Lewis et al.[1] concluded that this physiologic block was caused by local asphyxia. Compression of an intermediate degree produces local conduction block with preservation of distal excitability that may take several weeks to recover.[2] Denny-Brown and Brenner[3,4] found the anatomic basis for this to be demyelination with preservation of axonal continuity, and concluded that this lesion was caused by local asphyxia of the nerve rather than by mechanical deformation. In support of this concept were the experimental observations of Grundfest,[5] who showed that very high pressures were necessary to abolish conduction in the excised nerves of frogs enclosed in an oxygenated pressure chamber.

More recent clinical and experimental work has emphasized the importance of direct mechanical compression. Gilliatt et al.,[6] using a cuff inflated to 1000 mm Hg for 1 to 2 hours around the legs of baboons, found that the anatomic lesions were concentrated under the edges of the cuff, with sparing in the center, where the lesions might have been expected to be maximal if ischemia had played an important role. The characteristic lesion produced in this experiment was damage to large myelinated fibers with displacement of the node of Ranvier from its usual position under the Schwann cell junction, accompanied by stretching of the paranodal myelin on one side of the node and invagination of the paranodal myelin on the other. This nodal lesion is followed by a breakdown of the paranodal myelin. Repetition of the experiment with nylon cords attached to peripheral nerves in animals with attached weights designed to simulate human pressure palsies produced the same characteristic anatomic lesions. Thus, displacement of the node of Ranvier accompanied by stretching of paranodal myelin on one side of the node and invagination of myelin on the other side, followed in time by paranodal or segmental demyelination, may be regarded as the characteristic anatomic lesion caused by an acutely evolving compression neuropathy.

Division of Neurosurgery, University of Vermont College of Medicine, Burlington, Vermont

Neary et al.,[7] by careful microscopic examination of segments of ulnar and median nerves in cadaver specimens without clinical evidence of entrapment neuropathy, found a characteristic set of microscopic lesions in ulnar nerve segments in the area of the cubital tunnel and in median nerve segments at the flexor retinaculum, both clinically common sites of entrapment. In a high percentage of nerve segments, they found that the appearance of internodes was altered as a result of bulbous swelling at one end and thinning and retraction of myelin at the other; in some nerves intercalated segments indicative of previous demyelination also were present. Previous studies[8] indicated that the distortion of internodes resulted from slippage of myelin lamellae away from the site of the pressure, the bulbous ends of the internodes consisting of redundant folds of myelin. This process is thought to represent the earliest change to occur in nerve fibers subject to chronic recurrent compression and thus is the anatomic substrate of chronic compressive neuropathy.

Both the early lesion of acutely evolving compression neuropathy (displacement of the node of Ranvier with stretching of paranodal myelin on one side and invagination of myelin on the other side) and the early lesion of chronic compressive neuropathy (bulbous swelling at one end of the internode and retraction at the other end) are followed by segmental demyelination, which has been shown to be the characteristic lesion in chronic compression neuropathy in experimental animals.[9] Given time and continued compression, the neurapractic lesion of segmental demyelination may evolve into axonotmetic and neurometic lesions, culminating in complete fibrosis of a segment of nerve.

The predominant role of mechanical compression in producing entrapment is not universally accepted. Sunderland[10] emphasized the importance of vascular factors in the production of a carpal tunnel syndrome. He visualizes the carpal tunnel syndrome as an entity passing through three stages. In Stage 1, chronic mechanical compression leads to increased intrafunicular pressure, eventually resulting in slowing of intrafunicular capillary circulation. The nerve fibers are afflicted by vascular insufficiency and become hyperexcitable, resulting often in pain and paresthesias. The pain and paresthesias are aggravated by venous stasis. Relief is obtained by vigorously exercising the hand or arm, which promotes venous return. In Stage 2, capillary circulation slows to the point that the capillary endothelium is damaged, with intrafunicular edema and leakage of proteinaceous exudate into funiculi. Enlargement of the nerve may be observed grossly at the level of the flexor retinaculum. In Stage 3, fibroblasts proliferate in the protein exudate, leading to intrafunicular fibrosis associated with destruction of increasing numbers of nerve fibers. Eventually, nutrient vessels are completely obliterated with conversion of the affected segment of nerve into a fibrous cord. Sunderland points out that this hypothesis applies only to the carpal tunnel syndrome. It appears, however, that both direct mechanical deformation of myelin and vascular factors may play a role in the production of entrapment neuropathy, although the precise role of each variable has not been precisely defined.

General Management of Compressive Nerve Lesions

Two systems of classification of peripheral nerve lesions are in use. Seddon uses the terms neurapraxia, axonotmesis, and neurotmesis, while Sunderland classifies nerve injury into five degrees of severity. The fifth-degree nerve lesion is not applicable to neural compression lesions. It occurs when a nerve is completely severed and the ends retract. A first-degree Sunderland lesion is equivalent to neurapraxia, while a second-degree lesion is equivalent to axonotmesis. The fourth-degree lesion is neurotmetic and implies a neuroma in continuity. In third-degree lesions, intrafunicular fibrosis is present. These lesions may be reversible or axonotmetic, but they also may be neurotmetic with irreversible intrafunicular fibrosis.

In neurapraxia the nerve fiber is physiologically transected at the point of compression. Wallerian degeneration does not occur, however, and the axonal basement membrane is intact. Neurapraxia may be due to the following anatomic and physiologic causes: (1) electrolyte imbalance, including disturbances of sodium, potassium, and adenosine triphosphatase function,[11] occur at the site of compression and can result in neurapraxia; (2) displacement of the node of Ranvier with stretching and invagination of internodal myelin, discussed above as the earliest anatomic change of acutely evolving compression neuropathy, results in neurapraxia; (3) bulbous swelling of myelin at one end of the internode with thinning and retraction at the other, the earliest change in chronic compression neuropathy, may produce neurapraxia; (4) processes (2) and (3) above result in segmental demyelination over time, which produces neurapraxia; (5) intrafunicular anoxia, thought by Sunderland to be the etiology of the carpal tunnel syndrome, also may play a role in the production of neurapraxia. If neural compression continues over time, neurapractic lesions may evolve into axonotmetic and neurotmetic lesions.

Axonotmesis is characterized by complete interruption of the axons and their myelin sheaths, but the stroma of the nerve remains in continuity—Schwann tubes, endoneurium, and epineurium. Electron microscopy has shown that even the Schwann basement membranes persist. Axonal damage and loss of function are as complete as that occurring after nerve transection. Distal to the level of axonotmetic compression, complete Wallerian degeneration occurs; however, regeneration can occur spontaneously and is often of good quality because intact endoneurial tubes guide outgoing streams of axoplasm toward appropriate peripheral connections. Classically, regeneration occurs at the rate of 1 mm per day, or roughly 1 inch per month, and this is the expected rate of clinical recovery, which exhibits a sequential pattern depending upon the distance from the point of compression to the point of reinnervation of muscle fiber or sensory end-organ.

Neurotmesis describes a nerve that either has been completely severed or is disorganized by scar tissue to the point that spontaneous regeneration is impossible. Neurotmetic compression lesions require resection and suture, with or without the interposition of nerve grafts.

A neural compression lesion persisting for 60 days with no improvement requires surgical therapy. If neurologic deficit is not rapidly progressive, a neural compression lesion may be followed for 60 days after the diagnosis and conservative measures adopted, such as splinting in the case of the carpal tunnel syndrome. Neurapractic lesions that will resolve without surgery will exhibit evidence of recovery during this period, while axonotmetic lesions that will not require surgery exhibit reinnervation proceeding distally at the rate of 2.5 cm or 1 inch per month. During this period of observation, evidence for return of function may be sought by serial physical examination and electrical testing. An advancing Tinel's sign provides evidence of reinnervation often before motor and sensory recovery, but many patients with the advancing Tinel's sign will nonetheless exhibit poor spontaneous functional recovery.[12] It is important to test the autonomous sensory zone of the damaged nerve so that sensory overlap from other peripheral nerves is not mistakenly interpreted as regeneration in the injured nerve. In performing serial motor and sensory examination, one should have a clear idea of the expected schedule of functional recovery. In neurapractic lesions, distal functions return simultaneously after resolution of conduction block in the area of compression. Neurapractic lesions caused by local nodal electrolyte imbalance may be corrected within several days, with sudden reappearance of all motor and sensory functions distal to the compressed area. Neurapractic lesions caused by local myelin damage in the area of compression—whether myelin paranodal intussusception or segmental demyelination—require a 60-day period for local remyelinization and resolution of conduction block to occur. Therefore, within a 60-day period of observation and conservative therapy, the bulk of neurapractic lesions responding to conservative therapy should exhibit evidence of recovery. Axonotmetic lesions exhibit a proximal-to-distal march of sensory and motor recovery that occurs at the rate of 1 mm per day or 1 inch per month, which roughly corresponds to the rate of axonal regeneration.

Serial electrical testing also may be used to confirm that reinnervation is proceeding at the desired rate. When regeneration is occurring, serial EMGs show a decrease in the number of fibrillations and denervation potentials, which are replaced by nascent motor action potentials. These findings, however, cannot predict the quality or completeness of regeneration. Serial conduction velocities across affected segments may be obtained, to test for resolution of conduction block. Simple percutaneous nerve stimulation also is a valuable test. Muscle contraction distal to the point of compression indicates that useful clinical function in that muscle will occur in several weeks. If, after a 60-day period of observation of a neural compression lesion, physical and electrical examination shows that the expected rate of recovery is not occurring, surgical exploration is necessary.

Preoperatively, careful clinical examination and electrical testing are necessary to localize the area of entrapment and to be certain that the nerve is not compressed in more than one place, i.e., the "double crush" syndrome.[13] For example, the ulnar nerve may be compressed both at Guyon's tunnel in the wrist and at the cubital tunnel in the elbow. Decompression at only one level in such a situation is of minimal value.

Surgical exposure must be generous because several centimeters of normal nerve should be identified proximal and distal to the area of entrapment. Dissection proceeds from the proximal and distal sides to separate the epineurium from surrounding scar, thickened fascia, and fibrous bands. Many times this external neurolysis alone provides adequate treatment and decompression.

Indications for internal neurolysis, with dissection of individual funiculi, are less well established. Extensive internal neurolysis may provoke fibrosis in all layers of the nerve.[14] Spinner[15] points out that internal neurolysis should be limited to those fasciculi that are clinically involved. In cases of carpal tunnel syndrome where pain and dysesthesias are most severe in the long finger, he has obtained excellent results by selective internal neurolysis of the medial two or three funiculi of the median nerve. He cautions against internal neurolysis of all fasciculi of the median nerve in this condition. Curtis and Eversmann,[16] reporting 96 cases of carpal tunnel syndrome treated with both external and internal neurolysis, found that internal neurolysis increased the success of surgery in a subgroup of patients with constant sensory loss or thenar atrophy or both. Brown[17] emphasized the value of internal neurolysis for a wide variety of lesions in continuity, including those resulting from chronic entrapment. He pointed out that many lesions in continuity are accompanied by intraneural scarring, which can only be treated definitively by internal as well as external neurolysis. No patient in his series was made worse by internal neurolysis.

An intraoperative finding that is frequently encountered, particularly in neural compression lesions of long standing, is a neuroma in continuity, the management of which has been well outlined by Kline and Nulsen.[18] Direct nerve stimulation proximal to the neuroma may be attempted first. If distal muscle contraction is elicited, the lesion may be treated by external and, if indicated, internal neurolysis. If no motor response is elicited, an attempt is made to record nerve action potentials. This procedure is done by placing bipolar stainless electrodes proximal to the neuroma in continuity and then attempting to evoke a nerve action potential distal to the neuroma after stimulating proximal to the neuroma. Evoked responses are obtained by means of bipolar electrodes placed distal to the neuroma and recorded by an amplifier and an oscilloscope. The presence of a nerve action potential distal to the lesion after proximal stimulation means that neurolysis is indicated. Inability to evoke a nerve-action potential through the neuroma after a 60-day period of conservative management of a neural compression lesion indicates that satisfactory regeneration is not occurring and that resection of the neuroma, with or without intrafascicular nerve grafting, is indicated.

All peripheral nerve entrapment surgery is performed with headlight illumination under 3.5–4.5X magnification. The microscope is reserved for internal neurolysis, intrafascicular nerve grafting, and suturing of individual fascicles after resection of neuromas in continuity.

A variety of anesthetic options is available: (1) General endotracheal intubation with or without tourniquet on the extremity. This type of anesthesia should be used whenever a procedure lasting more than several hours is anticipated, particularly if the microscope will be required. (2) General anesthesia without intubation with or without tourniquet. This is of value in apprehensive patients when the procedure is of short duration. (3) Local anesthesia alone. This limits the scope of the procedure, particularly if unexpected intraoperative findings are encountered. It is seldom adequate for anything more complicated than simple carpal tunnel release. (4) Intravenous regional anesthesia is an excellent technique, which can be used in both the upper and the lower extremities. It provides adequate analgesia and, in addition, tourniquet effect. The maximal duration of a procedure with such anesthesia is approximately 2 hours. In general, we prefer systematic meticulous hemostasis to the use of tourniquet. Bleeding after tourniquet release must be thoroughly controlled to prevent postoperative wound hematoma, which can predispose to neural scarring and thus give a poor surgical result. A tourniquet must be used carefully in elderly patients and in those with a history of peripheral vascular insufficiency. We usually prefer general anesthesia to local and intravenous regional anesthesia because it is often difficult to tell preoperatively if a prolonged procedure with intrafascicular dissection and nerve grafting under the microscope will be necessary.

Individual Nerve Compression Lesions

Median Nerve Entrapment

Median nerve entrapment occurs distally in the carpal tunnel, or, less commonly, in the proximal forearm.

Entrapment of the median nerve at the wrist results in the carpal tunnel syndrome. The disease occurs more frequently in females, with the peak incidence between the ages of 40 and 60 years. The syndrome most often is caused by narrowing of the carpal tunnel. A history of repeated occupational trauma to the hand and wrist often may be elicited. Carpal tunnel syndrome also may be associated with a wide variety of systemic diseases. Amyloid infiltration of the transverse carpal ligament due to either primary or secondary amyloidosis (as in multiple myeloma) may produce a carpal tunnel syndrome. Diseases such as rheumatoid arthritis, acromegaly, and hypothyroidism, which result in thickening of connective tissue, may thicken the transverse carpal ligament sufficiently to result in median nerve compression.

The most common presentation of the syndrome is pain and paresthesias in the radial 3.5 fingers, often more severe at night and relieved by shaking of the hand. Diagnosis is easily arrived at when a complete set of signs and symptoms of the fully evolved syndrome is present— positive Tinel's and Phalen's signs, hypesthesia in the radial 3.5 digits, thenar atrophy, and EMG abnormalities in the distal median nerve. The disease, however, may present atypically as pain in the proximal upper extremity and shoulder.[19] Unexplained shoulder or proximal upper extremity pain is a clear indication for a detailed physical and electromyographic examination of the median nerve at the wrist. At times the diagnosis must be made purely on clinical grounds because EMG and nerve conduction time at the wrist are normal in up to 25 percent of cases.[15]

Conservative therapy consists of splinting the wrist in a neutral position. Local injections of xylocaine or steroid have not been useful in our experience. Indications for surgery include motor weakness, persistent arm and hand discomfort or paresthesias, and lack of response to conservative therapy.

The procedure of carpal tunnel release, including the skin incision preferred by the author, taking into account the position of the motor branch of the median nerve, is illustrated in Figure 93-1. After the incision is made, dissection is continued through the antebrachial fascia. The palmaris longus tendon is retracted, and the underlying median nerve is identified as it enters the carpal tunnel between the flexor digitorum superficialis and the flexor carpi radialis tendons. The transverse carpal ligament is divided along its entire length parallel to the median nerve, and the nerve is freed of all ligamentous structures as far as the proximal crease of the hand. Incomplete division of the transverse carpal ligament is a major cause of failure of this procedure to relieve symptoms.

Several special points regarding carpal tunnel surgery must be noted. Injury to the medial

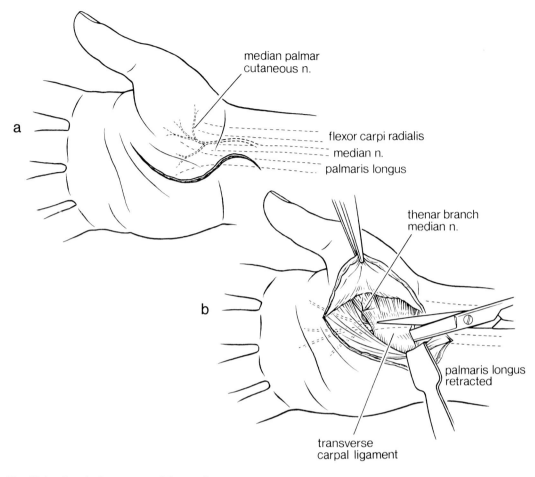

Fig. 93-1. Surgical exposure of the median nerve at the wrist. A curvilinear incision avoiding the branches of the medial palmar cutaneous nerve is utilized.

palmar cutaneous nerve recently has been emphasized as a cause of postoperative pain. This nerve arises 5.5 cm proximal to the radial styloid from the radial aspect of the median nerve. It then crosses the space between the median nerve and the flexor carpi radialis tendon and attaches to the undersurface of the antebrachial fascia under the ulnar margin of the flexor carpi radialis tendon. From this point it continues ulnarward to enter the transverse carpal ligament and passes via a tunnel of its own through the ligament 9–16 mm within the ligament.[20] Transverse incisions for carpal tunnel release should be avoided because of the possibility of injuring the main trunk of the medial palmar cutaneous nerve. At the level of the heel of the hand, the incision is best placed ulnar to the longitudinal axis of the fourth metacarpal to avoid injury to the distal branches of the nerve. At the wrist the skin incision may be curved either radially or ulnarward in an S configuration, which is helpful in avoiding contracture.

The presence of significant thenar atrophy is an indication for operative exposure and examination of the thenar branch of the median nerve. This recurrent branch usually arises distal to the transverse carpal ligament from the radial portion of the median nerve trunk. Frequently, however, the thenar branch may pass through a foramen of its own in the distal portion of the transverse carpal ligament,[15] which may constitute an area of neural compression and require release.

A less common but significant area of median nerve entrapment is the proximal forearm. In its course down the arm, the median nerve initially lies lateral to the brachial artery, but it gradually crosses the ventral surface of the artery in the lower part of the arm and lies medial to it at

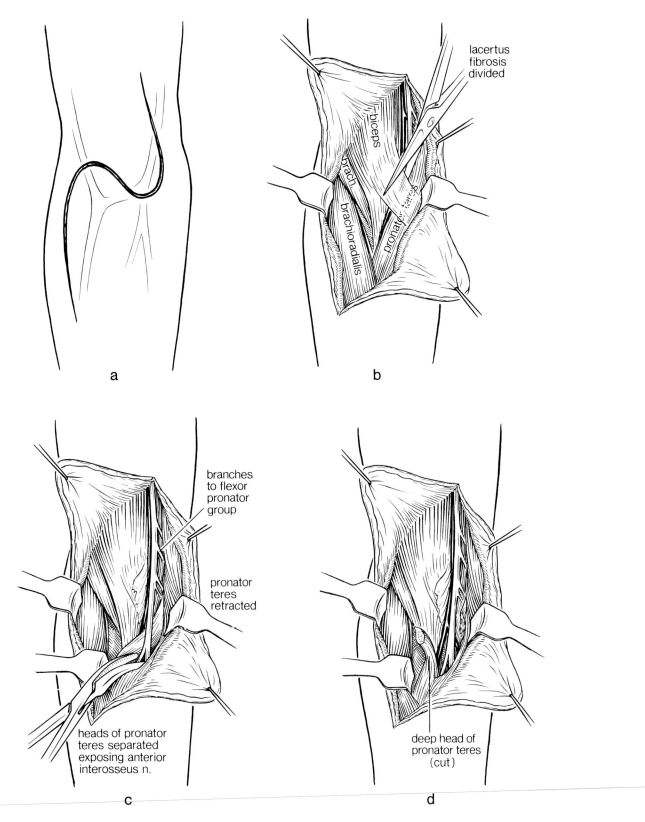

a

b

lacertus
fibrosis
divided

biceps

brach.

brachioradialis

pronator teres

c

branches
to flexor
pronator
group

pronator
teres
retracted

heads of pronator
teres separated
exposing anterior
interosseus n.

d

deep head of
pronator teres
(cut)

Fig. 93-2. Steps in the operative exposure of the median nerve and its anterior interosseous branch at the elbow.

the bend of the elbow, where it is deep to the lacertus fibrosus and superficial to the brachialis. In the forearm it passes between the two heads of the pronator teres and continues distally between the flexor digitorum sublimis and profundus. The median nerve branches innervating the flexor-pronator group originating from the medial epicondyle arise from the medial aspect of the nerve. The anterior interosseous nerve arises from the lateral aspect of the nerve as it passes between the heads of the pronator teres. The anterior interosseous nerve innervates the flexor pollicis longus, the radial half of the flexor digitorum profundus, and the pronator quadratus. It is important to preserve all of these branches.

The surgical approach to the median nerve in the proximal forearm is illustrated in Figure 93-2. A Z-shaped incision overlying the pronator teres is used. The incision begins 5 cm above the medial epicondyle, continues transversely following a flexion crease across the antecubital fossa, and then is carried distally along the medial margin of the brachioradialis muscle. The median nerve is identified as it lies on the brachialis muscle proximal to the lacertus fibrosus and then is traced distally. The lacertus fibrosus is divided and the nerve traced distally as it passes medial to the bicipital tendon into the antecubital fossa. The nerve then is traced distally as it passes between the two heads of the pronator teres. The tendinous origin of the deep head is divided when exploring the anterior interosseous nerve.

Two different types of median nerve compression syndrome prevail in the proximal forearm: (1) the pronator syndrome, and (2) the anterior interosseous syndrome. The pronator syndrome consists of a pain in the proximal volar aspect of the forearm, exacerbated on pronation of the forearm, weakness of intrinsic muscles innervated by the median nerve, paresthesias in the radial 3.5 digits, and normal function of the flexor pollicis longus, pronator quadratus, and flexor digitorum profundus of the second and third fingers—all of which are innervated by the anterior interosseous nerve. The most important cause of pronator syndrome is median nerve compression by a hypertrophic pronator teres and adhesions within the pronator teres. Less frequent causes include compression by the lacertus fibrosus or by a thickened flexor superficialis arch as well as passage of the median nerve posterior to both heads of the pronator teres. The anterior interosseous syndrome results in selective paralysis of the flexor digitorum profundus of the second and third fingers, the pronator quadratus, and the flexor pollicis longus. There are no sensory changes. The patient is unable to pinch the distal phalanges of the thumb and index finger together (Fig. 93-3). The most common cause of selective anterior interosseous compression neuropathy is compression by the tendinous origin of the deep head of the pronator teres. Treatment is by release of the tendinous origin of the deep head.

Ulnar Nerve Compression

Ulnar nerve compression occurs most commonly at the elbow, and, less often, at the wrist. The ulnar nerve in the arm runs medial to the axillary artery within the medial intermuscular septum. In the middle of the arm it angles dorsally, pierces the medial intermuscular septum, and follows the medial head of the triceps through the groove between the olecranon and medial epicondyle. In passing from the extensor surface behind the humerus to the forearm flexor surface, the nerve passes through the elliptical cubital tunnel bounded laterally by the elbow joint and its transverse ligament, and medially by the aponeurosis between the two heads of the flexor carpi ulnaris. It enters the forearm between the two heads of the flexor carpi ulnaris and continues distally between this muscle and the flexor digitorum profundus. A significant anatomic variation is the arcade of Struthers, a thickening of muscle and connective tissue passing medial to the nerve between the medial intermuscular septum and the medial head of the triceps. It is present in 70 percent of cadaver specimens.[21]

Ulnar nerve compression in the vicinity of the elbow has many causes. The nerve can be compressed at the cubital tunnel where it enters the forearm between the heads of the flexor carpi ulnaris because there is a fascial connection between the two muscle heads that can act as a compressing force, particularly during flexion. Within the ulnar groove repetitive frictional forces

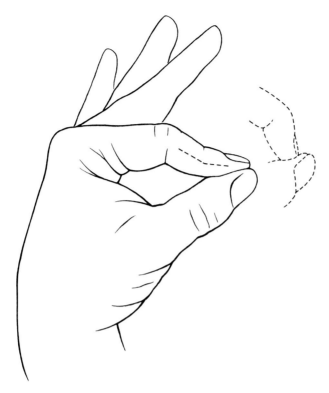

Fig. 93-3. The patient with anterior interosseous palsy is unable to pinch the distal phalanges of the first and second fingers together because of paralysis of the flexor pollicis longus and of the flexor digitorum profundus of the index finger.

may damage the nerve, since the nerve may elongate as much as 0.5 cm during flexion.[22] Local elbow pathology such as ganglion cysts, rheumatoid synovitis, osteoarthritis, and old medial epicondyle fractures may injure the nerve by direct local compression.

Medial epicondylectomy has been advocated for ulnar compression at the elbow,[23] and recent publications also claim success for simple division of the fibrous arch between the heads of the flexor carpi ulnaris.[24] Our surgical approach to the ulnar nerve at the elbow (Fig. 93-4) combines anterior translocation with division of the arcade of Struthers and the medial intermuscular septum proximally, and division of the aponeurosis between the heads of the flexor carpi ulnaris distally. This approach provides complete decompression above and below the elbow, and anterior translocation effectively removes the nerve from frictional forces in the ulnar groove. After translocation, the nerve lies subcutaneously at the elbow crease. Major causes of recurrent symptoms after anterior transposition include kinking caused by incomplete division of the medial intermuscular septum, compression at the entrance to the cubital tunnel by scar or incomplete division of the heads of the flexor carpi ulnaris, dense scarring of the nerve bed, and constriction where the fascial sling is created to hold the nerve in its anterior position. Submuscular transposition of the ulnar nerve[25] requires division of the flexor-pronator group of muscles close to their origin from the medial epicondyle, rerouting of the nerve deep to them, and resuturing of the muscles over the nerve. This technique is useful for reoperation,[26] especially when dense scarring has occurred after anterior subcutaneous transposition, because the nerve can be redirected deep to the flexor-pronator group into an unscarred bed.

At the wrist the ulnar artery and nerve pass superficial to the flexor retinaculum and under a thickened aponeurosis, which is an extension of the flexor carpi ulnaris. The area of passage under this aponeurosis is called Guyon's tunnel. Ulnar nerve entrapment in this area occurs at Guy-

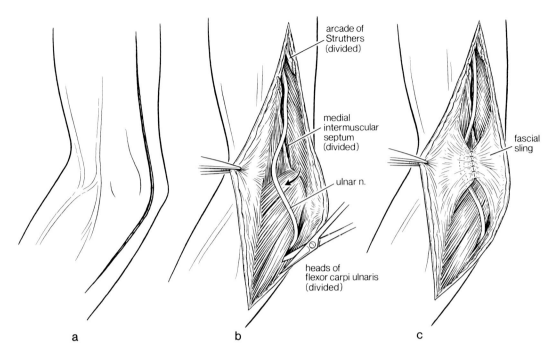

Fig. 93-4. Steps in the anterior transposition of the ulnar nerve at the elbow.

on's tunnel, or at the pisiform or hook of the hamate. Ulnar nerve entrapment at the wrist may result from anomalous muscles, ganglia, osteoarthritic bony spurs, or ligamentous thickening. Treatment consists of division of the aponeurosis forming the roof of the tunnel (Fig. 93-5). The underlying ulnar nerve then can be identified and neurolysis carried out. A diligent search also should be made for compression by bony spurs and anomalous muscles.

Radial Nerve Entrapment

The radial nerve is most susceptible to acute injury when fracture of the midshaft of the humerus occurs, injuring the nerve within the musculospiral groove. Chronic spontaneous entrapment is more likely to occur below the level of the elbow, where the nerve divides into superficial and deep (posterior interosseous) branches. After piercing the lateral intermuscular septum in the lower arm, the radial nerve runs between the brachialis and brachioradialis to the front of the lateral epicondyle and divides into superficial and deep portions. The superficial branch runs along the lateral border of the forearm under the brachioradialis and supplies sensation to the dorsal portions of the radial 3.5 fingers. The deep posterior interosseous branch passes between the two heads of the supinator and continues dorsolaterally around the neck of the radius.

Posterior interosseous entrapment occurs most commonly as the nerve passes between the heads of the supinator. The nerve enters the supinator through an inverted arch—the ''arcade of Frohse''—formed by the edge of the proximal border of the superficial head of the supinator. The arcade may compress the nerve just as the carpal ligament compresses the median nerve at the wrist.

Complete posterior interosseous palsy has the following features: (1) inability to extend the fingers at the metacarpophalangeal joints; (2) dorsiflexion of the wrist in a radial direction because of paralysis of the extensor carpi ulnaris; (3) inability to extend the thumb in a metacarpal plane; and (4) no sensory abnormalities.

The operative approach to the posterior interosseous nerve involves a curvilinear incision that avoids the cubital flexion crease (Fig. 93-6). The nerve is identified as it runs between the

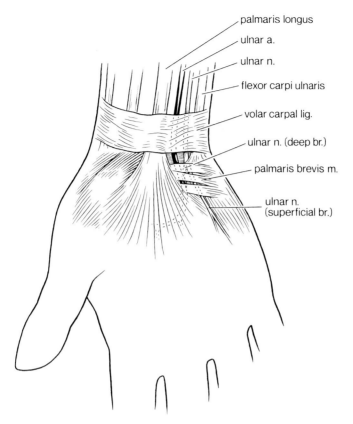

Fig. 93-5. In decompressing the ulnar nerve at the wrist, it is necessary to divide the volar carpal ligament and the palmaris brevis.

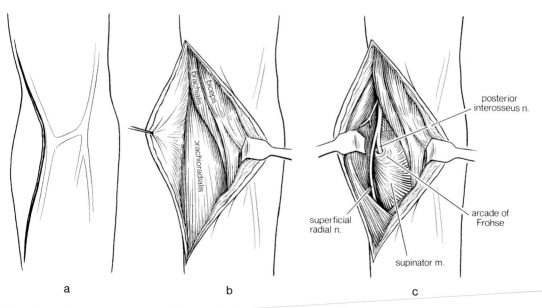

Fig. 93-6. Operative exposure of the posterior interosseous nerve. The arcade of Frohse, which runs between the heads of the supinator, may compress the posterior interosseous nerve just as the transverse carpal ligament compresses the median nerve at the wrist.

brachialis and brachioradialis and is followed along its course beneath the brachioradialis to its point of division into superficial and deep branches. The posterior interosseous branch then is traced through the arcade of Frohse between the two heads of the supinator. Surgical treatment consists of division of the arcade of the Frohse. If clear evidence of compression by the arcade is absent intraoperatively, the nerve should be traced within the supinator muscle itself because adhesions within the supinator muscle may rarely cause posterior interosseous entrapment.

Suprascapular Nerve Entrapment

Suprascapular nerve entrapment may occur as the nerve passes under the transverse scapular ligament through the suprascapular foramen[27] (Fig. 93-7). Arising from the upper trunk of the brachial plexus, the suprascapular nerve runs laterally, deep to the trapezius and omohyoid muscles, and, passing under the transverse scapular ligament through the suprascapular foramen, enters the supraspinous fossa. In the supraspinous fossa, the nerve gives branches to the supraspinatus muscle and then curves around the lateral border of the spine of the scapula to enter the infraspinous fossa, where it gives branches to the infraspinatus muscle. The nerve is relatively fixed at the level of the suprascapular foramen beneath the transverse scapular ligament, but the foramen constantly moves because of motion of the scapular during arm movement. Inflammatory reaction and swelling of the nerve beneath the ligament within the foramen may result.

Patients usually give a history of trauma to the shoulder area, either direct trauma, repetitive shoulder movements, or exaggerated shoulder movements. Pain is dull and aching and may radiate into the neck, medially into the interscapular area, or laterally down the arm. Wasting of the spinati muscles, pain on shoulder movement, and marked weakness on external rotation of the arm are prominent features. There are no sensory changes. The most accurate diagnostic test is EMG, showing denervation of the spinati muscles.

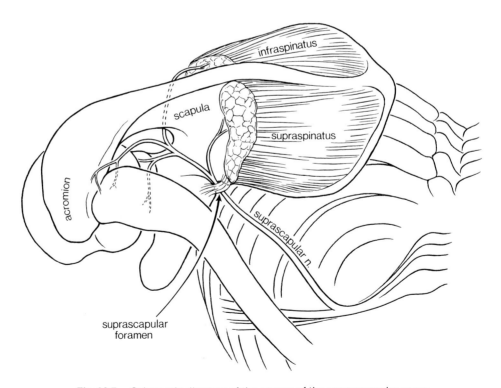

Fig. 93-7. Schematic diagram of the course of the suprascapular nerve.

Surgical therapy consists of division of the transverse scapular ligament. The surgical procedure is as follows. With the patient in lateral position, a transverse incision is made parallel to and 1 inch above the spine of the scapula. The trapezius muscle is identified and divided along the length of its fibers. After identification of the underlying supraspinatus muscle, the upper border of the scapula is identified just medial to the origin of the omohyoid muscle. The transverse scapular ligament then is identified, and a flat dissector is inserted between the ligament and the underlying nerve. The ligament then is divided by cutting down on the dissector. When neural compression has been severe and of long standing, the nerve bulges into the defect. Relief of pain is prompt following surgery, while recovery of motor function proceeds more slowly.

Thoracic Outlet Syndrome

Compression of the neurovascular bundle in the area of the thoracic outlet is the neuroanatomic common denominator for a variety of conditions described in the literature as hyperabduction syndrome,[28] scalenus anticus syndrome,[29] costoclavicular syndrome,[30] and Paget-Schroetter syndrome (subclavian-axillary vein thrombosis of effort).[31] All of these conditions are in reality merely special cases of thoracic outlet syndrome. The condition is best viewed as a special variety of peripheral entrapment neuropathy. Symptoms are more complex because they may be neural, vascular, or both. The same compressive force may affect the brachial plexus, the subclavian artery, and the subclavian vein. Successful surgical treatment requires adherence to several major principles: (1) The anatomic basis of neurovascular compression at the thoracic outlet must be thoroughly understood. (2) Diagnostic work-up must rule out a wide variety of other conditions often confused with thoracic outlet syndrome. Detailed inquiry must be made for vascular symptoms, since the vascular complications of the disease are potentially disastrous. (3) Successful surgical treatment involves complete decompression and a search for multiple areas of compression.

The anatomy of the thoracic outlet is illustrated in Figure 93-8. Neurovascular compression may have multiple causes: (1) The brachial plexus may be compressed at the interscalenic hiatus by the scalene muscles. Common insertion of the scalenus anticus and medius, posterior displacement of the normal scalenus anterior insertion, and unusually broad costal insertions of the scalenus minor and minimus all are anatomic variations that narrow the scalenic hiatus and may contribute to brachial plexopathy.[32] The upper cords of the brachial plexus may pass directly through the fibers of the scalene muscle.[33] The C7, C8, and T1 nerve roots may pass through the belly of the middle scalene muscle.[34] Gage and Parnell[33] postulated that trauma of the scalene muscle was a major cause of symptoms of thoracic outlet syndrome and reported microscopic changes in the scalene muscles including hypertrophy, inflammation, and degeneration. Sanders et al.,[34] however, detected microscopic changes in only 18 percent of cases in a large series of scalenectomies. Scalenus muscle spasm alone, in the absence of other predisposing anatomic causes, is now thought incapable of producing compressive symptoms.[35] (2) A wide variety of ligamentous structures and adhesions may cause neurovascular compression. Costocostal bands may originate from the anterolateral surface of the first rib and pass directly across the thoracic outlet to insert behind the scalene tubercle of the first rib. Fibrous bands are frequently associated with cervical ribs or elongated cervical transverse processes and extend from the tip of the first rib or elongated transverse process behind the brachial plexus to insert on the first rib. Scalenopleural bands[32] have been reported to cause compression of the lower roots of the brachial plexus. (3) A cervical rib may readily compress the overlying neurovascular bundle, both because of direct compression and because of the frequent presence of ligamentous bands between cervical ribs and the first rib. (4) The first rib is an extremely important structure because it forms part of the superior thoracic outlet, the scalenic hiatus, and the costoclavicular passage. Any abnormality of the first rib—thickening, unusual angulation, or bony exostoses—may compress the neurovascular bundle at any of these levels. Cadaveric dissection of asymptomatic patients[36] has demonstrated that the lower trunk of the brachial plexus composed of C8 and T1 makes con-

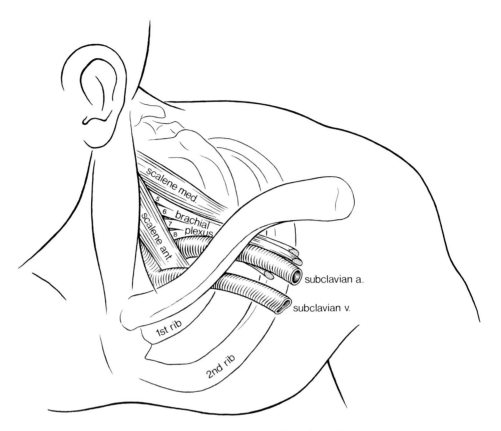

Fig. 93-8.   Anatomy of the thoracic outlet.

tact with the first rib in all cases. Frequently the seventh cervical nerve makes contact with the first rib as well. (5) The costoclavicular hiatus is a potential site of neurovascular compression because of the repetitive scissoring action of the clavicle against the neurovascular bundle. The costoclavicular syndrome, pain and paresthesias in the upper extremity first described in soldiers carrying knapsacks in the military position, is due to this mechanism. Subclavian vein thrombosis at the costoclavicular passage, often occurring after extreme exercise or heavy labor, also is thought to be caused by shearing of the vein at the costoclavicular passage between the first rib and the subclavian muscle and costoclavicular ligament.[37](6) Hyperabduction syndrome consists of pain and paresthesias and fatigability of the upper extremities produced upon hyperabduction of the arms. It often occurs in patients whose occupation entails prolonged abduction of the arms. The point of neurovascular compression is thought to be where the pectoralis minor tendon inserts on the coracoid process. Treatment is conservative, often by change of occupation.

The most common symptoms of thoracic outlet syndrome are supraclavicular pain, arm pain, and paresthesias, often in the fourth and fifth digits or in the entire hand, and, less often, in the first three fingers. Only 10 percent of patients have vascular symptomatology such as obliteration of the brachial or radial pulses, edema, peripheral cyanosis, and claudication. Physical examination often reveals supraclavicular tenderness, a fullness to palpation in the supraclavicular area, and tenderness over the brachial plexus, where evidence of a Tinel's sign may be sought. Placing the upper extremity in provocative positions is of value. When the arm is abducted and externally rotated, it often is possible to reproduce the patient's symptoms. The shoulder also may be placed in the military position and the arms pulled forcefully downward, with production of paresthesias and pain. Adson's maneuver is no longer used because it is often positive in normal subjects. Evidence of Tinel's signs at the wrist and elbow should be sought to exclude a carpal tunnel or cubital tunnel syndrome, and local orthopedic pathology such as bicipital tendonitis and shoulder bursitis excluded.

Detailed electromyelography of the upper extremities is performed to rule out associated carpal tunnel syndrome, cubital tunnel syndrome, or cervical radiculopathy—any of which may mimic thoracic outlet syndrome. Ulnar nerve conduction studies across the thoracic outlet may be slowed in up to 61 percent of cases,[38] but are often only minimally depressed. Normal ulnar conduction across the outlet in no way excludes the diagnosis of thoracic outlet syndrome. Where necessary, cervical myelography is performed to exclude a herniated cervical disc when this diagnosis remains a possibility. Apical lordotic views of the chest are done to exclude a tumor of the pulmonary apex infiltrating the brachial plexus. Cervical spine films and plain x-rays of the upper ribs are useful to exclude osseous abnormalities such as cervical rib and elongated transverse processes. Doppler ultrasonography[39] will detect significant arterial obstruction with the arm in provocative positions. The presence of vascular symptomatology is a definite indication for subclavian angiography and venography. Vascular complications of thoracic outlet syndrome occur in less than 10 percent of cases but are extremely serious. Poststenotic dilatation, aneurysm, mural thrombus with distal embolization, and total occlusion of the subclavian artery have been reported.[40] Retrograde thrombosis of the subclavian artery may result in a stroke.[41] These arterial complications may endanger the life of the patient and the viability of the extremity. Although these arterial complications may be due to compression by fibrous bands or adhesions, they are more often associated with osseous abnormalities[42] such as cervical rib, hypoplastic first ribs joining the second rib at the insertion of the anterior scalene muscle, osseous exostoses of the first rib, or elongated seventh cervical transverse processes with associated fibrous bands. The presence of arterial symptomatology demands a detailed radiographic search for bony abnormalities. Positional angiography[43] has to be interpreted cautiously, since normal subjects may obliterate their pulses in provocative positions.

Indications for surgery include significant vascular pathology, and, among patients with primarily neural symptoms, lack of response to conservative therapy such as heat, massage, and exercises to strengthen the musculature of the shoulder girdle. Scalenectomy alone is often but not invariably an inadequate procedure, carrying up to a 50 percent recurrence rate.[44] This procedure ignores the important restraining influence of the first rib at the superior thoracic outlet, scalene hiatus, and costoclavicular passage. The infraclavicular and posterior thoracoplasty approaches to the thoracic outlet are now rarely used. Two major approaches to the thoracic outlet are used in most centers: (1) transaxillary resection of the first rib combined with scalenectomy,[45] and (2) a supraclavicular approach. Advantages of the transaxillary procedure are that the first rib may be more completely removed posteriorly than through the supraclavicular approach. Also, the second rib may act to compress the neurovascular bundle even after the first rib is removed; the second rib may be inspected after removal of the first rib to see if it is compressing the brachial plexus, and, if necessary, resected—all of which is not possible through the supraclavicular approach. We prefer the supraclavicular approach, however, because the pathologic anatomy is better displayed, the phrenic nerve can be identified fully and protected, the brachial plexus can be thoroughly inspected for the presence of fibrous bands, and the plexus and axillary vessels can be viewed directly as the first rib is removed. When causalgic symptoms accompany thoracic outlet syndrome, sympathectomy of the lower stellate ganglion and the first three thoracic sympathetic ganglia can be performed through either approach.

Our own surgical approach emphasizes complete decompression (Fig. 93-9). Scalenectomy and resection of the first rib are performed, cervical ribs are resected if they are compressing the brachial plexus, and the plexus is explored in detail for evidence of fibrous bands. We use a supraclavicular incision over the lateral aspect of the sternocleidomastoid. After the deep cervical fascia is incised, the phrenic nerve and the anterior scalene muscles are identified. The phrenic nerve and accessory phrenic nerves are dissected free from the fascia investing the anterior scalene muscle. On the left side the thoracic duct and associated lymphatic channels pass in a loop toward the angle formed by the subclavian and internal jugular veins. These should be treated gently, and the thoracic duct should be protected with wet cottonoids. The scalene muscles then may be divided close to the first rib. The anterior and middle scalene muscles are sectioned and allowed to retract so that the scalene hiatus is completely free. The undersurface of the brachial

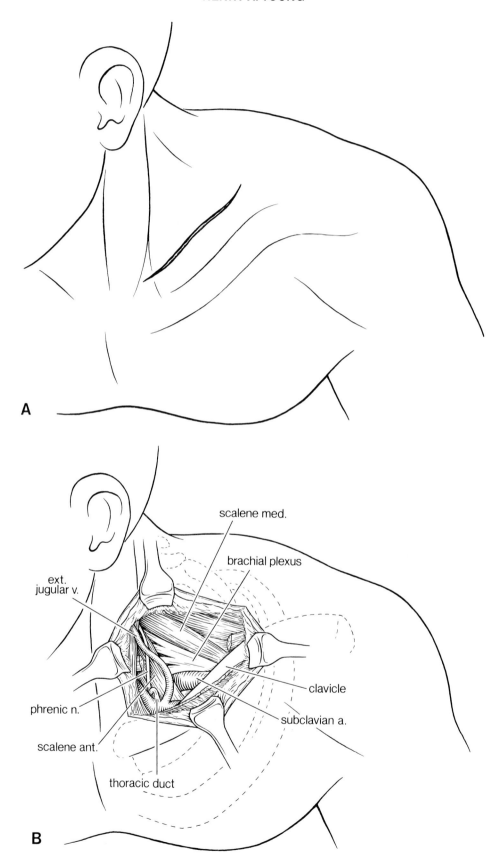

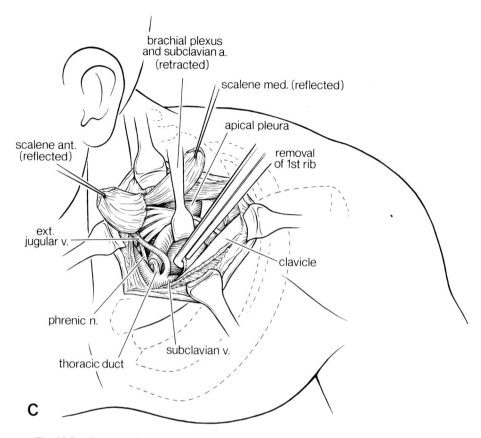

Fig. 93-9.   Steps in the supraclavicular approach to thoracic outlet decompression.

plexus then is explored for the presence of aberrant muscle fibers and restricting bands inserting on the first rib. The first rib then is removed with Kerrison rongeurs from the costochondral junction to the transverse process posteriorly. Cervical ribs are resected if they are adjudged to be causing neurovascular compression. Any fascial tissue extending from transverse processes of cervical vertebrae or from cervical ribs over the cupola of the lung is divided. By this procedure, the neurovascular bundle is freed of fibrous bands and osseous restraints, and, in addition, a patulous passage for the neurovascular bundle from the cervical to the axillary regions is created by removal of the first rib. Thrombectomy and vascular reconstruction, if indicated, are performed by vascular surgeons. If necessary, the supraclavicular incision may be extended below the clavicle and claviculectomy performed if it is necessary to trace the axillary vessels into the axilla for major vascular reconstruction.

Lateral Femoral Cutaneous Nerve Entrapment

The lateral femoral cutaneous nerve, which supplies sensation to the lateral aspect of the thigh, arises from the roots of L2 and L3 and, after running under the iliac fascia, passes through an opening in the lateral attachment of the inguinal ligament at the anterior superior pubic spine into the subcutaneous tissue of the thigh (Fig. 93-10). Entrapment neuropathy occurs where the nerve pierces the inguinal ligament and results in burning dysesthesias in the anterolateral aspect of the thigh—"meralgia paresthetica."

The condition most often presents without antecedent history of trauma. The mechanism of nerve injury is probably a pulling of the nerve by fascial attachments in the thigh against the opening for the nerve at the lateral edge of the inguinal ligament. Conservative therapy consists

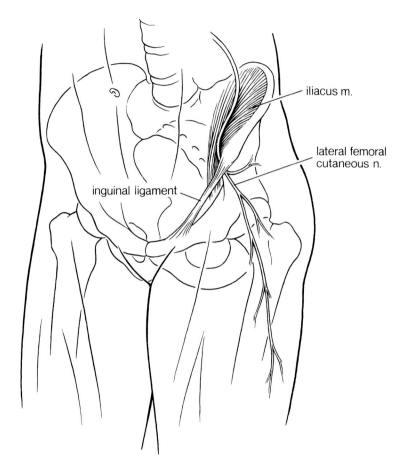

iliacus m.

lateral femoral
cutaneous n.

inguinal ligament

Fig. 93-10. Schematic diagram of the course of the lateral femoral cutaneous nerve.

of weight reduction and anti-inflammatory medication. If these fail, surgical neurolysis, involving decompression of the nerve as it passes through its canal within the inguinal ligament, is indicated. The nerve is approached through an incision beginning 2 to 3 cm above the anterior
superior iliac spine, passing along the edge of the ilium, and extending around and medial to the
anterior superior iliac spine down toward the thigh, overlying the interspace between the sartor-
ius and tensor fascia lata muscles. The nerve is identified distally as it passes beneath the tensor
fascia lata and penetrates the fascia lata; it then can be traced to the area of entrapment within
the inguinal ligament. Neurolysis is carried out several centimeters proximal to the point where
the nerve penetrates the inguinal ligament, in order to free the nerve proximally from its fascial
investments.

Posterior Tibial Nerve Entrapment

Entrapment neuropathy of the posterior tibial nerve may occur immediately below and behind the medial malleolus. The neurovascular bundle, accompanied by the tendons of the ti-
bialis posterior, flexor digitorum longus, and flexor hallucis longus, occupies a groove behind
the medial malleolus. The lancinate ligament provides a roof under which these structures pass
through a tunnel known as the tarsal tunnel (Fig. 93-11). Entrapment neuropathy at this point is
called the tarsal tunnel syndrome and is analogous to the carpal tunnel syndrome at the wrist.
Beyond the edge of the lancinate ligament the nerve branches into medial plantar, lateral plantar, and calcaneal branches. They supply the sole of the foot, the plantar surface of the toes, and
the plantar intrinsic musculature.

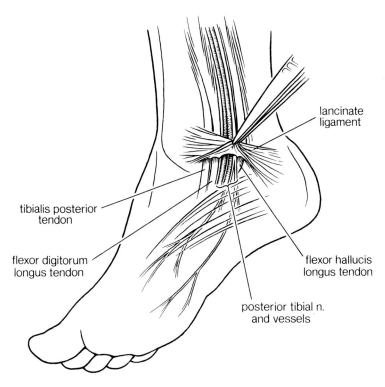

Fig. 93-11. Schematic diagram of the tarsal tunnel.

Compression at the level of the lancinate ligament results in pain and dysesthesias in the toes and sole of the foot, progressing to sensory and motor loss. Pain may be referred retrograde along the sciatic axis to the buttock. When motor disturbance occurs, the foot assumes a pes cavus position and clawing of the toes occurs. Pressure over the retromalleolar region often results in pain radiating into the sole of the foot. Putting the ankle in the valgus position aggravates the pain, while the varus position lessens the pain because it slackens the lancinate ligament. Electromyographic and nerve conduction studies are useful in diagnosis, but muscle sampling in the foot is extremely painful.

The condition may occur as a sequela of fracture, posttraumatic edema with resultant fibrosis, tenosynovitis, or venous engorgement of the posterior tibial veins due to peripheral vascular insufficiency. It also may be caused by thickening of the lancinate ligament secondary to systemic connective tissue diseases.

Conservative therapy consists of anti-inflammatory agents and correction of abnormal foot mechanics by use of a support, when necessary. Potential causative factors such as tenosynovitis or venous insufficiency should be corrected by medial or surgical means if they are present. Neurosurgical intervention becomes necessary when persistent pain or motor deficit occurs, or when conservative measures fail. Satisfactory relief is obtained by section of the lancinate ligament and external neurolysis of the nerve. It is advisable to trace the nerve distally to its trifurcation and to visualize the entrance of each of the plantar nerves into the foot so that compressive lesions of these branches distal to the lancinate ligament are not overlooked.

Common Peroneal Nerve Compression

The common peroneal nerve is vulnerable to compression neuropathy in the area of the fibular neck. The common peroneal nerve is derived from the bifurcation of the sciatic nerve in the lower thigh. It runs down the lateral aspect of the popliteal fossa and passes between the biceps femoris tendon and the lateral head of the gastrocnemius. It then pierces the deep fascia and

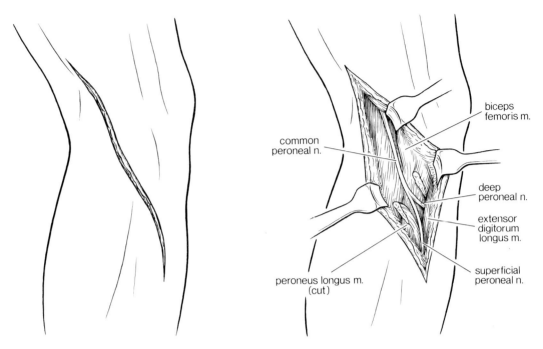

Fig. 93-12. Operative exposure of the common peroneal nerve at the fibular head. Surgical decompression is achieved by division of the superficial portion of the peroneus longus.

passes around the neck of the fibula through an opening in the origin of the peroneus longus muscle. This opening is essentially a gap between the sites of attachment of the peroneus longus to the head and to the body of the fibula. At or immediately beyond the opening in the origin of the peroneus longus, the nerve divides into its superficial and deep components.

The nerve is extremely vulnerable to injury as it crosses the fibula through the opening in the peroneus. Usually a history of trauma is elicited. Direct blunt trauma may injure the nerve at this level by impacting it against the fibula. Fibular fracture places the nerve at risk because of the possibility of both laceration by bony fragments and fibrosis secondary to local soft tissue edema. Trauma producing sudden, strong inversion at the ankle may produce a traction injury of the nerve as it passes over the fibular head through the origin of the peroneus longus. Pressure palsy is quite common at the fibular neck and may occur when patients lie on their side. Structural lesions in the popliteal fossa—such as laterally located popliteal cysts—may produce the lesion.

Pain in the lateral aspect of the leg and foot is a common presenting symptom. Pain may radiate up the sciatic axis to the buttock. Sensory loss in the dorsum of the foot and weakness of dorsiflexion and eversion of the foot may result.

So vulnerable is the common peroneal nerve as it curves around the fibular head that exposure of the nerve in this area is the most common neural decompression procedure in the lower extremity. The surgical procedure is illustrated in Figure 93-12. The incision extends from proximal to distal along the medial border of the biceps femoris, to the level of the fibular neck, and over the peroneal compartment distally. After opening the fascia lata, the biceps femoris is identified, and medial and deep to it the common peroneal nerve is found. It is then traced distally as it passes between the tendinous insertion of the biceps femoris and the lateral portion of the gastrocnemius. The lateral sural cutaneous nerve, arising high from the medial portion of the common peroneal nerve, should be identified and protected. The nerve is traced as it passes behind the biceps femoris toward the fibular neck. After the nerve has been identified as it passes through the peroneus longus, the more superficial portion of the peroneus longus may be divided and detached and the superficial and deep peroneal branches identified. The division of the small superficial portion of the peroneus and resultant close approximation of the nerve to the subcutaneous tissues carry no significant complication.

REFERENCES

1. Lewis T, Pickering GW, Rothschild P: Centripetal paralysis arising out of arrested blood flow to the limb, including notes on a form of tingling. *Heart 16*: 1–32, 1931
2. Seddon HJ: Three types of nerve injury. *Brain 66*:237–288, 1943
3. Denny-Brown D, Brenner C: Paralysis of nerve induced by direct pressure and by tourniquet. *Arch Neurol Psychol (Chicago) 51*:1–26, 1944
4. Denny-Brown D, Brenner C: Lesions in peripheral nerve resulting from compression by spring clip. *Arch Neurol Psychol (Chicago) 52*:1–19, 1944
5. Grundfest H: Effects of hydrostatic pressures upon the excitability, the recovery, and the potential sequence of frog nerve. *Cold Spring Harbor Symp Quant Biol 4*:179–187, 1936
6. Gilliatt RW, Ochoa J, Rudge P, et al: The cause of nerve damage in acute compression. *Trans Am Neurol Assoc 99*:71–74, 1974
7. Neary D, Ochoa J, Gilliatt RW: Subclinical entrapment neuropathy in man. *J Neurol Sci 24*: 283–298, 1976
8. Ochoa J, Marotte L: The nature of the nerve lesion caused by chronic entrapment in the guinea pig. *J Neurol Sci 19*:491–495, 1973
9. Fullerton PM, Gilliatt RW: Median and ulnar neuropathy in the guinea pig. *J Neurol Neurosurg Psychiatry 30*:393–402, 1967
10. Sunderland S: The nerve lesion in the carpal tunnel syndrome. *J Neurol Neurosurg Psychiatry 39*:615–626, 1976
11. Kuczynski K: Functional micro-anatomy of the peripheral nerve trunks. *Hand 6*: 1–10, 1974
12. Woodhall B, Nulsen F, White J, et al: *Neurosurgical Implications in Peripheral Nerve Regeneration.* Washington, D.C., Veterans Administration Monograph, 1957, pp 569–638
13. Upton ARM, McComas AJ: The double-crush in nerve entrapment syndromes. *Lancet 2*: 359–362, 1973
14. Rydevik B, Lundborg G, Nordborg C: Intraneural tissue reactions induced by internal neurolysis. *Scand J Plast Reconstr Surg 10*: 3–8, 1976
15. Spinner MS: *Injuries to the Major Branches of Peripheral Nerves of the Forearm.* Philadelphia, W. B. Saunders, 1978, p 37
16. Curtis RM, Eversmann WW: Internal neurolysis as an adjunct to the treatment of the carpal tunnel syndrome. *J Bone Joint Surg 55A*: 733–740, 1973
17. Brown BA: Internal neurolysis in traumatic peripheral nerve lesions in continuity. *Surg Clin North Am 52*: 1167–1175, 1972
18. Kline DG, Nulsen FE: The neuroma in continuity. Its preoperative and operative management. *Surg Clin North am 52*: 1189–1209, 1972
19. Kummel BM, Zazanis GA: Shoulder pain as the presenting complaint in carpal tunnel syndrome. *Clin Orthop 92*: 227–230, 1973
20. Taleisnik J: The palmar cutaneous branch of the median nerve and the approach to the carpal tunnel. *J Bone Joint Surg 55A*: 1212–1217, 1973
21. Kane E, Kaplam EB, Spinner M: Observations on the course of the ulnar nerve in the arm. *Ann Chir 27*: 487–496, 1973
22. Apfelberg DB, Larson SJ: Dynamic anatomy of the ulnar nerve at the elbow. *Plast Reconstr Surg 51*: 76–81, 1973
23. Neblett C, Ehni G: Medial epicondylectomy for ulnar palsy. *J Neurosurg 32*: 55–62, 1970
24. Osborne G: Compression neuritis of the ulnar nerve at the elbow. *Hand 2*: 10–13, 1970
25. Learmonth JR: Technique for transplanting the ulnar nerve. *Surg Gynecol Obstet 75*: 792–793, 1942
26. Broudy AS, Leffert RD, Smith RJ: Technical problems with ulnar nerve transposition at the elbow: findings and results of operation. *J Hand Surg 3*: 85–89, 1977
27. Rengachary SS, Burr D, Lucas S, et al: Suprascapular entrapment neuropathy: a clinical, anatomical, and comparative study. Part 2: anatomical study. *Neurosurgery 5*: 447–451, 1979
28. Wright IS: The neurovascular syndrome produced by hyperabduction of the arms; immediate changes produced in 150 normal controls, and effects on some persons of prolonged hyperabduction of arms as in sleeping, and in certain occupations. *Am Heart J 29*: 1, 1945
29. Adson AW, Coffey JR: Cervical rib, method of anterior approach for relief of symptoms by division of the scalenus anticus. *Ann Surg 83*: 839, 1927
30. Falconer MA, Weddel G: Costoclavicular compression of the subclavian artery and vein; relation to the scalenus anticus syndrome. *Lancet 2*: 539, 1943

31. Hughes ESR: Collective review, venous obstruction in the upper extremity (Paget-Schroetter's syndrome), review of 320 cases. *Surg Gyn Obstet (Suppl)*: 88-89, 1949
32. Pollak EW: Surgical anatomy of the thoracic outlet syndrome. *Surg Gynecol Obstet 150*: 97-102, 1980
33. Gage M, Parnell H: Scalenus anticus syndrome. *Am J Surg 73*: 252-267, 1947
34. Sanders RJ, Monsour JW, Gerber WF, et al: Scalenectomy versus first rib resection for treatment of the thoracic outlet syndrome. *Surgery 85*: 109-121, 1979
35. Clagett OT: Presidential address: research and prosearch. *J Thorac Cardiovasc Surg 44*: 153, 1962
36. Williams HT, Carpenter NH: Surgical treatment of the thoracic outlet compression syndrome. *Arch Surg 113*: 850-852, 1978
37. Etheredge S, Wilbur B, Stoney RJ: *Am J Surg 138*: 175-181, 1979
38. McGough EC, Pearce MB, Byrne JP: *J Thorac Cardiovasc Surg 77*: 169-173, 1979
39. Pisko-Dubienski ZA, Hollingsworth J: *Can J Surg 21*: 145-150, 1978
40. Judy KL, Heymann RI: Vascular complications of thoracic outlet syndrome. *Am J Surg 123*: 521, 1972
41. Samiy E: Thrombosis of the internal carotid artery caused by a cervical rib. *J Neurosurg 12*: 181, 1955
42. Dorazio RA, Ezzet F: Arterial complications of the thoracic outlet syndrome. *Am J Surg 138*: 246-250, 1979
43. Winsor T, Borw R: Costoclavicular syndrome, diagnosis and treatment. *JAMA 196*: 697, 1966
44. Raaf J: Surgery for cervical rib and scalenus anticus syndrome. *JAMA 157*: 219-223, 1955
45. Roos DB: Experience with first rib resection for thoracic outlet syndrome. *Ann Surg 173*: 429-442, 1971

CHAPTER 94
The Laser and Ultrasonic Aspirator in Neurosurgery

Steven L. Wald   Henry H. Schmidek

DEVELOPMENT OF NEW NEUROSURGICAL INSTRUMENTATION including the laser and the high-speed ultrasonic aspirator, have provided the neurosurgeon with a choice of tools for the performance of delicate and intricate procedures. These instruments are particularly suitable for the removal of central nervous system neoplasms. Each instrument has specific advantages. Technical proficiency and familiarity are major determinants in the choice of instrumentation.

The Laser

The application of laser technology to neurosurgical procedures has enjoyed ever-increasing popularity since its development by Maiman in 1959.[1] The unique properties of the carbon dioxide laser that make it particularly suitable for neurosurgical application are its ability to both vaporize and coagulate tissue. An additional advantage of the laser is that it may be integrated with the operating microscope.

Standard neurosurgical technique for the removal of neoplastic processes requires an adequate cerebral exposure, a line of demarcation between tumor and brain, suction, and thermoelectrical coagulation of vessels. Retraction of adjacent brain also is required and can produce serious neurologic sequelae, in spite of the emphasis on gentle cerebral retraction and manipulation facilitated by hyperosmolar agents and cerebrospinal fluid drainage. Dissection of tumor tissue near vital neural or vascular structures is fraught with danger and often results in incomplete resection of tumor tissue. In addition, blood loss is a major consideration during tumor excision. The introduction of laser technology provides the neurosurgeon with the means by which to resect tumor tissue while minimizing both retraction of normal brain tissue and the blood loss attendant upon these procedures.

Laser Physics

Laser, an acronym for *L*ight *A*mplification by the *S*timulated *E*mission of *R*adiation, is a form of light or radiant energy. All light is emitted by atoms according to physical principles. Every atom has a characteristic nucleus and a unique arrangement of electrons in surrounding shells. When energy is absorbed by an atom in its ground or stationary state, an electron shifts to a higher shell or orbit. When the electron returns to its stable configuration, energy is emitted as

Division of Neurosurgery, University of Vermont College of Medicine, Burlington, Vermont

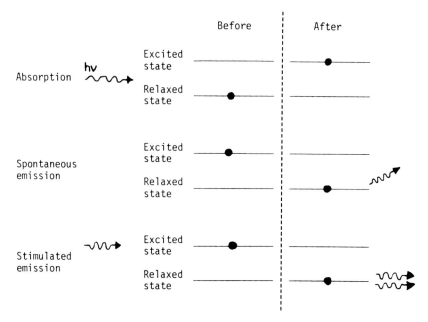

Fig. 94-1. Absorption of energy (photon) raises an atom in the ground state to an excited state. The photon can be spontaneously emitted. When an atom in the excited state is struck, two identical photons are emitted.

a photon. The stable state of an atom or molecule may thus be excited by adding energy to it, and it may then spontaneously emit energy as it returns to its ground state. Energy is conserved. If an already excited atom is struck by another photon, it will stimulate the emission of two identical photons (Fig. 94-1). Within the laser chamber, energy is added to raise the active element or compound to an excited state. Amplification then occurs with the addition of further energy. The emitted radiation of the laser is unique because the light waves are of a single length (monochromatic), parallel to each other (collimated), and in phase (coherent). The specific wavelength of the radiation produced depends on the active element or compound incorporated in the device.

Waves have four different physical characteristics: *wavelength* (distance from one peak to the next peak), *frequency* (number of waves per unit of time), *velocity,* and *amplitude* or displacement. Classification of electromagnetic waves on the basis of wavelength results in the classic electromagnetic spectrum (Fig. 94-2).

Biological Effects of the Laser

The laser is a form of light. It can be absorbed, reflected, or transmitted by tissue. Tissue absorption by any given laser is dependent on the wavelength generated by the active element or compound. The argon laser produces a visible green light and is selectively absorbed by red pigmented tissues and melanin. The energy produced by the carbon dioxide laser is invisible and is absorbed by water within tissue and converted to heat. Flash boiling of intracellular and extracellular water results in vaporization of the tissue. A useful comparison is shown in Table 94-1. Since the brain has a very high water content, nearly complete absorption of the carbon dioxide laser energy is achieved at surface levels. The microscopic appearance of tumor excised with the laser is characteristic.[2] An outer layer of charred debris covers a second deeper layer of destroyed, pyknotic cells and empty spaces. A third layer, partially destroyed by coagulation necrosis, is evident immediately above viable tumor cells. Little edema is seen in normal tissue adjacent to tumor. The entire depth of these changes ranges from 3 to 8 cells in thickness, significantly less than 1

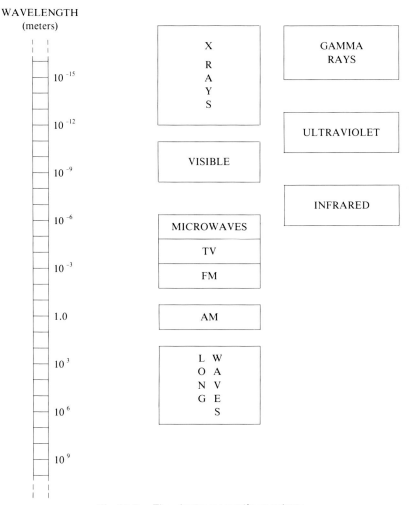

Fig. 94-2. The electromagnetic spectrum.

mm of penetration. The lack of heat conduction and destruction away from the point of impact further increases the precision of this instrument.

Experimental studies confirm the precise control and histopathologic effects of the carbon dioxide laser on neural structures. Stellar et al. created laser lesions in the cat brain and spinal cord and demonstrated a precise zone of normal tissue within 1 mm or less of totally destroyed cells.[2] Electron micrographs revealed well-preserved neurons immediately adjacent to the lesion. Saunders et al. compared laser-induced lesions of the cat brain to a similar lesion with coagulation of the pial margins, made with a scalpel.[3] Cerebral edema, as determined by a density gradient method, was consistently less in the hemisphere with the laser lesion. Takizawa also emphasized the more precise, localized demarcation produced by the laser compared to that created by electrosurgical units.[4] Laser skin incisions and subcutaneous and fascial dissection have demonstrated normal healing in all studies. Miller et al. reviewed the long-term effects of intraocular photocoagulation in albino rabbits.[5] Major retinal vessels were occluded without involvement of the underlying orbital structures. Lesions adjacent to the optic nerve exhibited no detectable involvement of the nerve on histologic review. The acute effects of CO_2 laser lesions on the cerebral microcirculation have been studied by Toya et al.[6] Using fluorescein angiography and varying the laser intensity from 14 to 60 W and the exposure time from 0.5 to 60 seconds, consistently sharp lines of demarcation were produced. Disturbances of the microcirculation were confined to within 3 mm of the center of the lesion.

Table 94-1. Characteristics of Lasers

Laser Type	Wavelength (microns)	Spectrum Location	Absorption* (mm)	Power output (watts)
Ruby	0.694	Visible	300	4
Argon	0.488 0.515	Visible	300	20
Neodymium-YAG	1.06	Infrared-near	60–100	Up to 50
Carbon dioxide	10.6	Infrared-far	0.3	Up to 100

*Absorption: Depth in water of 90 percent of radiant energy

Laser Systems

Commercially available laser units consist of a generating unit and a delivery system. The generating unit is composed of a portable console and a laser tube; the delivery system includes an articulated arm and either a free handpiece or an adaptor for use with the operating microscope. The console houses the laser medium, the control functions, the gas cylinders, and the electrical circuits. A laser tube extends from the console and incorporates a series of mirrors necessary to transmit laser energy. Two lasers are actually generated; a helium-neon laser beam is used to guide or track the operational high-energy carbon dioxide laser. The laser is turned on and off with a foot pedal.

Mode structure refers to the characteristics of beam divergence and power distribution within the laser spot. The fundamental mode, designated TEM_{00}, for Transverse Electromagnetic Mode, has a gaussian profile. Power is maximum at the center and decays at the edges. Higher-order modes have multiple peaks and cold spots within the spot diameter. The mode is predetermined by the manufacturer and cannot be changed.

The carbon dioxide laser is an efficient source of energy. The argon laser requires nearly 10,000 W of power to generate 1 W of laser power, while the carbon dioxide laser can produce 1 W of laser power with only 10 W of power input.

Technique

Manipulation of four variables determines the effect of laser energy on tissue. *Power output*, expressed in watts, is altered by adjusting the control panel. Current specifications allow for a power range of 1 to 80 W depending on the laser model being used. Actual delivery to tissue will decay from 5 to 10 W because of conduction through the articulating arm. Twenty watts of power is necessary to vaporize 10 mm^3 of tissue with an 80 percent water content.[7] *Spot size* is limited by manufactured standards and ranges from 0.1 mm to 2 mm for carbon dioxide lasers. At comparable power outputs, a smaller spot size will produce more energy at the point of impact. The extent of the laser's penetration is also controlled by the *length of time* tissue is exposed to the radiant energy. Lasers are programmed to emit light either continuously or at predetermined time intervals. Finally, by adjusting the available lens systems or by moving the free handpiece, the surgeon can *focus* or *defocus* the laser light. A defocused beam will vaporize larger areas of tissue; while a focused beam will act as a laser scalpel. The central goal of laser neurosurgery is to achieve an optimal thermal effect with the briefest amount of laser energy.

When laser energy strikes a tissue, producing vaporization, a plume of smoke is emitted. The plume is composed of vaporized water, carbon, and cellular debris. Continuous suction is necessary to remove the smoke and provide an unobstructed view. The laser lenses are kept clean by a continuous flow of nitrogen across their surfaces. Carbonization on the surface of the tissue or on either side of an incision will be seen. These carbon particles are harmless and may be left in place.

The use of the carbon dioxide laser in neurosurgery allows for significant reduction in the size of the craniotomy flaps. The neurosurgeon will be debulking neoplasms from within the mass, requiring exposure of only the tumor and an adjacent rim of compressed but normal brain.

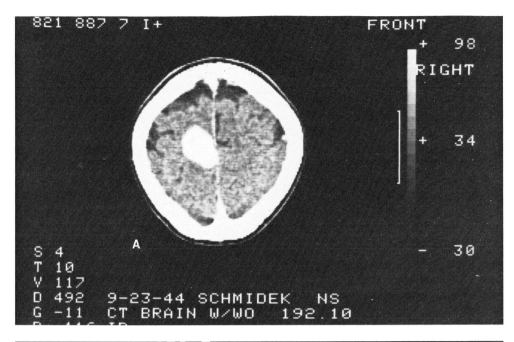

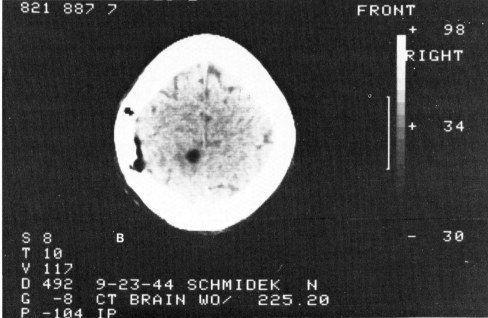

Fig. 94-3. **A.** A contrast-infused CT scan shows an enhancing parasaggital mass with adjacent edema. **B.** A contrast-enhanced CT scan performed several hours after operative excision reveals no residual tumor. Edema is unchanged from preoperative studies. No hematoma or bleeding from the tumor bed is evident.

With the laser, vessels up to 0.5 mm in diameter are simultaneously coagulated, which results in hemostatic control and reduction of blood loss during surgery. Larger vessels require conventional coagulation. Surface bleeding from tumor vessels must be evacuated or the energy from the laser will be absorbed by the blood rather than the tissue.

Deep-seated lesions require a small corticectomy followed by laser vaporization of the tumor mass. As the cavity enlarges, lateral exposure can be obtained without lengthening the cortical incision. Special reflective mirrors have been devised to direct the laser beam around the tumor cavity.

Certain safety precautions are instituted when using the laser. Signs are posted at each entrance to the operating room. Direct impact or reflected light can cause serious eye injuries and inflict third-degree burns. These injuries are less likely to occur with laser microneurosurgery. Metal retractors should be covered with moist cottonoid strips, which absorb the energy before it can strike the reflective surface. Eye protection is provided by wrap-around glasses of either plastic or glass. The surgeon will be protected by the various lenses of the operating microscope. The laser can ignite flammable gases or liquids, such as ether, alcohol, and acetone.

Clinical Application

The carbon dioxide laser is the most useful system for removing central nervous system neoplasms. Encouraging results are now appearing in the literature for both benign and malignant tumors.[8-16] Any solid intracranial or intramedullary spinal tumor is amenable to laser excision (Figs. 94-3 and 94-4). Lesions near vascular or neural structures can be removed "layer by layer" with fine adjustment of power to dissect tumor off these structures. Intraventricular lesions can be excised after cerebrospinal fluid has been evacuated. Tumors of the brainstem and posterior fossa can be excised by laser evaporation without manipulating the surrounding structures, which can cause the cerebrospinal fluid to be seeded with neoplastic cells. Although there was initial concern regarding the use of the laser in the pediatric patient, no evidence has been forthcoming to support this concern.[17] Tumor masses adjacent to or within peripheral nerves can be excised or vaporized with the laser.

Future Developments

Techniques have now been reported that combine the benefits of laser surgery with data derived by computerized tomography (CT) in order to perform stereotactic laser microsurgery.[18] Sophisticated computer programs are necessary, and complete removal currently is limited because the computer is unable to detect precisely the margins of a tumor.

Photoradiation therapy for malignant tumors has been reported by Laws et al.[19] Following intravenous administration of a hematoporphyrin derivative, which concentrates within tumor tissue, a probe is placed stereotactically within the tumor and is coupled to an argon laser unit. Empirically, the goal of the therapy is to administer red light at a wavelength of 630 nm for 45 minutes. Prior studies have shown that this system is effective in killing tumor cells in cell cultures and have suggested that hematoporphyrins accumulate in the cytoplasm and on cell membranes.[20] Although both clinical improvement and CT evidence of tumor regression were seen in 3 of the 5 patients, these are preliminary results only.

Progressive occlusion of experimentally-induced aneurysms was reported by Maira, using an argon laser, without effect on the parent vessel.[21] Jain and Gorisch employed a neodymium-YAG laser to seal experimental arterotomies and venotomies without producing mechanical or thermoelectric damage to the vessel.[22] The potential application of the laser to vascular lesions includes microanastamosis without suture.

Wet-field carbon dioxide laser surgery, which allows tissue vaporization through a fluid-filled compartment, is a neurosurgical application yet to be explored.[23,24]

Currently, endoscopic laser surgery is limited to use with nonflexible systems.[25] An impor-

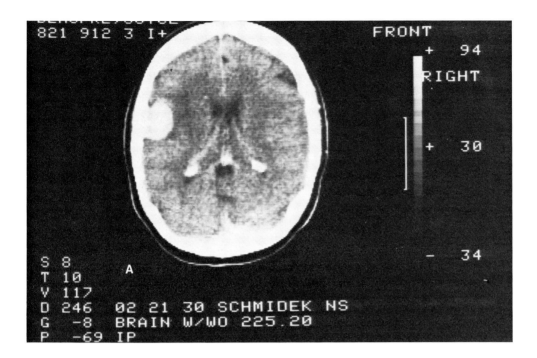

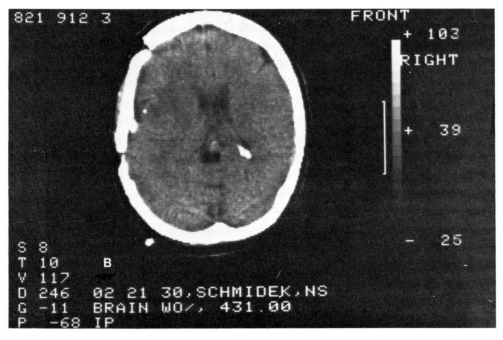

Fig. 94-4. **A.** A preoperative contrast-enhanced CT scan shows a mass over the left cerebral convexity. Minimal edema is detected. **B.** Postoperative CT scan performed 4 hours after surgery demonstrates no evidence of residual tumor. Bleeding within the operative site is negligible. There has been no change in the degree of cerebral edema. An epidural pressure monitor is present at the tumor site.

tant advance will be the development of fiberoptic systems for the transmission of carbon dioxide laser beams.[26]

Since the laser has the exquisite ability to create a discrete lesion, it probably will be employed in transphenoidal, functional, and spinal cord surgery, as well as in the laboratory, to study the effects of ablations within the nervous system.

The Ultrasonic Surgical Aspirator

Ultrasonic energy can be used to fragment and emulsify tissue. The success of this technique in ophthalmologic surgery prompted neurosurgeons to investigate its usefulness within the central nervous system. With the addition of suction and irrigation into a hand-held, self-contained unit, it is possible to excise and evacuate tumor tissue simultaneously.

The System

The surgical aspirator consists of a portable control and a power console connected to a handpiece. The tip of the device vibrates at a frequency of 23 kHz through a range of 100 μ or 0.004 inches. The vibration is imperceptible to the surgeon. Fragmentation and aspiration of tissue occurs within 1 to 2 mm of the vibrating tip. The flow rate of the irrigating solution, the magnitude of the vacuum, and the intensity of the vibration are adjustable. As currently designed, the vibrating tip must make contact with the tissue, precluding direct integration with the operating microscope.

Biological Effects of Ultrasonic Aspiration

The histologic characteristics of cortical and white matter resections performed with the ultrasonic aspirator have been studied by Flamm using the cat brain and spinal cord.[27] Microscopic sections were compared with those obtained by the techniques of standard suction and cautery, cutting loop cautery, and rongeur removal. Characteristic areas of hemmorhage and necrosis were seen in the areas of resection, surrounded by edema and swelling of axonal sheaths. No quantitative difference could be detected in the lesions created by the ultrasonic aspirator and those created by the other standard techniques. Prolonged ultrasonic exposure of the spinal cord without actual tissue resetion produced significant alterations of the evoked potentials. White matter edema, petechial hemorrhages, and cavitation were seen in microscopic sections of spinal cord. The spinal cord exposure experiment, as the authors comment, does not, however, mimic clinical application of this instrument.

Young et al. conducted simultaneous physiologic measurements of the rat sciatic nerve and spinal cord without actual tissue resection produced significant alterations of the evoked potenduct normal action potentials until contact was made with the vibrating tip of the probe. Reduction of ultrasonic intensity produced a momentary action potential degradation followed by a slow recovery that disappeared after 5 minutes. Small lesions created in the spinal cord did not produce alterations of white matter blood flow in adjacent regions or alter evoked potential responses.

Clinical Applications

The primary advantages of ultrasonic emulsification and aspiration are the lack of mechanical manipulation of normal tissue, the preservation of tissue planes, the lack of thermal effects, and the ability to aspirate and irrigate.

Clinical experience with the ultrasonic aspirator has led neurosurgeons to conclude that it is a useful tool for resection of firm, fibrous types of lesions not readily resectable by standard techniques.[29,30]

Table 94-2 compares the two systems described in this chapter.

Table 94-2. Comparative Surgical Characteristics of the Carbon Dioxide Laser and the Ultrasonic Aspirator

	Carbon dioxide laser	Ultrasonic aspirator
Hemostasis	Very good	Poor
Integration with microsurgical technique	Excellent	Fair
Speed of excision	Very good	Excellent
Lack of adjacent mechanical trauma	Excellent	Excellent
Cost	Expensive	Moderately expensive
Depth perception	Reduced	Very good
Ability to remove calcified or fibrous tissue	Excellent	Fair
Mechanism of action	Vaporization (thermal)	Emulsification
Safety precautions	Required	None
Reliability	Excellent	Excellent
Adaptability (stereotaxis, endoscopy, vascular)	Excellent	Fair
Reduction of operative time	Very good	Excellent

REFERENCES

1. Maiman TH: Stimulated optical radiation in ruby. *Nature* 187:493–494, 1960
2. Stellar S, Polanyi TG, Bredemeier HC: Experimental studies with the carbon dioxide laser as a neurosurgical instrument. *Med Biol Eng Comput* 8:549–558, 1970
3. Saunders ML, Young HF, Becker DP, et al: The use of the laser in neurological surgery. *Surg Neurol* 14:1–10, 1980
4. Takizawa T: Comparison between the laser surgical unit and the electrosurgical unit. *Neurol Med Chir (Tokyo)* 17:95–105, 1977
5. Miller JB, Smith MR, Pincus F, et al: Intraocular carbon dioxide laser photocautery. Part I. Animal experimentation. *Arch Ophthalmol* 97:2157–2162, 1979
6. Toya S, Kawase T, Iisaka Y, et al: Acute effect of the carbon dioxide laser on the epicerebral microcirculation. Experimental study by fluorescein angiography. *J Neurosurg* 53:193–197, 1980
7. Verschueren R: *The CO2 Laser in Tumor Surgery.* Assen, The Netherlands: Van Gorcum, 1976
8. Ascher PW: The use of the CO2 laser in neurosurgery, in Kaplan I (ed): *Laser Surgery II.* Jerusalem, Israel, Jerusalem Academic Press, 1978, pp 76–78
9. Ascher PW, Ingolitsch E, Walter G, et al: Ultrastructural findings in CNS tissue with CO2 laser, in Kaplan I (ed): *Laser Surgery II.* Jerusalem, Israel, Jerusalem Academic Press, 1978, pp 81–90
10. Hara M, Okada J, Takeuchi K, et al: Evaluation of laser surgery to treat brain tumor. *Neurol Surg (Tokyo)* 8:363–369, 1980
11. Hudgins R, Moody J, Sanders M, et al: Microsurgical laser vaporization of inaccessible tumors of the central nervous system. *Dallas Med J* 76:245–250, 1981
12. Kelly PJ, Alker GJ jr, Goerss S: Computer-assisted stereotactic laser microsurgery for the treatment of intracranial neoplasms. *Neurosurg* 10:324–331, 1982
13. Kosary IZ, Shacked I, Farine I: Use of surgical laser in the removal of an osteoma of the skull. *Surg Neurol* 8:151–153, 1977
14. Salcman M, Kaplan RS, Ducker TB, et al: Effects of age and reoperation on survival in the combined modality treatment of malignant astrocytoma. *Neurosurg* 10:454–463, 1982
15. Strait TA, Robertson JH, Clark WC: Use of the carbon dioxide laser in the operative management of intracranial meningiomas: a report of twenty cases. *Neurosurg* 10:464–467, 1982
16. Takizawa T, Yamazaki T, Miura N, et al: Laser surgery of basal, orbital, and ventricular meningiomas which are difficult to extirpate by conventional means. *Neurol Med Chir (Tokyo)* 20:719–737, 1980
17. Henderson BM, Goldman L, Martin LW, et al: The laser in pediatric surgery. *J Pediatr Surg* 3:263–270, 1968

18. Kelly PJ, Alker GJ jr: A stereotactic approach to deep-seated central nervous system neoplasms using the carbon dioxide laser. *Surg Neurol 5*:331–334, 1981
19. Laws ER, Cortese DA, Kinsey JH, et al: Photoradiation therapy in the treatment of malignant brain tumors: a phase I (feasibility) study. *Neurosurg 9*:672–678, 1981
20. Dougherty TJ, Kaufman JE, Goldfarb A, et al: Photoradiation therapy for the treatment of malignant tumors. *Cancer Res 38*:2628–2635, 1978
21. Maira G, Mohr G, Panisset A, et al: Laser photocoagulation for treatment of experimental aneurysms. *J Microsurg 1*:137–147, 1979
22. Jain KK, Gorisch W: Repair of small blood vessels with the neodymium-YAG laser. A preliminary report. *Surgery 85*:684–688, 1979
23. Miller JB, Smith MR, Pincus F, et al: Transvitreal carbon dioxide laser photocautery and vitrectomy. *Ophthalmol 85*:1195–1200, 1978
24. Smith MR, Miller JB: New trends in carbon dioxide laser microsurgery. *J Microsurg 1*:354–363, 1980
25. Strong MS, Jako GJ: Laser surgery in the larynx. Early clinical experience with continuous CO2 laser. *Ann Otol Rhinol Laryngol 81*:791–798, 1972
26. Pinnow DA, Gentile AL, Standlee AG, et al: Polycrystalline fiber optical wave guides for infrared transmission. *Appl Phys Letter 33*:28–29, 1978
27. Flamm ES, Ransohoff J, Wuchinich D, et al: Preliminary experience with ultrasonic aspiration in neurosurgery. *Neurosurg 2*:240–245, 1978
28. Young W, Cohen AR, Hunt CD, et al: Acute physiological effects of ultrasonic vibrations on nervous tissue. *Neurosurg 8*:689–694, 1981
29. Boggan JE, Edwards MSB: The resection of central nervous system tumors using the CUSA TM and surgical lasers, in *Surgical Update.* Mountain View, Calif., Cooper Medical Devices Corp., 1982, pp 2–4
30. Wisoff JH: Surgical management of spinal cord astrocytomas, in *Surgical Update.* Mountain View, Calif., Cooper Medical Devices Corp., 1982, pp 8–9

Subject Index

aorta and intercostal and anomalous arteries in relation
to, 1469
artery of Adamkiewicz and, 1460
case histories in, 1462, 1467, 1472–1473
cautery of feeding arteries in, 1470
clinical presentation and natural history of,
1462–1463
CT scans in, 1465
decompressive laminectomy in, 1472
diagnosis of, 1464–1466
dura opening in, 1468
embolization in, 1466–1467
lateral tomogram of midthoracic spine in, 1465
low thoracic myelogram in, 1471–1472
lumbar thoracic myelogram of, 1466
microsurgical obliteration of, 1467
myelography in diagnosis of, 1464
nidus excision in, 1467
onset of, 1462
operative exposure of, 1464
pain in, 1463
preoperative aortogram of, 1468
sex factor in, 1462
subarachnoid hemorrhage in, 1462–1463
surgery preparation for, 1467–1470
surgical excision of, 1467–1473
surgical position in, 1467–1468
surgical results in, 1473
treatment in, 1466–1473
Spinal cord compression
cervical myelogram of, 1254
cervical spondylotic myelopathy in, 1239
ligamentum flavum and, 1243
in spinal trauma, 1410
Spinal cord cysts, syringomyelia and, 104
Spinal cord decompression, posterior laminectomy in,
1269
Spinal cord dysplasia, 87
Spinal cord injuries
emergency surgery for, 1401
laminectomy in, 1417
pediatric anesthesia for, 14–15
spastic paraplegia from, 1177
transthoracic surgical decompression in, 1410
Spinal cord opiates, future potential of, 1208
Spinal cord position, variability of, 1465
Spinal cord structures, identification of at C2 by
threshold electrical stimulation, 1146
Spinal cord tumors, *see also* Intramedullary tumors
cervical myelograms of, 1450–1454
intramedullary, *see* Intramedullary spinal cord tumors
Spinal cord width variations, in open cordotomy,
1123–1124
Spinal deformity, *see also* Spinal cord arteriovenous
malformations
following cervical laminectomy, 64–65

CT scans of, 63
in meningomyelocele patients with malfunctioning
shunts, 66–67
myelography in diagnosis of, 63
after neurological procedures in children, 63–68
neurological deficits following correction of, 68
polytomography in diagnosis of, 63
postoperative management and prevention of,
65–66
radiation therapy in, 66
radiological studies of, 63
surgical treatment of, 67–68
Spinal dura ligation, malfunctioning shunt and, 67
Spinal dysraphism
air myelography in, 97
Arnold–Chiari malformation in, 90
clinical presentation in, 94–96
conus in, 88–90, 94–95
defined, 87
dermoid tumor in, 95–100
diagnostic assessment and surgery indications in,
96–98
diastematomyelia and, 89
equinus deformities in, 94
"fawn's tail" in, 93
female predominance in, 94
fibrous bands in, 91
intraspinal lipoma in, 97–99
leptomyelolipoma and, 88
lipomyelomeningocele in, 88
occult, *see* Occult spinal dysraphism
pathology of, 88–94
prophylactic surgery for, 96
radiographic studies in, 96–97
results and follow-up in, 101
skin abnormality in, 93–94
spine abnormalities in, 91–92
surgery of, 99–101
Spinal extradural abscess, 220–222
Spinal fracture-dislocation, ankylosing spondylitis
and, 1487–1488
Spinal fusion, 1321–1337
anterior lumbar discectomy and, 1373
for cervical spine, 1322–1324
decompressive laminectomy and, 1333
extraperitoneal, 1327
Harrington-rod thoracolumbar fusion in, 1332
incomplete conus lesion and, 1333
lateral extrapleural form of, 1327, 1331–1332
lateral retropleural approach in, 1328–1330
lateral thoracic extrapleural fusion in, 1327–1330
lumbar, *see* Lumbar spinal fusion; Posterior lumbar
interbody fusion
posterolateral or intertransverse fusion in, 1327
postoperative care in, 1334–1337
pseudoarthrosis in, 1334–1337

Spontaneous intracerebral hemorrhage, 749
Spontaneous nontraumatic carotid cavernous fistulas, 795
SSEPs, *see* Somatosensory evoked responses
STA−MCA bypass, *see* Superficial temporal artery−middle cerebral artery bypass
Staphylococcus, in bacterial endocarditis, 934
Staphylococcus aureus
   in brain abscess, 218
   in osteomyelitis of skull, 215, 222−223
   in spinal extradural abscess, 220−222
Stenosis
   of carotid artery, 672
   of subclavian-carotid junction, 695−698
Stereo endoscope, 421−422
Stereotactic amygdalotomy, 1033
Stereotactic apparatus, types of, 995−996
Stereotactic atlas, of human brain, 995
Stereotactic biopsy
   advantages and disadvantages of, 398
   angiography and, 393
   criteria for, 392−393
   CT scans in, 391−392
   glioblastoma multiforme from, 395−396
   in intracranial gliomas, 458
   morbidity and mortality in, 398
   operative procedure in, 394−396
   preoperative evaluation of, 393
   results in, 396−398
Stereotactic campotomy, tremor and, 1019
Stereotactic clipping
   of aneurysm neck, 780
   of arteriovenous malformations, 771−786
   case histories in, 779−784
   clinical results for, 777−784
   consecutive stages in, 775
   equipment for, 772−774
   indications for, 784
   operative technique in, 776−777
   preoperative calculations for, 774−776
   terms used in, 776
Stereotactic computerized tomography
   biopsy technique in, 405−417
   of pineal germinosa, 415
Stereotactic coordinates, determination of, 404, 993−994
Stereotactic head holder, in CT scanning, 409
Stereotactic laser microsurgery, 1546
Stereotactic mesencephalotomy, in cancer pain, 1008
Stereotactic rhizotomy, of trigeminal nerve, 1084
Stereotactic ring, in neurologic endoscopy, 425−426
Stereotactic surgery, 993−999
   for affective disorders, 1026−1032
   apparatus used in, 995−996
   Cartesian coordinates in, 404, 993−994
   CNS lesions in, 999

   contraindications in, 1019
   cryoprobe in, 999
   CT-guided, 405−417, 1034−1035
   CT scans in, 405, 409, 411, 1034−1035
   vs. electroconvulsive therapy, 1028
   electrode in, 993
   electrode guidance in, 1137
   electrode placement in, 998−999
   for epilepsy, 1032−1033
   for histologic diagnosis, 391−398
   Horsley-Clark apparatus in, 993−994
   in Huntington's chorea, 1020
   procedure in, 997−999
   radiologic considerations in, 996−997
   single-unit recording in, 998
   Talairach apparatus in, 1032
Stereotactic techniques, recent development of, 771
Stereotactic thalamotomy, 1019
   in choreathetosis, 1023
Stereotactic thermal hypophysectomy, 351−356
   anesthesia in, 351
   complications in, 356
   hemorrhage in, 356
   local infection in, 356
   methods in, 351−355
   operating room arrangement in, 352
   postoperative management in, 355
   radiofrequency electrode in, 353, 1137
   replacement therapy in, 355
Stereotactic vision, "true" vs. "pseudo," 421−422
Sternocleidomastoid muscle
   in cervical spondylosis surgery, 1244
   clamping of, 693
   in spinal trauma, 1406
   transection of, 701
Sternomastoid muscle, *see* Sternocleidomastoid muscle
Stimulation-produced analgesias, 1003
Stimulation techniques, in functional neurosurgery, 999−1001
Störz pediatric-type endoscope, 421
Streptococcal infection
   in brain abscess, 218
   in spinal extradural abscess, 220−221
Streptococcus, in bacterial endocarditis, 934
Stroke, *see also* Cerebral thrombosis; Intracerebral hemorrhage; Thrombosis
   direct brain revascularization following, 713
   hemorrhage and, 759
   mortality in, 747
   STA−MCA bypass graft for, 724−725
   in traumatic intracranial aneurysms, 941
Stryker frame
   in spinal trauma, 1402
   in thoracic/thoracolumbar fractures, 1272−1273, 1277−1280
Subarachnoid electrode, in multiple sclerosis evaluation, 1025

a
2 b
3 c
4 d
5 e
6 f
7 g
8 h
9 i
8 0 j